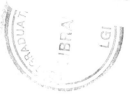

# Prognosis of Neurological Disorders
## Second Edition

# Prognosis of Neurological Disorders

## Second Edition

*Edited by*

## Randolph W. Evans, M.D.
Clinical Associate Professor of Neurology
University of Texas Medical School at Houston
Houston, Texas

## David S. Baskin, M.D., F.A.C.S.
Professor of Neurosurgery and Anesthesiology
Baylor College of Medicine
Houston, Texas

## Frank M. Yatsu, M.D.
Emeritus Professor of Neurology
University of Texas Medical School at Houston
Houston, Texas

*New York      Oxford*
OXFORD UNIVERSITY PRESS
*2000*

Oxford University Press

Oxford   New York

Athens   Auckland   Bangkok   Bogóta   Buenos Aires   Calcutta
Cape Town   Chennai   Dar es Salaam   Delhi   Florence   Hong Kong   Istanbul
Karachi   Kuala Lumpur   Madrid   Melbourne   Mexico City   Mumbai
Nairobi   Paris   São Paulo   Singapore   Taipei   Tokyo   Toronto   Warsaw

*and associated companies in*

Berlin   Ibadan

Published by Oxford University Press, Inc.
198 Madison Avenue, New York, New York, 10016
http://www.oup-usa.org

Oxford is a registered trademark of Oxford University Press

Library of Congress Cataloging-in-Publication Data
Prognosis of neurological disorders / edited by Randolph W. Evans,
David S. Baskin, Frank M. Yatsu. — 2nd ed.
p.   cm.      Includes bibliographical references and index.
ISBN 0-19-511936-3
1. Nervous system—Diseases—Prognosis.      I. Evans, Randolph W.
II. Baskin, David S.      III. Yatsu, Frank M.
[DNLM:   1. Nervous System Diseases—diagnosis.      2. Prognosis.      WL
141 P9845 2000]      RC346.P76 2000
616.8—dc21          99-19078

9      8      7      6      5      4      3      2      1

Printed in the United States of America
on acid-free paper

# Preface

We have been delighted with the warm reception of the first edition, which was published in 1992, the first book devoted to prognosis in neurology. Since then, there have been numerous new treatments and outcome studies. In cerebrovascular disease, the indications and risk/benefit of carotid endarterectomy for the treatment of symptomatic and asymptomatic carotid stenosis have now become well defined. Tissue plasminogen activator (t-PA) is an important treatment for many persons with acute cerebral ischemia. In multiple sclerosis, the dynamic nature of multiple sclerosis plaques demonstrated on serial magnetic resonance imaging studies has modified our concept of this disease. Immunotherapies have now been shown to improve the outlook. In human immunodeficiency virus (HIV) disorders, new protease inhibitors have made dramatic differences in the lives of many. Selective 5-HT$_1$ agonists, the triptans, have revolutioned migraine management. There are many areas where our knowledge of prognosis is still incomplete but slowly increasing.

The second edition has been reduced from 50 to 43 chapters by consolidation of the infectious disease chapters from nine to five and deletion of separate chapters on open heart surgery and normal pressure hydrocephalus. There are 19 new chapters with fresh authorship including the new topics of medicolegal issues and economics outcomes research. The chapters from the first edition have been revised and updated, 13 with new coauthors.

We appreciate the outstanding work of our 76 distinguished contributors. We thank our knowledgeable, enthusiastic editor at Oxford, Fiona Stevens. We also wish to give special thanks to our spouses, Marilyn Evans, Juli Baskin, and Mich Yatsu and our children, Elliott, Rochelle, and Jonathan Evans, Danielle and Alexandra Baskin, and Libby Yatsu Shu.

*Houston, Texas*                                                                                             RWE
September, 1999                                                                                              DSB
                                                                                                            FMY

# Preface to the First Edition

There are three fundamental questions that we address in clinical neurology and neurosurgery: What is the diagnosis? What is the treatment, medical and/or surgical? What is the prognosis? We deal with prognosis on a daily basis. Our patients and colleagues frequently request prognotic information which is also critical for developing treatment protocols. In years to come, outcome analysis will be of increasing importance as beleaguered health care providers and payors attempt to provide the most cost-effective treatment possible. In medical-legal cases, we are often asked as experts to predict the future with reasonable medical probability.

This volume is designed as a compendium of neurological disorders discussed from the viewpoint of prognosis. The information it provides can be found scattered among various other sources. For example, any of the standard textbooks on neurology and neurosurgery address prognosis to some extent. However, their coverage is not always complete or well-referenced. For many diseases, it is difficult to find any systematic, comprehensive discussions of prognosis. Since there is no single reference that covers neurological disorders from this standpoint, we hope that this book will be useful to neurologists and neurosurgeons.

The book begins with an introductory section discussing the ethical implications of prognosis from the viewpoint of a medical ethicist. A psychologist explores the effect on the patient of giving a prognosis. A critique of natural history studies completes the overview section.

In each chapter, the natural history of a given disease and its subgroups is explored. Clinical prediction rules and prognostic factors, as appropriate, are reviewed. A discussion then follows of how medical and/or surgical therapy alters natural history. Each chapter has full references of the important literature in that area.

This book is a practical guide for the neurologist and the neurosurgeon that can be used on a daily basis as a reference source when discussing prognosis with patients and their families, colleagues, and other interested parties. It may also be of interest to psychiatrists, internists, physiatrists, neuropsychologists, and attorneys as well. Looking at the whole of neurological disease, the many inadequacies in our predictive abilities are apparent. We hope that this volume will act as an impetus to acquire increasingly complete prognostic information.

We are grateful to our many outstanding contributors. We appreciate the encouragement and advice of our editor at Oxford University Press, Jeffrey W. House. The support of the Departments of Neurology and Neurosurgery at Baylor College of Medicine and the Department of Neurology at the University of Texas Medical School at Houston has been invaluable. Dr. Yatsu appreciates the ongoing support of the Clayton Foundation for Research. Finally, we wish to give special thanks to our spouses, Marilyn Evans, Juli Baskin, and Mich Yatsu, and our children, Elliott, Rochelle, and Jonathan Evans, and Libby Yatsu

*Houston, Texas*                                                         R.W.E.
May, 1992                                                                D.S.B.
                                                                         F.M.Y.

# Contents

# Contributors

Nada G. Abou-Fayssal, MD
*Department of Neurology*
*The Mount Sinai Medical Center*
*New York, New York*

Stanley H. Appel, MD
*Department of Neurology*
*Baylor College of Medicine*
*Houston, Texas*

Robert W. Baloh, MD
*Department of Neurology*
*UCLA School of Medicine*
*Los Angeles, California*

Albert Bandura, Ph.D.
*Department of Psychology*
*Stanford University*
*Stanford, California*

David S. Baskin, MD, FACS
*Department of Neurosurgery and*
  *Anesthesiology*
*Baylor College of Medicine*
*Houston, Texas*

John Booss, MD
*Department of Veterans Affairs*
*West Haven, Connecticut*
*Departments of Neurology*
  *and Laboratory Medicine*
*Yale University School of Medicine*
*New Haven, Connecticut*

Paul W. Brazis, MD
*Department of Neurology*
*Mayo Clinic, Jacksonville*
*Jacksonville, Florida*

Baruch A. Brody, Ph.D.
*Center for Medical Ethics*
  *and Health Policy*
*Baylor College of Medicine*
*Houston, Texas*

P. K. Coyle, MD
*Department of Neurology*
*State University of New York*
  *at Stony Brook*
*Stony Brook, New York*

Antonio Culebras, MD
*Neurology Services*
*Veterans Affairs Medical Center*
*SUNY Health Science Center*
*Community General Hospital*
*Syracuse, New York*

Jeffrey L. Cummings, MD
*Department of Neurology*
*UCLA School of Medicine*
*Los Angeles, California*

Josep O. Dalmau, MD, PhD
*Department of Neurology*
*Memorial Sloan-Kettering Cancer Center*
*New York, New York*

Andrew M. Demchuk, MD
*Department of Neurology*
*University of Texas Medical School*
   *at Houston*
*Houston, Texas*

Randolph W. Evans, MD
*Department of Neurology*
*University of Texas Medical School*
   *at Houston*
*Houston, Texas*

Nancy R. Foldvary, DO
*Department of Neurology*
*The Cleveland Clinic Foundation*
*Cleveland, Ohio*

Jason E. Garber, MD
*Department of Neurosurgery*
*Baylor College of Medicine*
*Houston, Texas*

Jane L. Gilmore, MD
*Department of Neurology*
*Emory University School of Medicine*
*Atlanta, Georgia*

Christopher G. Goetz, MD
*Department of Neurological Sciences*
*Rush-Presbyterian-St. Luke's Medical*
   *Center*
*Chicago, Illinois*

Donald E. Goodkin, MD
*USCF/Mount Zion Multiple*
   *Sclerosis Center*
*San Francisco, California*

Morris D. Groves, MD, JD
*Department of Neuro-Oncology*
*The University of Texas*
   *MD Anderson Cancer Center*
*Houston, Texas*

Raymond W. Grundmeyer, III, MD
*Department of Neurosurgery*
*Baylor College of Medicine*
*Houston, Texas*

David H. Gutmann, MD, PhD
*Neurofibromatosis Program*
*St. Louis Children's Hospital*
*Washington University School of Medicine*
*St. Louis, Missouri*

Lanny J. Haverkamp, PhD
*Department of Neurology*
*Baylor College of Medicine*
*Houston, Texas*

Robert G. Holloway, MD
*Department of Neurology*
*University of Rochester Medical Center*
*Rochester, New York*

Robert J. Jackson, MD
*Department of Neurosurgery*
*Baylor College of Medicine*
*Houston, Texas*

Jack I. Jallo, MD
*Department of Neurosurgery*
*Temple University School of Medicine*
*Philadelphia, Pennsylvania*

Praful Kelkar, MD
*Department of Neurology*
*University of Minnesota Medical School*
*Minneapolis, Minnesota*

Andrew Kertesz, MD, FRCP
*Department of Clinical Neurological
    Sciences*
*University of Western Ontario*
*Lawson Research Institute*
*St. Joseph's Health Centre*
*London, Ontario, Canada*

Afshan M. Khan, MD
*Department of Neurology and Pediatrics*
*Lincoln Medical and Mental Health
    Center and*
*Beth Israel Hospital and Medical Center*
*New York, New York*

David G. Kline, MD
*Department of Neurosurgery*
*Louisiana State University School of
    Medicine*
*New Orleans, Louisiana*

Robert L. Knobler, MD, PhD
*Department of Neurology*
*Thomas Jefferson University Hospital*
*Philadelphia, Pennsylvania*

Thomas D. Koepsell, MD, MPH
*Departments of Epidemiology
    and Health Services*
*University of Washington*
*Seattle, Washington*

Max Kole, MD
*Department of Neurosurgery*
*Henry Ford Hospital*
*Detroit, Michigan*

Eugene C. Lai, MD, PhD
*Department of Neurology*
*Baylor College of Medicine*
*Houston, Texas*

John T. Langfitt, PhD
*Department of Neurology*
*University of Rochester Medical Center*
*Rochester, New York*

Andrew G. Lee, MD
*Departments of Ophthalmology, Neurology,
    and Neurosurgery*
*Baylor College of Medicine*
*Houston, Texas*

Victor A. Levin, MD
*Department of Neuro-Oncology*
*The University of Texas MD Anderson
    Cancer Center*
*Houston, Texas*

W.T. Longstreth, Jr, MD, MPH
*Departments of Neurology
    and Epidemiology*
*University of Washington*
*Seattle, Washington*

Thomas J. Mampalam, MD
*Private Practice*
*Neurosurgery*
*Pinole, California*

Elliott L. Mancall, MD
*Department of Neurology*
*Thomas Jefferson University Hospital*
*Philadelphia, Pennsylvania*

Mario F. Mendez, MD, PhD
*Department of Neurology*
*UCLA School of Medicine*
*Los Angeles, California*

Alireza Minagar, MD
*Department of Neurology*
*University of Miami School of Medicine*
*Miami, Florida*

Patricia M. Moore, MD
*Department of Neurology*
*University of Pittsburgh School of Medicine,*
*Pittsburgh, Pennsylvania*

Dennis R. Mosier, MD, PhD
*Department of Neurology*
*Baylor College of Medicine*
*Houston, Texas*

Raj K. Narayan, MD
*Department of Neurosurgery*
*Temple University School of Medicine*
*Philadelphia, Pennsylvania*

Ewell L. Nelson, MD
*Department of Neurosurgery*
*Baylor College of Medicine*
*Houston, Texas*

Lorene M. Nelson, PhD
*Department of Health Research*
  *and Policy*
*Stanford University*
*Stanford, California*

Hans E. Neville, MD
*Department of Neurology*
*University of Colorado School of Medicine*
*Denver, Colorado*

Lois Margaret Nora, MD, JD
*Department of Neurology*
*University of Kentucky*
*Lexington, Kentucky*

Robert E. Nora, JD
*Hinshaw & Culbertson, Attorneys*
*Chicago, Illinois*

Gareth J. Parry, MD
*Department of Neurology*
*University of Minnesota Medical School*
*Minneapolis, Minnesota*

Page B. Pennell, MD
*Department of Neurology*
*Emory University School of Medicine*
*Atlanta, Georgia*

Fred Plum, MD
*Department of Neurology*
*New York Presbyterian*
  *Hospital-Cornell Campus*
*New York, New York*

Melissa C. Pulver, MD
*Department of Neurology*
*New York Presbyterian*
  *Hospital-Cornell Campus*
*New York, New York*

Isabelle Rapin, MD
*Department of Neurology*
*Albert Einstein College of Medicine*
*Bronx, New York*

Vincent M. Riccardi, MD
*American Medical Consumers*
*La Crescenta, California*

Steven P. Ringel, MD
*Department of Neurology*
*University of Colorado School of Medicine*
*Denver, Colorado*

Karen L. Roos, MD
*Department of Neurology*
*Indiana University School of Medicine*
*Indianapolis, Indiana*

Norbert Roosen, MD
*Department of Neurosurgery*
*Louisiana State University*
  *School of Medicine*
*New Orleans, Louisiana*

Mark L. Rosenblum, MD
*Department of Neurosurgery*
*Henry Ford Hospital*
*Detroit, Michigan*

Todd D. Rozen, MD
*Department of Neurology*
*Thomas Jefferson University Hospital*
*Philadelphia, Pennsylvania*

S. Clifford Schold, Jr, MD
*Director of Neuroscience*
*Duke Clinical Research Institute*
*Durham, North Carolina*

Lisa M. Shulman, MD
*Department of Neurology*
*University of Miami School of Medicine*
*Miami, Florida*

Lori A. Shutter, MD, PT
*Moss Rehabilitation Research Institute and*
  *Department of Rehabilitation Medicine*
*University of Pennsylvania*
*Philadelphia, Pennsylvania*

Stephen D. Silberstein, MD
*Department of Neurology*
*Thomas Jefferson University Hospital*
*Philadelphia, Pennsylvania*

David M. Simpson, MD
*Department of Neurology*
*The Mount Sinai Medical Center*
*New York, New York*

R. Glenn Smith, MD, PhD
*Department of Neurology*
*Baylor College of Medicine*
*Houston, Texas*

Barney J. Stern, MD
*Department of Neurology*
*Emory University School of Medicine*
*Atlanta, Georgia*

S. H. Subramony, MD
*Department of Neurology*
*The University of Mississippi*
*    School of Medicine*
*Jackson, Mississippi*

Alex C. Tselis, MD, PhD
*Department of Neurology*
*Wayne State University/Detroit Medical*
*    Center*
*Detroit, Michigan*

Gerald van Belle, PhD
*Department of Biostatistics and*
*    Environmental Health*
*University of Washington*
*Seattle, Washington*

Jacqueline Washington, MD
*Department of Neurology*
*Emory University School of Medicine*
*Atlanta, Georgia*

C. Peter N. Watson, MD, FRCP(C)
*Department of Medicine*
*The Irene Eleanor Smythe Pain Clinic*
*University of Toronto*
*Toronto, Ontario, Canada*

Emmanuelle L. Waubant, MD
*USCF/Mount Zion Multiple*
*    Sclerosis Center*
*San Francisco, California*

Theodore H. Wein, MD
*Department of Neurology*
*University of Texas Medical School*
*    at Houston*
*Houston, Texas*

William J. Weiner, MD
*Department of Neurology*
*University of Miami School of Medicine*
*Miami, Florida*

Anthony J. Windebank, MD
*Department of Neurology*
*Mayo Medical School and Mayo Clinic*
*Rochester, Minnesota*

Elaine Wyllie, MD
*Pediatric Epilepsy Program*
*The Cleveland Clinic Foundation*
*Cleveland, Ohio*

Frank M. Yatsu, MD
*Department of Neurology*
*University of Texas Medical School*
*    at Houston*
*Houston, Texas*

PART I

# ISSUES IN PROGNOSIS

# 1

# Ethical Issues Raised by the Clinical Use of Prognostic Information

BARUCH A. BRODY

The development of prognostic indicators and of reliable prognostic information can be of great value for many reasons. First, such information can be used in quality assurance activities. If the outcome of the management of patients of a certain type in a given institution is significantly worse than the outcome that would be expected given reliable prognostic information derived from general experience, then the institution in question has reason to examine carefully its management of those patients to see whether that management is substandard. Efforts funded by the Health Care Financing Administration (HCFA) in the late 1980s (Daley et al. 1988) to develop reliable prognostic indicators for stroke patients are an example of efforts to develop reliable prognostic information for quality assurance purposes. Second, such information can be used in helping to assess the impact of new interventions when a randomized trial to test the impact is impossible or inappropriate. Thus, if the outcome of the management of patients of a certain type following a new intervention is significantly better than the outcome that would be expected given reliable prognostic information derived from experience just prior to the introduction of the new intervention, then this provides the best form of a historically controlled study, a type of study that the

Food and Drug Administration (FDA) has approved (Kessler 1989). Finally, such information can be used in helping to make clinical decisions about the management of patients. For example, reliable prognostic information about persistent vegetative patients has been recommended (Multi-Society Task Force 1994; Ramsay 1996) as the basis for withholding and/or withdrawing life-prolonging care from such patients. It is this third type of use (particularly as applied to decisions to withhold and/or to withdraw such care) that we will examine in this chapter, for it is that use which raises the most pressing ethical issues.

What degree of certainty about prognosis is required before decisions about withholding and/or withdrawing life-prolonging care are appropriate? Is this prognostic certainty about mortality or about severe morbidity? What decisional processes must be undergone, and how should the information about prognosis be used in those decisional processes? These are the ethical questions that must be dealt with before we can use reliable information about prognosis as a basis for clinical decisions about withdrawing and/or withholding such care.

It is difficult to assess these issues in the abstract. Therefore, a particular example (prognostic information about the neurological outcome

3

of postarrest patients suffering from hypoxic–ischemic coma) will be used to make the discussion concrete. In the first section, three approaches are presented, one used by a Belgian collaborative group (Mullie et al. 1988), another used by a group based in New York (Levy et al. 1985), and a more recent approach developed by the BRCT I Study Group (Edgren et al. 1994). In the next two sections, fundamental features common to all of these approaches to developing adequate prognostic indicators are identified, and some of these features are challenged. In the final section, the ways in which more appropriately constructed processes could be used clinically are discussed. The goal in all of this is not primarily to criticize these approaches to a difficult problem (which have been chosen precisely because of their relatively sophisticated results), but rather to develop a better understanding of how reliable prognostic information should be factored into ethically appropriate clinical decision making about the level of care to be provided to patients who have undergone severe neurological damage.

## Three Approaches

The Belgian group used the Glasgow coma scale (GCS) as the basis for its prognostic scheme. Its scheme was developed solely for out-of-hospital cardiac arrest patients who were successfully resuscitated (there was an initial restoration of spontaneous circulation) and who were fully treated in accordance with accepted standards for advanced cardiac life support and for cardiopulmonary cerebral resuscitation. A patient was judged as a treatment failure if he or she died within 14 days or remained vegetative without regaining consciousness at the end of the 14 days, and was judged as a treatment success otherwise, even if the patient was severely disabled. The group developed its predictive rule based on an analysis of 216 patients seen in 1983 to 1984 and tested the rule in a cohort of 133 patients seen in 1985.

The predictive rule used the patient's best GCS score in the first 2 days as its basis for making initial predictions. Patients with a score of 4 or less were predicted to be treatment failures, while patients with a score of 10 or better were predicted to be treatment successes. Patients whose best score was 5 to 9 were considered not yet predictable, and predictions were deferred for 4 ad-

ditional days. At that point, a prediction was made based upon their best GCS score. If it was less than 8, the patient was predicted to be a treatment failure; if it was 8 or greater, the patient was predicted to be a treatment success.

The results were quite impressive. Of the 73 predicted to be treatment failures (54 on day 2 and 19 on day 6), only two did better by day 14, but one died on day 35 and the other survived with "substantial neurological damage." Of the 60 patients predicted to be treatment successes (49 on day 2 and 11 on day 6), 14 actually were failures (12 deaths and two vegetative patients). While the negative predictive value (97%) was clearly better than the positive predictive value (77%), the authors felt that this was appropriate: "Whereas an incorrect positive prediction has no adverse consequences for the patient, an incorrect negative prediction is unacceptable" (Mullie et al. 1988). The authors concluded that their results were very encouraging, but that a prospective study in a larger number of patients was needed before their rule could be safely used in daily clinical practice.

The New York group used a variety of specific neurological findings as the basis for its prognostic scheme. Its scheme was developed for patients suffering from hypoxic–ischemic coma as a result of cardiac arrest, respiratory failure, or profound hypotension. Outcomes were not divided just into failures and successes. Instead, outcomes were judged as best if patients recovered some independent function, as poorer if they were severely disabled and dependent upon others for daily living activities, and as poorest if they remained comatose or vegetative, and all of this was assessed in terms of best recovery in the first year independent of length of survival (even though better than 90% died in the first year). The group developed its predictive rules based on an analysis of 210 patients; it was not tested in an additional cohort of patients.

The predictive rules use the presence or absence of specific neurological findings at specified periods of time after the coma-inducing event as the basis for making predictions. For example, absence of pupillary reflexes at initial examination was very prognostic of the poorest neurological outcome, since none of the 52 patients meeting that description ever became independent and only three (6%) even regained consciousness. By contrast, presence at initial examination of preserved pupillary reflexes, motor responses that were extensor or better, and roving conjugate or better spontaneous eye movements was predictive of a much better neurological outcome, as 11 of the 27 patients (41%) meeting these criteria regained independent function. Similar rules were developed for neurological findings further down the road after the coma-inducing event.

As no attempt was made in this second group's published work to test the rules derived from a retrospective review of one cohort of patients on a different cohort of patients, one cannot present negative or positive predictive values. The authors do suggest, however, in contrast to the Belgian group, that both types of errors may be costly. Much as patients suffer if they are inappropriately predicted to do badly (since they may die as a result of withheld care when they could have survived with a good neurological outcome), so they suffer if they are inappropriately predicted to do well (since they may as a result of treatment survive as a vegetative patient for a prolonged period of time, something they may not have wanted).

The BRCT I Study Group used both coma scales (Glasgow and Glasgow-Pittsburgh) and specific neurological findings at specific times as the basis for its prognostic study. Patients involved in the study were comatose survivors of cardiac arrest who received a standardized protocol of life support at least for the first few days of the coma. A patient was judged as a treatment failure if the best result in 12 months was severe cerebral disability, persistent vegetative state, or death, and was judged as a treatment success otherwise. The group developed predictive rules based on an analysis of 262 patients; in the study under review, the rules were not tested in an additional cohort of patients.

The best of the predictive rules they developed used specific neurological findings at day 3 (their results did not support the New York rules for initial examinations, probably because their protocol required full life support for a period of time). On day 3, GCS score less than 5, Glasgow-Pittsburgh score less than 22, lack of response to pain, and lack of pupillary reflexes were all 100% predictive of a treatment failure, although the number of patients studied were less than 60 for each finding.

The group announced at the end of the article that further studies were being conducted that would test their predictive rules in a different cohort of patients. They suggested, however, that "after 3 days of observation under intensive care, a sufficiently precise clinical prediction of poor neurological outcome can be made to satisfy stringent ethical criteria for decision-making concerning limitation of life support in comatose survivors of cardiac arrest" (Edgren et al. 1994).

## Common Features of the Three Approaches

Having introduced the three approaches, the following is a discussion of the features they have in common. These features are usually—but not always—present in most other prognostic systems. These features are as follows: They are based upon a retrospective review of earlier cases; they involve controversial definitions of successful and nonsuccessful care; and they yield predictions of less than 100% certainty as to whether care in future cases will be successful.

The first feature of these approaches is that their predictive rules are built upon analyzing the results of treating patients in the past, often quite far in the past. This is most obvious for the New York group (their study, published in 1985, was based on patients admitted in the period 1973 through 1977) and the BRCT I Study Group (their study, published in 1994, was based on patients admitted in the period 1979 through 1983). It is less true of the Belgian group, whose study, published in 1988, was based on patients admitted to their hospitals in 1983 through 1985. Nevertheless, their predictive rule is based on data that, however current when published, are now more than a decade old. Moreover, until now, all of these approaches have been developed by retrospective analysis and testing. The significance of all of these limitations will emerge below.

A second feature of these approaches is that each incorporates a definition of treatment failure and success that is controversial because it is not shared with the others. Consider the case of a patient who is alive and conscious from day 14 to the end of the first year but suffers major intellectual deficits and is severely handicapped physically. This patient is a treatment success according to the Belgian group (since he is alive and conscious by day 14), a treatment failure according to the BRCT I Study Group (since his best functioning involves severe cerebral disabilities), and somewhere in between according to the New York group. Such disagreements on whether a particular case is a success or a failure are not mere academic possibilities; the case we are considering is a variation on case number 10 in the Andrews case series (Andrews 1993) of delayed recoveries. The significance of these controversies about the definition of success will also emerge below.

The third feature of each of these approaches is that their predictive rules make predictions that have less than 100% certainty. Consider the Belgian group. Even on their deliberately chosen conservative approach to predicting treatment failure, there were two incorrect predictions of treatment failure out of 73 predictions of treatment failure. Because they were extremely conservative in predicting treatment failure, they had few errors in predicting failure, but they paid a high price in a considerable percentage of errors (14 of 60 or 23%) in predicting treatment success. This trade-off will be discussed later, but it should be noted that there is no 100% certainty of prediction in their approach. It might appear that the New York approach is better in this respect. After all, of their 52 patients with no pupillary reflexes at initial examination, none ever fully recovered and became independent in their activities of daily living. Still, it should be noted that 3 of these 52 patients did regain consciousness (so treatment was to some degree successful). Moreover, as they themselves note, their data means only that we can be 95% confident that the percentage of patients with this prognostic indicator who recover independent function is somewhere between 0% and 7%. The importance of this cautionary note about the 95% confidence interval was reinforced by the BRCT I finding that predictions based upon initial examination were not that accurate. Moreover, like the Belgian approach, the New York indicators of success are much less certain. Patients with their best neurological findings at initial examination were a treatment success in only 41% of cases. Similar points can be made about the predictive rules developed in the BRCT I study. The significance of this lack of certainty will also emerge below.

Three crucial features of these approaches have been noted in this section. In the next section, the implications of these features for the clinical use of these approaches to prognosis is discussed.

## Clinical Implications of the Three Features

The first of these three features (the use of past data) is the most inevitable, and unfortunately it raises problems of variable magnitude from one prognostic indicator to the next. To understand why this is so, a review of some elementary observations about outcomes is necessary.

Clinical outcomes for a given class of patients are a function of two features: the condition of the patients when they present and the efficaciousness of the care given to these patients after they present. Over a period of time, changes in medical knowledge (and resulting changes in care) can clearly affect both. As a result, the clinical outcome for patients with the same presenting features can vary over time. Systems of prognostic indicators inevitably use past outcome data to predict future outcomes and are therefore vulnerable to the possibility that changes in treatment may mean that future outcomes will be very different from past outcomes. The degree of vulnerability is a function of the importance in treatment changes from the time the system was developed to the time it is being used, and this will vary from one indicator to another. Thus, one must recognize an inevitable uncertainty about the usefulness of prognostic indicators as one approaches a new patient.

Returning to the Belgian study (similar points could also be made about both of the other studies), the class of patients they examined were out-of-hospital cardiac arrests in the period 1983 through 1985 who were successfully resuscitated and admitted to a hospital. The management of such patients has changed since 1985. What does all of this mean for the prognostic indicator they proposed, the best GCS score in the first two days? It is hard to be sure. Does being a postarrest patient with a given GCS score mean the same thing clinically in 1999 that it meant in 1985? Do the changes in follow-up treatment make a difference as well? Might improvements in care mean that there are now more survivors who are seriously disabled, thereby producing more incorrect predictions of treatment failure, given the study's definition of treatment failure?

It is interesting to note that the authors of the study are not unaware of this problem. At one crucial point, they make the following observation:

To exclude the possibility that secular changes during the study could have affected the data, and to show the timeless character of the predictive rule, we also analyzed the patient data in randomly selected subsets; we constructed the predictive rule on a randomly selected subset of two thirds of the whole data set and tested it on the remaining third. The results obtained were identical. (Mullie et al. 1988)

None of this, unfortunately, shows the timeless character of the predictive rule. It merely shows that changes in 1983 through 1985 were not that important. It says nothing about changes since then, or about future changes in the period in which the rule might be used to guide patient management.

Conclusions from this first point should be drawn cautiously. The correct conclusion is not the global skeptical conclusion that prognostic indicators cannot be used because future outcomes may be different than past outcomes. It is, rather, that there is always a degree of uncertainty present in the use of such indicators, a degree that varies from one use to another, and that a correct decisional process must take that uncertainty into account. This will be discussed further in the section, Decisional Processes for the Clinical Use of Prognostic Information.

The second feature (the presence of a controversial definition of success in each study) gives rise to another set of issues but leads to a similar concluding point. The importance of the concept of appropriate decisional processes is highlighted again.

The authors of each of these approaches rightly understand that quality of life, as opposed to mere survival, is crucial in adequately defining success and failure. In this respect, all are improvements over other prognostic systems such as APACHE III (Knaus et al. 1991) which define success and failure solely in terms of in-hospital survival or death. Nevertheless, fundamental difficulties exist with each approach's definition of success.

One way to approach these issues and these difficulties is to consider a series of examples in which the approaches classify the results differently given the differing definitions of success adopted by these approaches. One example of their differing conclusions about success is the modified version of Andrews's patient number 10 discussed in the previous section. Another, his actual patient number 10, is the patient who regains full consciousness but lives dependent upon others for all activities of daily living. Is the treatment of such a patient a treatment success as the Belgians and the BRCT I Study Group would classify it, a minimal success (second lowest group) as the New York group would classify it, or a failure as many might think because it produced a long period of dependence for the patient and of suffering for the patient and the patient's family? Some might even say that this is worse than being vegetative because of the suffering caused to the patient by an awareness of dependency. Many more such questions could be raised, and it is hard to see how they are to be answered.

This leads to a deeper analysis of these issues, one that challenges this second feature at an even more fundamental level. Can there be a universal objective resolution of these issues that would enable a study to objectively classify some outcomes as successes and others as failures or which enables a study to classify objectively some outcomes as greater successes and others as lesser successes? Or would it be better to consider that successes and failures, or greater and lesser successes, are subjective, individually determined classifications? Thus, for some people, survival as a conscious individual for a prolonged period of time is of great value, even if one is functionally very dependent; for others, prolonged dependence on others is a horrendous prospect (perhaps out of a love for those others, perhaps out of a sense of self-dignity). In the extreme example of the vegetative patient, many would judge such a continued existence to be of no value, and some would even judge it to be a negative value; however, others would judge it to be of some positive value. For example, a 1987 statement (May et al. 1987) about vegetative patients argues that continued biological survival is of positive value.

Again, one needs to be careful about the conclusions that are drawn from these observations. The conclusion is certainly not that we should eschew considerations of quality of life as we attempt to define successful outcomes and failures; any return to a definition solely in terms of survival would be a mistake. It is rather that there is a fundamentally subjective character to judgments about quality of life, and that a correct decisional process must take into account the fundamental subjectivity of judgment about the success and/or failure of treatment. This will be examined again in the section, Decisional Processes for the Clinical Use of Prognostic Information.

The final feature (prognoses based on less than certainty) gives rise to a final set of issues and leads to similar observations about appropriate decisional processes. There is a fundamental problem about risks of different types that must be confronted as one develops a prognostic system. The system may mistakenly predict a bad outcome, and may lead (if life-prolonging care is withheld on the basis of the prediction) to the death of a patient who would have otherwise survived with a good outcome. A high negative predictive value means that there is a low likelihood that this will occur. All other things being equal, we want to have as high a negative predictive value as possible. The system may mistakenly predict a good outcome, and this may lead (because aggressive care is provided) to a long, painful dying process or to the survival of a patient in very bad condition (severely disabled or vegetative). A high positive predictive value means that there is a low likelihood that this will occur. All other things being equal, we want to have as high a positive predictive value as possible. In an ideal world, it would be possible to develop a system of prognostic indicators with perfect negative and positive predictive values. In the real world, one must often settle for less, making prognostications with known error rates, and we must choose between which rate we want to improve at the expense of the other rate. A better negative predictive value is possible by only predicting treatment failures in cases where the evidence of failure is overwhelming. This will avoid more false predictions of failure, but usually results in a lower positive predictive value because many more treatment successes are falsely predicted. On the other hand, a better positive predictive value is possible by predicting failures when the evidence of failure is less overwhelming, but this will result in a lower negative predictive value because more treatment failures are falsely predicted. How is the choice between these two options made?

The view of the Belgian group (that the highest priority must be given to attaining a very high negative predictive value because an incorrect negative prediction is unacceptable, while an incorrect positive prediction has no adverse consequences for the patient) has been quoted. Such a position cannot serve as the basis for developing a prognostic system in a world of uncertainty. In a world in which a false-negative prediction is unacceptable while a false-positive prediction has no adverse effects, a negative outcome should never be predicted, and one should wait until it occurs before acting on it; until then, only positive predictions should be made. It is precisely because false-positive predictions have adverse effects on patients, families, and the health care system that we try to make predictions, both negative and positive. The following is a quote from the New York group:

Perhaps the best answer is that if one waits until patients either awaken or die, their medical condition will have stabilized. The result can be prolonged survival for vegetative patients who might otherwise have died. For most of us this is an undesirable state. . . . The ability to predict outcome could also spare families the emotional and financial burden of prolonged care of patients with a hopeless prognosis. (Levy et al. 1985)

The BRCT I Study Group has also adopted the view that we need to balance the avoidance of both types of errors.

Therefore, it will be necessary to make trade-offs between improvements in negative predictive values and in positive predictive values. It will have to be decided what price is appropriate in lowering one predictive value to get what sort of improvement in raising the other predictive value. To do that, however, a value comparison must be made between the two types of mistakes. The more one emphasizes the harmful effects of the false-positive prediction, the more one will be prepared to accept some additional false-negative predictions to get an improvement in the positive predictive rate. The more one believes that such effects are insignificant in comparison to the harmful effects of the false-negative prediction, the more one will demand a high negative predictive rate even at the price of a considerable lowering in the positive predictive rate. The trade-offs are value choices, and they are just as much subjective individually determined choices as other value choices. There will not be any objectively correct sets of trade-offs.

Once again, conclusions should be drawn cautiously from these final observations. The conclusion is not that such trade-offs should be eschewed because they are based on subjective choices; in a world of uncertainty, any prognostic system must involve such trade-offs. Rather, it is that correct decisional processes involving prognostications of outcomes must take into account the subjectivity of the trade-offs made. Therefore, as mentioned previously, the conclusion is that the ability of decisional processes to incorporate these subjectively will be crucial for success when using prognostic information.

## Decisional Processes for the Clinical Use of Prognostic Information

The literature of medical ethics and medical jurisprudence has been dominated in the last 30 years by a canonical picture of medical decision making that involves a far more active role for patients and/or for the surrogates who speak for them. This theme is central to the legal doctrine of informed consent, with its implication that competent patients (or the surrogates of incompetent patients) can refuse care recommended by physicians, and to discussions of the ethics of decision making (Faden and Beauchamp 1986).

This canonical picture is based on two fundamental moral themes. The first is the theme of the rights of patients. Physicians may intervene on a patient only with the consent of that patient because it is the patient's body and he or she has a right to determine what is done. The second theme is that medical decisions are based on medical facts and on individual values, that the physician has expertise only about the former while the patient has expertise only about the latter, and that decision making must grow out of this joint expertise rather than from unilateral physician recommendations. Both themes are valid, and they often produce the same consequences for medical decision making. Of course there are occasions on which the consequences are different, which raises some of the most difficult questions for medical ethics. (For additional information on this topic, see Brody 1988.) The second theme is used here as the basis for developing a proper process for decision making using prognostic information.

Consider a patient who has suffered an out-of-hospital cardiac arrest, has been successfully resuscitated, and is in a coma 72 hours after the arrest. Obviously, the patient cannot now participate in any decisional process. Any necessary decisions will have to be made by the physicians caring for the patient and the surrogates of that patient (a guardian, someone with durable power of attorney, or a close family member). The crucial decision that has to be made is whether to treat the patient vigorously to avoid further arrests and to produce the best neurological outcome or to keep the patient comfortable and allow nature to take its course (whatever that may be). Naturally, there are many variations on each of these basic approaches, but the focus here is on the crucial fundamental decision.

The physician brings considerable expertise to this decision even before the development of prognostic indicators. He or she is aware of the details of the patient's condition and of what would be required to give the patient the best chance of surviving with improved neurological functioning. With prognostic indicators, he or she is better aware of the patient's likelihood of surviving and of recovering varying levels of neurological functioning. The physician brings this expertise to the decisional process. However, none of this expertise answers certain crucial questions: What outcomes would this patient judge as a success, and what outcomes would this patient judge as a failure? Would living in a severely disabled fashion, physically or mentally, be something that this patient prefers to dying or is this something that the patient would want to avoid, even at the cost of dying? Given these preferences, how would this patient want to make the trade-off between the possibility of erring and being alive but disabled versus the possibility of erring and dying when he or she could have recovered? These are value questions, and the answers will vary from individual to individual. The patient is, of course, the best authority on these matters, and any advance directives left by the patient should be consulted for guidance. When directives are not available or when the patient was silent on these issues, the next best source of information is surrogates who know the patient and the patient's values. They must use their expertise for the decisions that must be made.

Prognostic information is just more information that the physician can use in the decisional process. The goal of developing prognostic schemes is to develop information that will be relevant, when combined with the patient's values, to decisions made about levels of care. Prognostic systems should describe outcomes and assign probabilities to them, but they should neither judge some to be successes and others failures nor assign cutoff points at which predictions of success or failure are made.

A physician using the Belgian approach needs to convey to the surrogate something like the following:

The extent of a patient's coma is measured by a Glasgow coma scale. Your patient has a score of $x$. A careful study of patients with such a score reveals that the likelihood, if that patient is treated vigorously, of surviving and recovering to former status is $n_1$%; of surviving but being moderately disabled is $n_2$%; of surviving but being seriously disabled is $n_3$%; of surviving but never regaining consciousness is $n_4$%; and of dying is $n_5$%. This is the best information we now have concerning outcome, but it is based on past experience, and things have changed since then. My hunch is that this change means that certain outcomes are now more likely. In particular, there may be fewer deaths but more survivals without regaining consciousness or with severe disabilities. We have a choice between helping the patient survive and recovering some functioning or keeping the patient comfortable and letting nature take its course. I cannot tell you what to decide because what we should do is determined in large measure by the values of the patient, and you know those better than I. What would the patient have judged as an acceptable outcome, and what would he or she have preferred not to undergo, even at the cost of death? How, for example, did he or she feel about dependence? With your help in answering these questions, we can jointly try to determine what would be the best choice for this patient in light of his or her values.

Similar remarks, suitably modified, need to be made by physicians using the New York approach or the BRCT I Study Group approach.

There are many questions that need to be explored when using this approach. Some questions concern the most effective way of conveying this information, asking the questions, and coming to mutually agreed on conclusions. Other questions concern assessing the ability of surrogates to understand and participate and determining what to do if they cannot understand or will not participate. Finally, other questions concern the horrendous difficulties that arise when multiple surrogates are in conflict. The many difficulties involved in adopting this approach should not be underestimated, but it is preferable to the alternative—physicians using prognostic schemes to make decisions without considering the values of the patients.

A conclusion can now be drawn about the general clinical use of prognostic information. In the real world, prognostic information does not lead to universal treatment decisions because such decisions are a function of both objective information and subjective values. Systems of prognostic information should therefore be developed in a way that recognizes this fact, eschewing decisions about successful outcomes and trade-offs among predictive values. However, this does not undermine the significance of the development of prognostic information systems. If prognostic information without values leads nowhere, values without prognostic information point everywhere and yield no grounded clinical decisions. Reliable prognostic information is a crucial component, if not the whole basis, of sound decision making.

## References

Andrews, K. Recovery of patients after four months or more in the persistent vegetative state. BMJ 306: 1597–1600; 1993.

Brody, B. Life and death decision making. New York: Oxford University Press; 1988.

Daley, J.; Jencks, S.; Draper, D.; Lenhart, G.; Thomas, T.; Walker, J. Predicting hospital-associated mortality for medicare patients. JAMA 260:3617–3624; 1988.

Edgren, E.; Hedstrand, U.; Kelsey, S.; Sutton-Tyrrell, K.; Safar, P.; and BRCT I Study Group. Assessment of neurological prognosis in comatose survivors of cardiac arrest. Lancet 343:1055–1059; 1994.

Faden, R.; Beauchamp, T. A history and theory of informed consent. New York: Oxford University Press; 1986.

Kessler, D. The regulation of investigational drugs. N. Engl. J. Med. 320:281–288; 1989.

Knaus, W.; Wagner, D.; Draper, E.; Zimmerman, J. The APACHE III prognostic system. Chest 100: 1619–1636; 1991.

Levy, D.; Caronna, J.; Singer, B.; Lapinski, R.; Frydman, H.; Plum, F. Predicting outcome from hypoxic-ischemic coma. JAMA 253:1420–1426; 1985.

May, W.; Barry, R.; Griese, O.; Grisez, G.; Johnstone, B.; Marzen, T.; McHugh, J.; Meilaender, G.; Siegler, M.; Smith, W. Feeding and hydrating the permanently unconscious and other vulnerable persons. Issues Law Med. 3:203–217; 1987.

Multi-Society Task Force. Medical aspects of the persistent vegetative state. N. Engl. J. Med. 330:1499–1508 and 1572–1579; 1994.

Mullie, A.; Buylaert, W.; Michem, N.; Verbruggen, H. Predictive value of Glasgow coma score for awakening after out-of hospital cardiac arrest. Lancet I:137–140; 1988.

Ramsay, S. British group presents vegetative-state criteria. Lancet 347:817; 1996.

# 2

# Psychological Aspects of Prognostic Judgments

ALBERT BANDURA

It is now widely acknowledged that the level of health functioning is governed by biopsychosocial processes rather than solely by biological factors (Bandura 1997; Engle 1977). Psychological determinants contribute to physical and functional status by their impact on habits that impair or enhance health and on biological systems that mediate health and physical dysfunction. Because psychosocial factors account for some of the variability in health functioning their inclusion in prognostic schemes can enhance their predictive power. Prognostic judgments activate psychosocial processes that can influence health outcomes rather than simply serve as nonreactive forecastings. This chapter examines some of the psychological mechanisms through which prognostic judgments and clinical interventions can alter the probabilities of health outcomes.

Psychosocial determinants of health status operate largely through the exercise of personal agency. Among the mechanisms of personal agency, none is more central or pervasive than people's beliefs in their ability to exercise some control over their own health. This self-belief of personal control is called perceived self-efficacy, and is the foundation of human agency. Unless people believe that they can produce desired results by their actions they have little incentive to act or to persevere in the face of difficulties. Evidence from diverse lines of research shows that perceived self-efficacy operates as a common psychological mechanism through which psychosocial influences affect physical and functional status (Bandura 1997).

Perceived self-efficacy has diverse effects, each of which can influence health outcomes and how well people use their physical and cognitive capabilities (Bandura 1997, 1998). Such self-beliefs affect what people choose to do. They avoid activities they believe exceed their capabilities and as a result fail to develop competencies or experience declines through disuse. However, they readily undertake activities they judge themselves capable of handling. Self-efficacy beliefs also play a central role in the self-regulation of motivation. They determine how much effort people will exert in an endeavor, how long they will persevere in the face of difficulties and setbacks, and their resilience to adversity. The stronger the belief in one's efficacy, the greater and more persistent are the efforts. When faced with obstacles and disabilities, people who are beset by self-doubts about their capabilities slacken their efforts or give up quickly. A resilient sense of personal efficacy thus provides the needed staying power for surmounting difficulties that inevitably arise in any undertaking. People's beliefs in their efficacy also affect how much stress and depression they experience in taxing situations as well as their level of motivation. Stress and depression take their toll on the quality of health functioning.

## Impact of Perceived Self-Efficacy on Health Functioning

There are two major lines of research on the psychosocial determinants of health outcomes in which perceived self-efficacy plays an influential role. The more basic level of research examines how psychosocial factors affect biological systems that mediate health and susceptibility to disease through the self-efficacy mechanism. Stress has been implicated as an important contributing factor to many physical dysfunctions. Controllability appears to be a key organizing principle regarding the nature of these biological stress effects. Exposure to stressors with a concomitant strong sense of coping efficacy has no adverse physiological effects. Exposure to the same stressors with weak coping efficacy, however, activates autonomic arousal and catecholamine and endogenous opioid systems (Bandura 1997).

Biological systems are highly interdependent. The types of physiological reactions that have been shown to accompany weak coping efficacy are involved in the regulation of immune systems. Hence, exposure to uncontrollable stressors tends to impair the function of the immune system in ways that can increase susceptibility to illness (Cohen et al. 1991; Herbert and Cohen 1993a; Kiecolt-Glaser and Glaser 1987; Maier et al. 1985; Shavit and Martin 1987). Lack of behavioral or perceived control over stressors increases susceptibility to bacterial and viral infections, contributes to the development of physical disorders, and accelerates the rate of progression of disease (Schneideman et al. 1992). Building people's capabilities to manage acute and chronic stressors increases immune functioning (Antoni et al. 1990; Gruber et al. 1988; Kiecolt-Glaser et al. 1985; Wiedenfeld et al. 1990). Depression has also been shown to reduce immune function (Herbert and Cohen 1993b). Depression is associated with increased infectious disease, development and spread of malignant tumors, and faster tumor cell growth. The effect of perceived efficacy on infectious disease may be partly mediated through it effects on depression.

Lifestyle habits can enhance or impair health. This enables people to exert some behavioral control over their vitality and quality of health. The second level of research is concerned with modifying habits that enhance or impair health and functional status. Self-efficacy beliefs affect every phase of behavioral change (Bandura 1997). They determine whether people even consider changing their health-related behavior, whether they enlist the motivation and perseverance needed to succeed should they choose to do so, and how well they maintain the changes they have achieved. Each of these change processes are discussed briefly in the sections that follow.

People's beliefs that they can exercise some control over their health determine whether they consider changing their health habits or pursuing rehabilitative activities. Those who believe they lack what it takes to succeed see little point in even trying (Beck and Lund 1981) or, if they make an attempt, give up easily in the absence of quick results. Effective self-regulation of health behavior is not achieved through an act of will. It requires development of self-regulatory skills. To build a sense of controlling efficacy, people must develop skills to influence their own motivation and behavior. In such programs, they learn how to monitor the behavior they seek to change, how to set short-range, attainable subgoals to motivate and direct their efforts, and how to enlist incentives and social supports to sustain the effort needed to succeed (Bandura 1986). Once equipped with skills and belief in their capabilities, people are better able to adopt behaviors that promote health and to eliminate those that impair it. They benefit more from treatments for physical disabilities and their psychological well-being is less adversely affected by chronic impairments.

A growing body of evidence reveals that the impact of different therapeutic interventions on health outcomes is partly mediated through their effects on perceived self-efficacy. The stronger the perceived efficacy they instill, the more likely are people to enlist and sustain the effort needed to adopt and maintain health-promoting behavior. This has been shown in such diverse areas of health as level of postcoronary recovery (Ewart et al. 1983; Schröder et al 1997; Taylor et al. 1985); recovery from coronary artery surgery (Allen et al. 1990; Bastone and Kerns 1995; Jensen et al. 1993; Mahler and Kulik 1998; Oka et al.

1996; Sullivan et al. 1998); coping with cancer (Berkham et al. 1997; Cunningham et al. 1991; Merluzzi and Martinez-Sanchez 1997) and end-stage renal disease (Devins et al. 1982); adherence to immunosuppressive medication in renal transplantation (Brus et al. 1999; DeGeest et al. 1995); coping with oral surgery (Litt et al. 1995) and gastrointestinal endoscopy (Gattuso et al. 1992); enhancement of pulmonary function in patients suffering from chronic pulmonary disease (Kaplan et al. 1984); countering the debilitating and distressing effects of chronic fatigue syndrome (Findley et al. 1998); decreasing the risk of osteoporosis through physical activity and calcium intake (Haran et al. 1998); reduction in pain and dysfunction in rheumatoid arthritis (Holman and Lorig 1992; Schiaffino et al. 1991); reduction of the pain of childbirth and electing vaginal over repeat cesarean delivery (Dilles and Beal 1997; Manning and Wright, 1983); elimination of tension headaches (Holroyd et al. 1984; Martin et al. 1993); management of chronic low back, neck, and leg pain and impairment (Council et al. 1988; Dolce 1987; Kawanto et al. 1995); modification of eating habits and disorders (Desmond and Price 1988; Glynn and Ruderman 1986; Love et al. 1985; Schneider et al. 1987); reduction of cholesterol through dietary means (McCann et al. 1995); adherence to medication and prescribed rehabilitative activities (Clark and Dodge 1999; Ewart et al. 1986b); adoption and adherence to programs of physical exercise (Desharnais et al. 1986; McAuley 1992; Oman and King 1998; Sallis et al. 1986); self-management of diabetes (Grossman et al. 1987; Hurley and Shea 1992); regulation of sexual erectile functioning (Bach et al. 1999) control of sexual practices that pose high risk for transmission of AIDS (Bengel et al. 1996; McKusick et al. 1989; Walsh and Foshee 1998; Witte 1992); and control of addictive habits that impair health (DiClemente et al. 1995; Marlatt et al. 1995; Stephens et al. 1995). Meta-analyses confirm the influential role of self-efficacy beliefs across diverse domains of health functioning (Gilles 1993; Holden 1991).

Habit changes are of little value unless they endure. It is one thing to get people to change their health-related behavior; it is another thing to maintain those changes over time. People preside constantly over their own behavior, so they are in the best position to exercise influence over it.

Maintenance of habit change relies heavily on self-regulatory capabilities and the functional value of the behavior. This requires instilling a resilient sense of efficacy as well as imparting skills. Experiences in overcoming troublesome situations serve as efficacy builders. This is an important aspect of self-management because, if people are not fully convinced of their personal efficacy, they rapidly abandon the skills they have been taught when they fail to get quick results or suffer reverses. Studies of habit change show that a low sense of perceived self-efficacy increases vulnerability to relapse (Bandura 1997; DiClemente et al. 1995; Marlatt et al. 1995). Efforts at relapse prevention must be extended beyond personal change to provision of social support and guidance during difficult times. The strategies for strengthening perceived self-efficacy to enhance maintenance of health-promoting behavior and to reduce vulnerability to relapse will be considered later.

## Self-Efficacy as a Prognostic Indicator

As the above research amply documents, health outcomes are not governed solely by biologically rooted factors. Psychological determinants are also contributors through their impact on both health-related behavior and biological systems that mediate health functioning. Perceived personal efficacy is a psychological prognostic indicator of the course that health outcomes are likely to take. Results of a program of research on enhancement of perceived physical and cardiac efficacy for postcoronary recovery may serve to illustrate several general issues regarding prognosis of health outcomes and the course they are likely to take.

About half the patients who experience myocardial infarctions have uncomplicated ones (DeBusk et al. 1983). The heart heals rapidly, and they are physically capable of resuming an active life. However, the psychological and physical recovery is slow for patients who believe they have an impaired heart. They avoid physical exertion; they fear that they cannot handle the strains in their vocational and social life; they give up recreational activities; and they fear that sexual activities will do them in. The recovery problems stem more from patients' beliefs that their cardiac system has been impaired than from physical debility. The rehabilitative task is to convince patients that they have a sufficiently robust cardiovascular system to lead productive lives.

The initial study in this program of research demonstrated that having patients master increasing workloads on the treadmill strengthen patients' beliefs in their physical capabilities (Ewart et al. 1983). The stronger their perceived physical efficacy, the more active they become in their everyday life. Maximal treadmill attainment, itself, is a weak predictor of patients' level and duration of activity. Treadmill experiences exert their influence indirectly, facilitating recovery by raising patients' beliefs about their physical and cardiac capabilities. Enhanced perceived efficacy, in turn, fosters more active pursuit of everyday activities.

Ewart and his colleagues have further shown that patients' beliefs about their physical efficacy predicts compliance with prescribed exercise programs, whereas actual physical capability does not (Ewart et al. 1986a). This corroborates the earlier findings that the effect of treadmill experiences on activity level is largely mediated by changes in perceived self-efficacy. Patients who have a high sense of efficacy tend to overexercise, whereas those who doubt their physical efficacy underexercise at levels that provide little cardiovascular benefit.

Psychological recovery from a heart attack is a social, rather than solely individual, matter. The patients in the study illustrating this point were males. The wives' judgments of their husbands' physical and cardiac capabilities can aid or retard the recovery process. The direction that social support takes is partly determined by perceptions of efficacy. Spousal support is likely to be expressed in curtailment of activity if the husband's heart function is regarded as impaired, but as encouragement of activity if his heart function is judged to be robust. In the program designed to enhance postcoronary recovery (Taylor et al. 1985), the treadmill was used to raise and strengthen spousal and patients' beliefs in their cardiac capabilities.

Several weeks after patients had a heart attack their beliefs about how much strain their heart could withstand were measured. They then performed a symptom-limited treadmill, mastering increasing workloads with three levels of spouse involvement in the treadmill activity. The wife was either uninvolved in the treadmill activity; she was present to observe her husband's stamina as he performed the treadmill under increasing workloads; or she observed her husband's performance, whereupon she performed the treadmill exercises herself to gain firsthand information of the physical stamina required. We reasoned that having the wives personally experience the strenuousness of the task, and seeing their husbands match or surpass them, would convince them that their husband has a robust heart.

After the treadmill activities, couples were fully informed by the cardiologist about the patients' level of cardiac functioning and their capacity to resume activities of daily life. If the treadmill is interpreted as an isolated task, its impact on perceived cardiac and physical capability may be limited. To achieve a generalized impact of enhanced self-efficacy on diverse spheres of functioning in daily life, the stamina on the treadmill was presented as a generic indicant of cardiovascular capability. The patients were informed that their level of exertion exceeded whatever strain everyday activities might place on their cardiac system. This would encourage them to resume activities in their everyday life that place weaker demands on their cardiac system than the heavy workloads on the treadmill. The patient's and spouse's beliefs concerning his physical and cardiac capabilities were measured before and after the treadmill activity and again after the medical counseling.

Figure 2-1 shows the patterns of change in perceptions of the patients' physical and cardiac capabilities at different phases of the experiment under varying degrees of spousal involvement in the treadmill activity. Treadmill performances increased patients' beliefs in their physical and cardiac capabilities. Initially, the beliefs of wives and their husbands were highly discrepant—husbands judged themselves moderately hearty, whereas wives judged their husbands' cardiac capability as severely impaired and incapable of withstanding physical and emotional strain. Spouses who were either uninvolved in, or merely observers of, the treadmill activity, continued to believe that their husbands' physical and cardiac capabilities were severely impaired. Even the detailed medical counseling by the cardiology staff did not alter their pre-existing beliefs of their husbands' cardiac debility. However, wives

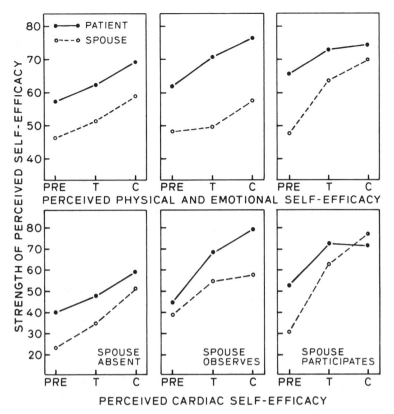

**Figure 2-1.** Changes in perceived physical and cardiac efficacy as a function of level of spouse involvement in the treadmill activity, patients' treadmill exercises, and the combined influence of treadmill exercises and medical counseling. Perceived efficacy was measured before the treadmill activity (*Pre*), after the treadmill activity (*T*), and after the medical counseling (*C*). One set of efficacy scales measured beliefs about the patient's capability to bear physical stressors (e.g., physical exertion, sexual activity) and strain of emotional stressors (e.g., anger arousal, social discord); cardiac efficacy measured beliefs about how much strain the patient's heart could withstand. (From Taylor et al. 1985).

who had personally experienced the strenuousness of the treadmill were persuaded that their husbands had a sufficiently robust heart to withstand the normal strains of everyday activities. The participant experience apparently altered spousal cognitive processing of treadmill information, giving greater weight to indicants of cardiac robustness than to symptomatic signs of cardiac debility. The change in perceived efficacy made the wives more accepting of the medical counseling. Following the medical counseling, couples in the participant spouse group had congruently high perceptions of the patients' cardiac capabilities.

The findings further show that beliefs of cardiac capabilities can affect the course of recovery from myocardial infarction. The higher the patients' and the spouses' beliefs in the patients' cardiac capabilities, the greater was the patients'

cardiovascular functioning as measured by peak heart rate and maximal workload achieved on the treadmill 6 months later. The joint belief in the patients' cardiac efficacy proved to be the best predictor of cardiac functional level. Initial treadmill performance did not predict level of cardiovascular functioning in the follow-up assessment when the influence of perceived efficacy is removed. But perceived cardiac efficacy predicted level of cardiovascular functioning when initial treadmill performance was partialled out.

Wives who believe that their husbands have a robust heart are more likely to encourage them to resume an active life than those who believe their husbands' heart is impaired and vulnerable to further damage. The positive relation between the wife's perceptions of her husband's cardiac capability and his treadmill accomplishments months later is, in all likelihood, partly mediated by spousal encouragement of activities during the interim period. Pursuit of an active life improves the patient's physical capability to engage in activities without overtaxing their cardiovascular system.

Coronary artery bypass surgery improves physical capacity; however, for some patients it produces little improvement or even deterioration in physical and social functioning. Studies of these diverse outcomes reveal that preoperative belief in one's physical efficacy is a good predictor of engagement in everyday physical and social activities, whereas physiological capacity, pre-operative severity of cardiac disability, number of coexisting medical problems, number of bypass grafts, age, or perceived exertion are nonpredictive (Allen et al. 1990; Oka et al. 1996). Intervention studies further corroborate that perceived self-efficacy is a common pathway through which psychosocial influences affect health outcomes across diverse types of diseases (Holman and Lorig 1992; Kaplan et al. 1984; O'Leary et al. 1988).

Prognostic judgments are not simply nonreactive forecasts of a natural history of a disease. Except in extreme pathologies that may be overwhelmingly determined by biological factors, the nature and course of clinical outcomes is partly dependent on psychological sources of influence. Strong belief in one's capability to exercise some control over one's physical condition serves as a psychological prognostic indicator of the probable level of health functioning. Thus, people with similar levels of physical impairment can achieve different functional outcomes depending on their self-beliefs of efficacy (Kaplan et al. 1984; Lorig et al. 1989; O'Leary et al. 1988). Even in the case of severe permanent impairment, where only partial recovery is possible, psychosocial factors will affect how much of the remaining functional capacity is realized. Because prognostic information can affect patients' beliefs in their physical efficacy, diagnosticians not only foretell but may partly influence the course of recovery from disease. This effect will be examined shortly in greater detail.

## Mode of Conveying Prognostic Information

Another important issue in the clinical management of patients concerns the way in which prognostic information is conveyed to them. This is usually done by describing possible outcomes and the probabilities associated with them. However, verbal prognostications alone may not have the intended impact, especially when they run counter to strong pre-existing beliefs, as is often the case. This is true even for positive prognostications if patients invest the medically prescribed restorative activities with grave risks. For example, in the study of postcoronary rehabilitation, wives were not in the least reassured of their husbands' cardiovascular hardiness by the positive prognostic judgments of the medical staff unless they had the benefit of direct confirmatory experiences.

To increase their persuasive influence, clinicians may have to convey positive prognostic information to their patients not only by word but also by structuring performance tasks for them that provide self-convincing experiences. This is an issue that will be explored later when discussing strategies for instilling a sense of personal efficacy and reducing vulnerability to relapse.

## Psychological Impact of Diagnostic Procedures

The manner in which diagnostic tests are conducted also can influence patients' beliefs about their efficacy, as in the cognitive processing of somatic information from the treadmill test. Treadmill activity produces a multitude of negative signs, such as fatigue, pain, shortness of breath, and other exercise-induced symptoms, which mount as the task continues. Patients who focus on their physical stamina as they master increasing workloads will judge their cardiac system as more robust than those who selectively attend to and remember the negative somatic signs. Positive indicants of capability can be made more salient by providing patients with ongoing feedback of their performance attainments as they master heavier workloads. Judgment of cardiac efficacy will vary depending on how this diverse symptom information and the indicants of cardiac robustness are weighted and integrated.

This is shown in a study with a group of healthy men and women who completed a symptom-limited treadmill before entering an exercise program (Juneau et al. 1986). Half the participants received concurrent feedback of the increasing workload they were attaining during the course of the treadmill task. The other half received the feedback about the workloads they attained just after they had completed the treadmill task. Their perceived cardiac efficacy was measured before and after the treadmill performance. They also recorded the physical signs they recall having experienced during the treadmill activity. Figure 2-2 shows how treadmill performances with and without concurrent feedback affect self-beliefs of cardiac capabilities.

In the absence of feedback of positive indicants of physical capability, exercise-induced symptoms completely dominate attention and memory representation of the treadmill experience. For healthy men, who generally have a more resilient conception of their cardiac capabilities, a taxing treadmill test without concurrent feedback did not alter their beliefs that they have a robust cardiac system. However, positive feedback that makes physical attainments on the treadmill more noticeable raised women's judgments of their cardiac capabilities. In the absence of such feedback, women read the mounting negative somatic sensations accompanying increasing exertion on the treadmill as indicants of cardiac deficiencies and lowered their judgments of their cardiac capabilities. Women did not experience any more nega-

tive somatic sensations than did men. The adverse impact of treadmill experiences without positive feedback stemmed from negative cognitive processing of symptom information rather than from greater amounts or salience of such symptoms.

Preconceptions tend to bias how information is weighted and integrated (Bandura 1986; Nisbett and Ross 1980). A similar process is indicated in women's reactions to delayed positive feedback regarding their treadmill performances. When told of their notable physical attainments, they raised their perceived cardiac efficacy to their pretreadmill level, but they achieved no net gain from the treadmill experience. Positive signs of cardiac capability are difficult to assimilate after conceptions of one's efficacy have already been formed under conditions in which negative signs clearly predominate. A coronary can markedly undermine beliefs concerning one's cardiac efficacy. A strong preconception of physical impairment makes negative physiological reactions to performance tests highly salient and recallable. Therefore, concurrent positive feedback of physical stamina would be especially important in countering beliefs of a frail cardiac capability in postcoronary patients who have not suffered clinical complications.

**Figure 2-2.** Impact of treadmill diagnostic performances on judgment of cardiac efficacy under conditions in which participants received concurrent feedback of the workloads they mastered or the feedback about their attainments was delayed until after the treadmill test was completed. (From Juneau et al. 1986.)

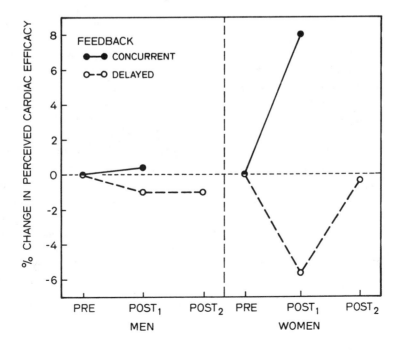

Any diagnostic procedure that gauges impairments and capabilities by testing the upper limits of performance will create a pattern of experiences reflecting both strengths and deficiencies. Patients who selectively notice and recall their performance deficiencies will judge their capabilities to be lower than those who notice their strengths as well. As shown in the preceding treadmill experiment, the adverse impact on perceived cardiac efficacy of diagnostic procedures that generate negative experiences can be reduced or counteracted by structuring performance tests in ways that give salience to one's remaining strengths. In addition to the type and timing of verbal feedback given to patients, there is some evidence to suggest that diagnostic tasks that create mounting failure by an ascending order of difficulty produce more adverse effects than if tasks of different levels of difficulty are intermixed to maintain a sense of attainment (Zigler and Butterfield 1968). Analysis of how the structure of diagnostic procedures and preconceptions of personal efficacy bias attention to, and cognitive processing of, somatic and behavioral information is of considerable clinical import as well as of theoretical interest (Cioffi 1991). The knowledge gained from these types of microanalytic studies would add greatly to our understanding of the psychological impact of experiences occasioned by diagnostic procedures.

## Scope of Prognostic Schemes

Another issue regarding prognosis concerns the range of factors included in a prognostic scheme, specifically whether health outcomes are viewed solely from a biomedical perspective or from a broader biopsychosocial perspective. As will be recalled from the earlier discussion, level of health functioning and quality of life are determined not only by the patients' physical status but also by a system of social influences that can enhance or impede the progress they make. For example, in the study of recovery from uncomplicated myocardial infarction, wives' beliefs in their husbands' cardiac robustness were better predictors of level of recovery of cardiac function than were physical indices of cardiovascular status as measured by the treadmill.

To the extent that the interpersonal influences contribute to health outcomes, giving these factors some weight in prognostic schemes will enhance their predictive utility. If no notice of them is taken, one is left with puzzling variability in the courses that health changes take and the unexplained differences in functional attainments of people who are equally physically impaired.

## Self-Validating Potential of Prognostic Judgments

Because prognostic information can affect patients' beliefs in their personal efficacy, diagnosticians not only foretell but may partly influence the course of recovery from disease. Health outcomes are related to predictive factors in complex, multidetermined, and probabilistic ways. Prognostic judgments, therefore, involve some degree of uncertainty. The predictiveness of a given prognostic scheme will depend on the number of relevant predictors it encompasses, the relative validities and interrelations of the predictors, and the adequacy with which they are measured. There is always leeway for expectancy effects to operate because prognostic schemes rarely include all of the relevant biological and psychosocial predictors and even the predictors that are singled out usually have less than perfect validity. Based on selected sources of information, diagnosticians form expectations about the probable course of a disease. The more confident they are in the validity of their prognostic scheme, the stronger are their prognostic expectations.

Prognostic expectations are conveyed to patients by attitude, word, and the type and level of care provided them. As alluded to earlier, prognostic judgments have a self-confirming potential. Expectations can alter patients' beliefs about their capabilities and their behavior in ways that confirm the original expectations. Evidence indicates that the self-efficacy mechanism operates as one important mediator of self-confirming effects. This is most clearly revealed in laboratory studies in which arbitrary information of personal capabilities is conveyed to people and its effects on their perceived self-efficacy and behavior are then measured. Self-management of pain provides a relevant example.

There are several ways by which perceived coping efficacy can facilitate the personal management of pain. People can exercise some control over their level of experienced pain through attentional and other cognitive activities that reduce conciousness of pain sensations or alter their aversiveness by how they are construed. People who believe they can alleviate pain enlist whatever ameliorative skills they have learned and persevere in their efforts. Those who judge themselves as inefficacious make no effort to do so or give up readily in the absence of quick relief. A sense of coping efficacy also reduces distressing anticipations that create aversive reactions and bodily tension, which only exacerbate pain sensations and discomfort.

Consciousness has a very limited capacity. It is hard to keep more than one thing in mind at the same time. If pain sensations are supplanted in consciousness, they are felt less. Dwelling on pain sensations only makes them more noticeable and thus more difficult to bear, whereas people can become oblivious to their bodily sensations when deeply engrossed in activities that command their attention. Perceived self-efficacy can lessen the extent to which painful stimulation is experienced as conscious pain by supporting engrossment in activities of high interest that can occupy one's consciousness for hours on end (Bandura 1997; McCaul and Malott 1984). Findings of studies of chronic clinical pain accord with this view (Jensen et al. 1991). Perceived self-regulatory efficacy predicts the use of behavioral and cognitive strategies to relieve pain after controlling for pain severity and outcome expectations. Lin and Ward (1996) provide further evidence that perceived efficacy can relieve pain by supporting palliative coping activities and creating the motivation to stick to them. People's beliefs in their pain-management efficacy reduced the intensity of low back pain and how much it interfered with daily life both directly and by fostering the use of cognitive and behavioral strategies that help to relieve pain.

The causal contribution of perceived efficacy to the self-management of pain has been verified experimentally. People given bogus feedback that they are good pain controllers raised their perceived self-efficacy and tolerance of cold pressor pain. In contrast, those led to believe that they were poor pain controllers lowered their perceived efficacy and found it hard to bear pain (Litt 1988). Instated perceived efficacy was a better predictor of pain tolerance than was past level of actual pain tolerance. A low sense of efficacy constrained efforts to ameliorate pain even when the opportunity to exercise some personal control ex-

isted. Arbitrarily altered efficacy beliefs also affected preference for personal or external control of pain. Those whose efficacy was raised preferred a strong personal role in the management of their pain; those whose efficacy was lowered wanted external interventions to stop their pain.

People who believe they can exercise some pain control are also likely to interpret unpleasant bodily sensations and states more benignly than those who believe them is nothing they can do to alleviate pain (Cioffi 1991). Focusing attention on the sensory, rather than the affective, aspects of pain also reduces distress and raises pain tolerance (Ahles et al. 1983). Even at an early age, some children discover effective pain control strategies on their own (Ross and Ross 1984). They often rely on engrossing attentional strategies when pain sensations are hard to displace from consciousness or they make them easier to bear by transforming their meaning.

Perceived efficacy mediates the analgesic potency of various psychological procedures. Cognitive techniques for alleviating pain, self-relaxation, and placebos all increase perceive efficacy both to endure and to reduce pain (Bandura et al. 1987; Reese 1983; Williams and Kinney 1991). The more self-efficacious people judge themselves to be, the less pain they experience in later cold pressor tests, and the higher is their pain threshold and pain tolerance.

Holroyd and his colleagues (1984) demonstrated with sufferers of recurrent tension headaches that the benefits of biofeedback training stem more from boosts in perceived coping efficacy than from the muscular exercises themselves. Perceived self-efficacy, created by bogus feedback that one is a skilled relaxer for controlling pain, predicted reduction in tension headaches, whereas the actual amount of change in muscle activity achieved in treatment was unrelated to the incidence of subsequent headaches.

Research on mechanisms governing self-management of pain focus heavily on ability to endure or alleviate experienced pain. Lackner and his associates extended the analysis to beliefs in efficacy to perform physical activities essential for everyday functioning that generate pain (Lackner et al. 1996). The patients were chronic pain sufferers with low back pain. Occupationally injured patients judged their efficacy for lifting, bending, carrying, pushing, and pulling objects. To test alternative regulatory mechanisms, the patients also rated their expectations that these physical activities would cause pain and reinjury. Perceived efficacy predicted performance of physical activities after controlling for pain and reinjury expectations. Neither expectations of pain intensity nor reinjury predicted level of physical function when the effects of efficacy beliefs were removed.

That perceived efficacy makes pain easier to manage is further corroborated by other studies of acute and chronic clinical pain (Council et al. 1988; Dolce 1987; Manning and Wright 1983; Holman and Lorig 1992). Treatment gains in perceived efficacy to control pain not only reduce intensity of experienced pain in long-term assessments but also increase physical functioning as measured by trunk strength and range of motion and flexion-extension movements in patients suffering from degenerative disc disease (Altmaier et al. 1993; Kaivanto et al. 1995). Belief that one can exercise some control over pain and one's physical functioning is also accompanied by fewer pain behaviors, less mood disturbance, better psychological well-being, and more active involvement in everyday activities (Affleck et al. 1987; Buescher et al. 1991; Buckelew et al. 1994; Jensen and Karoly 1991). Perceived coping efficacy predicts level of pain after controlling for disease severity, demographic factors, and depression. A strong sense of postoperative efficacy to manage pain similarly predicts use of pain medication during recovery from coronary artery surgery (Bastone and Kerns 1995).

The findings of experiments in which efficacy beliefs are raised or lowered by bogus feedback should not be taken to mean that arbitrary persuasory influence is a good way of enhancing beliefs of personal efficacy to reduce functional impairments associated with clinical conditions. Rather, such studies have special bearing on the self-confirming potential of prognostic judgments because efficacy beliefs are altered independently of actual physical status. In clinical practice, personal efficacy is strengthened by providing patients with the knowledge, coping skills, and self-assurance to make optimal use of their capabilities.

The preceding experimental analyses of self-confirming processes focused solely on how people's self-beliefs of efficacy and behavior are affected by what they are told about their capabilities. Other evidence suggests that prognostic judgments may bias how people are treated as well as what they are told. In these experiments, instructors are arbitrarily led to form either high or low expectations for those they serve. The studies generally reveal that instructors treat others differently under high than under low expectations in ways that tend to confirm the original expectations (Jones 1977; Jussim 1986). Although there is some variation in results, the findings generally show that under induced positive expectations instructors pay more attention to those in their charge, provide them with more emotional support, create greater opportunities for them to build their competencies, and give them more positive feedback than under induced low expectations.

Differential care that promotes in patients different levels of personal efficacy and skill in managing health-related behavior can exert stronger impact on the trajectories of health functioning than simply conveying prognostic information. The effects of verbal prognostications alone may be short-lived if they are repeatedly disconfirmed by personal experiences due to deficient capabilities. However, a sense of personal efficacy rooted in enhanced competencies fosters functional attainments that create their own experiential validation. Clinical transactions operate bidirectionally to shape the course of change. The functional improvements in patients fostered by positive expectancy influences further strengthen clinicians' beneficial expectations and their sense of efficacy to aid progress. In contrast, negative expectations that breed functional declines can set in motion a downward course of mutual discouragement.

## Conception of Ability

In recent years, major changes have occurred in the conception of human ability (Bandura 1990; Sternberg and Kolligian 1990). Ability is not a fixed entity that one does or does not have in one's behavioral repertoire. Rather, it involves a generative capability in which cognitive, social, emotional, and motivational factors govern the translation of knowledge and skills into performance attainments. There is a marked difference between possessing subskills and being able to integrate them into appropriate courses of action for varied purposes and to execute them well under difficult circumstances. Thus, with the same set of skills people may perform poorly, adequately, or extraordinarily depending on their thinking patterns, emotional states, and level of motivation.

The variable utilization of capabilities is illustrated in research on the impact of self-efficacy beliefs on level of memory functioning with advancing age (Bandura 1989; Berry 1987; Berry et al. 1989; Lachman et al. 1987). Human memory is an active constructive process in which information is semantically elaborated, transformed, and reorganized into meaningful cognitive representations that aid recall. People differ in how they construe memory and its changes with age (Lachman et al. 1995). Some view memory as a biological capacity that inevitably shrinks with age and is not personally controllable. Others view it as a set of cognitive skills that can be developed and maintained with effort. Those different conceptions of memory affect memory performance, with belief in memory as an improvable cognitive skill facilitating memory performance and belief in memory as a shrinking capacity impairing it. The stronger people believe in their memory capabilities, the more time they devote to cognitively processing memory tasks. Higher processing effort, in turn, produces better memory performance. Perceived self-efficacy affects actual memory performance both directly and indirectly through level of cognitive effort. Those who regard memory as simply a biologically shrinking capacity have little reason to try to exercise any control over their memory functioning. They are quick to read instances of normal forgetting as indicants of declining cognitive capacity. The more they disbelieve their memory capabilities, the poorer use they make of their cognitive capabilities.

The undermining efforts of disbelief in one's capabilities may also be mediated through depression. A low sense of personal efficacy to fulfill desired goals and to secure things that bring satisfaction to one's life creates depression. Despondent mood further diminishes beliefs in one's capabilities (Kavanagh and Bower 1985) in ways that can debilitate memory functioning. Indeed, West et al. (1983). found that depression is accompanied by a low sense of memory efficacy which, in turn, is associated with deficient memory performances.

Perceived memory efficacy predicts degree of improvement in memory performance following training in mnemonic aids (Rebok and Balcerak 1989). Self-efficacy retains its predictiveness when prior level of memory performance is controlled (Bandura 1989). However, young adults are more likely than older adults to raise their beliefs in their memory efficacy and to use the memory aids they have been taught in other types of memory tasks. Memory training in the elderly clearly requires more persuasive demonstrations that they can exercise some control over their memory in their everyday life by using cognitive strategies. This can be achieved by efficacy demonstration trials in which the elderly perform memory tasks with and without cognitive aids and observe that their memory improves when they use them. Modeling influences can be used to demonstrate how others have been able to improve their memory by habitual use of mnemonic aids. Persuasory influences that instill beliefs conducive to the use of memory skills can also help to raise elderly people's beliefs in their memory capabilities.

There are different types of memory. Significant advances in understanding memory functioning, therefore, require multifaceted measures of people's beliefs in their memory efficacy rather than a general measure. Evidence from diverse lines of research are consistent in showing that global measures sacrifice explanatory and predictive power (Bandura 1997).

Efficacy beliefs similarly contribute to level of physical functioning. This is most strikingly revealed in experiments in which beliefs of physical efficacy are raised in some people and lowered in others by bogus information unrelated to their actual physical capabilities (Weinberg et al. 1979). The higher the induced beliefs in one's physical efficacy, the greater are the physical attainments. Deficient performances spur those with a high sense of efficacy to even greater physical effort, but further impair the performances of those whose efficacy had been undermined. Self-beliefs of physical efficacy arbitrarily heightened in females and arbitrarily weakened in males obliterate large pre-existing sex differences in physical strength. As in the cognitive domain, viewing physical ability as an inherent attribute lowers perceived self-efficacy, retards skill development, and saps interest in such activities (Jourden et al. 1991). The nonability determinants of functional attainments have now been amply documented in diverse domains of activity (Bandura 1990).

## Ways of Instilling Resilient Self-Efficacy

People's beliefs about their efficacy can be developed and strengthened in four principal ways (Bandura 1986, 1997a): The most effective means is through *mastery experiences.* Successes build a robust sense of efficacy. Failures undermine it, especially if failures occur often early in the course of developing competencies. Self-efficacy is best developed by tackling challenges in successive attainable steps that serve to expand competencies. Subgoal attainments provide indicants of mastery for enhancing a sense of personal efficacy and help to sustain motivation along the way. If subgoal challenges are set too high, most performances prove disappointing and reduce motivation to continue the pursuit. People who have a low sense of efficacy are especially easily discouraged by failure and are quick to attribute it to personal incapacities.

Neurological injuries that produce severe permanent impairments can be devastatingly demoralizing to patients and their families. Patients have to reorganize their perspective to learn alternative ways of regaining as much control as possible over their life activities. Goals need to be restructured in ways that capitalize on remaining capacities. Ozer (1988) illustrates effective ways of structuring goals couched in functional terms to minimize disabilities created by chronic neurological impairment. Focus on achievement of functional improvements rather than on degree of organic impairments helps to counteract self-demoralization. Making difficult activities easier by breaking them down into graduated attainable steps helps to prevent self-discouragement of rehabilitative efforts.

Development of resilient self-efficacy requires some experience in mastering difficulties through perseverant effort. If people experience only easy successes they come to expect quick results. Their sense of efficacy is easily undermined by failure. Some setbacks and difficulties in human pursuits serve a useful purpose in teaching that success usually requires sustained effort. People develop resilience by learning how to manage failure, how to recover from failed attempts and setbacks, and how to enlist social support for their efforts. After they become convinced they have what it takes to succeed, they persevere in the face of adversity and quickly rebound from setbacks. By sticking it out through tough times, they emerge from adversity with a stronger sense of efficacy.

The second way of enhancing personal efficacy is through *social modeling.* People partly judge their capabilities in comparison with others (Bandura 1991). Seeing people similar to oneself regain, by perseverant effort, some control over their life activities despite impairment raises observers' beliefs about their own capabilities to lessen their disabilities. The failures of others coping with similar problems instill self-doubts about one's own ability to manage similar tasks. Having ex-patients exemplify the active lives they are leading can be especially influential in strengthening beliefs that functional improvements are realizable. Seeing how others manage difficult conditions can alter beliefs of personal efficacy through ways other than social comparison. Efficacious models can teach competencies and effective strategies for dealing with taxing situations. Adoption of serviceable strategies raises perceived self-efficacy. People also draw inspiration from seeing others change their lives for the better.

*Social persuasion* is the third mode of influence. People try to talk others into believing they possess the capabilities to achieve what they seek. Realistic boosts in efficacy can lead people to exert greater effort, which increases their chances of success. However, to raise unrealistic beliefs of personal capability runs the risk of inviting failure. Successful efficacy builders, however, do more than express faith in people's capabilities. They structure tasks for them in ways that are likely to bring improvements and avoid placing them prematurely in situations where they are likely to fail. By maintaining an efficacious attitude that functional gains are attainable when patients are beset with self-doubts, clinicians can help them to sustain their coping efforts in the face of reverses and discouraging obstacles. Through these various means clinicians can help patients to make the best use of their capacities.

People also rely partly on their physiological state in judging their capabilities. They read their anxiety arousal and tension as signs of vulnerability to dysfunction. In activities involving strength and stamina, people interpret their fatigue, aches, and pains as indicants of physical inefficacy. The fourth way of modifying personal efficacy is to equip patients with skills to reduce aversive physiological reactions or alter how they interpret somatic information. The meanings assigned to bodily sensations and states can have significant health consequences (Bandura 1991; Cioffi 1991).

The health benefits of a sense of personal efficacy do not arise simply from the incantation of capability. Saying something should not be confused with believing it to be so. Simply saying that one is capable is not necessarily self-convincing, especially when it contradicts firm pre-existing beliefs. No amount of declaration that one can fly, will persuade one that he or she has the efficacy to become airborne. Self-efficacy beliefs are the product of a complex process of self-persuasion that relies on cognitive processing of diverse sources of efficacy information conveyed behaviorally, vicariously, socially, and physiologically. Their strength is affected by the authenticity of the efficacy information on which they are based. Self-efficacy beliefs that are firmly established are resilient to adversity. In contrast, weakly held self-beliefs are highly vulnerable to change and negative experiences readily reinstate disbelief in one's capabilities.

## Reduction of Vulnerability to Relapse

Each of the methods for enhancing efficacy can be used to develop the resilient sense of perceived efficacy needed to override difficulties that inevitably arise from time to time. With regard to the performance mode, a resilient belief in one's personal efficacy is built through repeated demonstration trials in the exercise of control over progressively more difficult tasks. For example, as part of instruction in cognitive pain control strategies, arthritic patients were given efficacy demonstration trials in which they performed pain-producing activities with and without cognitive control and rated the level of pain they experienced (O'Leary et al. 1988). Explicit evidence that they achieved substantial reduction in experienced pain by cognitive means provided persuasive demonstrations that they could exercise some control over pain by enlisting cognitive-control strategies. Efficacy validating trials not only serve as efficacy builders, but put to trial the value of the techniques being taught.

Modeling influences, in which other patients demonstrate how to cope with difficulties and setbacks and show that success usually requires tenacious effort, can further strengthen perceived self-efficacy. Moreover, modeled perseverant success can alter the diagnosticity of failure experiences. Eventual accomplishments indicate that earlier failures partly reflect difficult task and situational factors rather than solely inherent personal deficiencies. Under this cognitive set, difficulties and setbacks prompt redoubling of efforts rather than breed self-discouraging doubts about one's capabilities. For example, pain threshold and tolerance is affected by modeling influences (Craig 1983). Thus, people who have seen others persevere despite pain function much more effectively when they themselves are in pain than if they had seen others give up quickly (Turkat and Guise 1983; Turkat et al. 1983).

Persuasory influences that instill self-beliefs conducive to optimal utilization of skills can also contribute to staying power. As a result, people who are persuaded they have what it takes to succeed and are told that the gains they achieved in treatment verify their capability are more successful in sustaining their altered health habits over a long time than those who undergo the same treatment without the efficacy-enhancing component (Blittner et al. 1978).

## Concluding Remarks

The present analysis addressed the issue of prognosis from a biopsychosocial perspective on health and human agentic capability. Converging lines of evidence indicate that perceived self-efficacy operates as an important prognostic indicator of level of functioning. Strength of perceived self-efficacy can influence the course of health outcomes and functional status through its intervening effects on cognitive, motivational, affective, and biological processes. In social cognitive theory (Bandura 1986, 1997), perceived efficacy is part of a larger set of sociocognitive factors that regulate human motivation, action, and well-being. People also motivate and guide their behavior by the physical, social, and self-evaluative effects they expect their efforts to produce. Personal goals and aspirations about the future one seeks to achieve and the intermediate plans and strategies for realizing that vision operate as another motivating force. Once people commit themselves to valued goals, they mount the effort needed to fulfill them. Perceived impediments, in the form of personal, social, and institutional barriers, further affect self-motivation and emotional well-being. Efficacy beliefs play a pivotal role in the exercise of personal agency because they not only operate on behavior in their own right, but through their impact on these other determinants. People's belief in their personal efficacy influence the goals and challenges they set for themselves, the outcomes they expect their actions to produce, and whether they view impediments as surmountable or as daunting obstacles over which they can exert little control.

Prognostic schemes that encompass sociocognitive determinants will have greater predictive power than those that ignore them. Moreover, prognostic evaluations have a self-confirming potential. Whether patients are expected to do well or to do poorly can affect their clinical management and beliefs in their capabilities in ways that confirm the original expectations. Patients are best served by prognosticians that enable them to realize their potential.

## References

Affleck, G.; Tennen, H.; Pfeiffer, C.; Fifield, J. Appraisals of control and predictability in adapting to a chronic disease. J. Pers. Soc. Psychol. 53:273–279; 1987.

Ahles, T. A.; Blanchard, E. B.; Leventhal, H. Cognitive control of pain: attention to the sensory aspects of the cold pressor stimulus. Cog. Ther. Res. 7:159–178; 1983.

Allen, J. K.; Becker, D. M.; Swank, R. T. Factors related to functional status after coronary artery bypass surgery. Heart Lung 19:337–343; 1990.

Altmaier, E. M.; Russell, D. W.; Kao, C. F.; Lehmann, T. R.; Weinstein, J. N. Role of self-efficacy in rehabilitation outcome among chronic low back pain patients. J. Counsel. Psychol. 40:1–5; 1993.

Antoni, M. H.; Schneiderman, N.; Fletcher, M. A.; Goldstein, D. A.; Ironson, G.; Laperriere, A. Psychoneuroimmunology and HIV-1. J. Consult. Clin. Psychol. 58:38–49; 1990.

Bach, A. K.; Brown, T. A.; Barlow, D. H. The effects of false negative feedback on efficacy expectancies and sexual arousal in sexually functional males. Behav. Ther. 30:79–95; 1999.

Bandura, A. Social foundations of thought and action: a social cognitive theory. Englewood Cliffs, NJ: Prentice-Hall; 1986.

Bandura, A. Regulation of cognitive processes through perceived self-efficacy. Dev. Psychol. 25:729–735; 1989.

Bandura, A. Reflections on nonability determinants of competence. In: Sternberg R. J.; Kolligian, J., Jr., eds. Competence considered. New Haven, CT: Yale University Press; 1990: p. 315–362.

Bandura, A. Self-efficacy mechanism in physiological activation and health-promoting behavior. In: Madden, J., IV, ed. Neurobiology of learning, emotion and affect. New York: Raven Press; 1991: p. 229–270.

Bandura, A. Self-efficacy: the exercise of control. New York: W. H. Freeman; 1997.

Bandura, A. Health promotion from the perspective of social cognitive theory. Psychol. Health 13:1–27; 1998.

Bandura, A.; O'Leary, A.; Taylor, C. B.; Gauthier, J.; Gossard, D. Perceived self-efficacy and pain control: opioid and nonopioid mechanisms. J. Pers. Soc. Psychol. 63:563–571; 1987.

Bastone, E. C.; Kerns, R. D. Effects of self-efficacy and perceived social support on recovery-related behaviors after coronary artery bypass graft surgery. Ann. Behav. Med. 17:324–330; 1995.

Beck, K. H.; Lund, A. K. The effects of health threat seriousness and personal efficacy upon intentions and behavior. J. Appl. Soc. Psychol. 11:401–415; 1981.

Beckham, J. C.; Burker, E. J.; Lytle, B. L.; Feldman, M. E.; Costakis, M. J. Self-efficacy and adjustment in cancer patients: a preliminary report. Behav. Med. 23: 137–142; 1997.

Bengel, J.; Belz-Merk, M.; Farin, E. The role of risk perception and efficacy cognitions in the prediction of HIV-related preventive behavior and condom use. Psychol. Health. 11:505–525; 1996.

Berry, J. M. A self-efficacy model of memory performance. Paper presented at the American Psychological Association meetings, New York, NY; 1987.

Berry, J. M.; West, R. L.; Dennehey, D. Reliability and validity of the memory self-efficacy questionnaire. Dev. Psychol. 25:701–713; 1989.

Blittner, M.; Goldberg, J.; Merbaum, M. Cognitive self-control factors in the reduction of smoking behavior. Behav. Ther. 9:553–561; 1978.

Brus, H.; vandeLaar, M.; Taal, E.; Rasker, J.; Wiegman, O. Determinants of compliance with medication in patients with rheumatoid arthritis: the importance of self-efficacy expectations. Patient Educ. Counsel. 36:57–64; 1999.

Buckelew, S. P.; Parker, J. C.; Keefe, F. J.; Deuser, W. E.; Crews, T. M.; Conway, R.; Kay, D. R.; Hewett, J. E. Self-efficacy and pain behavior among subjects with fibromyalgia. Pain 59: 377–384; 1994.

Buescher, K. L.; Johnston, J. A.; Parker, J. C.; Smarr, K. L.; Buckelew, S. P.; Anderson, S. K.; Walker, S. E. Relationship of self-efficacy to pain behavior. J. Rheumatol. 18:968–972; 1991.

Clark, N. M.; Dodge, J. A. Exploring self-efficacy as a predictor of disease management. Health Educ. Behav. 26:72–89; 1999.

Cioffi, D. Beyond attentional strategies: a cognitive-perceptual model of somatic interpretation. Psychol. Bull. 109:25–41; 1991.

Cohen, S.; Tyrrell, D. A. J.; Smith, A. P. Psychological stress and susceptibility to the common cold. N. Engl. J. Med. 325:606–612; 1991.

Council, J. R.; Ahern, D. K.; Follick, M. J.; Kline, C. L. Expectancies and functional impairment in chronic low back pain. Pain 33:323–331; 1988.

Craig, K. D. A social learning perspective on pain experience. In: Rosenbaum, M.; Franks, C. M.; Jaffe, Y., eds. Perspectives on behavior therapy in the eighties. New York: Springer; 1983: p. 311–327.

Cunningham, A. J.; Lockwood, G. A.; Cunningham, J. A. A relationship between perceived self-efficacy and quality of life in cancer patients. Patient Educ. Counsel. 17:71–78; 1991.

DeBusk, R. F.; Kraemer, H. C.; Nash, E. Stepwise risk stratification soon after acute myocardial infarction. Am. J. Cardiol. 12:1161–1166; 1983.

DeGeest, S.; Borgermans, L.; Gemoets, H.; Abraham, I.; Vlaminck, H.; Evers, G.; Vanrenterghem, Y. Incidence, determinants, and consequences of subclinical non-compliance with immunosuppressive therapy in renal transplant recipients. Transplantation 59:340–346; 1995.

Desharnais, R.; Bouillon, J.; Grodin, G. Self-efficacy and outcome expectations as determinants of exercise adherence. Psychol. Rep. 59:1155–1159; 1986.

Desmond, S. M.; Price, J. H. Self-efficacy and weight control. Health Educ. 19:12–18; 1988.

Devins, G. M.; Binik, Y. M.; Gorman, P.; Dattel, M.; McCloskey, B.; Oscar, G.; Briggs, J. Perceived self-efficacy, outcome expectations, and negative mood states in end-stage renal disease. J. Abnorm. Psychol. 91:241–244; 1982.

DiClemente, C. C.; Fairhurst, S. K.; Piotrowski, N. A. Self-efficacy and addictive behaviors. In Maddux J. E., ed. Self-efficacy, adaptation, and adjustment: theory, research and application. New York: Plenum; 1995: p. 109–141.

Dilles, F. M.; Beal, J. A. Role of self-efficacy in birth choice. J. Perinatol. Neonat. Nurs. 11:1–9; 1997.

Dolce, J. J. Self-efficacy and disability beliefs in behavioral treatment of pain. Behav. Res. Ther. 25:289–300; 1987.

Engle, G. L. The need for a new medical model: a challenge for biomedicine. Science 196: 129–136; 1977.

Ewart, C. K.; Stewart, K. J.; Gillilan, R. E.; Kelemen, M. H. Self-efficacy mediates strength gains during circuit weight training in men with coronary artery disease. Med. Sci. Sports Exerc. 18:531–540; 1986a.

Ewart, C. K.; Stewart, K. J.; Gillilan, R. E.; Kelemen, M. H.; Valenti, S. A.; Manley, J. D.; Kalemen, M. D. Usefulness of self-efficacy in predicting overexertion during programmed exercise in coronary artery disease. Am. J. Cardiol. 57:557–561; 1986b.

Ewart, C. K.; Taylor, C. B.; Reese, L. B.; DeBusk, R. F. Effects of early post-myocardial infarction exercise testing on self-perception and subsequent physical activity. Am. J. Cardiol. 51:1076–1080; 1983.

Findley, J. C.; Kerns, R.; Weinberg, L. D.; Rosenberg, R. Self-efficacy as a psychological moderator of chronic fatigue syndrome. J. Behav. Med. 21:351–362; 1998.

Gattuso, S. M.; Litt, M. D.; Fitzgerald, T. E. Coping with gastrointestinal endoscopy: self-efficacy enhancement and coping style. J. Consult. Clin. Psychol. 60:133–139; 1992.

Gillis, A. J. Determinants of a health-promoting lifestyle: an integrative review. J. Adv. Nurs. 18:345–353; 1993.

Glynn, S. M.; Ruderman, A. J. The development and validation of an eating self-efficacy scale. Cog. Ther. Res. 10:403–420; 1986.

Grossman, H. Y.; Brink, S.; Hauser, S. T. Self-efficacy in adolescent girls and boys with insulin-dependent diabetes mellitus. Diabetes Care 10:324–329; 1987.

Gruber, B.; Hall, N. R.; Hersh, S. P.; Dubois, P. Immune system and psychologic changes in metastatic cancer patients using relaxation and guided imagery: a pilot study. Scand. J. Behav. Thera. 17:25–46; 1988.

Herbert, T. B., Cohen, S. Stress and immunity in humans: a meta-analytic review. Psychosom. Med. 55:364–379; 1993a.

Herbert, T. B.; Cohen, S. Depression and immunity: a meta-analytic review. Psychol. Bull. 113:472–486; 1993b.

Holden, G. The relationship of self-efficacy appraisals to subsequent health related outcomes: a meta-analysis. Soc. Work Health Care. 16:53–93; 1991.

Holman, H.; Lorig, K. Perceived self-efficacy in self-management of chronic disease. In: Schwarzer R., ed. Self-efficacy: thought control of action. Washington, DC: Hemisphere; 1992: p. 305–323.

Holroyd, K. A.; Penzien, D. B.; Hursey, K. G.; Tobin, D. L.; Rogers, L.; Holm, J. E.; Marcille, P. J.; Hall, J. R.; Chila, A. G. Change mechanisms in EMG biofeedback training: cognitive changes underlying improvements in tension headache. J. Consult. Clin. Psychol. 52:1039–1053; 1984.

Horan, M. L.; Kim, Katherine K.; Gendler, P.; Froman, R. D.; Patel, M. D. Development and evaluation of the osteoporosis self-efficacy scale. Res. Nurs. Health 21:395–403; 1998.

Hurley, C. C.; Shea, C. A. Self-efficacy: strategy for enhancing diabetes self-care. Diabetes Educ. 18:146–150; 1992.

Jensen, K.; Banwart, L.; Venhaus, R.; Popkess-Vawter, S.; Perkins, S. B. Advanced rehabilitation nursing care of coronary angioplasty patients using self-efficacy theory. J. Adv. Nurs. 18:926–931; 1993.

Jensen, M. P.; Karoly, P. Control beliefs, coping efforts, and adjustment to chronic pain. J. Consult. Clin. Psychol. 59:431–438; 1991.

Jensen, M. P.; Turner, J. A.; Romano, J. M. Self-efficacy and outcome expectancies: relationship to chronic pain coping strategies and adjustment. Pain 44:263–269; 1991.

Jones, R. A. Self-fulfilling prophesies: social, psychological, and physiological effects of experiences. Hillsdale, NJ: Erlbaum; 1977.

Jourden, F. J.; Bandura, A.; Banfield, J. T. The impact of conceptions of ability on self-regulatory factors and motor skill acquisition. J. Sport Exerc. Psychol. 8:213–226; 1991.

Juneau, M.; Rogers, F.; Bandura, A.; Taylor, C. B.; DeBusk, R. Cognitive processing of treadmill experiences and self-appraisal of cardiac capabilities. Stanford University, Stanford, CA; 1986.

Jussim, L. Self-fulfilling prophecies: a theoretical and integrative review. Psychol. Rev. 93:429–445; 1986.

Kaplan, R. M.; Atkins, C. J.; Reinsch, S. Specific efficacy expectations mediate exercise compliance in patients with COPD. Health Psychol. 3:223–242; 1984.

Kavanagh, D. J.; Bower, G. H. Mood and self-efficacy: impact of joy and sadness on perceived capabilities. Cog. Ther. Res. 9:507–525; 1985.

Kawvanto, K. K.; Estlander, A-M.; Moneta, G. B.; Vanharanta, H. Isokinetic performance in low back pain patients: the predictive power of the self-efficacy scale. J. Occup. Rehab. 5:87–99; 1995.

Kiecolt-Glaser, J. K.; Glaser, R. Behavioral influences on immune function: evidence for the interplay between stress and health. In: Field, T., McCabe, P. M., Schneiderman, N., eds. Stress and coping across development. Vol. 2. Hillsdale, NJ: Erlbaum; 1987: p. 189–206.

Kiecolt-Glaser, J. K.; Glaser, R.; Strain, E. C.; Stout, J. C.; Tarr, K. L.; Holliday, J. E.; Speicher, C. E. Modulation of cellular immunity in medical students. J. Behav. Med. 9:5–21; 1986.

Kiecolt-Glaser, J. K.; Glaser, R.; Williger, D.; Stout, J.; Messick, G.; Sheppard, S.; Ricker, D.; Romisher, S. C.; Briner, W.; Bonnell, G.; Donnerberg, R. Psychosocial enhancement of immunocompetence in a geriatnic population. Health Psychol 4:25–41; 1985.

Lachman, M.; Bandura, M.; Weaver, S. L.; Elliott, E. Assessing memory control beliefs: the memory controllability inventory. Aging Cog. 2:67–84; 1995.

Lachman, M. E.; Steinberg, E. S.; Trotter, S. D. Effects of control beliefs and attributions on memory self-assessments and performance. Psychol. Aging 2:266–271; 1987.

Lackner, J. M.; Carosella, A. M.; Feuerstein, M. Pain expectancies, pain, and functional self-efficacy expectancies as determinants of disability in patients with chronic low back disorders. J. Consul. Counsel. Psychol. 64:212–220; 1996.

Lin, C.; Ward, S. E. Perceived self-efficacy and outcome expectancies in coping with chronic low back pain. Res. Nurs. Health 19:299–310; 1996.

Litt, M. D. Self-efficacy and perceived control: cognitive mediators of pain tolerance. J. Pers. Soc. Psycol. 54:149–160; 1988.

Litt, M. D.; Nye C.; Shafer, D. Preparation for oral surgery: evaluating elements of coping. J. Behav. Med. 18:435–459; 1995.

Lorig, K.; Seleznick, M.; Lubeck, D.; Ung, E.; Chastain, R. L.; Holman, H. R. The beneficial outcomes of the arthritis self-management course are not adequately explained by behavior change. Arthritis Rheuma. 32:91–95; 1989.

Love, S. Q.; Ollendick, T. H.; Johnson, C.; Schlezinger, S. E. A preliminary report of the prediction of bulimic behavior: a social learning analysis Bull. Soc. Psychol. Addict. Behav. 4:93–101; 1985.

Mahler, H. I. M.; Kulik, J. A. Effects of preparatory videotapes on self-efficacy beliefs and recovery from coronary bypass surgery. Ann. Behav. Med. 20:39–46; 1998.

Maier, S. F.; Laudenslager, M. L.; Ryan, S. M. Stressor controllability, immune function, and endogenous opiates. In: Brush, F. R., Overmier, J. B., eds. Affect, conditioning, and cognition: essays on the determinants of behavior. Hillsdale, NJ: Erlbaum; 1985: p. 183–201.

Manning, M. M.; Wright, T. L. Self-efficacy expectancies, outcome expectancies, and the persistence of pain control in childbirth. J. Pers. Soc. Psychol. 45:421–431; 1983.

Marlatt, G. A.; Baer, J. S.; Quigley, L. A. Self-efficacy and addictive behavior. In: Bandura, A., ed. Self-efficacy in changing societies. New York: Cambridge University Press; 1995: P. 289–315.

Martin, N. J.; Holroyd, K. A.; Rokicki, L. A. The headache self-efficacy scale: adaptation to recurrent headaches. Headache J. 33:244–248; 1993.

McAuley, E. Understanding exercise behavior: a self-efficacy perspective. In: Roberts, G. C., ed. Motivation in sport and exercise. Champaign, IL: Human Kinetics; 1992: P. 107–127.

McCann, B. S.; Bovbjerg, V. E.; Brief, D. J.; Turner, C.; Follette, W. C; Fitzpatrick, V; Dowdy, A.; Retzlaff, B.; Walden, C. E.; Knopp, R. H. Relationship of self-efficacy to cholesterol lowering and dietary change in hyperlipidemia. Ann. Behav. Med. 17:221–226; 1995.

McCaul, K. D.; Malott, J. M. Distraction and coping with pain. Psychol. Bull. 95:516–533; 1984.

McKusick, L.; Coates, T. J.; Morin, S. F. Longitudinal predictors of reductions in high risk sexual behaviors among gay men in San Francisco: the AIDS behavioral research project. Am. J. Public Health 80:978–983; 1989.

Merluzzi, T. V.; Martinez-Sanchez, M. A. Assessment of self-efficacy and coping with cancer: development and validation of the cancer behavior inventory. Health Psychol. 16: 163–170; 1997.

Nisbett, R.; Ross, L. Human inference: strategies and shortcomings of social judgment. Englewood Cliffs, NJ: Prentice-Hall; 1980.

Oka, R. K.; Gortner, S. R.; Stotts, N. A.; Haskell, W. L. Predictors of physical activity in patients with chronic heart failure secondary to either ischemic or idiopathic dilated cardiomyopathy. Am. J. Cardiol. 77:159–163; 1996.

O'Leary, A.; Shoor, S.; Lorig, K.; Holman, H. R. A cognitive-behavioral treatment for rheumatoid arthritis. Health Psychol. 7:527–544; 1988.

Oman, R. F.; King, A. C. Predicting the adoption and maintenance of exercise participation using self-efficacy and previous exercise participation rates. Am. J. Health Promot. 12:154–161; 1998.

Ozer, M. N. The management of persons with spinal cord injury. New York: Demos; 1988.

Rebok G. W.; Balcerak, L. J. Memory self-efficacy and performance differences in young and old adults: effect of mnemonic training. Dev. Psychol. 25:714–721; 1989.

Reese, L. Coping with pain: the role of perceived self-efficacy. Unpublished doctoral dissertation, Stanford University, Stanford, CA; 1983.

Ross, D. M.; Ross, S. A. Childhood pain: the school-aged child's view. Pain. 20:179–191; 1984.

Sallis, J. F.; Haskell, W. L.; Fortmann, S. P.; Vranizan, M. S.; Taylor, C. B.; Solomon, D. S. Predictors of adoption and maintenance of physical activity in a community sample. Prev. Med. 15:331–341; 1986.

Schiaffino, K. M.; Revenson, T. A.; Gibofsky, A. Assessing the impact of self-efficacy beliefs on adaptation to rheumatoid arthritis. Arthritis Care Res. 4:150–157; 1991.

Schneider, J. A.; O'Leary, A.; Agras, W. S. The role of perceived self-efficacy in recovery from bulimia: a preliminary examination. Behav. Res. Ther. 25:429–432; 1987.

Schneiderman, N.; McCabe, P. M.; Baum, A., eds. Stress and disease processes: perspectives in behavioral medicine. Hillsdale, NJ: Erlbaum; 1992.

Schröder, K. E. E.; Schwarzer, R.; Endler, N. S. Predicting cardiac patients' quality of life from the characteristics of their spouses. J. Health Psychol. 2:231–244;1997.

Shavit, Y.; Martin, F. C. Opiates, stress, and immunity: animal studies. Ann. Behav. Med. 9:1–20; 1987.

Stephens, R. S.; Wertz, J. S.; Roffman, R. A. Self-efficacy and marijuana cessation: a construct validity analysis. J. Consult. Clin. Psychol. 63:1022–1031;1995.

Sternberg, R. J.; Kolligian, J., Jr., eds. Competence considered: perceptions of competence and incompetence across the lifespan. New Haven, CT: Yale University Press; 1990.

Sullivan, M. D.; Andrea, Z.; LaCroix, A. Z.; Russo, J.; Katon, W. J. Self-efficacy and self-reported functional status in coronary heart disease: a six-month prospective study. Psychosom. Med. 60:473–478; 1998.

Taylor, C. B.; Bandura, A.; Ewart, C. K.; Miller, N.H.; DeBusk, R. F. Exercise testing to enhance wives' confidence in their husbands' cardiac capabilities soon after clinically uncomplicated acute myocardial infarction. Am. J. Cardiol. 55:635–638; 1985.

Turkat, I. D.; Guise, B. J. The effects of vicarious experience and stimulus intensity of pain termination and work avoidance. Behav. Res. Ther. 21:241–245; 1983.

Turkat, I. D.; Guise, B. J.; Carter, K. M. The effects of vicarious experience on pain termination and work avoidance: a replication. Behav. Res. Ther. 21:491–493; 1983.

Walsh, J. F.; Foshee, V. Self-efficacy, self-determination and victim blaming as predictors of adolescent sexual victimization. Health Educ. Res. 13:139–144; 1998.

Weinberg, R. S.; Gould, D.; Jackson, A. Expectations and performance: an empirical test of Bandura's self-efficacy theory. J. Sport Psychol. 1:320–331; 1979.

Wiedenfeld, S. A.; O'Leary, A.; Bandura, A.; Brown, S.; Levine, S.; Raska, K. Impact of perceived self-efficacy in coping with stressors on components of the immune system. J. Pers. Soc. Psychol. 59:1082–1094; 1990.

West, R. L.; Berry, J. M.; Powlishta, K. K. Self-efficacy and prediction of memory task performance. Washington University, St. Louis, MO; 1983.

Williams, S. L.; Kinney, P. J. Performance and non-performance strategies for coping with acute pain: the role of perceived self-efficacy, expected outcomes, and attention. Cog. Ther. Res. 15:1–19; 1991.

Witte, K. The role of threat and efficacy in AIDS prevention. Int. Q. Community Health Educ. 12:225–249; 1992.

Zigler, E.; Butterfield, E. C. Motivational aspects of changes in IQ test performance of culturally deprived nursery school children. Child Dev. 39:1–14; 1968.

# 3

# Medical Legal Issues in the Prognosis of Neurologic Disorders

ROBERT E. NORA AND LOIS MARGARET NORA

A number of medical legal issues arise in the consideration of prognosis in neurological disorders. This chapter will introduce several issues that practicing physicians who deliver information about prognosis should be aware of. The chapter begins with an exploration of informed consent. Informed consent is an ethical and legal doctrine which states that competent patients have the right to make informed decisions about their own medical treatment based upon adequate information provided by the physician. Obviously, the physician's opinion about prognosis, and any changes in prognosis related to medical or surgical interventions, is relevant to informed decision making. The issue of misdiagnosis is then addressed. What happens when a physician's prognostic statements are incorrect because the patient's diagnosis is incorrect? Finally, the emerging issue of medical futility is discussed. A decision that a particular intervention will be futile for a patient frequently relates to a prognostic conclusion that the physician has made and sometimes impacts the patient's prognosis.

Laws regarding informed decision making and medical malpractice vary significantly from state to state. Consequently, while the attempt has been made to provide a helpful overview, it is important that any reader consult with experts in his or her own jurisdiction on specific issues that arise.

## Informed Consent

According to the Presidential Commission for the Study of Ethical Problems in Medicine and Biomedical and Behavioral Research (1982), 90% of physicians surveyed in 1961 preferred not to inform their patients of a diagnosis of cancer. In contrast, by 1977, 97% of physicians surveyed said they relayed diagnoses of cancer to their patients on a routine basis (Presidential Commission 1982). These statistics reflect "a revolution in attitudes among patients and physicians alike regarding the desirability of frank and open disclosure of relevant medical information" (Presidential Commission 1982). This revolution in attitudes was both a cause and an effect of the legal doctrine of informed consent.

The present-day informed consent doctrine represents the legal system's attempt to balance the patient's philosophical right to control his or her medical treatment with the physician's need for some professional discretion and freedom of action in treating the patient. The doctrine has evolved alongside society's recognition of the patient's right to control his or her medical treatment, the increasing sophistication of medicine, medical technology and the health care delivery system, and the increasing interplay of medicine and the courts.

The scope and extent of the informed consent doctrine has changed quickly and haphazardly, leaving different standards in effect in different jurisdictions. This section will define informed consent, provide historical background of the legal doctrine, and describe its current status.

## Defining Informed Consent

An informed consent can be broadly defined as "a person's agreement to allow something to happen (e.g., a surgical procedure, a lumbar puncture, beginning anticonvulsant medication) that is based on a full disclosure of facts needed to make the decision intelligently" (Black's Law Dictionary 1979). Unfortunately, a more specific definition cannot be obtained, since the more specific definitions used in the cases all incorporate the doctrinal standards used in the applicable jurisdictions. Three basic concepts are incorporated by the law as necessary to a person giving informed consent: The patient must have information sufficient to reach a decision in his best interest; the patient must be reasonably competent to evaluate all his or her options; and, the patient must be reasonably competent to evaluate all the risks and consequences of all his or her options (*Brown v. Murphy* 1996).

## Background

Initially, a patient's claim that his physician had failed to properly advise him or her or get his or her consent for treatment was analyzed as a battery (Prosser and Keaton 1984). Battery is an intentional tort, defined as a harmful or offensive contact with the person resulting from an act intended to cause such contact or fear of it (Second Restatement of Torts). Obviously, a physician operating on a patient made and intended contact with the patient. Harm was found in the patient's pain and suffering, disability, disfigurement, lost wages, and medical expenses. The nature, extent, and duration of the injuries and any aggravation of a previous condition also affected the award of damages. In cases of nominal injuries, damages were presumed from the interference with the patient's autonomy. Since battery was an intentional tort, punitive damages were sometimes available.

At the beginning of the 20th, consent was very strictly construed against the physician. If, however, the patient consented to the physician's treatment, there was no offensive touching and no

battery as a matter of definition. Consent was implied in cases of emergency. Moreover, courts recognized that patients sometimes gave very general consent vesting the physician with great discretion. Eventually, the law recognized the complex and inexact nature of medicine, and became more liberal in construing consent in favor of the physician.

Over the past 50 years, legal analysis of consent cases has shifted from intentional tort theory and recognized that giving consent was really a matter of professional judgment. Accordingly, the cases began to be seen as a form of professional negligence cases (*Natanson v. Kline* 1960). The importance of battery as a cause of action declined. Today, battery is only recognized in limited circumstances: where treatment is completely unauthorized; where the consent is for one type of treatment and the physician performs another substantially different treatment; or where the patient consents to treatment by one physician and a second physician, who the patient has not consented to, actually performs the procedure (*Trogrun v. Fruchtman* 1973; *Cobbs v. Grant* 1972; *Guebard v. Jabaay* 1983).

## Present-Day Informed Consent

The plaintiff in a medical malpractice case must prove three things: the (1) standard of care that applies to his physician (the physician's duty); (2) that a deviation from that standard occurred (breach of duty); and (3) that the deviation proximately caused plaintiff's injuries. (*Borowski v. Von Solbrig* 1975). An informed consent case is a medical malpractice case. In this type of case, the plaintiff must prove (1) the standard of information disclosure that applies to his or her physician (the physician's duty); (2) that the physician deviated from that standard; and (3) that the deviation proximately caused plaintiff's injuries. The standard of disclosure varies from jurisdiction to jurisdiction and affects the type of evidence necessary to establish a breach of the standard of disclosure. Additionally, two standards are used to determine if a breach has proximately caused injuries.

The foundation for the modern doctrine of informed consent has four bases. First, a patient generally knows much less about medical science than his or her physician. Second, a competent adult has the right to decide whether or not to submit to medical treatment. Third, a patient's consent to treatment is effective only it is an informed consent. Fourth, a patient must depend upon and trust in his or her physician for the information needed to decide whether to undergo medical treatment. From these bases, the law derives the physician's duty "of reasonable disclosure of the available choices with respect to proposed therapy and of the dangers inherently and potentially involved in each" (*Arato v. Avedon* 1973).

Prognosis is one type of information that might be expected to be presented to a patient. However, courts do not prescribe the exact form of information physicians must supply their patients. In the *Arato* case, Arato's family sued his physician after his death, claiming that Arato only underwent chemotherapy for pancreatic cancer because the doctor failed to disclose to him the dismal statistical life expectancy of patients with pancreatic cancer (*Arato v. Avedon* 1973). The family claimed that Arato would have foregone the chemotherapy, got his business affairs in order, and lived out his final days in peace if the dire statistics had been disclosed to him. His doctor admitted he did not provide the statistics, but stated he told his patient that pancreatic cancer was usually fatal. He also advised the patient that the chemotherapy he recommended was unproven. The jury returned a verdict for the physician. The appellate court reversed, holding as a matter of law that the disclosure was inadequate, since the statistics were not provided the patient. The Supreme Court of California, in bank, held physicians do not need to provide survival or mortality percentages to their patients as a matter of law. The court recognized that physicians need leeway in giving advice and recommending treatment so that they do not needlessly alarm their patients. Thus, a verdict for a physician was affirmed on appeal.

### The Physician's Duty

The duty to obtain informed consent rests with the physician. While a nurse can present the patient with the informed consent form, the duty to give proper disclosure to a patient remains with the physician. This duty is given to the physician due to his special relationship with the patient and his specialized knowledge and training (*Pickle v. Curns* 1982). Generally, hospitals and hospital nurses do not have a duty to provide informed consent. A hospital may have a duty to provide a method to be sure that physicians properly disclose information to their patients in the hospital (*Pickle v. Curns* 1982). However, at least two jurisdictions, Pennsylvania and Illinois, have created an exception to the general rule and held that federal regulations covering experimental trials and devices required hospitals to provide informed consent to pursuant to federal regulations (*Kus v. Sherman Hospital* 1995; *Friter v. Jolab* 1992). Generally, a physician's negligence in failing to provide informed consent will not be imputed to a hospital unless the physician is an agent of the hospital (*Pickle v. Curns* 1982).

Virtually all physicians are familiar with informed consent forms used in hospitals and completed before patients undergo invasive procedures, tests, or treatments. These forms are required by the hospitals pursuant to written procedures. The use of such a system provides strong evidence that a *hospital* has provided a method to ensure that physicians provide informed consent (*Wintus v. Podzamski* 1993). However, the use of such forms provides strong evidence that a physician obtained informed consent only if the forms are clearly filled out and document a detailed informed consent discussion. The use of forms as a substitute for a detailed informed consent discussion does not meet the duty to provide meaningful disclosure. Some physicians mistakenly believe that if a patient filled out a consent form, then the patient cannot claim a lack of informed consent. Nearly all courts hold that while such forms are evidence that a physician provided some disclosure, the presence of a form is not dispositive evidence (*Guebard v. Jabaay* 1983). Plaintiff may be allowed to present evidence that the disclosure was not complete or specific enough, that he or she signed the form only because he or she was told to sign it, that the form was filled out after he or she signed it, or that he or she signed the form without having it explained.

Informed consent doctrine is not limited to occasions when an invasive procedure is contemplated. When a physician prescribes medication for a patient, the physician is responsible for providing the patient with proper disclosures concerning the medication, since the extent of disclosure is a question of medical judgment (*Hatfield v. Sandoz-Wander, Inc.* 1984). Since the prescribing physician has the duty of providing the patient with informed consent concerning the medication, any alleged negligence in warning the patient is chargeable against the physician, not against a hospital or pharmacist (*Kirh v. Michael Reese Hospital and Medical Center* 1994).

### The Contemplated Disclosure

What sort of information must the physician give the patient as part of informed consent? The reasonable disclosure contemplated consists of advising a patient of these elements: his or her diagnosis; the nature and purpose of the proposed treatment; the risks and consequences of the treatment; the probability of success of the treatment; alternative treatments and their nature and purpose; risks and consequences of the alternative treatments; the probability of success of alternative treatments; and the patient's prognosis if treatment is not given (Louisell and Williams 1981).

Some jurisdictions require a physician to advise the patient of any personal stake the physician has in having the patient undergo the treatment, unrelated to the patient's health, whether economic or research, such as when a physician will later sell any harvested cells (*Moore v. Regents of University of California* 1990). Finally, some jurisdictions require a physician to inform his patients if he has contracted human immunodeficiency virus (HIV) (*Doe v. Northwestern University* 1997).

The goal of the disclosure is effective communication. All these elements should be explained in simple, nontechnical terms so they can be understood by the patient. The terms risks and consequences, used interchangeably in common parlance, have similar but distinct meanings here. A risk is something that might occur, a known complication. For example, aseptic necrosis of the femoral head is a risk of steroid use. A consequence is something that can be expected to occur. For example, a consequence of a tubal ligation is sterility. The physician is required to disclose only the risks he knows or reasonably should know. A physician should be sure to disclose the risks of foregoing treatment or tests (*Truman v. Thomas* 1980).

### Measuring the Adequacy of Disclosure

The standard used by courts to judge whether disclosure complies with a physician's duty to disclose available choices to his patient has been changing and varies from jurisdiction to jurisdiction. Traditionally, physicians were judged by the material risk standard. Under this standard, a physician had to disclose to a patient those risks disclosed by other qualified physicians acting reasonably under similar circumstances. In other words, a physician had to disclose to his patient those risks that other similarly qualified physicians told their patients under similar circumstances (*Fuller v. Starnes* 1980; *Rush v. Miller* 1981). The material risk standard continues to be applied in a majority of jurisdictions.

Recently, courts concerned that the material risk standard inappropriately gives physicians the right to choose which information tho patient receives have adopted the reasonable patient standard. In these jurisdictions, a physician must furnish a patient with all the information a reasonable patient would require to make an informed decision on whether to undergo treatment. Under the reasonable patient standard, the focus of disclosure changes from what a reasonable physician should tell the patient to what a reasonable patient would consider significant information from his physician (*Crain v. Allison* 1982; *Canterbury v. Speace* 1972). Generally, those courts that have adopted the reasonable patient standard have done away with the requirement that a plaintiff present expert testimony as to the propriety of the physician disclosure. In other words, the patient will not need to present a physician expert to criticize the disclosure made by the defendant physician. On a practical level, more cases go to trial in jurisdictions using a reasonable patient standard, since they are not dismissed prior to trial because of plaintiff's failure to obtain an expert.

Some patients might not fit the "reasonable patient" model. At least one court has held that a physician who has or should have special knowledge that a patient has special concerns or fears about risks not normally considered material by the physician should discuss these risks with his patient (*Kinikin v. Heupel* 1981).

An interesting hybrid approach to the standard of disclosure occurs in Texas. In that state, a Medical Disclosure Panel has determined what risks should be disclosed to patients for a number of different interventions (Texas Medical Liability and Insurance Improvement Act 1977). For each of these interventions, the panel has determined which risks need to be disclosed and the form of the disclosure. A physician who discloses to the patient the established risks for one of these interventions is entitled to a rebuttable presumption that he gave adequate disclosure. If a physician fails to disclose these risks to his patient, the patient is entitled to a rebuttable presumption that adequate disclosure was not given.

The Medical Disclosure Panel has not defined risks and required disclosure for all medical interventions, however. For those that are not included in the Panel's materials, a reasonable patient standard of disclosure is used.

## Causation Standards

As in all negligence cases, the plaintiff must show that his injuries were proximately caused by the physician's alleged negligence. In informed consent cases, plaintiff must show not only that his injuries were caused in fact by the treatment, but also that he or she would not have undergone the treatment if adequate disclosure had been given. An objective reasonable patient standard is usually applied here. A plaintiff must show that a reasonable patient would not have undergone the treatment if proper disclosure had been made (*Guebard v. Jabaay* 1983).

A minority of jurisdictions have adopted the subjective particular patient standard. The jurisdictions that have adopted this standard frame the issue of causation as whether the particular plaintiff would have foregone treatment if proper disclosure had been made. This causation standard is very easy for the plaintiff to meet, since the plaintiff is the particular plaintiff in each case. This causation standard provides a defense to the physician only in cases where the treatment is obviously needed to prevent serious injury or death. The particular plaintiff standard is justified by these jurisdictions with an argument that the right to decide for oneself cannot be tempered by a standard based on what others might do (*Scott v. Bradford* 1979).

## An Illustration

The recent Texas case *Weidner v. Marlin* (1997) provides an excellent illustration on how the different disclosures and causation standards affect the trial of an informed consent case. Briefly, the facts, as set forth in the opinion are as follows: plaintiff was born with a lipoma at the base of his spinal cord. The lipoma got larger and plaintiff suffered neurological symptoms by age 9. Plaintiff

was referred to defendant Marlin, a pediatric neurosurgeon, at age 10 because of urinary dribbling and neurological deficit of the lower extremities. Dr. Marlin diagnosed lipomeningocele with a tethered spinal cord. Surgery was performed, the condition was corrected, further neurological injury was prevented, and there were no major complications. Six years later, plaintiff complained of numbness in his right foot. He returned to Dr. Marlin, who confirmed an increase in neurological deficits. Magnetic resonance images (MRIs) revealed a retethering of the spinal cord. Marlin recommended immediate surgery to plaintiff and his parents (note that the patient was just 17 years old), and told them that plaintiff could lose bladder control if surgery were not performed. Plaintiff weighed his decision for several months, noted further deterioration, and, through his parents, consented to the surgery.

Dr. Marlin advised plaintiff and his father of these risks of the spinal surgery: (1) pain, numbness, or clumsiness; (2) impaired muscle function; (3) incontinence or impotence; (4) unstable spine; (5) recurrence or continuation of the condition that required the operation; and (6) injury to major blood vessels. Plaintiff's father signed a consent form that listed all these risks before the surgery. The risks are those set forth by the Texas Medical Disclosure Panel for spinal surgery.

Plaintiff suffered permanent paralysis below his knees, which Marlin concluded was due to stretching of the nerves during surgery. Plaintiff sued Dr. Marlin, claiming, among other things, that Marlin negligently performed the surgery and failed to obtain his informed consent. Plaintiff and his father claimed they did not understand that "impaired muscle function" might include paralysis.

At trial, the plaintiff was not able to find an expert to testify that Dr. Marlin had made any errors during surgery that caused plaintiff's injury. Plaintiff's expert conceded that the nerves could be stretched without any negligence and could not say that any unskilled act by Marlin caused the paralysis. Marlin was granted a direct verdict on the negligent performance of surgery claim.

Plaintiff's expert gave the opinion that Marlin was negligent in not explaining adequately that "impaired muscle function" included a possibility of paralysis. The criticism created a question of fact sending the case to the jury. However, because Marlin had advised plaintiff in compliance with the requirements set forth by the Texas Medical Disclosure Panel, the jury was instructed that plaintiff's father's signature on the consent form created a presumption that adequate disclosure of risks was given. This presumption could be overcome if the jury found that Marlin failed to explain the meaning of "impaired muscle function" to plaintiff's parents. The jury returned a verdict in favor of Marlin that was affirmed on appeal.

Defendant clearly benefited from Texas's statutory disclosures panel scheme. Because plaintiff's father signed a consent form that listed the risks of spinal surgery set forth by the panel, the jury had to presume he had given adequate disclosure. The panel's judgment is a substitute for the physician's judgment, even though the patient never meets with the panel or discusses his surgery with it. Consider how this might have been handled in other jurisdictions. If the material risk standard were applied, the jury would have heard testimony about whether a reasonably qualified neurosurgeon performing the surgery under similar circumstances would have customarily advised the patient of the risk of paralysis, and would not have been instructed to presume that adequate disclosure had been made. Finally, if the Texas Medical Disclosure Panel had not written guidelines about consent for spinal surgery, then a reasonable person standard would have been applied in the case. Would a reasonable person in plaintiff's position have wanted to know that he risked paralysis by having the surgery? Since plaintiff mulled his decision over for some months before deciding to go ahead with surgery, it is clear he was concerned about the risks.

Turning to the issue of causation, would a reasonable plaintiff have foregone spinal surgery and risked bladder incontinence? Unfortunately, the decision does not mention whether plaintiff was warned he might end up paralyzed if he turned down surgery. Trying to answer whether the particular plaintiff would have foregone surgery here is not difficult, since plaintiff's decision undoubtedly was influenced by his neurological deterioration and continued urinary dribbling. Plaintiff would be hard pressed to prevail on the issue of causation, since he had gone forward with surgery when faced with suffering lesser or equal injuries during his decision-making waiting period. Generally, this is not the case unless disability or fatality can result.

## Futility

In recent years, medical futility has emerged as an important issue in patient care and in the medical legal arena. Treatment that has no benefit to the patient is considered futile. Consequently, futility conclusions lead to decisions to not initiate, or in some cases to discontinue, certain medical therapies. Frequently, these decisions are made without consultation with the patient or the patient's surrogate, and sometimes these decisions are made against their wishes (Asch et al. 1995). Neurologic conditions figure prominently in many cases involving futility, and prognosis is an implicit, if not explicit, issue in these decisions. When there is general agreement of all parties that a particular intervention is futile, it is not pursued.

A number of medical legal issues relate to treatment decisions based on futility. The first and most fundamental issue is what definition of futility is being used. A second issue is whether or not patients or their surrogates need to consent to decisions to limit care on the basis of futility. A third issue is whether patients or their surrogates need to be informed, even if their assent is not required. A final issue is the implication of futility policies on medical practice in hospitals and long-term care facilities. This section will begin with a few sample cases that illustrate how legal issues arise in futility cases, and then each of the four issues will be discussed in detail.

Lawsuits that have arisen related to futility tend to be of many types: medical malpractice, allegations that informed consent was not obtained, attempts to change patient guardianship, and pleas for prospective decisions about the limits of care (Johnston et al. 1997). However, the cases can be broadly categorized into two groups based upon whether the case goes to court before or after the futility decision is implemented. The first group of case occurs when there is conflict between the patient (or surrogate) and the physician/health care team over a decision to limit treatment based on futility, and the court is asked to resolve the conflict before the decision is carried out. The second group of cases occurs when treatment has been limited on the basis of a futility decision, and subsequent litigation claims of negligence for that limitation are made.

*In re Helga Wanglie* (1991) is a well-known example in the first group of cases. Mrs. Wanglie was an 85-year-old woman with persistent vegetative state who was maintained on a ventilator in an intensive care setting for a prolonged period of time. Her physicians sought to discontinue aggressive care, including ventilatory support, on the basis that it was futile care. Her diagnosis of persistent vegetative state and its associated prognosis were key factors in their determination that the therapy was futile. Mrs. Wanglie's husband, her legal surrogate, disagreed with the medical conclusions. He remained hopeful that she would improve, but also stated that Mrs. Wanglie would have identified her current condition as worthy of continued aggressive therapy. When the conflicting opinions could not be resolved in the hospital setting, and transfer to another facility was not possible, the hospital went to court seeking to replace Mr. Wanglie with another surrogate decision maker. This lawsuit was unsuccessful, and Mr. Wanglie was retained as surrogate.

The *Baby K* case is another example of an attempt at judicially sanctioned prospective limits on care based on futility (*In re Baby K* 1993). Baby K is an anencephalic child. Traditionally, anencephaly has been viewed as an obvious case in which any therapy other than comfort care is futile. There is no therapy that will replace the missing cerebral hemispheres and death invariably occurs. However, Baby K's mother insisted upon aggressive therapy feeling strongly that any life was of value. When the hospital sought to obtain a prospective determination that they could limit treatment, the court found that the Emergency Medical Treatment and Active Labor Act (EMTALA) required physicians to intervene with assistive therapy if the child presented to the emergency department. This decision was upheld on appeal, although many medical commentators find the appellate dissent the most thoughtful opinion in the case.

The arguments presented by plaintiffs, and the reasoning used by the courts in these and other prospective cases, differ from case to case. (*In re Helga Wanglie* 1991; *In re Baby K* 1993; *In re Matter of Finn* 1995). In general, however, courts have tended to find for the party requesting that the treatment be offered or continued. Consequently, when there is a prospective disagreement about whether or not a treatment is futile and should be limited, courts have not supported the noninitiation or discontinuation of therapy.

The second group of futility-related cases have arisen when a physician has made a determination that treatment is futile, and has acted on this decision (*Morgan v. Olds* 1987; *Hartsell v. Fort Sanders Regional Medical Center* 1995; *La Salle National Trust v. Swedish Covenant Hospital* 1995; Johnson et al. 1997). When plaintiffs have subsequently sued on the grounds of medical malpractice, they have been largely unsuccessful. For example, in *Morgan v. Olds* (1987), the patient was resuscitated from multiple cardiac arrests, but became ventilator dependent in a persistent vegetative state (PUS). The physician proposed weaning him from the ventilator and wrote an order that he should not be resuscitated in the event of another arrest. Whether the patient's wife assented to this plan was a matter of contention. After weaning, he deteriorated and was not resuscitated. His widow subsequently sued on multiple grounds, including medical malpractice. She was unsuccessful.

Several cases of this nature have involved physicians who did not institute aggressive care for very premature newborns on the basis that it would be futile to do so (*Hartsell v. Fort Sanders Regional Medical Center* 1995; *La Salle National Trust v. Swedish Covenant Hospital* 1995). When the newborns continued to breathe after a matter of hours, aggressive therapies were instituted. The children survived but with significant disabilities. Later suits against the physicians were unsuccessful.

In these retrospective claims of malpractice, defendant physicians have tended to prevail. There appear to be several reasons. The first is the relative difficulty in proving a medical malpractice claim. Physicians have been able to successfully argue that discontinuation of care, or noninitiation of care, was within appropriate medical judgment and standard of care. In several cases, hospital futility policies have been used to support the appropriateness of physician judgment. It also appears that discussion of scientific data supporting the medical decision is more successful in the second group of cases.

## What Definition of Futility is Used?

A critical issue in futility debates is what futility definition is being used. It is interesting to note that the words futile and futility are not defined in recent editions of medical and legal dictionaries

(Black's Law Dictionary 1979; Stedman 1984). In medical practice, multiple definitions of futility have been advanced. In general, these definitions can fit into one of two broad categories. The first category of futility definitions are quantitative and tend to be based in the physiologic effects of the contemplated treatment. The second category of futility definitions are qualitative and tend to be based on an analysis of overall benefit to the patient. These two categories are very different from each other. Distinguishing what type of definition is being used is important not only in conversation with patients, but also in determining what information should be given to patients, and how courts tend to view resulting conflicts. It appears that many hospital futility policies are moving towards definitions of futility that include both quantitative and qualitative components.

Quantitative futility definitions define futility as a situation in which it is impossible that a contemplated therapy will achieve its desired effect according to some standard probability estimate. Some commentators limit the effects that can be considered to the immediate physiologic effects of the interventions (Truog et al. 1992). With this narrow construct, for example, the only effects of ventilation that should be considered are whether or not tissue oxygenation occurs and the only effects of artificial nutrition to be considered would be whether or not it would support the nutritional needs of the patient's tissues. Because only the physiologic effect of an intervention is considered, the definition is quite narrow. The advantages of using such definitions include their clarity, scientific basis, and ease of defense. In fact, some commentators suggest that such narrowly defined physiologic futility is the only appropriate definition that can be used (Truog et al. 1992).

Definitions limited to immediate physiologic effect have been criticized on the basis of being too narrow. In fact, these definitions cover only a tiny portion of the cases where futility issues arise, and are not very helpful. Other quantitative definitions focus on the overall outcome intended to be achieved by the therapy. Hence, this broader definition would allow one to consider the probability that the effect of artificial nutrition or ventilation would be to restore a PVS patient to cognitive functioning.

Whether the effect is limited to the immediate physiologic or a broader notion, no consensus has been reached as to what the probability estimate must be. However, Schneiderman, et al. (1990) have proposed one definition that has attained many adherents. They propose that when the physician concludes that in the last 100 cases, a particular medical treatment has not resulted in the desired outcome (interpreted more liberally than immediate physiologic effect), they should regard the treatment as futile.

While not completely eliminating value judgments, quantitative definitions tend to minimize them. The conclusion is more scientific and data-driven. Many suggest that these are strengths of quantitative futility definitions, but others suggest that such definitions eliminate critical information about the patient, the patient's choices, and the patient's situation that should be incorporated into the analysis of the situation.

The second type of futility definition is one that is largely qualitative in nature. Qualitative definitions focus on the benefits of the intervention to the patient, rather than the effects of the intervention. Qualitative definitions are less data driven and more dependent on the particular patient's condition, including prognosis. Value judgments of both the patient and the physicians are likely to impact the definition, and underlying assumptions of all parties must be considered.

One advantage of qualitatively based futility definitions is the broader range of cases that can be addressed. Also, these definitions allow patient, caregiver, and societal input into decisions about how benefit should be defined. However, numerous disadvantages also arise. There tend to be multiple definitions of futility when benefit is the operative meaning. Society has not yet addressed the difficult question of what constitutes benefit; the situation lends itself to everyone having their own construct of what constitutes beneficial futility. There are worrisome possibilities that qualitative definitions of futility may devalue individuals with physical and mental disabilities, the poor, and other disadvantaged members of our communities. (Truog et al. 1992; Cranford and Gostin 1992).

It is important in futility considerations that the physician be clear about what sort of futility definition is being used. Frequently, discussions about futile care for patients with advanced neurologic disease are qualitative in nature, focusing on benefits of therapy rather than on the effects of that therapy. Understanding the differences between the types of futility definitions that can be used provides a segway into the next area of medical legal discussion, whether or not patients must assent to treatment decisions made on the basis of futility determinations.

## Must Patients Consent to Treatment Limitations Based on Futility?

Must patients acquiesce to treatment limitations based on futility or can they require physicians to offer therapy that physicians determine to be futile? There is a remarkable amount of debate on both these issues. The medical community has reached consensus that there is no moral obligation to continue such therapy once physicians have made the judgment that it is futile (Schnederman and Jecker 1993; Smith 1995; Paris et al. 1990; Council on Ethical and Judicial Affairs 1991). Several court cases have implied that consent is not necessary, stressing that futility decisions are really decisions in the province of medical practitioners and out of the competence of others (*In re Dinnerstein* 1973; *Barber v. Superior Court of California* 1993). Some medical and legal commentators have gone so far as to suggest that physicians who continue futile therapies are acting in an unprofessional manner (Smith 1995; Jecker and Schneiderman 1992). However, there is far from societal and legal consensus on this issue, as exemplified in the *Wanglie* case above (*In re Helga Wanglie* 1991).

Arguments in favor of requiring patient assent are particularly strong when a qualitative definition of futility is being used. Benefits-based futility decisions involve values and priorities. Patients and physicians may not share the same understanding of what constitutes a worthwhile benefit. For example, a physician might reasonably decide that a medical therapy that can be expected only to provide a patient with a few more days of life that will be spent in pain is futile. However, the patient might find that the mere benefit of living an additional period of time, even with pain and a diminished quality of life, might be worthwhile if there is potential to get his or her affairs in order, see a loved one who has not yet come to the hospital, or accomplish some other goal that has benefit to the patient.

Consequently, while professional standards suggest that physicians need not gain patient assent to such decisions, it would be a mistake to suggest that this would be a risk-free maneuver from a legal perspective. This is particularly the case when many commentators (even those who believe strongly that futile interventions should be limited) and increasing numbers of hospital futility policies call for patients to be given information about futility decisions, even if the patient's consent is not considered necessary to limit therapy.

## Should Patients be Informed About Limitations of Therapy Related to Futility?

A related issue is whether or not patients should be informed when the medical team concludes a therapy is futile. When patient consent is obtained, the patient clearly will be informed. But what about those situations in which patient assent is either not obtained or not considered necessary? Should patients be informed when medical treatments available to them will be limited because of futility? In answering this question, we will first consider the specific issue of cardiopulmonary resuscitation (CPR), and then consider other therapies.

CPR has achieved a unique status among medical treatments and is treated differently than other medical interventions. When CPR is successful it is quite remarkable; when employed unsuccessfully, the patient's death occurs. It is a therapy that is frequently performed out of the hospital by nonphysician medical personnel, and oftentimes by laypersons. There is a general social expectation that CPR is performed on patients dying in the hospital unless a specific decision has been made not to perform it. Indeed, CPR is the only medical therapy that requires an order that it *not* be performed when a patient is admitted into the hospital. In some ways, CPR has achieved status as a "rite of passage" above and beyond its usefulness medically.

The special status of CPR contributes to the current consensus (albeit not unanimous) that patients should be informed when do-not-resuscitate (DNR) orders are entered fschneiderman et al. 1990; Council on Ethical and Judicial Affairs 1991; Tomlinson and Brody 1991. This applies whether the decision to make a patient "DNR" is based on physiologic futility criteria or benefit-based futility.

Apart from decisions about CPR, there is great debate about whether patients should be informed that therapies deemed to be futile will not be offered. Arguments in favor of informing patients include the following. Our society places a high value on patient autonomy and the patient's right to make informed decisions about him/herself. These decisions should be treated as pertinent information that the patient may have strong opinions about and which may impact other decisions that the patient will make. Informing patients of these decisions and allowing their input will build trust in physicians by patients. This may be particularly important as patients become more concerned about who (e.g., physician, insurance program) is making decisions about what therapies are offered them, and as patients consider physician incentives in managed health care systems. The arguments for requiring patient consent to limitations of therapy mentioned above also apply to this question.

On the other hand, there are arguments against informing patients about decisions not to institute care based on futility. We do not routinely inform patients about therapies that are unrelated to, and hence futile, for their clinical condition. An expectation that patients be informed about all futile therapies could be carried to an illogical conclusion where patients are given information about many medical interventions that have absolutely no relevance to their clinical condition. Related in part to this is the concern that information overload may be as detrimental to patients as conveying too little information. A final argument is that the mere suggestion of a therapy by a physician to a patient lends a veneer of possibility. One commentator has suggested that it would be cruel and unusual punishment for physicians to advise patients of therapies that are not indicated (Smith 1995).

The arguments for informing the patient are weakest when a decision is being made on the basis of a narrowly constructed quantitative futility definition. Otherwise, informing patients appears more appropriate for several reasons. The communication may identify information that the physician was unaware of. It can help prepare patients and their families. It can identify disagreements early and allow opportunities for conflict resolution that avoid later litigation.

**The Role of Institutional Futility Policies**

As this chapter has suggested, conflict can occur related to futility decisions. Conflict that has occurred between patient (or surrogate) and physician has been presented, but it should be noted that conflicts can occur between other members of the health care team, various consulting physicians, family members, and others. This chapter presented some of the legal cases that have resulted from this conflict. It is in the interest of all parties to attempt to resolve these conflicts without going to court.

One of the means for conflict resolution that is increasingly available in hospitals are "futility policies." Although there is great variation among the various futility policies that hospitals have developed, these policies generally attempt to provide a definition of futility that will be used locally in the hospital, explicitly state what information is to be provided to patients related to futility decisions, and provide a procedure for conflict resolution when the patient and physician do not agree. (Johnston et al. 1997; Smith 1993; Murphy and Finucane 1993; Halevy and Brody 1996; Murphy 1994; Tomlinson and Czlonka 1995).

From a risk management perspective, physicians should be aware of any futility policies in place at hospitals and long-term care facilities in which they practice. Because there is little standardization among policies, it would not be unusual for physicians in practice at multiple locations to have different policies at the different locations. Conforming one's behavior to hospital policies is a powerful indication that the physician met the professional standard of behavior. This can be helpful if there is related malpractice litigation. On the other hand, activities out of conformance with hospital policy can be problematic from a risk management perspective. Ignorance of policy is not an adequate defense.

One advantage of having a futility policy is the possibility of defining, at least on an institution-wide basis, what futility means. There is no reason that institutions need to limit themselves to one definition, and many definitions incorporate quantitative and qualitative components. Similarly, the policy may indicate differing expectations for patient assent and/or the provision of patient information depending on specific situations.

Typically, futility policies have conflict resolution procedures that go into effect when the patient (or surrogate) disagrees with a medical decision. If discussion with the physician does not yield a result that both patient and physician are comfortable with, other avenues for conflict resolution are necessary.

Many institutions have a first level of appeal to an ethics committee or ethics consultation service. This can be beneficial in terms of enhancing the dialogue and may also be wise from a risk management perspective. If agreement between the physician and patient (or surrogate) is not reached at this level, transfer of care to another physician or another institution may be possible. If these options are not possible, an additional level of extrainstitutional appeal should be available. This will typically be to the traditional legal system, although alternative dispute resolution mechanisms are increasingly being put in place in various jurisdictions.

## Conclusion

In sum, informed consent and futility are two important issues that may arise in the consideration of the prognosis of neurological disorders. It is important that physicians be aware of the standards of care in both of these areas, are cognizant of any local policies, and conform their behavior to those policies to the greatest degree possible.

## References

*Arato v. Avedon,* 5 Cal. 4th 1172, 858 P.2d 598 (Cal. Supreme Court, in bank, 1973).

Asch, D. A.; Hansen-Flaschen, I.; Lanken, P. N. Decisions to limit or continue life-sustaining treatment by critical care physicians in the United States: conflicts between physicians' practices and patients' wishes. Am. J. Respir. Crit. Care Med. 151:288–292; 1995.

*Barber v. Superior Court of California,* 195 Cal. R. 484 (Ct. App. 1983). Black's Law Dictionary, 5th Edition, Minneapolis: West Publishing Co.; 1979.

*Borowski v. von Solbrig,* 60 Ill. 2d 418, 328 N.E.2d 301 (1975).

*Brown v. Murphy,* 278 Ill. App.3d 981, 664 N.E.2d 186 (1st Dist. 1996).

*Canterbury v. Spence,* 464 F.2d 772 (D.C. Cir. 1972).

*Cobbs v. Grant,* 8 Cal. 3d 229, 502 P.2d 1 (1972).

Council on Ethical and Judicial Affairs. Guidelines for the appropriate use of do-not-resuscitate orders. JAMA. 265(14):1868–1871; 1991.

*Crain v. Allison,* 443 A.2d 558 (D.C. App. 1982).

Cranford, R.; Gostin, L. Futility: a concept in search of a definition. Law Med. & Health Care 20(4):307–309; 1992.

*Doe v. Northwestern University,* 289 Ill. App.3d 39, 682 N.E.2d 145 (1st Dist. 1997).

*Friter v. Jolab,* 414 Pa.Super. 622, 607 A.2d 1111 (1992).

*Fuller v. Starnes,* 268 Ark. 476, 597 S. W. 88 (1980).

*Guebard v. Jabaay,* 117 Ill. App.3d 1, 72 Ill. Dec. 498, 452 N.E.2d 751, at 755 (2d Dist. 1983).

Halevy, A.; Brody, B. A. A multi-institution collaborative policy on medical futility. JAMA 276(7): 571–574; 1996.

*Hartsell v. Fort Sanders Regional Medical Center* 905 S.W.2d 944 (Tenn Ct. App. E Sect. 1995).

*Hatfield v. Sandoz-Wander, Inc.,* 124 Ill. App.3d 780, 464 N.E.2d 1105 (1st Dist. 1984).

*In re Baby K* 832 F.Supp. 1022 (E.D. Va. 1993), aff'd 16 F.3d 590 (4th Cir. 1994).

*In re Dinnerstein,* 380 N.E.2d 134 (Mass. App. 1978).

*In re Helga Wanglie,* Fourth Judicial District (Dist. Ct., Probate Ct. Div). PX-91-283, Minnesota, Hennepin County (1991).

*In re Matter of Finn,* 625 N.Y.S. 2d 809 (Sup. Ct. 1995).

Jecker, N. S.; and Schneiderman, L. J. Futility and rationing. Am. J. Med. 92:189–196; 1992.

Johnston, S. H.; Gibbons, V. P.; Goldner, J. A.; et al. Legal and institutional policy responses to medical futility. J. Health Hosp. Law 30(1):2–21; 1997.

*Kinikin v. Heupel,* 305 N.W.2d 589 (Minn. 1981).

*Kirk v. Michael Reese Hospital and Medical Center,* 117 Ill. 2d 507, 513 N.E.2d 387 (1st Dist. 1984).

*Kus v. Sherman Hospital,* 268 Ill. App.3d 771, 780, 644 N.E.2d 1214 (2d Dist. 1995).

*LaSalle National Trust v. Swedish Covenant Hospital* 273 Ill. App.3d 780, 210 Ill. Dis. 113, 652 N.E.2d 1089 (1st Dist. 1995).

Louisell & Williams, Medical Malpractice, 1981, section 22.01 at 594.44.

*Moore v. Regents of University of California,* 51 Cal. 3d 120, 271 Cal. Rptr. 146, 793 P.2d 479 (1990).

*Morgan v. Olds,* 417 N.W.2d 232 (Iowa 1987).

Murphy, D. J. Can we set futile care policies? Institutional and systemic challenges. J. Am. Geriatr. Soc. 42(8): 890–893; 1994.

Murphy, D. J.; Finucane, T. E. New do-not-resuscitate policies. A first step in cost control. Arch. Intern. Med. 153:1641–1648; 1993.

*Natanson v. Kline,* 186 Kan. 393, 350 P.2d 1093 (1960).

Paris, J. J.; Crone, R. K.; Reardon, F. Physicians refusal of requested treatment. N. Engl. J. Med. 322:1012–1015; 1990.

*Pickle v. Curns,* 106 Ill. App.3d 734, 62 Ill. Dec. 79, 435 N.E.2d 877 (2d Dist. 1982).

Presidential Commission for the Study of Ethical Problems in Medicine and Biomedical and Behavioral Research, Making Health Care Decisions, the Ethical and Legal Implications of Informed Consent in the Patient—Practitioner Relationship. Vol. 1. Footnote 14 (1982), cited in *Arato v. Avedon,* 5 Cal. 4th 1172, 858 P.2d 598 (Cal. Supreme Court, in bank, 1973).

Prosser and Keaton on the Law of Torts, section 32 (1984).

*Rush v. Miller,* 648 F.2d 1075 (Sixth Cir. 1981).

Schneiderman, L. S.; Jecker, N. Futility in practice. Arch. Intern. Med. 153:437; 1993.

Schneiderman, L. J.; Jecker, N. S.; Jonsen, A. R. Medical futility: its meaning and ethical implications. Ann. Intern. Med. 1112:949–954; 1990.

*Scott v. Bradford,* 606 P.2d 554 (Okla. 1979).

Second Restatement of Torts, section 12.

Smith, M. L. Futile medical treatment and patient consent. Cleve. Clin. J. Med. 60(2):151–154; 1993.

Smith, G. P. Utility and the principle of medical futility: safeguarding autonomy and the prohibition agains cruel and unusual punishment. J. Contemp. Health Law Policy 12(1):1–39; 1995. [See particularly footnote #1.]

Stedman, T. L. Stedman's Medical Dictionary. 24th edition. Baltimore: Williams & Wilkins; 1984.

Texas Medical Liability and Insurance Improvement Act, Tex, Rev. Civ. Stat. Annot. article 4590i, subchapter F., sections 6.01–6.07 (Vernon Supp. 1977).

Tomlinson, T; Brody, H. Futility and the ethics of resuscitation. JAMA 264(10):1276–1280; 1990.

Tomlinson, T.; Czlonka, D. Futility and hospital policy. Hastings Cent. Rep. 3:28–35; 1995.

*Trogrun v. Fruchtman,* 58 Wis. 2d 569, 207 N. W. 297 (1973).

*Truman v. Thomas,* 27 Cal. 3d 285, 165 Cal. Rptr. 308, 611 P.2d 902 (Supreme Court Cal., in bank, 1980).

Truog, R. D.; Brett, A. S.; Frader, J. The problem with futility. N. Engl. J. Med. 326(23):1560–1564; 1992.

*Weidner v. Marlin* 1997 WL 531129 (Tex. App. San Antonio).

*Winters v. Podzamski,* 252 Ill. App.3d 821, 621 N.E.2d 72 (3d Dist. 1993).

*Ziegert v. South Chicago Community Hospital,* 99 Ill. App. 3d 83, 425 N.E.2d 450 (1st Dist. 1981).

# 4

# Prognosis: Keystone of Clinical Neurology

W. T. LONGSTRETH, JR., THOMAS D. KOEPSELL,
LORENE M. NELSON, AND GERALD VAN BELLE

Classic epidemiology deals with groups of people, risk factors, and etiology, while clinical epidemiology concentrates on groups of patients, prognostic factors, and outcomes (Weiss 1986). Central to understanding clinical epidemiology is the study of prognosis. Prognosis can be regarded as a set of outcomes and their associated probabilities following the occurrence of some condition that can be a symptom (amaurosis fugax), a sign (asymptomatic bruit), a laboratory finding (high-grade stenosis of the internal carotid artery), or a disease (ischemic stroke) (Longstreth et al. 1987b).

Clinical neuroepidemiology attempts to address important questions in clinical neurology that practitioners and researchers face on a regular basis. First is the issue of diagnosis (Longstreth et al. 1987a). However, a diagnosis that has no prognostic implications does little more than describe a constellation of patient characteristics. Prognosis links diagnoses to outcomes. In addition, study of prognosis identifies the diseases that warrant treatment. Treatment itself becomes an intervention intended to modify prognosis. Thus, in clinical neurology, the concepts of diagnosis, prognosis, and treatment are inseparable, with prognosis being the keystone.

This review describes a set of principles and guidelines that can be useful in designing, ana-

lyzing, and evaluating studies of prognosis. In the first section, different types of study designs used to address questions of prognosis are presented. The cohort design is the strongest and will be discussed in greatest detail. In the second section, the approach to data analysis in studies of prognosis is reviewed, specifically addressing the time-linked nature of clinical observations and the necessity of examining multiple variables simultaneously. In the third section, how evidence-based medicine can be applied to prognosis is described (Evidenced-Based Medicine Working Group 1992; Sackett et al. 1997). Often, factors in the design and analysis that strengthen a study and the conclusions that can be drawn from it about the subjects actually investigated (internal validity) paradoxically limit the ease with which the results can be generalized to other groups of patients (external validity) (Moses 1985). The question of internal and external validity will be revisited on several occasions.

## Design of Studies of Prognosis

Except in the restricted domain of randomized trials of therapy, studies of prognosis do not lend themselves to an experimental design in which factors of interest can be randomly assigned. Many patient characteristics of potential prognostic importance are not subject to manipulation, much less to random assignment. The typical study of prognosis involves patients to whom various diagnostic and therapeutic maneuvers are applied in the course of clinical care. The ideal study of prognosis would seek to describe the natural history of a condition, from its biological start to its end and without interventions that could influence outcome.

The two broad classes of nonexperimental or observational studies used to investigate prognosis are descriptive and analytic. Descriptive studies tally the outcomes for some condition. Analytic studies attempt to test hypotheses about whether certain potential prognostic factors are associated with particular outcomes. The types of clinical study most commonly encountered in the neurologic literature are the case report and case series. These descriptive studies have the weakest design. Their importance rests in describing events that can occur or characteristics that may coexist, without necessarily providing any information on frequency. They indicate possibilities rather than probabilities. Case reports also can provide important exceptions to prognostic rules. Imagine the importance of a single well-documented case of a patient diagnosed with brain death who subsequently underwent full neurologic recovery. Less dramatic examples exist, such as cases of recovery after cardiac arrest when prognostic factors indicated otherwise (Rosenberg et al. 1977; Snyder et al. 1983; Ringel et al. 1988).

In the next two sections, two designs that are stronger than case reports and case series are discuss in detail, cohort and case-control studies.

## Cohort Design

Perhaps the most natural design for an investigation of prognosis is the cohort study. It entails assembling a group of patients with a specific condition. Information on potential prognostic factors at baseline and details on the occurrence of one or more outcomes over time are collected or are available for review. The essential ingredients of a cohort study are listed in Table 4-1 and are similar to the components of a good clinical trial. A cohort study enables the investigator to determine the absolute risk of an outcome. This absolute risk is termed *incidence* and is the fre-

**Table 4-1.** Design and Evaluation of Studies of Prognosis

| |
|---|
| Define condition of study explicitly |
| Assemble inception cohort |
| Describe referral pattern |
| Define prognostic factors explicitly |
| Assess prognostic factors equally in all groups |
| Achieve complete follow-up |
| Define outcomes explicitly |
| Assess outcomes equally in all groups |
| Adjust for extraneous prognostic factors |

Modified from Sackett et al. (1991).

quency of specific outcome events over some time period in a defined population of patients (Rothman 1986). An important prognostic factor will split the cohort into groups whose incidence for a particular outcome differ. One measure of this difference is the *absolute risk*. This is the difference between the incidence in patients with the prognostic factor and the incidence in patients without the factor. Another measure of this difference is the *relative risk*. This is the ratio of, rather than the difference between, the incidence in patients with and without the prognostic factor.

For investigation of prognosis, cohort studies are used for two broad purposes. First, they can be used to compare persons with the condition of interest to persons without the condition in order to determine whether the observed incidence of adverse outcomes exceeds what would be expected in the absence of the condition. For example, a comparison of stroke incidence among persons with and without carotid bruits helped characterize the prognostic implications of a bruit (Heyman et al. 1980; Wolf et al. 1981). Second, cohort studies can be used to identify subgroups of persons with a given condition who may face different prognoses. For example, the incidence of unprovoked seizures was compared between two groups of patients following recovery from encephalitis and meningitis. One group consisted of patients who had early seizures complicating their infections and the other group consisted of patients who did not have early seizures. Patients with early seizures were at greater risk for future unprovoked seizures (Annegers et al. 1988).

Cohort studies can be prospective or retrospective. In a prospective study, patients with a certain condition are identified and characterized at the start of the study and are followed for the outcomes of interest as the study proceeds in time. None of the outcomes to be measured has yet occurred at the start of a prospective cohort study. The Framingham Study is a prime example of an ongoing prospective cohort study (Wolf et al. 1978). A retrospective cohort study is similar in design except that the outcome events have already occurred by the time the study is initiated. Its success depends upon the information on diagnosis, prognostic factors and outcome having been collected in a complete and comparable fashion in the past and being available for review. The investigator should strive to achieve the same completeness of prognostic information on patients who develop the outcome of interest as on those who do not. Many retrospective cohort studies have been possible with the records linkage system maintained at the Mayo Clinic, serving Olmsted County, Minnesota (Kurland and Brian 1978).

### Assembly of Inception Cohort

A cohort study of prognosis entails the investigation of a well-defined group of patients. A specific diagnosis defines who will comprise the cohort. To ensure homogeneity and to allow comparison with other groups of patients, the criteria for diagnosis must be explicitly stated. Often this is not a trivial task. Consider defining primary lateral sclerosis, multiple sclerosis, migraine headache, or carpal tunnel syndrome.

Once the criteria for diagnosis are established, then patients meeting these criteria are assembled into an *inception cohort.* This means that the study groups should consist of patients followed from a comparable time point in the course of their condition, usually the onset or diagnosis. The beginning of the disease must be defined the same way for all members of the cohort. Otherwise, the prognosis may differ substantially depending on when in the clinical course the cohort is assembled. In some situations the prognosis may improve. For example, consider the relatively good outcomes in a cohort of patients assembled 3 months after their subarachnoid hemorrhage or transient ischemic attack compared to a cohort assembled immediately following the onset of first symptoms. In some conditions, the onset of disease may be difficult to define. Consider, for example, the effect that advances in neuroimaging have had on the diagnosis

of brain tumors; the diagnosis may be made earlier. Thus the time to certain outcomes, such as death, will be longer (Miles et al. 1981). The same may hold for imaging and multiple sclerosis. Because of early imaging, the apparent change in prognosis reflects the change in the definition of when the disease began and is sometimes referred to as *lead time bias* (Weiss 1986). Feinstein and colleagues (1985) have used the phrase, the Will Rogers phenomenon, to describe this "zero-time shift" and "stage migration" produced by new diagnostic techniques.

Besides leading to an earlier diagnosis, imaging may lead to a different diagnosis and thus alter apparent prognosis. Such an effect is demonstrated with primary intracerebral hemorrhage (Drury et al. 1984). Prior to the widespread availability of computed tomographic (CT) scanning of the head, the diagnosis of intracerebral hemorrhage rested on a devastating clinical picture and often autopsy confirmation. Not surprisingly, with the introduction of CT scanning more benign bleeds have been identified among patients who previously would likely have been classified as having had ischemic strokes. Thus the introduction of CT scanning has resulted in an apparent fall in case fatality rates for intracerebral hemorrhages. More mild cases are now included in the denominator of these rates but not in the numerator because they survive.

Designs that include patients from a certain population without regard to when the condition began, prevalent cases, risk yielding misleading results. This is because patients with the condition have different probabilities of being included in the study, depending on the chronicity of their illness. Figure 4-1 illustrates a hypothetical study of patients with malignant brain tumors in a population. Choosing a prevalent sample of such patients involves selecting all such patients whose disease is active at a particular point in time, as indicated by the vertical line in Figure 4-1. The consideration of prevalent cases, rather than all newly diagnosed or incident cases, results in an overrepresentation of patients with long survivals. Patients with short survivals are less likely to be included in a sample of prevalent cases because they may have died before or been diagnosed after the sampling is done. If incident cases of disease had been included at the time of diagnosis, then an inception cohort would have been assem-

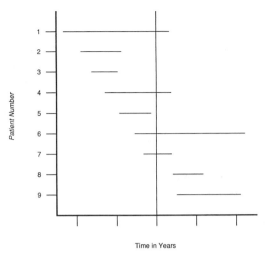

Figure 4-1. Incident versus prevalent cases. The start of the horizontal line for each patient with a malignant brain tumor represents the time of diagnosis, and the end of the line, the time of death.

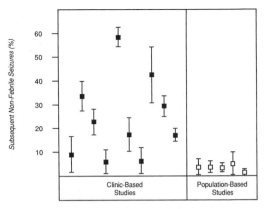

Figure 4-2. Rate of nonfebrile seizures following febrile convulsion. Closed squares represent studies from referral centers and open squares from population-based surveys. Rates and their 95% confidence intervals are shown. (Modified from Ellenberg and Nelson 1980; Sackett et al. 1991; and Longstreth et al. 1987b.)

bled and individual cases of short survival would not have been missed.

In all cohort studies of prognosis, the selection of patients has a profound effect on prognosis. A bias can result when more severe cases are referred to academic centers where they are more likely to be described in the literature (Motulsky 1978). Examples of this referral bias would include the higher rate of epilepsy following febrile convulsions in studies from referral centers rather than population-based studies, (Fig. 4-2) (Ellenberg and Nelson 1980), the higher rates of mental retardation with tuberous sclerosis reported from referral centers (Nagib et al. 1984), the more malignant course of multiple sclerosis reported from referral centers (Nelson et al. 1988), and the shorter survival of Friedreich's disease reported from referral centers (Leone et al. 1988).

Other types of selection bias that can affect how the cohort is assembled have been described by Sackett and colleagues (1991). Specific cases being referred to a specific expert leads to "centripetal" bias; interesting cases being more completely evaluated than more mundane cases, "popularity" bias; only certain cases being able to pass through several screening procedures, "referral filter" bias; and the types of diagnostic evaluations varying from institution to institution, "diagnosis access" bias. All of these biases can make the cohort being studied so unique that even if the study is internally valid, the results cannot be applied to other patients: that is, external validity is lacking. The challenge for a clinician is to find a study of prognosis whose cohort most closely resembles the type of patients that he or she sees or is likely to see. In this respect, a complete ascertainment of cases for a defined population, as in the door-to-door search in Copiah County, Mississippi, for patients with strokes (Schoenberg et al. 1986), may be less useful for the clinician than for the public health official because 20% of stroke survivors in that study were never hospitalized. The outcomes in that cohort are unlikely to reflect a neurologist's experience with stroke patients.

### Maximizing Internal Validity

Besides using an inception cohort, the internal validity of a cohort study can be strengthened with explicit and standardized definitions of potential prognostic factors and outcomes. Ideally in cohort studies the outcomes should be determined in such a way that outcome data cannot be biased by knowledge of prognostic factors. Even when blinding or other measures are employed as protection against the biased assessment of outcome, the possibility still exists, especially with potentially fatal illnesses, that decisions about medical support were based on the prognostic factors of interest and that a self-fulfilling prophecy resulted. Thus, if physicians already consider a large clot and reduced level of consciousness to be indicators of a poor outcome after intracerebral bleed, they may limit medical support in patients with these factors. Not surprisingly, a retrospective study of prognostic factors in intracerebral hemorrhage may find these two factors important predictors of outcome, namely, survival (Tuhrim et al. 1988). Instead, they may be important predictors of a physician's behavior, namely, withdrawing medical support, which in turn determines outcome.

Prospective studies would ideally keep information on prognosis from physicians making medical decisions that could influence outcome. In many clinical settings, the deliberate withholding of important prognostic information from clinicians cannot be achieved; the physicians cannot be made ignorant of the findings on the physical examination or the imaging studies. An alternative, to provide maximal support to all patients, is neither practical nor ethical in most clinical situations. Sometimes when a new prognostic test is first introduced it can be evaluated without the results influencing researchers' or practitioners' determination of outcome. For example, investigators of cerebrospinal fluid enzymes after cardiac arrest withheld the results of the test from the treating physicians and from themselves until the outcome was determined (Longstreth et al. 1984).

The choice of outcome to assess depends in part on what disease is being studied and what information is available. Life versus death is not always an appropriate outcome to measure, but other outcomes dealing with morbidity may be difficult to quantify. For example, Fletcher and colleagues (1996) describe six categories of outcome: disease, death, disability, discomfort, dissatisfaction, and destitution. As discussed by Patrick and Deyo (1989), some outcomes are disease specific, such as the Glasgow Coma Outcome Scale (Jennett and Bond 1975), the Kurtzke Disability Status Scale (Kurtzke 1989), or the NIH Stroke Scale (Lyden et al. 1994). Other instruments are designed to be broader measures of health status and quality of life such as the Sickness Impact Profile (Bergner et al. 1981) or the Medical Outcome Study Short Form (Stewart et al. 1988). These generic measures of outcome are only rarely used in studies of neurologic illnesses. Their use in clinical neurology is likely to increase given patients', physicians', and society's growing concerns with medicine's ability to prolong life at the expense of quality. As Fries and colleagues (1989) stated, "add life to

your years, not years to your life." Consider the vegetative or severely impaired survivors of a serious head injury, cardiac arrest, or subarachnoid hemorrhage. Instead of these generic measures, outcomes in studies of prognosis are most commonly measured by diagnostic test results, physical signs, or symptoms (Fletcher and Fletcher 1979).

Complete follow-up of the cohort is also required and is one of the most challenging aspects of a cohort study. The greater the number of patients lost from the cohort, the greater the compromise of the study's internal validity and of the conclusions that can be drawn from the study. Depending on which patients were lost to follow-up, the effect on the results can be either positive or negative. For example, patients with paralysis in the distribution of the facial nerve might fail to return for follow-up if their condition spontaneously improves (Katusic et al. 1986). Alternatively, patients with brain tumors who are doing poorly might be lost to follow-up because they seek medical treatment elsewhere or because they die. If the rate at which patients are lost differs substantially among the different comparison groups, then the results of the study may be subject to bias. The magnitude of these effects can sometimes be estimated by alternately assuming the worst and the best outcomes for the patients who are lost to follow-up.

### Clinical Trials of Treatment and Prognosis

A unique and increasingly important type of prospective cohort study of prognosis is that nested within a randomized, controlled clinical trial of treatment. Particularly when one arm of the trial is a no-treatment, or placebo, control group, the variation in outcomes within this group may provide insight into the prognostic importance of factors measured on entry into the trial. Except for the treatment being randomized, inferences about potential prognostic factors are based on observational comparisons that do not involve the random allocation. On the other hand, the control and standardization of other treatments in randomized trials helps to minimize the mixing of treatment effects with the effects of other potential prognostic factors. Also, information on patient characteristics and outcomes are compiled in a prospective and standardized fashion, which is the exception in most studies dealing solely with issues of prognosis. The reason that information on prognostic factors is typically collected as part of treatment trials is because often these factors have a greater potential effect on outcomes than the treatments being tested (Sather 1986). Knowledge of prognosis is essential for clinical trials for several reasons: to ensure that randomization has resulted in treatment groups that are balanced with respect to prognostic factors; to obtain a more precise estimate of treatment effects by controlling for prognostic factors in the analysis; and to examine treatment effects in different prognostic subgroups.

In a clinical trial, the treatment groups can be examined separately to assess potential prognostic factors whose effects may be modified by the treatment given. Information measured at baseline or around the time of randomization is most useful. For example, important information about prognosis in Guillain-Barre syndrome has emerged from a multicenter clinical trial (McKhann et al. 1988), and data about prognosis after cardiac arrest have come from the Brain Resuscitation Clinical Trials (Edgren 1987). Given the difficulty in funding studies that deal solely with prognosis, clinical trials will likely remain an important source of prospective information on prognosis.

An important limitation of using clinical trials is that only a select group of patients are studied. Typically, clinical trials have specific inclusion and exclusion criteria in order to select those patients who have the greatest likelihood of receiving benefit from the intervention being tested or who may be the least likely to suffer adverse effects of the treatment. In one trial of heparin after ischemic stroke (Duke et al. 1986), over 3000 patients were screened to enroll 225 subjects for the study. In another trial of a calcium channel blocker for ischemic stroke (Gelmers et al. 1988), 20% of the placebo group died in the first month following the stroke, suggesting that the patients included in this trial may have had a more grave prognosis than if all patients with ischemic strokes had been considered. In this trial, more patients with infarctions in the left side of the brain ($n = 116$) than in the right side of the brain ($n = 70$) were included, reflecting the greater ease by which an aphasic patient could meet entrance criteria for stroke severity.

## Case-Control Design

The case-control design is another nonexperimental analytic method often used in epidemiology. In the context of prognosis, the case-control design involves the comparison of a group of patients known to have had a poor outcome from a certain condition with another group known to have had a good outcome from the same condition. It relates these differences in outcome to prognostic factors measured at an earlier time in the clinical course of each patient. Advantages of the case-control study include its being relatively inexpensive, requiring a relatively brief time to perform, being especially efficient for rare outcomes, and being suitable for the study of multiple potential predictors of an outcome. More commonly it is used to address questions of etiology in classic epidemiology by allowing identification of risk factors for disease. Its use to address questions of prognosis in clinical epidemiology is unusual. In one such example, investigators identified a group of patients with multiple sclerosis whose disease ran a malignant course and another group whose course was more benign (Clark et al. 1982). They then sought to determine which factors in the patients' past were different between the groups and thus might be important prognostic factors. Another study used a similar design to try to identify important prognostic factors in Parkinson's disease (Goetz et al. 1988).

The major disadvantages of the case-control study are that it involves retrospective assessment of the prognostic factors of interest and may be susceptible to bias, which is often difficult to detect or control. It also does not yield data on the absolute risk, or incidence, of particular outcomes as does the cohort study. Although the cohort study yields actual absolute and relative risks, as discussed in the previous section, the case-control study yields an odds ratio, which is only an estimate of the relative risk of good versus poor outcomes in persons with or without a particular characteristic. In addition, the odds ratio computed from case-control data is a good estimate of the relative risk only if the outcome of interest is rare (Feinstein 1985). In this context, "rare" is usually meant to indicate about 10% or less. For many outcomes of disease, this assumption may be violated. Consider the occurrence of a malignant course in patients with multiple sclerosis or Parkinson's disease. Thus, the major advantage of case-control studies, the ability to investigate rare outcomes, makes this design less appealing than the cohort design for conditions with the outcome of interest being common.

Clinical situations do exist, however, in which the case-control study is a valid and efficient method to investigate prognosis. Its uncommon use in studies of prognosis may indicate under-utilization of an important study design. Consider conditions in which an important outcome is rare. Sudden death is a rare outcome that can complicate the clinical course of patients with epilepsy (Jay and Leestma 1981). A case-control design may be an appropriate method to try to identify those factors associated with sudden death. After establishing specific diagnostic criteria, a group of epileptic patients with sudden death (cases) and a group of epileptic patients without sudden death (controls) would be compared with respect to potential prognostic factors. Information on the factors would be obtained retrospectively by reviewing medical records or by interviewing people who knew the patients. Note that such a study would not address the question of the absolute risk of sudden death in patients with epilepsy. A cohort study would be needed to answer such a question but would be extremely difficult to do because the outcome of interest, sudden death, is so rare. Other examples of uncommon outcomes suited to the case-control designs would include studies of very good outcomes after a diagnosis of glioblastoma multiforme, amyotrophic lateral sclerosis, or severe head injury or studies of the very poor outcomes after Guillain-Barre syndrome, unruptured aneurysms, or aseptic meningitis. Finally, depending on how the sampling of controls is done, the rare disease assumption of a case-control study may not be required for valid estimation of the relative risk (Greenland and Thomas 1982).

## Analysis of Studies of Prognosis

The goal of data analysis is usually to describe the incidence of one or more outcomes and to identify associations between potential predictors and outcomes that are not just accidental. The potential predictors or prognostic factors are sometimes termed the *independent variables;* and the outcomes, *dependent variables.*

The most important prognostic factors to identify are those that may have a causal link to the outcomes. Such a causal relationship can teach us about the pathophysiology of the condition and suggest possible avenues of treatment, if the factor can be modified. For instance, if some im-

munologic change predicts progression in a patient with multiple sclerosis (Garren et al. 1998), could manipulation of the change prevent progression? Elevated blood glucose levels may exacerbate brain ischemia and result in worse outcomes for ischemic stroke (Woo et al. 1988). Is this finding a cause or an effect? Could lowering of blood glucose levels result in an improved outcome?

Just because a prognostic factor is associated with an outcome does not mean that a causal relationship exists. Other features of the association are relevant in seeking to establish causality. Some features concern the study data, such as whether a dose–response relationship can be demonstrated and whether the temporal sequence is correct. Other considerations go beyond the study data, such as consistency of findings with other clinical studies and biological plausibility. Even if evidence for a causal link is lacking, a strong association between predictor and outcome identifies an important prognostic factor capable of predicting outcomes. Cerebrospinal fluid creatine kinase isoenzymes are strongly associated with outcome after cardiac arrest (Vaagenes et al. 1988; Tirschwell et al. 1997). No one would argue that the enzymes are causing brain damage. Rather, their leakage into the cerebrospinal fluid is a result of brain damage. The lack of a causal relation does not obviate their usefulness as predictors of outcome.

Analyses in studies of prognosis aim to describe outcomes and identify predictors. Often they involve striking a balance between deriving an understandable summary measure of a prognostic factor and trying to capture as much information about the disease as possible. Clinicians find simple summaries most appealing, but much information can be lost. The simplest approach is to pick some dichotomous outcome—life or death, ambulatory or not, recurrent seizure or not—and to ignore time altogether, assuming that enough time has transpired for all the outcomes of interest to have occurred. Progression to a certain stage, remission, or recurrence can define the endpoint. For example, 14% of patients with myasthenia gravis had their disease remain clinically localized to the extraocular muscles (Grob et al. 1987). Alternatively, a single time may be selected at which to assess outcome. For example, the 5-year survival of patients with an oligodendroglioma was 34% (Mørk et al. 1985). If the outcomes are examined at more than one time, more information is captured. For instance, the 2-year survival after the diagnosis of subarachnoid hemorrhage and amyotrophic lateral sclerosis may be similar at about 50%, but the shape of the two survival curves would be very different as shown in Figure 4-3. Note that, in these hypothetical curves, the time at which 50% of the cohort has died is the median survival. For both illnesses the median survival is 2 years. Median survival is often used as a summary measure in studies because its calculation does not require that all members of the cohort have died, as would be necessary to calculate mean survival.

## Survival Analysis

Survival analysis is a powerful technique to study prognosis (Peto et al. 1977). For it to be applicable, the outcome must be dichotomous, or made

**Figure 4-3.** Survival curves for a hypothetical cohort of patients with subarachnoid hemorrhage and another with amyotrophic lateral sclerosis.

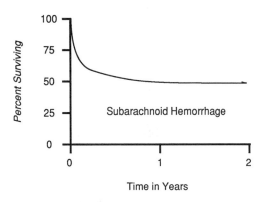

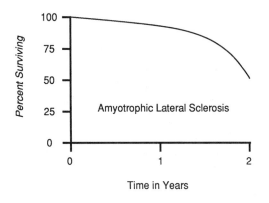

to be dichotomous, and it must be an event that a patient can experience only once. Any such dichotomous outcome can be used, not just life and death. Recurrent events such as seizures can be studied by considering only the first occurrence. Separate curves can be constructed for patients with particular prognostic factors, and statistical tests can be applied to decide whether the curves are significantly different. The information from the curve can be summarized numerically by using a specific time point at which the heights of the curves are compared, such as 5-year survival, or by determining the amount of time required for a given survival curve to reach a certain height, such as median survival time. Alternatively, the curves can be assessed visually or quantified by calculating the area under the curve or the person-years lived by the cohort.

Ideally, the survival curve would include information on the entire cohort followed completely until all its members had experienced the outcome of interest. Rarely is such an ideal achieved in a clinical study. Instead, members of the cohort are often lost to follow-up or are *censored* for some other reason. One of the strengths of survival analysis is that it uses as much of the information available on each patient as possible. Assumptions need to be made about those censored or lost to follow-up. Consequently, the curves are estimates and become increasingly so as the number of persons under observation continues to fall as one moves from left to right on the time axis. Key to the use of information on all cases, even those subsequently censored or lost to follow-up, is the assumption that those who are lost from the cohort share the same survival experience as the entire cohort with respect to the outcome of interest. Situations can be easily imagined where this assumption is violated. As suggested previously, patients with a brain tumor who are doing poorly may seek help elsewhere and may be lost to follow-up. Their survival experience may be much worse than the remainder of the cohort. A survival curve that assumes that their survival experience is the same will give an overly optimistic picture of the clinical course of this cohort. One simple and conservative method for setting bounds on the extent of the bias is to reconstruct the curves under the pessimistic assumption that all those lost to follow-up had a poor outcome at the time of last contact.

As an example of the technique, consider a hypothetical study in which patients with a diagnosis of epilepsy who have been free of any seizures for 2 years are advised to consider stopping their antiseizure medications. The study runs for 4 years during which time ten such patients who want to stop their medications are enrolled and followed as indicated in Figure 4-4A. Patients number 3 and 5 stop coming to the clinic for follow-up, and neither can be located after the times indicated. Patient number 9 was killed in a motor vehicle accident. He was the driver, but otherwise the details of the accident were unknown. The next step in the analysis is to change the time scale in Figure 4-4A to 4-4B so that all cases line up against the vertical axis at time zero. This is tantamount to establishing an inception cohort, as described previously, in which all patients are followed from an equivalent temporal milestone. Now a survival curve can be constructed. It begins at 100% on the vertical axis, indicating that all the patients are initially seizure free. It continues horizontally until one of the patients being followed experiences a first recurrent seizure. Dropouts, such as patients number 3, 5, and 9 with incomplete follow-up information, have no immediate effect on the height of the curve. When a patient suffers his or her first recurrent seizure, the curve drops. The new height of the curve, new percentage remaining seizure free, is given by the following formula:

$$\text{(old percent remaining seizure free} \times \frac{(N-1)}{N}$$

where $N$ is the number of subjects under observation just before the time of the seizure and the old percent refers to the height of the curve also just before the time of the seizure. Figure 4-4C shows the resulting survival curve and the appropriate calculations. For this example, based on so few patients, the survival curve is made up of a few large steps; for larger cohorts, it adopts a smoother shape.

The curve in Figure 4-4C assumes that the two patients who were lost to follow-up and the one patient who was censored because of death experienced the same rate of seizure recurrence as the entire cohort. A critic might argue that the two patients lost to follow-up probably both had seizures but, because they were disgruntled about the advice that they had received in the clinic, did not return and sought treatment for their epilepsy elsewhere. The patient who died in the motor vehicle accident could also have had a seizure, which could have been the cause of the accident. With these considerations the curve can be redone under the possibly extreme assumption that all three patients with missing information experienced a recurrent seizure around the time of their last contact for patients number 3 and 5 or at the time of the motor vehicle accident for patient number 9.

Time-linked analysis of outcomes that are not dichotomous are not as well developed and are less commonly used. Often an outcome that will be measured as a continuous variable in a study will need to be made a dichotomous variable for survival analysis. Consider, for example, the use of a device to assess grip strength in a patient with amyotrophic lateral sclerosis. The results are read from the device as a continuous variable. For purposes of a survival analysis, however, a particular level of weakness has to be used to dichotomize the continuous variable and then a survival curve can be constructed on the basis of this dichotomous outcome. Growth curve analysis allows a continuous outcome measure to be examined over time (Zerbe 1979). It is used most commonly to examine change in height of children over time. It is rarely applied to studies of outcome, but would seem to be well suited to many situations in clinical medicine.

## Confounding and Effect Modification

Other efforts in the analysis of prognosis studies are directed at dealing with confounding and effect modification (Miettinen 1974; Hennekens and Buring 1987). Confounding occurs because a factor is related to both a prognostic factor and the outcome. Such confounding factors can cause the association between a prognostic factor and an outcome to be over- or underestimated. In an extreme situation, confounding can cause an association to appear present when one is in fact lacking, or vice versa. Consider an obvious example is one in which gray hair is proposed to be associated with a worse outcome from head trauma. A cohort of patients with head trauma are separated into those with and without gray hair and outcomes in the two groups are compared. If a statistically significant association were found, one would hesitate to conclude that the presence of gray hair is linked to outcome from head trauma

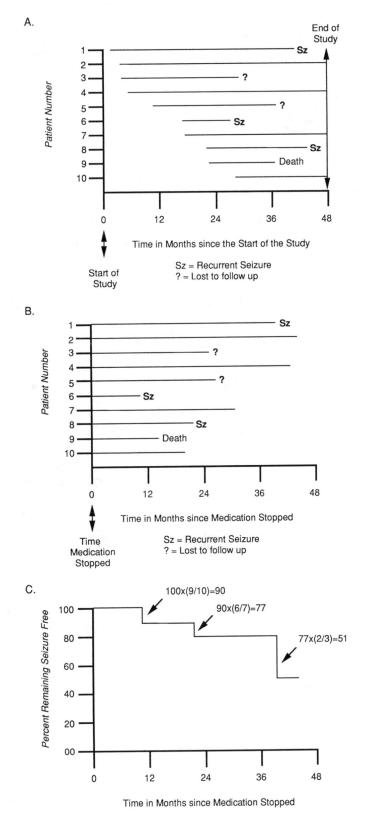

**Figure 4-4.** Hypothetical example of survival analysis for recurrence of seizures after stopping antiseizure medications. See text for complete explanation

without first examining the effects of age. Age is likely related to both gray hair and to outcome from head trauma and must then be taken into account in the analysis. Confounding is typically more subtle and can easily invalidate conclusions drawn from a study that is trying to establish a causal link between a prognostic factor and an outcome. If causation is not an issue, then neither is confounding. Thus in the example above, regardless of any confounding by age, gray hair may still be an important predictor of outcome.

An important and difficult issue in many cohort studies is a phenomenon called confounding by indication. This problem arises when an objective of the study is to determine the effects of a particular form of evaluation or treatment from observational data, or to determine the effect of some patient characteristic that is itself an indication (or contraindication) for a certain form of intervention. Under these circumstances, the form of evaluation or treatment a patient receives may be so closely linked to a particular feature of his or her clinical status that the effect of the evaluation or treatment cannot be separated from the effect of the underlying indication (or contraindication) for it. For example, the case fatality rate for patients in an intensive care unit who have a neurology consult may be higher than the case fatality rate for patients in an intensive care unit who do not have a neurology consult. The consultation does not cause the patients' death. Rather, the indication for a neurology consult is what places a patient at high risk for death. Again, confounding applies only to the attempt to assign causality. Even though a causal relationship does not exist, a neurology consult on a patient in the intensive care unit may still be a marker for a poor outcome.

Several techniques exist to search for and control confounding, but the most generally useful analytic methods are stratification and multivariate modeling. Stratification involves forming subgroups of patients who are similar with respect to the confounding factor. Then the association between the potential prognostic factor and outcome is evaluated in each subgroup or stratum. So for the example above, the association between gray hair and outcome after head trauma could be examined by age strata. Although a strong association may exist for the entire group, none may be present when considering separately the subgroups of young patients and older patients. Techniques

to combine evidence across strata include direct and indirect standardization (Fleiss 1986; Hennekens and Buring 1987) and the Mantel-Haenszel method (1959). Such approaches to control confounding are most useful when the number of confounding factors is small. Unfortunately, the situation in a clinical setting often becomes complicated with several potential predictors and confounders.

Effect modification or interaction occurs when the strength of the association between a prognostic factor and an outcome differs among subgroups formed according to a third factor. Unlike with confounding where the associations are similar in all subgroups, with effect modification the associations differ by subgroup. With confounding, the estimate of the association derived from the subgroups is better than the unadjusted estimate derived from the entire group. With effect modification, the estimate of the association derived from the subgroups differ so much that combining them as would be done to control for confounding would be inappropriate. When effect modification is present, subgroups should not be lumped together. For example, the prognosis of patients with cryptococcal meningitis is worsened by concomitant infection with immunodeficiency virus (Rosenblum et al. 1988). To summarize the prognosis of cryptococcal meningitis and not consider human immunodeficiency virus (HIV) status is to ignore an important effect modifier. A single summary is not appropriate. Rather the prognosis has to be presented separately for those with and without concomitant infection with HIV.

An increasingly recognized source of effect modification relates to the interaction of genetic and environmental factors. Thus a genetic factor may define subgroups of patients with a particular neurological condition that have different prognoses. For example, having the ε4 allele of apolipoprotein E identifies a subgroup of patients with worse outcomes after intracerebral hemorrhage (Alberts et al. 1995) and after head injury (Teasdale et al. 1997).

## Multivariate Models

Multivariate models allow the investigator to look at the relation of many variables to outcome (Rothman 1986; Feinstein 1996). These models can be used to help identify the most important predictor variables and to allow the creation of clinical predictive rules (Wasson et al. 1985). Such models have been used to predict outcomes after cardiac arrest (Levy et al. 1985), intracranial hemorrhage (Tuhrim et al. 1988), subarachnoid hemorrhage (Longstreth et al. 1993), acute stroke in general (Fullerton et al. 1988), febrile convulsions (Annegers et al. 1987), acute idiopathic neuropathy (Winer et al. 1988), Bell's palsy (Katusic et al. 1986), Alzheimer's disease (Heyman et al. 1987), and many other conditions. Most of the multivariate techniques listed in Table 4-2 are available in statistical packages that are widely distributed. Methods exist to address both confounding and effect modification with these multivariate models.

Often little understanding of multivariate modeling is needed to perform the analysis, but because many pitfalls exist, a biostatistician experienced with these techniques should be consulted. A danger exists of finding some idiosyncrasy of the data set rather than true variations in outcomes for the disease in question. This danger increases as the number of predictor variables examined increases. A general rule is to have at least ten patients with the outcome of interest for each variable that is included in the model. Often the validity of the model can be tested. One simple approach is to generate prognostic rules on one randomly chosen half of the data set and then test them on the remaining half. As mentioned previously, an internally valid study or model may still have limited external validity as a result of the characteristics of the cohort under study.

**Table 4-2.** Multivariate Models

| Method | Nature of Predictor Variables | Nature of Outcome Variable |
|---|---|---|
| Multiple linear regression | Categorical or continuous | Continuous |
| Discriminant analysis | Continuous, with normal distribution | Dichotomous |
| Multiple logistic regression* | Categorical or continuous | Dichotomous |
| Log-linear modeling* | Categorical | Categorical, with two or more categories |
| Cox proportional hazards model* | Categorical or continuous | Survival time |

* Can be used to obtain adjusted relative risk estimates for predictor variables.

Logistic regression is the multivariate method of choice when prognostic data have been collected according to a case-control design. Logistic regression is a favorite of epidemiologists because adjusted odds ratio estimates can be calculated from the coefficients of the predictor variables. These estimates of relative risk are useful summaries of the strength of the relation between a predictor and an outcome controlling for other factors included in the model. As with survival analysis, the outcome variable in logistic regression must be dichotomous.

One of the more sophisticated models used in studies of outcome is the Cox proportional hazards model (Cox 1972). This allows multiple variables that can be time-dependent to be considered simultaneously in an analysis of survival. As in logistic regression, the coefficients from the Cox proportional hazards model can be converted to adjusted relative risk estimates. For example, when this type of analysis was applied to seizure recurrence following a febrile convulsion (Annegers et al. 1987), the adjusted relative risk for seizure recurrence was 3.6 if the febrile convulsion had focal features. Thus, patients whose febrile convulsion had focal features would be 3.6 times as likely to have a seizure recurrence per unit of time as those whose febrile convulsion lacked focal features. A relative risk of 1.0 would indicate no relation between potential predictors and outcome. A relative risk less than 1.0 would indicate a favorable prognosis with the factor present.

From the standpoint of data analysis, clinical trials of treatments can be seen as studies of prognosis where the treatments are just another potential predictor of outcome. Many prognostic factors cannot be modify such as age, gender, or race. Treatments are simply prognostic factors that can be modified. Consider, for example, the cooperative study investigating the treatment of Guillain-Barre syndrome (McKhann et al. 1988) and the one studying treatment of coma after cardiac arrest (Brain Resuscitation Clinical Trial I Study Group 1986). Despite both being randomized, double-blind trials, analyses included the Cox proportional hazards model with several potential predictors of outcome including treatment. After controlling for the effects of the other predictors of outcome, the analyses yielded a coefficient for the treatment variable that was significant for plasmapheresis for Guillain-Barre syndrome and insignificant for pentobarbital for coma after cardiac arrest.

Another type of model that has been used in studies of prognosis is the Markov process (Beck and Pauker 1983). Various stages of disease progression are defined, and probabilities are assigned for moving from one stage to another. This technique has been used to model the clinical course of patients with headaches (Leviton et al. 1980) and multiple sclerosis (Wolfson and Confavreux 1987). Another type of model has been used to try to characterize the nonrandom occurrence of seizures in patients with epilepsy (Hopkins et al. 1985). Artificial neural networks have also been suggested for predicting medical outcomes (Tu 1996). Finally, another technique called recursive partitioning is especially useful for identifying interactions and appealing in the ease of understanding the results (Feinstein 1996). Unlike the models listed in Table 4-2 that yield predictive equations, recursive partitioning results in a classification tree. At each split, the prognostic factor is identified that does the best at separating the patients into two groups with different outcomes. An example of the technique is a study of predictors of outcome after cardiac arrest (Levy et al. 1985).

All of these statistical techniques help investigators to decide which prognostic factors are the most important. The importance of a predictor can be established on the basis of statistical significance, clinical usefulness, or both. Patients who do and do not regain consciousness after out-of-hospital cardiac arrest have admission temperatures that differ by an average of 0.2°C, being lower in those who did not regain consciousness (Longstreth et al. 1983). Although this is a statistically significant difference ($p = .026$), it lacks clinical usefulness. For a prognostic factor to be useful, the relation between predictor and outcome must be clinically convincing, not just statistically significant.

## Evidence-Based Medicine

The practice of evidence-based medicine, or for neurologists evidence-based neurology, entails "integrating individual clinical expertise with the best available external evidence from systematic research" (Sackett et al. 1996). It is a supplement, not a substitute, for intuition, clinical experience, and an understanding of pathophysiology. It can

be applied to many areas of medicine including prognosis. Guidelines exist to help physicians use this problem-oriented method to answer questions about prognosis (Laupacis et al. 1994).

The technique begins with a physician, a patient, and a question about prognosis. The first step is to find the evidence related to the specific question about prognosis. Sometimes readily available books provide the needed answers but, with the exception of this text, good prognostic information is often difficult to find in books (McKibbon et al. 1995). Often, the physician needs to search the literature to identify pertinent articles. Suggestions exist on the most effective searching strategies to identify articles about prognosis (McKibbon et al. 1995). When using MEDLINE, the searcher will simply combine the disease of interest with text words such as "prognosis" or "mortality" or "natural" or "history" or "predict" or "course." Each article is also indexed by the type of study design, so the best articles on prognosis can often be identified by seeking those also indexed as "cohort studies."

Once the pertinent articles are identified, the next step is to critically appraise the articles and judge the internal validity of the individual studies. Specific guidelines have been proposed (Laupacis et al. 1994), and the key elements are summarized in Table 4-3. Note that these are a distillation of the essential ingredients listed in Table 4-1, now aimed at the person reading the article rather than the investigator designing the study. If the study is valid, the results are examined for the size and precision of the effects. The size of effect is often summarized as a relative risk, median survival, or 5-year survival. The precision is often estimated with 95% confidence intervals.

The final step is the most difficult and asks if results from internally valid studies have external

**Table 4-3.** Guides to Critically Evaluate an Article About Prognosis

| |
| --- |
| Are the results of the study valid? |
| Primary Guides |
|   Was the sample of patients representative and well defined at a similar point in the course of the disease? |
|   Was follow-up sufficiently long and complete? |
| Secondary Guides |
|   Were objective and unbiased outcome criteria used? |
|   Were adjustments made for important prognostic factors? |

Modified from Laupacis et al. 1994.

validity. Should the results be applied to the patient who was the source of the physician's question about prognosis? Most important in deciding the external validity is the similarity of the physician's patient to the patients who were subjects of the internal valid study. Important prognostic information will help the physician in selecting or avoiding therapy and in counseling and reassuring the patient.

## Conclusions

One of the major tasks of a neurologist is to render an accurate prognosis. Many of the patients that neurologists care for have grave diseases for which treatments are lacking or are ineffective, so prognosis becomes even more important. With the nervous system at risk, patients and families insist that neurologists "avoid expressing prognosis with vagueness when it is unnecessary, and with certainty when it is misleading" (Fletcher et al. 1996). Armed with an understanding of prognosis, the neurologist can appropriately counsel patients, families, and other physicians. Even with this understanding, the neurologist is challenged by having to translate probabilities that range from 0 *to* 1 in groups of patients to 0 *or* 1 for a specific patient. If the prognosis is known, the clinician can identify situations where aggressive or dangerous treatments are indicated because of the poor outcomes that follow the usual clinical course. If the prognosis is certain enough, such as with brain death or a persistent vegetative state, decisions to withdraw therapy can be considered.

Sometimes studies of prognosis are all clinicians have to try to judge the external validity of a trial of some treatment (Weiss 1986). If lowering blood pressure in white and black men results in reduced cardiovascular disease outcome events (Hypertension and Detection Follow-up Program Cooperative Group 1979), will the same conclusions apply to women or Asians? If the clinical course of all these patients with hypertension is similar, then the results of the trial are assumed to apply to women and Asians. If a drug could be shown to prevent post-traumatic epilepsy, it would probably be used in other situations where a brain injury can lead to later epilepsy such as following meningitis or following surgery on the brain.

For investigators, studies of prognosis may indicate which diseases have an important impact on function and thus require further investigation. In addition to indicating which diseases require treatments, the search for prognostic factors may yield clues as to the pathophysiology of the disease and its treatment.

Many studies of prognosis in neurology fall far short of the ideal study. Nevertheless, each study provides some information and helps to reduce the mystery that surrounds many neurologic illnesses. Ignorance about clinical course and prognosis can potentially cause more harm than good with some patients. Examples include the discovery of an asymptomatic bruit on physical examination and an unidentified bright object on a magnetic resonance imaging study. Sometimes in our haste to intervene and treat, the clinical course or prognosis of certain conditions remains vague and ill-defined. Detailed studies of prognosis should precede studies of treatment, but such a sequence is often reversed.

In this chapter, the basic elements of studies of prognosis have been presented. Some necessary skills for researcher and clinician to master to be able to perform and interpret such studies have been outlined. Prognosis is the keystone to clinical neurology, and a better understanding of prognosis leads to a better understanding of clinical neurology. This chapter has dealt in generalities and methodologies. The subsequent chapters turn to the prognosis of specific conditions.

## References

Alberts, M. J.; Graffagnino, C.; McClenny C.; DeLong, D.; Strittmatter, W.; Saunders A. M.; Roses, A. D. ApoE genotype and survival from intracerebral hemorrhage. Lancet 346:575; 1995.

Annegers, J. F.; Hauser, W. A.; Beghi, E.; Nicolosi, A.; Kurland, L. T. The risk of unprovoked seizures after encephalitis and meningitis. Neurology 38:1407–1410; 1988.

Annegers, J. F.; Hauser, W. A.; Shirts, S. B.; Kurland, L. T. Factors prognostic of unprovoked seizures after febrile convulsions. N. Engl. J. Med. 316:493–498; 1987.

Beck, J. R.; Pauker, S. G. The Markov process in medical prognosis. Med. Decis. Making 3:419–458; 1983.

Bergner, M.; Bobbitt, R. A.; Carter, W. B.; Gilson, B. S. The Sickness Impact Profile: development and final revision of a health status measure. Med. Care 19:787–805; 1981.

Brain Resuscitation Clinical Trial I Study Group. Randomized clinical study of thiopental loading in comatose survivors of cardiac arrest. N. Engl. J. Med. 314:397–403; 1986.

Clark, V. A.; Detels, R.; Visscher, B. R.; Valdiviezo, N. L.; Malmgren, R. M.; Dudley, J. P. Factors associated with a malignant or benign course of multiple sclerosis. JAMA 248:856–860; 1982.

Cox, D. R. Regression models and life tables (with discussion). J. R. Stat. Soc. Series B 34:187–220; 1972.

Drury, I.; Whisnant, J. P.; Garraway, W. M. Primary intracerebral hemorrhage: impact of CT on incidence. Neurology 34:653–657; 1984.

Duke, R. J.; Bloch, R. F.; Turpie, A. G. G.; Trebilcock, R.; Bayer, N. Intravenous heparin for the prevention of stroke progression in acute partial stable stroke: a randomized controlled trial. Ann. Intern. Med. 105:825–828; 1986.

Edgren, E. The prognosis of hypoxic-ischaemic brain damage following cardiac arrest. Acta Univ. Ups. (Comprehensive summaries of Uppsala dissertations from the faculty of medicine) 89. 1–44; 1987.

Ellenberg, J. H.; Nelson, K. B. Sample selection and the natural history of disease: studies of febrile seizures. JAMA 243:1337–1340; 1980.

Evidence-Based Medicine Working Group. Evidence-based medicine. A new approach to teaching the practice of medicine. JAMA 268:2420–2425; 1992.

Feinstein, A. R. Clinical epidemiology: the architecture of clinical research. Philadelphia: W. B. Saunders Co.; 1985.

Feinstein, A. R.; Sosin, D. M.; Wells, C. K. The Will Rogers phenomenon: stage migration and new diagnostic techniques as a source of misleading statistics for survival in cancer. N. Engl. J. Med. 312:1604–1608; 1985.

Feinstein, A. R. Multivariable analysis: an introduction. New Haven, CT: Yale University Press; 1986.

Fleiss, J. L. The design and analysis of clinical experiments. New York: John Wiley & Sons; 1986.

Fletcher, R. H.; Fletcher, S. W. Clinical research in general medical journals: a 30-year perspective. N. Engl. J. Med. 301:180–183; 1979.

Fletcher, R. H.; Fletcher, S. W.; Wagner, E. H. Clinical epidemiology: the essentials. 3rd ed. edition. Baltimore: Williams & Wilkins; 1996.

Fries, J. F.; Green, L. W.; Levine, S. Health promotion and the compression of morbidity. Lancet 1:481–483; 1989.

Fullerton, K. J.; Mackenzie, G.; Stout, R. W. Prognostic indices in stroke. Q. J. Med. 66:147–162; 1988.

Garren, H.; Steinman, L.; Lock, C. The specificity of the antibody response in multiple sclerosis. Ann. Neurol. 43:4–6; 1998.

Gelmers, H. J.; Gorter, K.; de Weerdt, C. J.; Wiezer, H. J. A. A controlled trial of nimodipine in acute ischemic stroke. N. Engl. J. Med. 318:203–207; 1988.

Goetz, C. G.; Tanner, C. M.; Stebbins, G. T.; Buchman, A. S. Risk factors for progression in Parkinson's disease. Neurology 38:1841–1844; 1988.

Greenland, S.; Thomas, D. C. On the need for the rare disease assumption in case-control studies. Am. J. Epidemiol. 116:547–553; 1982.

Grob, D.; Arsura, E. L.; Brunner, N. G.; Namba, T. The course of myasthenia gravis and therapies affecting outcome. Ann. N. Y. Acad. Sci. 505:472–499; 1987.

Hennekens, C. H.; Buring, J. E. Epidemiology in medicine. Boston: Little, Brown & Co.; 1987.

Heyman, A.; Wilkinson, W. E.; Heyden, S.; Helms, M. J.; Bartel, A. G.; Karp, H. R.; Tyroler, H. A.; Hames, C. G. Risk of stroke in asymptomatic persons with cervical arterial bruits: a population study in Evans County, Georgia. N. Engl. J. Med. 302:838–841; 1980.

Heyman, A.; Wilkinson, W. E.; Hurwitz, B. J.; Helms, M. J.; Haynes, C. S.; Utley, C. M.; Gwyther, L. P. Early-onset Alzheimer's disease: clinical predictors of institutionalization and death. Neurology 37:980–984; 1987.

Hopkins, A.; Davies, P.; Dobson, C. Arch. Neurol. 42:463–467; 1985.

Hypertension and Detection Follow-up Program Cooperative Group. Five-year findings of the hypertension detection and follow-up program: II. Mortality by race, sex and age. JAMA 242:2572–2577; 1979.

Jay, G. W.; Leestma, J. E. Sudden death in epilepsy: a comprehensive review of the literature and proposed mechanism. Acta. Neurol. Scand. 63(suppl. 82):1–66; 1981.

Jennett, B.; Bond, M. Assessment of outcome after severe brain damage: a practical scale. Lancet 1:480–484; 1975.

Katusic, S. K.; Beard, C. M.; Wiederholt, W. C.; Bergstralh, E. J.; Kurland, L. T. Ann. Neurol. 20:622–627; 1986.

Kurkland, L. T.; Brian, D. D. Contributions to neurology from records linkage in Olmsted County, Minnesota. Adv. Neurol. 19:93–105; 1978.

Kurtzke, J. F. The Disability Status Scale for multiple sclerosis: apologia pro DSS sua. Neurology 39(2Pt1):291–302; 1989.

Laupacis, A.; Wells, G.; Richardson, W. S.; Tugwell, P. Users' guides to the medical literature: V. How to use an article about prognosis. JAMA 272:234–237; 1994.

Leone, M.; Rocca, W. A.; Rosso, M. G.; Mantel, N.; Schoenberg, B. S.; Schiffer, D. Friedreich's disease: survival analysis in an Italian population. Neurology 38:1433–1438; 1988.

Leviton, A.; Schulman, J.; Kammerman, L.; Porter, D.; Slack, W.; and Graham, J. R. A probability model of headache recurrence. J. Chron. Dis. 33:407–412; 1980.

Levy, D. E.; Caronna, J. J.; Singer, B. H.; Lapinski, R. H.; Frydman H.; Plum, F. Predicting outcome from hypoxic-ischemic coma. JAMA 253:1420–1426; 1985.

Longstreth, W. T., Jr.; Clayson, K. J.; Chandler, W. L.; Sumi, S. M. Cerebrospinal fluid creatine kinase activity and neurologic recovery after cardiac arrest. Neurology 34:834–837; 1984.

Longstreth, W. T., Jr.; Diehr, P.; Inui, T. S. Prediction of awakening after out-of-hospital cardiac arrest. N. Engl. J. Med. 308:1378–1382; 1983.

Longstreth, W. T., Jr.; Koepsell, T. D.; van Belle, G. Clinical neuroepidemiology: I. Diagnosis. Arch. Neurol. 44:1091–1099; 1987a.

Longstreth, W. T., Jr.; Koepsell, T. D.; van Belle, G. Clinical neuroepidemiology: II. Outcomes. Arch. Neurol. 44:1196–1202; 1987b.

Longstreth, W. T., Jr.; Nelson, L. M.; Koepsell, T. D.; van Belle, G. Clinical course of spontaneous subarachnoid hemorrhage: a population-based study in King County, Washington. Neurology 43:712–718; 1993.

Lyden, P.; Brott, T.; Tilley, B.; Welch, K. M. A.; Mascha, E. J.; Levine, S.; Haley, E. C.; Grotta, J.; Marler, J. Improved reliability of the NIH Stroke Scale using video training. Stroke 25:2220–2226; 1994.

Mantel, N.; Haenszel, W. Statistical aspects of the analysis of data from retrospective studies of disease. J. Natl. Cancer Inst. 22:719–748; 1959.

McKhann, G. M.; Griffin, J. W.; Cornblath, D. R.; Mellits, E. D.; Fisher, R. S.; Quaskey, S. A. Plasmapheresis and Guillain-Barré syndrome: analysis of prognostic factors and the effect of plasmapheresis. Ann. Neurol. 23:347–353; 1988.

McKibbon, K. A.; Walker-Dilks, C.; Haynes, R. B.; Wilczynski, N. Beyond ACP Journal Club: how to harness MEDLINE for prognosis problems. ACPJ Club Jul–Aug, A-12–A-14; 1995.

Miettinen, O. S. Confounding and effect modification. Am. J. Epidemiol. 100:350–353; 1974.

Miles, I.; Mitchelson, M.; Morgan, R.; Michaelides, C.; Staurt, G.; Jayasinghe, L.; Baddeley, H. Improved survival of patients with glioma in the CT era. Diagn. Imaging 50:313–320; 1981.

Moses, L. E. Statistical concepts fundamental to investigations. N. Engl. J. Med. 312:890–987; 1985.

Motulsky, A. G. Biased ascertainment and natural history of diseases. N. Engl. J. Med. 298:1196–1197; 1978.

Mørk, S. J.; Lindegaard, K-F.; Halvorsen, T. B.; Lehmann, E. H.; Solgaard, I.; Hattevoll, R.; Harvei, S.; Ganz, J. Oligodendroglioma: incidence and biological behavior in a defined population. J. Neurosurg. 63:881–889; 1985.

Nagib, M. G.; Haines, D. J.; Erickson, D. L.; Mastri, A. R. Tuberous sclerosis: a review for the neurosurgeon. Neurosurgery 14:93–98; 1984.

Nelson, L. M.; Franklin, G. M.; Hamman, R. F.; Boteler, D. L.; Baum, H. M.; Burks, J. S. Referral bias in multiple sclerosis research. J. Clin. Epidemiol. 41:187–192; 1988.

Patrick, D. L.; Deyo, R. A. Generic and disease-specific measures in assessing health status and quality of life. Med. Care 27(suppl. 3):S217–S332; 1989.

Peto, R.; Pike, M. C.; Armitage, P.; Breslow, N.; Cox, D. R.; Howard, S. V.; Mantel, N.; McPherson, K.; Pete, J.; Smith, P. G. Design and analysis of randomized clinical trials requiring prolonged observation of each patient: II. Analysis and examples. Br. J. Cancer 35:1–39; 1977.

Ringel, R. A.; Riggs, J. E.; Brick, J. F. Reversible coma with prolonged absence of pupillary and brainstem reflexes: an unusual response to a hypoxic-ischemic event in MS. Neurology 38:1275–1278; 1988.

Rosenberg, G. A.; Johnson, S. F.; and Brenner, R. P. Recovery of cognition after prolonged vegetative state. Ann. Neurol. 2:167–168; 1977.

Rosenblum, M. L.; Levy, R. M.; and Bredesen, D. E. AIDS and the nervous system. New York: Raven Press; 1988.

Rothman, K. J. Modern epidemiology. Boston: Little, Brown & Co.; 1986.

Sackett, D. L.; Haynes, R. B.; Guyatt, G. H.; Tugwell, P. Clinical epidemiology: a basic science for clinical medicine. 2nd ed. Boston: Little, Brown & Co.; 1991.

Sackett, D. L.; Rosenberg, W. M.; Gray, J. A. M.; Haynes, R. B.; Richardson, W. S. Evidence-based medicine: what is it and what it isn't. BMJ 312:71–72; 1996.

Sackett, D. L.; Richardson, W. S.; Rosenberg, W.; Haynes, R. B. Evidence-based medicine: how to practice and teach EBM. New York: Churchill Livingstone; 1997.

Sather, H. N. The use of prognostic factors in clinical trials. Cancer. 58:461–467; 1986.

Schoenberg, B. S.; Anderson, D. W.; Haerer, A. F. Racial differentials in the prevalence of stroke: Copiah County, Mississippi. Arch. Neurol. 43:565–568; 1986.

Snyder, B. D.; Cranford, R. E.; Rubens, A. B.; Bundlie, S.; Rockswold, G. E. Delayed recovery from post anoxic persistent vegetative state (abstract). Ann. Neurol. 14:152; 1983.

Stewart, A. L.; Hays, R. D.; Ware, J. F. The MOS shortform general health survey. Med. Care 26:724–735; 1988.

Teasdale, G. M.; Nicoll, J. A. R.; Murray, G.; Fiddes, M. Association of apolipoprotien E polymorphism with outcomes after head injury. Lancet 350:1069–1071; 1997.

Tirschwell, D. L.; Longstreth, W. T., Jr.; Rauch-Mathews, M. E.; Chandler, W. L.; Rothstein, T.; Wray, L.; Eng, L. J.; Fine, J.; Copass, M. K. Cerebrospinal fluid creatine kinase BB isoenzyme activity and neurologic prognosis after cardiac arrest. Neurology 48:352–357; 1997.

Tu, J. V. Advantages and disadvantages of using artificial neural networks versus logistic regression for predicting medical outcomes. J. Clin. Epidemiol. 49:1225–1231; 1996.

Tuhrim, S.; Dambrosia, J. M.; Price, T. R.; Mohr, J. P.; Wolf, P. A.; Heyman, A.; Kase, C. S. Prediction of intracerebral hemorrhage survival. Ann. Neurol. 24:258–263; 1988.

Vaagenes, P.; Safar, P.; Diven, W.; Moosy, J.; Rao, G.; Cantadore, R.; Kelsey, S. Brain enzyme levels in CSF after cardiac arrest and resuscitation in dogs: markers of damage and predictors of outcome. J. Cereb. Blood Flow Metab. 8:262–275; 1988.

Wasson, J. H.; Sox, H. C.; Neff, R. K.; Goldman, L. Clinical prediction rules: applications and methodological standards. N. Engl. J. Med. 313:793–799; 1985.

Weiss, N. S. Clinical epidemiology: the study of the outcome of illness. New York: Oxford University Press; 1986.

Winer, J. B.; Hughes, R. A. C.; Osmond, C. A prospective study of acute idiopathic neuropathy: I. Clinical features and their prognostic value. J. Neurol. Neurosurg. Psychiatry 51:605–612; 1988.

Wolf, P. A.; Kannel, W. B.; Dawber, T. R. Prospective investigations: the Framingham Study and the epidemiology of stroke. Adv. Neurol. 19:107–120; 1978.

Wolf, P. A.; Kannel, W. B.; Sorlie, P.; McNamara, P. Asymptomatic carotid bruit and risk of stroke: The Framingham Study. JAMA 245:1442–1445; 1981.

Wolfson, C.; Confavreux, C. Improvements to a simple Markov model of the natural history of multiple sclerosis: I. Short-term prognosis. Neuroepidemiology 6:101–115; 1987.

Woo, E.; Ma, J. T. C.; Robinson, J. D.; Yu, Y. L. Hyperglycemia is a stress response in acute stroke. Stroke 19:1359–1364; 1988.

Zerbe, G. O. Randomization analysis of the completely randomized design extended to growth and response curves. J. Am. Stat. Assoc. 74:215–221; 1979.

# 5

# Economic Prognosis: Evaluating Economic Outcomes of Health Care

JOHN T. LANGFITT AND ROBERT G. HOLLOWAY

Physicians provide information about prognosis so that patients, families, and colleagues can decide how to treat or cope with disease in an individual patient. Answers to questions such as "What is the natural history?" "What interventions (medical, surgical or environmental) alter natural history?" and "How do certain patient characteristics predict natural history and response to available treatments?" play a central role in individual-level decision making. For this audience, descriptions of prognosis focus on patient-centered outcomes, such as symptom frequency, severity, course, treatment effects, and quality of life.

In the past 20 years, a growing audience of policymakers has begun to demand new prognostic information, information about the *economic* outcomes of diseases and their treatments. Public health officials, managed care organizations, hospital formulary directors, and others responsible for policy-level decisions need to know about the economic consequences of diseases and their treatments, in order to ensure that important health problems continue to be addressed, but that increasingly scarce health care resources are allocated efficiently. When health care resources become limited, it is increasingly important that they be allocated efficiently if the overall health of the population is to be maintained.

From 1980 through 1990, U.S. national health care expenditures grew from 9.2% to 13.5% of gross domestic product (GDP) (Levit et al. 1998a). The annual rate of growth has slowed substantially during the 1990s. Nevertheless, U.S. health care spending exceeded $1 trillion in 1996 (Levit et al. 1998b). The percentage of U.S. GDP spent on health care continues to exceed that of other industrialized nations (Anderson 1997). The expansion of managed care and the prominence of debates about Medicare funding reflect the scale of private and public demands to further stabilize or reduce health care spending.

In response to these concerns, a new, multidisciplinary, research methodology has emerged to provide information about the costs of illness and how efficiently the health care system uses available resources. Cost-of-illness studies and economic evaluations (cost-minimization, cost-effectiveness, cost-utility, and cost-benefit analyses) have become ubiquitous in the medical and health policy literature, yet there remain many unresolved issues about their appropriate roles and methods. This chapter provides an overview of the basic principles, methods, roles, and current limitations of economic outcomes research.

## Defintions, Principles, and a Typology

Economic outcomes research provides a comprehensive account of the economic costs and health consequences of disease and how these change with natural history and different treatments (Drummond et al. 1997). "Cost" may be defined as "the loss or penalty incurred, especially in gaining something." In this sense, *direct medical costs* are the monetary benefits that are given up in order to provide for the organization and operation of the health sector (e.g., funds to pay for provider fees, medicines and supplies, equipment, overhead). *Direct, nonmedical costs* include costs incurred outside the health sector that are attributable to the disease (e.g., patient out-of-pocket expenses for travel to obtain medical care, special education services, child care). Direct medical and nonmedical costs also include *time costs* (e.g., caregiver time, patient time in seeking treatment), since that time could be spent productively or in leisure. *Productivity costs* are losses of economic productivity due to inefficiency at work as a result of illness, days off work, unemployment, and premature mortality.*

The health consequences of disease (i.e., premature mortality, morbidity, disability, pain, and suffering) can also be considered *costs,* insofar as they represent the loss of something valued (i.e., life and health). However, these consequences are not commonly thought of in monetary terms, in part because many people are uncomfortable with the notion of placing a monetary value on human life, pain, and suffering. Nevertheless, the fact that resources (which can be valued monetarily) are expended to improve health necessarily implies an underlying value structure that (at least theoretically) can be expressed in monetary terms (Phelps and Mushlin 1991). Throughout this chapter, we use the term "health effect" to refer to any consequences to health that are a result of disease or intervention.

## Cost-of-Illness Studies

Cost-of-illness studies describe the overall direct and productivity costs attributable to a disease. Their goal is to focus policymakers' attention on

---

* Productivity costs are sometimes referred to as "indirect" costs. We use "productivity costs" throughout, because "indirect" costs in other contexts frequently refers to fixed economic costs of production (i.e., overhead).

diseases with the greatest financial costs. Among neurologic disorders, cost-of-illness studies have been published for epilepsy, stroke, and multiple sclerosis (Begley et al. 1994; Cockerell et al. 1994; Bourdette et al. 1993; Taylor et al. 1996). Cost-of-illness studies are a valuable first step in identifying policy priorities. However, they are inherently limited in guiding specific policy decisions. Effective interventions may not yet exist for high-burden diseases (e.g., human immunodeficiency virus [HIV] vaccines), or the health sector may have limited power to implement ones that do (e.g., airbag and handgun legislation). Even when effective interventions are available, cost-of-illness studies cannot provide information about which treatments are most efficient in reducing overall disease burden, given a limited amount of resources (Davey and Leeder 1993).

## Economic Evaluations

Economic evaluations of health care are designed to inform specific, resource allocation decisions at the policy level. They determine how efficiently specific, alternative interventions improve health in specific populations. They attempt to answer the question, "How can a limited amount of resources be distributed in order to maximize the overall health of the population?" Economic evaluations are called by different names (cost-minimization, cost-effectiveness, cost-utility, and cost-benefit analysis), depending on how health effects are summarized and valued.

For example, a health maintenance organization (HMO) might consider whether they should replace an established drug for treating multiple sclerosis (MS) (β-interferon) with a new one (Copolymer 1). If the net health effects are known to be the same (i.e., the two medicines have similar side effects and effects on MS symptoms), then only the net direct costs of treating with the two drugs would be compared in a cost-minimization analysis. Here, the question is simply "If we consider all the costs of treatment and any savings in future costs as a result of improving health, does treating with the new drug (Copolymer 1) cost less than treating with the old drug (β-interferon)?"

Typically, however, interventions differ in side effects and/or effectiveness. In this situation, the policymaker is faced with the decision matrix shown in Table 5-1.

**Table 5-1.** Decision Alternatives Comparing Copolymer 1 to β-Interferon in Terms of Costs and Health Effects

|  | Direct/Productivity Costs Lower with Copolymer 1 | Direct/Productivity Costs Greater with Copolymer 1 |
|---|---|---|
| Health effects *greater* with Copolymer 1 | Copolymer 1 *dominates* β-interferon<br>**Adopt Copolymer 1** | Is the benefit of Copolymer 1 worth the additional cost?<br>**Yes—adopt Copolymer 1**<br>**No—do not adopt Copolymer 1** |
| Health effects *lower* with Copolymer 1 | Are the savings with Copolymer 1 worth the lost benefits?<br>**Yes—adopt Copolymer 1**<br>**No—do not adopt Copolymer 1** | β-Interferon *dominates* Copolymer 1<br><br>**Do Not Adopt Copolymer 1** |

If Copolymer 1 produces both greater health effects and lower costs (upper left quadrant), then it clearly is the best to adopt. In economic parlance, it is said to "dominate" the other. For example, in one study, plasma exchange favorably influenced the course of acute Guillain-Barr syndrome in addition to reducing overall health costs compared to conservative management (Osterman et al. 1984). Similarly, if Copolymer 1 produces both greater costs and *lower* health effects, it is equally clear that it should *not* replace β-interferon. More commonly, a new intervention is more expensive, but produces superior health effects (upper right quadrant). In this case, it must be determined whether the additional health effects provided are "worth" the additional costs. When health effects are expressed in natural units (e.g., percent reduction of MS exacerbations), the analysis is termed a cost-effectiveness analysis.

The incremental cost-effectiveness ratio (CER) is a commonly used metric for the efficiency gained by choosing one intervention over the other. The CER is the ratio of the difference in resource costs to the difference in health effects between the two interventions. It is a direct expression of the incremental cost per unit of health effect resulting from choosing a new intervention over an established one. For the MS example, the CER could be expressed as:

$$\frac{\text{Costs}_{\text{Copolymer 1}} - \text{Costs}_{\beta\text{-interferon}}}{\text{Reduced exacerbation}_{\text{Copolymer 1}} - \text{Reduced exacerbation}_{\beta\text{-interferon}}}$$

When allocating scarce resources, interventions with low CERs should be viewed favorably. By producing health effects more efficiently, they free up resources to be used in other ways. By the same token, interventions with high CERs require justification on other grounds because they are a less efficient use of resources.

Often, interventions affect health in multiple ways (e.g., life expectancy, side effects, symptom relief) that cannot easily be expressed in a single metric. In such cases, net health effects are expressed as individual preferences, or "utilities" for the quality of the health states resulting from each intervention. In this case, the analysis is a cost-utility analysis and efficiency is expressed as the incremental cost-utility ratio.

Finally, in cost-benefit analysis, an explicit monetary value is placed on health effects. For example, respondents might be presented with a scenario describing MS symptoms and the side effects and symptoms typically experienced following treatment with β-interferon and Copolymer 1. They might then be asked how much of an additional health insurance premium they would be willing to pay in order to have access to each drug (should they need it) (O'Brien and Gafni 1996). If the net costs are lower than the net benefits (expressed monetarily as what the population would be willing to pay for them), then the intervention should be adopted.

## Methodology

The principles of economic outcomes research outlined above are relatively straightforward. In practice, the methodology is complicated by the same biases and sources of random error found in other areas of clinical research. In addition, there are methodologic challenges peculiar to economic evaluations.

## Planning ("Framing") the Economic Evaluation

As with any clinical research question, an early conceptualization phase helps to focus the study on relevant research questions (Torrance et al. 1996).

### Audience for the Study

Economic evaluations answer questions for an intended audience. A growing number of countries including Australia and Canada are requiring cost-effectiveness information as part of the drug approval process (Neumann and Johannesson 1994). In addition to government formularies, an audience may include managed care organizations, individual health care providers, or other governmental entities such as Congress and the Public Health Service. At times, there may not be a well-defined audience. Rather, it may be the general medical community, since the primary purpose of the analysis may be to influence opinion or to stimulate additional scientific inquiry.

### Perspective of the Analysis

One of the most important decisions to make in the early planning phases of a study is to determine the study perspective (Davidoff and Powe 1996). An economic evaluation can be conducted from a number of different perspectives. The perspective chosen will dictate the scope of costs and health effects to collect and how to value them. The most comprehensive perspective is the societal perspective. In this case, all direct and productivity costs and health effects are collected, regardless of who incurs them. Narrower perspectives are possible, particularly when the intended audience has a more focused viewpoint. For example, the HMO analyzing β-interferon and Copolymer 1 from their own (i.e., payor's) perspective would include only the direct medical costs for which they are responsible. Analyses conducted from the provider and patient perspective will include a different set of costs and health effects.

### Defining the Target Intervention

The intervention under study (the "target" intervention) must be specified so that the audience can assess whether the results will apply to their own setting. Specific characteristics to consider when defining the intervention include the technology (e.g., carotid endarterectomy), personnel deliver-

ing the services (e.g., vascular surgeons), the site of delivery (e.g., academic medical centers), and the timing of the services (e.g., after a transient ischemic attack).

### Target Population for the Intervention

The target population is the population of patients for whom the intervention is intended. Consideration should be given to traditional patient characteristics and variables, as well as the geographic region where they live. For example, a study assessing the cost-effectiveness of a screening program to identify asymtomatic carotid stenosis included a population of asymptomatic 65-year-old men with a 5% prevalence of 60% carotid stenosis (Lee et al. 1997).

### Comparator Intervention

Studies should compare the new intervention to existing practices since the relevant question is, "What is the cost effectiveness of replacing existing practices with the new intervention?" Clearly defining a "comparator" intervention is extremely important, since artificial comparisons can lead to inappropriate conclusions. For example, comparing a new dopamine agonist to placebo for treating Parkinson's disease would produce a very favorable CER, since treating with a dopamine agonist is likely to produce considerably better health effects compared to no treatment. In practice, however, the question typically is whether to replace an existing dopamine agonist with the new one. If the new agent is considerably more costly, but only slightly more effective than the comparator, then the CER will be considerably less favorable than it was in the placebo comparison. This partly explains why placebo-controlled clinical trials have limited application in economic evaluations. It may be appropriate, however, to have a "no-treatment" comparison. In the carotid stenosis screening study, the comparison program was the "no-screening" strategy (Lee et al. 1997).

### Time Horizon

The time horizon refers to the length of time needed to capture the relevant health and economic outcomes. Since economic evaluations often use distal health endpoints (i.e., life expectancy), long time horizons are required for which sufficient primary data may not exist. This often requires that long-term outcomes be modeled, using existing epidemiological data and/or expert opinion. In the study assessing the cost-effectiveness of screening for carotid stenosis, the investigators used 5-year follow-up data from the Asymptomatic Carotid Artery Surgery trial (Executive Committee for the Asymptomatic Carotid Atherosclerosis Study 1995). To assess the lifetime cost-effectiveness of the screening program, however, the investigators had to use modeling techniques to extrapolate beyond the available trial data.

## Research Designs

Performing an economic evaluation is compatible with many different research designs (Torrance et al. 1996). Primary research designs include those studies where the majority of economic data collection is expressly collected as part of the research (i.e., primary data collection). Secondary research designs use data from existing databases collected for other purposes (e.g., insurance claims) or from existing data published in the literature. Often, for any given evaluation, data will be obtained from a number of secondary sources. Primary research designs can have a secondary data collection component, but the emphasis is on primary data collection.

The two types of primary research designs are cost-effectiveness trials and "piggyback" trials. Cost-effectiveness trials prospectively collect data on the costs and effects of competing interventions in a randomized controlled trial (RCT) under real-world conditions. Since differences in the costs and effectiveness of the target and comparator programs are the primary clinical endpoints, costs and effects can be derived directly from the studies themselves. Cost-effectiveness trials are rare, mainly due to the cost of the trial itself. Economic data frequently have large variances, requiring large samples to obtain sufficient power to test the economic hypotheses. Interventions frequently have long-term cost and health implications, requiring a long follow-up period to capture the relevant health and economic outcomes.

A more common primary research design is to perform an economic evaluation "piggybacked" onto an existing RCT protocol (Powe and Griffiths 1995; Drummond 1995; Adams et al. 1992). Piggyback studies prospectively collect economic data along with the clinical data and are now common in clinical trial programs. Although relatively efficient, they may have insufficient power to test economic hypotheses, since sample sizes have been calculated to provide sufficient power to test the clinical hypotheses only. Since they are usually trials of efficacy (i.e., "Can it work under ideal circumstances?"), rather than overall effectiveness ("Does it work in real life circumstances?"), generalizability may be limited. Other problems include how to handle protocol-induced costs and the lack of consensus regarding statistical techniques (O'Brien et al. 1994).

Many economic evaluations employ some form of mathematical modeling to represent the clinical and economic event pathways (Mandelblatt et al. 1996). Decision-analytic, economic models calculate the total expected costs of alternative interventions by combining the conditional probabilities of all possible clinical events with their associated costs. Reliance on the modeling can vary, depending upon the intensity of the primary data collection effort and the time horizon of the study. For studies using mainly secondary data, the model may be the primary focus of the study (i.e., modeling designs), such as in a recent study assessing the cost-effectiveness of temporal lobectomy in intractable epilepsy (Langfitt 1997). For primary research designs, combination designs are often employed. This hybrid approach obtains data from an RCT and extrapolates over a longer time horizon by using epidemiological data and modeling techniques, such as in a recent RCT assessing the cost-effectiveness of automatic implantable defibrillators (Mushlin et al. 1997).

In hybrid and secondary designs, differences in effectiveness must often be estimated from uncontrolled, observational studies; from RCTs of populations that differ in potentially important respects from the target population; and from a variety of synthesis methods including meta-analyses, consensus panels, and expert opinion. The error inherent in these approaches is a strong argument for conducting economic evaluations in the context of RCTs, using the target population. For example, hybrid studies of the cost-utility of epilepsy surgery have estimated effectiveness of the comparator strategy (medical management) from the results of randomized controlled, add-on trials of anticonvulsants in intractable patients (Wiebe et al. 1995; Langfitt 1997; King et al. 1997). However, using data from patients in add-on trials may underestimate effectiveness of medical management in the population eligible for surgery. Add-on trials often include many patients who have been rejected for surgery because of characteristics that also may make them more difficult to control medically.

## Assessing Health Effects

Assessing health effects is a three-step process of identifying, summarizing, and valuing all relevant effects of the interventions (e.g., on mortality, morbidity, health-related quality of life.) Health effects that are relevant to the perspective of the study are identified by consulting the literature, clinical experts, and groups of affected patients.

### Health Effects as Natural Units

The simplest case is cost-effectiveness analysis, where all relevant effects can be summarized in natural units (e.g., alive vs. dead, number of MS exacerbations, identified vs. missed by a screening test). There is no methodological necessity to value the effects, as long as it is clear that more (or fewer) natural units are better.

### Health Effects as Preferences for Multiattribute Health States

Frequently, interventions affect multiple aspects, or attributes of health status that cannot be easily summarized and valued along a single dimension. Effects of surgery range from death to cure, with gradations of disability in between. Drugs that alleviate the motor symptoms of Parkinson's disease also alleviate symptoms or cause side effects outside the motor system. If a person's seizures are better controlled with a novel anticonvulsant, but they are more sedated, is that better or worse than having more seizures, but being more alert? The answer depends on how the person values the various combinations of these attributes of health states.

Preference measures suitable for valuing multiattribute health states include visual analog scale, standard-gamble, time trade-off, person trade-off, magnitude estimation, and willingness to pay (Nord 1992a). Most determine the relative value of health states by eliciting the point at which a person is indifferent in a trade-off between life in a suboptimal health state and some alternative. The methods differ primarily in the kinds of alternatives that are traded. For example, the time trade-off method uses peoples' attitudes toward length

of life as a measure of their preferences for a certain health state. Suppose a person would be willing to trade off 5 of her remaining 20 years of living in a suboptimal health state (e.g., frequent complex partial seizures [CPS]) for the opportunity to live that reduced life expectancy in perfect health. The value to her of living with frequent CPS is a function of the proportion of life expectancy she would give up, or trade-off: specifically, $1- (5/20)$, or 0.75. A person who dreaded living with frequent CPS might be willing to trade 15 of their remaining years in exchange for perfect health. The value of living with frequent CPS to that person would be correspondingly lower: $1- (15/20)$, or 0.25. Willingness-to-pay methods determine how much money a person would forgo (i.e., trade-off) to obtain a health effect.

### Standardized Preference Measures

It is often difficult to compare results of economic outcomes studies because methods of preference assessment vary across studies. Also, preference values for the same health state vary, depending on the method used (Nord 1992a; Richardson 1994; Sackett and Torrance 1978; Tversky and Kahneman 1981). Recently, standardized, multiattribute health classification systems have been developed that yield preference values for a wide range of health problems. Two of them, the Health Utilities Index (HUI) and EuroQOL, have been used extensively in population surveys and in studies of clinical populations (Gold, Franks et al. 1996; Statistics Canada 1994; van Agt et al. 1994; Busschbach et al. 1994; Whitton et al. 1997). These systems have the considerable advantage of having demonstrated reliability and validity in different populations. They are likely to detect large differences with sufficiently large sample sizes. However, they may be limited in their ability to detect smaller yet clinically significant effects in specific populations. True group differences will be missed if they are small compared to the differences the instrument was designed to detect. For example, the EuroQOL classifies anxiety/depression on a 3-point scale (none, moderate, extreme), so it may not detect changes from milder levels of depression to normal functioning. True group differences also may be missed if they involve disease-specific symptoms that are not included in the more generic instrument. In a study of children experiencing remission of asthma, the

HUI failed to detect changes in self-reported health status symptoms that were detected by a measure designed to measure asthma-specific symptoms (Juniper et al. 1997).

Preference measures differ in important ways from health status and health-related quality-of-life (HRQOL) measures (e.g., Sickness Impact Profile, Rand Short Form 36)(Bergner et al. 1981; Ware et al. 1993). Health status and HRQOL measures systematically place a person at a specific point on a descriptive continuum of health. Preference measures assess the value a person places on being at that point on the continuum (Froberg and Kane 1989; Revicki and Kaplan 1993). Since the purpose of economic evaluation is to determine whether health effects are "worth the cost" of the interventions that produce them, economic evaluations need to use preference measure that capture information about how differences in health status are valued.

### Combining Quality and Quantity of Life— The Quality-Adjusted Life-Year

A complete valuation of health effects requires that preferences for health states (quality of life) be combined with effects on longevity (quantity of life). The quality-adjusted life-year (QALY) is a common metric used in cost-utility analyses to combine preferences for specific health states with years lived in those health states. The concept of the QALY is illustrated in Figure 5-1.

Quality of life is expressed as a preference measure on a 0 to 1 scale, where 1 represents optimal health and 0 represents worst possible health (usually death). Life expectancy (quantity of life) is expressed as years on the horizontal axis. Over the course of a life, a person experiences transient illnesses that temporarily reduce the quality of his or her life. This is followed by a serious illness. Without the intervention, the person experiences a chronically reduced quality of life and premature death. With the intervention, the quality of his or her life is restored to near-perfect health and a more normal life expectancy. The dashed area under the curve represents the total, QALYs gained for this person by the intervention. Alternatives to the QALY have been proposed that value an entire lifetime pathway of health states or the output of an entire program in terms of its equivalence to saving a young healthy life. (Mehrez and Gafni 1989; Nord 1992b). Although they have conceptual advantages, they have enjoyed less broad usage in the research literature because they have been developed more recently and are more difficult to implement.

### Cost Assessment

To assess costs, it is necessary to identify, describe, summarize, and value all direct medical, nonmedical, and productivity costs affected by each intervention.

### Identifying and Describing Resources

Cost-identification studies are essential first steps in identifying all relevant resource utilization. The categories of resource utilization that are in-

**Figure 5-1.** Quality-adjusted life-years gained from an intervention.

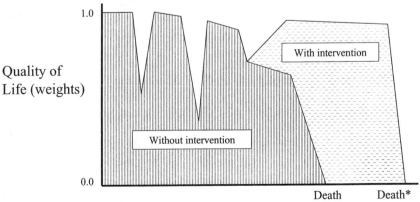

Quality of Life (weights)

1.0

0.0

With intervention

Without intervention

Death    Death*

Duration of Life (years)

cluded in any given study will depend on the perspective and clinical situation. Analyses should include all relevant costs that are hypothesized to differ between interventions. Occasionally, it is appropriate to include only a few types of costs. For example, Lloyd et al. conducted a cost-minimization analysis of initial treatment of deep vein thrombosis from the payor's perspective (Lloyd et al. 1997). They compared intravenous administration of unfractionated heparin (a low-cost drug) to subcutaneous administration of low-molecular-weight heparin (a more expensive drug that does not require intravenous administration and monitoring of clotting time). Because RCTs had shown that the treatments are equally efficacious, the authors included only the costs associated with the different medications and the time and material costs of administration and laboratory monitoring.

How best to gather medical utilization data in a clinical trial remains an area open for empirical research. A variety of techniques have been used to date, including patient and provider interviews (i.e., face-to-face and telephone) as well as health care utilization diaries (Powe and Griffiths 1995). Alternatively, medical utilization can be abstracted from patient medical records and administrative billing databases. Nationalized health care systems and closed-panel HMOs with comprehensive, computerized accounting systems are well suited to this approach. Despite the growth of managed care and integrated delivery systems, access to information systems is still limited. As new bridges are built between the research community and managed care corporations, opportunities for accessing comprehensive medical resource databases will increase.

Existing databases can also provide secondary data on medical resource consumption. Major national data sources on medical resource use include the National Ambulatory Medical Care Survey, the National Hospital Discharge Survey, and the National Medical Expenditure Survey. Last, expert consensus opinion can provide estimates on the type and frequency of resources used over a particular time period.

### Summarizing and Valuing Costs

The assignment of dollar values to units of resource consumption is a potential source of bias and error in economic evaluations. From an econ-omist's perspective, the value of a resource is its "opportunity cost," or the value of the best alternative use to which the resource could have been put. For goods and services traded in an unrestricted market, the opportunity cost is the market price. However, medical resource prices (e.g., charges) are poor estimates of their opportunity cost, because markets for direct medical resources are distorted by insurance subsidies and other market imperfections[†] (Finkler 1982). Therefore, a detailed costing analysis is often required to determine true opportunity costs.

Micro-costing uses time-and-motion studies to identify differences in resource utilization between interventions. Then, a market price is assigned to each unit of utilization to determine the difference in cost. Micro-costing provides the most valid data on cost differences. It is also feasible if the interventions being compared differ only in the utilization of a small number of resources to be costed. When a large number of different resources must be costed, gross-costing is a more feasible approach, since performing the requisite time- and motion studies is prohibitively time consuming. Gross-costing assigns dollar values to units of utilization derived from hospital accounting systems, the Medicare Fee Schedule, and/or the Medicare DRG payment (Lave et al. 1994). However, gross-costing may provide biased estimates of true opportunity costs. Cost-accounting systems rarely assign costs to procedures at a sufficiently detailed level to reflect the actual amount of resources consumed (Finkler 1982). For example, if the costs of operating room use are based on the average cost across procedures, this will underestimate the true cost of more resource-intensive procedures (e.g., heart transplant) relative to less resource-intensive procedures (e.g., hernia repair). There are also variations in how so-called hotel costs (e.g., housekeeping, laundry) are allocated across institutions, limiting generalizability.

Data on productivity loss due to premature mortality can be captured by determining mortality rates associated with each intervention, usually via literature review. Productivity loss due to morbidity can be obtained via structured interviews that assess time lost from work, reductions in produc-

[†] An exception to this is when the analysis is conducted from the perspective of the payor. Dollar reimbursement to the provider is an appropriate measure of cost from the payor perspective.

tivity while at work, and periods of unemployment. The dollar value of productivity loss is frequently taken to be the wage rate of an individual (Luce et al. 1996). Although this can be a practical and valid valuation of the opportunity cost of time, it reflects labor market biases against certain groups (e.g., women, minorities, and the elderly), raising concerns about equity. For example, if analyses showed that screening for prostate cancer was more cost-effective than screening for cervical cancer, and that this difference arose because screening for prostate cancer averted a larger productivity loss due to gender-based wage differences, it is questionable whether acting on these results would be acceptable policy.

## Roles of Economic Evaluations

There is growing interest in the role that economic evaluations play in insurance coverage decisions, the Food and Drug Administration (FDA) approval process, and in practice guideline development and application (Garber 1994). Many European countries are already using cost-effective criteria (Neumann and Johannesson 1994). Since January 1993, Australia has required information about cost-effectiveness in applications for new drugs to help guide national reimbursement decisions.

The dominant health care theme of the 1990s, "value", has increased the demand for economic information. Those who pay for medical care (e.g., patients, employers, government, and insurers) want to pay for cost-effective care. Those who can profit from medical care (e.g., pharmaceutical companies) want to demonstrate that their products are cost-effective. Those who are vulnerable to funding cuts (e.g., medical specialists) want to prove their worth. One proposed use of information from economic evaluations has been "league tables." A league table is a rank-order list of incremental cost-effectiveness or cost-utility ratios from lowest to highest. An example of a league table is shown in Table 5-2.

Every program or technology in the left column represents a published economic evaluation in which the health care or other social intervention was incrementally compared with an alternative program. The comparison program is often not present on these tables and is shown in parenthesis for only the automobile occupant restraint

**Table 5-2.** Example of a League Table

| Technology* | Cost/Life-Year Gained (1993/4 $US) |
|---|---|
| Polio immunization for children (Sisk et al. 1983) | <$0 |
| CT in patients with severe headaches (Knaus et al. 1980) | $4,809 |
| Air bag/lap belts (vs. lap/shoulder belts) (Zechauser and Shepard 1976) | $17,129 |
| Zidovudine for people with AIDS (Scitovsky et al. 1990) | $26,261 |
| Dialysis for end-stage renal disease (Churchill et al. 1984) | $50,542 |
| Captopril for people age 35–65 with no heart disease and >95 mm Hg (Edelson et al. 1990) | $92,537 |
| Intensive care for patients undergoing neurosurgery for head trauma (Barnes 1977) | $492,568 |
| Seat belts for passengers in school buses (Transportation Research Board National Research Council 1989) | $2,760,050 |

* References are taken from Tengs et al. (1995).

system. For example, for the polio immunization intervention, the alternative strategy was a "no-vaccination approach." The right column contains the incremental cost-effectiveness ratios calculated from each study. Ratios for the two non medical interventions are presented, since interventions by the medical sector may compete with interventions from outside the medical sector for societal resources.

The common interpretation of a league table is that technologies near the top of the list represent better investments in resources; it costs less money to gain 1 year of life. Theoretically, a policy maker charged with maximizing the health of a population under a fixed budget would start investing in those technologies at the top of the list, and continue down the list until the budget is exhausted. In practice, this approach is complicated by the fact that research methods vary across studies (as discussed above) and efficiency is only one of many factors that need to be considered when broadly allocating health care resources. These factors include, but are not limited to, the concept of distributive justice and the value society attaches to saving an identified life (Hadorn 1991).

Another use of information from economic evaluations is to improve efficiency by identifying when the incremental effects of applying specific interventions within specific populations reach a point of significantly diminishing returns on the investment. For example, it is known that hormone replacement therapy (HRT) in peri-menopausal women reduces the risk of future osteoporotic hip fracture. Tosteson et al. (1990) used an economic evaluation to address questions immediately relevant to decisions about treatment in this group: Will reducing future costs by avert-ing hip replacement and premature death offset the costs of a bone density screening program and treatment? Since screening is expensive, should all perimenopausal women have HRT, or just those with documented bone loss? At what level of bone loss should HRT be instituted? They con-structed a decision model, using published data on the prevalence of hip fracture; prevalence of levels of severity of bone mineral density (BMD) loss; the associated relative risks of hip fracture and premature death; and the costs of screening, hormone treatment, hip replacement, and nursing home placement. Selected results of the analysis are graphed in Figure 5-2.

Treating only the most severely affected women (with BMD of less than 0.9 g/cm²) would result in a relatively low (i.e., favorable) cost-effectiveness ratio of $11,700 per life-year saved. Treatment costs are relatively low due to the low prevalence of severe bone loss. Treatment costs are also substantially offset by averting high fu-ture costs of hip fracture in this high-risk sub-group. As women with lesser degrees of BMD loss are treated, the curve on the graph flattens out, reflecting the principle that it is most efficient

to treat those most likely to benefit (i.e., "the sick-est of the sick"). A strategy of universal treatment raises treatment costs substantially, but with more modest future cost savings and health effects, since treatment prevents few fractures in the women with a low baseline risk. This results in a much higher incremental cost-effectiveness ratio of $349,000 per life-year saved. This kind of analysis is valuable to decision makers because it identifies the specific point(s) at which the curve flattens out, or where the return on investments in health care begins to diminish substantially. Data from such studies may be used to inform cost-relevant guidelines for the many resource alloca-tion decisions that are made "at the margin."

## Limitations

Economic evaluations offer an intuitively appeal-ing way to measure how efficiently different sectors of the health care system produce health effects. However, there is surprisingly little evi-dence that the results of economic evaluations have had a substantial impact on policy decisions, to date. In a recent European survey, economic evaluation experts estimated that of 66 studies re-viewed, less than one-third were believed to have influenced policy (Davies et al. 1994). There may be a number of reasons for this.

### Ethical Problems

The use of economic evaluations to guide policy decisions may be objected to on ethical grounds. Although it is recognized that policymakers need to limit resources, providers who respond to these pressures find themselves in an ethical dilemma. For example, in response to variations in practice patterns, many areas of medicine have developed guidelines to promote best medical practice for specific conditions, based on the best available medical evidence (Davis and Taylor-Vaisey 1997; Grimshaw and Russel 1993). A physician who believes the validity of such guidelines and treats a patient accordingly is fulfilling his or her ethical obligation to the patient, because the outcome cri-teria used to inform the guidelines are typically limited to patient outcomes. In other words, guidelines typically take only health effects into account. However, when guidelines are based on costs that are not relevant to the patient perspec-tive, the physician who implements them may not

**Figure 5-2.** Cost-effectiveness of screening for osteo-porosis in perimenopausal women BMD, bone mineral density. (Adapted from Tosteson et al. 1990.)

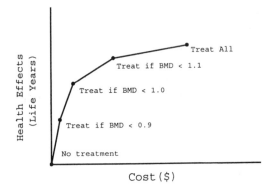

be acting solely in the patient's best interests. The prospect of being placed in this dual role of agent for the patient and for the policymaker is likely to explain the resistance of many clinicians to applying the results of economic evaluations. There does not appear to be a simple solution to this problem.

## Method Heterogeneity

Methods for summarizing and valuing costs and health effects are evolving rapidly, so published studies vary considerably in the methods they employ. Consequently, it is often impossible to compare results across studies. Experts differ over whether effectiveness or efficacy studies are the most appropriate sources of data. Randomized trials are the best *controlled* comparisons of alternative interventions, but assessing the true cost-effectiveness of an intervention requires an understanding of the incremental costs and effects gained or lost in a real-world setting. The more one deviates from real-world practices, as in a placebo-controlled trial with protocol-driven resource use, the less generalizable the study results become. Studies also vary in the types of costs considered and the sources of data. In the past 20 years, studies estimating the cost of epilepsy have varied in whether they used primary or secondary source data and whether they included or excluded direct medical, direct nonmedical, and productivity costs (Commission for the Control of Epilepsy and its Consequences 1978; Lewin-ICF 1992; Begley et al. 1994; Cockerell et al. 1994; Begley et al. 1998). The earlier studies relied exclusively on secondary-source, prevalence data or expert opinion to calculate direct medical costs. Only recently have population-based, incidence data been collected. A particular problem for studies of epilepsy is whether to include direct, nonmedical costs for institutionalized, mentally retarded persons with epilepsy, since it is unclear whether these costs truly are attributable to the epilepsy or to the mental retardation.

For evaluations where a long time horizon is appropriate, long-term epidemiological and experimental data on many diseases and interventions are very limited. The long-term economic stream of events for clinical conditions is even less well documented than are the clinical outcomes. Finally, most published cost-effectiveness or cost-utility ratios represent point estimates and do not incorporate variability in the different data sources to produce confidence limits around these estimates. Although researchers are beginning to develop the requisite statistical techniques, the field is young and far from application in routine research efforts (Eddy 1992).

## Bias

Lack of standardization in the design and conduct of economic evaluations means that investigators have considerable discretion in study design, measurement, and interpretation of their results. Indeed, a structured review of published CEAs noted only a fair adherence to certain fundamental principles (Udvarhelyi et al. 1992). Expertise in a clinical area may be essential to identifying the full range of costs and intervention effectiveness, but self-interest (e.g., on the part of specialists, pharmaceutical companies, and medical device manufacturers trying to "prove" the value of their enterprise) may be a potent obstacle to performing impartial assessments. Recognizing this potential, the *New England Journal of Medicine* has placed a moratorium on publishing reports of economic evaluations of pharmaceuticals or medical devices where the project is solely funded by the manufacturer or major stakeholder (Kassirer and Angell 1994). In the European survey that assessed the impact of economic evaluations on health policy, approximately one-half of the studies funded by government ministries were felt to have affected policy, compared to fewer than 20% of studies that were funded explicitly to promote commercial interests (Davies et al. 1994). Finally, it has been suggested that the health care community would have more confidence in the results of economic evaluations if those who perform them were subject to the same scrutiny and ethical and methodological standards applied to the accounting profession (Reinhardt 1997). The financial community is willing to base their decisions on accountants' valuations of corporate assets and liabilities in part because the accounting profession enforces consistency in valuation methods and access to the raw data upon which the analyses are based.

Proposals have been made to standardize the conduct and reporting of economic evaluations. The expert Panel on Cost-Effectiveness in Health and Medicine convened by the U.S. Public Health

Service recently published extensive guidelines for the conduct and reporting of cost-effectiveness analyses (Gold, Siegel et al. 1996). One recommendation was that published CEAs include sufficient data and analysis so that an estimate of cost-effectiveness from the societal perspective can be derived. Given the data and design requirements for a full societal perspective analysis, this is a rigorous standard. It remains to be seen how broadly it will be applied by the research community.

## Conclusions

The economic evaluation of health care is a young, rapidly maturing field of inquiry. By identifying areas of inefficient and efficient resource allocation, it has substantial potential to improve the efficiency of the health care system and save health care dollars while maintaining the quality of health care. Like any new field, many conceptual and methodological issues require further study and standardization for this potential to be realized. The publication of guidelines by the Panel on Cost-Effectiveness in Health and Medicine and the ongoing development of standardized preference methods grounded firmly in economic and psychometric theory represent significant, recent progress toward this goal (Gold, Siegel et al. 1996; Feeny et al. 1995; van Agt et al. 1994).

Clinicians have an important role to play as this methodology evolves. As health care resources become scarce, policymakers will be forced to make more choices among competing technologies. Economic evaluations designed to inform these choices will be performed from perspectives with implicit values that do not always reflect the values of clinicians and the patients for whom they care. By being actively involved in study design and implementation, clinicians can ensure that economic evaluations validly reflect the complexity of the disease treatment process and the value of health effects. Clinicians can also evaluate economic evaluations critically to ensure methodological rigor and identify inherent biases. As systems for financing and delivering medical care continue to evolve, the clinician's input will be critical to preserve the long-term perspective needed to maintain high quality and broad access to care.

## References

Adams, M. E.; McCall, N. T.; Gray, D. T.; Orza, M. J.; Chalmers, T. C. Economic analysis in randomized controlled trials. Med Care 30:231–243; 1992.

Anderson, G. F. In search of value: an international cost comparison of cost, access and outcomes. Health Affairs 16:163–171; 1997.

Barnes, B. A. Cost-benefit analysis of surgery: current accomplishments and limitations. Am. J. Surg. 133:438–446; 1977.

Begley, C. E.; Annegers, J. F.; Lairson, D. R.; Reynolds, T. F. Estimating the cost of epilepsy in the United States (abstract). Epilepsia, 38(S8):242–243, 1998.

Begley, C. E.; Annegers, J. F.; Lairson, D. R.; Reynolds, T. F.; Hauser, W. A. Cost of epilepsy in the United States: a model based on incidence and prognosis. Epilepsia 35:1230–1243; 1994.

Bergner, M.; Bobbitt, R. A.; Carter, W. B.; Gilson, B. S. The Sickness Impact Profile: development and final revision of a health status measure. Med. Care 19:787–805; 1981.

Bourdette, D. N.; Prochazka, A. V.; Mitchell, W.; Licari, P.; Burks, J. Health care costs of veterans with multiple sclerosis: implications for the rehabilitation of MS. VA Multiple Sclerosis Rehabilitation Study Group. Arch. Phys. Med. Rehab. 74:26–31; 1993.

Busschbach, J. J.; Horikx, P. E.; van den Bosch, J. M.; Brutel de la Riviere, A.; de Charro, F.T. Measuring the quality of life before and after bilateral lung transplantation in patients with cystic fibrosis. Chest 105:911–917; 1994.

Churchill, D. N.; Lemon, B. C.; & Torrance, G. W. A cost-effectiveness analysis of continuous ambulatory peritoneal dialysis and hospital hemodialysis. Med. Decis. Making 4:489–500; 1984.

Cockerell, O. C., Hart, Y. M.; Sander, J. W.; Shorvon, S. D. The cost of epilepsy in the United Kingdom: an estimation based on the results of two population-based studies. Epilepsy Res. 18:249–260; 1994.

Commission for the Control of Epilepsy and its Consequences. Economic cost of epilepsy. In: Anonymous, ed. Plan for Nationwide Action on Epilepsy. 4th ed. Washington, DC: (NIH): DHEW Publication no. 78–279; 1978: p. 117–148.

Davey, P. J.; Leeder, S. R. The cost of cost-of-illness studies. Med. J. Aust. 158:583–584; 1993.

Davidoff, A. J.; Powe, N. R. The role of perspective in defining economic measures for the evaluation of medical technology. Int. J. Technol. Assess. Health Care 12:9–21; 1996.

Davies, L.; Coyle, D.; Drummond, M. Current status of economic appraisal of health technology in the European community: report of the network. Soc. Sci. Med. 38:1601–1607; 1994.

Davis, D. A.; Taylor-Vaisey, A. Translating guidelines into practice: a systematic review of theoretic concepts, practical experience and research evidence in the adoption of clinical practice guidelines. Can. Med. Assoc. J. 157:408–416; 1997.

Drummond, M. F. Economic analysis alongside clinical trials: problems and potential. J. Rheumatol. 22:1403–1407; 1995.

Drummond, M. F.; O'Brien, B.; Stoddart, G. L.; Torrance, G. W. Methods for the economic evaluation of health care programmes. 2nd ed. New York: Oxford University Press; 1997.

Eddy, D. M. Clinical decision making: from theory to practice. Cost-effectiveness analysis. A conversation with my father. JAMA 267:1669–1675; 1992.

Edelson, J. T.; Weinstein, M. C.; Tosteson, A. N. A.; Williams, L.; Lee, T. H. Long term efficacy and cost-effectiveness of various initial monotherapies for mild to moderate hypertension. JAMA 264:41–47; 1990.

Executive Committee for the Asymptomatic Carotid Atherosclerosis Study. Endarterectomy for aymptomatic carotid artery stenosis. JAMA 273:1421–1428; 1995.

Feeny, D.; Furlong, W.; Boyle, M.; Torrance, G. W. Multi-attribute health status classification systems. Pharmacoeconomics 7:490–502; 1995.

Finkler, S. A. The distinction between costs and charges. Ann. Intern. Med. 96:102–109; 1982.

Froberg, D. G.; Kane, R. L. Methodology for measuring health-state preferences—I: measurement strategies. J. Clin. Epidemiol. 42:345–354; 1989.

Garber, A. M. Can technology assessment control health spending? Health Affairs 115–126; 1994.

Gold, M.; Franks, P.; Erickson, P. Assessing the health of the nation. The predictive validity of a preference-based measure and self-rated health. Med. Care 34:163–177; 1996.

Gold, M. R.; Siegel, J. E.; Russell, L. B.; Weinstein, M. C. Cost-effectiveness in health and medicine. New York: Oxford University Press; 1996.

Grimshaw, J. M.; Russel, I. T. Effect of clinical guidelines on medical practice: a systematic review of rigorous evaluations. Lancet 342:1317–1322; 1993.

Hadorn, D. C. Setting health care priorities in Oregon: cost-effectiveness meets the rule of rescue. JAMA 265:2218–2225; 1991.

Juniper, E. F.; Guyatt, G. H.; Feeny, D. H.; Griffith, L. E.; Ferrie, P. J. Minimum skills required by children to complete health-related quality of life instruments for asthma: comparison of measurement properties. Eur. Respir. J. 10:2285–2294; 1997.

Kassirer, J. P.; Angell, M. The journal's policy on cost-effectiveness analyses. N. Engl. J. Med. 331:664–670; 1994.

King, J. T.; Sperling, M. R.; Justice, A. C.; O'Connor, M. J. A cost-effectiveness analysis of anterior temporal lobectomy for intractable temporal lobe epilepsy. J. Neurosurg. 87:20–28; 1997.

Knaus, W. A.; Wagner, D. P.; Davis, D. O. CT for headache: cost-benefit for sub-arachnoid hemmorhage. AJNR Am. J. Neuroradiol. 1:567–572; 1980.

Langfitt, J. T. Cost-effectiveness of anterotemporal lobectomy in medically intractable complex partial epilepsy. Epilepsia 38:154–163; 1997.

Lave, J. R.; Pashos, C. L.; Anderson, G. F.; et al. Costing medical care: using Medicare administrative data. Med. Care 32:JS77–JS89; 1994.

Lee, T. T.; Solomon, N. A.; Heidenreich, P. A.; Oehlert, J.; Garber, A. M. Cost-effectiveness of screening for carotid stenosis in asymptomatic patients. Ann. Intern. Med. 126:337–346; 1997.

Levit, K.; Cowan, C.; Braden, B.; Stiller, J.; Sensenig, A.; Lazenby, H. National health care expenditures in 1997: More slow growth. Health Affairs 17:99–110; 1998a.

Levit, K. R.; Lazenby, H. C.; Braden, B. R.; the National Health Accounts Team. National health spending trends in 1996. Health Affairs 17:35–51; 1998b.

Lewin-ICF. The costs of disorders of the brain. Washington, DC: National Foundation for Brain Research; 1992.

Lloyd, A. C.; Aitken, J. A.; Hoffmeyer, U. K.; Kelso, E. J.; Wakerly, E. C.; Barber, N. D. Economic evaluation of the use of nadroparin in the treatment of deep-vein thrombosis in Switzerland. Ann Pharmacother. 31:842–846; 1997.

Luce, B. R.; Manning, W. G.; Siegel, J. E.; Lipscomb, J. Estimating costs in cost-effectiveness analysis. In: Gold, M. R.; Siegel, J. E.; Russell, L. B.; Weinstein, M. B., eds. Cost-effectiveness in health and medicine. New York: Oxford University Press; 1996: p. 176–213.

Mandelblatt, J. S.; Fryback, D. G.; Weinstein, M. C.; Russell, L. B.; Gold, M. R.; Hadorn, D. C. Assessing the effectiveness of health interventions. In: Gold, M. R.; Siegel, J. E.; Russell, L. B.; Weinstein, M. C., eds. Cost-effectiveness in health and medicine. New York: Oxford University Press; 1996: p. 135–175.

Mehrez, A.; Gafni, A. Quality-adjusted life years, utility and healthy-year equivalents. Med. Decis. Making 9:142–149; 1989.

Mushlin, A. I.; Zwansiger, J.; Gajary, E.; Andrews, M.; Marron, R. Approach to cost-effectiveness assessment in the MADIT trial. Am. J. Cardiol. 80:33F–41F; 1997.

Neumann, P. J.; Johannesson, M. From principle to public policy: using cost-effectiveness analysis. Health Affairs 13:206–214; 1994.

Nord, E. Methods for quality adjustment of life years. Soc. Sci. Med. 34:559–569; 1992a.

Nord, E. An alternative to QALYs: the saved young life equivalent (SAVE) [see comments]. BMJ 305:875–877; 1992b.

O'Brien, B.; Gafni, A. When do the "dollars" make sense: toward a conceptual framework for contingent valuation studies in health care. Med. Decis. Making 16:288–299; 1996.

O'Brien, B. J.; Drummond, M. F.; Labelle, R. F.; Willan, A. In search of power and significance: issues in the design and analysis of stochastic cost-effectiveness studies in health care. Med. Care 32:150–163; 1994.

Osterman, P. O.; Lundemo, G.; Pirskanen, R.; Fagius, P.; Siden, A. Beneficial effects of plasma exchange in acute inflammatory polyradiculoneuropathy. Lancet 2:1296–1298; 1984.

Phelps, C. E.; Mushlin, A. I. On the (near) equivalence of cost-effectiveness and cost-benefit analyses. Int. J. Technol. Assess. Health Care 7:12–21; 1991.

Powe, N. R.; Griffiths, R. I. The clinical-economic trial: promise, problems, and challenges. Control. Clin. Trials 16:377–394; 1995.

Reinhardt, U. E. Making economic evaluations respectable. Soc. Sci. Med. 45:555–562; 1997.

Revicki, D. A.; Kaplan, R. M. Relationship between psychometric and utility-based approaches to the measurement of health-related quality of life (review). Qual. Life Res. 2:477–487; 1993.

Richardson, J. Cost utility analysis: what should be measured? (review). Soc. Sci. Med. 39:7–21; 1994.

Sackett, D. L.; Torrance, G. W. The utility of different health states as perceived by the general public. J. Chron. Dis. 31:697–704; 1978.

Scitovsky, A. A.; Cline, M. W.; Abrams, D. I. Effects of the use of AZT on the medical care costs of persons with AIDS in the first 12 months. J. Acquir. Immune Defie. Syndr. 3:904–912; 1990.

Sisk, J. E.; Sanders, C. R. Analyzing the cost-effectiveness and cost-benefit of vaccines. World Health Forum 4:83–88; 1983.

Statistics Canada. Health status of Canadians: report of the 1991 General Social Survey. Ottawa: Statistics Canada; 1994.

Taylor, T. N.; Davis, P. H.; Torner, J. C.; Holmes, J.; Jacobson, M. F. Lifetime cost of stroke in the United States. Stroke 27:1459–1466; 1996.

Tengs, T. O., Adams, M. E., Pliskin, J. S.; et al. Five-hundred life-saving interventions and their cost-effectiveness. Risk Anal. 15:369–390; 1995.

Torrance, G. W.; Siegel, J. E.; Luce, B. R. Framing and designing the cost-effectiveness analysis. In: Gold, M. R.; Siegel, J. E.; Russell, L. B.; Weinstein, M. C., eds. Cost-effectiveness in health and medicine. New York: Oxford University Press; 1996: p. 54–81.

Tosteson, A. N.; Rosenthal, D. I.; Melton, L. J., III; Weinstein, M. C. Cost effectiveness of screening perimenopausal white women for osteoporosis: bone densitometry and hormone replacement therapy. Ann. Intern. Med. 113:594–603; 1990.

Transportation Research Board National Research Council. Improving school bus safety. Special Report #22:1989.

Tversky, A.; Kahneman, D. The framing of decisions and the psychology of choice. Science 211:453–458; 1981.

Udvarhelyi, I. S.; Colditz, G. A.; Rai, A.; Epstein, A. M. Cost-effectiveness and cost-benefit analyses in the medical literature. Are the methods being used correctly?. Ann. Intern. Med. 116:238–244; 1992.

van Agt, H. M.; Essink-Bot, M. .; Krabbe, P. F.; Bonsel, G. J. Test-retest reliability of health state valuations collected with the EuroQOL questionnaire. Soc. Sci. Med. 39:1537–1544; 1994.

Ware, J. E., Jr.; Snow, K. K.; Kosinski, M.; Gandek, B. SF-36 health survey: manual and interpretation guide. Boston: Health Institute, New England Medical Center; 1993.

Whitton, A. C.; Rhydderch, H.; Furlong, W.; Feeny, D.; & Barr, R. D. Self-reported comprehensive health status of adult brain tumor patients using the Health Utilities Index. Cancer 80(2):258–265; 1997.

Wiebe, S.; Gafni, A.; Blume, W. T.; Girvin, J. P. An economic evaluation of surgery for temporal lobe epilepsy.. J Epilepsy 8:227–235; 1995.

Zechauser, R.; Shepard, D. Where now for saving lives? Law Contemp. Probl. 40:4–45; 1976.

PART II

# CEREBROVASCULAR DISORDERS

# 6

# Prognosis of Stroke

THEODORE H. WEIN, ANDREW M. DEMCHUK, AND FRANK M. YATSU

Stroke is the leading cause of long-term disability in North America; there are, for example, an estimated 3 million stroke survivors in the United States (American Heart Association 1992). While in 1992 the American Heart Association estimated that 500,000 new cases of stroke occurred annually in the United States, more recent data suggest this number may be as high as 750,000 (American Heart Association 1992; Broderick et al. 1998). Each year approximately 140,000 individuals are transferred to nursing homes following nonfatal stroke. The total cost for stroke consisting of both direct health care expenses and indirect personal financial loss have been estimated to range from $30 to $40 billion per year (American Heart Association 1992; Lanska and Kryscio 1995; Matchar and Duncan 1994; Dobkin 1995). Given the devastating physical and financial toll stroke plays on victims and the health care system, maximal effort should be placed on preventive therapy and more effective therapies. Prognostic information on stroke subtypes, detailed in this chapter, is a vital step in understanding the disease and in defining the best prevention and treatment options.

## Prognosis of Ischemic Stroke

### Prognosis by Etiology

#### Large Artery Atherosclerosis

Atherosclerotic disease of the aortic arch and carotid arteries has been associated with increased stroke risk. To date, several studies have confirmed the benefit of carotid endarterectomy (CEA) in symptomatic carotid stenosis of greater than 70%. The North American Symptomatic Carotid Endarterectomy Trial (NASCET) demonstrated that CEA decreased 2-year risk of ipsilateral stroke from 26% to 9% ($p < .001$), when compared to best medical therapy (aspirin) a relative risk reduction of 65% (North American Symptomatic Carotid Endarterectomy Trial collaborators 1991). Surgical mortality was 0.6%, and all 30-day perioperative stroke or death was 5.8 percent. Any major stroke or death was 18.1% in the medical group and 8% in the surgical patients. Comparable results have been reported in the European Carotid Surgery Trial (ECST) as well as the Veterans Affairs Cooperative Trial with relative risk reductions of stroke from 39% and 60%, respectively (European Carotid Surgery Trialists' Collaborative Group 1991; Mayberg et al. 1991). Individuals with an ulcerated carotid plaque may be at increased risk of stroke compared to patients with nonulcerated plaques, although this remains controversial (Eliasziw et al. 1994). This risk more than doubles at higher degrees of stenosis; there is a 26.3% risk of ipsilateral stroke at 24 months with 75% stenosis, and a risk of 73.2% with 95% stenosis. When recurrent ipsilateral events occur, the risk of stroke at 2 years was increased to 41.2% compared to 18.6% in patients who had only one ipsilateral cerebrovascular event (Paddock-Eliasziw et al. 1996). An occluded contralateral artery doubles one's risk of ipsilateral stroke; in addition, this subgroup also carries an increased risk of perioperative stroke (4%) as do individuals with a mild to moderate contralateral stenosis (5.1%) (Gasecki et al. 1995).

The NASCET trial waited 6 weeks prior to CEA after cerebral infarction. A worrisome sign for physicians are strokes and a high-grade stenosis or "string" sign on angiography of the carotid artery. One year risk for these patients in the medically treated arm was 35.1%; if stenosis was between 90% and 94%, however, this risk decreased to 11.1% in patients with near occlusion (Morgenstern et al. 1997). The risk at 1 month of stroke with high-grade stenosis was 1.7%, implying that emergent endarterectomy may not be indicated.

The preliminary NASCET results for carotid stenosis of 50% to 69% was recently presented. An absolute risk reduction of 6.5% in favor of CEA was found (22.3% vs. 15.7%). This infers that 15 patients must undergo CEA in order to prevent one stroke. This benefit was only found, however, in males who were not diabetic, had experienced hemispheric and not retinal events, and had been treated with high-dose aspirin. When carotid stenosis was less than 50%, a marginal trend was present for CEA being advantageous (18.7% vs. 14.9%); the number of CEAs required to prevent one recurrent stroke was 26. Follow-up in the NASCET trial confirmed the continued benefit of CEA at 8 years in the greater than 70% stenosis; on the other hand, the benefit of CEA with 50% to 69% stenosis was lost after 2 to 3 years.

Much controversy remains as to the role of surgery in asymptomatic carotid stenosis, and some authorities have even suggested that there is no role for surgery (Mayberg et al. 1991; Executive Committee for the Asymptomatic Carotid Atherosclerosis Study 1995; CASANOVA Study Group 1991; Perry et al. 1997). The Asymptomatic Carotid Atherosclerotic Study (ACAS) randomized 1662 patients with a carotid stenosis of greater than 60%. The aggregate risk of ipsilateral stroke, perioperative stroke, or death over 5 years was 5.1% for patients undergoing CEA and 11.0% for patients treated with best medical therapy. This confers a 1.2% absolute risk reduction per year or a relative risk reduction of 53%. No benefit was found for women. The low complication rate of 2.4% in the study may make the study less generalizable. Other studies have shown no benefit for surgery because of a low stroke risk in this population (Mayberg et al. 1991; CASANOVA Study Group 1991).

*Summary of Prognosis for CEA.* CEA is clearly beneficial in symptomatic individuals with greater than 70% stenosis and a subset of those with 50% to 69% stenosis. Surgery for asymptomatic carotid stenosis has been documented to be beneficial in one large trial with a low complication rate and should be reserved for younger individuals with few comorbidities and progressing stenosis as determined by serial ultrasound.

Little data are available on the natural history and progression of intracranial stenosis of the major arteries. In a retrospective multicenter trial of 151 patients, Coumadin reduced to nearly 50% the relative risk reduction of myocardial infarction, stroke, or sudden death (Chimowitz et al. 1995). Stroke in the same vascular territory occurred in 10% of the aspirin-treated and in 2% of the warfarin treated patients. This study is limited by its sample size and the low number of events. Currently, the Warfarin-Aspirin Symptomatic Intracranial Disease Study (WASID) is underway to address whether antiplatelet or anticoagulation therapy is superior in preventing recurrent stroke. Until these prospective data become available, symptomatic patients with intracranial arterial stenosis can be treated with Coumadin.

### Aortic Embolism

The aorta is one the first vessels to exhibit signs of atherosclerosis. The advent of transesophageal echocardiography (TEE) has allowed visualization of this structure and has permitted extensive investigation of atherosclerosis in this location (Tunick and Kronzon 1990). Aortic atherosclerosis has recently been identified as an independent risk factor for stroke. Amarenco et al. identified a high incidence (14.4%) of raised plaque (≥4 mm) in the transverse aorta by transesophageal echocardiography among stroke patients compared to controls (2%) (Amarenco et al. 1994). Jones et al. confirmed these results in a similar case-control study (Jones et al. 1995). This group found complex aortic atheroma (>5 mm thick, mobile or ulcerated) in 22% of stroke patients but only 4% of control patients.

Aortic atherosclerosis has also been identified as an important cause of embolic stroke related to invasive cardiac interventions, such as coronary artery bypass graft (CABG) surgery, coronary angiography during catheterization, intra-aortic balloon-pump placement, or cross-clamping and cannulation of the aorta for heart (Katz et al. 1992). Surgical modifications by avoiding these aortic lesions or using hypothermic circulatory arrest with aortic arch atherectomy have led to a lower complication rate of stroke (Duda et al. 1995; Trehan et al. 1997).

Studies have demonstrated aortic atheroma to be an important predictor of future embolic risk (French Study of Aortic Plaques in Stroke Group 1996; Tunick et al. 1994). The annual risk of recurrent stroke among stroke patients with aortic atheroma greater than or equal to 4 mm thick is 11.9%. The annual risk of stroke, MI, systemic embolization, or death is a staggering 26%. Specific features of aortic plaque morphology on TEE have prognostic value. In patients with brain infarction, aortic plaque greater than or equal to 4 mm thick with no plaque calcification was associated with a dramatic 63.4 per 100 patient-years incidence of stroke, myocardial infarction, systemic emboli, or death (Cohen et al. 1997). This finding confirms aortic atheroma as a powerful prognostic marker of overall vascular risk. In comparison, symptomatic internal carotid artery stenosis was associated with a 16.1% annual risk of stroke or death in the medically treated arm of the NASCET study (North American Symptomatic Carotid Endarterectomy Trial Collaborators 1991). A recent study has demonstrated complex (ulcerated or mobile) morphology to be a more potent risk factor for stroke than atheroma

thickness (Di Tullio et al. 1998). Follow-up of 109 patients with aortic atherosclerotic plaques identified a higher risk of vascular events with mobile plaques (von Sohsten et al. 1998). Aortic atheroma should be considered in patients with carotid stenosis if symptoms are discordant with the side of stenosis (Demopoulos et al. 1995). Aortic atheromas frequently coexist with severe carotid disease.

Aortic atherosclerosis is closely linked to coronary artery atherosclerosis. Identifying aortic atherosclerosis by transesophageal echocardiography may predict the presence of severe coronary artery disease (Fazio et al. 1993). The absence of aortic atheroma visualized by TEE appears to be a powerful predictor for the absence of significant coronary artery disease (Tribouilloy et al. 1997; Parthenakis et al. 1996).

The optimal preventive stroke treatment for aortic arch disease has not been determined, although recent information may suggest a benefit from anticoagulation. Recently, a study of patients with a previous systemic embolic event and mobile aortic atheroma revealed a 32% annual incidence of stroke in those patients not receiving warfarin versus 0% in the warfarin-treated group (Dressler et al. 1998). Aortic plaque is a common finding in patients with atrial fibrillation. Causes of stroke in patients with atrial fibrillation may be due to aortic plaque in some instances. In the SPAF-III study adjusted-dose warfarin (INR 2 to 3) decreased stroke risk by 75% compared to combination therapy (low-dose warfarin and aspirin) in patients with atrial fibrillation and complex aortic plaque (The Stroke Prevention in Atrial Fibrillation Investigators Committee on Echocardiography 1998). Until a prospective randomized study of anticoagulation for aortic plaque is performed, current evidence would suggest that patients with greater than or equal to 4 mm noncalcified aortic plaque may benefit most from long-term anticoagulation.

## Patent Foramen Ovale

Stroke of unclear etiology or so-called cryptogenic stroke has been reported to account for up to 40% of all ischemic strokes (Sacco et al. 1989). Several recent studies have reported a higher incidence of patent foramen ovale (PFO) in patients with cryptogenic stroke, although a causal relationship remains to be firmly established and is currently a subject of debate (Lechat et al. 1988; Mas and Zuber for the French Study Group on Patent Foramen Ovale and Atrial Septal Aneurysm 1995; Hanna et al. 1994). The natural history of stroke rates in patients with PFOs as well as the long-term prognosis for recurrent stroke in this population remains poorly understood. The pathogenesis of ischemic stroke in patients with PFO remains unclear, as the source of the presumed paradoxical embolus is frequently not identifiable.

The incidence of PFO in an autopsy series of 965 normal hearts was reported as ranging from 27.3% to 34.3%, although in other series in the general population the incidence was as low as 15% (Hagen et al. 1984; Thompson and Evans 1930). Lechat et al. compared 60 adults with ischemic strokes under 55 years of age with 100 normal controls (Lechat et al. 1988). PFO was prevalent in 40% of stroke patients versus 10% of controls. In patients with an identifiable cause for their stroke the prevalence of PFO was 21%. Patients with no identifiable risk factors had a prevalence of PFO of 54%. Another French study retrospectively identified 132 patients with cryptogenic strokes who were found to have PFO or atrial septal aneurysms (ASA) (Mas and Zuber for the French Study Group on Patent Foramen Ovale and Atrial Septal Aneurysm 1995). With a mean follow-up of 22.6 months, an annual stroke recurrence of 1.2% was observed while the annual cumulative risk of transient ischemic attack (TIA) or stroke rate was 3.4%. This rate increased to 4.4% when individuals had concomitant PFO and atrial septal aneurism. Hanna et al. found no recurrent infarcts in a mean follow-up period of 28 months in 15 patients with cryptogenic stroke and PFO (Hanna et al. 1994). The Lausanne study of 140 consecutive nonselected patients with stroke and PFO showed a stroke or death rate of 2.4% per year and a TIA or stroke rate of 3.8% per year (Bogousslavsky et al. 1996). The stroke recurrence rate was 1.9% during a follow-up of 3 years.

Predictors of subsequent embolic events have not been clearly defined. Multivariate analysis in the Lausanne study found that independent risk factors for stroke recurrence were interatrial communication, history of recent migraine, posterior cerebral artery infarct, and a coexisting cause of stroke (Bogousslavsky et al. 1996). No correlation was found between treatment (antiplatelet, anticoagulant, or surgical closure) and stroke recurrence. These factors must be interpreted cautiously, as only eight recurrences occurred. Other reported risk factors have been increased right-to-left shunting (>20 bubbles on transesophageal echocardiography) as well as larger PFOs (Homma et al. 1994; Stone et al. 1996). The variations in physiologic morphology may account for the differences in stroke rates seen in individuals with and without symptomatic PFOs.

Currently, there is no consensus on the optimal therapeutic modality for PFOs. The small number of events in these studies preclude a meaningful comparison of the efficacy of various medical therapies for stroke prevention. Aspirin as an initial therapy proved effective in preventing stroke recurrence in 15 patients followed by Hanna et al. (1994). The authors suggested that warfarin or surgical closure be reserved as therapy only in individuals who are aspirin failures. A study of 17 patients, however, reported a 50% recurrence rate in patients treated with aspirin, suggesting that aspirin may not be the optimal medical therapy, as no events were recorded in the warfarin group (Sharma et al. 1991). In contrast, Bridges et al. (1992) reported that 12 of 32 patients treated with warfarin experienced neurological events and subsequently underwent surgical procedures. et al.

No surgical complications were found with direct surgical closure of 28 patients with prior strokes (Homma et al. 1997). One stroke and three TIAs were reported in a mean follow-up of 19 months. The actuarial rate of recurrence was 19.5%, with no recurrence reported in patients younger than 45. In this study 11 of 28 patients were placed on aspirin after the procedure and two of four patients with recurrent stroke had been receiving an antiplatelet agent. Zhu et al. found stroke recurrence in two of six patients undergoing surgical closure, with a mean follow-up of 3.9 years (Zhu et al. 1992). A series of 30 patients undergoing direct surgical closure by Devuyst et al. did not experience any neurological events, with a mean follow-up of 2 years (Devuyst et al. 1996). The absence of cerebrovascular events following surgical closure has also been reported by Harvey et al., although this study was of limited sample size (Harvey et al. 1986).

A transcatheter closure using a double umbrella device in 36 patients with presumed paradoxical right-to-left shunt was performed by Bridges et al. (1992). Following closure, four

TIAs and no strokes were reported over a mean follow-up period of 34 months. No complications were reported by Ende et al. following transcatheter closure of ten patients over a mean follow-up period of 32 months (Ende et al. 1996). The clinical course of 179 consecutive patients with atrial septal defects (ASDs) diagnosed after the age of 40 found that no difference in stroke incidence was seen in patients who underwent surgical closure when compared to medical therapy (Konstantinides et al. 1995). However, a decreased mortality from all causes (relative risk, 0.31; 95% CI, 0.11 to 0.85) was seen in patients who had undergone surgical repair of their ASD.

The role of PFOs in the genesis of cryptogenic stroke still remains debated. The available data are highly suggestive of a correlation; however, larger trials are needed to establish the etiology of cryptogenic stroke with PFO as well as to further explore criteria for optimal medical and surgical treatments. To date, neither antiplatelets nor anticoagulants have been proven superior to one another. Surgical or transcatheter closures can be performed with relatively few complications; however, their overall effectiveness in reducing stroke recurrence remains unclear.

Although the precise prognosis for stroke occurrence or recurrence is uncertain, one approach to consider is the implementation of anticoagulation therapy with large PFOs or interarterial shunt. Should anticoagulation therapy fail, closure of the PFO would be indicated. It is hoped that these questions will be addressed in the long-awaited Warfarin Aspirin Recurrent Stroke Study (WARSS), which is analyzing PFO in Cryptogenic Stroke (PICSS) to identify its relationship to stroke as well as establish whether antiplatelet or anticoagulation therapy is superior for secondary prevention.

### Cardioembolism

Cardioembolism accounts for 15% to 30% of all ischemic strokes (Mohr and Sacco 1982). The Trial of Org 10172 in Acute Stroke Treatment (TOAST) study group recently defined cardiac abnormalities as either high risk or medium risk for embolization (Adams et al. 1993). High-risk cardiac abnormalities include atrial fibrillation, prosthetic valve disease, rheumatic heart disease, bacterial endocarditis, atrial myxoma, and dilated cardiomyopathy.

The prognosis of stroke due to cardiogenic causes is generally worse than by other etiologies. Cardioembolism is associated with larger infarcts, likely secondary to larger sized thromboemboli (Timsit et al. 1993) and to the abrupt onset of vascular occlusion, which may not allow for the development of adequate collateral supply. These embolic strokes may also be associated with more frequent hemorrhagic transformation, sometimes leading to massive intracerebral hemorrhage (Alexandrov et al. 1997). Autopsy findings revealed hemorrhagic transformation in 51% to 71% with embolic strokes and 2% to 21% with nonembolic strokes. This high hemorrhagic transformation rate may be due to late reperfusion of ischemic brain commonly seen with cardioemboli.

The risk of re-embolization soon after cardioembolic stroke has always been thought to be high. Previous studies have reported that 2% to 21% of untreated patients have recurrent events in the first 2 weeks (Pessin et al. 1993). Recent results from the TOAST trial refute this high risk. Only 1% of patients with cardioembolic strokes suffered recurrent stroke in the first 7 days in this randomized trial (Publication Committee for the Trial of ORG 10172 in Acute Stroke Treatment [TOAST] Investigators 1998). No reduction in recurrent stroke was seen with anticoagulation, suggesting a limited role for early anticoagulation to prevent recurrent stroke.

Mitral valve prolapse has been considered a risk factor for stroke, particularly in young patients (Barnett et al. 1980). The Olmsted County population-based study, however, did not demonstrate an increased risk of stroke (Orencia, Petty et al. 1995). A subset of mitral valve prolapse with redundant leaflets identified on echocardiography may be associated with a substantially higher risk of cerebral embolic events, infective endocarditis, and sudden death (Nishimura et al. 1985).

Mitral annular calcification (MAC) is a degenerative process commonly encountered in the elderly population. The Framingham Study reported a doubled risk of stroke among 1159 patients after adjusting for multiple vascular risk factors in the presence of MAC by echocardiography. The incidence of stroke increased with the severity of MAC measured by millimeters of calcification (Boon et al. 1997). A cohort of 657 revealed MAC to only be a marker for other vascular risk factors (Eicher et al. 1997). The exact role for

MAC in thrombus formation has not been established to date. The mechanism for stroke may be related to the presence of pedunculated thrombi of the mitral annulus (Benjamin et al. 1992).

Cryptogenic stroke patients with MAC identified by transthoracic echocardiography should be further evaluated by transesophageal echocardiography, as this modality is better able to identify thrombus on the calcified portion of the mitral valve. More definitive information is required to understand the importance of this abnormality.

An embolic stroke due to bacterial endocarditis is associated with very poor prognosis. Transesophageal echocardiography is more sensitive at detecting vegetations than transthoracic echocardiography. TEE is also better able to identify complications such as mitral valve perforation, abscess, and subaortic complications, which may benefit from timely surgery (Liu et al. 1995). Mitral valve vegetations, large vegetation size (≥10 mm) (Magge et al. 1989), and spontaneous echo contrast (Rohmann et al. 1992) are TEE-defined abnormalities associated with a worse prognosis. Early visualization of echocardiographic findings provides valuable prognostic and therapeutic information for this condition.

Atrial myxoma is rare but is also associated with a very high rate of systemic embolization (30% to 40%). Although a serious condition, surgical removal may be curative with a 0% to 3% operative mortality (Reynen 1995).

Atrial fibrillation is the most common cardiac source of emboli and affects 2% of the population. The annual risk of stroke is approximately 5% without anticoagulation (Anonymous 1994). Atrial fibrillation has been associated with increased stroke severity, disability, and mortality (Lin et al. 1996), and as a result these patients have longer hospital stays and lower discharge rates to their homes (Jørgensen et al. 1996). Risk factors predicting stroke with atrial fibrillation include advanced age, hypertension, congestive heart failure (CHF), and previous thromboembolism. Left ventricular systolic dysfunction identified by transthoracic echocardiography is also an independent predictor of stroke in patients with atrial fibrillation (Atrial Fibrillation Investigators 1998). TEE predictors of thromboembolism include left atrial thrombus, left atrial spontaneous echo contrast, and complex aortic plaque (Zabalgoitia et al. 1998). The presence of left atrial spontaneous echo contrast ("smoke") is associated with 14% of stroke compared to 4% in the absence of "smoke" (Leung et al. 1994). Recently, the SPAF-III investigators determined a low-risk group of patients with atrial fibrillation. Patients without the risk factors are at particularly low risk for disabling stroke (0.5% per year). These risk factors are CHF, left ventricular (LV) dysfunction (evection fraction [EV] <25%), systolic blood pressure (BP) greater than 160 mm Hg, hypertension, female gender, and age over 75 years (SPAF III Writing Committee for the Stroke Prevention in Atrial Fibrillation Investigators 1998). Clinical and echocardiographic findings offer substantial prognostic information in patients with atrial fibrillation. This information can now help guide appropriate therapy for these patients.

Stroke is a common sequela of myocardial infarction (MI). The reported incidence of stroke after MI ranges between 1% and 4% within the first year (Tanne et al. 1995; Mooe et al. 1997; Loh et al. 1997). Stroke most commonly occurs in the first 5 days after MI (Mooe et al. 1997). Typically, anteriorly located MIs are more strongly associated with future embolic events. Risk factors for stroke after MI include advanced age, atrial fibrillation, poor LV function, previous MI, or previous stroke. A recent study suggests a decreasing incidence of stroke in the myocardial infarction population that may be due to thrombolytic therapy (Sloan et al. 1998). A substantial percentage of strokes in this population are not directly a consequence of the myocardial infarction but due to concomitant carotid atherosclerosis or small vessel disease (Martin and Bogousslavsky 1993).

## Prognosis by Therapy

### Antiplatelet Therapy

Medical therapy has had a significant impact on prognosis after TIA and/or stroke (Barnett et al. 1995). It is now accepted, after numerous prospective studies, that aspirin plays an effective role in primary and secondary stroke prevention. Aspirin reduces the risk of stroke after cerebrovascular symptoms by approximately 20% to 30% in patients not thought to have symptoms secondary to a cardioembolic source (Antiplatelet Trialists' Collaboration 1988; 1994; Barnett et al. 1995). Subsequent meta-analysis of 145 randomized trials of antiplatelet therapy versus control found that among 10,000 patients with either stroke or TIA, 18% of individuals treated with aspirin had recurrent events compared to 22% in controls (Antiplatelet Trialists' Collaboration 1994). These findings translate to preventing 40 strokes per 1000 individuals treated or a relative risk reduction of 23% for nonfatal strokes. The overall relative risk reduction for vascular events was 25%. The optimal dose of aspirin remains debated, as effective stroke prevention has occurred with doses ranging from 50 to 1300 mg. Higher doses of aspirin (900 mg every day) have been documented to be associated with arrest of carotid plaque progression and decreased risk of perioperative stroke after endarterectomy (650 mg twice daily), although this treatment may carry a higher risk of side effects (Ranke et al. 1993; North American Symptomatic Carotid Endarterectomy Trial Collaborators 1991; Dyken et al. 1992).

Prophylactic aspirin therapy in high-risk patients for stroke but without symptoms of TIA or stroke has not been proven beneficial, although it is customary to treat individuals with 325 mg of aspirin a day for prevention of coronary artery disease. This treatment has been shown beneficial (Barnett et al. 1995; Steering Committee of the Physicians' Health Study Research Group 1989; Peto et al. 1988). While the Physicians Health Study and the British Doctors Study both showed significant decreases in myocardial infarction, both had increases in the number of hemorrhagic strokes, though these were not statistically significant. Nonetheless, the trend is concerning and, more recently, similar data have been reported by Kronmal et al., who emphasized the need for prospective studies (Kronmal et al. 1998). Two large randomized trials recently explored the role of aspirin in acute ischemic stroke. In the International Stroke Trial (IST) 19,435 patients were randomized to receive either 300 mg/d of aspirin versus no aspirin within 48 hours of an acute ischemic stroke (International Stroke Trial Collaborative Group 1997). While no significant reduction in mortality was found, patients in the aspirin arm of the study had a reduced risk of recurrent stroke (ischemic and hemorrhagic) when compared to controls (3.7% vs. 4.6%; $p < .01$). Recurrent ischemic stroke was decreased in the aspirin group when compared to controls (2.8% vs. 3.96%; $p < .001$). The reduction in death or nonfatal recurrent

stroke favored aspirin treatment (11.3% vs. 12.4%; $p < .05$). Follow-up at 6 months revealed a nonsignificant trend of fewer individuals in the aspirin group being dead or dependent (62.2% vs. 63.5%; $p = .07$). The Chinese Acute Stroke Trial (CAST) compared 160 mg of aspirin to placebo administered within 48 hours of acute stroke in 21,106 patients (CAST [Chinese Acute Stroke Trial] Collaborative Group 1997). While aspirin reduced the incidence of recurrent stroke (1.6% vs. 2.1%; $p = .01$), there was a slight increase in hemorrhagic strokes (1.1% vs. 0.9%; $p > .1$). A 14% relative risk reduction in mortality was observed in the aspirin-treated group in the first4 weeks (3.3% vs. 3.9%; $p = .04$), while death or non-fatal stroke was diminished by 12% (5.3% vs. 5.9%), giving an absolute difference of 6.8 fewer cases per 1000. Less death or dependency was also found in the aspirin-treated group (30.5% vs. 31.6%; $p = 0.08$), translating into 11.4 fewer patients per 1000 treated. The combined results of the IST and the CAST showed that aspirin reduced the rate of death or nonfatal stroke recurrence by 10 per 1000 patients treated and decreased death or dependency by about 13 per 1000 patients treated.

Prophylactic stroke therapy with ticlopidine (TICLID) has been investigated in two large studies. The Ticlopidine Aspirin Stroke Study (TASS) randomized patients to receive either 500 mg/d of ticlopidine versus 1300 mg/d of aspirin and reported a 21% relative risk reduction in fatal or nonfatal stroke (10% vs. 13%) and a 12% relative risk reduction of nonfatal stroke or death from any cause at 3 years (17% vs. 19%) (Hass et al. 1989). Further subgroup analysis suggested that ticlopidine was more effective in women and in posterior circulation strokes (Grotta et al. 1992). The Canadian American Ticlopidine Study compared 500 mg of ticlopidine to placebo (Gent et al. 1989). There was a relative risk reduction of 30% in combined yearly rates of stroke, myocardial infarction, or death from any vascular cause (15% vs. 11%). Combination of aspirin and ticlopidine has been shown to decrease the incidence of myocardial infarction, vascular events, and the need for repeat intervention following coronary artery angioplasty and stenting (Schomig et al. 1996).

Clopidogrel, a drug similar to ticlopidine in action but with fewer side effects, was compared to 325 mg of aspirin in 19,185 high-risk patients. There was a slight reduction in stroke, myocardial infarction, or vascular death (5.32% vs. 5.83%) in the clopidogrel-treated group, yielding a relative risk reduction of 8.7% in comparison to aspirin (CAPRIE Steering Committee 1996).

Studies investigating dipyridamole as monotherapy and in combination with aspirin have had conflicting results (ESPS Group 1987; American-Canadian Cooperative Study Group 1983; Bousser et al. 1983; Diener et al. 1996). These studies have been criticized for not thoroughly evaluating the etiology of stroke and establishing stroke subtype (Barnett et al. 1995). While the ESPS-2 trial demonstrated reductions in recurrent stroke, TIA, and stroke or death with dipyridamole in monotherpay and even greater benefit with combination therapy with aspirin, there are several limitations to the study. A higher dose of aspirin was not compared to the very low dose of aspirin (50 mg/d) with ticlopidine, which may have been equally as efficacious. Furthermore, this study included patients with atrial fibrillation who may have benefited from anticoagulation.

In treating acute stroke patients, a reasonable approach is to treat individuals with 325 mg of aspirin as soon as possible. Aspirin failures should be switched to ticlopidine or clopidigrel. Should these agents fail, combinations of aspirin and clopidegrel or ticlopidine should be considered, although supportive data are not available.

### Anticoagulation Therapy

Anticoagulation therapy is frequently used for secondary stroke prevention in patients with cardiac sources of embolism. In several atrial fibrillation trials, anticoagulation has substantially reduced the risk of stroke. Pooling the results of five atrial fibrillation trials identified an 84% stroke risk reduction among women and 60% stroke risk reduction among men receiving warfarin. The annual rate of stroke was 4.5% in the control group and 1.4% in the Coumadin group. Risk factors in atrial fibrillation patients predicting stroke were previous TIA or stroke, increasing age, history of hypertension, and diabetes (Anonymous 1994). Recently, the SPAF-III trial evaluated two regimens in a high-risk group of elderly atrial fibrillation patients with at least one thromboembolic risk factor. Patients with CHF or EF below 25%, previous thromboembolism, systolic BP above 160, or who were females above 75 years old were randomized to adjusted-dose Coumadin or low-intensity fixed-dose warfarin and aspirin. This trial was prematurely terminated because of a high rate of stroke in the combination low-intensity warfarin and aspirin arm. The annual rate of stroke was 7.9% with this regimen and only 1.9% using adjusted-dose warfarin (Anonymous 1996). Adjusted-dose anticoagulation reduced the risk of stroke or systemic embolism from 11.9% to 3.4% in the previous thromboembolism group. This regimen prevented most cardioembolic strokes or stroke of unknown cause (2 vs. 15, 3 vs. 15, respectively). Rates of major hemorrhage did not differ between treatment groups. Anticoagulation reduced the rate of stroke particularly among patients with TEE findings of dense echo contrast or complex aortic plaque (Stroke Prevention in Atrial Fibrillation Investigators Committee on Echocardiography 1998). A target INR between 2 and 3 should be the standard approach to treatment of atrial fibrillation patients with prior stroke unless risks of anticoagulation are excessive. Although anticoagulation is well established and efficacious in atrial fibrillation, prosthetic valve disease, dissection, and dilated cardiomyopathies, it has not been established as the optimal therapy for other causes of stroke.

Anticoagulation was recently studied in a large post–MI population. Although warfarin substantially reduced the rate of ischemic stroke, the incidence of intracranial bleeding increased more than eightfold (17 vs. 2 intracranial bleeds). Most intracranial bleeding occurred when the INR was greater than 3 (Azar et al. 1996).

The SPIRIT study examined the role of high-intensity anticoagulation (INR, 3.0 to 4.5) in patients with recent minor stroke or TIA with noncardiac causes. This trial was terminated prematurely due to high rates (ninefold increase) of intracranial bleeding in the anticoagulation arm of the study. The bleeding incidence increased by 43% per 0.5 increase in INR (Stroke Prevention in Reversible Ischemia Trial [SPIRIT] Study Group 1997). Systemic and intracranial bleeding are potential serious complications of anticoagulation. The major prognostic indicators for bleeding include intensity of anticoagulation (INR > 4) (Hylek and Singer 1994; Cannegieter et al. 1995); older age; concurrent medications; and presence of comorbid diseases such as renal, hepatic, or cardiac diseases. The frequency of bleeding is reduced by less intense therapy (INR 2 to 3) which is still efficacious for most indications (Landefeld and Beyth 1993). A recent case-control study identified that excessive acetaminophen ingestion, new medications known to potentiate warfarin, advanced malignancy, recent diarrheal illness, and decreased oral intake contribute to excessive anticoagulation with warfarin (INR > 6) (Hylek et al. 1998).

### *Angioplasty and Stenting of the Intracranial and Extracranial Vessels*

The advent in the past decade of smaller diameter catheters, angioplasty balloons, and stents has provided interventional radiologists, cardiologists, neurologists, and neurosurgeons an alternative technique to establish revascularization of the extracranial and intracranial vessels. Cerebral percutaneous transluminal angioplasty (PTA) and intravascular stenting of the cervicocephalic vessels are currently under investigation in several multicenter trials to help establish their feasibility, safety, long-term durability, and effectiveness in preventing stroke.

There are numerous reports of small series of patients who have undergone angioplasty and/or stenting; however, it is difficult to ascertain complication rates and patency rates due to the small sample size of individual studies, limited follow-up time, evolving stent technology, and varying anticoagulation and antiplatelet regimens following stenting, which clearly play a role in stent endothelialzation as well as alter restenosis rates (Kachel 1996; Theron 1992; Higashida et al. 1996; Dietrich et al. 1996; Yadav et al. 1997). Wholey et al. identified 24 interventional centers in Europe, North and South America, and Asia all of which completed questionnaires in order to establish the current status of carotid angioplasty and stenting (Wholey et al. 1998). A total of 2048 carotid angioplasties and stentings had been done, with a success rate of 98.6%. A 30-day postprocedure mortality rate was 1.37%. Complication rates at 30 days included a 3.08% risk of minor stroke and a 1.32% risk of major stroke. Restenosis rates at 6 months were 4.80%, but more extensive follow-up was not available. These results compare favorably to the NASCET trial in which 30-day complication rates were: 0.6% surgical mortality, 3.7% minor stroke, 1.8% major stroke, 2.1% major stroke or death, and 5.8% all perioperative stroke or death (North American

Symptomatic Carotid Endarterectomy Trial Collaborators 1991). One must note that the majority of the angioplasty and stenting studies included both symptomatic and asymptomatic patients with carotid stenosis, which may skew results in favor of endovascular approaches; however, the NASCET group of patients are highly selected and have minimal surgical comorbidity. The benefit of PTA and stenting in high-risk patients with both symptomatic and asymptomatic stenosis was reported by Yadav et al. in 107 patients who underwent 126 carotid stent placements (Yadav et al. 1997). Mean stenosis diameter was reduced from 78% to 2%. Complications consisted of two major strokes, seven minor strokes, and one death during the first 30 days, yielding a combined endpoint for stroke and death of 7.9%. Ipsilateral incidence of stroke and death was 1.6%. Mean stenosis at 6 months in 81 patients was 18%. Asymptomatic restenosis occurred in 4.9% of patients, and five patients required repeat interventions (two PTAs for restenosis, two PTAs for stent deformity, and one CEA for restenosis). Mathur et al. stented 271 extracranial carotid arteries in 231 high-risk patients who had either symptomatic or asymptomatic carotid disease. Coronary artery disease was present in 71% of subjects, 12% had contralateral occlusion, and 39% had bilateral disease (Mathur et al. 1998). Only 14% of these subjects would have been eligible for the NASCET trial, as the remaining 86% would have been excluded secondary to comorbidities. Complication rates in the first 30 days following the procedure were 6.2% minor strokes and 0.7% major strokes. Patients that met NASCET entry criteria had a 2.7% risk of postprocedure stroke, a complication rate comparable to the ACAS trial (Executive Committee for the Asymptomatic Carotid Atherosclerosis Study 1995). Age and the presence of multiple or lengthy stenoses were found to be independent predictors of procedural strokes.

PTA of the intracranial vessels has had mixed success secondary to variation in lesion location and the risk of occluding vital arterial perforators and branches, technical feasibility of gaining access to the lesion, and vessel tortuosity. Clark et al. reported 17 patients who underwent intracranial PTA with a success rate of 82% (Clark et al. 1995). Mean stenosis diminished from 72% to 43%, and the complication rate was 11.8% (two patients suffered strokes). A much higher complication rate was encountered by Higashida et al. (Higashida et al. 1996). Despite PTA, 30% (10 of 33) of patients suffered strokes, of whom four died. A further 21% (7 of 33) suffered TIAs during the procedure. The higher complication rate was attributed to the marked tortuosity of the intracranial vasculature as well as its smaller luminal diameter. A restenosis rate at 3 months of 29.6% was reported by Mori et al. in 35 patients who underwent PTA of the intracranial vessels (Mori et al. 1997). Restenosis occurred in severe, eccentric or angulated lesions and lower restenosis rates were seen in concentric and short lesions. In a smaller series of 15 patients who had failed warfarin therapy, with a mean 2-year follow-up, Callahan and Berger reported complications in 2 of 15 patients undergoing angioplasty of the intracranial vessels. One patient suffered rupture of the vessel and the second suffered a brain stem stroke, likely secondary to occlusion of a small perforating vessel off of the basilar (Callahan and Berger 1997). In contrast, Takis et al. had a technical failure in two of ten patients. Of the remaining eight patients, five suffered from vasospasm and developed strokes (Takis et al. 1997).

Despite the results reported in the numerous series above, conclusions on prognosis with angioplasty and stenting are confounded by numerous factors such as the presence of symptomatic versus asymptomatic disease, concomitant medical conditions, type of stent used, and whether antiplatelet or anticoagulation therapy was instituted. Several recent coronary artery trials have shown decreased complication and restenosis rates in stenting patients who are treated with a regimen of combined aspirin and ticlofidine therapy or the newer antiglycoprotein IIb/IIIa agents, which have been shown to be superior to combinations of heparin, warfarin, and aspirin ((Schomig et al. 1996; EPILOG Investigators 1997; EPIC Investigators 1994; IMPACT-II Investigators 1997; Tcheng et al. 1995).

Angioplasty and stenting may offer a noninvasive means of treating cerebrovascular disease. However, this technique is still in its infancy and conclusions may not be made regarding prognosis pending completion of well-controlled, randomized trials as well as a standardization of stent technology and use of antiplatelet or anticoagulation protocols.

### Thrombolytic Therapy

Thrombolytic therapy has been studied intensively for several years. Recent large multicenter trials have clearly demonstrated no benefit with streptokinase (Multicenter Acute Stroke Trial—Europe Study Group 1996; Donnan et al. 1995; Multicenter Acute Stroke Trial—Italy (MAST-I) Group 1995). Mortality and intracerebral hemorrhage were substantially increased with this therapy given within 6 hours of symptom onset. Alternatively, intravenous recombinant tissue plasminogen activator (rt-PA) appears beneficial. It is currently the only approved therapy for acute stroke in the United States. The first intravenous rt-PA study, the European Cooperative Acute Stroke Study (ECASS) trial, demonstrated improved neurologic outcome in a defined subgroup of stroke patients with moderate or severe neurologic deficits. Unfortunately, several ineligible patients were randomized, resulting in an inconclusive overall effect compared to placebo. Twenty percent of the rt-PA–treated patients developed parenchymal hematomas compared to 7% in the placebo arm of this trial (Hacke et al. 1995). The NINDS rt-PA trial demonstrated 0.9 mg/kg intravenous rt-PA to be superior to placebo in patients with stroke symptoms developing less than 3 hours earlier. Intravenous rt-PA led to a 30% to 50% increase in the number of patients returning to full independence by 3 months. This benefit was not at a cost of increased mortality. The mortality rate in this trial was 17% in the rt-PA arm and 21% in the placebo arm. The only concerning result was a 6.4% risk of symptomatic intracerebral hemorrhage (ICH) compared to 0.6% with placebo (NINDS rt-PA Stroke Study Group 1995). Methodological differences including a higher dose and longer time window for treatment in the ECASS trial may have explained the difference in results. A follow-up trial in Europe, ECASS-II, is attempting to confirm the NINDS rt-PA trial results using the 0.9 mg/kg dose.

The ideal route for administering thrombolytic therapy has not yet been established. Intravenous thrombolysis offers the advantage of earlier treatment and simplified administration. Local intra-arterial thrombolysis affords direct delivery of thrombolytic and mechanical disruption of clot. Local delivery is invasive and associated with a substantial delay in therapy. One nonrandomized thrombolytic study did compare routes of administration. Intra-arterial therapy was associated with superior recanalization rates in occlusions of proximal vessels such as the distal internal carotid artery (ICA), middle cerebral artery (MCA) stem, and basilar artery, and therefore may prove more beneficial in these occlusions than intravenous therapies (Sasaki et al. 1995). An angiographic study of intravenous rt-PA identified poor recanalization particularly with terminal ICA or MCA stem occlusion (del Zoppo et al. 1992).

Previous studies using intra-arterial thrombolytic therapy have demonstrated good outcomes from early recanalization (Mori et al. 1988; Hacke et al. 1988; Brandt et al. 1996; Huemer et al. 1995; Wijdicks et al. 1997). Ongoing trials are addressing the role of this therapy in patients with occlusion of major cerebral arteries. The first randomized, double-blind, placebo-controlled study, PROACT, revealed a reduction in mortality and improvement in good outcome in those stroke patients with MCA stem occlusions receiving intra-arterial therapy up to 6 hours after symptom onset (del Zoppo et al. 1998). A larger trial, PROACT-II, is currently recruiting patients.

The recent Food and Drug Administration (FDA) approval of intravenous rt-PA (0.9 mg/kg dose) within 3 hours of symptom onset should result in some improvement of stroke prognosis. Unfortunately, only a fraction (1% in the United States) of stroke patients arrive and are treated within this short time period. Intense community education is required to increase awareness of the symptoms of stroke to increase effectively the impact of thrombolytic therapy in acute stroke.

## Prognosis of Intracerebral Hemorrhage

Except for intracerebellar hemorrhage, which can respond gratifyingly to surgical decompression, other areas of ICH have proved to be a daunting problem both for therapeutic options and for prognosis. Since no consensus exists on the optimum, effective treatment of ICH, either medical or surgical, recent reports have attempted to quantify factors prognosticating outcome. It is the hope and expectation that predictable identification of viable patients, who later deteriorate, will provide a basis for interventional therapies, such as hematoma evacuation. A recurrent theme in the various recent reports emphasize ICH size and the general

functional status as measured, for example, by the Glasgow coma scale (GSC).

In a retrospective study of 75 ICH patients seen in an emergency room in an average of slightly over 3 1/2 hours from onset, Lisk et al. (1994) found that hemorrhage volume, intraventricular extension, GCS score, age, and gender contributed to prognosis. Two models and a formula including these factors were developed. For the models predicting good outcome with Rankin scores of 0 to 2 without need for surgery, the key factors were age, hemorrhage diameter, and ventricular extension. This group is important to identify for any prospective study, as other authors have pointed out, because interventional measures such as hematoma evacuation are unnecessary and potentially hazardous. It is of note that virtually all of these patients had a hemorrhage diameter of less than 3.3 cm; the single outlier was a patient with an arteriovenous malformation. For the second model predicting poor outcome with a Rankin of 5 to 6 (6 representing death), a stepdown logistic regression analysis was performed, and the factors of GCS score, hemorrhage volume, plus the patient's age and gender were important. Interestingly, neither the site of the hemorrhage nor blood pressure were prognostic factors, unlike other series discussed below. In a word, this study's data suggest that large ICH in patients who are awake will likely be the best candidates for hematoma evacuation.

In a 9-year review ending in 1990, of 896 ICH patients, Rosenow et al. (Rosenow et al. 1997) found a correlation with good outcome with lower mortality when the etiology was arteriovenous malformations and the ICH was localized in the cerebral hemispheres or polar regions, as opposed to the other locations such as thalamus, brain stem, or cerebellum. On the other hand, a worse prognosis correlated with ventricular extension of the ICH, increasing age (in this case ≥65), surgical intervention, basal ganglia ICH, and hypertension as cause of ICH. While these statistical correlations with digitized outcomes of either being alive or dead provide the extremes of subjects who require no intervention and those with lethal injuries, absence of information on hematoma volume or neurological status, such as GCS, and its change over time make it difficult to develop parameters for intermediate subjects who might benefit from surgical intervention.

To address the issue regarding ICH volume, several papers specifically address that, in addition to the one noted above by Lisk et al. (1994). In a study of 188 cases of ICH, Broderick et al. (1993) found that ICH volume, measured by an eliptical formula, plus the GSC score predicted the 30-day mortality. Specifically, three categories of volumes were analyzed (namely, ≤30 ml, 30 to 60 ml, and ≥61 ml), and GCS scores were segregated between either greater than or equal to 9 or less than or equal to 8. For the largest ICH (≥60 ml and GCS of ≤8), the 30-day mortality was 91%. For those between 30 and 60 ml, only 1% was independent at 30 days, while 81% of those with ICH of less than or equal to 30 ml and a GCS of 9 or higher were alive. Thus, ICH volumes of less than or equal to 30 ml and 60 ml or more either recover, by and large, or die, respectively; therefore, considerations for intervention would be primarily directed to ICH volumes between 30 and 60 ml plus GCS of moderate level.

Supporting the importance of ICH volume and GCS is the report by Zorzon et al. (1995). They reviewed 138 cases of ICH, also calculating the volume using the elipsoid formula of 4/3 abc, and correlated 17 clinical and five computed tomographic (CT) abnormalities with prognosis. In their multivariate logistic regression analysis, they found three factors that independently predicted 30-day mortality; they were ICH volume, GCS score, and intraventricular hemorrhage. Interestingly, site of hemorrhage and volume of ICH separately predicted outcome, although ICH volume greater than approximately 47 cc was more lethal.

In the large Stroke Data Bank Study, Mayer et al. (1994) evaluated factors contributing to neurological deterioration following ICH. Of the total cohort of 1805 strokes, 237 (13%) had supratentorial ICH, and of that latter group, 46 noncomatose (GCS of 8) ICH subjects were analyzed. Neurological deterioration occurred in one-third, particularly over the first day after ICH and was correlated with ICH volume (e.g., >45 ml), occasional rebleeding, and midline shift with evidences of edema. The 30-day mortality for this group was nearly one-half at 47%. Deterioration was not associated with factors considered risks in others series, such as GCS score, hypertension, location of ICH, intraventricular spread, age, gender, race, and stroke-risk factors, including glucose level. Thus, for the important issue of progression, which may signal patients requiring urgent intervention, ICH volume was the most crucial factor.

To simplify the approach to ICH prognosis, Tuhrim et al. (1995) applied two logistic regression models to determine the prognosis of 129 supratentorial ICH patients. The first model contains only three elements to measure: ICH size, GCS score, and pulse pressure, which is a surrogate for intracranial pressure (ICP). The second and more complex model included the above three factors and a total of 18 risk factors commonly believed relevant. In their analysis, the first simple model accurately prognosticated outcome, which again reflects the power of a few parameters. In the African American population, believed to have an increased incidence of ICH, a study by Qureshi et al. (1995) found similar risk factors for early deterioration, namely, ICH volume, especially greater than 30 ml, GCS score less than 12, and intraventricular spread.

From an analysis of the recent literature on ICH prognosis, no consensus exists on the precise identification of factors predicting outcome in an individual case. However, it can be concluded that large-volume ICH, particularly 30 to 60 ml, reduced GCS, especially less than 8, and progression augur poorly for 30-day outcome, with mortality at nearly 50% and morbidity with lack of functional independence at over 90%.

Since hypertension and its degree of elevation are etiologically related to ICH occurrence, it is surprising that hypertension itself does not necessarily portend a bad prognosis, although it may in univariate analyses (Qureshi et al. 1995; Zorzon et al. 1995; Mayer et al. 1994). However, in a large study of 1701 ICH patients in Tokyo, Terayama et al. (1997) found a significant relationship with both ICH volume and elevated blood pressure. However, this association existed primarily with putaminal and thalamic ICH, not polar, pontine, or cerebellar ICH. For example, the mean arterial pressure (MAP) of 592 putaminal ICH who survived was $123.8 \pm 20.6$ mm Hg, while that of 184 who died was significantly higher at $136.0 \pm 36.3$ mm Hg. And for the fatal ICH volume, it was an average of $58.2 \pm 24.4$ ml compared to the nonfatal group with an average of $27.0 \pm 11.4$ ml. Thus, under certain circumstances for particular hemorrhage sites, higher blood pressures may be detrimental, particularly in provoking presumed cerebral edema. Although this issue is not directly answered by this paper by Terayama et al., the report by Dandapani et al. (1995) helps to answer this important question. They retrospectively analyzed 87 hypertensive ICH and divided them into those with initial MAPs greater than 145 mm Hg ($n = 34$) and those with MAPs less than or equal to 145 mm Hg ($n = 53$). Subjects who were hypertensive on admission (approximately 90%) were treated with antihypertensive agents, particularly oral nifedipine. Also used for control were intravenous sodium nitroprusside, labetalol, clonidine, and angiotensin-converting enzyme inhibitors. The patients were categorized into those whose MAP was greater than 125 mm Hg ($n = 40$) or less than or equal to 125 mm Hg ($n = 47$) within the 2- to 6-hour post-treatment period and then correlated with outcomes. Unfortunately, CTs were not generally available to quantititate ICH volume, a crucial factor as noted above and a factor that can directly affect the ability to control blood pressure. Nonetheless, this study supports a growing body of evidence supporting reduction of elevated MAP with ICH to reduce complications of rebleeding and brain edema and to improve outcome.

As for risk factors for ICH that may prognosticate outcome, it is of interest that the customary ones for ischemic strokes due to atherosclerosis of age and smoking also increase the risk for ICH. Thus, smoking has the same lethal implications for ICH (Jørgensen et al. 1995). Of further prognostic importance for ICH is anticoagulation and its degree, a commonly recognized hazard and concern. In a study of 77 patients with ICH, Hylek and Singer (1994) found that a 0.5 increase in prothrombin time ratio, particularly of ratios greater than 2.0, caused a doubling for ICH risk. The occurrence of ICH increased with odds ratios near or greater than 2.0 with previous history of stroke, prosthetic valve replacement, age 80 years or older, plus duration of anticoagulation more than 5 years.

In summary, the prognosis of ICH is largely dependent on the size of the ICH and the GCS score, but other factors such as the initial elevated MAP and its control, plus intraventricular spread of blood, may be important and will require further study.

## Prognosis of Subarachnoid Hemorrhage

Prognosis of subarachnoid hemorrhage (SAH) from a ruptured aneurysm is related to clinical status at onset plus complications related to well-known factors such as recurrent hemorrhage, vaso-spasm, hydrocephalus, ease of obliterating the aneurysm surgically or by other interventional techniques, plus other medical and surgical factors. The natural history of SAH forms the basis of developing prognostic guidelines, but since the focus of this chapter is on prognosis, natural history alone is beyond the scope of this chapter; however, a review by Barrow and Reisner on natural history is recommended (Barrow and Reisner 1993). In perhaps the longest follow-up series published, with minimum follow-up of 24 years (range 24 to 32.5 years), Olafsson et al. (1997) reported on a modest number of 86 subjects with confirmed aneurysms seen in Iceland between 1958 and 1968. Although early mortality of 47% is similar to other study cohorts with SAH, this report provides an unusually long follow up period to assess long-term survivorship and risk of recurrent hemorrhages. For long-term prognosis, survivorship following SAH was primarily dependent on the degree of neurological disability, with the vast majority (>95%) having surgery. In subjects surviving 6 months past the initial SAH that were either normal neurologically or minimally impaired, survivorship was virtually identical to the general population of Iceland. In those with moderate or severe neurological deficits, a nearly 20-fold increase in mortality occurred, but primarily in the 5- to 9-year post-SAH period. The excess mortality could not be explained on their disabilities; recurrent hemorrhage occurred in approximately 10% of these cases. Thus, if patients with SAH can survive the first 6 months following extirpation of the offending aneurysm and have little or no neurological deficits, the prognosis for survivorship is excellent and coincides with the general population. Efforts to prognosticate outcome on the basis of coma rating scales, such as the GCS or the Innsbruck coma scale, are commonly used to follow patients in the early stages of SAH when they may be stuporous or comatose (Diringer and Edwards 1997). But while the extremes of the scale are of prognostic value, the intermediate ranges are more difficult and require the aggregation of multiple factors that will impact prognosis, as discussed below on factors influencing vasospasm.

## Prognosis After SAH Related to Clinical Grading

The issue of early versus late surgery for ruptured intracranial aneurysms was resolved in favor of intermediate timing of surgery in patients who are relatively stable neurologically, without active vasospasm, and who demonstrate an operable aneurysm (Kassell et al. 1990). Nonetheless, complication rates are distressingly similar for both good and poor neurological grades. In a retrospective review of 355 SAH patients from the anterior circulation seen over a 10-year period ending in 1993 at the Harborview Medical Center in Seattle, Le Roux and colleagues (1996) found that except for cerebral swelling associated with intracerebral hemorrhage, the complications of failure to occlude the aneurysm, major vascular occlusion, intraoperative aneurysm rupture, or surgical contusion were similar in the two groups. These results suggest that neither early nor late surgery conferred any advantages in averting various neurosurgical complications, but the authors nonetheless conclude that early surgery is preferable because the known complications of rebleeding, vasospasm, brain edema, and hydrocephalus can be addressed more aggressively with interventions not available otherwise, such as volume expansion and hypertension (Le Roux et al. 1996).

## Vasospasm

As noted above, two major factors contributing to the poor prognostic outcome of SAH are vasospasm and rebleeding. To identify factors contributing to the former, Shimoda et al. (1997) reviewed their 10-year experience ending in 1994 of 605 patients with aneurysmal SAH. Of this number, 137 had surgery with neck obliteration within 3 days following SAH, and the authors analyzed factors believed contributory to vasospasm. In the last 4 years of the study, all patients received either intravenous nicardipine or diltiazem for 7 to 21 days postoperatively for prophylaxis against delayed ischemic deficits. In addition, at 3 to 5 days postoperatively, patients were given a single intracisternal injection of 30,000 to 60,000 units urokinase to achieve thrombolysis (since the thrombus is believed to provoke vasospasm), and hypervolemia was instituted in all patients with delayed ischemic deficits, along with dobutamine with or without dopamine therapy. Delayed ischemic deficits were diagnosed by clinical signs and symptoms of focal neurological nature plus CT evidence for infarction; angiography was not performed. In their analysis of factors contributing to delayed ischemic deficits, they found the following relating to the poor clinical status of the patients: older age (though a mean age difference be-

tween the two groups is roughly 59 vs. 54); poorer neurological status as measured by the World Federation of Neurological Surgeons grading scale; Fisher's scale of 4, a semiquantitative means of measuring the amount of blood load in the subarachnoid spaces; delayed ischemic deficits following rebleeding, the latter an ominous and foreboding sign with high associated morbidity and mortality regardless; alteration of consciousness associated with rebleeding complications with surgical intervention; lack of any improvement following hypervolemic therapy; and, finally, intracranial complications following the administration of hypervolemic therapy. Although not subjected to multivariate analysis, the unfavorable prognostic aspect of vasospasm might be reduced to its occurring predominantly in subjects who are of poorer neurological grade. Thus, while Le Roux et al. did not find outcome to vary with clinical status, delayed ischemic deficits presumed to be caused by vasospasm appear to be related to neurological impairment. What this study by Shimoda et al. does not answer is whether the use of the calcium channel blocker nimodipine might have averted more effectively delayed isch-emic deficits as shown in a number of prospective, randomized, double-blind studies. While factors provoking vasospasm are yet undetermined, by indirection and obliquely, use of nimodipine can be supported by this study to improve prognosis against delayed ischemic deficits.

## Blood Load on CT and Vasospasm

The problem of general neurological status at the time of SAH and the occurrence of vasospasm is further supported by studies of Grosset et al. from Glasgow (Grosset et al. 1994). In their study of 121 SAH patients, the authors correlated CT evidence for the blood load quantitated by the technique of Fisher et al., noted above, with evidence of vasospasm, documented by transcranial Dopper velocities taken every 2 days following SAH. For example, in patients with Fisher's Grade 1, 2, and 3 showing no visible blood, diffuse sheets of blood of less than 1-mm thickness, and diffuse blood of greater than 1-mm thickness, respectively, the peak velocity went up significantly from $149 \pm 9$, $164 \pm 7$, $176 \pm 6$ cm/s (mean $\pm$ SE), respectively. In terms of those developing delayed ischemic deficits, 57% of Fisher's grade 3 did, while 35% of Fisher's grade 2 did. Although not all series show a parallel correlation between the amount of blood load with clinical deficits and impaired outcome, these more recent studies support the general notion that the more serious the insult with SAH, the more devastating the outcome.

One poor prognostic feature after SAH is vasospasm. Since multiple studies have documented the value of using the calcium channel blocker nimodipine in doses of approximately 60 mg orally four times daily in minimizing vasospasm, or at least the occurrence of ischemic episodes (Pickard et al. 1989), this has become standard prophylaxis therapy. However, in patients with apparent normal cerebral blood flow (CBF) by xenon CT or by transcranial Doppler following SAH, a novel application of acetazolaminde to determine impaired vascular reserve may predict those who will develop spasm and allow more aggressive interventions. In a study of 50 SAH patients whose CBF was measured by stable xenon-enhanced CT, Yoshida et al. (1996) could not predict which patient would develop vasospasm on the basis of the xenon CT CBF values taken within 4 days of SAH onset. However, with acetazolamide, the authors identified those who did and did not develop vasospasm, based on either showing or not showing vascular reactivity. While the exact mechanism accounting for vasospasm is uncertain, the authors speculate that either lactic acidosis or increased intracranial pressure caused nonreactivity. Although these may prove to be surrogate markers for future occurrence of vasospasm and the need for aggressive interventions, including angioplasty, vascular reactivity provides another prognostic indicator for SAH outcome.

## Posterior Circulation Aneurysmal Rupture

As opposed to anterior circulation aneurysms reviewed above by Le Roux et al., the posterior circulation aneurysms with SAHs generally result in poorer prognoses. In a review by Schievink et al. (1995) from the Mayo Clinic of a survey of all SAH mortality over a 30-year period ending in 1984, the characteristics of all first-time SAHs, numbering 136 cases, were analyzed. In this group of 99 women and 37 men, with a mean age of 55 years, survival to 48 hours was only 32% for the 19 posterior circulation aneurysms as opposed to 77% for 87 with anterior circulation aneurysms or 70% for those with an unidentified aneurysm site. Survivals to 30 days were 11%, 57%, and 53%, respectively, with a substantially significant difference for early mortality with posterior aneurysmal SAH. With

multivariate analyses, it is clear that posterior circulation aneurysmal SAHs present with poorer clinical conditions, (i.e., Hunt and Hess grades IV and V, substantially greater "sudden death" syndromes, and rebleeding). The authors reasoned that the lethal nature of posterior SAH is the vulnerability of the brain stem structures in the compacted space. Because of the strikingly poor prognosis for posterior SAH, the authors recommend a more aggressive approach to the obliterative treatment of unruptured posterior circulation aneurysms.

## Prognosis of Hydrocephalus Associated With SAH

Hydrocephalus resulting from blockage of resorptive capacities for cerebrospinal fluid (CSF) by clotted blood is determined to a large extent by the amount of subarachnoid blood, similar to blood's effect in provoking vasospasm. In a series of 660 Veterans Administration Hospital patients with demonstrable aneurysms seen over a 15-year period in Rotterdam reported by Vermeij et al. (1994), multivariate analysis using the Cox proportional hazards model showed a correlation between cisternal and ventricular blood, hydrocephalus on initial CT, plus the use of the antifibrinolytic agent tranexamic acid with hydrocephalus development. In their careful analysis, the amount of blood was quantitated by assigning a score of 0 to 3 for the amount of blood in each of ten cerebral cisterns. A maximum score is 30, but 18 was considered high blood load score. Hydrocephalus was measured as the bicaudate index using the width of the frontal horns at the foramen of Monro divided by the width of the brain at the junction and compared to normal control data. Although multiple other factors have been proposed as being causative of hydrocephalus and discussed by Vermeij et al., their multivariate analysis shows a strong correlation with the amount of blood load and the use of tranexamic acid. Since impaired consciousness and vasospasm correlate with hydrocephalus and thereby impair prognosis after SAH, these data support the continued need to treat hydrocephalus aggressively with shunting or draining in order to improve neurological prognosis.

## Aneurysm Size and Rupture

The issue of an aneurysm's size and its propensity to rupture has been controversial, with authorities for or against the ominousness of aneurysms less than 10 mm in diameter. Two recent reports appear to put to rest this issue by showing persuasively that aneurysms of 5 to 10 mm in diameter are prone to rupture and are therefore not benign. In the 5-year Danish Aneurysm Study ending in 1983, authored by Rosenorn and Eskesen (1997), a total of 1076 subjects with SAH were studied; 19% had a maximum diameter of less than 5 mm, while 51% had a diameter of 5 to 10 mm. Although the neurological impairment and amount of CT blood load were greater with larger (>10 mm) aneurysms, the mortality in the small, medium, and large aneurysms was 47%, 39%, and 51%, respectively. Return to previous occupation and mental activities was, however, better with smaller aneurysms. On the basis of their findings, the authors conclude that asymptomatic small aneurysms should be operated on because these have a high probability of bleeding.

In a similar 5-year review of their experiences, Orz et al. (1997) reported on 1558 aneurysms operated on, 1248 with and 310 without rupture. Of the ruptured aneurysms, 475 (38%) were small, with a maximum diameter of less than 6 mm. These authors, like those of the Danish Aneurysm Study, conclude that small aneurysms are not innocuous and should be operated on electively.

### SAH Without Detectable Aneurysm

This subject is extensively reviewed by Rinkel et al. (1993), who point out that in 15% to 20% of SAH subjects, the initial angiogram will show no aneurysm, but that to approach these patients clinically, they should be divided into two groups, depending on the CT findings. (1) perimesencephalic hemorrrhage with blood confined to the cistern around the midbrain and (2) diffusely or anteriorly located blood. The former, accounting for about 10% of all SAH and two-thirds of all those with negative angiograms, is relatively benign. These patients are over age 20 but typically in their sixth decade, and they usually have only a mild, slow-onset headache without an acute, severe one. Loss of consciousness is rare and focal neurological deficits do not occur. About 20% will show mild hydrocephalus but are relatively asymptomatic from it. The recovery period is short, and the patients customarily resume their previous activities. It is believed that venous bleeding accounts for this SAH. Thus, for this group of subjects with perimesencephalic SAH, the prognosis is excellent.

In subjects with diffuse or anteriorly located blood in the basal cisterns on CT, the prognosis is quite different and depends on the primary cause of bleeding. These patients, unlike the perimesencephalic patients, may be drowsy or stuporous and have symptomatic hydrocephalus. In these patients, a repeat angiogram is essential, and the repeat study may show an aneurysm in a high percentage. However, other conditions that predispose to bleeding must be considered and include the following: dissection, both vertebral and carotid; dural and spinal arteriovenous malformations; trauma; mycotic aneurysms; cocaine abuse; sickle cell anemia; coagulation disorders; pituitary apoplexy; and a few other miscellaneous disorders such as neoplasms.

### Multiple Aneurysms

Multiple cerebral aneurysms occur in 18% to 30% of SAH cases, and while the prognosis with multiplicity reflects the same factors contributing to outcome with single aneurysms, certain distinctions occur as reported by Cervoni et al. (1993). In their 5-year experience from "La Sapienza" University of Rome, 41 (9%) of 450 patients with SAH had aneurysms that were multiple and primarily in the anterior circulation. Prognosis was related to not only clinical status and timing of surgery, but importantly whether the aneurysms were unilateral or bilateral. Of note in this series, and relevant to concerns regarding aneurysm size, is the following: those that bled were larger and greater than 1 cm in diameter. The likely reason for the graver prognosis for bilateral aneurysms is the necessary staged procedures, which meant time delay and greater chances for vasospasm. The mortality in this series was 15%—mortality from others ranged from 9% to 20%—whereas single aneurysm mortality ranges from 8% to 14%. Thus, the prognosis for life with multiple aneurysms is worse by about 5% compared to single aneurysms, and bilateral aneurysms make that prognosis even worse.

### Prognostic Value of Brainstem Auditory Evoked Potentials, Somatosensory Evoked Potentials, and Pupillary Reaction

In a study of 64 SAH cases reported by Hojer and Haupt (1993), both brain stem auditory evoked potentials (BAEP) and somatosensory evoked potentials (SEP) correlated with the clinical grade of the patients. Patients with normal studies had a favorable outcome, whereas patients with lower Hunt-Hess grades (such as IV to V) had impairment or loss of BAEP or SEP. For pupillary reactions, Yoshimoto et al. (1997) found that in a study of 68 gravely ill SAH patients seen over a greater than 7-year period ending in 1995, bilateral unreactive pupils were associated with a 95% mortality rate. This high figure compares to a 64% mortality rate when these patients exhibit abnormal or no motor responses. The authors postulate that the unreactive pupils reflect relative brain stem hypoperfusion from severely increased intracranial pressure resulting from massive and often lethal SAH. Thus, these two surrogates for the prognosis of SAH, namely, absence of pupillary reaction and impaired or absent evoked potentials, indicate a grave or lethal outcome.

# References

Adams J. H.; Bendixen B. H.; Kappelle L. J.; Biller, J.; Love, B. B.; Gordon, D. L., Marsh, E. E. Classification of subtype of acute ischemic stroke. Definitions for use in a multicenter clinical trial. TOAST. Trial of Org 10172 in Acute Stroke Treatment. Stroke 24:35–41; 1993.

Alexandrov, A. V.; Black, S. E.; Ehrlich, L. E.; Caldwell, C. B.; Norris, J. W. Predictors of hemorrhagic transformation occurring spontaneously and on anticoagulants in patients with acute ischemic stroke. Stroke 28:1198–1202; 1997.

Amarenco, P.; Cohen, A.; Tzourio C.; Bertrand, B.; Hommel, M.; Besson, G.; Chauvel, C.; Touboul, P. J.; Bousser, M. G. Atherosclerotic disease of the aortic arch and the risk of ischemic stroke. N. Engl. J. Med. 331:1474–1479; 1994.

American-Canadian Cooperative Study Group. Persantine aspirin trial in cerebral ischemia. Part II: endpoint results. Stroke 16:406–415; 1983.

American Heart Association. 1992 Heart and stroke facts. Dallas: American Heart Association; 1992.

Anonymous. Adjusted-dose warfarin versus low-intensity, fixed-dose warfarin plus aspirin for high-risk patients with atrial fibrillation: Stroke Prevention in Atrial Fibrillation III randomized clinical trial. Lancet 348:633–638; 1996.

Anonymous. Risk factors for stroke and efficacy of antithrombotic therapy in atrial fibrillation. Analysis of pooled data from five randomized controlled trials. Arch. Intern. Med. 154:1449–1457; 1994.

Antiplatelet Trialists' Collaboration. Collaborative overview of randomized trials of antiplatelet therapy I: prevention of death, myocardial infarction and stroke by prolonged antiplatelet therapy in various categories of patients. BMJ 308:81–106; 1994.

Antiplatelet Trialists' Collaboration. Secondary prevention of vascular disease by prolonged antiplatelet treatment. BMJ 296:320–331; 1988.

Atrial Fibrillation Investigators. Echocardiographic predictors of stroke in patients with atrial fibrillation. Arch Intern. Med. 158:1316–1320; 1998.

Azar, A. J.; Koudstaal, P. J.; Wintzen, A. R.; van Bergen, P. F.; Jonker, J. J.; Deckers, J. W. Risk of stroke during long-term anticoagulant therapy in patients after myocardial infarction. Ann. Neurol. 39:301–307; 1996.

Barnett, H.; Eliasziw, M.; Meldrum, H. Drugs and surgery in the prevention of ischemic stroke. N. Engl. J. Med. 332:238–248; 1995.

Barnett, H.; for the North American Symptomatic Carotid Endarterectomy Trial (NASCET). Collaborative Group Results from NASCET—patients with moderate disease (abstract). Cerebrovasc. Dis. 8:21; 1998.

Barnett, H. J.; Boughner, D. R.; Taylor, D. W.; Cooper, P. E.; Kostuk, W. J.; Nichol, P. M. Further evidence relating mitral valve prolapse to cerebral ischemic events. N. Engl. Med. 302:139–144; 1980.

Barrow, D. L.; Reisner, A. Natural history of intracranial aneurysms and vascular malformations. Clin. Neurosurg. 40:3–39; 1993.

Benjamin, E. J.; Plehn, J. F.; D'Agostino, R. B.; Belanger, A. J.; Comai, K.; Fuller, D. L.; Wolf, P. A.; Levy, D. Mitral annular calcification and the risk of stroke in an elderly cohort. N. Engl. J. Med. 327: 374–379; 1992.

Bogousslavsky, J.; Garazi, S.; Jeanrenaud, X.; Aebischer, N.; Van Melle, G.; for the Lausanne Stroke with Paradoxical Embolism Study Group. Stroke recurrence in patients with patent foramen ovale: the Lausanne study. Neurology 46:1301–1305; 1996.

Boon, A.; Lodder, J.; Cheriex, E.; Kessels, F. Mitral annulus calcification is not an independent risk factor for stroke: a cohort study of 657 patients. Neurol 244:535–541; 1997.

Bousser, M.; Eschwege, E.; Hagenah, M.; Lefauconnier, J.; et al. AICLA controlled trial of aspirin and dipyridamole in the secondary prevention of atherothrombotic cerebral ischemia. Stroke 14:5–14; 1983.

Brandt, T.; von Kummer, R.; Muller-Kuppers, M. M.; Hacke, W. Thrombolytic therapy of acute basilar artery occlusion: variables affecting recanalization and outcome. Stroke 27:875–881; 1996.

Bridges, N.; Hellenbrand, W.; Latson, L.; Filiano, J.; Newburger, J.; Lock, J. Transcatheter closure of patent foramen ovale after presumed paradoxical embolism. Circulation 86:1902–1908; 1992.

Broderick, J. P.; Brott, T. G.; Duldner, J. E.; Tomsick, T.; Huster, G. Volume of intracerebral hemorrhage. A powerful and easy-to-use predictor of 30-day mortality. Stroke 24: 987–993; 1993.

Broderick, J.; Brott, T.; Kothari, R.; Miller, R.; et al. The greater Cincinnati/Northern Kentucky stroke study. Preliminary first ever and total incidence rates of stroke among blacks. Stroke 29:415–421; 1998.

Callahan, A.; Berger, B. Balloon angioplasty of intracranial arteries for stroke prevention. J. Neuroimaging 7:232–235; 1997.

Cannegieter, S. C.; Rosendaal, F. R.; Wintzen, A. R.; van der Meer, F. J. M.; Vandenbroucke, J. P.; Briet, E. Optimal oral anticoagulant therapy in patients with mechanical heart valves. N. Engl. J. Med. 333:11–17; 1995.

CAPRIE Steering Committee. A randomised, blinded trial of clopidogrel versus aspirin in patients at risk of ischaemic events (CAPRIE). Lancet 348:1329–1339; 1996.

CASANOVA Study Group. Carotid surgery versus medical therapy in asymptomatic carotid stenosis. Stroke 22:1229–1235; 1991.

CAST (Chinese Acute Stroke Trial) Collaborative Group. CAST: randomised placebo-controlled trial of early aspirin use in 20 000 patients with acute ischaemic stroke. Lancet 349:1641–1649; 1997.

Cervoni, L.; Delfini, R.; Santoro, A.; Cantore, G. Multiple intracranial aneurysms: surgical treatment and outcome. Acta Neurochir (Wien) 124:66–70; 1993.

Chimowitz, M. I.; Kokkinos, J.; Strong, J.; Brown, M. B.; Levine, S. R.; Silliman, S.; Pessin, M. S.; Weichel, E.; Sila, C. A.; Furlan, A. J.; et al. The warfarin-aspirin symptomatic intracranial disease study. Neurology 45:1488–1493; 1995.

Clark, W.; Barnwell, S.; Nesbit, G.; O'Neill, O.; Wynn, M.; Coull, B. Safety and efficacy of percutaneous transluminal angioplasty for intracranial atherosclerotic stenosis. Stroke 26:1200–1204; 1995.

Cohen, A.; Tzourio, C.; Bertrand, B.; Chauvel, C.; Bousser, M.-G.; Amarenco, P. Aortic plaque morphology and vascular events. A follow-up study in patients with ischemic stroke. Circulation 96:3838–3841; 1997.

Dandapani, B. K.; Suzuki, S.; Kelley, R. E.; Reyes-Iglesias, Y.; Duncan, R. C. Relation between blood pressure and outcome in intracerebral hemorrhage. Stroke 26:21–24; 1995.

del Zoppo, G.; Higashida, T.; Furlan, A.; Pessin, M.; Rowley, H.; Gent M.; and the PROACT investigators. PROACT: a phase II randomized trial of recombinant pro-urokinase by direct arterial delivery in acute middle cerebral artery stroke. Stroke 29:4–11; 1998.

del Zoppo, G. J.; Poeck, K.; Pessin, M. S.; Wolpert, S. M.; Furlan, A. J.; Ferbert, A.; Alberts, M. J.; Zivin, J. A.; Wechsler, L.; Busse, O.; Greenlee, R.; Brass, L.; Mohr, J. P.; Feldmann, E.; Hacke, W.; Kase, C. S.; Biller, J.; Gress, D.; Otis, S. M. Recombinant tissue plasminogen activator in acute thrombotic and embolic stroke. Ann. Neurol. 32:78–86; 1992.

Demopoulos, L. A.; Tunick, P. A.; Bernstein, N. E.; Perez, J. L.; Kronzon, I. Protruding atheromas of the aortic arch in symptomatic patients with carotid artery disease. Am. Heart J. 129:40–44; 1995.

Devuyst, G.; Bogousslavsky, J.; Ruchat, P.; Xavier, J.; et al. Prognosis after stroke followed by surgical closure of patent foramen ovale: a prospective follow up study with brain MRI and simultaneous transesophageal and transcranial Doppler ultrasound. Neurology 47:1162–1166; 1996.

Di Tullio, M. R.; Sacco, R. I.; Savoia, M. T.; Sciacca, R. R.; Mendoza, L. M.; Titova, I. V.; Garcia, M.; Zwas, D. R.; Fard, A.; Takuma, S.; Homma, S. Aortic arch atheromas complexity as a risk factor for ischemic stroke in the elderly. Cerebrovasc. Dis. 8 (suppl. 4):1–103; 1998.

Diener, H.; Cunha, L.; Forbes, C.; Sivenius, J.; et al. European Stroke Study 2, dipyridamole and acetylsalicylic acid in the secondary prevention of stroke. J. Neurol. Sci. 143:1–13; 1996.

Dietrich, E. B.; Ndiaye, M.; Reid, D. B. Stenting in the carotid artery: initial experience in 110 patients. J. Endovasc. Surg. 3:42–62; 1996.

Diringer, M. N.; Edwards, D. F. Does modification of the Innsbruck and the Glasgow coma scale improve their ability to predict functional outcome? Arch. Neurol. 54: 606–611; 1997.

Dobkin, B. The economic impact of stroke. Neurology 45(suppl. 1):S6–9; 1995.

Donnan, G. A.; Davis, S. M.; Chambers, B. R.; Gates, P. C.; Hankey, G. J.; McNeil, J. J.; Rosen, D.; Stewart-Wynne, E. G.; Tuck, R. R. Trials of streptokinase in severe acute ischemic stroke. Lancet 345:578–579; 1995.

Dressler, F. A.; Craig, W. R.; Castello, R.; Labovitz, A. J. Mobile aortic atheroma and systemic emboli: efficacy of anticoagulation and influence of plaque morphology on recurrent stroke. J. Am. Coll. Cardiol. 31:134–138; 1998.

Duda, A. M.; Letwin, L. B.; Sutter, F. P.; Goldman, S. M. Does routine use of aortic ultrasonography decrease the stroke rate in coronary artery bypass surgery? Vasc. Surg. 21:98–107; 1995.

Dyken, M.; Barnett, H. J. M.; Easton, D.; Fields, W.; et al. Low dose aspirin and stroke: "it ain't necessarily so." Stroke 23:1395–1399; 1992.

Eicher, J.-C.; Soto, F.-X.; DeNadai, L.; Ressencourt, O.; Falcon-Eicher, S.; Giroud, M.; Louis, P.; Wolf, J.-E. Possible association of thrombotic, nonbacterial vegetations of the mitral ring—mitral annular calcium and stroke. Am. J. Cardiol. 79:1712–1715; 1997.

Eliasziw, M.; Streifler, J.; Fox, A.; Hachinski, V.; et al. Significance of plaque ulceration in symptomatic patients with high grade carotid stenosis. Stroke 25:304–308; 1994.

Ende, D.; Chopra, S.; Rao, P. Transcatheter closure of atrial septal defect or patent foramen ovale with the buttoned device for prevention of recurrence of paradoxic embolism. Am. J. Cardiol. 78:233–236; 1996.

EPIC Investigators. Use of monoclonal antibody directed against the platelet glycoprotein IIb/IIIa receptor in high risk coronary angioplasty. N. Engl. J. Med. 330:956–961; 1994.

EPILOG Investigators. Platelet glycoprotein IIb/IIIa receptor blockade and low dose heparin during percutaneous coronary revascularization. N. Engl. J. Med. 336:1689–1696; 1997.

ESPS Group. The European Stroke Prevention Study (ESPS): principal endpoints. Lancet 2:1351–1354; 1987.

European Carotid Surgery Trialists' Collaborative Group. MRC European Carotid Surgery Trial: interim results of symptomatic patients with severe (70–99%) or with mild (0–29%) carotid stenosis. Lancet 337: 1235–1245; 1991.

Executive Committee for the Asymptomatic Carotid Atherosclerosis Study. Endarterectomy for asymptomatic carotid artery stenosis. JAMA 273:1421–1428; 1995.

Fazio, G. P.; Redberg, R. F.; Winslow, T.; Schiller, N. B. Transesophageal echcardiographically detected atherosclerotic aortic plaque is a marker of coronary artery disease. J. Am. Coll. Cardiol. 21:144–150; 1993.

French Study of Aortic Plaques in Stroke Group. Atherosclerotic disease of the aortic arch as a risk factor for recurrent ischemic stroke. N. Engl. J. Med. 334: 1216–1221; 1996.

Gasecki, A.; Aliasziw, M.; Ferguson, G.; Hachinski, V.; et al. Long-term prognosis and effect of endarterectomy in patients with symptomatic severe carotid stenosis and contralateral carotid stenosis or occlusion: results from NASCET. J. Neurosurg. 83: 778–782; 1995.

Gent, M.; Easton, J.; Hachinski, V.; Panak, E.; et al. The Canadian American ticlopidine study (CATS) in thromboembolic stroke. Lancet 1:1215–1220; 1989.

Grosset, D. G.; McDonald, I.; Cockburn, M.; Straiton, J.; Bullock, R. R. Prediction of delayed neurological deficit after subrachnoid haemorrhage: a CT blood load and Doppler velocity approach. Neuroradiology 36:418–421; 1994.

Grotta, J.; Norris, J.; Kamm, B.; et al. Prevention of stroke with ticlopidine: who benefits most? Neurology 42:111–15; 1992.

Hacke, W.; Kaste, M.; Fieschi, C.; Toni, D.; Lesaffre, E.; von Kummer, R.; Boysen, G.; Bluhmki, E.; Hoxter, G.; Mahagen, M. G.; Hennerici, M. G.; for the ECASS Study Group. Intravenous thrombolysis with recombinant tissue plasminogen activator for acute hemispheric stroke: the European Cooperative Acute Stroke Study (ECASS). JAMA 274:1017–1025; 1995.

Hacke, W.; Zeumer, H.; Ferbert, A.; Bruckmann, H.; del Zoppo, G. J. Intra-arterial thrombolytic therapy improves outcome in patients with acute vertebrobasilar occlusive disease. Stroke 19:1216–1222; 1988.

Hagen, P. T.; Schotz, D. G.; Edwards, W. D. Incidence and size of patent foramen ovale during the first 10 decades of life: an autopsy study of 965 normal hearts. Mayo Clin. Proc. 59:17–20; 1984.

Hanna, J. P.; Sun, J. P.; Furlan, A. J.; Stewart, W. J.; Sila, C. A.; Tan, M. Patent foramen ovale and brain infarct: echocardiographic predictors, recurrence and prevention. Stroke 25:782–786; 1994.

Harvey, J.; Teague, S.; Anderson, J.; Voyles, W.; Thadani, U. Clinically silent atrial septal effects with evidence for cerebral embolization. Ann. Intern. Med. 105:695–697; 1986.

Hass, W.; Easton, J.; Adams, H.; Pryse-Phillips, W.; et al. A randomized trial comparing ticlopidine with aspirin for the prevention of stroke in high risk patients. N. Engl. J. Med. 321:501–507; 1989.

Higashida, R. T.; Tsai, F. Y.; Hallbach, V. V.; Dowd, C. F.; Heishima, G. B. Transluminal angioplasty, thrombolysis and stenting for extracranial and intracranial cerebral vascular disease. J. Intervent. Cardiol. 9:209–214; 1996.

Hojer, C.; Haupt, W. F. Prognostic ranking of AEP and SEP findings in subarachnoid haemorrhage. Analysis of 64 patients. Neurochirurgia 36:110–116; 1993.

Homma, S.; Di Tullio, M.; Sacco, R.; Mihalatos, D.; Li Mandri, G.; Mohr, J. P. Characteristics of patent foramen ovale associated with cryptogenic stroke. A biplane transesophageal echocardiographic study. Stroke 25:582–586; 1994.

Homma, S.; Di Tullio, M.; Sacco, R.; Sciacca, R.; Smith, C.; Mohr, J. Surgical closure of patent foramen ovale in cryptogenic stroke patients. Stroke 28:2376–2381; 1997.

Huemer, M.; Niederwieser, V.; Ladurner, G. Thrombolytic treatment for acute occlusion of the basilar artery. J. Neurol. Neurosurg. Psychiatry 58:227–228; 1995.

Hylek, E. M.; Heiman, H.; Skates, S. H.; Sheehan, M. A.; Singer, D. E. Acetaminophen and other risk factors for excessive warfarin anticoagulation. JAMA 279:657–662; 1998.

Hylek, E. M.; Singer, D. E. Risk factors for intracranial hemorrhage in outpatients taking warfarin. Ann. Intern. Med. 120:897–902; 1994.

IMPACT-II Investigators. Randomised placebo controlled trial of effect of eptifibatide on complications of percutaneous coronary intervention: IMPACT-II. Lancet 349:1422–1428; 1997.

International Stroke Trial Collaborative Group. The International Stroke Trial (IST): a randomised trial of aspirin, subcutaneous heparin, both, or neither among 19 435 patients with acute ischaemic stroke. Lancet 349:1569–1581; 1997.

Jones, E. J.; Kalman, J. M.; Calafiore, P.; Tonkin, A. M.; Donnan, G. A. Proximal aortic atheroma: an independent risk factor for cerebral ischemia. Stroke 26: 218–224; 1995.

Jørgensen, H. S.; Nakayama, H.; Raaschou, H. O.; Olsen, T. S. Intracerebral hemorrhage versus infarction: stroke severity, risk factors, and prognosis. Ann. Neurol. 38:45–50; 1995.

Jørgensen, J. S.; Nakayama, H.; Reith, J.; Raaschou, H. O.; Olsen, T. S. Acute stroke with atrial fibrillation. The Copenhagen Stroke Study. Stroke 27:1765–1769; 1996.

Kachel, R. Results of balloon angioplasty in the carotid arteries. J. Endovasc. Surg. 3:76–79; 1996.

Kassell, N. F.; Torner, J. C.; Jane, J. A.; et al. The International Cooperative Study on the Timing of Aneurysm Surgery. Part 2: surgical results. J. Neurosurg. 73:37–47; 1990.

Katz, E. S.; Tunick, P. A.; Rusinek, H.; Ribakove, G.; Spencer, F. C.; Kronzon, I. Protruding aortic atheromas predict stroke in elderly patients undergoing cardiopulmonary bypass: experience with intraoperative transesophageal echocardiography. J. Am. Coll. Cardiol. 20:70–77; 1992.

Konstantinides, S.; Geibel, A.; Olschewski, M.; Gornandt, L.; et al. A comparison of surgical and medical therapy for atrial septal defect in adults. N. Engl. J. Med. 333:469–73; 1995.

Kronmal, R.; Hart, R.; Manolio, T.; Talbert, R.; et al. Aspirin use and incidence of stroke in the cardiovascular health study. Stroke 29:887–894; 1998.

Landefeld, C. S.; Beyth, R. J. Anticoagulant-related bleeding clinical epidemiology, prediction, and prevention. Am. J. Med. 95:315–328; 1993.

Lanska, D.; Kryscio, R. Geographic distribution of hospitalization rates, case fatality and mortality from stroke in the United States. Neurology 45:634–640; 1995.

Le Roux, P. D.; Elliott, J. P.; Newell, D. W.; Grady, M. S.; Winn, H. R. The incidence of surgical complications is similar in good and poor grade patients undergoing repair of ruptured anterior circulation aneurysms: a retrospective review of 355 patients. Neurosurgery 38:887–895; 1996.

Lechat, P.; Mas, J. L.; Lascault, G.; Loron, P.; et al. Prevalence of patent foramen ovale in patients with stroke. N. Engl. J. Med. 318:1148–1152; 1988.

Leung, D. Y. C.; Black, I. W.; Cranney, G. B.; Hopkins, A. P.; Walsh, W. F. Prognostic implications of left atrial spontaneous echo contrast in nonvalvular atrial fibrillation. J. Am. Coll. Cardiol. 24:755–762; 1994.

Lin, H. J.; Kelly-Hayes, M.; Beiser, A. S.; Kase, C. S.; Benjamin, E. J.; D'Agostino, R. B. Stroke severity in atrial fibrillation. The Framingham Study. Stroke 27:1760–1764; 1996.

Lisk, D. R.; Pasteur, W.; Rhoades, H.; Putnam, R. D.; Grotta, J. C. Early presentation of hemispheric intracerebral hemorrhage: prediction of outcome and guidelines for treatment allocation. Neurology 44: 133–139; 1994.

Liu, F.; Ge, J.; Kupferwasser, I.; Meyer, J.; Mohr-Kahaly, S.; Rohmann, S.; Erbel, R. Has transesophageal echocardiography changed the approach to patients with suspected or known infective endocarditis? Echocardiography 12:637–650; 1995.

Loh, E.; St. John Sutton, M.; Wun, C.- C. C.; Rouleau, J. L.; Flaker, G. C.; Gottlieb, S. S.; Lamas, G. A.; Moye, L. A.; Goldhaber, S. Z.; Pfeffer, M. A. Ventricular dysfunction and the risk of stroke after myocardial infarction. N. Engl. J. Med. 336:251–257; 1997.

Magge, A.; Daniel, W. G.; Frank, G.; et al. Echocardiography in infective endocarditis: reassessment of prognostic implications of vegetation size determined by the transthoracic and the transesophageal approach. J. Am. Coll. Cardiol. 14:631–638; 1989.

Martin, R.; Bogousslavsky, J. Mechanisms of late stroke after myocardial infarct: the Lausanne Stroke Registry. J. Neurol. Neurosurg. Psychiatry 56:760–764; 1993.

Mas, J. L.; Zuber, M.; for the French Study Group on Patent Foramen Ovale and Atrial Septal Aneurysm. Recurrent cerebrovascular events in patients with patent foramen ovale, atrial septal aneurysm, or both and cryptogenic stroke or transient ischemic attack. Am. Heart J. 130:1083–1088; 1995.

Mase, G.; Zorzon, M.; Biasutti, E.; Tasca, G.; Vitrani, BI.; Cazzato, G. Immediate prognosis of primary intracerebral hemorrhage using an easy model for the prediction of survival. Acta Neurol. Scand. 91: 306– 309; 1995.

Matchar, D.; Duncan, P. Cost of stroke. Stroke Clin. Updates 5:9–12; 1994.

Mathur, A.; Roubin, G.; Iyer, S.; Piamsonboon, C.; et al. Predictors of stroke complicating carotid artery stenting. Circulation 97:1239–1245; 1998.

Mayberg, M. R.; Wilson, S. E.; Yatsu, F.; et al. Carotid endarterectomy and prevention of cerebral ischemia in symptomatic carotid stenosis. JAMA 266:3289– 3294; 1991.

Mayer, S. A.; Sacco, R. L.; Shi, T.; Mohr, J. P. Neurologic deterioration in noncomatose patients with supratentorial intracerebral hemorrhage. Neurology 44:1379–1384; 1994.

Mohr, J. P.; Sacco, R. L. Classification of ischemic strokes. In: Barnett, H. J. M.; Mohr, J. P.; Stein, B.; Yatsu, F. M., eds. Stroke. New York: Churchill Livingstone; 1982: p. 272

Mooe, T.; Eriksson, P.; Stegmayr, B. Ischemic stroke after acute myocardial infarction. Stroke 28:762–767; 1997.

Morgenstern, L.; Fox, A.; Sharpe, B.; Eliasziw, M.; et al. The risk and benefits of carotid endarterectomy in patients with near occlusion of the carotid artery. North American Symptomatic Carotid Endarterectomy Trial (NASCET) Group. Neurology 48:911–915; 1997.

Mori, E.; Tabuchi, M.; Yoshida, T.; Yamdori, A. Intracarotid urokinase with thromboembolic occlusion of the middle cerebral artery. Stroke 19:802–812; 1988.

Mori, T.; Mori, K.; Fukuoka, M.; Arisawa, M.; Honda, S. Percutaneous transluminal cerebral angioplasty: serial angiographic follow-up after successful dilation. Neuroradiology 39(2):111–116; 1997.

Multicenter Acute Stroke Trial—Italy (MAST-I) Group. Randomized controlled trial of streptokinase, aspirin, and combination of both in treatment of acute ischemic stroke. Lancet 346:1509–1514; 1995.

Multicenter Acute Stroke Trial—Europe Study Group. Thrombolytic therapy with streptokinase in acute ischemic. N. Engl. J. Med. 335:145–150; 1996.

NINDS rt-PA Stroke Study Group. Tissue plasminogen activator for acute ischemic stroke. N. Engl. J. Med. 333:1581–1587; 1995.

Nishimura, R. A.; McGoon, M. D.; Shub, C.; Miller, F. A., Jr.; Ilstrup, D. M.; Tajik, A. J. Echocardiographically documented mitral-valve prolapse. Long term follow-up of 237 patients. N. Engl. J. Med. 313: 1305–1309; 1985.

North American Symptomatic Carotid Endarterectomy Trial Collaborators. Beneficial effect of carotid endarterectomy in symptomatic patients with high-grade carotid stenosis. N. Engl. J. Med. 325:445– 453; 1991.

Olafsson, E.; Hauser, W. A.; Gudmundsson, G: A population-based study of prognosis of ruptured cerebral aneurysm: mortality and recurrence of subarachnoid hemorrhage. Neurology 48:1191–1195; 1997.

Orencia, A. J.; Petty, G. W.; Khandheria, B. K.; Annegers, J. F.; Ballard, D. J.; Sicks, J. D.; O'Fallon, W. M.; Whisnant, J. P. Risk of stroke with mitral valve prolapse in population-based cohort study. Stroke 26:7–13; 1995.

Orencia, A. J.; Petty, G. W.; Khandheria, B. K.; Annegers, J. F.; Ballard, D. J.; Sicks, J. D.; O'Fallon, W. M.; Whisnant, J. P. Mitral valve prolapse and the risk of stroke after initial cerebral ischemia. Neurology 45:1083–1086; 1995.

Orz, Y.; Kobayashi, S.; Osawa, M.; Tanaka, Y: Aneurysm size: a prognostic factor for rupture. Br. J. Neurosurg. 11:144–149; 1997.

Paddock-Eliasziw, L.; Eliasziw, M.; Barr, H.; Barnett, H.; for the North American Symptomatic Carotid Endarterectomy Group. Long-term prognosis and the effect of carotid endarterectomy in patients with recurrent ipsilateral ischemic events. Neurology 47:1158–1162; 1996.

Parthenakis, F.; Skalidis, E.; Simantirakis, E.; Kounali, D.; Vardas, P.; Nihoyannopoulos, P. Absence of atherosclerotic lesions in the thoracic aorta indicates absence of significant coronary artery disease. Am. J. Cardiol. 77:1118–1121; 1996.

Perry, J. R.; Szalai, J. P.; Norris, J. W.; for the Canadian Stroke Consortium. Consensus against both endarterectomy and routine screening for asymptomatic carotid artery stenosis. Arch. Neurol. 54:25–28; 1997.

Pessin, M. S.; Estol, C. J.; Lafranchise, F.; Caplan, L. R. Safety of anticoagulation after hemorrhagic infarction. Neurology 43:1298–1303; 1993.

Peto, R.; Gray, R.; Collins, R.; Wheatley, K.; et al. Randomized trial of prophylactic daily aspirin in British male doctors. BMJ 296:313–316; 1988.

Pickard, J. D.; Murray, G. D.; Illingworth, R.; et al. Effect of oral nimodipine on cerebral infarction and outcome after subarachnoid haemorrhage: British Aneurysm Nimodipine Trial (BRANT). BMJ 298:636–642; 1989.

Publication Committee for the Trial of ORG 10172 in Acute Stroke Treatment (TOAST) Investigators. Low molecular weight heparinoid, ORG 10172 (Danaparoid), and outcome after acute ischemic stroke. A randomized controlled trial. JAMA 279:1265–1272; 1998.

Qureshi, A. I.; Safdar, K.; Weil, J.; Barch, C.; Bliwise, D. L.; Colohan, A. R.; Mackay, B.; Frankel, M. R. Predictors of early deterioration and mortality in black Americans with spontaneous intracerebral hemorrhage. Stroke 26:1764–1767; 1995.

Ranke, C.; Hecker, H.; Creutzig, A.; Alexander, K. Dose dependent effect of aspirin on carotid atherosclerosis. Circulation 87:1873–1879; 1993.

Reynen, K. Cardiac myxomas. N. Engl. J. Med. 333:1610–1617; 1995.

Rinkel, G. J. E. ; van Gijn, J.; Wijdicks, E. F. M. Subarachnoid hemorrhage without detectable aneurysm: a review of the causes. Stroke 24:1403–1409; 1993.

Rohmann, S.; Erbel, R.; Darius, H.; et al. Spontaneous echo contrast imaging in infective endocarditis: a predictor of complications? Int. J. Card. Imaging 8:197–207; 1992.

Rosenorn, J.; Eskesen, V. Patients with ruptured intracranial saccular aneurysms: clinical features and outcome according to size. Br. J. Neurosurg. 8:73–78; 1994.

Rosenow, F.; Hojer, C.; Meyer-Lohmann, C.; Hilgers, R. D.; Muhlhofer, H.; Kleindienst, A.; Owega, A.; Koning, W.; Heiss, W. D. Spontaneous intracerebral hemorrhage. Prognostic factors in 896 cases. Acta Neurol. Scand. 96:174–182; 1997.

Sacco, R.; Ellenberg, J.; Mohr, J.; Tatemichi, T.; Hier, D.; Price, T.; Wolf, P. Infarcts of undetermined cause: the NINCDS Stroke Data Bank. Ann. Neurol. 25:383–390; 1989.

Sasaki, O.; Takeuchi, S.; Koike, T.; Koizumi, T.; Tanaka, R. Fibrinolytic therapy for acute embolic stroke: intravenous, intracarotid, and intra-arterial local approaches. Neurosurgery 36:246–253; 1995.

Schievink, W. I.; Wijdicks, E. F. M.; Piepgras, D. G.; Chu, C.-P.; O'Fallon, W. M.; Whisnant, J. P. The poor prognosis of ruptured intracranial aneurysms of the posterior circulation. J. Neurosurg. 82:791–795; 1995.

Schomig, A.; Neumann,: Kastrati, A.; Schuhlen, H.; et al. A randomized comparison of antiplatelet and anticoagulation therapy after placement of coronary-artery stents. N. Engl. J. Med. 334:1084–1089; 1996.

Sharma, A.; Ofili, E.; Castello, R.; Sullivan, N.; Labovitz, A. Effect of treatment on recurrent embolic events with atrial septal aneurysm and associated right to left shunting (abstract). J. Am. Soc. Echocardiogr. 43:294; 1996.

Shimoda, M.; Oda, S.; Tsugane, R.; Sato, O. Prognostic factors in delayed ischaemic deficit with vasospasm in patients undergoing early aneurysm surgery. Br. J. Neurosurg. 11:210–215; 1997.

Sloan, M. A.; Pirzada, S. R.; Ornato, J. P.; Gurwitz, J. H.; Gore, J. M.; Tiefenbrunn, A. J.; French, W. J.; Weaver, W. D.; Rogers, W. J. The rate of ischemic stroke following acute myocardial infarction is decreasing. The national registry of myocardial infarction experience. J. Am. Coll. Cardiol. 31:406A; 1998.

SPAF III Writing Committee for the Stroke Prevention in Atrial Fibrillation Investigators. Patients with nonvalvular atrial fibrillation at low risk of stroke during treatment with aspirin. JAMA 279:1273–1277; 1998.

Steering Committee of the Physicians' Health Study Research Group. Final report on aspirin component of the ongoing Physicians' Health Study. N. Engl. J. Med. 321:129–135; 1989.

Stone, D. A.; Godard, J.; Corretti, M. C.; Kittner, S. J.; Sample, C.; Price, T. R.; Plotnick, G. D. Patent foramen ovale: association between the degree of shunt by contrast transesophageal echocardiography and the risk of future ischemic neurologic events. Am. Heart J. 131:158–161; 1996.

Stroke Prevention in Atrial Fibrillation Investigators Committee on Echocardiography. Transesophageal echocardiography correlates of thromboembolism in high-risk patients with nonvalvular atrial fibrillation. Ann. Intern Med. 128:639–347; 1998.

Stroke Prevention in Reversible Ischemia Trial (SPIRIT) Study Group. A randomized trial of anticoagulants versus aspirin after cerebral ischemia of presumed arterial origin. Ann. Neurol. 42:857–865; 1997.

Takis, C.; Kwan, E.; Pessin, M.; Jacobs, D.; Caplan, L. Intracranial angioplasty: experience and complications. AJNR Am. J. Neuroradiol. 18:1661–1668; 1997.

Tanne, D.; Reicher-Reiss, H.; Boyko, V.; Behar, S. Stroke risk after anterior wall acute myocardial infarction. Am. J. Cardiol. 76:825–826; 1995.

Tcheng, J.; Harrington, R.; Kotke-Marchant, K.; Kleiman, N.; et al. Multicenter randomized, double blind, placebo-controlled trial of platelet integrin glycoprotein IIb/IIIa blocker Integrelin in elective coronary intervention. Circulation 91:2151–2157; 1995.

Terayama Y.; Tanahashi, N.; Fukuuchi, Y.; Gotoh, F. Prognostic value of admission blood pressure in patients with intracerebral hemorrhage. Keio Cooperative Stroke Study. Stroke 28: 1185–1188; 1997.

Theron, J. Angioplasty of brachiocephalic vessels. In: Vinuela, V.; Halbach, V. V.; Dion, J. E., eds. Interventional neuroradiology: endovascular therapy of the central nervous system. New York: Raven Press, 1992: p. 167–180.

Thompson, T.; Evans, W. Paradoxical embolism. Q. J. Med. 23:135–150; 1930.

Timsit, S. G.; Sacco, R. L.; Mohr, J. P.; Foulkes, M. A.; Tatemichi, T. K.; Wolf, P. A.; Price, T. R.; Hier, D. B. Brain infarction severity differs according to cardiac or arterial embolic source. Neurology 43:728–733; 1993.

Trehan, N.; Mishra, M.; Dhole, S.; Mishra, A.; Karlekar, A.; Kohli, V. M. Significantly reduced incidence of stroke during coronary artery bypass grafting using transesophageal echocardiography. Eur. J. Cardio-thorac. Surg. 11:234–242; 1997.

Tribouilloy, C.; Peltier, M.; Colas, L.; Rida, Z.; Rey, J.-L.; Lesbre, J.-P. Multiplane transoesophageal echocardiographic absence of thoracic aortic plaque is a powerful predictor for absence of significant coronary artery disease in valvular patients, even in the elderly. Eur. Heart J. 18:1478–1483; 1997.

Tuhrim, S.; Horowitz, D. R.; Sacher, M.; Godbold, J. H. Validation and comparison of models predicting survival following intracerebral hemorrhage. Crit. Care Med. 23:950–954; 1995.

Tunick, P. A.; Kronzon, I. Protruding atherosclerotic plaque in the aortic arch of patients with systemic embolization: a new finding seen by transesopha-geal ecocardiography. Am. Heart J. 120:658–660; 1990.

Tunick, P. A.; Rosenzweig, B. P.; Katz, E. S.; Freedberg, R. S.; Perez, J. L.; Kronzon, I. High risk for vascular events in patients with protruding aortic atheromas: a prospective study. J. Am. Coll. Cardiol. 23:1085–1090; 1994.

Vermeij, F. H.; Hasan, D.; Vermuelen, M.; Tanghe, H. L. J.; van Gijn, J. Predictive factors for deterioration from hydrocephalus after subarachnoid hemorrhage. Neurology 44:1851–1855; 1994.

von Sohsten, R.; Ahmar, W.; Dawan, R.; Ren, J.; Jyotinagaram, M.; Daralis, D.; Chaudhry, F. Prognostic implication of mobile vs. complex aortic plaque: a transesophageal echocardiographic study (abstract). J. Am. Coll. Cardiol. 31(suppl. C): 1366; 1998.

Wholey, M.; Wholey, M.; Bergeron, P.; Diethrich, E.; et al. Current global status of carotid artery stent placement. Cathet. Cardiovasc. Diagn. 44:1–6; 1998.

Wijdicks, E. F. M.; Nichols, D. A.; Thielen, K. R.; Fulgham, J. R.; Brown, R. D.; Meissner, I.; Meyer, F. B.; Piepgras, D. G. Intra-arterial thrombolysis in acute basilar artery thromboembolism: the initial Mayo Clinic experience. Mayo Clin. Proc. 72:1005–1013; 1997.

Yadav, S.; Roubin, G.; Iyer, S.; et al. Elective stenting of the extracranial carotid arteries. Circulation 95: 376–381; 1997.

Yoshida, K.; Nakamura, S.; Watanabe, H.; Kinoshita, K. Early cerebral blood flow and vascular reactivity to acetazolamide in predicting the outcome after ruptured cerebral aneurysm. Acta Neurol. Scand. 166(suppl):131–134; 1996.

Yoshimoto, Y.; Wakai, S.; Ochiai, C.; Nagai, M. Significance of pupillary reactivity in poor-grade aneurysm patients as a prognostic factor and an indication for active treatment. Br. J. Neurosurg. 11: 25–31; 1997.

Zabalgoitia, M.; Halperin, J. L.; Pearce, L. A.; Blackshear, J. L.; Asinger, R. W.; Hart, R. G. Transesophageal echocardiographic correlates of clinical risk of thromboembolism in nonvalvular atrial fibrillation. J. Am. Coll. Cardiol. 31:1622–1626; 1998.

Zhu, W.; Khandheria, B.; Warnes, C.; Seward, J.; Danielson, G. Closure of patent foramen for cryptogenic stroke in you patients: long term follow-up (abstract). Circulation 86:I-147; 1992.

Zorzon, M. G.; Biasutti, M.; Tasca, G.; Vitrani, B.; Cassato, G. Immediate prognosis of primary intracerebral hemorrhage using an easy model for the prediction of survival. Acta Neurol. Scand. 91:306–309; 1995.

# PART III

# CRANIAL NERVES AND BRAIN STEM

# 7

# Neuro-Ophthalmology

ANDREW G. LEE AND PAUL W. BRAZIS

Neuro-ophthalmology is the specialty dealing with neurologic diseases affecting the visual system. The subspecialty bridges the gap between the disciplines of neurology, ophthalmology, and neurosurgery. Unfortunately, the prognosis for the majority of neuro-ophthalmologic problems has often been poor and patients have historically had very few treatment options. Nevertheless, there are some notable exceptions that are highlighted in this chapter (e.g., optic neuritis). In addition, although traditionally neuro-ophthalmology has been a diagnostic rather than therapeutic subspecialty, recent advances in the understanding of basic disease pathophysiology, neuroimaging, and neurosurgical techniques have improved visual outcomes in many patients with neuro-ophthalmic conditions. We review the prognosis for some of the more common neuro-ophthalmic diseases.

## Optic Neuritis

Optic neuritis (ON) is an immune-mediated, demyelinating disease of the optic nerve that typically presents with the following clinical profile: (1) acute, usually unilateral loss of visual acuity, color vision, and/or visual field that usually progresses over 7 days or less, and begins to improve over the following 30 days; (2) a relative afferent pupillary defect in unilateral or bilateral, but asymmetrical cases; (3) periocular pain, especially with eye movement in 90% of patients; (4) usually normal (i.e., retrobulbar) in 65%, but sometimes swollen (i.e., papillitis) optic nerve head in 35% of patients, occasionally with eventual optic disc atrophy after 4 to 6 weeks; and (5) often a young adult female (but may affect patients of any age and either gender).

Although corticosteroids have been the mainstay of therapy for acute ON, well-controlled data to support treatment efficacy until recently have been lacking. The Optic Neuritis Treatment Trial (ONTT) was subsequently developed to evaluate the efficacy of corticosteroid treatment for acute ON and investigate the relationship between ON and multiple sclerosis (MS). The ONTT was a National Eye Institute–sponsored randomized, controlled clinical trial that enrolled 457 patients at 15 clinical centers in the United States between the years 1988 and 1991 (Beck and Trobe 1992). The ONTT entry criteria included:

1. Patients who were between the ages of 18 and 46 years.
2. Patients had an afferent pupillary defect and a visual field defect in the affected eye consistent with the clinical diagnosis of ON.

3. Patients were examined within 8 days of the onset of visual symptoms of a first attack of acute unilateral ON.

The patients were randomly assigned to one of three treatment arms in the study:

1. Intravenous (IV) methylprednisolone sodium succinate (250 mg every 6 hours for 3 days) followed by oral prednisone (1 mg/kg/d for 11 days).
2. Oral prednisone (1 mg/kg/d for 14 days).
3. Oral placebo for 14 days.

The major conclusions of the ONTT related to treatment are summarized as follows:

1. High-dose IV followed by oral corticosteroids accelerated visual recovery, but provided no long-term benefit to vision.
2. "Standard dose" oral prednisone alone did not improve the visual outcome, and was associated with an increased rate of new attacks of ON.
3. IV corticosteroids followed by oral corticosteroids reduced the rate of development of clinically definite MS during the first 2 years, particularly in patients with signal abnormalities on brain magnetic resonance imaging (MRI), but by 3 years the treatment effect had subsided.

Based on these results, the authors recommended that treatment with oral prednisone in standard doses be avoided in ON, and that treatment with IV methylprednisolone be considered in patients with abnormal MRI of the brain or a particular need (such as a monocular patient or occupational requirement) to recover visual function more rapidly. Although brain MRI may not be necessary for diagnosis of ON, neuroimaging may be valuable for prognostic purposes. In the ONTT, patients with multiple signal abnormalities on MRI most clearly benefited from IV corticosteroid therapy in terms of the development of MS, but the rate of development of MS was too low in the patients with normal MRI to assess. An improved short-term effect on vision and lack of long-term influence on vision of IV corticosteroids has been supported by other randomized studies (Sellebjerg, 1999; Wakakura,1999).

1. Patients in the IV corticosteroid group started to recover vision sooner than those in the other two groups. Median visual acuity improved to 20/25 by 4 days after entry in the IV group and by 15 days in the other two groups. By 30 days, difference among groups were sufficiently small to be of little visual consequence.
2. Eighty-eight percent of patients improved at least 1 Snellen line by day 15 after study entry and 96% improved at least 1 Snellen line by 30 days.
3. For most patients, recovery of visual acuity was nearly complete by 30 days after study entry. Among the patients with incomplete recovery by 30 days, most showed slow gradual improvement for up to 1 year.
4. Visual acuity worsened after discontinuation of treatment in only ten (2%) patients.
5. Visual recovery generally begins within the first 2 weeks after the onset of visual symptoms. Much of the recovery occurs by the end of 1 month; thereafter, a slow continued recovery of any remaining deficit occurs for several months. Patients with incomplete recovery at 6 months may continue to improve slightly between 6 months and 1 year follow-up. Lack of at least 1 line of visual acuity improvement within the first 3 weeks after the onset of visual symptoms should be considered atypical (although the cause may still be due to optic neuritis, if there is no definite MS history, then consider inflammatory, infectious, or compressive causes for the optic neuropathy). Worsening of vision after termination of steroid course is also atypical and requires further investigation regarding etiology.
6. The only predictor of poor visual outcome was poor visual acuity at the time of study entry. Even so, of 160 patients starting with visual acuity 20/200 or worse, all had at least some improvement and only eight (5%) had visual acuities that were still 20/200 or worse at 6 months. Of 30 patients whose initial visual acuity was light perception or no light perception, 20 (67%) recovered to 20/40 or better. Baseline acuity was the best predictor of 6-month visual acuity outcome; older age was statistically associated with a slightly worse outcome but this appeared to be of no clinical importance.

At 5-year follow-up for 347 (87%) of 545 patients in the ONTT (Optic Neuritis Study Group 1997a), most affected eyes had normal or only slightly abnormal visual acuity and the results did not significantly differ by treatment group. Visual acuity in affected eyes was 20/25 or better in 87%, 20/25 to 20/40 in 7%, 20/50 to 20/190 in 3%, and 20/200 or worse in 3%. Recurrence of ON in either eye occurred in 28% of patients and was more frequent in those with MS and in patients without MS who were in the prednisone treatment group. Most eyes with a recurrence retained normal or almost normal visual function. Thus, most patients retain good or excellent vision 5 years following an attack of ON, even if the ON recurred. In African American patients, visual acuities with ON may be more severely affected at onset and after 1 year of follow-up compared to white patients (Phillips et al. 1998).

Thus, although most patients with idiopathic or demyelinating ON recover visual function within 30 days, some patients do not experience complete recovery. Other patients, despite 20/20 Snellen visual acuity, complain of subjective visual loss that may correspond with persistent defects of color vision, contrast sensitivity, depth perception, visual field, or motion perception (Cleary et al. 1997). In the ONTT, visual acuity was 20/40 or better in 93% of patients at 12 months, but 3% of patients had 20/200 or worse visual acuity.

Patients with idiopathic ON (especially those with multiple periventricular white matter abnormalities on MRI) are at risk for the development of MS. The rate of development of MS following ON is quite variable in the literature. For example, Rizzo and Lessell, in a study of 60 New England Caucasians with optic neuritis, noted that the risk of developing clinical MS by 15 years was 69% for women and 33% for men (Rizzo and Lessell 1988). Rodriguez et al., incorporating life-table analysis, showed that 39% of 95 patients with isolated optic neuritis in an incidence cohort had progressed to clinically definite MS by 10 years of follow-up, 49% by 20 years, 54% by 30 years, and 60% by 40 years (Rodriguez et al. 1995). These latter authors noted no difference in developing MS between men and women.

In the ONTT, the 5-year cumulative probability of clinically definite MS (CDMS) was 30% and did not differ by treatment group (Optic Neuritis Study Group 1997b). Neurological impairment in the patients who developed CDMS was generally mild. Brain MRI performed at study entry was a strong predictor of CDMS, with the five–year risk of CDMS ranging from 16% in the 202 patients with no MRI lesions to 51% in 89 patients with three or more MRI lesions. Independent of brain MRI, the presence of prior nonspecific neurological symptoms was also predictive of the development of CDMS. Lack of pain, the presence of disc swelling (particularly if severe or associated with hemorrhages or exudate), and mild visual acuity loss (20/40 or better) were features of the ON associated with a low risk of CDMS among the 189 patients who had no brain MRI lesions and no history of neurological symptoms or ON in the fellow eye. CDMS developed by 5 years in 0 of 19 patients whose visual loss was painless, 8 of 90 patients (9%) whose visual acuty at entry was 20/40 or better, and in 6 of 78 (8%) who had swollen optic discs. Among patients with swollen disc, CDMS did not develop in any patient who had severe disc edema, disc or peripapillary hemorrhages, or macular exudates. Thus, the 5-year risk of CDMS following optic neuritis is highly dependent on the number of lesions present on brain MRI. However, even a normal brain MRI does not preclude the development of CDMS. In these patients with no brain MRI lesions, certain clinical features identify a subgroup with a low 5-year risk of CDMS.

The presence of oligoclonal bands in the cerebrospinal fluid (CSF) is associated with development of CDMS (Cole et al. 1998). However, the results suggest that CSF analysis is only useful in the risk assessment of ON patients when the MRI is normal and not predictive when MRI lesions are present at the time of ON. CDMS developed within 5 years in 22 of 76 patients (29%), 16 of 38 (42%) patients with oligoclonal bands present and 6 of 38 (16%) without bands. Among the 39 patients with normal MRI, CDMS developed in 3 of 11 (27%) with bands present but in only one patient (4%) without bands. In contrast, among 37 patients with abnormal MRIs, CDMS developed in 13 of 27 (48%) with bands and five of ten (50%) without bands.

In summary, factors that increase the risk of MS in patients with ON include abnormal MRI, prior nonspecific neurological symptoms, increased CSF IgG or the presence of oligoclonal bands, the use of oral corticosteroids, and a previous history of ON; factors that decrease the subsequent risk of MS include a normal MRI, absence of eye pain, marked disc swelling, bilateral simultaneous ON at onset, and childhood onset of ON (Frederiksen 1997; Jacobs et al. 1997; Lucchinetti et al. 1997).

## Nonarteritic Anterior Ischemic Optic Neuropathy

Anterior ischemic optic neuropathy (AION) is typically characterized clinically by the acute onset of usually painless unilateral visual loss in a middle-aged to older patient (usually age >50 years); an ipsilateral afferent pupillary defect; and swelling of the optic nerve head with or without peripapillary hemorrhages (Arnold and Hepler 1994). The presence of optic disc edema in the acute phase allows the diagnosis of AION to be made. Later, the optic disc usually develops sector or diffuse pallor or may develop glaucomatous like cupping.

Although it is rare for nonarteritic AION (NA-AION) to recur in the same eye, it may involve the fellow eye in 10.5% to 73% of cases, with most authors citing contralateral eye involvement in 25% to 40% of cases. In patients with bilateral disease, the final outcome between the eyes is similar for acuity, color vision, and visual fields (visual acuity in 81% within 3 Snellen lines, color vision in 69% within three plates, and computerized visual field in 75% within 5 dB of the mean deviation) (Boone et al. 1996).

The visual loss in AION is often acute and usually remains static, but may deteriorate after onset. For example, Arnold and Helper (1994) studied visual acuity and perimetry in the acute (<3 days after onset) and convalescent (>3 months after onset) phases of diseases in 27 patients with NA-AION. Six of the patients had progressive visual loss while 21 remained stable. Overall, significant worsening occurred in 11.1% for visual acuity and 22.2% for visual field. In the Ischemic Optic Neuropathy Decompression Trial (see below), 45% of patients reported worsening (subjective) of vision between the onset of visual symptoms and baseline exam (Ischemic Optic Neuropathy Decompression Trial Study Group 1996). Although vision may deteriorate in patients with NA-AION after the initial ictus, progression in patients with presumed AION, in our opinion, should prompt further evaluation, including neuroimaging, to exclude other causes of a progressive optic neuropathy.

Patients with typical features of AION (acute onset unilateral visual loss and ipsilateral optic disc edema in an older patient) do not require neuroimaging. The major entity that needs to be excluded in AION is giant cell arteritis (GCA). An erythrocyte sedimentation rate (ESR) and other appropriate evaluation for GCA should be performed in all cases of AION in which there is a clinical possibility for GCA. Patients with atypical features should be evaluated for other etiologies of an optic neuropathy.

Unfortunately, although corticosteroids (systemic, retrobulbar, subtenon), anticoagulation, acetazolamide, hemodilution, vasodilators, vasopressors, atropine, norepinephrine, diphenylhydantoin, and hyperbaric oxygen have been tried in the past, there remains no proven therapy for NA-AION. Most patients with NA-AION are left with significant residual impairment of visual acuity and/or visual fields. The natural history of NA-AION in the past has been difficult to define. In the Ischemic Optic Neuropathy Decompression Trial (Ischemic Optic Neuropathy Decompression Trial Group 1995), there was an unexpectedly high rate of spontaneous improvement (defined as ≥3 lines improvement of visual acuity from baseline at 6 months) in 42.7% of patients. This rate of improvement is higher than the previous literature on AION before 1989 (<10%). However, even with this improvement, many patients are left with significant visual impairment.

NA-AION is associated with an increased risk of subsequent stroke or myocardial infarction (Sawle et al. 1990) but is not a marker for atherosclerotic carotid artery stenosis (Fry et al. 1993). Medical control of underlying hypertension, diabetes, and other presumed etiologic vasculopathic risk factors (such as smoking cessation) has been recommended, but there are no well-controlled data on the efficacy of such measures. Aspirin is often given to patients following the development of NA-AION, but there does not seem to be any beneficial effect of treatment on eventual visual outcome. Some authors, however, have suggested that aspirin therapy might reduce the risk of AION in the fellow eye (Kupersmith et al. 1995).

The well-designed, masked, prospective, randomized Ischemic Optic Neuropathy Decompression Trial (IONDT) at 25 clinical centers was initiated with the support of the National Eye Institute. The study inclusion criteria included a clinical syndrome consistent with NA-AION (i.e., acute, unilateral visual loss, afferent pupillary defect, swollen optic nerve), age greater than 50 years, visual symptoms for less than 14 days from onset, and visual acuity of 20/64 or worse. Patients were randomly assigned to either optic nerve sheath fenestration (ONSF) (119 patients) or a control group (125 patients). Surgery was performed by experienced, protocol-certified study surgeons. The primary outcome measure was a 3 or more line improvement of visual acuity after 6 months, and visual field mean deviation on the Humphrey Field Analyzer (Program 24-2) was a secondary outcome measure. In the study population, initial visual acuities were 20/200 or worse in 34% of the patients. Recruitment was halted in September 1994 on the recommendation of the study's Data and Safety Monitoring Committee. After 6 months, 32.6% of the ONSF (surgery) group had improved 3 or more lines of visual acuity compared with 42.7% of the control group; but 23.9% of the ONSF group had lost 3 or more lines of visual acuity compared with only 12.4% of the control group. Likewise, visual field data confirmed a lack of benefit for surgery. The 3-month and 12-month data were confirmed by the findings of the 6-month data. In addition, there was no indication of benefit from ONSF in the subgroup of patients with progressive visual loss. The authors concluded that "ONSF is not effective and may be harmful in NA-AION", but were careful to state that they could "offer no recommendation regarding the safety and efficacy of this surgery for other conditions" (Ischemic Optic Neuropathy Decompression Trial Group 1995). We agree that ONSF should not be performed for NA-AION.

## Giant Cell Arteritis

Giant cell (temporal or cranial) arteritis is an inflammatory vasculopathy of the elderly affecting medium- to large-sized arteries. GCA may present with numerous systemic and ocular manifestations. GCA usually causes visual loss as the result of AION. All patients older than age 50 with AION should be suspected of having GCA (McDonnell et al. 1986).

In 1990, the American College of Rheumatology analyzed 33 criteria for GCA. The highest sensitivity criteria were:

1. Age greater than 50 years old
   Mean age 69 years old
   90% greater than 60 years

2. Westergren ESR greater than 50 mm/h
3. Abnormal temporal artery biopsy (TAB)

The highest specificity criteria were:

1. Jaw, tongue claudication
2. Visual abnormalities (e.g., AION, amaurosis, optic atrophy)
3. Temporal artery abnormalities (e.g., decreased pulse, tenderness or nodules)

If at least three or more criteria of the following five were met, the specificity of diagnosis was 91.2% and the sensitivity was 93.5%:

1. Age greater than 50 years
2. New headache (localized)
3. Temporal artery abnormality (e.g., tender or decreased pulse)
4. Elevated ESR (>50 mm/h)
5. Abnormal TAB (e.g., necrotizing arteritis, multinucleated giant cells)

The TAB is a relatively easy and safe procedure to perform with low morbidity. Patients in whom a unilateral TAB is negative and a strong clinical suspicion for GCA exists should undergo a TAB on the contralateral side. In order to minimize cost, some authors have advocated that a frozen section be performed on the symptomatic side TAB, and if it is normal, proceed at the same sitting with a contralateral TAB. Unilaterally positive TABs have been demonstrated in 8% to 14% of retrospective bilateral TAB series.

Untreated GCA may result in significant visual loss in one or both eyes. Therefore, it is imperative that corticosteroid therapy begin immediately upon clinical suspicion of GCA to prevent visual loss (i.e., before the diagnostic TAB and laboratory confirmation). Most authors have recommended an initial dose of prednisone of 1.0 mg/kg to 1.5 mg/kg/d (60 to 100 mg/d).

The visual loss with arteritic AION is often more profound than that with NA-AION. Without treatment, the second eye is affected in approximately 75% of cases (simultaneous bilateral visual loss is highly suggestive of arteritic AION). If the fellow eye becomes affected, approximately one-third will do so within 24 hours, another one-third within 1 week, and most of the remainder within 4 weeks.

The visual morbidity in GCA was studied by Liu et al. (1994), who studied 45 patients with biopsy-proven GCA who had visual symptoms and 41 patients (63 eyes) who lost vision (mean follow-up, 50 weeks). The authors observed the following:

1. Visual loss was unilateral in 19 patients (46%), sequential in 15 patients (37%) (mean interval between eyes, 23 days; range, 1 to 219 days; median, 5 days), and simultaneous in 7 patients (17%).
2. The etiology of visual loss (63 eyes) was AION in 55 patients (88%), posterior ischemic optic neuropathy in 2 patients (3%), central retinal artery occlusion in three patients (5%), branch retinal artery occlusion in three patients (5%), choroidal infarction in four patients (6%), and optic atrophy of unclear etiology in three patients (5%).
3. The temporal profile of visual loss was sudden in 46 eyes (73%) and gradual or stepwise over 2 days to 3 weeks in 11 eyes (15%).
4. AION developed in 88% of eyes. In these patients, visual acuity was 20/200 or worse in 70%, 21% had no light perception, and the majority of field defects in testable eyes, aside from central scotomas associated with loss, showed altitudinal or arcuate patterns.
5. Six patients lost vision during steroid treatment for systemic symptoms of GCA, whereas in 39 patients visual symptoms prompted steroid treatment.
6. For visual symptoms, 25 patients received IV methylprednisolone (250 mg 4 times daily for 3 to 5 days), whereas 20 received oral prednisone alone. In the 41 patients with visual loss, vision was unchanged in 20 (49%), worsened in seven (17%), and improved in 14 (34%). Subsequent fellow eye involvement was observed only with oral therapy, and a greater percentage of patients (9 of 23 [39%] vs. 5 of 18 [28%]) improved with IV treatment.

The authors concluded that in patients with visual loss due to GCA, there was a 34% chance for some improvement in visual function after steroid treatment. IV therapy may diminish the likelihood of fellow eye involvement and was associated with a slightly better prognosis for visual improvement. Other authors have, however, documented progressive visual loss from GCA despite high-dose intravenous methylprednisolone (Cornblath and Eggenberger 1997).

Thus, although some patients note improvement in symptoms within 1 to 2 days of starting steroid therapy, other patients may experience visual loss, despite adequate corticosteroid therapy. Too rapid or early reduction of steroid therapy in GCA may also precipitate visual loss. Most patients can be tapered off steroids within 1 year, but some patients (especially those with neurological symptoms) may require prolonged (years) or indefinite therapy and recurrences may occur years later.

## Traumatic Optic Neuropathy

Traumatic optic neuropathy (TON) is a clinical diagnosis characterized by (1) a history of direct or indirect impact injury to the head, face, or orbit; (2) unilateral or bilateral visual loss; (3) variable loss of visual acuity (range 20/20 to no light perception); (4) variable loss of visual field; (5) an afferent pupillary defect (unilateral or bilateral but asymmetrical cases); and (6) normal or less commonly swollen optic nerve. Other etiologies of visual loss in the setting of trauma (e.g., open globe, traumatic cataract, vitreous hemorrhage, retinal detachment) must be excluded.

Once the clinical diagnosis of TON is made, neuroimaging should be performed if possible. The incidence of visible canal fracture in TON is variable and does not correlate well with the severity of visual loss. Computed tomography (CT) scans may be the best test in the setting of trauma for the evaluation of the emergent patient with TON, for detailed examination for bone fractures, for evaluation of the bone anatomy, and for the detection of acute hemorrhage.

The natural history of TON is unknown. Hughes described 56 cases of untreated TON, of which 44% were permanently blind and 16% gained useful vision (Hughes 1962). There are, however, no large, well-controlled, randomized, prospective data regarding the treatment of TON. The literature on medical and surgical treatment of TON is thus difficult to summarize accurately due to the variations in clinical presentation, treatment modalities (e.g., steroids alone, steroids with surgery, surgery alone), variable surgical techniques and approaches, variable study inclusion criteria, recruitment bias, small sample sizes, and different outcome measures. Cook et al. in 1996 reviewed all cases of TON published in the English language literature and performed a meta-analysis of treatment results (Cook et al. 1996). Recovery of vision was significantly better in patients who underwent treatment than in those having observation alone. No significant difference in improvement was noted among patients treated with corticosteroids alone, surgical decompression alone, or combination of these modalities. The prognosis for visual recovery worsened with increasing severity of grade. Recovery of vision was better in patients without orbital fractures, and was better in patients with anterior rather than posterior fractures.

Chou et al. in 1996 summarized the treatment results from the literature (28 reports) and found improvement in 94 (53%) of 176 medical treatment patients; 219 (46%) of 477 surgical treatment patients; and 25 of 81 (31%) patients without treatment (Chou et al. 1996).

Although the mainstay of medical treatment for TON has been corticosteroids, there are no prospective data to support the efficacy of treatment or validity of the various steroid preparations, dosage, or duration of therapy.

Since there are no double-masked, placebo-controlled, prospective, randomized data for the treatment of TON, many authors have advocated extrapolating data on the use of higher dose methylprednisolone (MP) for central nervous system (CNS) injury. The first National Acute Spinal Cord Injury Study (NASCIS 1) (Bracken and Holford 1993) was a non–placebo-controlled study that concluded that there was no beneficial effect of MP 1000 mg bolus then 1000 mg/d for 10 days ("high dose") compared with MP 100 mg bolus then 100 mg/d for 10 days ("standard dose"). NASCIS 2 was a multicenter, placebo-controlled, randomized, double-masked study of acute spinal cord injury that showed treatment within 8 hours with MP 30 mg/kg bolus followed by 5.4 mg/kg/h for 24 hours resulted in significant improvement in motor and sensory function compared to placebo. MP delivered after 8 hours did not improve neurologic outcome. It was felt that MP in the 15 to 30 mg/kg dose range has a different pharmacologic effect on CNS injury parameters including blood flow, calcium homeostasis, energy metabolism, and clinical outcome.

Multiple surgical approaches (e.g., lateral facial, transantral, transconjunctival/intranasal endoscopic, sublabial transnasal, transfrontal, trans-

ethmoidal, or combination approaches, extracranial vs. intracranial) and surgical indications have been offered for the treatment of TON. Unfortunately, there is no prospective evidence to support the use of any one surgical approach to the optic nerve over another.

Joseph et al. reported 14 patients in a retrospective, nonconsecutive study with TON treated with transethmoidal-sphenoidal canal decompression and dexamethasone pre- and postoperatively. Eleven of the 14 patients improved, including three of five patients who presented with no light perception vision (Joseph et al. 1990). Unfortunately, until a randomized, prospective, double-masked, placebo-controlled clinical trial is performed the treatment of TON will remain controversial.

## Ocular Motor Cranial Nerve Palsies

Ocular motor cranial nerve palsies may occur in isolation or associated with other localizing neurologic signs and symptoms (nonisolated). The ocular motor cranial nerves travel from their respective nuclei in the brainstem, pass important neurologic structures in the brainstem, enter the subarachnoid space, travel within the cavernous sinus, and finally enter the orbit through the superior orbital fissure to innervate their target organs. Thus, most nonisolated ocular motor cranial neuropathies can be topographically localized by the "company they keep" (e.g., a third-nerve palsy in association with brain stem signs, such as a contralateral hemiparesis, or a sixth-nerve palsy in association with cavernous sinus signs, such as a Horner's syndrome). The etiologies of an ocular motor cranial neuropathy include neoplastic (e.g., benign or malignant tumors), traumatic, congenital, vascular (e.g., aneurysm), or ischemic. The prognosis of recovery of an ocular motor cranial neuropathy depends in part upon treatment of the underlying etiology.

A long-standing palsy due to congenital, traumatic, infectious, inflammatory, or compressive etiologies may require prism therapy or strabismus surgery to alleviate diplopia. Alternatively, a palsy due to these same etiologies may resolve spontaneously or resolve following treatment of the underlying disorder. The variable recovery rate for these palsies makes it difficult to estimate prognosis for these conditions. Vasculopathic isolated ocular motor cranial neuropathies, on the other hand, do not require any initial neuroimaging studies, and observation for improvement over the next 6 to 8 weeks is recommended. Patients with vasculopathic palsy often resolve spontaneously within 4 to 6 months. Rush and Younge (1981) reported a recovery rate for fourth-nerve palsy of 53.5% in 172 nonselected cases, and a higher recovery rate of 71% in 166 patients with diabetes mellitus, hypertension, or atherosclerosis. Ksiazek et al. (1981) reported improvement in 90% of 39 patients with microvascular and idiopathic fourth-nerve palsies within 6 months' time. Vasculopathic sixth-nerve palsies (SNPs) may be observed (without neuroimaging) for improvement for 4 to 12 weeks. Some authors have recommended observing vasculopathic isolated SNP beyond a 3-month interval of recovery if the esotropia and the abduction deficit were decreasing. Nonvasculopathic SNPs have a significant (27%) chance of harboring an underlying malignant neoplasm.

Vasculopathic palsies usually improve within a few months, and patients with progressive or unresolved signs, or patients with new neurological signs or symptoms, should have neuroimaging. Patients with spontaneously resolving palsies do not require any further neuroimaging. It is recommended that elderly patients who present with headache, scalp tenderness, jaw claudication, or visual loss undergo an appropriate evaluation for GCA, including an ESR and a TAB. Evaluation for myasthenia gravis should be particularly considered in any patient with a painless, nonproptotic, pupil-spared ophthalmoplegia.

## Horner's Syndrome

Interruption of the ocular sympathetic pathway is known as Horner's syndrome (HS). HS is characterized most frequently by the following clinical signs: ipsilateral mild ptosis; "upside-down ptosis" and apparent enophthalmos; anisocoria due to ipsilateral miosis; dilation lag (slow dilation of the pupil with the HS after the lights are dimmed); and variable facial anhidrosis (due to preganglionic lesions). The syndrome may result from a lesion anywhere along a three-neuron pathway that arises as a first-order (central) neuron from the posterolateral hypothalamus, descends the brain stem and lateral column of the spinal cord to exit at the cervical (C8)–thoracic (T2) level (cilio-

spinal center of Budge) of the spinal cord as a second-order neuron. This second-order (intermediate) preganglionic neuron exits the ventral root and arches over the apex of the lung and ascends the cervical sympathetic chain to synapse in the superior cervical ganglion and exits as a third-order neuron. The neural fibers for sweating of the face travel with the external carotid artery and the third-order postganglionic neuron travels with the carotid artery into the cavernous sinus, onto the abducens nerve for a short course, and then with the ophthalmic division of the trigeminal nerve join the nasociliary branch, pass through the ciliary ganglion, and reach the eye as long and short ciliary nerves.

The evaluation of HS includes two stages: (1) recognition of the clinical syndrome and (2) confirmation and localization by pharmacologic testing. We divide HS into several types and discuss the management recommendations for each type.

The HS per se usually does not result in any symptomatic deficit. The prognosis, however, is related to the underlying etiology. Patients with a clear temporal association of the onset of a HS with trauma (neck, chest), iatrogenic (e.g., central lines, neck or chest surgery, chest tubes), or intentional surgical damage (e.g., sympathectomy) to the sympathetic chain do not require any further evaluation.

Patients with an HS that cannot be localized by clinical examination alone should undergo pharmacologic confirmation and topographical localization to the preganglionic or postganglionic level. Cocaine inhibits the reuptake of norepinephrine at the neuromuscular junction. Therefore, topical 5% to 10% cocaine will dilate a normal pupil (the mydriatic effect is small and is usually about 1 mm) but will not dilate a pupil with an HS (regardless of the location of the affected sympathetic neuron). Minimal or no dilation of the pupil after topical cocaine confirms that an HS exists but does not localize to preganglionic or postganglionic lesion. Hydroxyamphetamine stimulates the release of norepinephrine from the junction and therefore will dilate a HS pupil if the lesion is preganglionic but will not dilate the pupil if the lesion is postganglionic.

Grimson and Thompson reported 120 patients with HS. Of these 120 patients, 41% were preganglionic HS, and one-half of these preganglionic HS were due to underlying neoplasm (Grimson and Thompson 1979). Maloney et al. reported an etiology in 270 (60%) of 450 cases of HS. Of the 180 cases without a defined etiology, 65 (35%) were re-examined (6 months to 28 years later) without a definite etiology and the authors believed that this indicated a benign and stable origin to the HS. The etiology of the remaining 270 cases included 60 (13%) tumors (23 benign lesions and 37 malignant lesions); 54 (12%) cluster headaches; 45 (10%) iatrogenic cases (e.g., neck surgery and carotid angiography); 18 (4%) Raeder's syndromes; 18 (4%) trauma; 13 (3%) cervical disc protrusions; 13 (3%) congenital cases; 13 (3%) vascular occlusions; nine (2%) vascular anomalies, and 27 (6%) miscellaneous (e.g., pneumothorax, herpes zoster, cervical rib, and mediastinal lymphadenopathy) cases. Of these 270 cases, 34 (13%) were central preganglionic HS, 120 (44%) were intermediate preganglionic HS, and 116 (43%) were peripheral postganglionic HS. Of particular interest, 13 patients in this series had undetected malignancy, and ten were due to primary or metastatic tumor involving the pulmonary apex. Nine of these ten (90%) patients had arm pain (due to presumed involvement of the adjacent sympathetic chain and C8–T2 nerves) as a complaint.

Giles and Henderson reported a 35.6% incidence (77 cases) of HS due to underlying neoplasm. Of these 77 cases, 58 were malignant (mostly bronchogenic carcinoma and metastatic disease) and 19 were benign (e.g., neurofibroma and thyroid adenoma) (Giles and Henderson 1958).

Patients with preganglionic lesions should have imaging directed towards the preganglionic sympathetic chain to exclude malignancy (especially chest neoplasms). Patients with a postganglionic HS and other neurological signs and symptoms (e.g., third, fourth, or sixth cranial neuropathy) should have imaging directed towards the postganglionic sympathetic pathway (i.e., cavernous sinus). Isolated postganglionic HS, on the other hand, are usually benign and do not require aggressive evaluation.

## Ocular Myasthenia Gravis

Myasthenia gravis (MG) is a clinical syndrome characterized by muscular weakness due to dysfunction of the neuromuscular junction. MG often affects the eyelids and extraocular muscles and may mimic any painless, pupil-spared, nonproptotic ophthalmoplegia. Ocular myasthenia (OM) is a form of MG confined to the extraocular, levator palpebrae superioris, and/or orbicularis oculi muscles. Variability and fatigability of ptosis or ophthalmoplegia are the hallmarks of OM. Additional signs of OM include enhancement of ptosis (worsening of contralateral ptosis with ipsilateral lid elevation), lid fatigue on sustained upgaze, orbicularis oculi weakness, and the Cogan's lid twitch sign (overshoot of the upper eyelids after refixation to primary from a downgaze position).

Intravenous edrophonium (Tensilon) may improve the signs and symptoms of OM (i.e., ptosis or ophthalmoplegia) as a diagnostic test. Acetylcholine receptor antibodies may be detected in the serum of up to 90% of patients with generalized MG but in only 50% of patients with OM. Electromyography (especially single-fiber or repetitive stimulation) may also be useful in confirming the diagnosis. The treatment of ocular MG includes patching to alleviate diplopia or medical treatments such as pyridostigmine, corticosteroids, or other immunosuppressive agents. Stable ocular deviations or ptosis due to ocular MG may be amenable to surgical treatment. Thymectomy may be indicated, especially in patients with thymic abnormalities (e.g., thymic hyperplasia or thymoma) and may improve the symptoms of ocular and generalized MG. Most patients with ocular MG improve with therapy over time.

Approximately 50% of patients with MG initially present with OM, but only 12% to 50% of these remain ocular (Grob 1953; Ferguson et al. 1955; Garland and Clark 1956; Schlezinger and Fairfax 1959; Perle et al. 1966; Simpson et al. 1966; Bever et al. 1983; Grob et al. 1987; Evoli et al. 1988; Oosterhuis 1988, 1989). Of the 50 to 80 percent of patients with purely ocular symptoms and signs at onset that go on to develop generalized, most, but not all, develop generalized symptoms within 2 to 3 years of onset of the disorder. Bever et al. (1983) performed a retrospective study and found that 226 (84%) of 269 myasthenics displayed ocular findings at onset of disease and 142 (53%) demonstrated only ocular involvement. Follow-up (average, 14 years; range, 1 to 39 years) of 108 patients with MG who had only ocular symptoms and signs at onset showed that 43 (40%) remained ocular and 53 (49%) became generalized. Of the 53 patients that became generalized, 44 (83%) did so within 2 years of onset of the disease. Age of onset in their patients was of prognostic significance. Patients older than 50 years at onset had a greater risk of generalized MG and severe complications, while patients younger at onset had a more benign outcome. In another study of 1487 myasthenic patients, 53% presented with ocular MG and 202 (15%) continued to demonstrate purely ocular involvement for up to 45 years of follow-up (mean, 17 years) (Grob et al. 1987). Of those patients with strictly ocular signs and symptoms during the first month after onset (400 of the 1487 patients), 66% subsequently developed clinically generalized disease; of these, 78% became generalized within 1 year after onset of symptoms and 94% within 3 years.

About 10% to 20% of patients with OM will undergo spontaneous remission, which may be temporary or permanent (Simpson et al. 1966). While corticosteroid treatment produces a higher incidence of remission and improvement, there is no evidence that anticholinesterase agents affect the course of the disease (Grob et al. 1987; Kupersmith et al. 1996). Kupersmith et al. reported a retrospective review of 32 patients with OM who were treated with corticosteroids and followed for a minimum of 2 years (Kupersmith et al. 1996). Patients were treated with one or more courses of daily prednisone (the highest initial dose, 40 to 80 mg) gradually withdrawn over 4 to 6 weeks. Subsequently, in six patients, 2.5 to 20 mg of prednisone was given on alternate days for more than 6 months. Two years after diagnosis, generalized MG had developed in three patients (9.4%); elevated acetylcholine receptor antibody levels and abnormal electrophysiologic studies were not predictive of worsening. Of the 16 patients that had follow-up for 3 years and the 13 that had follow-up for 4 or more years, ocular motility was normal in 56% at 3 years and 62% at 4 years with two additional patients developing generalized MG at 4 years. The authors concluded that moderate dose daily prednisone for 4 to 6 weeks, followed by low-dose alternate-day therapy as needed, can control the diplopia of OM and that the frequency of deterioration to generalized MG at 2 years may be reduced. Sommer et al. retrospectively analyzed 78 patients with OM with a mean disease duration of 8.3 years (Sommer et al. 1997). In 54 patients (69%) symptoms and

signs remained confined to the extraocular muscles during the observation period, while the remaining 24 patients (31%) developed symptoms of generalized myasthenia (50% of them within 2 years and 75% within 4 years after onset). A somewhat reduced risk of generalization was found in those with mild symptoms, normal repetitive stimulation studies, and low or absent acetylcholine receptor antibodies at the time of diagnosis.

Patients receiving immunosuppressive treatment (corticosteroids and/or azathioprine) rarely developed generalized myasthenia (6 of 50, or 12%). Those without such treatment, usually due to uncertain diagnosis and late referral, converted into generalized myasthenia significantly more often (18 of 28, or 64%). The authors concluded that short-term corticosteroids and long-term azathioprine seemed adequate to achieve remission in most patients. The proportion of patients developing generalized myasthenia gravis was smaller in this population compared to previously published groups and early immunosuppressive treatment was thought to be at least partially responsible for this finding. Thymectomy (performed in 12 patients with an abnormal chest CT) also correlated with a good outcome, but had no apparent advantage over medical treatment alone (Sommer et al. 1997).

Until a prospective clinical trial of corticosteroids or other immunosuppressive is performed in patients with OM, the value of these agents in the prevention of the development of generalized MG remains undefined.

## Pseudotumor Cerebri

Pseudotumor cerebri (PTC) is a clinical syndrome characterized by (1) signs and symptoms limited to increased intracranial pressure (e.g., headache, papilledema, sixth-nerve palsy); (2) a normal neuroimaging study; and (3) normal cerebrospinal fluid content with an elevated opening pressure. The major complications of PTC are headache and visual loss due to papilledema.

PTC typically occurs in obese, young females and the diagnosis should be considered atypical in thin, male, or elderly patients. Evaluation for exposure to exogenous agents that may cause PTC (e.g., lithium, tetracycline) or sinus thrombosis should he performed in these individuals. Thus, in patients with an atypical presentation or course, in addition to standard neuroimaging studies (preferably MRI) and cerebrospinal fluid analysis (with opening pressure) consideration should be given to ruling out sinus thrombosis (e.g., MR venogram).

Visual field loss, with or without visual acuity loss, may occur in patients with PTC (Wall and George 1991; Corbett et al. 1982). The exact incidence of visual loss in patients is unknown. Some authors have noted that 13% of eyes of patients at initial visit have acuity greater than 20/20 with 10% abnormal at final visit. Visual field loss in at least one eye (other than enlarged blind spot) was found in 96% of patients with Goldmann perimetry and 92% with automated perimetry (Wall and George 1991; Corbett et al. 1982). The loss of vision in patients with PTC may be indolent and progressive leading to blindness. Occasionally, acute visual loss may occur due to ischemic optic neuropathy, subretinal hemorrhage from neovascular membrane, central retinal artery occlusion, branch retinal artery occlusion, or central retinal vein occlusion. The only risk factor for visual loss in the series of Corbett et al. (1982) was systemic hypertension.

The treatment of PTC includes medical and surgical options. Weight loss in obese individuals is a reasonable and safe treatment and gastric reduction surgery has been reported to improve PTC in selected obese individuals (Sugerman et al. 1995). Acetazolamide is first-line therapy, but other second-line medications have been used with anecdotal success including furosemide, methazolamide, and digoxin. Corticosteroids may be a useful adjunctive therapy in patients with acute visual loss but may increase weight gain, and corticosteroid use/withdrawal has been associated with PTC.

Patients who fail, are intolerant to, or are noncompliant with medical therapy may be treated surgically. Repeat lumbar punctures have not proven to be effective, may be poorly tolerated, and have little theoretical basis for success, since the rapid rate of cerebrospinal fluid formation would preclude any short-term benefit. Optic nerve sheath decompression is generally safe and effective and usually results in rapid resolution of ipsilateral disc edema and improvement in visual loss (Spoor et al. 1991). Lumboperitoneal shunting may also improve papilledema and visual loss.

# References

Arnold, A. C.; Hepler, R. S.. Natural history of nonarteritic anterior ischemic optic neuropathy. J. Neuroophthalmol 14:66; 1994.

Beck, R. W.; Trobe, J. D. What we have learned from the optic neuritis treatment trial. Ophthalmology 102:1504; 1992.

Bever, C. T., Jr.; Aquino, A. V.; Penn, A. S.; et al. Prognosis of ocular myasthenia gravis. Ann. Neurol. 14:516–519; 1983.

Boone, M. I.; Massry, G. G.; Frankel, R. A.; et al. Visual outcome in bilateral nonarteritic ischemic optic neuropathy. Ophthalmology 103:1223–1228; 1996.

Bracken, M. B.; Holford, T. R. Effects of timing of methylprednisolone or naloxone administration on recovery of segmental and Ion-tract neurologic function in NASCIS 2. J. Neurosurg. 79:500–507; 1993.

Bracken, M. B.; Shepard, M. J.; Hellenbrand, K. G.; et al. Methylprednisolone and neurological function 1 year after spinal cord injury. Results of the National Acute Spinal Cord Injury Study. J. Neurosurg. 63:713; 1985.

Chou, P. J.; Sadun, A. A.; Chen, Y. C.; Su, W. Y.; Lin, S. Z.; Lee, C. C. Clinical experiences in the management of traumatic optic neuropathy. Neuroophthalmology 18:325–336; 1996.

Cleary, P. A.; Beck, R. W.; Bourque, L. B.; et al. Visual symptoms after optic neuritis. Results from the ONTT. J. Neuroophthalmol. 17:18–28; 1997.

Cole, S. R.; Beck, R. W.; Moke, P. S.; et al. The predictive value of CSF oligoclonal banding for MS 5 years after optic neuritis. Neurology 51:885–887; 1998.

Cornblath, W. T.; Eggenberger, E. R. Progressive visual loss from giant cell arteritis despite high-dose intravenous methylprednisolone. Ophthalmology 104:854–858; 1997.

Cook, M. W.; Levin, L. A.; Joseph, M. P.; Pinczower, E. F. Traumatic optic neuropathy. A meta-analysis. Arch. Otolaryngol. Head Neck Surg. 122:389–392; 1996.

Corbett, J. J.; Savino, P. J.; Thompson, H. S.; et al. Visual loss in pseudotumor cerebri. Follow-up of 57 patients from five to 41 years and a profile of 14 patients with permanent severe visual loss. Arch. Neurol. 39:461; 1982.

Evoli, A.; Tonali, P.; Bartoccioni, A. P.; Lo Monaco, M. Ocular myasthenia: diagnostic and therapeutic problems. Acta Neurol. Scand. 77:31–35; 1988.

Ferguson, F. R.; Hutchinson, E. C.; Liversedge, L. A. Myasthenia gravis: results of medical management. Lancet 2:636–639; 1955.

Frederiksen, J. L. Bilateral acute optic neuritis: prospective clinical, MRI, CSF, neurophysiological and HLA findings. Neuroophthalmology 17:175–183; 1997.

Fry, C. L.; Carter, J. E.; Kanter, M. C.; et al. Anterior ischemic optic neuropathy is not associated with carotid artery atherosclerosis. Stroke 24:539–542; 1993.

Garland, H.; Clark, A. N. G. Myasthenia gravis: a personal study of 60 cases. Br. Med. J. 2:1259–1262; 1956.

Giles, C. L.; Henderson, J. W. Horner's syndrome: an analysis of 216 cases. Am. J. Ophthalmol. 46:289–296; 1958.

Grimson, B. S.; Thompson, H. S. Horner's syndrome: overall view of 120 cases. In: Thompson, H. S.; ed. Topics in neuro-ophthalmology. Baltimore: Williams & Wilkins; 1979: 151–156.

Grob, D. Course and management of myasthenia gravis. JAMA 153:529–532; 1953.

Grob, D.; Arsura, E.; Brunner, N.; Namba, T. The course of myasthenia and therapies affecting outcome. Ann. N. Y. Acad. Sci. 505:472–499; 1987.

Hughes, B. Indirect injury of the optic nerve and chiasm. Bull. Johns Hopkins Hosp. 111:98–126; 1962.

Ischemic Optic Neuropathy Decompression Trial Research Group. Optic nerve decompression surgery for nonarteritic anterior ischemic optic neuropathy (NAION) is not effective and may be harmful. JAMA 273:625; 1995.

Ischemic Optic Neuropathy Decompression Trial Study Group. Characteristics of patients with non-arteritic anterior ischemic optic neuropathy eligible for the Ischemic Optic Neuropathy Decompression Trial. Arch. Ophthalmol. 114:1366–1374; 1996.

Jacobs, L. D.; Kaba, S. E.; Miller, C. M.; et al. Correlation of clinical, magnetic resonance imaging, and cerebrospinal fluid findings in optic neuritis. Ann. Neuol. 41:392–398; 1997.

Joseph, M. P.; Lessell, S.; Rizzo J., Momose, K. J. Extracranial optic nerve decompression for traumatic optic neuropathy. Arch. Ophthalmol. 108:1091–1093; 1990.

Ksiazek, S.; Behar, R.; Savino, P. J.; et al. Isolated acquired fourth nerve palsies. Neurology 38 (suppl. 1):246; 1988.

Kupersmith, M. J.; Frohman, I. P.; Sanderson, M. C.; et al. Aspirin reduces second eye anterior ischemic optic neuropathy. Ophthalmology 102:104; 1995.

Kupersmith, M. J.; Moster, M.; Bhuiyan, S.; et al. Beneficial effects of corticosteroids on ocular myasthenia gravis. Arch. Neurol. 53:802–804; 1996.

Liu, G. T.; Glaser, J. S.; Schatz, N. J.; Smith, J. L. Visual morbidity in giant cell arteritis. Clinical characteristics and prognosis for vision. Ophthalmology 101:1779–1785; 1994.

Lucchinetti, C. F.; Kiers, L.; O'Duffy, A.; et al. Risk factors for developing multiple sclerosis after childhood optic neuritis. Neurology 49:1413–1418; 1997.

McDonnell, P. J.; Moore, G. W.; Miller, N. R.; et al. Temporal arteritis: a clinicopathologic study. Ophthalmology 93:518; 1986.

Optic Neuritis Study Group. Visual function 5 years after optic neuritis. Experience of the Optic Neuritis Treatment Trial. Arch. Ophthalmol. 115:1545–1552; 1997a.

Optic Neuritis Study Group. The 5-year risk of MS after optic neuritis. Experience of the Optic Neuritis Treatment Trial. Neurology 49:1404–1413; 1997b.

Oosterhuis, H. J. G. H. Long-term effects of treatment in 374 patients with myasthenia gravis. Monogr. Allergy 25:75–85; 1988.

Oosterhuis, H. J. G. H. The natural course of myasthenia gravis: a long term follow up study. J. Neurol. Neurosurg. Psychiatry 52:1121–1127; 1989.

Perlo, V. P.; Poskanzer, D. C.; Schwab, R. S.; et al. Myasthenia gravis: evaluation of treatment in 1,335 patients. Neurology 16:431–439; 1966.

Phillips, P. H.; Newman, N. J.; Lynn, M. J. Optic neuritis in African Americans. Arch. Neurol. 55:186–192; 1998.

Rizzo, J. F., III; Lessell, S. Risk of developing multiple sclerosis after uncomplicated optic neuritis: a long-term prospective study. Neurology 38: 185–190; 1988.

Rodriguez, M.; Siva, A.; Cross, S. A.; et al. Optic neuritis: a population-based study in Olmsted County, Minnesota. Neurology 45:244–250; 1995.

Rush, J. A.; Younge, B. R. Paralysis of cranial nerves III, IV, and VI. Arch. Ophthalmol. 99:76–79; 1981.

Sawle, G. V.; James, C. B.; Russell, R. W. The natural history of non-arteritic ischemic optic neuropathy. J. Neurol. Neurosurg. Psychiatry 53:830–833; 1990.

Schlezinger, N. S.; Fairfax, W. A. Evaluation of ocular signs and symptoms in myasthenia gravis. Arch. Ophthalmol. 62:985–990; 1959.

Sellebjerg, F.; Nielsen, S.; Frederiksen, J. L.; Olesen, J. A randomized, controlled trial of oral high-dose methylprednisolone in acute optic neuritis. Neurology 52:1479–1484; 1999.

Simpson, J. A.; Westerberg, M. R.; Magee, K. R. Myasthenia gravis: an analysis of 295 cases. Acta Neurol. Scand. 42:1–27; 1966.

Sommer, N.; Sigg, B.; Melms, A.; et al. Ocular myathenia gravis: response to long term immunosuppressive treatment. J. Neurol. Neurosurg. Psychiatry 62:156–162; 1997.

Spoor, T. C.; Ramocki, J. M.; Madion, M. P.; et al. Treatment of pseudotumor cerebri by primary and secondary optic nerve sheath decompression. Am. J. Ophthalmol. 112:177; 1991.

Sugerman, H. J.; Felton, W. L., III; Salvant, J. B., Jr.; et al. Effects of surgically induced weight loss on idiopathic intracranial hypertension in morbid obesity. Neurology 45:1655–1659; 1995.

Wakakura, M.; Minei-Higa, R.; Oono, S.; et al. Baseline features of idiopathic optic neuritis as determined by a multicenter treatment trial in Japan. Jpn. J. Ophthalmol. 43:127–132; 1999.

Wall, M.; George, D. Idiopathic intracranial hypertension (pseudotumor cerebri): a prospective study of 50 patients. Brain 114:155; 1991.

# 8

# Neuro-Otology

ROBERT W. BALOH

Since vertigo and other forms of dizziness have so many different causes, the key in determining treatment and prognosis is to make a correct diagnosis. Vertigo always indicates an imbalance in the vestibular system. Determining early on whether the vertigo is of central or peripheral origin is critically important because some central causes are life threatening and may require immediate intervention. Vertigo of peripheral origin (labyrinth and/or eight nerve) usually resolves over hours to days whereas, if the central lesion is the cause, the vertigo will typically persist and nearly always is accompanied by other neurological signs. This chapter describes the prognosis and treatment of the common peripheral causes of vertigo.

## Vestibular Neuritis

Vestibular neuritis (vestibular neuronitis) presents with a gradual onset of vertigo, nausea, and vomiting for several hours (Dix and Hallpike 1952; Schuknecht and Kitamura 1981; Silvoniemi 1988; Baloh et al. 1996). The symptoms usually reach a peak within 24 hours and then gradually resolve after several days. During the first day, the patient is off-balance and has difficulty focusing because of spontaneous nystagmus. These acute symptoms typically resolve within 2 to 3 days, but

often it takes several weeks before the patient feels well enough to return to normal activities. About two-thirds of patients have a benign course with complete recovery within 1 to 3 months. There are important exceptions to this rule, however. Occasionally, patients, particularly the elderly, will have intractable dizziness that persists for years. At least one recurrent bout of vertigo (usually less severe than the initial bout) occurs in 20% to 30% of patients. This may represent reactivation of a latent virus because it is often associated with a systemic viral illness. A small percentage of patients will have multiple recurrent episodes of vertigo, leading to a profound bilateral vestibulopathy (called bilateral sequential vestibular neuritis) (Schuknecht and Witt 1985). The episodic vertigo eventually is replaced by a persistent disequilibrium and oscillopsia (Baloh et al. 1989).

## Management

The optimum management of patients with vestibular neuritis is controversial because the pathophysiology is uncertain. Unless there is convincing evidence to suspect a vascular or nonviral infectious cause, the patient should be managed as a case of presumed viral neuritis (i.e., symptomatic treatment of the acute vertigo with antivertiginous medication). Although steroids have been recommended for their anti-inflammatory effect (Ariyasu et al. 1990), there have been no controlled studies to assess the risk-benefit ratio for these drugs. Although approximately one-third of patients with vestibular neuritis have a permanent loss of vestibular function (as documented by serial caloric examinations), the central nervous system (CNS) is able to adapt to the vestibular loss, and residual symptoms usually are minimal once the compensation has occurred (Böhmer 1996). Vestibular exercises should be started immediately after the acute vomiting and nausea subside, and they should be continued until the dizziness and imbalance are minimal (Herdman 1996).

## Bacterial Labyrinthitis

Two types of labyrinthitis are associated with bacterial infections of the temporal bone: (1) serous or toxic labyrinthitis in which bacterial toxins or chemical products invade the inner ear and (2) suppurative labyrinthitis in which bacteria invade the inner ear. The former often leads to only subtle symptoms, such as an insidious high-frequency sensorineural hearing loss, whereas the latter typically leads to a profound combined auditory and vestibular loss with little or no recovery.

Serous labyrinthitis is probably the most common complication of acute or chronic middle ear infection. The toxins or inflammatory cells penetrate the basilar membrane and invade the endolymph at the basal turn of the cochlea. Damage to this region of the cochlea explains the high incidence of high-frequency sensorineural hearing loss in patients with chronic otitis media (Paparella et al. 1980). Acute suppurative labyrinthitis is manifested by the sudden onset of severe vertigo, nausea, vomiting, and unilateral deafness. The infection originates in the middle ear or the cerebrospinal fluid (CSF). When the labyrinthitis is a direct complication of middle ear disease, it is more likely to occur from chronic otitis media and mastoiditis than from an acute middle ear infection. The most common port of entry of bacteria into the inner ear, however, is from the spinal fluid in patients with meningitis (Dichgans et al. 1999). Meningogenic bacterial labyrinthitis is usually bilateral, whereas direct invasion from a chronic otitic infection is almost always uni-

lateral. Endolymphatic hydrops can be a sequela of both serous and suppurative labyrinthitis (Schuknecht 1978).

## Management

Management of bacterial labyrinthitis is directed at the associated infection of the middle ear, mastoid and, if present, meninges. A patient with acute or chronic bacterial ear disease associated with sudden or rapidly progressive inner ear symptoms should be hospitalized and treated with local cleansing and topical antibiotic solutions to the affected ear and parenteral antibiotics capable of penetrating the blood-brain barrier (Neely 1993). Surgical intervention to eradicate the middle ear and mastoid infection usually is required after a few days of antibiotic treatment. If the labyrinthitis is secondary to a primary meningitis, it is best to treat the underlying meningitis. A resistant or recurrent meningitis may result from an unrecognized posterior fossa epidural abscess with dural perforation or from a congenital direct communication with the CSF.

## Viral Labyrinthitis

Of the thousands of infants born deaf every year, approximately 20% are thought to be the result of congenital viral infections of the inner ear (Pappas 1983). More than 4000 people are stricken each year with "sudden deafness," a unilateral, infrequently bilateral, sensorineural hearing loss of acute onset, presumed to be of viral origin in most cases (Wilson et al. 1983). An acute onset of intense vertigo (some due to viral vestibular neuritis, others to labyrinthitis) strikes a similar number of people. The most convincing evidence for a viral cause of these isolated auditory and vestibular syndromes comes from the temporal bone studies of Schuknecht (1985) and Schuknecht et al. (1986) in Boston. These pathological studies are supported by experimental studies in animals in which it has been shown that several viruses will selectively infect the labyrinth or the eighth nerve (Davis and Johnson 1983; Nomura et al. 1985).

Viral labyrinthitis can present with sudden deafness (usually unilateral and rarely bilateral), acute vertigo (with associated autonomic symptoms), or a combination of auditory and vestibular symptoms. Although the term *sudden deafness* is commonly used, the hearing loss due to viral infection usually takes several hours and may evolve over several days (Wilson et al. 1983). The sudden hearing loss reverses, at least partially, in most cases. It returns to normal in more than 50% of patients (with or without treatment). Tinnitus and fullness in the involved ear also are common.

## Management

As in vestibular neuritis, management of viral labyrinthitis is directed at the symptoms. Vestibular exercises are begun as soon as possible to accelerate the compensation process (Herdman 1996). Antiviral agents, such as cytosine arabinase and acyclovir, have been used for treating systemic viral illnesses in children; however, it is unclear whether the hearing loss often associated with disorders such as cytomegalovirus and rubella infections is altered by this treatment. There have been no reports of the efficacy of antiviral agents in adults with presumed viral labyrinthitis.

## Syphilitic Labyrinthitis

Syphilitic infections remain an important cause of vertigo and hearing loss despite the general availability of penicillin. Syphilitic infections produce auditory and vestibular symptoms by two mechanisms: meningitis with involvement of the eight nerve and osteitis of the temporal bone with associated labyrinthitis. The former typically occurs as an early manifestation of acquired syphilis, whereas the latter occurs as a late manifestation of both congenital and acquired syphilis. With early acquired syphilis, the predominant pathological finding is basilar meningitis affecting the eighth nerve, particularly the auditory branch. The hearing loss typically occurs with the rash and lymphadenopathy of secondary syphilis (Saltiel et al. 1983). Usually it is abrupt in onset, tends to be bilateral, and is rapidly progressive. Vestibular symptoms often are absent. Patients may demonstrate symptoms and signs of meningitis, including headache, stiff neck, cranial nerve palsies, and optic neuritis.

Both congenital and acquired syphilitic infections produce temporal bone osteitis and labyrinthitis as a late manifestation. The congenital variety is approximately three times as common as the acquired variety (Morrison 1975). The time of onset of congenital syphilitic labyrinthitis is anywhere from the first to seventh decades, with the peak incidence in the fourth and fifth decades. Acquired syphilitic labyrinthitis rarely occurs before the fourth decade and has a peak incidence in the fifth and sixth decades. The natural history of syphilitic labyrinthitis is a slow, relentless progression to profound or total bilateral loss of vestibular and auditory function (Morrison 1975; Steckelberg and McDonald 1984). This progression is marked by episodes of sudden deafness, vertigo, and fluctuation in the magnitude of hearing loss and tinnitus.

## Management

Penicillin is the treatment of choice for the otological manifestations of syphilis. Because CSF infection accompanies the early manifestations of acquired syphilis, high-dose intravenous penicillin is recommended. If the penicillin is begun early, the prognosis is excellent; complete recovery of hearing and vestibular function usually occurs (Saltiel et al. 1983). For the late manifestations of congenital and acquired syphilitic labyrinthitis, the combination of steroids and penicillin is superior to penicillin alone (Morrison 1975; Steckelberg and McDonald 1984). Numerous penicillin regimens have been used, but the most popular is benzathine penicillin (2.4 million U) given weekly for 6 weeks to 3 months. Along with the penicillin, prednisone, beginning at a dose of 60 mg/d on an alternate-day regimen, is given for 3 months followed by slow tapering. If symptoms recur during the tapering, a maintenance dose of prednisone may be required. Most patients can be expected to stabilize or improve on this therapeutic regimen.

## Benign Positional Vertigo

Patients with benign positional vertigo (BPV) develop brief episodes of vertigo with position change, typically turning over in bed, getting in and out of bed, bending over and straightening up, and extending the neck to look up. "Top-shelf" vertigo, in which a patient experiences an episode of vertigo while reaching for something on a high shelf, is nearly always due to benign positional vertigo. The diagnosis is based on the finding of the characteristic torsional upbeat paroxysmal positional nystagmus with rapid positional testing (the Dix-Hallpike test) (Baloh et al. 1996).

In a review of 240 cases of benign positional vertigo (Baloh et al. 1987), no episodes of positional vertigo lasted longer than 1 minute. Often after a flurry of episodes, however, patients complained of prolonged nonspecific dizziness (lightheaded, motion sick) and nausea that lasted for hours to days. Typically, bouts of positional vertigo were intermixed with variable periods of remission. The mean age of onset was 54 years with a range of 11 to 84 years. At the time of examination, one-third of the patients reported benign positional vertigo (including remissions) lasting longer than 1 year, and seven reported them lasting longer than 10 years.

In slightly more than one-half of the cases, a likely diagnosis was determined. The two largest diagnostic categories were post-traumatic and postviral labyrinthitis or viral neuritis. In patients with the former, onset of positional vertigo occurred immediately after major head trauma. Patients with viral neuritis or labyrinthitis reported a prior episode of acute vertigo gradually resolving over 1 to 2 weeks. Episodes of benign positional vertigo began as soon as 1 week and as long as 8 years after the acute attack. Women outnumbered men by a ratio of 1.6 : 1, combining all diagnostic categories. This ratio was approximately 2 : 1 if only the idiopathic and miscellaneous groups were considered. Others have reported an even higher female-to-male preponderance with idiopathic benign positional vertigo (Katsarkas and Kirkham 1978). The age of onset peaked in the sixth decade in the idiopathic group and in the fourth and fifth decades in the postviral group, and it was evenly distributed during the second to sixth decade in the post-traumatic group.

## Management

Benign positional vertigo results from debris (calcium carbonate crystals) moving freely within the semicircular canals (usually the posterior semicircular canal) (Laska and Remler 1997). It can be cured at the bedside with a simple positioning maneuver designed to remove the debris from the semicircular canal (Fig. 8-1). If one identifies the characteristic fatigable, torsional positioning nystagmus after the Dix-Hallpike test and the nystagmus disappears after performing the maneuver then the diagnosis of benign positional vertigo is confirmed (Baloh 1996). A small percentage of patients (1% or 2%) are not cured by this maneuver, possibly due to the fact that the debris becomes lodged in the canal and cannot easily be

moved out. The lack of success after the positional maneuver, therefore, does not rule out a benign peripheral origin if other features of the nystagmus are typical.

The particle-repositioning maneuver moves the patient from one head-hanging position to another so that the clot rotates around the posterior semicircular canal and into the utricle (Fig. 8-1). Once the particles enter the utricle, they presumably are cleared through the endolymphatic duct and sac so that they can no longer interfere with semicircular canal dynamics. The patient is instructed to avoid lying flat for at least 2 days after the maneuver is performed to prevent the clot from re-entering the posterior canal orifice. Herdman et al. (1992) compared the Epley (1992) and Semont et al. (1988) maneuvers for treating BPV and found a comparable cure rate of 70% to 90% with both. Most workers recommend performing the maneuver several times in repetition until the positional vertigo and nystagmus disappear. Between 10 % and 20% of patients have an exacerbation within a week or two of performing the maneuver and about 50% of patients will eventually have a recurrence of positional vertigo (Herdman et al. 1992).

For rare patients with prolonged intractable benign positional vertigo unresponsive to the particle-repositioning maneuver, surgical procedures may be considered. The ampullary nerve can be sectioned from the posterior semicircular canal crista or the posterior semicircular canal can be blocked with a bone plug (Gacek 1978; Parnes and McClure 1990). These procedures are nearly always effective in relieving the benign positional vertigo, but there is a significant risk (5% to 10%) of a sensorineural hearing loss.

## Meniere's Disease

Meniere's disease (endolymphatic hydrops) is characterized by fluctuating hearing loss and tinnitus, episodic vertigo, and a sensation of fullness or pressure in the ear. The underlying problem is progressive endolymphatic hydrops caused by impaired resorption of the endolymph; all symptoms and signs result from this increased endolymph pressure. Typically the patient develops a sensation of fullness, pressure, and decreased hearing and tinnitus in one ear. Vertigo rapidly follows, reaching a maximum intensity within

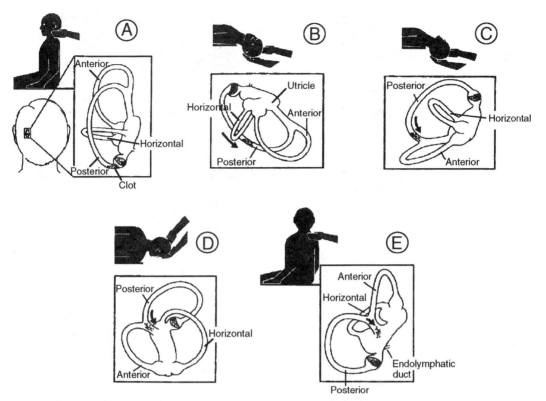

**Figure 8-1.** Positional maneuver designed to remove debris from the posterior semicircular canal. (Adapted from Epley 1992.) In the sitting position (*A*) the clot of calcium carbonate crystals lies at the bottommost position within the posterior canal. Movement to the head-hanging position (*B*) causes the clot to move away from the cupula producing an excitatory burst of activity in the ampullary nerve from the posterior canal (ampullofugal displacement of the cupula). Movement across to the other head-hanging position (*C*) causes the clot to move further around the canal. The patient then rolls onto the side facing the floor (*D*), causing the clot to enter the common crus of the posterior and anterior semicircular canals. Finally the patient sits up (*E*) and the clot disperses in the utricle. The maneuver is repeated until no nystagmus is induced and the patient is instructed not to lie flat for 48 hours (to prevent the debris from re-entering the canal).

minutes and then slowly subsiding during the next several hours. The patient usually is left with a sense of unsteadiness and dizziness for days after the acute vertiginous episode. In the early stages, the hearing loss is completely reversible, but in later stages, a residual hearing loss remains. Tinnitus may persist between episodes but usually increases in intensity immediately before or during the acute episode. It is typically described as a roaring sound (the sound of the ocean or a hollow sea shell). The patient prefers to lie in bed until the acute symptoms pass. The episodes occur at irregular intervals for years, with periods of remission unpredictably intermixed (Eggermont and Schmidt 1985). Approximately 50% will have at least one major remission within the first 2 years of onset (Silverstein et al. 1989). Even-

tually, severe permanent hearing loss develops and the episodic nature spontaneously disappears ("burned-out phase"). In about one-third of patients, bilateral involvement eventually will occur (Wladislavosky-Waserman et al. 1984).

Delayed endolymphatic hydrops develops in an ear that has been damaged years before usually by viral or bacterial infection (Nadol et al. 1975; Schuknecht, 1978). With this disorder, the patient reports a history of hearing loss since early childhood, followed many years later by typical symptoms and signs of endolymphatic hydrops. If the hearing loss is profound, as it often is, the episodic vertigo will not be accompanied by fluctuating hearing levels and tinnitus. Delayed endolymphatic hydrops can be unilateral or bilateral, depending on the extent of damage of the original insult.

## Management

Medical management of Meniere's disease consists of symptomatic treatment of the acute spells with antivertiginous medications, such as meclizine and phenergan (25 to 50 mg) and long-term prophylaxis with salt restriction and diuretics. The mechanism by which a low-salt diet decreases the frequency and severity of attacks with Meniere's disease is unclear, but there is extensive empiric evidence for its efficacy (Boles et al. 1975; Jackson et al. 1981). The author recommends salt restriction in the range of 1 g of sodium per day with a minimal therapeutic trial of 2 to 3 months. Diuretics (acetazolamide, 250 mg; or hydrochlorothiazide, 50 mg) provide additional benefit in some patients, but generally they cannot replace a salt-restriction diet.

Two types of surgery have been used for treating Meniere's disease: endolymphatic shunts and ablative procedures. Although shunts are logical because of the presumed pathophysiology of Meniere's syndrome, it is difficult to achieve a long-standing functional shunt (Schuknecht 1986). Furthermore, recent clinical trials have questioned seriously the efficacy of these surgical shunt procedures (Silverstein et al. 1989; Thomsen et al. 1981). The rationale for ablative surgery in the treatment of Meniere's disease is that the nervous system is better able to compensate for complete loss of vestibular function than for loss that fluctuates in degree. Ablative procedures are most effective in patients with unilateral involvement with no functional hearing on the damaged side. Severe vertigo is expected during the immediate postoperative period, but most patients who follow a structured vestibular exercise program can return to normal activity within 1 to 3 months. Ablative surgical procedures generally should be avoided in elderly patients because they have great difficulty adjusting to a vestibular imbalance. Tinnitus is usually not helped by surgery.

## Perilymph Fistula

The classic presentation of an acute perilymph fistula is a sudden audible pop in the ear immediately followed by hearing loss, vertigo, and tinnitus. The key to diagnosis is to identify the characteristic precipitating factors: head trauma, barotrauma, cough, sneeze, straining, vigorous exercise, chronic otitis with cholesteatoma, post-stapedectomy surgery, and congenital malformations. Nonspecific imbalance and disequilibrium aggravated by quick head movements or sudden turning may result from a chronic perilymph fistula. Patients may prefer to sleep on one side rather than the other to avoid an ill-defined uncomfortable dizzy sensation. The latter feature may suggest benign positional vertigo, although the positional dizziness with perilymph fistula is not as intense and is more persistent than that associated with benign positional vertigo.

## Management

The majority of perilymph fistulae spontaneously heal without innervation. For this reason, most authors advocate conservative management with an initial period of bed rest, sedation, head elevation, and measures to decrease straining (Gacek 1993). One exception to this conservative approach is acute barotrauma, in which immediate exploration has been advocated (Pullen et al. 1979). Persistent fluctuating auditory and vestibular symptoms indicate exploration of the middle ear after an initial trial of conservative management. Even in these cases, however, only about one-half to two-thirds of ears are found to have fistulae. The goal of surgery for chronic fistulae is to stabilize hearing loss and relieve vestibular symptoms. The middle ear typically is explored through a posterior tympanotomy. Often the fistula is in the area of the oval window. Recurrence of symptoms after repair occurs in at least 10% of cases; rarely, intractable symptoms will necessitate ablative surgery with labyrinthectomy or nerve section.

## Acoustic Neuromas

The most common symptom associated with an acoustic neuroma is slowly progressive unilateral hearing loss (Erickson et al. 1965; Mattox 1987). Often patients will complain of an inability to understand speech when using the telephone before they are aware of a loss in hearing. Unilateral tinnitus is the next most common symptom. Vertigo occurs in less than 20% of patients, although approximately one-half will complain of some mild impairment of balance. Next to the auditory nerve, the most commonly involved cranial nerves (by compression) are the seventh and fifth, producing facial weakness and numbness, respectively. Involvement of the sixth, ninth, tenth, eleventh, and twelfth nerves occurs only in the late stages of disease with massive tumors. Large acoustic neuromas also may produce increased intracranial pressure from obstruction of CSF outflow, resulting in severe headaches and vomiting.

## Management

With few exceptions, management of an acoustic neuroma is surgical. Occasionally, a patient with a small acoustic neuroma may be followed, particularly if the patient is elderly or has underlying medical problems (Wazen et al. 1985). These tumors may remain confined to the internal auditory canal for years, and symptoms may be restricted to those of the eighth nerve.

There are three general surgical approaches to the cerebellopontine angle: translabyrinthine, suboccipital, and middle fossa (Mattox 1987). The translabyrinthine approach destroys the labyrinth, but often it allows complete removal of the tumor without endangering nearby neural structures, particularly the facial nerve. This is the procedure of choice for a patient with severe hearing loss and a tumor of less than 3 cm (Kim and Jenkins 1996). With the suboccipital and middle fossa approaches, residual hearing can be saved because the labyrinth is not destroyed (Tator and Nedzelski 1985). Traditionally, the suboccipital approach is performed by neurosurgeons, while the middle fossa approach is performed by otologic surgeons.

## References

Ariyasu, L.; Byl, F. M.; Sprague, M. S.; Adour, K. K. The beneficial effect of methylprednisone in acute vestibular vertigo. Arch. Otolaryngol. Head Neck Surg. 116:700; 1990.

Baloh, R. W. Benign positional vertigo. In: Baloh, R. W.; Halmagyi, G. M., eds. Disorders of the vestibular system. New York: Oxford University Press; 1996: p. 328.

Baloh, R. W.; Honrubia, V.; Jacobson, K. Benign positional vertigo. Clinical and oculographic features in 240 cases. Neurology 37:371; 1987.

Baloh, R. W.; Jacobson, K.; Honrubia, V. Idiopathic bilateral vestibulopathy. Neurology 39:272; 1989.

Baloh, R. W.; Lopez, I.; Ishiyama, A.; Wackym, P. A.; Honrubia, V. Vestibular neuritis: clinical-pathological correlation. Otolaryngol. Head Neck Surg. 114:586;1996.

Böhmer, A. Acute unilateral peripheral vestibulopathy. In: Baloh, R. W.; Halmagyi, G. M., eds. Disorders of the vestibular system. New York: Oxford University Press; 1996: p. 318.

Boles, R.; Rice, D. H.; Hybels, R.; Work, W. P. Conservative management of Meniere's disease: Furstenberg regimen revisited. Ann. Otol. Rhinol. Laryngol. 84:513; 1975.

Davis, L. E.; Johnsson, L. G. Viral infections of the inner ear: clinical, virologic and pathologic studies in humans and animals. Am. J. Otolaryngol. 4:347; 1983.

Dichgans, M.; Jäger, L.; Mayer, T.; Schorn, K.; Pfister, H. W. Bacterial meningitis in adults. Neurology 52:1003;1999.

Dix, M.; Hallpike, C. The pathology, symptomatology and diagnosis of certain common disorders of the vestibular systems. Ann. Otol. Rhinol. Laryngol. 61:987;1952.

Eggermont, J. J.; Schmidt, P. H. Meniere's disease: a long-term follow-up study of hearing loss. Ann. Otol. Rhinol. Laryngol. 94:1;1985.

Epley, J. M. The canalith repositioning procedure: for treatment of benign paroxysmal positional vertigo. Otolaryngol. Head Neck Surg. 107:399;1992.

Erickson, L.; Sorenson, G.; McGavran, M. A review of 140 acoustic neurinomas (neurilemmomas). Laryngoscope 75:601; 1965.

Gacek, R. R. Perilymphatic fistula. In: Cummings, C. W.; Fredrickson, J. M.; Harker, L. A.; Krause, C. J.; Schuller, D. E., eds. Otolaryngology—head and neck surgery. St. Louis: C. V. Mosby; 1993: p. 3017.

Gacek, R. R. Further observations on posterior ampullary nerve transection for positional vertigo. Ann. Otol. Rhinol. Laryngol. 87:300; 1978.

Herdman, S. J. Vestibular rehabilitation. In: Baloh, R. W.; Halmagyi, G. M., eds. Disorders of the vestibular system. New York: Oxford University Press; 1996: p. 583.

Herdman, S. J.; Tusa, R. J.; Zee, D. S.; Proctor, L. R.; Mattox, D. E. Single treatment approached to benign positional vertigo. Arch. Otolaryngol. Head Neck Surg. 119:450; 1992.

Jackson, C. G.; Glasscock. M. E.; Davis, W. E.; Hughes, G. B.; Sismanis, A. Medical management of Meniere's disease. Ann. Otol. 90:142; 1981.

Katsarkas, A.; Kirkham, T. H. Paroxysmal positional vertigo: a study of 255 cases. J. Otolaryngol. 7:320; 1978.

Kim, H. N.; Jenkins, H. A. Vestibular schwannomas and other cerebellopontine angle tumors. In: Baloh, R. W.; Halmagyi, G. M., eds. Disorders of the vestibular system. New York: Oxford University Press; 1996: p. 461.

Laska, D. J.; Remler, B. Benign paroxysmal positioning nystagmus: classic descriptions, origins of the provocative positioning technique, and conceptual developments. Neurology 48:1167; 1997.

Mattox, D. E. Vestibular schwannomas. Otolaryngol. Clin. North Am. 20:149; 1987.

Morrison, A. W. Late syphilis. In: Morrison, A., ed. Management of sensorineural deafness. Boston: Butterworths; 1975: p. 109–144.

Nadol, J. B.; Weiss, A. D.; Parker, S. W. Vertigo of delayed onset after sudden deafness. Ann. Otol. 84: 841; 1975.

Neely, J. G. Complications of temporal bone infection. In: Cummings, C. W.; Fredrickson, J. M.; Harker, L. A.; Krause, C. J.; Schuller, D. E., eds. Otolaryngology—head and neck surgery. St. Louis: C. V. Mosby; 1993: p. 2840.

Nomura, Y.; Kurata, T.; Saito, K. Sudden deafness: human temporal bone studies and an animal model. In: Nomura, Y., ed. Hearing loss and dizziness. Tokyo: Igaku-Shoin; 1985: p. 58.

Paparella, M. M.; Goycoolea, M. V.; Meyerhoff, W. L. Inner ear pathology and otitis media: a review. Ann. Otol. Rhinol. Laryngol. 89:249; 1980.

Pappas, D. G. Hearing impairments and vestibular abnormalities among children with subclinical cytomegalovirus. Ann. Otol. Rhinol. Laryngol. 92:552; 1983.

Parnes, L. S.; McClure, J. A. Posterior semicircular canal occlusion for benign paroxysmal positional vertigo. Ann. Otol. Rhinol. Laryngol. 99:330; 1990.

Pullen, F. W.; Rosenberg, G. H.; Cabeza, C. H. Sudden hearing loss in divers and others. Laryngoscope 84: 1373; 1979.

Saltiel, P.; Melmed, C. A.; Portnoy, D. Sensorineural deafness in early acquired syphilis. Can. J. Neurol. Sci. 10:114; 1983.

Schuknecht, H. F. Delayed endolymphatic hydrops. Ann. Otol. 87:743; 1978.

Schuknecht, H. F. Endolymphatic hydrops: can it be controlled? Ann. Otol. Rhinol. Laryngol. 95:36; 1986.

Schuknecht, H. F. Neurolabyrinthitis. Viral infections of the peripheral auditory and vestibular systems. In: Nomura, Y., ed. Hearing loss and dizziness. Tokyo: Igaku-Shoin; 1985: p. 1.

Schuknecht, H. F., Kimura, R. R.; Nanfal, P. M. The pathology of idiopathic sensorineural hearing loss. Arch. Otorhinolaryngol. 243:1; 1986.

Schuknecht, H. F.; Kitamura, K. Vestibular neuritis. Ann. Otol. Rhinol. Laryngol. 90(suppl.):l; 1981.

Schuknecht, H. F.; Witt, R. L. Acute bilateral sequential vestibular neuritis. Am. J. Otolaryngol. 6:255; 1985.

Semont, A.; Freyss, G.; Vitte, E. Curing the BPPV with a liberatory maneuver. Adv. Otorhinolaryngol. 42: 290; 1988.

Silverstein, H.; Smouha, E.; Jones, R. Natural history vs. surgery for Meniere's disease. Otolaryngol. Head Neck Surg. 100:6; 1989.

Silvoniemi, P. Vestibular neuronitis. Acta. Otolaryngol. 453(suppl.):9; 1988.

Steckelberg, J. M.; McDonald, T. J. Otologic involvement in late syphilis. Laryngoscope 94:753; 1984.

Tator, C. H.; Nedzelski, J. M. Preservation of hearing in patients undergoing excision of acoustic neuromas and other cerebellopontine angle tumors. J. Neurosurg. 63:168; 1985.

Thomsen. J.; Brettan, P.; Tos, M.; Johnsen, N. J. Placebo effect of surgery for Meniere's disease. Arch. Otolaryngol. 107:271; 1981.

Wazen, J.; Silverstein, H.; Norrell, H.; Besse, B. Preoperative and postoperative growth rates in acoustic neuromas documented with CT scanning. Otolaryngol. Head Neck Surg. 93:151; 1985.

Wilson, W. R.; Veltri, R. W.; Larid, N.; et al. Viral and epidemiologic studies of idiopathic sudden hearing loss. Otolaryngol. Head Neck Surg. 91:653; 1983.

Wladislavosky-Waserman, P.; Facer, G. W.; Mokri, B.; Kurland, L. T. Meniere's disease: a 30-year epidemiologic and clinical study in Rochester, MN, 1951–1980. Laryngoscope 94:1098; 1984.

# PART IV

# PAIN DISORDERS

# 9

# Spinal Spondylosis and Disc Disease

RAYMOND W. GRUNDMEYER, III, JASON E. GARBER,
EWELL L. NELSON, AND DAVID S. BASKIN

## Cervical Spine Disease

Cervical spondylosis and cervical disc disease are the most common and significant disorders affecting the cervical spine. They can each lead to myelopathy, radiculopathy, or myeloradiculopathy. The pattern of the deficit depends on the anatomy of the underlying lesion, and its effect on the neural elements through both static and dynamic actions.

The cervical spine is biomechanical elegance—it is uniquely capable of providing a high degree of mobility balanced by the equally important constraint of stability. The cervical spine is in constant motion and is therefore especially prone to degenerative changes. This process begins with desiccation of the intervertebral discs (Naylor 1976), which causes the disc space to collapse, altering the cervical anatomy. In an attempt to provide stability, the cervical spine responds with a series of changes that have collectively been termed *spondylosis*. They include hypertrophy of facet joints, thickening of intralaminar and interbody ligaments, narrowing of neural foramina, fissuring of the annulus fibrosus, and osteophyte formation. In fact, Weinstein et al. (1977) defined spondylosis as "vertebral osteophytosis secondary to degenerative disk disease."

When the term *disc degeneration* is used in the absence of spondylosis, it refers to the presence of a disc bulge, prolapse, extrusion, or sequestration—a classification scheme that was developed by Macnab (Masaryk et al. 1988). The last of these three, disc prolapse, extrusion, and sequestration are often considered disc "herniations." The pathophysiology of this type of disc disease is different than the pathophysiology of disc desiccation. In fact, as one ages, desiccation of the discs helps to prevent new disc herniations, particularly for those over the age of 50 (Kramer 1990).

Changes in the cervical spine are common in the adult population (Friedenberg and Miller 1963; Hitselberger and Witten 1968; Teresi et al. 1987; Lawrence et al. 1966). At least 80% of males and females older than 55 years of age have some radiographic evidence of spondylosis (Lawrence et al. 1966). In 100 asymptomatic patients, Teresi et al. (1987) found that 57% of patients over age 64 had disc protrusions, and 26% had spinal cord impingement. Spinal cord compression (with obliteration of the posterior subarachnoid space) occurred in 7%. In those less than 64 years of age, 20% had disc protrusions, and 16% had spinal cord impingement.

Neck and arm pain are also common in the adult population (Robertson 1993). The most important step in understanding the prognosis for patients who suffer from neck and arm pain with or without myelopathy is to approach the problem with an appropriate differential diagnosis. The presentation of spondylotic disease can be easily confused with neurodegenerative diseases like amyotrophic lateral sclerosis or multiple sclerosis, intraspinal tumors, and peripheral nerve entrapment.

## Pathophysiology of Cervical Degeneration

Cervical degeneration is a multifaceted process involving the intervertebral discs, the facet joints, the vertebral bodies, and the intraspinal and paraspinal soft tissues. While the interactions between each of these regions are complex, most authors emphasize the importance of the intervertebral disc.

The intervertebral disc accounts for 20% of the height of the cervical spine. It is composed of a central gelatinous structure, the nucleus pulposus, surrounded by concentric lamellae of collagen fibrils, the annulus fibrosus, and bounded above and below by cartilaginous endplates. It is an avascular structure with a sparse connective tissue cell population that receives its nutrients via pores in the outermost calcified layer of the endplates (the lamina cribosa) and capillaries surrounding the annulus. While it is able to resist both transverse and rotational shear, as well as some distraction, its most significant functional characteristic is the ability to sustain a compressive load. The nucleus pulposus distributes the load across the vertebral endplate, and is contained by the action of the annulus fibrosus.

The disc's ability to load share decreases as it ages, and the temporal relationship of these developments leads to a window during the fourth and fifth decades during which disc herniations peak and then progressively decrease after age 50 (Kramer 1990). The bulging annulus, however, persists and is attached firmly to the periosteum of the vertebral body by strong collagen fibrils called Sharpey's fibers. These attachments lift the periosteum off of the vertebral body. This change coupled with the increased mobility of the involved segments promotes the formation of subperiosteal osteophytic spurs (Brain et al. 1952). As the disc collapses, the facet joints override one another and hypertrophy (Dunsker 1981; White and Panjabi 1988), while the interlaminar tissue buckles and hyper-

trophies leading to the development of posterior canal compromise. These changes in the cervical spine serve to restore stability to the aging segment.

## Cervical Spondylosis and Myelopathy

Cervical spondylosis leads to myelopathy through a combination of vascular phenomena (Parke 1988; Panjabi and White 1988; Al-Mefty et al. 1993; Breig et al. 1966), and static and dynamic compression (Parke 1988; Epstein et al. 1969; Stoltmann and Blackwood 1964; Hoff and Wilson 1977; Burrows 1963; Taylor 1953; Wilkinson 1960). While radiographic evidence of degeneration may be found in asymptomatic patients (Gore et al. 1986), the combination of a narrow spinal canal (under 12-mm sagittal axis) combined with osteophytosis and ligamentous hypertrophy commonly leads to cervical spondylitic myelopathy (CSM) (Adams and Logue 1971).

Although Clarke and Robinson recognized myelopathy associated with cervical spondylosis in 1956, the disorder was reported to cause five distinct syndromes in the paper by Crandall and Batzdorf at UCLA (Crandall and Batzdorf 1966). These syndromes were a transverse lesion syndrome with corticospinal, dorsal column, and spinothalamic involvement (47%); a motor system syndrome with corticospinal and anterior horn cell involvement (19%); a central cord syndrome with distal arm weakness (13%); a Brown-Sequard's syndrome (13%); and a brachalgia and cord syndrome causing arm pain and long tract signs (8%). The long-term study at UCLA revealed that 90% of patients with CSM had gait disturbance, and approximately 70% and 75% had sphincter dysfunction and lower extremity weakness, respectively (Gregorius et al. 1976). The signs present on admission included lower extremity spasticity (80%) and weakness (70%) and spinothalamic and posterior column deficits (40% to 50%) (Gregorius et al. 1976).

## Natural History of Myelopathy

The natural history of cervical CSM is poorly understood, due in part to the historical nature of much of the literature, which predates modern neuroimaging and current sophisticated neurosurgical practice, including the use of the operative microscope. Recent advances in neuroradiology have paralleled the progression of the clinical neurosciences. Together, these have led to better patient selection and operative outcomes in patients who suffer from CSM today.

The onset of CSM is typically insidious, and progression is common. Many patients are symptomatic for several years before seeking medical attention. The clinical picture is dominated by periods of stability and episodic progression (Clarke and Robinson 1956; Lees and Turner 1963; Campbell and Phillips 1960; Hukuda et al. 1988; Nurick 1972a, 1972b; Symonds 1953; Gregorius et al. 1976). Clarke and Robinson found that 75% of patients treated nonoperatively will show deterioration, and that motor signs are more progressive than the sensory signs. While 50% of their patients who were treated with a neck brace alone had improvement in pain, brachialgia, and ability to dress, they note that patients' adaptation to disability, particularly during periods of stability, was interpreted as improvement.

Lees and Turner in their 1963 study discussed the natural history of the disorder in 44 patients with spondylotic myelopathy. They argue for a conservative approach to treatment. They found that most patients with mild disease either improved or remained stable at follow-up (there were four patients in this group and three had a follow-up of <10 years). Fifteen patients were classified as having moderate disease at presentation (considerable difficulty performing everyday tasks). At follow-up, none had improved to the mild category, and one progressed to the severe group (could hardly walk; was unable to work; and was often confined to a chair, bed, or house). Twenty-five patients were in the severe category when first evaluated. At follow-up, one had no disability, but 17 remained severely disabled, and the remainder had improved a grade to moderate disability. In 1976, Gorter reviewed five prior studies to examine the nature of CSM managed with conservative treatment. His review of these 164 patients treated conservatively found that 49% improved, but none were cured; 36% remained stable, and 15% worsened (Gorter 1976).

Nurick, in another classic paper (Nurick 1972b), examined the natural history of CSM. He agreed with the findings of Lees and Turner that in most cases of CSM, there was an initial phase of deterioration followed by a static period lasting a number of years. Nurick's premise was that CSM was "generally benign and non-progressive in nature." However, he argues that patients who are less severely affected—grade 1 or 2 (signs of disease but no trouble walking or slight difficulty in walking)—benefit from laminectomy. He concluded that the long-term prognosis is dependent on both the severity of the myelopathy at presentation, as well as the age of the patient.

Ball and Saunders in 1992 were critical of Nurick's premise and point out that in his series, 5 of the 12 patients (41%) who presented in the grade 1 category deteriorated at least one grade, and 40% of those treated conservatively in the grade 2 group deteriorated at least one grade (Ball and Saunders 1992). They also go on to show that if Nurick's own data are analyzed by nonparametric analysis of covariance rather than by chi-square analysis, patients who were treated surgically had a better outcome than those treated conservatively, with a $p$ value of .016 for those who presented in grade 1 or 2 initially and a $p$ value of .027 for all grades initially. Others have also found that the natural history of CSM is not one of improvement, and have even reported progression of myelopathy without precipitating cause (Wilberger and Chedid 1988).

Clark and Robinson wrote about the progressive nature of CSM, and found that the motor system was most likely to show deterioration. In contrast, Lees and Turner's argument for conservative treatment is not convincing, as it was based on what they observed in only four patients who presented with mild disease. Although Nurick's premise was that the disease was benign and non-progressive, Ball and Saunders's analysis of Nurick's data demonstrates the clear benefit of surgery. Since many of these earlier surgical series for CSM reported approximately 50% favorable outcome, which was comparable to the natural history of the disease (Rowland 1992), conservative management was thought to be appropriate, except in the presence of severe or progressive deficits. The results of the most recent series have been far superior to the earlier studies, with improved outcomes ranging from 85% to 100% (Phillips 1973; Whitecloud and LaRocca 1976; Zhang et al. 1983; Mann et al. 1984; Boni et al. 1984; Hukuda et al. 1985; Yonenobu et al. 1985; Hanai et al. 1986; Wiberg 1986; Bernard and Whitecloud 1987; Yang et al. 1987; Kojima et al.

1989; Zdelblick and Bohlman 1989; Seifert and Stolke 1991; Saunders et al. 1991; Okada, Shirasaki et al. 1991; Burger et al. 1996). Patients who have a shorter duration of preoperative symptoms have superior results from surgery (Peserico et al. 1962; Phillips 1973; Hamanishi and Tanaka 1996; Guidetti and Fortuna 1969; Yang et al. 1985; Hukuda et al. 1985; Saunders et al. 1991; Ebersold et al. 1995; Fox and Onofrio 1994; Lee et al. 1997; Wiberg 1986; Wohlert et al. 1984; Guidetti et al. 1980; Bertalanffy and Eggert 1988).

Therefore, it is now clear that CSM is a disease that can and should be treated by surgical intervention in most cases. Early intervention is indicated especially in patients who do not have coexisting complicating disease states.

A recent study by Wada et al. (1999) suggests that there are radiographic features that can predict the outcome of surgical intervention in patients with CSM. The best prognostic factor was the transverse area of the spinal cord at the site of maximum compression. The presence of high signal intensity areas on $T_2$-weighted images also correlated poorly with the recovery rate.

**Anterior Surgical Results**

In CSM, the bony compression is located anteriorly in 75% of patients (Cusick 1991). The recent trend within neurosurgical practice has been to address the anatomy of spondylotic disease directly from an anterior approach. The anterior approach to CSM offers the advantage of allowing both a decompression and osteosynthesis with a single operation. In doing so, the surgeon is able to treat the compressive lesion in addition to eliminating one of its primary etiologies. While most anterior cervical operations can be fundamentally categorized as either a single or multisegmental discectomy with osteosynthesis (i.e., anterior cervical discectomy with fusion [ACDF], or multilevel subtotal corpectomy and discectomy with strut grafting), it is helpful to simply consider just the anterior approach versus the posterior approach. There is no literature to suggest that any one of the variations of the anterior approach is superior to the others. The specific indications for the use of one versus the other are discussed in neurosurgical and spine textbooks elsewhere.

In 1976, Whitecloud and LaRocca presented the first published results of subtotal corpectomy with strut grafting. In their series of 18 patients,

100% improved, with significant pain relief, functional recovery, and improvement of overall neurological status. While they do not report the details of the recovery, they did note that complete resolution of preoperative symptoms was not achieved (Whitecloud and LaRocca 1976). In the same year, Gorter reviewed the literature to compare conservative treatment versus an anterior approach, versus two different posterior approaches. He concluded that surgical treatment was superior to conservative treatment, but no one surgical approach was shown to be superior to the others. In his review, 345 patients had undergone an anterior approach, and at follow-up, 73% were either cured or improved, 19% were unchanged, 7% were worse, and 1% had died (Gorter 1976).

These impressive results were tempered by the papers to follow in the 1980s in which only about 50% of patients improved after anterior surgery for CSM (Lunsford et al. 1980a, 1980b; Mosdal 1984; Wohlert et al. 1984). Lunsford et al. found that in their series of 32 patients who underwent an anterior procedure for CSM, only 50% were improved at follow-up, which varied from 1 to 7 years. The series was small and no statistical link could be made between results and the patients' age, duration of symptoms, severity of myelopathy, cervical canal size, or the number of levels the operation spanned. Patients who were younger and who had symptoms less than 6 months tended to be more likely to improve, however. In their series, the surgical microscope was not used (Lunsford et al. 1980a, 1980b). Like Lunsford, Mosdal in his review of 755 patients who received an anterior operation for cervical spondylosis found that postoperatively 81% experienced either total or partial relief of symptoms. At late follow-up, only 42% of those with myelopathy benefited, while 71% benefited with regard to neck pain, brachialgia, and neuropathy (Mosdal 1984).

The mediocre results of Lunsford et al. are the exception in the modern literature. There are many reports that indicate a greater than 90% improvement rate for patients who undergo anterior surgery for CSM (Phillips 1973; Zhang et al. 1983; Mann et al. 1984; Boni et al. 1984; Hanai et al. 1986; Zdelblick and Bohlman 1989; Seifert and Stolke 1991; Burger et al. 1996). Zhang et al. found that in their series of 121 patients with CSM, 91% improved and 73% were able to resume normal activity (Zhang et al. 1983). Similarly, Yang et al., in a series of 214 cases of cervical spondylotic myelopathy that were treated by anterior multilevel decompression and fusion using the Robinson technique, demonstrated an improvement rate of 88%. At an average follow-up of 47 months, 59.3% experienced good or excellent results, 29% fair, 7.8% no change, and 3.8% deteriorated. Of those who had disease for less than 1 year prior to operation (111 patients), 74% had good or excellent results, whereas of those with disease more than 2 years prior to operation, only 36% had good or excellent results. The average number of discs removed was 3.1 (Yang et al. 1985). Another paper that addressed multisegmental cervical spondylotic myelopathy by Boni et al. in 1984 found that 98% were improved with surgery. Of their 29 cases of spondylotic myelopathy, 51% experienced a good outcome and 47% had moderate outcomes. Follow-up was from 6 months to 13 years (Boni et al. 1984).

Hukuda et al., in their 1985 series of 191 patients who received either an anterior or a posterior procedure for myelopathy, found that the results of the procedure were dependent on the clinical syndrome present. The syndromes were classified according to Crandall and Batzdorf's classification of 1966 (1) brachialgia and cord, (2) central, (3) transverse, (4) Brown-Sequard, and (5) (motor). According to the Japanese Orthopaedic Association (JOA) grading criteria, in which 17 points represents the normal person, patients with brachialgia and cord syndrome improved by 2 points, central syndrome by 1.8 points, transverse syndrome by 4.9 points, Brown-Sequard syndrome by 3.8 points, and motor syndrome by 3 points. Thus the greatest improvement was seen in those with the transverse, Brown-Sequard, or the motor group, but these three groups had a more severe preoperative grade (9.5 points) as compared to those with brachialgia and cord and central syndromes (14.2 points). These authors also found that patients who had experienced symptoms for less than a year prior to operation did much better than patients who had a duration of symptoms greater than 1 year. For patients under 50 years of age, the average point gain was 3.9 in those who received their operation promptly versus 2.9 for those who had symptoms for more than a year. For those over the age of 50 the corresponding average

point gain was 4.2 versus 2.2. They concluded, therefore, that early surgical intervention yields better results and that these results are even more significant in older patients. Their data also suggest that an anterior procedure is optimal in those who have involvement at one or two levels without stenosis of the spinal canal, and in those who suffer from signs and symptoms involving the arms rather than the trunk and the legs. In a similar paper that year, Yonenobu et al. reported on 95 patients with CSM due to multisegmental disease treated by either extensive laminectomy, multilevel ACDF, or subtotal corpectomy. They found that subtotal corpectomy was superior to laminectomy or multilevel ACDF for multilevel disease up to three involved levels, and that the average point gain (by the JOA grading system) for subtotal corpectomy was 6 points as compared to 3.3 points for multilevel ACDF and 3.3 points for laminectomy. This corresponded to a rate of recovery (percentage gain of points based on the JOA grading system) of 67% for subtotal corpectomy, 53% for multilevel ACDF, and 49% for laminectomy. The average follow-up was 50 months (Yonenobu et al. 1985). Senegas et al. in 1985 saw a 73% improvement rate in their 45 cases of CSM treated by corpectomy. Mean follow-up was 48 months (Senegas et al. 1985).

During the late 1980s, a number of papers continued to report excellent results. In 1986, Hanai et al. saw marked improvement at short follow-up in 100% of their 30 patients who underwent corpectomy for CSM. None were worse at final follow-up (mean, 36 months) (Hanai et al. 1986). Bernard and Whitecloud in 1987 demonstrated significant improvement in 19 of their 21 patients (90%) with multisegmental cervical spondylotic myelopathy (MSCSM) treated by corpectomy. At 1 year, they continued to see improvement in 76% (Bernard and Whitecloud 1987). Kojima et al.'s 1989 paper examined the results of patients who were myelopathic due to multisegmental cervical spondylosis (MSCS) or ossification of the posterior longitudinal ligament (OPLL). Their 45 patients were treated with corpectomy. Of those with MSCSM alone, 16 of 19 (84%) had a good result. Those with OPLL alone had a good result 92% of the time (11 of 12 patients). Those with myelopathy due both to OPLL and MSCS had a good result 86% of the time (12 of 14 patients). Overall results for anterior decompression was

87% (Kojima et al. 1989). Zdelblick and Bohlman in 1989 reported 100% improvement in their eight cases of cervical kyphosis and myelopathy treated by corpectomy (Zdelblick and Bohlman 1989). Rengachary and Redford in 1989 reported improvement in 86% of their 22 cases of CSM by corpectomy and fibular strut grafting (Rengachary and Redford 1989).

The impressive reports of anterior surgery continued with the Seifert and Stolke report of 1991, with improvement in 100% of their patients with multilevel cervical spondylosis, with an average follow-up of 21 months. They had excellent results (symptom-free or nearly symptom-free) from an anterior decompressive procedure in 77% of their patients, while another 14% continued to suffer some nuchal or cervicobrachial pain (alleviated by analgesics or soft collar at night) and the remaining 9% continued to have myelopathic symptoms that they reported as improved following surgery. Of those (15 patients) who were employed but unable to perform their regular work duties preoperatively, 87% were able to return to work full-time, while one (6.5%) returned to work half-time and one retired as a result of the spondylosis (Seifert and Stolke 1991). In that same year, Saunders et al. reported improvement in 85% of their series of 40 patients treated by subtotal corpectomy. Their patients experienced a long-term cure rate of 57.5% (follow-up, 2 to 5 years) after an initial cure rate of 62.5%. Two patients accounted for the regression of improvement and both demonstrated inadequate decompression by magnetic resonance imaging (MRI). They regressed at 18 and 36 months. Only 45% of those with symptoms longer than 1 year experienced cure, while 70% of those with symptoms shorter than 1 year experienced cure. Sixty percent of their patients were considered severely impaired preoperatively and they experienced a cure rate of 50%. The failure rate (failure being no improvement in preoperative symptoms or regression of improvement) was 15%—accounted for by the two patients whose cure regressed, one patient who was an error in diagnosis (multiple sclerosis), and three patients with severe syndromes of long duration who experienced only minimal improvement. No patients experienced worsening of their myelopathy. Their data also demonstrate the need for early operative intervention, preferably within a year of the onset of symptoms (Saunders et al. 1991).

In 1991, Okada et al. reported satisfactory results in 78% of their 37 patients with CSM, but they noted that 97% had improvement in their ability to walk after surgery. At follow-up, one patient reverted to his preoperative status and three deteriorated due to new spondylotic stenosis (Okada, Shirasaki et al. 1991). In Ebersold et al.'s 1995 review of 84 patients treated for CSM with a mean follow-up of 7.35 years, 33 patients underwent anterior decompression with fusion. Of these, 24 (73%) showed immediate functional improvement and nine were unchanged. One patient demonstrated early deterioration. Late deterioration was defined as occurring from 2 to 68 months postoperatively. Four required additional posterior procedures. At last follow-up, 18 (55%) of the 33 were improved, nine (27%) were unchanged, and six had deteriorated. The only poor prognostic sign was duration of preoperative symptoms. They concluded that even with adequate decompression and initial improvement there exists a group of patients who will experience late functional deterioration (Ebersold et al. 1995). In 1996, Burger et al. detailed their surgical results by reporting the rate of improvement in 17 patients treated by cervical corpectomy according to their preoperative symptoms. Paresis was improved in 92%, spasticity in 73%, sensory deficits in 60%, and pain in 100% of their patients (Burger et al. 1996). The following year, Banerji et al. reviewed 26 patients who were treated by multilevel corpectomy for OPLL or CSM and found that 80% had a good result (Banerji et al. 1997). Emery et al. (1998) reviewed 108 cases of patients with CSM who had been managed with anterior decompression and arthrodesis, and reported that 46% of those with an abnormal gait preoperatively had a completely normal gait after surgery. Another 40% noted significant improvement, with only one patient noting worsening. Fessler et al. (1998) have also reported improvement in 86% of patients with CSM treated with anterior cervical corpectomy, with superior results compared to historical control subjects receiving either no treatment or laminectomy.

In summary, the anterior approach for treatment of CSM is usually the best surgical approach to utilize. Clinicians who evaluate these patients are urged to consider early surgical intervention, regardless of surgical approach, because the disease is progressive, and because the outcome of surgical treatment is best when intervention occurs within a year after the onset of symptoms.

## Posterior Surgical Results

While the anterior approach to spinal cord decompression has gained favor, the use of the posterior approach continues to be an effective solution for the treatment of cervical spondylotic myelopathy in the appropriate patient. The posterior approach does allow one to address cord compression due to buckling of the ligamentum flavum and the posterior elements (Taylor 1953; Wilkinson 1960; Parke 1988; Epstein et al. 1969; Stoltmann and Blackwood 1964; Hoff and Wilson 1977; Panjabi and White 1988). It is appropriate in patients with a congenitally or developmentally narrow spinal canal (Galera and Tovi 1968), but is contraindicated in patients in whom the normal cervical lordosis has given way to a kyphotic deformity (Batzdorf and Batzdorf 1988). Some authors have found that those with a more severe myelopathy or those with transverse lesions, the Brown-Sequard syndrome, or the motor syndromes are best treated by the posterior approach (Hukuda et al. 1985). Some advantages of the posterior approach are that it avoids the operative risks associated with the anterior dissection and that it allows for more rapid postoperative mobilization by virtue of its lack of a fusion procedure. Disadvantages include greater postoperative discomfort due to the extensive dissection of the posterior neck muscles, and a higher incidence of late neurologic deterioration due to instability (Hanai et al. 1986; Mikawa et al. 1987; Oiwa et al. 1985; Sim et al. 1974; Yasuoka et al. 1981, 1982; Yonenobu et al. 1985, 1986; Saito et al. 1991).

In general, the results of posterior operations for CSM have been inferior to those of anterior operations, although no randomized prospective study has been done to compare the two approaches; therefore, definitive conclusions as to which method is superior cannot be drawn. The posterior approach has been successful, however, and is clearly superior to conservative management, as demonstrated by the results of Stoops and King (1962), who reported an 80% favorable outcome rate in their 42 patients treated with laminectomy. None were worse after surgery. They did not identify any prognostic factor that was associated with outcome including age, sex, duration of symptoms, severity of symptoms, myelographic findings, or decompression of osteophytes (Stoops and King 1962). The study of Crandall and Batzdorf in 1966 sought to compare the results of anterior versus posterior decompressive procedures in a series of 62 patients that were followed from 1 to 10 years. Twenty-one patients were treated with ACDF and 71% had either excellent or improved symptoms, but 19% were worse at follow-up. Eleven patients underwent laminectomy with opening of the dura and dural grafting. They had similar outcomes, as 82% had either excellent results or were improved, while 18% were worse. Twenty-three patients underwent laminectomy alone. Here the results were disappointing, as only 31% were categorized as excellent or improved, while 39% were worse. Seven patients underwent a laminectomy that was followed by ACDF when they failed to improve, and of this group, 71% were improved and 29% were worse at follow-up (Crandall and Batzdorf 1966).

Symon and Lavender in 1967 reported favorable results in 71% of their 41 patients treated with extensive laminectomy without foraminotomy, while 24% were unchanged and 5% were worse at follow-up. They concluded that the extent of the laminectomy rather than foraminotomy or dentate ligament sectioning was prone to better results (Symon and Lavender 1967). In Epstein's 1969 series of 37 patients treated by a posterior approach (laminectomy, foraminotomy, and osteophytectomy), 78% had a good to excellent result, while 89% were improved with surgery; 8% were unchanged and one patient continued to have progressive disease that was indicative of spinal cord and motor neuron disease independent of spondylosis. Average follow-up was 42 months (Epstein et al. 1969). Most would not advocate such an aggressive anterior osteophytectomy via a posterior approach since the report of Allen (1952), who had disastrous outcomes when trying to remove the ventral osteophytes extradurally through a posterior laminectomy.

In 1973, Fager demonstrated favorable results in 68% of his 35 patients treated with extensive laminectomy with sectioning of the dentate ligament. Another 26% had disease arrest. Remarkably, five of the eight most severely affected were significantly improved, but he comments that they had a more acute course than the moderately severe group in whom only 10 of 17 improved. Two worsened postoperatively during follow-up from 1 to 6 years (Fager 1973). Despite Fager's favorable results with sectioning of the dentate ligament, Piepgras in 1977 compared denticulate ligament sectioning versus no sectioning in two groups of patients who underwent extensive laminectomies and found no significant difference in outcome (Piepgras 1977).

In 1992, Yonenobu et al. published their results for posterior surgery (laminoplasty in this case). While they fail to report the number of patients who were improved by the surgery, they demonstrated an average rate of functional recovery of 45% in patients who underwent laminoplasty for CSM at a minimum follow-up of 2 years. The average preoperative score of function based on the JOA scoring system was 9.3 and the average postoperative score after minimum follow-up was 12.8. The spinal alignment in 14% of their patients worsened, but had no neurologic consequences at the time point of assessment (Yonenobu et al. 1992).

Fox and Onofrio report good results in all seven of their patients with multilevel cervical spondylotic myelopathy and superimposed central soft disc herniation treated with decompressive laminectomy and transdural excision of the ventral disc herniation. At mean follow-up of 51 months, two patients had a full neurological recovery, and the other five were improved. No perioperative morbidity or mortality occurred and none had developed kyphotic deformity. They comment that their dramatic results may be the result of a preoperative duration less than a year, younger age (mean, 46.7), and relatively mild neurologic disease (Fox and Onofrio 1994).

In Ebersold et al.'s 1995 review of 84 patients treated for CSM with a mean follow-up of 7.35 years, 51 patients underwent posterior laminectomy. Of these, 35 (69%) showed immediate functional improvement, 11 (21%) were unchanged, and five (10%) were worse. Five patients demonstrated early deterioration. Late deterioration was defined as occurring from 2 to 68 months postoperatively. At last follow-up, 19 (37%) of the 51 were improved, 13 (26%) were unchanged, and 19 (37%) had deteriorated. The only poor prognostic sign was duration of preoperative symptoms. They concluded that even with adequate decompression and initial improvement, there exists a group of patients who will experience late functional deterioration (Ebersold et al. 1995).

Lee et al. in 1997 demonstrated good results with the use of cervical laminoplasty for the treatment of CSM. In their series of 25 patients, 100% had gait disturbance with long tract signs and 52% had bowel/bladder or sexual dysfunction preoperatively. With a minimum of 18 months' follow-up, 84% of their patients had gait improvement following the procedure, and bowel/bladder function improved in 77% of those with preoperative dysfunction. Hand numbness and tingling were improved in 87%. Four patients had concomitant radiculopathy that was treated simultaneously with posterior foraminotomy, and the radiculopathy was alleviated in each of these four. The only complication in this series was a single case of anterior scalene syndrome postoperatively. The predictors of a poor surgical outcome in this series were age greater than 60 years at presentation, duration of symptoms greater than 18 months prior to surgery, preoperative bowel or bladder dysfunction, and lower extremity dysfunction. Even in this group of patients, 70% experienced gait improvement (Lee et al. 1997).

A recent study by Saruhashi et al. (1999) supports the value of laminoplasty, with good clinical results, even in patients with poor preoperative alignment. Indeed, the supporters of this surgical technique believe that it is superior to simple laminectomy, because after the decompression is completed, the laminae are realigned and ultimately fuse, thus theoretically producing less instability. Variations of the basic technique, utilizing less bony removal, also appear promising (Hidai et al. 1999). Superiority compared to simple laminectomy remains to be proven, as there are no good prospective randomized clinical trials comparing the two techniques.

In summary, both the anterior and posterior approaches have a place in the treatment of CSM. Although differences in surgical techniques complicate precise comparison of studies, most agree that the anterior approach is usually preferable.

**Natural History of Radiculopathy**

The most common sign of degenerative disc disease is radiculopathy (Hoff et al. 1977; Hoff and Wilson 1977), which is present in up to 90% of cases where myelopathy is found (Clarke and Robinson 1956; Hoff et al. 1977; Hoff and Wilson

1977). However, patients who present with radiculopathy rarely develop myelopathy (Nurick 1972a). Symptoms are usually present for 3 to 4 weeks prior to seeking medical attention (Scoville et al. 1976), yet many patients with disc disease will improve over time and neurological complications are rare (Arnasson et al. 1987; Clark 1991; Lees and Turner 1963; Zeidman and Ducker 1992). In most cases, conservative management yields good results and only a minority of patients will require operative intervention (Beck 1991). The most commonly affected root is C6 and C7 (Clements and O' Leary 1990; Lunsford et al. 1980a; Friedenberg and Miller 1963; Henderson et al. 1983; Radhakrishnan et al. 1994) and the Spurling maneuver may exacerbate or produce radicular pain (Spurling and Scoville 1944). Nonoperative management is appropriate initially in most patients. Those with severe unrelenting pain, progressive neurological deficits, or vocational requirements that prohibit neurological deficits should be offered surgical treatment early, as well as those who have persistent pain or neurological deficit after an appropriate trial of conservative management (usually 6 to 12 weeks).

Blades and Cooper (1996) comment on the 1965 article by DePalma and Subin that studied the natural history of cervical radiculopathy, by reporting on a group of 255 patients that were managed nonoperatively for 3 months. Twenty-nine percent obtained complete pain relief, 49% improved and could be employed to some degree, and 22% failed to improve (DePalma and Subin 1965). At 1 year, however, 27% (68) were considered failures of nonoperative management. This group was observed for a total of 5 years, at which time 55% had a poor outcome with significant pain and limitation of activity. The remainder experienced satisfactory pain relief and activity. Thus, the majority of patients improved without operative intervention, but of the original group, 15% were failures of nonoperative treatment at 5 years (Blades and Cooper 1996).

Gore et al. (1987) followed 205 patients for neck pain without neurological dysfunction for 10 years and found that with conservative management 79% were improved, 43% were free of pain, and 32% continued to have moderate to severe pain, the degree of which was not related to degenerative changes, anteroposterior (AP) diameter of the spinal canal, degree of cervical lordosis, or changes in these measurements (Gore et al. 1987). The authors agree with Rothman's statement that "it does not appear that cervical disc degeneration is a brief self-limiting disorder, but rather a chronic disease, productive of significant pain and incapacity over an extended period of time" (Rothman 1982).

Persson et al. (1997) found no difference in long-term outcome (approximately 12 months) in their prospective randomized series of 81 patients suffering for at least 3 months from cervical radicular pain due to a spondylotic spur with or without a bulging disc between surgery (Cloward procedure), physiotherapy, or cervical collar. Their endpoints were pain intensity, function, and mood. In the short term, the surgery group did better with regard to pain, and both surgery and physiotherapy did better in the short term with regard to function. Sherk (1997), in response to this article, points out that it blurred the distinction between each of the three groups in that some patients who underwent surgery were treated subsequently with physiotherapy, that some patients who were treated with either a collar or physiotherapy underwent subsequent surgery, and that some patients in the surgery group did not undergo surgery because of preoperative subjective improvement. The authors also failed to discuss the anatomic lesion, patient motivation, secondary gain factors, litigation, workers' compensation or litigation status, smoking habits, and level of alcohol consumption in each of the three groups. The study also arbitrarily limited surgery to a single level and reported that a number of patients required further surgery for additional levels after the original operation (Sherk 1997).

While a trial of nonoperative therapy is usually appropriate, the results of surgery for cervical radiculopathy are excellent. A favorable surgical outcome can be expected in more than 90% of patients in whom there is radiological evidence of nerve root compression (Fager 1978; Gore and Sepic 1984; Herkowitz 1988; Henderson et al. 1983). Improvement can be expected in over 90% of those not involved in litigation or workers' compensation claims (Cloward 1962; Smith and Robinson 1958; Murphy and Gado 1972; Robinson 1964; Lees and Turner 1963; Batzdorf and Flannigan 1991; Aronson et al. 1970; Martins 1976; Riley et al. 1969; Aldrich 1990; Henderson et al. 1983; Krupp et al. 1990; Murphey et al. 1973; Scoville et al. 1976; Williams 1983; Zeidman and Ducker 1993). Additionally, patients with radicular pain have the highest probability of pain relief from surgery (Gore and Sepic 1984; Riley 1978; White et al. 1973; Williams et al. 1968). The development of outpatient surgery for cervical radiculopathy is another recent and positive development (Silvers et al. 1996; Tomaras et al. 1997).

## Anterior Surgery for Radiculopathy

The anterior approach for treatment of cervical disc disease was first described by Robinson and Smith in 1955 and with slight modification by Cloward in 1962 (Robinson and Smith 1955; Cloward 1962). Since this time, surgical treatment by the anterior approach has been shown by many authors to be very successful with low morbidity (Aronson et al. 1970; Brigham and Tsahakis 1995; Murphy and Gado 1972; Gore and Sepic 1984; Tegos et al. 1994; Riley et al. 1969; Pointillart et al. 1995; Benini et al. 1982; Bertalanffy and Eggert 1988; Hankinson and Wilson 1975; Robertson 1973; Wilson and Campbell 1977; Martins 1976; Herkowitz et al. 1990; Romner et al. 1994; Bosacco et al. 1992; Brodke and Zdeblick 1992).

In 1966, Rosomoff and Rossman found that in their 50 patients who underwent cervical discectomy and fusion, all patients (100%) with radicular pain obtained complete relief whereas 88% of patients with nonradicular discomfort became asymptomatic. Ninety-seven percent of patients with motor deficits due to root compression improved, whereas 79% of those with a sensory deficit improved (Rosomoff and Rossman 1966).

Riley et al. in 1969 reported on 93 patients treated by ACDF (Smith-Robinson technique) for arm paresthesias, brachialgia, and neck pain, with neck pain being the most common symptom (92% of patients had posterior neck pain). In 72% of patients they achieved a good or excellent result, with improvement in 90%. If two or fewer levels were fused, then 75% had good or excellent results, whereas those with three or more levels had a good or excellent result only 58% of the time. There was no correlation between final result and the patient's age, duration of symptoms, gender, or maintenance of interspace height. Nonunion occurred in 14% of the 166 disc spaces. Overall, 93% benefited from the operation (Riley et al. 1969).

Aronson et al. in 1970 had good results in the 35 patients who received an anterior operation (Smith-Robinson) for a soft disc protrusion or extrusion. Of the 44 patients who received the operation, 35 responded to the questionnaire. All of their patients (100%) were improved. Sixty-nine percent had complete relief of arm pain, while 29% had partial relief and one patient had no change in arm pain. With regard to neck pain, again, all were improved, with 54% experiencing complete relief and 46% experiencing partial relief. Cases that were not in litigation did better (Aronson et al. 1970). That same year, Jacobs et al. reported that 82% of their 65 patients with cervical radiculopathy had good or excellent results (Jacobs et al. 1970). Two years later, Murphy and Gado had good results in 92% of their 26 patients with radiculopathy treated by anterior discectomy without fusion. Twelve of their patients had posterior osteophytes and 50% of these demonstrated remodeling after a year following the surgery (Murphy and Gado 1972).

The anterior procedure is considered safe, and most complications are due to bone graft harvesting. Graft donor site problems are usually minor, but occur in as many as 20% of patients (Whitecloud 1989). They include persistent donor site pain, hematoma, anterior superior iliac spine fracture, bowel injury, and lateral femoral cutaneous nerve injury (Gore et al. 1987; Hukuda et al. 1985). To avoid complications at the graft site, some surgeons prefer to avoid fusion altogether and perform discectomy alone for patients whose suffering is attributed to a single level alone. A more recent trend has been to use banked bone, which completely avoids graft site problems, and likely has a fusion rate similar to autologous bone grafts. In an attempt to compare anterior operations with and without fusion, Martins in 1976 reported the results of 51 patients treated either by the Cloward procedure or by radical discectomy and foraminotomy without fusion and found that the outcomes were no different between the two groups in relieving preoperative symptoms. Almost all patients (92%) expressed satisfaction with the results of the operation. Sixty-four percent of those with the Cloward procedure had good to excellent results, while 65% of those with discectomy and foraminotomy alone had good to excellent results (Martins 1976).

Lunsford et al. in 1980 reported good results with an anterior operation for both hard (83% improvement in 168 cases) and soft discs (87% improvement in 85 cases). Overall, improvement was seen in 84% of patients with surgery. Seventy-two percent of those with soft discs and 65% of those with hard discs had either a good or an excellent result. There was no statistical difference in results, however, between those with hard versus soft discs. Neither the type of anterior procedure (Cloward vs. Smith-Robinson) nor the addition of a fusion versus simple discectomy resulted in better outcomes. Those in the fusion group had higher perioperative morbidity due to complications of the graft and graft site. The number of levels operated on did not affect outcome. Thirty-eight percent reported a recurrence of one or more symptoms during the follow-up period that were most often intermittent in nature and were almost always treated with conservative means (Lunsford et al. 1980a). In 1981, Kooijman and Bossers found that a good or satisfactory result was achieved in 89% of their 62 patients suffering from cervicobrachial syndrome (Kooijman and Bossers 1981). Later, Kooijman reported the long-term results of 154 patients with cervicobrachialgia who had been treated by the anterior approach and were then followed for an average of 12 years. Seventy-five percent of these patients had relief of their pain and paresthesias (Kooijman 1991).

Benini et al. in 1982 reported their results in 25 patients who received an anterior operation without fusion for cervical disc herniation. Overall, 88% of their patients experienced relief of pain, with immediate relief in 76% and delayed relief (4 to 6 months) in 12%. Only 8% continued to have paresthesias in one to two fingers (Benini et al. 1982). Similarly, Tegos et al. in 1994 had excellent results in their series of patients who were treated by anterior discectomy without fusion. Ninety-five percent of their patients experienced improvement in radiculopathy (Tegos et al. 1994). The following year, Pointillart et al. reviewed 68 patients who received an anterior cervical discectomy without fusion and were able to achieve follow-up in 57 of these cases. The average time to follow-up was 23 months and 92% were found to have excellent or good clinical results (Pointillart et al. 1995).

Gore and Sepic in 1984 reported a 96% incidence of complete or near-complete resolution of symptoms after anterior discectomy and fusion in their 146 patients. Mean follow-up was 5 years. Of those with arm pain alone, 86% had complete relief; versus 80% for those with neck and arm pain; versus 56% for those with neck, arm, and head pain. Patients who had a shorter preoperative duration of symptoms did better, which led Gore and Sepic to agree with others (Herzberger et al. 1962; Hirsch et al. 1964) that those with surgically correctable problems should have surgery promptly following a trial of conservative measures. They also found, as did others (De Palma et al. 1972; Robinson et al. 1962), that the osteophytes would spontaneously resorb after solid fusion in most cases and that pain relief would usually occur prior to osteophyte resorption. They did not, therefore, advocate removal of osteophytes (Gore and Sepic 1984). In that same year, Mosdal published his review of 755 patients who received an anterior discectomy and fusion (Cloward technique) for neck pain, radiculopathy, and myelopathy. Eighty-one percent experienced relief following surgery, but at follow-up only 71% had benefited with regard to neck pain or radiculopathy. The operative complication rate was 4% (Mosdal 1984).

In 1990, Clements and O'Leary reported in retrospective fashion their results of 94 patients treated by an anterior operation for posterolateral spondylosis and/or disc herniation. Only symptomatic levels were treated even though in 23 patients additional asymptomatic levels of spondylosis were present. In those with only symptomatic levels, 88% had either a good or excellent result, whereas in those with asymptomatic levels that were left untreated only 60% had a good or excellent result. Despite this, they recommend surgery for the levels that are symptomatic rather than all levels with spondylosis, as those with additional levels will have good to excellent results 60% of the time and that when the procedure is deemed a failure, a salvage operation is always possible. The rate of pseudoarthrosis in this series was 4% (Clements and O'Leary 1990). The same year, Herkowitz et al. in their series of 17 patients with soft disc herniation treated by the anterior approach, 94% noted good or excellent results (Herkowitz et al. 1990).

In 1992, Bosacco et al. found that satisfactory results were achieved in 87% of 232 patients who underwent anterior cervical discectomy and fusion and were followed for an average of 6.8 years (Bosacco et al. 1992). That same year, Brodke and Zdeblick reported excellent results in 51 patients who were treated by anterior discectomy and fusion and followed for an average of 1 year. Excellent or good results were obtained in 92% of cases, and 88% of those with a soft disc as opposed to 100% of those with a hard disc had good or excellent results. The patients with radiculopathy had better outcomes than those whose chief complaint was only pain (95% excellent to good vs. 78%, respectively) (Brodke and Zdeblick 1992).

Romner et al. in 1994 reported on 52 patients who had undergone an anterior operation for cervical radiculopathy and found that in 94% an excellent outcome was achieved (Romner et al. 1994). Brigham and Tsahakis in 1995 reported their results in 43 patients who underwent an anterior operation for cervical radiculopathy and reported good to excellent results in 77% to 14%, respectively. Three patients (7%) had no relief, but none were worse. All of their patients expressed satisfaction, with 72% being very satisfied and 28% being somewhat satisfied. Relief of radicular pain was achieved in all (100%) patients with single-level spondylosis or herniated disc, whereas relief of neck pain was seen in 32 of the 36 patients (89%) who described neck pain as a component of their chief complaint. The rate of bony fusion in this study was 93% (Brigham and Tsahakis 1995).

## Posterior Approaches for Radiculopathy

The classic papers by Spurling and Scoville in 1944 and by Frykholm in 1947 describe the posterior approach for decompression of the foramen (Spurling and Scoville 1944; Frykholm 1947). Since publication of these two papers, numerous investigators have found the posterior approach to yield good or excellent results in over 90% of cases (Aldrich 1990; Henderson et al 1983; Krupp et al. 1990; Murphey et al. 1973; Scoville et al. 1976; Williams 1983; Zeidman and Ducker 1993; Simeone and Dillin 1986; Fager 1977, 1978; Rothman and Simeone 1992; Tomaras et al. 1997; Kumar et al. 1998). In large part, the great success of the following papers is due to the careful selection of patients. Posterior microdiscectomy is particularly useful for posterolateral disc hernia-

tions, whereas the anterior approach for central disc herniation is more appropriate.

Murphey et al. in 1973 reported a large series of 648 patients who received an operation for a laterally ruptured cervical disc. They were able to obtain a follow-up on 380 of these patients. They reported improvement in 100% of their patients after surgery, with 37% experiencing 100% relief, 90% obtained a good or excellent result, 90% were able to keep the same job as preoperatively, and only 4% had to change jobs as a result of pain. Follow-up was from 1 to 28 years. In their large series, there was less than a 1% chance of an adverse event (Murphey et al. 1973). Five years later, Fager reported a 97% incidence of excellent outcome in his patients treated by a posterior approach (Fager 1978).

Henderson et al. in 1983 reviewed the posterior approach to cervical radiculopathy in 846 consecutive operative cases in 736 patients: 96% experienced relief of significant arm pain or paresthesias, 98% experienced resolution of motor deficit, 92% considered themselves to have had either a good or excellent result, 103 patients (13.9%) required an additional posterior procedure but only 3.3% were considered recurrence (same side, same level), and seven patients (1%) required three procedures. Mean follow-up was 2.8 years and their was no significant difference in outcomes between those with a hard versus a soft disc. The mean length of time to return to work or normal activity was 9.4 weeks (Henderson et al. 1983). Simeone and Dillin in 1986 had similar results with a good or excellent outcome in 96% of their patients treated by a posterior laminoforaminotomy (Simeone and Dillin 1986).

Aldrich (1990) reported excellent results in his series of 36 patients treated by the posterior approach. All had acute monoradiculopathy caused by soft cervical disc herniation. Pain relief and motor-power improvement was immediate in all (100%) patients. Sensory and residual motor loss improved dramatically and normalized at approximately 6 months. No complications are reported, mean hospital stay was 2 days, and mean follow-up was 26 months. The author comments that the disadvantages of the posterior approach, which include postoperative neck pain and instability, can be avoided by using microsurgical techniques with a small midline incision and a limited facetectomy. He also agrees with the comments of Fager (1977) and Murphey et al. (1973) that this is one of the most gratifying of all neurosurgical procedures (Aldrich 1990). That same year, Herkowitz et al. reported that in their series of 16 patients with soft disc herniation treated by the posterior approach, 75% noted good or excellent results while 93% reported improvement (Herkowitz et al. 1990).

Zeidman and Ducker in 1993 reported excellent results in their series of 172 patients who were treated by the posterior approach for lateral nerve root compression over a 7-year period: 97% (167) of patients reported relief of radicular pain, and 93% of those with weakness who underwent a laminoforaminotomy with discectomy (36 of 39 patients) experienced improvement to baseline function (Zeidman and Ducker 1993).

Davis in 1996 studied 163 patients who had been treated by the posterior approach for cervical radiculopathy due to either hard or soft discs with a mean follow-up of 15 years and found an 86% success rate. Only ten patients (6%) had poor outcomes, and seven of these did strenuous work and had workers' compensation claims, two were at psychologic risk or were addicted to medications, and one had a legal claim (Davis 1996).

Woertgen et al. (1997) performed a prospective study of prognostic factors for 54 patients with lateral cervical disc herniations treated with dorsal foraminotomy. At 1 year of follow-up 94% were either completely recovered or improved. A short duration of preoperative complaints and unequivocal radicular radiation were associated with better outcomes. They also make an argument for early surgery in those with motor or sensory loss because the risk of an unsuccessful outcome increases when these signs are present and the surgery is delayed more than 2 to 3 months.

Tomaras et al. (1997) reported that a series of 200 healthy patients treated for cervical radiculopathy on an outpatient basis by the posterior approach obtained excellent results. In those cases where workers' compensation claims were not involved, 93% of patients obtained either an excellent or good result and were able to return to work at a mean of 2.9 weeks. In cases that involved workers' compensation claims, 78% of patients reported an excellent or good outcome and were able to return to work at a mean of 7.6 weeks postoperatively. Seven patients (3.8%) had a poor outcome, and two of these underwent an additional posterior procedure and reported a good outcome

at follow-up. There was follow-up in 183 patients and the mean follow-up was 19 months. No patients were readmitted in the immediate postoperative period.

## Spondylosis and Disc Disease in the Thoracic Spine

Although long recognized as a disease entity, degenerative disease involving the thoracic spine is rare, compared to spondylosis, stenosis, and disc herniation affecting the cervical and lumbar regions. The understanding of the thoracic spine, its biomechanics, and the diseases that affect it has improved over the last several decades. Much of this change can be attributed to improvements in radiologic techniques, including computed tomography (CT)-myelography and especially MRI. Technological innovations have also led to the development of new ways to surgically access these areas, including endoscopic assisted approaches. These changes have resulted in improvement in the prognosis for individuals suffering from degenerative thoracic spine disease.

### Thoracic Disc Herniation

Thoracic disc herniation is the most common degenerative disorder involving the thoracic spine. While it was previously thought that these herniations comprise approximately 1% of all clinically symptomatic spinal disc herniations (Arce and Dorhmann 1985), the advent of MRI and CT-myelography has suggested that thoracic disc herniations occur in 11% to 14% of patients (Awwad et al. 1991). Some studies suggest a slight female preponderance (1.4 : 1). The age at onset is predominantly in the fourth through sixth decades. Although disc herniations have been found at all thoracic interspaces, the most common areas of involvement are T8–T11. As many as 75% may be found below the T8 level (Arce and Dorhmann 1985). The next most common region involves T1 and T2, with rare occurrences from T3–T7 (Stillerman and Weiss 1992). It is postulated that these common areas of involvement are the result of biomechanical forces acting at the thoracolumbar and cervicothoracic junctions (Haley and Perry 1950). The relatively immobile midthoracic region is stabilized additionally by the rib cage.

An unusual presentation is it that of intradural disc herniation. It is thought to be secondary to dense adhesions between the posterior longitudinal ligament and the ventral dura mater (Blikra 1969). Although results can be favorable, the majority of reported cases have poor long-term results. Thus it must be considered as a problem with a poor prognosis when encountered (Isla et al. 1988); three of four sited case reports resulted in long-term paraparesis or paraplegia.

There is no pathognomonic clinical presentation for a herniated thoracic disc. They commonly present with back pain. Antecedent trauma was found in association in all 14 patients reviewed by Carson et al. (1971). However, trauma is not a consistent finding, as only 35% of patients reviewed by Le Roux et al. in 1993 had such a history. The pain is more often found in the mid to upper spinal region. A radiating radicular component along a rib border is common, due to impingement on the exiting intercostal nerve root. Although sensory findings are common, they usually are not as useful as pain for determining level of herniation. In one study, 80% of patients had radicular pain that correctly localized the level of the herniation (Le Roux et al. 1993). Because the thoracic spinal canal is so narrow, even small herniations can prove symptomatic. Myelopathic symptoms, including hyper-reflexia, gait abnormalities, or bladder dysfunction indicate spinal cord or high conus medullaris compression. Close examination may also reveal Brown-Sequard symptomatology. Myelopathy is usually a late sign. Retrospective analysis will often reveal a protracted course of vague symptoms often extending over years preceding the development of myelopathy. High thoracic disc herniation is rare (<4% of all thoracic disc herniations) and may present with radicular medial arm pain, intrinsic hand weakness, and an associated Horner's syndrome (Alberico et al. 1986). Surgical access for treatment of these lesions is more complicated than other approaches. Good outcome and a low rate of morbidity is generally encountered when the procedure is performed by experienced surgeons (Sundaresan et al. 1984).

Myelography was the mainstay of diagnosis for years, and this technique has been significantly improved with the advent of CT. MRI has also been found extremely helpful in revealing spinal cord changes resulting from compression (Francavilla et al. 1987). Unlike lumbar and most cervical herniations, thoracic herniations will often become calcified. This has led some to recommend plain films as an initial tool for evaluation (Baker et al. 1965). Although plain radiographs may uncover other abnormalities including compression fractures or kyphosis, it cannot reliably distinguish such calcified herniations. The development of CT-myelography and MRI has also led to the diagnosis of many lesions that are asymptomatic (Awwad et al. 1991). Despite some lesions being large and others small, no radiological features have been found to reliably predict neurologic findings (Le Roux et al. 1993).

The nonsurgical approach to treatment is most often recommended initially, unless motor weakness or bladder dysfunction is present, associated with cord compression. Rest in association with nonsteroidal anti-inflammatory agents can often relieve symptoms of radiculopathy. Persistence of symptoms or myelopathy often indicates the need for surgical intervention. A better prognosis following surgical treatment has been found for those who have noncalcified disc herniations, symptoms lasting less than 1 month, and an association with a traumatic event (Arce and Dorhmann 1985) (Table 9-1).

For many years, posterior approaches were considered the standard of care. The results following decompressive laminectomy for thoracic disc herniation have been disappointing due to the need for significant cord manipulation to access the disc protrusion (Arseni and Nash 1960). Only 42.5% had fair results; an additional 57.5% were left with paraplegia or paraparesis when only laminectomy was performed. To avoid cord manipulation, anterior and lateral approaches were devised (transthoracic, lateral extracavitary, and the transpedicular approach), and results are now

**Table 9-1.** Prognostic Factors for Treatment of Thoracic Disc Herniation

| Favorable Prognostic Signs | Poor Prognostic Signs |
| --- | --- |
| Strong correlation between radiographic images and symptoms | Weak correlation between radiographic images and symptoms |
| Short duration (<1 month) | Long duration |
| Radiculopathy only | Acute paraplegia/bladder dysfunction/myelopathy |
| Traumatic etiology | Nontraumatic etiology |
| Soft disc herniation | Calcified disc herniation |
| Low thoracic level of involvement (T8–T12) | High thoracic lesion (T1–T2) |

much improved (Arce and Dorhmann 1985). A thoracic laminectomy supplemented by a transpedicular approach is the most commonly utilized procedure to surgically treat these lesions; it allows posterolateral access, thus avoiding cord manipulation. It also avoids the risks associated with transthoracic surgery, and fusion is rarely indicated (Sekhar and Jannetta 1983). Although calcified disc herniations were once a poor prognostic sign, specialized curettes are now available that enable easier removal of all herniations (Le Roux et al. 1993). The lateral extracavitary approach has been described for treatment of thoracic fractures (Larson et al. 1976). For the well-trained surgeon, the more technically demanding extracavitary approach can be as effective as the transpedicular approach with less cord manipulation (Maiman et al. 1984). Despite this advantage, the results are not significantly different than the more simply performed transpedicular approach. The transthoracic approach may be employed successfully in skilled hands but generally is associated with a higher rate of morbidity compared to the other approaches (Ransohoff et al. 1969). However, recent improvements have allowed transthoracic approaches to be performed more safely. The incorporation of endoscopic assisted thoracic procedures may prove to change the standard of surgical approach in the future. However, until most spinal surgeons become familiar with the equipment and the anatomy, the posterior transpedicular approach will remain the most often performed procedure.

## Thoracic Stenosis

Thoracic spinal stenosis is more unusual than thoracic disc herniation. Myelopathy is generally the predominant symptom rather than pain. Symptoms may include motor or sensory complaints, but often are vague and rarely relate to a specific nerve root involvement. Like stenosis in other regions of the spine, canal narrowing is secondary to facet arthropathy, ligamentum hypertrophy, as well as disc degeneration. When stenosis is secondary to facet arthropathy and laminar thickening, laminectomy with medial facetectomy yields good results. In one series, five of seven patients showed stabilization or improvement of myelopathy (Yamamoto et al. 1988). Long-standing myelopathy resulting from spondylosis alone can respond favorably to decompressive laminectomy

(Marzluff et al. 1979); one patient was followed for 6 years before appropriate diagnosis was made and surgery performed.

OPLL can occur in the thoracic spine and may cause stenosis. Because the pathology is anterior, many suggest that it be approached surgically via a transthoracic or trans-sternal approach. The results have been favorable, but are limited in numbers. One study reported three patients treated for progressive myelopathy including gait disturbance; two had improvement of lower extremity strength, while one developed paraplegia that returned to preoperative levels over 3 months (Kojima et al. 1994). Calcified dural adhesions create a high risk for CSF leak, and the need for interbody fusion makes the long-term prognosis less favorable than other causes of stenosis treated by posterior decompression. Ossification of the ligamentum flavum (OLF) can also significantly affect the thoracic spine. OLF has been found to affect primarily the T10–T12 regions (Okada et al. 1991). It can be identified by its typical beak-like projection into the dorsal spinal canal as seen by lateral radiographs; however, it is best viewed by CT (Miyasaka 1982). Surgical complications including iatrogenic kyphosis and poor results with laminectomy alone have been found; 10 of 14 patients had laminectomy with fair results in 40% and neurological deterioration in 30%. More favorable results were found when decompression in association with laminoplasty was performed; four of four patient had improvement in lower extremity strength (Okada et al. 1991).

Although relatively rare, thoracic degenerative disease is becoming a more readily identified disorder especially with the more frequent use of MRI and CT-myelography to evaluate patients with possible spinal disorders. Prognosis is good for disc herniations when symptoms are radicular in nature, they are of relatively short duration (less than several months), and they are clearly related to a low thoracic level (Table 9-2). Although a traumatic etiology is also associated with favorable prognosis, this may be because patients sought medical attention at an earlier time. In skilled hands, all surgical approaches have good results. The transpedicular approach incorporates low morbidity with effective decompression. Poor prognosis is found when symptoms correlate poorly with radiographic findings, when symptoms have been present for years, and when myelopathy has developed. Although surgically accessible, high thoracic lesions tend to have poorer results due to a higher morbidity with surgery. Thoracic spinal stenosis most often presents with myelopathic symptoms present for years. Surgical treatment is especially required to halt the natural history of progressive myelopathy. Nonoperative therapy alone has poor results with thoracic stenosis. When stenosis is secondary to spondylosis, the results are very good; however, the association of ossification of the ligamentum flavum or posterior longitudinal ligament significantly worsens surgical outcome (Table 9-2).

## Spondylosis and Disc Disease in the Lumbar Spine

Low back pain is experienced by nearly all individuals at some point in their lives. The discomfort may be isolated to the low back, or the pain may radiate down the leg. For most, the resolution is rapid, often only requiring a short period of rest or diminished activity level. For some, however, the pain becomes severe and functionally incapacitating. For these individuals, recovery may require not only rest but significant changes in work, the need for medication, and possibly surgical intervention.

The most common cause of lumbar dysfunction lies in the degenerative changes that occur in all of us as we age (Mooney 1987). For some, this natural process can be very debilitating. For others, the aging process may only create anatomical changes without development of symptoms. As common degenerative changes occur throughout the spine, various anatomical changes are produced, and often symptom complexes develop.

**Table 9-2.** Prognostic Factors in Thoracic Stenosis

| Favorable Prognostic Signs | Poor Prognostic Signs |
| --- | --- |
| Spondylotic stenosis | Nonoperative therapy |
| Short duration of symptoms | Long duration of myelopathy |
| Clear association of symptoms with radiographic findings | Stenosis secondary to ossification of the ligamentum flavum (OLF) |
| | Stenosis secondary to ossification of the posterior longitudinal ligament (OPLL) |

The prognosis for improvement via either medical or surgical intervention is dependent on a multitude of factors. The two most important prognostic factors relating to successful treatment of lumbar spinal pathology are accurate diagnosis and appropriate patient selection.

## Lumbar Disc Herniation

Lumbar disc herniation is one of the most common degenerative spinal disorders. The pathophysiology of disc rupture is based on the development of small tears in the annulus fibrosus, typically in the dorsolateral region. Compressive, flexive, and rotational forces associated with disc dehydration and degeneration found with aging lead to prolapse and herniation of the nucleus pulposus through these small openings (Gordon et al. 1991). The subsequent impingement of the adjacent nerve root leads to radiculopathy. Treatment for symptomatic disc herniations accounts for the majority of lumbar spinal surgery. Because the most common disc spaces involved are L4–L5 and L5–S1, L5 and S1 radiculopathy are the common clinical findings. The symptoms can be subtle, including mild weakness or numbness, or they may be severe including foot drop or bladder incontinence. Severe pain radiating down the posterior aspect of the leg (i.e., sciatica) is the symptom that causes most patients to seek medical attention (Pappas et al. 1992).

Although disc herniation can be found in the pediatric population, it is quite rare. More often it is found in 30- to 50-year-old individuals, with a preponderance in males. Heavy lifting or vigorous physical activity is often antecedent in the history, but many patients have an otherwise sedentary lifestyle (Pappas et al. 1992). Physical examination is important because often signs of radiculopathy are found that have gone unnoticed by the patient. Physical exam maneuvers including the straight leg raise or lateral bending can also help with diagnostic decision making (Smith et al. 1993). Because lumbar radiculopathy is nonspecific, it can be caused by various other etiologies including facet arthropathy, nerve sheath tumors, or rarely metabolic abnormalities such as diabetic mononeuropathy (Zahrawi 1988). Lumbar radiculopathy can also be found in various lumbar degenerative disorders including disc herniation, stenosis, spondylosis, and spondylolisthesis (Paine and Haung 1972). Therefore, to confirm the diagnosis, radiographic tests including CT-myelography and MRI have become standard (Hashimoto et al. 1990). Difficulty develops with appropriate diagnosis when the imaging does not confirm the clinical findings (i.e., wrong level or wrong side of nerve root involvement, many herniated discs, or no disc herniation). The first step toward successful treatment is accurate diagnosis of a symptomatic herniated disc.

The prognosis of symptomatic disc herniation is such that a several-week course of bedrest associated with analgesics will result in complete resolution of symptoms in 32%. An additional 44% will benefit from prolonged physiotherapy. Incapacitating pain or acute profound neurologic deficit are findings that warrant early surgical intervention, and can occur in up to 24% of patients (Weber 1983). Another subset of patients often benefits from conservative care, but has residual symptoms. Among 280 patients in Weber's prospective randomized study, 44% still had significant symptoms at 2 weeks. These patients were randomized into surgery versus further conservative care with the addition of physical therapy. In the ensuing year, 10% randomized to conservative care developed recurrent symptoms so severe they required surgery. At 1 year, the conservatively treated patients had a 25% good result and 50% fair result. Those randomized to surgery had a 66% good and 25% fair result. Recurrence of symptoms was twice as common among the conservatively treated patients in the first 4 years at 25% compared to 13% for those surgically treated. However, in the next 6 years, this trend reversed and those originally randomized to surgery had a 30% recurrence compared to only 20% for the conservatively randomized patients. Despite the recurrence rate, symptoms were severe enough to require reoperation in only 7% randomized to surgery. At 10 years, surgery resulted in 60% good and 33% fair results compared to 57% and 36%, respectively, for conservative care. While the difference in outcome is not statistically significant at 10-year follow-up, the data suggest that surgery may be better treatment when symptoms are persistent. Furthermore, in properly selected patients, surgery produces more rapid improvement, permitting earlier return to work and a more normal lifestyle.

Sensory deficits were found in 35% at 10 years, and were evenly distributed between the two groups. Motor deficits were found in only 7%; they also were evenly distributed. The natural history with conservative treatment alone is, therefore, very similar over a 10-year time span compared to surgical treatment. The only significant changes were noted in those with persistent symptoms treated with surgery during the first year following diagnosis (Weber 1983).

Surgery should usually be reserved for those with neurological deficits, although there is a role for surgery in those with persistent pain without neurological deficit following extensive conservative care. Most agree that disabling pain that is clearly radicular and correlates with findings on diagnostic imaging is a relative indication for surgery, if conservative measures fail, even without the presence of a neurological deficit.

Lumbar microdiscectomy currently is the surgery of choice. Standard surgical technique includes a small laminotomy to access the spinal canal and the disc space allowing removal of the disc fragment (lumbar microdiscectomy) (Wilson and Harbaugh 1981). A foraminotomy to enlarge the neural foramen, and thus further decompress the nerve root is also often performed (Panjabi et al. 1983). Today this should be performed under loupe or microscopic magnification. The standard lumbar laminectomy with discectomy and without neurodissection has been found to increase hospital stay. Standard hospital stays range from 3 to 6 days in most studies with standard laminectomy. Comparing the two surgeries, time to discharge was decreased 2.63 days and the mean time to return to work was 4.8 days with microdiscectomy versus 11.76 days for the standard procedure (Wilson and Harbaugh 1981). Ambulatory surgery is now safely being performed, with same-day discharges in 91% of patients undergoing microdiscectomy; of these patients, 92% had relief of back pain and 96% had relief of radicular pain (Bookwalter et al. 1994).

Some have suggested that minimal disc fragment removal versus radical disc space curettage leads to a higher rate of recurrence (Semmes 1960). A 4% recurrence following curettage has been stated, although a 10% recurrence is most commonly reported (Maroon and Abla 1985). Microdiscectomy with disc fragment removal has been shown to have a 7% recurrence (Williams 1978).

In today's society, cost is an ever-increasing concern. Cost analysis studies have shown the long-term monetary costs to be similar comparing surgical ($56,054) to nonsurgical therapy ($53,638) over a 5-year period. Significantly more work was missed with the nonsurgically treated patients (97.4 weeks) compared to the surgically treated patient (78.9 weeks) over this 5-year period, accounting for nearly 1 month extra lost work per year (Shvartzman et al. 1992).

Results of surgical procedures are difficult to standardize, because they must include improvement of symptoms as well as return to activity and return of function. Typically, results are defined as excellent if symptoms are completely resolved, associated with only occasional back pain, there is return to prior occupation, and if the prior general activity level is maintained. Good results are described when intermittent back or leg pain remains requiring medications, but the patient is able to return to their prior occupation. However, usually there is a general decline in the level of physical activity. Fair results occur when there is improvement in symptoms but not a complete return to baseline function, there is a continued need for pharmaceutical treatment, and the patient can work but has changed occupations. Poor results and failure occur when symptoms persist, the patient cannot return to work, and activity level declines significantly (Zahrawi 1988).

Poor prognosis is frequently the case when inappropriate treatment strategies are utilized. In the past, chemonucleosis was a treatment option, but the results and potential complications have eliminated it as a viable treatment choice (Van Alphen et al. 1989; Deburge et al. 1985). Watters et al. in 1988 compared standard lumbar discectomy to chemonucleosis and found only 64% with good to excellent results for chemonucleosis compared to 84% with surgery. Return to work was also earlier in the surgery group (Watters et al. 1988). In the past, an anterior approach for symptomatic disc rupture was also considered a treatment option. Blumenthal et al. in 1987 stated that this was successful in 74% of his patients (Blumenthal et al. 1988). Despite his relative success, the disadvantages are substantially higher, including complications such as abdominal injury as well as the need for successful fusion (Blumenthal et al. 1988). The posterior approach with laminotomy and microdiscectomy has become

the standard, well-recognized surgical approach (Williams 1978). With the advent of new technological advances, percutaneous endoscopic assisted microdiscectomy may become the standard surgical strategy in the future (Mayer and Brock 1991). Regardless of surgical technique, accurate diagnosis is of utmost importance. Multiple prior operations suggest inappropriate diagnosis or patient selection, and reoperation has a much lower chance for successful outcome.

Poor prognostic factors include acute motor paralysis, urinary retention, associated litigation, age greater than 50, and comorbid medical conditions (Pappas et al. 1992). Other studies have not revealed such results. Weber in 1983 showed male gender and physical activity to be prognostically important for good outcome at 4 years but only age to be important at 10-year follow-up (mean age in good outcome, 40.3 years; mean age in poor outcome, 46.9 years). Workers' compensation cases tend to have worse results; 100% of noncompensation patients improved compared to 88.2% of compensation cases (Zahrawi 1988). Good prognosis for improvement is dependent on many variables (Table 9-3). A short symptom period with a clearly diagnosable radiculopathy leads to appropriate diagnosis without chronic neuropathic changes. Motor and sensory symptomatology are often significantly improved with surgery, but long-term studies reveal 7% residual weakness and 35% sensory abnormalities at 10-year follow-up (Weber 1983). Most single-level, first-time operations for lumbar disc disease will have good or excellent results; Zahrawi in 1988 described 10% good and 83% excellent initial postsurgical outcomes. Men tended to have better outcomes than women (Zahrawi 1988); this trend seen in Weber's study at 4-year follow-up was not seen at 10-year follow-up. Interestingly, no prognostic correlation was found with occupation, duration of symptoms,

**Table 9-3.** Prognostic Factors for Treatment of Lumbar Disc Herniation

| Favorable Prognostic Signs | Poor Prognostic Signs |
| --- | --- |
| Age <40 | Age >40 |
| Associated with non-industrial accident | Industrial accident |
| No prior surgery | Multiple prior operations |
| Self-employed | Workers' compensation |
| No premorbid medical conditions | litigation |
|  | Multiple other medical problems |

or level of disease. At 10-year follow-up, only age was statistically significant (Weber 1983). Of importance is the fact that in both the surgically treated group and in those with conservative treatment, the recurrence rate was approximately equal (20%) over the 10-year follow-up period. Symptoms were also found to be so debilitating in 20% treated conservatively that they went on to have surgery within 1 year of initiating conservative therapy (Zahrawi 1988). Pappas et al. in 1992 showed a more favorable result in individuals with a higher level of education and in those patients who were self-employed. Nonindustrial injuries were found to have a 96% success rate (i.e., good to excellent result) compared to 74% for those suffering industrial accidents (Pappas et al 1992). Padua et al. (1999) confirm the fact that most patients without complicating factors continue to enjoy good to excellent outcomes from hemilaminectomy as long as 15 years after surgery.

Despite the excellent results seen following surgery, many will respond to conservative treatment and this should be initially recommended. Ten-year follow-up in most studies shows similar results between conservative and surgical treatment. Better results are seen from surgical treatment after 1 year. The results favor surgery but are closer 4 years following surgery (Weber 1983). Appropriate diagnosis, patient selection, and proper surgical technique ultimately are the most important factors contributing to successful surgical treatment.

## Far Lateral Disc Herniations

Far lateral disc herniations comprise approximately 10% of all lumbar disc herniations (Hood 1996). They occur in the far lateral region of the disc space resulting in foraminal or extraforaminal nerve root compression. Typical lumbar disc herniations appear in the dorsolateral portion of the annulus and subsequent caudal displacement causes compression on the inferior nerve root (i.e., a L5 radiculopathy from an L4–L5 disc herniation). The far lateral disc herniation impinges on the superior root; displacement is rostral rather than caudal. Severe pain often is associated with such pathology. It is speculated that this finding is the result of compression near the dorsal root ganglion (Maroon et al. 1990). Most far lateral disc herniations occur above the L5–S1 level and therefore present as an L2–L4 radicular syndrome (Abdullah

et al. 1988). Pain with straight leg raising (SLR) occurs in approximately 10% suffering far lateral disc herniation. Lateral bending maneuvers can elicit symptoms in up to 83% of cases (Abdullah et al. 1988). Because the fragment is outside the spinal canal and often beyond the root sleeve, it can be difficult if not impossible to detect by myelography. The introduction of CT helped better identify lateralized disc herniations (Godersky et al. 1984). Before MRI this entity was substantially underreported, accounting for less than 2% of lumbar disc operations (Macnab 1971). Although some advocate the use of discography with or without CT to help identify far lateral disc herniation, most spinal surgeons utilize MRI solely or in combination with CT-myelography (Angtuaco et al. 1984). Most studies now recognize that with the advent of MRI, the occurrence is approximately 10%.

The approaches to lateral disc herniation include a standard laminectomy combining an intraspinal approach to the disc space with an extracanalicular approach (Jane et al. 1990). Occasionally, an entirely extraspinal approach is utilized with a paramedian incision rather than a midline incision; this approach is advocated without facetectomy to decrease risk of spinal instability (Maroon et al. 1990). Due to the association of lateral recess stenosis with many disc herniations, CT-myelography, which shows bony anatomy better than MRI, has been found valuable by some surgeons in determining the appropriate surgical approach (Epstein et al. 1990). The outcome of surgery for these herniations is generally good. Complete pain relief was found in 81% and only mild back discomfort was found in 15% 3 months following surgery (Abdullah et al. 1988).

## Lumbar Stenosis

Lumbar stenosis is a degenerative condition in which narrowing of the spinal canal in the lumbar region leads to compromise of the neurovascular structures, resulting in low back and leg pain (Watanabe and Parke 1986). It is often related to position due to dynamic changes in canal size. This syndrome occurs primarily with walking and is relieved with rest. Because these symptoms are similar to vascular symptoms in those with peripheral vascular disease, it is referred to as neurogenic claudication due to its neurological origin (Epstein and Epstein 1996). This complex may also be associated with a distinct radiculopathy.

Many patients are susceptible to this disease due to congenital narrowing of the sagittal diameter of the canal (Pappas and Sonntag 1996). Facet arthropathy (spondylosis), disc herniation, and thickening of the ligamentum flavum often contribute to canal compromise (Kirkaldy-Willis et al. 1978). Bilateral canal disease diffusely or at a single level will tend to create concentric circumferential narrowing and generalized symptoms. Lateral recess stenosis secondary to facet arthropathy contributes to development of radicular symptoms (Epstein et al. 1972). With all forms of stenosis, small acute disc herniations may lead to severe neurological deficits due to the compromised canal space. Approximately 15% of lumbar stenosis patients will have an associated disc herniation.

Biomechanical studies have shown that the general shape of the canal is similar to a triangle with variability of both the height and base. Those with congenital narrowing show symptoms earlier in life due to small sagittal diameter. They will often have short pedicles contributing to general loss of sagittal diameter. Relative stenosis occurs with a diameter of 12 mm, whereas absolute stenosis is felt to occur at 10 mm. Nearly all will show symptoms of cauda equina or nerve root involvement with this degree of stenosis. Those with otherwise normal canal size become symptomatic usually when degenerative changes in the facets lead to hypertrophy; this is therefore described as secondary or acquired stenosis (Verbiest 1972, 1980). The facets narrow the canal both in a sagittal and axial manner to such an extent they often touch (kissing facets). Studies in dogs have revealed both neural and vascular changes due to relative degrees of stenosis (Delamarter et al. 1990). With 25% compression, venous congestion and mild changes in cortical evoked potentials were found. With 50% compromise, major evoked potential changes were seen, as well as edema, major venous congestion, and demyelination in the nerve roots. At 75% compromise, axoplasmic flow was severely impaired, wallerian degeneration was seen in both motor and sensory roots, and changes were seen in the dorsal columns at superior levels in the spinal cord. Thus, vascular compromise as well as direct neural compression leads to the varied symptoms found with stenosis. Biomechanically, standing and walking leads to hyperlordosis, in-

buckling of the ligamentum flavum and, thus, canal narrowing precipitating symptoms.

Patients with congenital stenosis will often present at an earlier age (e.g., 30 to 40 years). Those with achondroplasia may present even earlier due to more severe congenital stenosis (Epstein 1955). The acquired form of lumbar stenosis tends to be seen at a later age, 50 to 60 years. Symptoms of neurogenic claudication are the presenting symptom complex in over 80% of patients. It is less frequent in patients with acquired stenosis; they often have radicular symptoms. The L5 root is the most commonly affected. Those with S1 involvement often will have significant lateral recess stenosis. Bowel and bladder incontinence is typically a rare and late finding in those with severe compromise, suggesting long-standing injury that is likely to show poor recovery following surgery (Epstein and Epstein 1996). Coexisting cervical disease is found in a significant number of individuals with lumbar stenosis; about 5% will have symptoms attributable to both regions (Epstein et al. 1984).

Because the symptoms are similar to other problems involving the lumbar region, radiographic evaluation is essential. Plain radiographs may reveal spondylotic changes, hyperlordosis, congenital stenosis, or other contributing abnormalities such as spondylolithesis. Myelography and now MRI have become essential to identify the nonosseous abnormalities, including disc herniation and ligamentum flavum hypertrophy, that often strongly contribute to canal narrowing. Although some have shown CT-myelography to be more accurate at identifying lumbar stenosis compared to MRI (92.3% to 88.5%, respectively), MRI is very accurate at identifying scar tissue when contrast is utilized (Jia and Shi 1991). MRI is, therefore, more valuable when the patient has undergone prior surgery. Dynamic flexion/extension studies utilizing MRI have been performed and show significant volume increase with flexion as well as increase in sagittal diameter (Dia et al. 1989). Dynamic studies utilizing myelography are felt to be more useful because they show complete contrast obstruction with severe stenosis during extension and release during flexion (Yamada et al. 1972). However, clinically this modality has not become widespread or entirely useful. One difficulty encountered is that many asymptomatic patients will also have significant stenosis.

Conservative therapy has been advocated as an initial treatment for those with neurogenic claudication secondary to lumbar stenosis (Johnsson et al. 1991). Follow-up at 3 years revealed 60% improvement (relief of neurogenic claudication) in the surgically treated group, with only 30% improvement in those conservatively treated. Walking capacity also increased in those treated surgically. However, no significant deterioration in function was seen in the untreated group over the 3-year follow-up period, whereas 25% of the surgically treated felt worse subjectively.

When presenting symptoms are severe, surgical intervention is warranted. Typically, complete laminectomy at the level of stenosis is performed to decompress central canal stenosis. Supplementation with medial facetectomy is performed when lateral recess stenosis and radicular symptomatology are found. When stenosis is severe over multiple levels, complete laminectomies can be performed. Postoperative instability, however, can be produced by too radical a decompression. Degenerative olithesis increased in 43% of patients (Johnsson et al. 1989; Johnson et al. 1986). Among those with instability, only 31% had good results. In the group showing no postoperative instability, 80% had good results. Due to the risk of postlaminectomy instability, some have advocated multilevel laminotomies (fenenstration procedures) (Arynpur and Ducker 1990; Young et al. 1988; Lin 1982). Total relief of symptoms occurred in 90% using multilevel lumbar laminotomies (Arynpur and Ducker 1990). This is felt to improve stability, especially in the younger patient who generally is more active and in whom spondylotic changes have not resulted in joint space fusion.

Single-level disease is most common at L4–L5. Multilevel disease, however, is more common (contributing to over 75% of symptomatic stenosis). Surgical treatment is successful (i.e., produces good or excellent results) in up to 80% of many studies. Nearly 70% of patients require two- to four-level decompression. Reoperation has only a 50% success rate. Lumbar stenosis associated with spondylolithesis is more common in women and occurs predominantly at the L4–L5 level (Alexander et al. 1985). Usually, facet arthropathy has led to in situ fusion and therefore surgical decompression is all that is required (Lee 1983). In one large series, posterolateral fusion with or without instrumentation was only recommended initially along with decompression in 4% of patients. Good to excellent results were seen in 80% of such patients. Surgical failure was felt to be secondary to inadequate decompression in most patients. Reoperation without fusion was performed in nearly all, with satisfactory results.

Many factors are involved in a successful outcome of surgical treatment (Table 9-4). Appropriate preoperative diagnosis, young age, and adequate decompression are very important in contributing to success. Overall, initial decompression in all age groups shows a 60% to 70% good or excellent outcome. In studies of patients less than 60 years of age, improvement may approach or surpass 80%. Some studies suggest that increasing age produces much poorer results. One study, however, reviewed 143 patients (average age, 74.9 years) and found a 77.3% good to excellent result during follow-up (Quigley et al. 1992). These patients were also found to have low morbidity and no increase in length of hospitalization compared to younger patients who had undergone lumbar decompression. Although intuitively it may seem that surgery for multilevel disease would be less successful than single-level stenosis, the outcomes tend to be similar in the early postoperative period. Those with radicular deficits tend to have better outcomes than those with neurogenic claudication alone. Those requiring fusion tended to have worse results. Only 3% of reoperated patients were fused. All of these patients had spondylolithesis. Only 5% of all patients with stenosis and grade I spondylolithesis, however, ultimately required fusion (Epstein and Epstein 1996). Therefore, degenerative grade I spondylolithesis and stenosis most often will not require fusion. In 1991, Herkowitz reviewed all

**Table 9-4.** Prognostic Factors for Treatment of Lumbar Stenosis

| Favorable Prognostic Signs | Poor Prognostic Signs |
| --- | --- |
| Young age (<60) | Old age (>60) |
| Neurogenic claudication with radiculopathy | Neurogenic claudication in association with bladder dysfunction |
| No prior operations | Multiple prior operation |
| No premorbid conditions | Many other medical problems |
| Complete laminectomy for decompression | Fenestration procedures |

preoperative studies in all those requiring reoperation for fusion due to postsurgical spondylolithesis. He found that disc degeneration at that level was common in all those individuals and could predict need for fusion at initial surgery (Herkowitz and Kurz 1991). Due to the overall low rate of postoperative instability, it is advocated that adequate decompression be performed. There is a slight increase in subluxation when more than three levels are decompressed, but it remains 5% to 15% in most studies. Symptomatic recurrence is most common at adjacent levels. Within 5 years of initial surgery, 27 percent have developed recurrent symptoms and at 10 years this approaches 50 percent (Epstein and Epstein 1996; Herkowitz and Kurz 1991).

## Spondylolithesis

Spondylolithesis has been a recognized spinal deformity for over a century. Kilian first described its appearance in 1854 as a subluxation of the lumbosacral joint (McPhee 1990). Lateral lumbar radiographs reveal a forward slippage of one vertebrae on its adjacent inferior vertebral body. This disorder can be found in individuals from adolescence through late adulthood. The most common levels of the spinal column involved are L4–L5 and L5–S1. Although radiologically the appearance is similar, the etiology and therefore the prognosis for improvement can be distinctly different (Bennet 1996; Baldwin 1996). Symptoms related to spondylolithesis can be very similar to those caused by many other spinal disorders (i.e., back pain with or without associated leg pain or weakness). Sensory loss or neurogenic claudication is very common. Therefore, accurate diagnosis is the first step toward improvement and leads to the best chance for symptomatic and functional recovery.

Classification of spondylolithesis grew into recognizable categories as the various etiological factors became better understood. The Meyerdig and Taillard classifications are the most widely used; however, they do not address etiology at all (Meyerding 1954; Taillard 1976). They only reflect upon the relations of the vertebral bodies as regarded by a lateral radiographs. If the slippage is one-fourth the endplate length, then it is graded type I by Meyerdig and 25% by Taillard. As the slippage increases, the grade changes similarly (type II or 50% slip, etc.). The importance of the classification is that it is simple and reflects the anatomical change over time. Progression of slippage worsens the long-term results.

Facet arthropathy (spondylosis) is the result of biomechanical stress on the facet joints leading to bone growth, and often subsequent canal narrowing and/or foraminal stenosis. This often occurs in conjunction with the dehydration and degeneration of the intervertebral discs. Disc degeneration can lead to accelerated facet arthropathy due to changes in biomechanical stress (Goel et al. 1985). Takahashi believes disc degeneration is so important in the cause of spondylolithesis that he advocates anterior interbody fusion (Takahashi et al. 1990). With such changes, the axis of downward force moves from the nucleus pulposus to the apophyseal joints, which results in their progressive hypertrophy as they try to withstand the biomechanical stress. Allbrook showed that L4 has the highest range of mobility (Allbrook 1957). The L4–L5 facet joint is obliquely oriented to the transverse plane. With arthropathic changes, this orientation can become sagittal, resulting ultimately in ventrodorsal slippage. The L5–S1 facet, on the other hand, is oriented in the coronal plane, and ventrodorsal slippage (spondylolithesis) only results from defects in the neural arch (i.e., malformation or fracture of the pars interarticularis).

Over time it was realized that spondylolithesis is a multifactorial occurrence and that the variety of etiologies and patient groups responded differently to treatment. Separating these etiological groups has led to the identification of specific factors, important for determining prognosis and appropriate treatment. It has been generally accepted that surgical stabilization combined with neural decompression is the treatment of choice in many patients with spondylolithesis whose symptoms are unresponsive to nonoperative measures (Bennet 1996; Baldwin 1996). Degenerative spondylolithesis results from long-standing spondylotic changes in the facet joints. Fracture of the pars interarticularis (or malformation, as it is regarded in the congenital form) can also lead to anterior subluxation. Spondylolysis is the result of fracture of the pars without lithesis. This entity can be asymptomatic but often is debilitating if occurring iatrogenically as a result of another posterior lumbar operation. Besides spondylolysis, lumbar stenosis also is commonly associated with spondylolithesis. Because isthmic (i.e., congenital) spondylolithesis is the result of a defect in the pars interarticularis, the neural arch does not accompany the vertebral body during its forward slip. Therefore, canal compromise (i.e., lumbar stenosis) is not found in conjunction with this entity until the slip is greater than 50%. On the other hand, degenerative spondylolithesis is almost always found with associated stenosis as a result of significant facet hypertrophy; lumbar decompression is a must for these individuals (Bennet 1996; Baldwin 1996). Scoliosis is often coexistent with spondylolithesis. In the lumbar region it is felt that it is the result of muscle spasm and often resolves following fusion of the lithesed segment (Seitsalo et al. 1988).

Congenital spondylolithesis anatomically is the result of progressive slip secondary to a loss of continuity of the pars interarticularis. The neural arch is not intact and symptoms may not become severe until marked lithesis has occurred. A study by Hanly in Pittsburg tried to identify various influences on outcome (Hanley and Levy 1989). For those with back pain alone, in situ posterolateral fusion of L4-sacrum was performed. Although direct repair of the pars defect has been performed, the long-term results are poor compared to standard posterolateral fusion (Bradford and Iza 1985; Hambly et al. 1989). For those with associated radicular symptoms, decompression also was done. Success was found not to be a function of degree of slippage. Those in litigation had satisfactory results only 39% of the time, whereas those not involved had an 83% satisfactory rate; 73% of patients with back pain alone improved, whereas only 50% with radicular symptoms were satisfied. Males and smokers did worse than women and nonsmokers. Satisfactory outcome was seen in 78% of women and only 53% of men. Smokers had 48% satisfactory rate compared to 74% for nonsmokers (Hanley and Levy 1989) (Table 9-5). Ultimately, it was shown that a workers' compensation–associated injury and pseudoarthrosis had profoundly negative influences on outcome. A trend toward unsatisfactory outcome was seen in males, smokers, and those with radicular symptoms (Hanley and Levy 1989). Advanced age did not predict outcome. Other studies have looked primarily at adolescents with spondylolithesis (Lindholm et al. 1990). Their results tend to be better. It is felt that symp-

toms in adolescents result primarily from instability, whereas in adulthood, disc degeneration and nerve root compression play a more significant role. Isthmic defects occur in approximately 5% of the white population and radiographically are not identifiable until 6 years of age (Lindholm et al. 1990). Most cases are asymptomatic, but it is felt to be the leading cause of back and sciatic pain in children and adolescents; gait abnormality and lumbar deformity also were frequent findings. The L5–S1 level is most commonly involved in adolescents (Lindholm et al. 1990).

Iatrogenic spondylolithesis results most often from damage to the pars interarticularis following wide decompression for lumbar stenosis (Shenkin and Hash 1979). In a group of individuals (mean age, 56.8 years) followed for 6 years, spondylolithesis occurred in 15% with three or more levels of decompression. There was a 6% rate for two or more levels of decompression. This study demonstrated an overall 10% rate of spondylolithesis at 6 years. Only two of the six patients (33%) were symptomatic from the slippage and both did well with relief of symptoms following posterolateral fusion.

Degenerative spondylolithesis results from facet arthropathy with an intact neural arch. This condition most often occurs in women at the L4–L5 level. The L5 nerve root becomes stretched and/or compressed resulting in radiculopathy. The L3–L4 level is the next most involved. Due to the intact neural arch, segmental stenosis and neurogenic claudication often accompany the symptoms (Matsunaga et al. 1990). An autopsy study revealed an L4–L5 spondylolithesis in 4.1%

**Table 9-5.** Prognostic Factors for Treatment of Spondylolithesis

| Favorable Prognostic Signs | Poor Prognostic Signs |
| --- | --- |
| Back pain without radiculopathy | Progressive slippage |
| Grade I spondylolithesis | >Grade I spondylolithesis |
| Degenerative spondylolithesis requiring decompression only | Iatrogenic spondylolithesis requiring reoperation for fusion |
| Adolescent congenital spondylolithesis requiring posterolateral fusion | Reoperation for pseudoarthrosis/ multiple prior operations |
| Nonsmokers | Smokers requiring fusion |
| Symptoms <4 years | Symptoms >4 years |
| Women | Males |
| No associated litigation | Workers' compensation case |

of the population. In a small study of 20 patients, all symptoms were relieved by laminectomy and medial facetectomy alone (Epstein et al. 1976). It was felt that posterolateral arthrodesis should be considered in younger individuals. Due to the intact neural arch, symptoms (i.e., cauda equina syndrome or radiculopathy) tend to occur before significant slip has occurred. The mainstay of surgical therapy has been laminectomy with medial facetectomy with or without fusion (Herron and Trippi 1989; Lombardi et al. 1985; Matsuzaki et al. 1990). Those in Epstein's study with intermittent neurogenic claudication were found to have the best response to surgery (Epstein et al. 1976). The degree and progression of slippage does not necessarily correlate with symptoms (Epstein et al. 1983).

In all individuals a period of conservative care including bedrest, diminished activities, and nonsteroidal anti-inflammatory agents is indicated prior to embarking on surgical treatment. Surgery is indicated when there has been no improvement with conservative measures. The patients with best results following surgery had predominantly preoperative complaints of intermittent neurogenic claudication. They also had symptoms for 4 or less years. The treatment included a two-level laminectomy with medial facetectomy. Among these patients, 60% were found to have spondylotic interbody fusion. Approximately 10% developed recurrence but improved with further decompression. Those who did worse has various associated risk factors including diabetes, obesity, and hip and knee arthropathy limiting functional ambulation (Epstein et al. 1983).

## Lumbar Fusion

Fusion may be required to maintain stability for a variety of spinal disorders. The rationale for lumbar fusion in cases of low back pain is based on the assumption that the fusion will eliminate motion at a degenerated and unstable spinal segment, thus relieving the back pain (McCormick 1996). Complications with bone graft harvest, fusion technique, or placement of instrumentation can affect successful outcome (Kurz et al. 1989; Whitecloud et al. 1989; Jones et al. 1989). With appropriate technique and rigid postoperative immobilization, posterolateral fusion occurs in 70% with isthmic spondylolithesis. An 88% fusion rate is attained when anterior interbody fusion is also performed. Degenerative spondylolithesis has a 95% fusion rate when posterolateral and anterior interbody fusion is performed. Poor indications are the strongest source for poor outcome. Fusion to halt the progressive slippage in spondylolithesis is the most commonly accepted and agreed-on indication (Laasonen and Soini 1989). Fusion for degenerative disc disease with or without discectomy and root decompression is controversial, although it has a role in selected patients. Recurrent pain following fusion is a challenge, as the etiology may be canal or foraminal stenosis, pseudoarthrosis, disc herniation, and/or facet arthropathy. Pseudoarthrosis has generally been considered a leading cause for poor results and persistent symptoms in patients following fusion. Lateral flexion/extension radiographs may reveal movement but are often false-positive for fusion (Dvorak et al. 1991; Hayes et al. 1989; Liyang et al. 1989). Excessive movement is felt to represent instability (Dupuis et al. 1985). Hairline fractures and fragmentation are better defined by CT scan (Laasonen and Soini 1989). The accuracy of radiological evaluation to determine adequacy of fusion is poor, however, with all modalities used (Brodsky et al. 1991). When symptoms persist, reoperation to fuse the pseudoarthrosis often is beneficial, although excellent results are rare. The leading cause of pseudoarthrosis is the number of levels involved, and a history of tobacco use (Silcox et al. 1995). A functional failure may occur with or without appropriate fusion (Prolo 1996).

Posterolateral fusion is predominantly utilized now but may be supplemented with anterior interbody fusion to help obtain a higher rate of fusion (Kim et al. 1990; Loguidice et al. 1988). Placement of instrumentation has inherent risks, but its use has led to improved rates of lumbar fusion (Farber et al. 1995; Vaccaro and Garfin, 1995). As with all surgical procedures, these risks are reduced when placement is performed by experienced surgeons (Weinstein et al. 1988).

There are three main fusion techniques in the lumbar spine: posterior, posterolateral, and anterior. Biomechanical studies have revealed that such fusions create different shifts in spinal stressors (Lee and Langrana 1984; Fraser 1995). In all cases, however, the center of gravity was moved posterior, creating stronger forces on the facet joints with the greatest effect on the level adjacent to the fusion. The load transmission was more evenly distributed with the anterior and posterolateral fusions. These studies showed the posterior fusion to have the greatest load changes, and many patients eventually developed adjacent-level facet hypertrophy and stenosis.

The development of adjacent-level disease following lumbar fusion is a significant problem. This incidence has been reported in 11% to 41% with all fusion types (Lee and Langrana 1984). One study revealed an average symptom-free interval of 8.5 years (Lee 1988), after which patients usually presented with recurrent back pain. All had hypertrophied facets with stenosis above the level of fusion except one, who had an L1–L4 fusion who subsequently developed L5 facet arthropathy. Treatment with improvement occurred with further decompression alone. Symptomatic degenerative disc disease was, however, found in only 5 of 143 fusions (Lee 1988). In four of five patients, pseudoarthrosis was found as well as osteoporosis. Hambly et al. (1998) present an opposing point of view. They followed 42 patients who had undergone a posterolateral fusion, with an average follow-up of 22.6 years. They found that there was no statistical difference between the study group and a cohort group, and that degenerative changes in the study group occurred at equal frequency two levels above the fusion as they did one level above the fusion. Utilization of instrumentation can significantly reduce the pseudoarthrosis rate (Whitecloud et al. 1994). There were no excellent results (i.e., returning to normal daily activities without pain) for these individuals (Lee 1988). Posterior lumbar interbody fusion was a technique used for many years to create a fusion between adjacent vertebral bodies without an additional anterior surgical approach. The results are encouraging in many short-term studies, but long-term results reveal higher rates of pseudoarthrosis and increased instability (Wetzel and LaRocca 1991). These worse results long term are felt to be secondary to the iatrogenic changes created in the posterior elements, enabling safe placement of the interbody bone grafts.

## Prognosis and Patient Selection

Identifying significant prognostic factors requires determining not only elements contributing to good outcome but also factors associated with poor results. The "failed back" patient can be defined as one who has undergone prior lumbar surgery with unsatisfactory long-term results, resulting in significant physical as well as psychological dysfunction (Sypert and Arpin-Sypert 1996). The main problem found in nearly all such patients is initial inappropriate patient selection (Fager and Freidberg 1980). In order to avoid such a situation, accurate diagnosis is essential. This must be followed by surgery aimed at correcting well-defined abnormalities that correlate with patient complaints and physical findings on examination. Iatrogenically introduced injury is also a factor contributing to poor outcome. It is essential that a surgeon can operate safely and effectively. Despite appropriate selection and good operative technique, surgical complications (e. g., infection, CSF leak, arachnoiditis, pseudoarthrosis) occur as well as recurrence and adjacent-level disease (Zeidman and Long 1996). Psychosocial factors including litigation have a strong influence on short-term and long-term improvement. Physiological factors such as premorbid status, osteoporosis, and even coexistent smoking can create profound problems. The period of pain-free interval following surgery is one of the most important prognostic factors when considering reoperation (Sypert and Arpin-Sypert 1996). No improvement following surgery suggests inappropriate selection initially, irreversible injury, or inadequate surgical treatment. A period of relief followed by gradual onset over several months can suggest scar tissue formation. A more rapid onset can suggest recurrence. Relief followed by recurrent symptoms years later likely represents the ongoing pathological process with or without adjacent-level disease or instability. Many factors are important, and careful attention to all will lead to the best likelihood for successful treatment of all the various lumbar degenerative processes.

**Acknowledgment.** This research was supported by grant R01 CA78912-01 from the National Cancer Institute, National Institutes of Health; by grant 004949-054 from the Texas Higher Education Coordinating Board; and by grants from The Taub Foundation, The Henry J. N. Taub Fund for Neurosurgical Research, The George A. Robinson, IV Foundation, The Blanche Greene Estate Fund of The Pauline Sterne Wolff Memorial Foundation, and The Seigo Arai Fund of The Neurological Research Foundation

# References

Abdullah, A.; Wolber, P.; Warfield, J. Surgical management of extreme lateral lumbar disc herniations: review of 138 cases. Neurosurgery 22:648–653; 1988.

Adams, C. B. T.; Logue, V. Studies in cervical spondylotic myelopathy. III. The movement and contour of the spine in relation to the neural complications of cervical spondylosis. Brain 94:569–586; 1971.

Alberico, A.; Sahni, S.; Hall, J. High thoracic disc herniation. Neurosurgery 19:449–451; 1986.

Aldrich, F. Posterolateral microdiscectomy for cervical monoradiculopathy caused by posterolateral soft cervical disc sequestration. J. Neurosurg. 72:370; 1990.

Alexander, E.; Kelly, D., Jr.; Davis, C., Jr. Intact arch spondylolisthesis. J. Neurosurg. 63:840–844; 1985.

Allbrook, D. Movements of the lumbar spinal column. J. Bone Joint Surg. 39B:339–345; 1957.

Allen, K. L. Neuropathies caused by bony spurs in the cervical spine with special reference to surgical treatment. J. Neurol. Neurosurg. Psychiatry 154:20; 1952.

Al-Mefty, O.; Harkey, H. L.; Marawi, I.; et al. Experimental chronic compressive cervical myelopathy. J. Neurosurg. 79:550–561; 1993.

Angtuaco, E.; Holder, J.; Boop, W. Computed tomographic discography in evaluation of extreme lateral disc herniation. Neurosurgery 14:350–352; 1984.

Arce, C.; Dorhmann, G. Thoracic disc herniation, improved diagnosis with computed tomographic scanning and a review of the literature. Surg. Neurol. 23:356–361; 1985.

Arnasson, O.; Carlsson, C. A.; Pellettieri, L. Surgery and conservative treatment of cervical spondylotic radiculopathy and myelopathy radiculopathy. Acta Neurochir. (Wien) 84:48–53; 1987.

Aronson, N.; Bagan, N.; Filtzer, D. L. Results of using the Smith-Robinson approach for herniated and extruded cervical discs. J. Neurosurg. 32:721; 1970.

Arseni, C.; Nash, F. Thoracic intervertebral disc protrusion: a clinical study. J. Neurosurg. 17:418–430; 1960.

Arynpur, J.; Ducker, T. Multilevel lumbar laminectomies: an alternative to laminectomy in the treatment of lumbar stenosis. Neurosurgery 26:429–433; 1990.

Awwad, E.; Martin, D.; Smith, K. Asymptomatic versus symptomatic herniated thoracic discs: their frequency and characteristics as detected by computed tomography after myelography. Neurosurgery 28:180–186; 1991.

Baker, H.; Love, J.; Uihlein, A. Roentgenologic featuress of protruded thoracic intervertebral disks. Radiology 84:1059–1065; 1965.

Baldwin, N. Lumbar spondylolysis and spondylolithesis. Principles of spinal surgery. New York: McGraw-Hill; 1996: p. 681–702.

Ball, P. A.; Saunders, R. L. Subjective myelopathy. In: Saunders, R. L.; Bernini, P. M., eds. Cervical spondylotic m24yleopathy. Boston: Blackwell; 1992: p. 48–55.

Banerji, D.; Acharya, R.; Behari, S.; Chhabra, D. K.; Jain V. K. Corpectomy for multi-level cervical spondylosis and ossification of the posterior longitudinal ligament. Neurosurg. Rev. 20(1):25–31; 1997.

Batzdorf, U.; Batzdorf, B. M. E. Analysis of cervical spine curvature in patients with cervical spondylosis. Neurosurgery 22:827–836; 1988.

Batzdorf, U.; Flannigan, B. D. Surgical decompressive procedures for cervical spondylotic myelopathy. A study using magnetic resonance imaging. Spine 16:123–127; 1991.

Beck, D. W. Cervical spondylosis: clinical findings and treatment. Contemp. Neurosurg. 13(23):1–6; 1991.

Benini, A.; Krayenbuhl, H.; Bruderl, R. Anterior cervical discectomy without fusion: microsurgical technique. Acta Neurochir. (Wien) 61:105–110; 1982.

Bennet, G. Spondylolysis and spondylolithesis. Neurological surgery. Philadelphia: W. B. Saunders Co.; 1996: p. 2416–2431.

Bernard, T. N.; Whitecloud, T. S., III. Cervical spondylotic myelopathy and myeloradiculopathy. Clin. Orthop. Rel. Res. 221:149–157; 1987.

Bertalanffy, H.; Eggert, H-R. Clinical long-term results of anterior discectomy without fusion for treatment of cervical radiculopathy and myelopathy: a follow-up of 164 cases. Acta Neurochir. 90:127–135; 1988.

Blades, D. A.; Cooper, P. R. Management of cervical disc herniation: anterior surgical approaches. In: Menezes, A. H.; Sonntag, V. K. H.; Benzel, E. C.; Cahill, D. W.; McCormick, P. C.; Papadopoulous, S. M., eds. Principles of spinal surgery. New York: McGraw-Hill; 1996: p. 517–529.

Blikra, G: Intradural herniated lumbar disc. J. Neurosurg. 31:676–679; 1969.

Blumenthal, S.; Baker, J.; Dossett, A. The role of anterior lumbar fusion for internal disc disruption. Spine 13:566–569; 1988.

Boni, M.; Cherubino, P.; Denaro, V.; et al. Multiple subtotal somatectomy: technique and evaluation of a series of 39 cases. Spine 9:358–361; 1984.

Bookwalter, J., III; Busch, M.; Nicely, D. Ambulatory surgery is safe and effective in radicular disc disease. Spine 19:526–530; 1994.

Bosacco, D. N.; Berman, A. T.; Levenberg, R. J.; et al. Surgical results in anterior cervical discectomy and fusion using a countersunk interlocking autogenous iliac bone graft. Orthopedics 15(8):923–925; 1992.

Bradford, D.; Iza, J. Repair of the defect in spondylolysis or minimal degrees of spondylolithesis by segmental wire fixation and bone grafting. Spine 10:673–678; 1985.

Brain, R. W.; Northfield, D.; Wilkinson, M. The neurologic manifestations of cervical spondylosis. Brain 75:187–225; 1952.

Breig, A.; Turnbull, I.; Hassler, O. Effects of mechanical stresses on the spinal cord in cervical spondylosis. J. Neurosurg. 25:45–56; 1966.

Brigham, C. D.; Tsahakis, P. J. Anterior cervical foraminotomy and fusion. Surgical technique and results. Spine 20(7):766–770; 1995.

Brodke, D.; Zdeblick, T. Modified Smith-Robinson procedure for anterior cervical discectomy and fusion. Spine 17:S427–S430; 1992.

Brodsky, A.; Kovalsky, E.; Khalil, M. Correlation of radiologic assessment of lumbar spine fusions with surgical exploration. Spine 16:S261–S265; 1991.

Brown, M. Pathophysiology of disc disease. Orthop. Clin. North. Am. 2:359–370; 1971.

Burger, R.; Tonn, J. C.; Vince, G. H.; Hofmann, E.; Reiners, K.; Roosen, K. Median corpectomy in cervical spondylytic multisegmental stenosis. Zentralbl. Neurochir. 57(2):62–69; 1996.

Burrows, E. H. The sagittal diameter of the spinal canal in cervical spondylosis. Clin. Radiol. 14:77–86; 1963.

Campbell, A. M. G.; Phillips, D. G. Cervical disk lesions with neurological disorder. Br. Med. J. 2: 481–485; 1960.

Carson, J.; Gumpert, J.; Jefferson, A. Diagnosis and treatment of thoracic intervertebral disc protrusions. J. Neurol. Neurosurg. Psychiatry 34:68–77; 1971.

Clark, C. R. Degenerative conditions of the spine. In: Frymoyer, J., ed. The adult spine: priciples and practice. New York: Raven Press; 1991: p. 1145–1164.

Clarke, E; Robinson, P. Cervical myelopathy: a complication of cervical spondylosis. Brain 79:483–510; 1956.

Clements, D. H.; O' Leary P. F. Anterior cervical discectomy and fusion. Spine 15(10):1023–1025; 1990.

Cloward, R. B. New method of diagnosis and treatment of cervical disc disease. Clin. Neurosurg. 8:93; 1962.

Crandall, P. H.; Batzdorf, U. Cervical spondylotic myelopathy. J. Neurosurg. 25:57–66; 1966.

Cusick, J. F. Pathophysiology and treatment of cervical spondylotic myelopathy. Clin. Neurosurg. 37: 661–681; 1991.

Davis, R. A. A long-term outcome study of 170 surgically treated patients with compressive cervical radiculopathy. Surg. Neurol. 46(6):523–533; 1996.

Deburge, A.; Rocelle, J.; Benoist, M. Surgical findings and results of surgery after failure of chemonucleosis. Spine 10:812–815; 1985.

Delamarter, R.; Bohlman, H.; Dodge, L., Experimental lumbar spinal stenosis: analysis of the cortical evoked potentials, microvasculature, and histopathology. J. Bone Joint Surg. 72:110; 1990.

De Palma, A. F.; Rothman, R. H.; Lewinnek, G. E.; Canale, S. T. Anterior interbody fusion for severe cervical disc degeneration. Surg. Gynecol. Obstet. 134:755–758; 1972.

De Palma, A.; Subin, D. Study of the cervical syndrome. Clin. Orthop. 38:135–141; 1965.

Dia, L.; Xu, Y.; Zhang, W. The effect of flexion-extension motion of the lumbar spine on the capacity of the spinal canal: an experimental study. Spine 14:523; 1989.

Dunsker, S. B. Cervical spondylotic myelopathy: pathogenesis and pathophysiology. In: Dunsker, S. B., ed. Cervical spondylosis. New York: Raven Press; 1981: p. 119–133.

Dupuis, P.; Yong-hing, K.; Cassidy, J. Radiologic diagnosis of degenerative lumbar spinal instability. Spine 10:262–276; 1985.

Dvorak, J.; Panjabi, M.; Novotny, J. Clinical validation of functional flexion-extension roentgenograms of the lumbar spine. Spine 16:943–950; 1991.

Ebersold, M. J.; Pare, M. C.; Quast, L. M. Surgical treatment for cervical spondylytic myelopathy. J. Neurosurg. 82(5):745–51; 1995.

Emery, S. E.; Bohlman, H. H.; Bolesta, M. J.; Jones, P. K. Anterior cervical decompression and arthrodesis for the treatment of cervical spondylotic myelopathy. Two to seventeen-year follow-up. J. Bone Joint Surg. Am. 80:941–951; 1998.

Epstein, J. Compression of the spinal cord and cauda equina in achondroplastic dwarfs. Neurology 5: 875–877; 1955.

Epstein, J. A.; Carras, R.; Lavine, L. S.; et al. The importance of removing osteophytes as part of the surgical treatment of myeloradiculopathy in cervical spondylosis. J. Neurosurg. 30:219–226; 1969.

Epstein, J.; Epstein, B.; Lavine, L. Degenerative lumbar spondylolithesis with an intact neural arch (pseudospondylolithesis). J. Neurosurg. 44:139–147; 1976.

Epstein, J.; Epstein, B.; Rosenthal, A. Sciatica caused by nerve root entrapment in lateral recess: the superior facet syndrome. J. Neurosurg. 36:584–589; 1972.

Epstein, N.; Epstein, J. Lumbar spinal stenosis. Neurol. Surg. 106:2390–2415; 1996.

Epstein, N.; Epstein, J.; Carras, R. Degenerative spondylolithesis with an intact neural arch: a review of 60 cases with an analysis of clinical findings and the development of surgical management. Neurosurgery 13:55–561; 1983.

Epstein, N.; Epstein, J.; Carras, R. Coexisting cervical and lumbar stenosis: diagnosis and management. Neurosurgery 15:489–495; 1984.

Epstein, N.; Epstein, J.; Carras, R. Far lateral lumbar disc herniations and associated structural abnormalities: evaluation in 60 patients of the comparative value of CT, MRI, and CT myelography in diagnosis and management. Spine 15:534–539, 1990.

Fager, C. Management of cervical disc lesions and spondylosis by posterior approaches. Clin. Neurosurg. 24:488–507; 1977.

Fager, C. A. Results of adequate posterior decompression in the relief of spondylotic cervical myelopathy. J. Neurosurg. 38:684–692; 1973.

Fager, C. A. Posterior surgical tactics for the neurological syndromes of cervical disc and spondylotic lesions. Clin. Neurosurg. 25:218–244; 1978.

Fager, C.; Freidberg, S. Analysis of failures and poor results of lumbar spine surgery. Spine 5:87–94; 1980.

Farber, G.; Place, H.; Mazur, R. Accuracy of pedicle screw placement in lumbar fusions by plain radiographs and computed tomography. Spine 20: 1494–1499; 1995.

Fessler, R. G.; Steck, J. C.; Giovanini, M. A. Anterior cervical corpectomy for cervical spondylotic myelopathy. Neurosurgery 43:257–265; 1998.

Fox, M. W.; Onofrio, B. M. Transdural approach to the anterior spinal canal in patients with cervical spondylotic myelopathy and superimposed central soft disc herniation. Neurosurgery 34(4):634–641; 1994.

Francavilla, T.; Powers, A.; Dina, T. MR imaging of thoracic disk herniations. J. Comput. Assist. Tomogr. 11:1062–1065; 1987.

Fraser, R. Interbody, posterior, and combined lumbar fusions. Spine 20:S167–S177; 1995.

Friedenberg, Z. B.; Miller, W. T. Degenerative disease of the cervical spine. J. Bone Joint Surg. 45A: 1171–1178; 1963.

Frykholm, R. Deformities of dural puches and strictures of dural sheaths in the cervical region producing nerve-root compression. A contribution to the etiology and operative treatment of brachial neuralgia. J. Neurosurg. 4:403; 1947.

Galera, G. R.; Tovi, D. Anterior disc excision with interbody fusion in cervical spondylotic myelopathy and rhizopathy. J. Neurosurg. 28:305–310; 1968.

Godersky, J.; Erikson, D.; Seljeskog, E. Extreme lateral disc herniation: diagnosis by computed tomographic scanning. Neurosurgery 14:549–552; 1984.

Goel, V.; Goyal, S.; Clark, C. Kinematics of the whole lumbar spine: effect of discectomy. Spine 10: 543–554; 1985.

Gordon, S; Yang, K.; Mayer, P. Mechanism of disc rupture. Spine 16:450–456; 1991.

Gore, D. R.; Sepic, S. B. Anterior cervical fusion for degenerated of protruded discs. A review of one hundred and forty-six patients. Spine 9:667–671; 1984.

Gore, D. R.; Sepic, S. B.; Gardner, G. M. Roentgenographic findings of the cervical spine in asymptomatic people. Spine 11:521–524; 1986.

Gore, D. R.; Sepic, S. B.; Gardner, G. M.; Murray, M. P. Neck pain: a long term follow-up of 120 cases. Spine 12:1–5; 1987.

Gorter, K. Influence of laminectomy on the course of cervical myelopathy. Acta Neurochir. (Wien) 33: 265–281; 1976.

Gregorius, F. K.; Estrin, T.; Crandall, P. H. Cervical spondylotic radiculopathy and myelopathy: a long-term follow-up study. Arch. Neurol. 33:618–625; 1976.

Guidetti, B.; Fortuna, A. Long-term results of surgical treatment of myelopathy due to cervical spondylosis. J. Neurosurg. 30:714–721; 1969.

Guidetti, B.; Fortuna, A.; Samponi, C.; Lunardi, P. P. Cervical spondylosis myelopathy. In: Grote, W.; Brock, M.; Clar, H. E.; Klinger, M.; Nau, H. E., eds. Advances in neurosurgery 8: surgery of cervical myelopathy. Berlin: Springer-Verlag; 1980: p. 104–111.

Haley, J.; Perry, J. Protrusions of intervertebral discs. Study of their distribution, characteristics and effects on the nervous system. Am. J. Surg. 80:394–404; 1950.

Hamanishi, C.; Tanaka, S. Bilateral wide laminectomy with or without posterolateral fusion for cervical spondylotic myelopathy: relationship to the type of onset and time until operation. J. Neurosurg. 85:447–451; 1996.

Hambly, M.; Lee, C.; Gutteling, E. Tension band wiring-bone grafting for spondylolysis and spondy-lolithesis: a clinical and biomechanical study. Spine 14:455–459; 1989.

Hambly, M. F.; Wiltse, L. L.; Raghavan, N.; et al. The transition zone above a lumbosacral fusion. Spine 23:1785–1792; 1998.

Hanai, K.; Fujiyoshi, F.; Kamei, K. Subtotal vertebrectomy and spinal fusion for cervical sppondylotic myelopathy. Spine 11(4):310–315; 1986.

Hankinson, H.; Wilson, C. B. Use of the operating microscope in anterior cervical discectomy without fusion. J. Neurosurg. 43:452–456; 1975.

Hanley, E., Jr.; Levy, J. Surgical treatment of isthmic lumbosacral spondylolithesis: analysis of variables influencing results. Spine 14:48–50; 1989.

Hashimoto, K.; Akahori, O.; Kitano, K. Magnetic resonance imaging of lumbar disc herniation: comparison with myelography. Spine 15:1166–1169, 1990.

Hayes, M.; Howard, T.; Gruel, C. Roentgenographic evaluation of lumbar spine flexion-extension in asymptomatic individuals. Spine 14:327–330; 1989.

Henderson, C. M.; Hennessey, R. G.; Shuey H. J.; Shackelford, E. G. Posterior-lateral foraminotomy as an exclusive operative technique for cervical radiculopathy: a review of 846 consecutively operated cases. Neurosurgery 13:504–512; 1983.

Herkowitz, H. N. A comparison of anterior cervical fusion, cervical laminectomy, and cervical laminaplasty for the surgical management of multiple level spondylotic radiculopathy. Spine 13:774–780; 1988.

Herkowitz, H.; Kurz, L. Degenerative lumbar spondylolithesis with lumbar stenosis: a prospective study comparing decompression with decompression and intertransverse process arthrodesis. J. Bone Joint Surg. 73:802–808; 1991.

Herkowitz, H. N.; Kurz, L. T.; Overholt, D. P. Surgical management of cervical soft disc herniation. A comparison between the anterior and posterior approach. Spine 15(10):1026–30; 1990.

Herron, L.; Trippi, A. L4-5 degenerative spondylolithesis: the results of treatment by decompressive laminectomy without fusion. Spine 14:534–538; 1989.

Herzberger, E. E.; Chandler, A.; Bear, N. E.; Kindschi, L. G. Anterior interbody fusion in the treatment of certain disorders of the cervical spine. Clin. Orthop. 24:83–93; 1962.

Hidai, Y.; Ebara, S.; Kamimura, M.; et al. Treatment of cervical compressive myelopathy with a new dorso-lateral decompressive procedure. J. Neurosurg. 90 (4 suppl.):178–185; 1999.

Hirsch, C.; Wickbom, I.; Lidstrom, A.; Rosengren, K. Cervical-disc resection. A follow-up of myelographic and surgical procedure. J. Bone Joint Surg. 46A:1811–1821; 1964.

Hitselberger, W. E.; Witten, R. M. Abnormal myelograms in asymptomatic patients. J. Neurosurg. 28: 204–208; 1968.

Hoff, J. T.; Nishimura, M.; Pitts, L.; et al. The role of ischemia in the pathogenesis of cervical spondylotic myelopathy. Spine 2:100–108; 1977.

Hoff, J. T.; Wilson, C. B. The pathophysiology of cervical spondylotic radiculopathy and myelopathy. Clin. Neurosurg. 24:474–487; 1977.

Hood, R. Management of the far lateral disk herniation. Principles of spinal surgery. New York: McGraw-Hill; 40:621–629; 1996.

Hukuda, S.; Mochizuki, T.; Ogata, M.; et al. Operations for cervical spondylotic myelopathy. A comparison of the results of anterior and posterior procedures. J. Bone Joint Surg. 67B:609–615; 1985.

Hukuda, S.; Ogata, M.; Katsuura, A. Experimental study on acute aggravating factors of cervical spondylotic myelopathy. Spine 13:15–20; 1988.

Isla, A.; Roda, J.; Bencosme, J. Intradural herniated dorsal disc: case report and review of literature. Neurosurgery 22:737–738; 1988.

Jacobs, B.; Krueger, E. G.; Leivy, D. M. Cervical spondylosis with radiculopathy. Results of anterior diskectomy and interbody fusion. JAMA 211(13): 2135–2139; 1970.

Jane, J.; Haworth, C.; Broaddus, W. A neurosurgical approach to far-lateral disc herniation. J Neurosurg. 72:143–144; 1990.

Jia, L.; Shi, Z. MRI and myelography in the diagnosis of lumbar canal stenosis and disc herniation: a comparative study. Chin. Med. J. 104:303; 1991.

Johnson, K.; Willner, S.; Johnsson, K. Postoperative instability after decompression for lumbar stenosis. Spine 11:107–110; 1986.

Johnsson, K.; Redlund-Johnell, I.; Uden, A. Preoperative and postoperative instability in lumbar spinal stenosis. Spine 14:591–593; 1989.

Johnsson, K. E.; Uden, A.; Rosen, I. The effect of decompression on the natural course of spinal stenosis. A comparison of surgically treated and untreated patients. Spine 16:615–619; 1991.

Jones, A.; Stambough, J.; Balderston, R. Long-term results of lumbar spine surgery complicated by unintended incidental durotomy. Spine 14:443–446; 1989.

Kim, S.; Francis, D.; Lonstein, J. Factors affecting fusion rate in adult spondylolisthesis. Spine 15:979–984; 1990.

Kirkaldy-Willis, W.; Wedge, J.; Yong-hing, K. Pathology and pathogenesis of lumbar spondylosis and stenosis. Spine 3:319–328; 1978.

Kojima, T.; Shiro, W.; Kubo, Y. Surgical treatment of ossification of the posterior longitudinal ligament in the thoracic spine. Neurosurgery 34:854–858; 1994.

Kojima, T.; Waga, S.; Kubo, Y.; et al. Anterior cervical vertebrectomy and interbody fusion for multi-level spondylosis and ossification of the posterior longitudinal ligament. Neurosurgery 24:864–872; 1989.

Kooijman, M. A. Anterior cervical spine fusion in treatment of cervicobrachialgia. Acta Orthop. Belg. 57(1):99–105; 1991.

Kooijman, M. A.; Bossers, G. T. Anterior cervical spine fusion in treatment of cervicobrachialgia. Acta Orthop. Belg. 47(1):140–149; 1981.

Kramer, J. Intervertebral disc disease. Causes, diagnosis, treatment, and prophylaxis. 2nd ed. New York: Thieme; 1990.

Krupp, W.; Schattke, H.; Muke, R. Clinical results of the foraminotomy as described by Frykholm for the treatment of lateral cervical disc herniation. Acta Neurochir. 107:22; 1990.

Kumar, G. R.; Maurice-Williams, R. S.; Bradford, R. Cervical foraminotomy: an effective treatment for cervical spondylotic radiculopathy, Br. J. Neurosurg. 12:563–568; 1998.

Kurz, L.; Garfin, S.; Booth, R., Jr. Harvesting autogenous iliac bone grafts: a review of complications and techniques. Spine 14:1324–1331; 1989.

Laasonen, E.; Soini, J. Low-back pain after lumbar fusion: surgical and computed tomographic analysis. Spine 14:210–213; 1989.

Larson, S; Holst, R.; Hemmy, D. Lateral extracavitary approach to traumatic lesions of the thoracic and lumbar spine. J. Neurosurg. 45:628–637; 1976.

Lawrence, J. S.; Bremmer, J. N.; Bier, F. Osteoarthrosis: prevalence in the population and relationship between symptoms and x-ray changes. Ann. Rheum. Dis. 25:1–24; 1966.

Le Roux, P.; Haglund, M.; Harris, A. Thoracic disc experience: experience with the transpedicular approach in twenty consecutive patients. Neurosurgery 33:58–66; 1993.

Lee, C. Lumbar spinal instability (olisthesis) after extensive posterior spinal decompression. Spine 8: 429–433; 1983.

Lee, C. Accelerated degeneration of the segment adjacent to a lumbar fusion. Spine 13:375–377; 1988.

Lee, C.; Langrana, N. Lumbosacral spinal fusion: a biomechanical study. Spine 9:574–580; 1984.

Lee, T. T.; Manzano, G. R.; Green, B. A. Modified open door cervical expansive laminoplasty for spondylotic myelopathy: operative technique, outcome, and predictors for gait improvement. J. Neurosurg. 86(1): 64–68; 1997.

Lees, F; Turner, J. W. A. Natural history and prognosis of cervical spondylosis. Br. Med. J. 2:1607–1610; 1963.

Lin, P. Internal decompression for multiple levels of lumbar spinal stenosis: a technical note. Neurosurgery 11:546–549; 1982.

Lindholm, T.; Ragni, P.; Ylikoski, M. Lumbar isthmic spondylolithesis in children and adolescents: radiologic evaluation and results of operative treatment. Spine 15:1350–1355; 1990.

Liyang, D.; Wenming, Z.; Zhihua, Z. The effect of flexion-extension motion of the lumbar spine on the capacity of the spinal canal: an experimental study. Spine 14:523–525; 1989.

Loguidice, V.; Johnson, R.; Guyer, R. Anterior lumbar interbody fusion. Spine 13:366–369; 1988.

Lombardi, J.; Wiltse, L.; Reynolds, J. Treatment of degenerative spondylolithesis. Spine 10:821–827; 1985.

Lunsford, L. D.; Bissonette, D. J.; Jannetta, P. J.; Sheptak, P. E.; Zorub, D. S. Anterior surgery for cervical disc disease. Part 1: treatment of lateral cervical disc herniation in 253 cases. J. Neurosurg. 53:1–11; 1980a.

Lunsford, L. D.; Bissonette, D. J.; Zorub, D. S. Anterior surgery for cervical disc disease. Part 2: treatment of cervical spondylotic myelopathy in 32 cases. J. Neurosurg. 53:12–19; 1980b.

Macnab, I. Negative disc exploration: an analysis of the causes of nerve-root involvement in sixty-eight patients. J. Bone Joint Surg. 53A:891–903; 1971.

Maigne, J.; Rime, B.; Deligne, B. Computed tomographic follow-up study of forty-eight cases of nonoperatively treated lumbar intervertebral disc herniation. Spine 17:1071–1074; 1992.

Maiman, D.; Larson, S.; Luck, E. Lateral extracavitary approach to the spine for thoracic disc herniation: report of 23 cases. Neurosurgery 14:178–186; 1984.

Mann, K. S.; Khosla, V. K.; Gulati, D. R. Cervical spondylotic myelopathy treated by single-stage multilevel anterior decompression. J. Neurosurg. 60:81–87; 1984.

Maroon, J.; Kopitnik, T.; Schulhof, L. Diagnosis and microsurgical approach to far-lateral disc herniation in the lumbar spine. J. Neurosurg. 72:378–382; 1990.

Maroon, J. C.; Abla, A. Microdiscectomy versus chemonucleolysis. Neurosurgery 16:644–649; 1985.

Martins, A. N. Anterior cervical discectomy with and without interbody bone graft. J. Neurosurg. 44:290–295; 1976.

Marzluff, J.; Hungerford, G.; Kempe, L. Thoracic myelopathy caused by osteophytes of the articular processes. J. Neurosurg. 50:779–783; 1979.

Masaryk, T.; Ross, J.; Modic, M.; et al. High resolution MR imaging of sequestered lumbar intervertebral discs. AJR Am. J. Roentgenol. 150:1155–1162; 1988.

Matsunaga, S.; Sakou, T.; Morizono, Y. Natural history of degenerative spondylolithesis: pathogenesis and natural course of slippage. Spine 15:1204–1210; 1990.

Matsuzaki, H.; Tokuhashi, Y.; Matsumoto, F. Problems and solutions of pedicle screw plate fixation of lumbar spine. Spine 15:1159–1165; 1990.

Mayer, H.; Brock, M. Percutaneous endoscopic discectomy: surgical technique and preliminary results compared to microsurgical discectomy. J. Neurosurg. 78:216–225; 1991.

McCormick, P. Indications and techniques of lumbar spine fusion. Neurological surgery. Philadelphia: W. B. Saunders Co.; 1996: p. 2461–2474.

McPhee, B. Spondylolithesis and spondylolysis. Neurological surgery. Philadelphia: W. B. Saunders Co.; 1990: p. 2749–2784.

Meyerding, H. W. Spondylolithesis. Surg. Gynecol. Obstet. 54:371–377; 1954.

Mikawa, Y.; Shikata, J.; Jamamuro, T. Spinal deformity and instability after multilevel cervical laminectomy. Spine 12:6–11; 1987.

Miyasaka, K.; Kaneda, K.; Ito, T. Ossification of spinal ligaments causing thoracic radiculomyelopathy. Radiology 143:463–468; 1982.

Mooney, V. Where is the pain coming from? Presidential address. Spine 12:754–759; 1987.

Mosdal, C. Cervical osteochondrosis and disc herniation. Eighteen years' use of interbody fusion by Cloward's technique in 755 cases. Acta Neurochir. (Wien) 70:207–225; 1984.

Murphey, F.; Simmons, J.; Brunson, B. Surgical treatment of laterally ruptured cervical disc. Review of 648 cases, 1939 to 1972. J. Neurosurg. 38:679–683; 1973.

Murphy, M. B.; Gado, M. Anterior cervical discectomy without interbody bone graft. J. Neurosurg. 37:71–74; 1972.

Naylor, A. Intervertebral disc prolapse and degeneration. The biochemical and biophysical approach. Spine 1:108–114; 1976.

Nurick, S. The pathogenesis of the spinal cord disorder associated with cervical spondylosis. Brain 95:87–100; 1972a.

Nurick, S. The natural history and the results of surgical treatment of the spinal cord disorder associated with cervical spondylosis. Brain 95:101–108; 1972b.

Oiwa, T.; Hirabayashi, K.; Uzawa, M.; Ohira, T. Experimental study on post-laminectomy deterioration of cervical spondylotic myelopathy: influences of intradural surgery and persistent spinal block. Spine 10:717–721; 1985.

Okada, K.; Oka, S.; Tohge, K. Thoracic myelopathy caused by ossification of the ligamentum flavum: clinicopathologic study and surgical treatment. Spine 16:280–287; 1991.

Okada, K.; Shirasaki, N.; Hayashi, H.; et al. Treatment of cervical spondylotic myelopathy by enlargement of the spinal canal anteriorly, followed by arthrodesis. J. Bone Joint Surg. 73A:352–364; 1991.

Padua, R.; Padua, S.; Romanini, E.; et al. Ten to 15-year outcome of surgery for lumbar disc herniation: radiographic instability and clinical findings. Eur. Spine J. 8:70–74; 1999.

Paine, K.; Haung, P. Lumbar disc syndrome. J. Neurosurg. 37:75–82; 1972.

Panjabi, M.; Takata, K.; Goel, V. Kinematics of lumbar intervertebral foramen. Spine 8:348–357; 1983.

Panjabi, M. M.; White, A. A. Biomechanics of nonacute cervical spinal cord trauma. Spine 13:838–842; 1988.

Pappas, C.; Harrington, T.; Sonntag, V. Outcome analysis in 654 surgically treated lumbar disc herniations. Neurosurgery 30:862–866; 1992.

Pappas, C.; Sonntag, V. Degenerative disorders of the spine: lumbar stenosis. Principles of spinal surgery. New York. McGraw-Hill 41:631–644; 1996.

Parke, W. W. Correlative anatomy of cervical spondylotic myelopathy. Spine 13:831–837; 1988.

Persson, L. C.; Carlsson, C. A.; Carlsson, J. Y. Long-lasting cervical radicular pain managed with surgery, physiotherapy, or a cervical collar. A prospective, randomized study. Spine 22(7):751–758; 1997.

Peserico, L.; Uihlein, A.; Baker, G. S. Surgical treatment of cervical myelopathy associated with cervica spondylosis. Acta Neurochir. 10:365–375; 1962.

Phillips, D. G. Surgical treatment of myelopathy with cervical spondylosis. J. Neurol. Neurosurg. Psychiatry 36:879–884; 1973.

Piepgras, D. G. Posterior decompression for myelopathy due to cervical spondylosis: laminectomy alone versus laminectomy with dentate ligament section. Clin. Neurosurg. 24:508–515; 1977.

Pointillart, V.; Cernier, A.; Vital, J. M.; Senegas J. Anterior discectomy without interbody fusion for cervical disc herniation. Eur. Spine 4(1):45–51; 1995.

Prolo, D. Morphology and metabolism of fusion of the lumbar spine. Neurological surgery. Philadelphia: W. B. Saunder Co.; 1996: p. 2449–2459.

Quigley, M.; Kortyna, R.; Goodwin, C. Lumbar surgery in the elderly. Neurosurgery 30: 672–674; 1992.

Radhakrishnan, K.; Litchy, W. J.; O'Fallon, M. W.; Kurland, L. T. Epidemiology of cervical radiculopathy—a population-based study from Rochester, Minnesota, 1976 through 1990. Brain, 117:325–335; 1994.

Ransohoff, J.; Spencer, F.; Siew, F. Transthoracic removal of thoracic disc: case reports and technical notes. J. Neurosurg. 31:459–461; 1969.

Rengachary, S.; Redford, J. Partial median vertebrectomy and fibular grafting in the management of cervical spondylotic myelopathy (abstract). J. Neurosurg. 70:325A; 1989.

Riley, L. H., Jr. Anterior cervical spine surgery. The American Academy of Orthopaedic Surgeons: instructional course lectures, vol. 27. St. Louis; C. V. Mosby; 1978: p.154–158. 1978.

Riley, L. H., Jr.; Robinson, R. A.; Johnson, D. A. The results of anterior interbody fusion of the cervical spine. Review of 93 consecutive cases. J. Neurosurg. 30:127; 1969.

Robertson, J. D. The rape of the spine. Surg. Neurol. 31:59–72; 1993.

Robertson, J. T. Anterior removal of cervical disc without fusion. Clin. Neurosurg. 20:259–261; 1973.

Robinson, R. A. Anterior and posterior cervical fusions. Clin. Orthop. 35:34; 1964.

Robinson, R. A.; Smith, G. W. Anterolateral cervical disc removal and interbody fusion for cervical disc syndrome (abstract). Johns Hopkins Hosp. Bull. 96:223–224; 1955.

Robinson, R. A.; Walker, A. E.; Ferlic, D. C.; Wiecking, D. K. The results of anterior interbody fusion of the cervical spine. J. Bone Joint Surg. 44A: 1569–1587; 1962.

Romner, B.; Due-Tonnessen, B. J.; Egge, A.; et al. Modified Robinson-Smith procedure for the treatment of cervical radiculopathy. Acta Neurol. Scand. 90(3):197–200; 1994.

Rosomoff, H. L.; Rossmann, F. Treatment of cervical spondylosis by anterior cervical diskectomy and fusion. Arch. Neurol. 14(4):392–398; 1966.

Rothman, R. H. The spine. 2nd ed. Philadelphia: W. B. Saunders Co.; 1982: p. 477.

Rowland, L. P. Surgical treatment of cervical spondylotic myelopathy: time for a controlled trial. Neurology 42:5–13; 1992.

Saito, T.; Yamamuro, T.; Shikata, J.; et al. Analysis and prevention of spinal column deformity following cervical laminectomy. I. Pathogenetic analysis of postlaminectomy deformities. Spine 16:494–502; 1991.

Saruhashi, Y.; Hukuda, S.; Katsuura, A.; et al. A long-term follow-up study of cervical spondylotic myelopathy treated by "French window" laminoplasty. J. Spinal Disord. 12:99–101; 1999.

Saunders, R. L.; Bernini, P. M.; Shirreffs, T. G., Jr.; et al. Central corpectomy for cervical spondylotic myelopathy: a consecutive series with long-term follow-up evaluation. J. Neurosurg. 74:163–170; 1991.

Scoville, W. B.; Dohrmann, A. M.; Corkill, A. R. Late results of cervical disc surgery. J. Neurosurg. 45: 203–210; 1976.

Seifert, V.; Stolke, D. Multisegmental cervical spondylosis: treatment by spondylectomy, microsurgical decompression, and osteosynthesis. Neurosurgery 29:498–503; 1991.

Seitsalo, S.; Osterman, K.; Poussa, M. Scoliosis associated with lumbar spondylolisthesis: a clinical survey of 190 young patients. Spine 13:899–904; 1988.

Sekhar, L.; Jannetta, P. Thoracic disc herniation: Operative approaches and results. Neurosurgery 12: 303–305; 1983.

Semmes, R. Ruptured intervertebral discs. Their recognition and surgical relief. Clin. Neurosurg. 8:78–92; 1960.

Senegas, J.; Guerin, J.; Vital, J. M.; et al. Decompression medullaire etendue par voie anterieure dans le traitmendes myelopathies par cervicarthrose. Rev. Chir. Orthop. 71:291–300; 1985.

Shenkin, H.; Hash, C. Spondylolithesis after multiple bilateral laminectomies and facetectomies for lumbar spondylosis. J. Neurosurg. 50:45–47, 1979.

Sherk, H. H. Point of view. Long-lasting cervical radicular pain managed with surgery, physiotherapy, or a cervical collar. A prospective, randomized study. Spine 22(7):758; 1997.

Shvartzman, L.; Weingarten, E.; Sherry, H. Cost-effectiveness analysis of extended conservative therapy versus surgical intervention in the management of herniated lumbar intervertebral disc. Spine 17: 176–182; 1992.

Silcox, D., III; Daftari, T.; Boden, S. The effect of nicotine on spinal fusion. Spine 20:1549–1553; 1995.

Silvers, H. R.; Lewis, P. J.; Suddaby, L. S.; Asch, H. L.; Clabeaux, D. E.; Blumeson, L. E. Day surgery for cervical microdiscectomy: is it safe and effective?. J. Spinal Disord. 9(4):287–93; 1996.

Sim, F. H.; Svien, H. J.; Bickel, W. H. Swan-neck deformity following extensive cervical laminectomy. A review of 21 cases. J. Bone Joint Surg. Am. 56: 564–580; 1974.

Simeone, F. A.; Dillin, W. Treatment of cervical disc disease: selection of operative approach. Contemp. Neurosurg. 8:1–6; 1986.

Smith, G. W.; Robinson, R. A. The treatment of certain cervical spine disorders by anterior removal of the intervertebral disc and interbody fusion. J. Bone Joint Surg. Am. 40A:607; 1958.

Smith, S.; Massie, J.; Chesnut, R. Straight leg raising. Spine 18:992–999; 1993.

Spurling, R.; Scoville, W. Lateral rupture of the cervical intervertebral discs. Surg. Gynecol. Obstet. 78:350–358; 1944.

Stillerman, C.; Weiss, M. Management of thoracic disc disease. Clin. Neurosurg. 38; 325–387, 1992.

Stoltmann, H. F.; Blackwood, W. The role of the ligamenta flava in the pathogenesis of myelopathy in cervical spondylosis. Brain 87:45–50; 1964.

Stoops, W. L.; King, R. B. Neural complications of cervical spondylosis: their response to laminectomy and foraminotomy. J Neurosurg. 19:986; 1962.

Sundaresan, N.; Shah, J.; Foley, K. An anterior surgical approach to the upper thoracic vertebrae. J. Neurosurg. 61:686–690; 1984.

Symon, L.; Lavender, P. The surgical treatment of cervical spondylotic myelopathy. Neurology 17: 117–127; 1967.

Symonds, C. The interrelation of trauma and cervical spondylosis in impression of the cervical cord. Lancet 264:451–454; 1953.

Sypert, G.; Arpin-Sypert, E. Evaluation and management of the failed back syndrome. Neurological surgery. Philadelphia: W. B. Saunders Co.; 1996: p. 2432–2447.

Taillard, W. F. Etiology of spondylolithesis. Clin. Orthop. 117:30–39; 1976.

Takahashi, K.; Kitahara, H.; Yamagata, M. Long-term results of anterior interbody fusion for treatment of degenerative spondylolithesis. Spine 15:1211–1215; 1990.

Taylor, A. R. Mechanism and treatment of spinal cord disorders associated with cervical spondylosis. Lancet 1:717–720; 1953.

Tegos, S.; Rizos K.; Papathanasiu, A.; Kyriakopulos, K. Results of anterior discectomy without fusion for treatment of cervical radiculopathy and myelopathy. Eur. Spine J. 3(2):62–65; 1994.

Teresi, L. M.; Lfkin, R. B.; Reicher, M. A., et al. Asymptomatic degenerative disc disease and spondylosis of the cervical spine: MR imaging. Radiology 164:83–88; 1987.

Tomaras, C. R.; Blacklock, J. B.; Parker, W. D.; Harper, R. L. Outpatient surgical treatment of cervical radiculopathy. J. Neurosurg. 87:41–43; 1997.

Vaccaro, A.; Garfin, S. Internal fixation (pedicle screw fixation) for fusions of the lumbar spine. Spine 20: S157–S165; 1995.

Van Alphen, H.; Braakman, R.; Bezemer, P. Chemonucleosis versus discectomy: a randomized multicenter trial. J. Neurosurg. 70:869–875; 1989.

Verbiest, H. Neurogenic intermittent claudication in cases with absolute and relative stenosis of the lumbar vertebral canal in cases with narrow lumbar intervertebral foramina, and in cases of both entities. Clin. Neurosurg. 20:204; 1972.

Verbiest, H. Stenosis of the lumbar vertebral canal and sciatica. Neurosurg. Rev. 3:75; 1980.

Wada, E.; Yonenobu, K.; Suzuki, S.; et al. Can intramedullary signal change on magnetic resonance imaging predict surgical outcome in cervical spondylotic myelopathy? Spine 24:455–461; 1999.

Watanabe, R.; Parke, W. Vascular and neural pathology of lumbosacral spinal stenosis. J. Neurosurg. 64:64–70; 1986.

Watters, W., III; Mirkovic, S.; Boss, J. Treatment of the isolated lumbar intervertebral disc herniation: microdiscectomy versus chemonucleosis. Spine 13: 360–361; 1988.

Weber, H. Lumbar disc herniation. Spine 8:131–139; 1983.

Weinstein, J.; Spratt, K.; Spengler, D. Spinal pedicle fixation: reliability and validity of roentgenogrambased assessment and surgical factors on successful screw placement. Spine 13:1012–1018; 1988.

Weinstein, P. R.; Ehni, G.; Wilson, C. B. Lumbar spondylosis: diagnosis, management and surgical treatment. Chicago: Year Book; 1977.

Wetzel, F.; LaRocca, H. The failed posterior lumbar interbody fusion. Spine 16:839–845; 1991.

White, A. A.; Panjabi, M. M. Biomechanical considerations in the surgical management of cervical spondylotic myelopathy. Spine 13:856–860; 1988.

White, A. A., III.; Southwick, W. O.; De Ponte, R. J.; Gainor, J. W.; Hardy, R. Relief of pain by anterior cervical spine fusion for spondylosis. A report of sixty five patients. J. Bone Joint Surg. 55A:525–534; 1973.

Whitecloud, T., III; Davis, J.; Olive, P. Operative treatment of the degenerated segment adjacent to a lumbar fusion. Spine 19:531–536; 1994.

Whitecloud, T. S., III. Management of radiculopathy and myelopathy by the anterior approach. In: The Cervical Spine Research Society Editorial Committee, eds. The cervical spine. 2nd ed. Philadelphia: J. B. Lippincott; 1989: p. 644–658.

Whitecloud, T. S., III; LaRocca, H. Fibular strut graft in reconstructive surgery of the cervical spine. Spine 1:33–43; 1976.

Whitecloud, T.; Butler, J.; Cohen, J. Complications with the variable spinal plating system. Spine 14: 472–476; 1989.

Wiberg, J. Effects of surgery on cervical spondylotic myelopathy. Acta Neurochir. 81(3–4): 113–117; 1986.

Wilberger, J. E., Jr.; Chedid, M. K. Acute cervical spondylotic myelopathy. Neurosurgery 22:145–146; 1988.

Wilkinson, M. The morbid anatomy of cervical spondylosis and myelopathy. Brain 83:589–616; 1960.

Williams, J. L.; Allen, M. B., Jr.; Harkess, J. W. Late results of cervical discectomy and interbody fusion: some factors influencing results. J. Bone Joint Surg. 50A:277–286; 1968.

Williams, R. Microlumbar discectomy: a conservative surgical approach. Spine 3:175–182; 1978.

Williams, R. W. Microcervical foraminotomy: a surgical alternative for intractable radicular pain. Spine 8:708–716; 1983.

Wilson, D.; Harbaugh, R. Microsurgical and standard removal of the protruded lumbar disc: a comparative study. Neurosurgery 8:422–427; 1981.

Wilson, D. H.; Campbell, D. D. Anterior cervical discectomy without bone graft. J. Neurosurg. 47: 551–555; 1977.

Woertgen, C.; Holzschuh, M.; Rothoerl, R. D.; Haeusler, E.; Brawanski, A. Prognostic factors of posterior cervical disc surgery: a prospective, consecutive study of 54 patients. Neurosurgery 40(4): 724–729; 1997.

Wohlert, L; Buhl, M.; Eriksen, E. F.; et al. Treatment of cervical disc disease using Cloward's technique. III. Evaluation of cervical spondylotic myelopathy in 138 cases. Acta Neurochir. 71:121–131; 1984.

Yamada, H.; Ohya, M.; Okada, T. Intermittent cauda equina compression due to narrow canal. J. Neurosurg. 37:83–88; 1972.

Yamamoto, I.; Matsumae, M.; Ikeda, A. Thoracic spinal stenosis: experience with seven cases. J. Neurosurg. 68:37–40; 1988.

Yang, K. C.; Lu, X. S.; Cai, Q. L.; Ye, L. X.; Lu, W. Q. Cervical spondylotic myelopathy treated by anterior multilevel decompression and fusion. Follow-up report of 214 cases. Clin. Orthop. 221:161–164; 1987.

Yang, K. Q.; Lu, X. S.; Cai, Q. L.; et al. Anterior multilevel decompression and fusion for cervical spondylotic myelopathy. Report of 214 cases. Chin. Med. J. 98:1–6; 1985.

Yasuoka, S.; Peterson, H. A.; Laws, E. R.; MacCarty, C. S. Pathogenesis and prophylaxis of postlaminectomy deformity of the spine after multiple level laminectomy: difference between children and adults. Neurosurgery 9:145–151; 1981.

Yasuoka, S.; Peterson, H. A.; MacCarty, C. S. Incidence of spinal column deformity after multilevel laminectomy in children and adults. J. Neurosurg. 57:441–445; 1982.

Yonenobu, K.; Fuji, T.; Ono, K.; et al. Choice of surgical treatment for multisegmental cervical spondylotic myelopathy. Spine 10:711–716; 1985.

Yonenobu, K.; Hosono, N.; Iwasaki, M.; Asano, M.; Ono, K. Laminoplasty versus subtotal corpectomy. A comparative study of results in multisegmental cervical spondylotic myelopathy. Spine 17(11): 1281– 1284; 1992.

Yonenobu, K.; Okada, K.; Fuji, T.; et al. Causes of neurologic deterioration following surgical treament of cervical myelopathy. Spine 11:818–823; 1986.

Young, S.; Veerapen, R.; O'Laoire, S. Relief of lumbar canal stenosis using multilevel subarticular fenestrations as an alternative to wide laminectomy: preliminary report. Neurosurgery 23:628–633; 1988.

Zahrawi, F. Microlumbar discectomy (MLD). Spine 13:358–359, 1988.

Zdeblick, T. A.; Bohlman, H. H. Cervical kyphosis and myelopathy. J. Bone Joint Surg. 71A:170–182; 1989.

Zeidman, S. M.; Ducker, T. B. Cervical disc diseases. Neurosurg. Q. 2:116–163; 1992.

Zeidman, S. M.; Ducker, T. B. Posterior cervical laminoforaminotomy for radiculopathy: review of 172 cases. Neurosurgery 33:356; 1993.

Zeidman, S.; Long, D. Failed back surgery syndrome. Principles of spinal surgery. New York: McGraw-Hill; 1996: p. 657–677.

Zhang, Z. H.; Yin, H.; Yang, K.; et al. Anterior intervertebral disc excision and bone grafting in cervical spondylotic myelopathy. Spine 8:16–19; 1983.

# 10

# Whiplash Injuries

RANDOLPH W. EVANS

Whiplash injuries are among the most controversial topics in medicine (Evans et al. 1994). The term *whiplash* may have been first introduced by Harold Crowe, an American orthopedist, in 1928 (Crowe 1964). However, the first use of the term may be in an article by Arthur G. Davis, another American orthopedist (Davis 1945). While many say that the term is unscientific (Yates and Smith 1994), whiplash has become well entrenched in the medical literature and the lay vocabulary in English and other languages. In Spanish (in Mexico and Chile, *latigazo*), Portuguese (*chicotada*), Italian (*colpo di frusta*), and Swedish (*pisksnartskada*), the term used for this injury is a literal translation of "whiplash" (Evans 1995a).

Many physicians use the term *whiplash injury* synonymously with acute or chronic cervical sprain, cervical myofascial pain syndrome, acceleration-deceleration injury, and hyperextension injury. Whiplash describes a biomechanical event: the typical mechanism of the hyperextension-flexion of the head and neck that occurs when an occupant of a motor vehicle is hit from behind by another vehicle. An injury may or may not result. Some clinicians also use the term to describe other types of collisions in which the neck is subjected to different sequences and combinations of flexion, extension, vertical, and lateral movement. Whiplash is best used only as a

description of the mechanism of injury and not as a description of the sequelae. Chronic or late whiplash syndrome refers to persistent symptoms present more than 6 months after the injury.

Because a significant percentage of these injuries results in lawsuits, insurance companies, attorneys, and courts frequently request prognostic information. Physicians estimate prognosis based on the perceived severity of the accident; symptoms; objective findings on examination and testing; duration and extent of treatment; credibility of the patient and concerns about compensation neurosis or malingering; their own clinical experience; and for some, doubts about whether chronic whiplash syndrome actually exists. For many, the prognostic literature has not been read or is considered unimportant in comparison to the other factors used in making prognostic judgments. In addition, specialists have a widespread cynicism about treating anxious and depressed patients with late whiplash syndrome who never seem to get well despite multiple physician opinions, extensive testing, and never-ending treatments.

## Epidemiology

The National Safety Council estimated that there were 13,800,000 motor vehicle accidents including 3,900,000 rear-end collisions in the United

States in 1997. Since there is no reporting system, the actual number of whiplash injuries per year is not known. However, if Dolinis' finding that 35% of Australian drivers in rear-end collisions sustained whiplash injuries (Dolinis 1997), then as many as 1 million persons in the United States may have whiplash injuries yearly.

Rear-end collisions are responsible for about 85% of all whiplash injuries (Hohl 1974; Deans et al. 1986). Neck pain develops in 56% of patients involved in a front or side impact accident (Deans et al. 1986). Seventy-three percent of patients wearing a seatbelt develop neck pain as compared to 53% of those not wearing seatbelts (Deans et al. 1987). However, proper use of headrests can reduce the incidence of neck pain in rear-end collisions by 24% (Nygren 1984; Morris 1989). Most studies have reported whiplash injuries occurring more often in females, especially in the 20- to 40-year old age group, with an overall male-female ratio of about 30% to 70% (Hohl 1974; Balla 1980; Skovron 1998). The greater susceptibility of females might be due to a narrower neck with less muscle mass supporting a head of roughly the same volume (Kahane 1982) or a narrower spinal canal compared with men (Pettersson et al. 1995).

According to one estimate, 94% of patients with late whiplash syndrome see more than one specialist (Balla 1980). Therefore, it is not at all surprising that the whiplash type of injury is one of the most common problems that neurologists and neurosurgeons evaluate and treat. According to a survey in the United States, neurologists see 10.3 and neurosurgeons 7.0 patients monthly with whiplash injuries (Evans et al. 1994).

## Etiology of Symptoms

### Controversies

The acute whiplash syndrome with complaints of neck stiffness, aching, and headaches is well accepted by the public and the medical profession. However, as the symptoms persist for months or years, some physicians argue that sprains should heal within a few weeks and there must be another reason why patients continue to complain. Nonorganic explanations offered for persistent complaints include emotional or psychological problems (Neck injury and the mind 1991); exposure to social or medical fashions that perpetuate pain (Ferrari and Russell 1997); a culturally conditioned and legally sanctioned illness, a man-made disease (Awerbuch 1992; Mills and Horne 1986); a result of social and peer copying (Livingston 1993); secondary gain and malingering (Schmand et al. 1998); and demanding an explanation outside the realm of organic psychiatry and neurology (Pearce 1994). In recent dueling editorials, two rheumatologists argue for psychological factors (Ferrari and Russell 1997), and a psychiatrist promotes organic reasons (Radanov 1997) for persistent complaints.

An epidemiological study challenges the organicity of chronic symptoms. Schrader et al. (1996) and Obelieniene et al. (1998, 1999) retrospectively examined the incidence of chronic symptoms after whiplash injuries in Lithuania, where few people are covered by insurance. Chronic neck pain and headache were no more common in accident victims than controls. The authors conclude that expectation of disability, a family history, and attribution of pre-existing symptoms to the trauma may be more important determinants for those who develop chronic symptoms. However, the study has significant sources of bias. The study cohort of 202 persons was drawn from police records of all those involved in a car accident rather than those who were injured. Previous studies followed patients who were injured and sought treatment after the accident. The power of this study is not sufficient to comment on the very small percentage of people who are involved in accidents, have symptoms, and then develop chronic problems. Only 23% of the study population was female. Since chronic symptoms develop more often in women, another source of bias is present.

Experimental studies also question the presence of persistent complaints of those involved in low-speed rear-end collisions. Volunteer subjects exposed to speed changes from 4 to 14 km/h do not have persistent complaints (Brault et al. 1998; Castro et al. 1997). However, the small study populations do not reflect the total population exposed to rear-end collisions who may have individual susceptibilities to persistent symptoms such as pre-existing spine pathology, older age, and previous medical history (Castro et al. 1997). Freeman et al. (1999) dispute the methodology of this and other types of studies claiming to refute the existence of whiplash syndrome.

This situation is very similar to doubts about the postconcussion syndrome both now and in the late 19th century when the controversy over functional versus organic etiology was about both the postconcussion syndrome and the whiplash-type injury, "railway spine" (Trimble 1981; Evans 1994; see also Chapter 23). Although the case for organicity is not quite as strong as the one for the postconcussion syndrome, the arguments are still quite compelling.

## Pathology

Animal and human studies have demonstrated structural damage from whiplash-type injuries (Barnsley et al. 1993, 1994; Rauschning and Jónsson 1998). Experimentally caused acceleration-deceleration injuries in primates have demonstrated multiple injuries including muscle damage, rupture of the anterior longitudinal and other ligaments, avulsion of disc from vertebral body, retropharyngeal hematoma, intralaryngeal and esophageal hemorrhage, cervical sympathetic nerve damage, and even various brain injuries including hemorrhages and contusions of brain and brain stem (MacNab 1964; Wickstrom et al. 1967; Ommaya et al. 1968).

Human studies have demonstrated similar lesions (Barnsley et al. 1994). A magnetic resonance imaging (MRI) study of selected patients within 4 months of whiplash injuries has revealed a variety of lesions: ruptures of the anterior longitudinal ligament, horizontal avulsion of the vertebral endplates, separation of the disc from the vertebral endplate, occult fractures of the anterior vertebral endplates, acute posterolateral cervical disc herniations, focal muscular injury of the longus colli muscle, posterior interspinous ligament injury, and prevertebral fluid collections (Davis 1991). Keith (1986) has described injury of the second cervical ganglion and nerve as the cause of unilateral neck and suboccipital area pain with decreased sensation in the C2 dermatome as a cause of symptoms in a small minority of patients following whiplash injury. Autopsy series have demonstrated clefts in the cartilage plates of the intervertebral discs, posterior disc herniations though a damaged annulus fibrosis, and hemarthrosis in facet joints (Taylor and Kakulas 1991; Taylor and Twomey 1993).

## Symptoms and Signs

Table 10-1 lists the sequelae of whiplash injuries, which include neck and back injuries; headache; dizziness; paresthesias; weakness; cognitive, somatic, and psychological sequelae; visual symptoms; and rare sequelae (Evans 1996). Although these symptoms are certainly common in the general population, those with whiplash injuries have an increased prevalence as compared with a control population with the following ratios: neck pain, 8:1; paresthesia, 16:1; neck and back pain, 32:1; and occipital headache, 11:1 (Bannister and Gargan 1993).

### Neck pain

Neck pain is usually due to myofascial and/or facet (zygapophyseal) joint injury. Cervical disc herniations, cervical spine fractures, and dislocations are uncommon. Facet joint injury at different levels can produce characteristic patterns of referred pain over various parts of the occipital, posterior cervical, shoulder girdle, and scapular regions (Dwyer et al. 1990). Neck pain may arise from at least one facet joint in 54% of patients with chronic pain from whiplash injuries (Barnsley et al. 1995).

### Headaches

Headaches following whiplash injuries are usually of the tension type and are often associated with greater occipital neuralgia (Magnusson 1994). Greater occipital neuralgia or referred pain from trigger points from suboccipital muscles can produce a pattern of radiating pain variably over the occipital, temporal, frontal, and retro-orbital distribution. Whiplash trauma can also injure the temporomandibular joint and cause jaw pain often associated with headache (Brooke and LaPointe 1993). Headache may be referred from the C2–C3 facet joint that is innervated by the third occipital nerve, so-called third occipital headache (Bogduk and Marsland 1986). C2–C3 facet joint injury can result in pain complaints in the upper cervical region extending into the occiput and at times toward the ear, vertex, forehead, or eye. Using third occipital nerve blocks to diagnose the condition, the prevalence of this type of headache among patients with persistent headaches after whiplash injury has been reported as 38% to 50% (Lord et al. 1994, 1996a). Occasionally, whiplash injuries can

**Table 10-1.** Sequelae of Whiplash Injuries

| | |
|---|---|
| Neck and back injuries | Weakness |
|   Myofascial |   Radiculopathy |
|   Fractures and dislocations |   Brachial plexopathy |
|   Disc herniation |   Entrapment neuropathy |
|   Spinal cord compression |   Reflex inhibition of muscle contraction by painful |
|   Spondylosis |     cutaneous stimulation |
|   Radiculopathy | Cognitive, somatic, and psychological sequelae |
|   Facet joint syndrome |   Memory, attention, and concentration impairment |
|   Increased development of spondylosis |   Nervousness and irritability |
| Headaches |   Sleep disturbances |
|   Muscle contraction headache |   Fatigue |
|   Greater occipital neuralgia |   Depression |
|   Temporomandibular joint injury |   Personality change |
|   Migraine |   Compensation neurosis |
|   Third occipital headache | Visual symptoms |
| Dizziness |   Convergence insufficiency |
|   Vestibular dysfunction |   Oculomotor palsies |
|   Brain stem dysfunction |   Abnormalities of smooth pursuit and saccades |
|   Cervical origin |   Horner's syndrome |
|   Barre syndrome |   Vitreous detachment |
|   Hyperventilation syndrome | Rare sequelae |
| Paresthesias |   Torticollis |
|   Trigger points |   Tremor |
|   Thoracic outlet syndrome |   Transient global amnesia |
|   Brachial plexus injury |   Esophageal perforation and descending mediastinitis |
|   Cervical radiculopathy |   Hypoglossal nerve palsy |
|   Facet joint syndrome |   Superior laryngeal nerve paralysis |
|   Carpal tunnel syndrome |   Cervical epidural hematoma |
|   Ulnar neuropathy at the elbow |   Internal carotid and vertebral artery dissection |

precipitate recurring migraine with and without aura and basilar migraines de novo (Winston 1987; Weiss et al. 1991).

## Dizziness

In a study of 262 patients with persistent neck pain and headaches for 4 months or longer after the injury, symptoms were reported as follows: vertigo, 50%; floating sensations, 35%; tinnitus, 14%; and hearing impairment, 5% (Oosterveld et al. 1991). Post-traumatic vertebral insufficiency and dysfunction of the vestibular apparatus, brain stem, cervical sympathetics (Barre syndrome), and cervical proprioceptive system have all been postulated as causing dizziness (Hinoki 1985; Chester 1991; Fischer et al. 1997). Hyperventilation syndrome can also occur in patients who are in pain and anxious, producing dizziness and paresthesias periorally and/or of the extremities either bilaterally or unilaterally (Evans 1995b).

## Paresthesias

In one study, 33% of patients with symptoms but no objective findings complained of paresthesias acutely, and 37% reported paresthesias after a mean follow-up of 19.7 months (Norris and Watt 1983). Paresthesias can be referred from trigger points, brachial plexopathy, facet joint syndrome, entrapment neuropathies, cervical radiculopathy, and spinal cord compression. Thoracic outlet syndrome is commonly caused by whiplash injuries, occurring four times more often in women than in men (Capistrant 1986). Thoracic outlet syndrome has been controversial, since at least 85% of cases are of the nonspecific neurogenic or so-called disputed type that is a diagnosis of exclusion. This nonspecific type may actually be a myofascial pain syndrome with referred pain from the anterior neck muscles such as the anterior scalene or from the shoulder area from the pectoralis minor and not due to neural or vascular compression (Hong and Simons 1993). Entrapment neuropathies can result from several mechanisms. Carpal tunnel syndrome can be caused by acute hyperextension of the wrist on the steering wheel (Label 1991). If the patient has a cervical radiculopathy or neurogenic thoracic outlet syndrome from the injury, a double crush syndrome resulting in carpal tunnel syndrome or cubital tunnel syndrome may ensue (Swenson 1994).

## Weakness

Complaints of upper extremity weakness, heaviness, or fatigue are common after whiplash injuries even when there is no evidence of cervical radiculopathy, myelopathy, brachial plexopathy, or entrapment neuropathy. The nonspecific type of thoracic outlet syndrome can produce these complaints. Alternatively, patients may have a sensation of weakness or heaviness because of reflex inhibition of muscle due to pain that can be overcome by more central effort (Aniss et al. 1988).

## Psychological and Cognitive Symptoms

In a study of patients with chronic symptoms after a whiplash injury, cognitive, psychological, and somatic symptoms occurred in the following percentages: nervousness and irritability, 67%; cognitive disturbances, 50%; sleep disturbances, 44%; fatigability, 40%; disturbances of vision, 38%; symptoms of depression, 37%; headache, 85%; neck pain, 100%; vertigo, 72%; and brachialgia, 60% (Kischka et al. 1991). These symptoms are nonspecific and are also common in patients with postconcussion syndrome, chronic pain syndrome, depression, and anxiety neurosis. Post-traumatic stress disorder may also be associated with whiplash injuries (Jaspers 1998).

It is controversial whether persistent neuropsychological deficits following whiplash injury are evidence for mild traumatic brain injury (Taylor et al. 1996). Deficits in tests of attention, concentration, cognitive flexibility, and memory have been described (Yarnell and Rossie 1988; Kischka et al. 1991; Ettlin et al. 1992). Although a 2-year prospective study did find that symptomatic subjects were impaired on tasks of divided attention but not on memory tests (Di Stefano and Radanov 1995), another prospective study of 39 patients found no evidence of cognitive deficits (Karlsborg et al. 1997). In a functional imaging study of 21 patients with late whiplash syndrome, Radanov et al. (1999) found no significant correlations between regional perfusion or metabolism in any brain area on single photon emission computed tomography (SPECT) or positron emission tomography (PET) studies and the scores of divided attention or working memory. There were significant relations between state anxiety and divided attention. Subjective cognitive complaints may be due to chronic pain, depression, stressful life events, and malingering (Smed 1997; Schmand et al. 1998).

Evidence of cerebral hypoperfusion has also been reported as supportive of a brain injury in some persons with whiplash injuries. In a small study of six patients compared to 12 controls, PET and SPECT evidence of parieto-occipital hypometabolism was reported (Otte et al. 1997). In another study, 13 patients with late whiplash syndrome and cognitive complaints were compared to 16 controls using hexamethylpropylene amine oxime (HmPAO) SPECT, [18]fluorodeoxyglucose (FDG) PET, and MRI (Bicik et al. 1998). The study group had significantly decreased FDG uptake in the frontopolar and lateral temporal cortex and in the putamen.

Although HmPAO and Tc-99m-bicisate (ECD) brain SPECT studies in patients with late whiplash syndrome and cognitive complaints have demonstrated parieto-occipital hypoperfusion (Otte et al. 1995, 1996), similar findings have also been seen in patients with nontraumatic chronic cervical pain (Otte et al. 1995). One possible explanation is stimulation of pain-sensitive afferents in the cervicotrigeminal system, which could have widespread effects on local vasoactive peptides and the cranial vascular system (Otte et al. 1997). Since depression can also cause perfusion abnormalities (Alexander 1998) and because FDG PET does not allow reliable diagnosis of metabolic disturbances for individual patients (Bicik et al. 1998), FDG PET and HmPAO SPECT should not be used as a diagnostic tool in the routine evaluation of patients with late whiplash syndrome (Bicik et al. 1998).

## Other Symptoms

A variety of other problems may follow whiplash injuries. Interscapular and low back pain are reported in 20% and 35%, respectively, of patients during the first months after the injury (Hohl 1974). In one study, 25% of patients reported persistent back pain after a mean follow-up of 2 years (Hildingsson and Toolanen 1990). Patients often report visual symptoms, especially blurred vision, usually due to convergence insufficiency, although oculomotor palsies can occasionally occur (Burke et al. 1992; Van Nechel et al. 1998). Rare sequelae include torticollis (Truong et al. 1991; Jankovic 1994), tremor (Ellis 1997), transient global amnesia (Fisher 1982), esophageal perforation (Stringer et al. 1980), descending mediastinitis (Totstein et al. 1986), superior laryngeal nerve paralysis (Brademann and Reker 1998), hypoglossal nerve palsy (Dukes and Bannerjee 1993), cervical epidural hematoma (Dougall et al. 1995), internal carotid artery dissection (Janjua et al. 1996), and extracranial vertebral artery dissection (Hinse et al. 1991; Viktrup et al. 1995).

## Radiographic Findings

Because asymptomatic radiographic findings are common, it is usually difficult to determine what findings are new and what findings are pre-existing unless recent preinjury studies are available. Cervical spondylosis and degenerative disc disease occur with increasing frequency with older age and are often asymptomatic (Friedenberg and Miller 1963; Irvine et al. 1965). Cervical disc protrusions are also common in the general population and are often asymptomatic. In a study of asymptomatic subjects, protrusions were present in 20% of patients ages 45 to 54 years and in 57% of patients older than 64 years (Teresi et al. 1987). Another study of those without symptoms found major abnormalities in 19% including 10% with herniated discs (Boden et al. 1990). In patients without radicular complaints or findings, cervical MRI studies have a low yield (Voyvodic et al. 1997). In another prospective study where most of the injured had neurological deficits, abnormal MRI studies were found in two-thirds, including 24% with herniated discs (Pettersson et al. 1994). Since there are no known morphological correlates, imaging studies cannot diagnose painful facet joints, which are diagnosed with the use of local anesthetic blocks (Bogduk et al. 1996).

## Prognostic Studies

Studies on the prognosis of whiplash injuries are fraught with methodological differences, including selection criteria of patients, patient attrition rates, prospective and retrospective designs, duration of follow-up, and treatment used. Some of the studies do not discuss the treatment modalities used, if any. Although the majority of patients studied probably have only soft tissue injuries, testing such as cervical myelography, computed tomography (CT) scan, or MRI studies have not been uniformly performed to exclude disc disease, cervical stenosis, and radiculopathy due to spondylosis. In general, patients are placed into study groups based on the relatively mild nature of the complaints and physical findings, as compared to patients with cervical fractures, myelopathy, and so forth.

In the first prognostic study, Gay and Abbott (1953) evaluated 50 patients who suffered a whiplash injury and concluded, "Characteristically, these patients were more disabled and remained handicapped for longer periods than was anticipated, considering the mild character of the accident." In addition, "The symptoms from this condition were so tenacious and the rate of recovery so slow that it was felt that every effort should be made by public authorities to prevent this kind of suffering." Gotten (1956) reviewed the chronic cases and stated, "in some instances there were indications that the injury was being used by the patient as a convenient lever for personal gain." What have we learned in the last 45 years?

## Neck Pain and Headaches

Neck pain and headaches commonly occur after whiplash injuries and may persist in significant numbers of patients, as multiple studies document (Table 10-2). After a motor vehicle accident, 62% of patients presenting to the emergency room complain of neck pain (Deans et al. 1986). The onset of neck pain occurs within 6 hours in 65%,

**Table 10-2.** Percentage of Patients With Persistence of Neck Pain and Headaches After a Whiplash Injury

|  | 1 Week | 1 Month | 2 Months | 3 Months | 6 Months | 1 Year | 2 Years | 10 Years |
|---|---|---|---|---|---|---|---|---|
| Neck pain (%) | 92[a] | 64[c] | 63[d] | 38[a] | 25[a] | 19[a] | 16[i] | 74[g] |
|  | 88[b] |  |  | 51[c] | 43[c] | 26[c] | 29[b,e] |  |
|  |  |  |  |  |  |  | 44[f] |  |
| Headaches (%) | 54[b] | 82[h] |  | 35[a] | 26[a] | 21[a] | 9[e] | 33[g] |
|  | 57[a] |  |  | 73[h] |  |  | 15[i] |  |
|  |  |  |  |  |  |  | 37[f] |  |

[a] Radanov et al. 1994b; [b] Hildingsson and Toolanen 1990; [c] Deans et al. 1987; [d] Greenfield and Ilfeld 1977; [e] Maimaris et al. 1988; [f] Norris and Watt 1983; [g] Gargan and Bannister 1990; [h] Balla and Karnaghan 1987; [i] Radanov et al. 1995.

within 24 hours in 28%, and within 72 hours in the remaining 7% of patients (Greenfield and Ilfeld 1977; Deans et al. 1987). In a prospective study of 180 patients seen within 4 weeks of the injury, 82% complained of headaches that were occipitally located in 46%, generalized in 34%, and in other locations in 20% (Balla and Karnaghan 1987). Fifty percent of the patients had headache present more than half the time.

Many studies have reported persistence of neck pain and headaches in significant numbers of patients. A well-designed prospective study reported the following percentages of patients with complaints of neck pain and headaches, respectively, at various times after the injury: 92% and 57%, 1 week, 38% and 35%, 3 months; 25% and 26%, 6 months; 19% and 21%, 1 year; and 16% and 15%, 2 years (Radanov et al. 1994b, 1995). In three other studies, neck pain present 2 years after injury has been variously reported in 29% (Maimaris et al. 1988; Hildingsson and Toolanen 1990) and 44% of patients (Deans et al. 1987). In two different studies with a mean time after the accident of 10 years and 13.5 years, neck pain was still present in 74% (Gargan and Bannister 1990) and 86% (Robinson and Cassar-Pullicino 1993) of subjects, respectively. Symptoms present 2 years after injury were still present 10 years after the injury (Gargan and Bannister 1990).

## Acceleration of Cervical Spine Disease

Trauma and whiplash injuries can accelerate the development of cervical spondylosis with degenerative disc disease. Persons with a history of a serious head or neck injury and miners under the age of 40 have an increased incidence of spondylosis (Irvine et al. 1965). Although two studies have reported that whiplash injuries can accelerate the development of cervical spondylosis with degenerative disc disease (Hohl 1974; Gargan and Bannister 1990), one did not show a relationship (Parmar and Raymakers 1993). A surgical series provides additional evidence that whiplash injury causes structural changes predisposing to premature degenerative disc disease (Hamer et al. 1993). The incidence of cervical disc disruption following whiplash injuries was twice that of a control population. The mean age at operation of those patients with a previous whiplash injury was significantly less than those patients without a previous injury.

## Prognostic Variables

There are numerous risk factors for persistent symptoms (Table 10-3). The age of the patient and occupational categories are important variables. The majority of patients who develop the chronic whiplash syndrome are between the ages of 21 and 50 (Balla 1980). Older age of patients is prognostically significant of persistent symptoms at various times after the injury including 6 months (Radanov et al. 1994b), 2 years (Maimaris et al. 1988), and 10 years (Gargan and Bannister 1990). Although one study reported that patients in upper middle compared to lower and higher occupational categories have an increased incidenceof symptoms persisting for longer than 6 months (Balla 1980), another found no relationship between persisting symptoms and the type of vocational activity (Radanov et al. 1994b).

Sturzenegger and colleagues (1994) reported on the relationship between accident mechanisms and initial findings: "Three features of accident mechanisms were associated with more severe symptoms: an unprepared occupant; rear-end collision, with or without subsequent frontal impact; and rotated or inclined head position at the moment of impact." A higher frequency of multiple symptoms especially of cranial nerve or brain stem dysfunction was associated with a rear-end collision. Other studies report only a minimal or no association of a poor prognosis with the speed or severity of the collision and the extent of vehicle damage (Kenna and Murtagh 1987; Parmar and Raymakers 1993).

**Table 10-3.** Risk Factors for Persistent Symptoms

Accident mechanisms
   Inclined or rotated head position
   Unpreparedness for impact
   Car stationary when hit
Occupant's characteristics
   Older age
   Female gender
   Stressful life events unrelated to the accident
Symptoms
   Intensity of initial neck pain or headache
   Occipital headache
   Interscapular or upper back pain
   Multiple symptoms or paresthesias at presentation
Signs
   Reduced range of movement of the cervical spine
   Objective neurological deficit
Radiographic findings
   Pre-existing degenerative osteoarthritic changes
   Abnormal cervical spine curves
   Narrow diameter of cervical spinal canal

The following are risk factors for a less favorable prognosis: interscapular or upper back pain (Greenfield and Ilfeld 1977; Maimaris et al. 1988); occipital headache (Maimaris et al. 1988); multiple symptoms or paresthesias at presentation (Gargan and Bannister 1990; Radanov et al. 1994b); reduced range of movement of the cervical spine (Norris and Watt 1983); the presence of an objective neurologic deficit (Norris and Watt 1983; Maimaris et al. 1988); and pre-existing degenerative osteoarthritic changes (Norris and Watt 1983; Miles et al. 1988; Borchgrevink et al. 1995; Voyvodic et al. 1997). Abnormal cervical spine curves have been variably reported as prognostic (Griffiths et al. 1995) and not prognostic (Maimaris et al. 1988) of a poor outcome. A history of pretraumatic headache and both the presence and intensity of neck pain are all risk factors for persistent headaches 6 months after the injury (Robinson and Cassar-Pullicino 1993). Cervical stenosis is a risk factor for the development of myelopathy after whiplash injuries both with cervical spine fractures or dislocations and without (Epstein et al. 1980). Narrow diameter of the cervical spinal canal is a risk factor for chronic neck pain (Pettersson et al. 1995). Stressful life events unrelated to the accident may increase the risk of persistent pain complaints (Karlsborg et al. 1997; Smed 1997).

A prospective study of 117 patients found 18% with injury-related symptoms at 2 years (Radanov et al. 1995). The study found the following risk factors:

Symptomatic patients were older, had higher incidence of rotated or inclined head position at the time of impact, had higher prevalence of pretraumatic headache, showed higher intensity of initial neck pain and headache, complained of a greater number of symptoms, had a higher incidence of symptoms of radicular deficit and higher average scores on a multiple symptom analysis, and displayed more degenerative signs (osteoarthrosis) on X ray.

Sturzenegger et al. (1995) also performed a 12-month follow-up study of 117 consecutive patients. Variables that predicted persistence of symptoms at 1 year are the following: intensity of initial neck pain and headache; rotated or inclined head position at the moment of impact; unpreparedness at the time of impact; and car stationary when hit.

## Psychological Factors

Although psychological factors such as neurosis are commonly cited as the cause of persistent symptoms, a prospective study of 78 consecutive patients with whiplash injuries demonstrated that psychosocial factors, negative affectivity, and personality traits were not significant in predicting the duration of symptoms (Radanov et al. 1991). Psychosocial factors and vocation were not predictive of persistent symptoms during a 1-year follow-up (Radanov et al. 1994b). Similarly, in another 1-year prospective study, baseline psychological variables were not associated with neck symptoms (Mayou and Bryant 1996).

Cognitive and psychological symptoms may be due to somatic symptoms (Radanov et al. 1994a; Wallis et al. 1998). In those with chronic neck pain due to a single painful facet joint following whiplash injuries, psychological distress resolved following successful radiofrequency neurotomy (Wallis et al. 1997). Based upon a comparison of psychological profiles of those with whiplash-associated headaches to those with nontraumatic headaches and controls, patients with whiplash-associated headache suffer psychological distress secondary to chronic pain and not from tension headache and generalized psychological distress (Wallis et al. 1998).

## Return to Work and Chronic Disability

A number of studies have investigated the issues of return to work and chronic disability. In a retrospective analysis of over 5000 cases of whiplash injury, 26% were not able to return to normal activities at 6 months (Balla 1988). In a retrospective study of 102 consecutive patients seen in the emergency department, patients in the good prognostic group (66% of total) had an average time off work of 2 weeks with a maximum of 16 weeks (Maimaris et al. 1988). One-third of these patients had no time off at all. In the poorer prognostic group patients, 20% had no time off work, 9% did not return to work by 2 years, and the average time off work was 6 weeks. In a series of consecutive medicolegal cases, 79% of patients returned to work by 1 month, 86% by 3 months, 91% by 6 months, and 94% by 1 year (Pearce 1989). Nygren (1984) reported that permanent medical disability occurred in 9.6% of patients involved in rear-end collisions and 3.8% involved in front or side impact accidents.

Radanov and colleagues performed a prospective study to assess psychological risk factors for disability (Radanov et al. 1993). At 6 months, 7%

had partial or complete disability. The disabled and nondisabled patients who were still symptomatic at 6 months did not differ with respect to psychosocial stress, negative affectivity, and personality traits, as evaluated at baseline. One year after the accident, 5% were still disabled (Radanov 1994b).

## Litigation and Symptoms

Many clinicians and certainly the insurance industry and defense attorneys believe that pending litigation is a major cause of persistent symptoms that promptly resolve once the litigation is completed (Livingston 1993). Eight studies have looked at the effect of settlement of litigation on symptoms (Table 10-4).

Gotten (1956), in Memphis, Tennessee, interviewed 100 patients 1 to 26 months after settlement of claims for injury. Fifty-four percent of the patients had no significant symptoms; 34% reported minor discomfort on damp, cloudy days or with exercises or lifting; and 12% continued to have severe symptoms. He concluded, "Once the psychoneurotic symptoms had developed, they persisted for many months and were refractory to treatment, being finally resolved to a great extent by settlement of the litigation."

MacNab (1964), in Toronto, Ontario, surveyed patients 2 or more years after settlement of litigation. Of the 145 patients of the original cohort of 266 available for follow-up, 121 were still having symptoms which for most were minor rather than a cause of significant disability. He also noted that in patients with concomitant injuries, the broken wrist or sprained ankle would heal as expected and yet the neck pain would persist:

It is difficult to understand why the patients' traumatic neurosis should be confined solely to their necks and not be reflected in continuing disability in relation to other injuries sustained at the same time. Moreover, if the symptoms resulting from an extension-acceleration injury of the neck are purely the result of a litigation neurosis, it is difficult to explain why 45 per cent of the patients should still have symptoms two years or more after settlement of their court action.

Schutt and Dohan (1968) studied 74 women with whiplash injuries in New Jersey. Symptoms and litigation status were assessed 6 to 26 months after the accident. Of the 5% with litigation pending, 75% had persisting symptoms. Of the 9.5%

with litigation settled, 71% had persisting symptoms. Of the 23% with no litigation at all, 82% had persisting symptoms. The remaining 9.5% had an unknown litigation status.

Norris and Watt (1983) reported a series of 61 patients with whiplash injuries from rear-end collisions in Sheffield, England. The average time from injury to settlement was 17.25 months for patients with symptoms but no signs. At a mean follow-up of 35.8 months, 50% had persisting symptoms and 50% had improved. Of the patients with symptoms and a reduced range of movement of the cervical spine but no neurological signs, 64% had not improved and the other 36% had improved after a mean follow-up of 43.4 months and an average time from injury to settlement of 15.9 months. Of the patients with symptoms, a reduced range of cervical movement, and evidence of objective neurological loss, 25% had improved, 50% had not changed, and 25% had worsened at a mean follow-up of 43 months and an average time from injury to settlement of 27.6 months. Symptoms present 2 years after injury were still present 10 years after injury (Gargan and Bannister 1990).

Maimaris et al. (1988) performed a retrospective study of 102 consecutive patients presenting to the emergency room with whiplash injuries with a follow-up of about 2 years. They reported: "The average time for settlement was 9 months, yet all these patients continued to have symptoms for between 2 and 2.5 years after injury. These results suggest that litigation does not influence the natural progression of symptoms."

Robinson and Casesar-Pullicino (1993) reported a retrospective study of 21 patients seen in an orthopedic office practice. After a mean follow-up of 13.5 years after injury, 86% still had neck complaints.

Finally, Parmar and Raymakers (1993) described 100 patients involved in rear-end collisions who were seen in medicolegal consultation. After a mean follow-up of 8 years after the injury, 55% reported neck pain and 14% described significant neck pain. If improvement after settlement of litigation does occur, the mean interval between settlement and even mild improvement is 72 weeks.

Litigants are similar to nonlitigants. Litigants and nonlitigants have similar recovery rates (Pennie and Agambar 1990) and similar response rates to treatment for facet joint pain (Lord et al. 1996a). Patients with ongoing litigation showed a statisti-

**Table 10-4.** Persistence of Neck Symptoms After Settlement of Litigation

| Study | No. of Patients | Selection of Patients | Time from Injury to Settlement | Length of Follow-up After Settlement | Neck Complaints (%) |
|---|---|---|---|---|---|
| Gotten, 1956; Memphis, TN | 100 | Neurosurgery office practice | Not reported | 1–26 months | 54 no "appreciable" symptoms<br>34 minor symptoms<br>12 severe symptoms |
| MacNab, 1964; Toronto, Ontario | 145 | Orthopedic office practice | Not reported | 2 or more years | 83 most with minor symptoms |
| Schutt and Dohan, 1968; Newark, NJ | 7, all women | Employees of Radio Corporation of America (RCA) plant | Not reported | Not reported Follow-up 6–26 months after injury | 71 |
| Hohl, 1974; Los Angeles, CA | 102, total not stated | Orthopedic office practice, patients without cervical degenerative changes | Within 6 months | 4.5 + years | 17 |
| Norris and Watt, 1983; Sheffield, England | | Prospective study of consecutive emergency room presentations | After 18 months | 3.5 + years | 62 |
| Symptoms, no signs | 14 | | 17.25 ± 11.9 months | 35.8 ± 8.4 months | 50 improved<br>50 no change |
| Symptoms, reduced range of motion | 14 | | 15.9 ± 11.2 months | 43.4 ± 9.4 months | 64 no change<br>36 improved |
| Symptoms, reduced range of cervical movement, and objective neurological loss | 8 | | 27.6 ± 6.5 months | 43 ± 10 months | 50 no change<br>25 improved<br>25 worse |
| Maimaris et al., 1988; Leicester, England | 10 | Retrospective study of consecutive emergency room presentations | Average 9 months | 15–20 months | 100 |
| Robinson and Caesar-Pullicino, 1993; Shropshire, England | 21 | Retrospective study of orthopedic office practice | Not reported | Mean follow-up 13.5 years after injury | 86 |
| Parmar and Raymakers, 1993; Leicester, England | 100, all in rear-end accidents | Retrospective study of orthopedic office practice | Not reported | Mean follow-up 8 years after injury | 55<br>14 significant pain |

cally significant improvement with multimodality treatment (Schofferman and Wasserman 1994). Mayou and Bryant (1996) evaluated consecutive patients who presented to the Accident and Emergency Department after whiplash injuries just after the accident (63 of 74 agreed to an interview) and at 3 months (61 subjects) and 1 year (57 subjects). Compensation was not a major determinant of any aspect of outcome. Litigation was a cause of considerable worry, anger, and frustration. In summary, the majority of plaintiffs who have persistent symptoms at the time of settlement of their litigation are not cured by a verdict (Mendelson 1982; Shapiro and Roth 1993).

Certainly, there are some patients who exaggerate or lie about persisting complaints to help or make their legal case. Neurotic, histrionic, or sociopathic patients may thrive on the attention and endless treatments recommended by some physicians and encouraged by some plaintiff attorneys. Since pain is subjective, the clinician is almost totally dependent on the word of the patient. Secondary gain, exaggeration, and malingering should be considered in all patients with persistent complaints after whiplash injuries. In one study of litigants, 88.7% were found to have inconsistent nongenuine abnormalities on examination (Peterson 1998). Schmand et al. (1998) performed neuropsychological studies of patients with late whiplash syndrome reporting memory or concentration problems. In the context of litigation, the prevalence of underperforming was 61% as defined by a positive score on the malingering test.

If the patient is considered credible, the physician should not be deterred from making a diagnosis. Using subjective criteria, clinicians diagnose most migraine and tension type headaches on a daily basis without any reservations. The clinician should evaluate the merits of each case individually (Conomy 1998). The available evidence does not support bias against patients just because they have pending litigation (Benoist 1998).

## Treatment

Most clinicians are appropriately skeptical about the effectiveness of the astounding array of available treatments for whiplash injuries (Evans et al. 1994). Most have been poorly studied in randomized prospective studies (Quebec Task Force on Whiplash-Associated Disorders 1995) without which placebo effects and the natural history of the disorder may be misattributed to an effect of treatment (Turner et al. 1994). Patients see both physicians and other healers who are unwitting partners in health care (Murray and Rubel 1992). In the United States, 42% of the adult population uses alternative therapy yearly, 12% for neck problems and 13% for headaches (Eisenberg et al. 1998). According to a patient survey in the United States, alternative medicine users find these approaches to be more congruent with their own values, beliefs, and philosophical orientations toward health and life (Astin 1998). The litigation process can also generate unnecessary consultations, testing, and treatment.

Prospective controlled studies indicate that early mobilization of the neck using the Maitland technique followed by local heat and neck exercises produces more rapid improvement after acute injuries than the use of a cervical collar and rest (Mealy et al. 1986) and is as effective as physical therapy performed during the first 8 weeks after the injury (McKinney et al. 1989). In another study, the outcome was better for patients who were encouraged to continue engaging in their normal, preinjury activities as usual than for patients who took sick leave from work and who were immobilized during the first 14 days after the injury (Borchgrevink et al. 1998). Cervical traction may be no more effective than exercises alone (Pennie and Agambar 1990). In a small prospective randomized study of patients with neck pain and musculoskeletal signs (75% of those treated) and others also with neurologic signs (25%), the administration of high-dose methylprednisolone within 8 hours of the injury prevented extensive sick leave as compared to the placebo controls at 6 months (Pettersson and Toolanen 1998).

Treatment of pain arising from facet joint injury is being increasingly studied. A controlled prospective study showed a lack of effect of intra-articular corticosteroid injections in the cervical facet joints for chronic pain after whiplash injuries (Barnsley et al. 1994). In a small study of patients with chronic facet joint pain confirmed with double-blind placebo-controlled local anesthesia, percutaneous radiofrequency neurotomy with multiple lesions of target nerves provided at least 50% relief for a median duration of 263 days compared to similar relief for 8 days in the control group (Lord et al. 1996b). Radiofrequency neurotomy of the C2–C3 joint was not included in this study because a pilot study showed significant technical problems (Bogduk 1998).

Other invasive and surgical treatments are sometimes recommended. Patients with radicular symptoms and signs may respond better to cervical epidural steroid injections than those with neck pain alone (Ferrante et al. 1993). Although complications are uncommon, the data for efficacy are largely anecdotal (Bogdux 1995). Surgery is sometimes inappropriately recommended for bulging discs and spondylosis. Even with appropriate indications, discectomy and anterior cervical fusion may produce unimpressive results in patients with chronic symptoms after whiplash injury (Algers et al. 1993).

According to uncontrolled studies, trigger point injections can be beneficial for acute and chronic myofascial injuries (Garvey et al. 1989). One group reports benefit from injection of sterile water in or subcutaneous to trigger points caused by whiplash injuries (Byrn et al. 1991, 1993). Case reports describe cervicogenic headache relief with injections of botulinum toxin in a trapezius muscle tender area (Hobson and Gladish 1997) and pericranial trigger points (Wheeler 1998). Transcutaneous electrical nerve stimulating (TENS) units may also be beneficial (Graff-Radford et al. 1989).

Routine treatment for acute injuries often consists of pain medications, nonsteroidal antiinflammatory medications, muscle relaxants, and the use of a cervical collar for 2 to 3 weeks. Neurologists frequently prescribe range-of-motion exercises and physical therapy with a variety of modalities. Standard treatments are provided for post-traumatic headache. Some patients with occipital neuralgia benefit from nerve blocks (Sjaastad 1990; Anthony 1992). For persistent complaints, tricyclic antidepressants are often prescribed. The chronic frequent use of narcotics, benzodiazepines, barbiturates, and carisprodol should be sparingly recommended because of the potential of habituation. Medication abuse headaches can also develop.

Clearly, adequately controlled prospective studies of conventional and unconventional treatments and more effective treatments for chronic pain are greatly needed (Newman 1990; Carette 1994; Quebec Task Force on Whiplash-Associated Disorders 1995). Until then, a compassionate, sympa-

thetic approach by the neurologist might result in greater patient satisfaction (Porter 1989) and reduce unnecessary expenditures from patients' therapeutic quests.

## References

Alexander, M. P. In the pursuit of proof of brain damage after whiplash injury. Neurology 51:336–340; 1998.

Algers, G.; Pettersson, K.; Hildingsson, C.; Toolanen, G. Surgery for chronic symptoms after whiplash injury. Follow-up of 20 cases. Acta Orthop. Scand. 64:654–656; 1993.

Aniss, A. M.; Gandevia, S. C.; Milne, R. J. Changes in perceived heaviness and motor commands produced by cutaneous reflexes in man. J. Physiol. 397:113–126; 1988.

Anthony, M. Headache and the greater occipital nerve. Clin. Neurol. Neurosurg. 94:297–301; 1992.

Astin, J. Why patients use alternative medicine. Results of a national study. JAMA 279:1548–1553; 1998.

Awerbuch, M. S. Whiplash in Australia: illness or injury? Med. J. Aust. 157:193–196; 1992.

Balla, J. I. The late whiplash syndrome. Aust. N. Z. J. Surg. 50:610–614; 1980.

Balla, J.; Karnaghan, J. Whiplash headache. Clin. Exp. Neurol. 23:179–182; 1987.

Bannister, G., Gargan, M. Prognosis of whiplash injuries: a review of the literature. Spine 7:557–569; 1993.

Barnsley, L.; Lord, S.; Bogduk, N. The pathophysiology of whiplash. Spine 7:329–353; 1993.

Barnsley, L.; Lord, S.; Bogduk, N. Whiplash injury. Pain 58:283–307; 1994.

Barnsley, L.; Lord, S. M.; Wallis, B. J.; Bogduk, N. The prevalence of chronic cervical zygapophyseal joint pain after whiplash. Spine 20:20–26, 1995.

Benoist, M. Natural evolution and resolution of the cervical whiplash syndrome. In: Gunzburg, R.; Szpalski, M., ed. Whiplash injuries: current concepts in prevention, diagnosis, and treatment of the cervical whiplash syndrome. Philadelphia: Lippincott-Raven; 1998: p. 117–126.

Bicik, I.; Radanov, B. P.; Schäfer, N.; et al. PET with [18]fluorodeoxyglucose and hexamethylpropylene amine oxime SPECT in late whiplash syndrome. Neurology 51:345–350; 1998.

Boden, S. D.; McCowin, P. R.; Davis, D. O. Abnormal magnetic resonance scans of the cervical spine in asymptomatic subjects. A prospective investigation. J. Bone Joint Surg. Am. 72:1178–1184; 1990.

Bogduk, N. Spine update. Epidural steroids. Spine 20:845–848; 1995.

Bogduk, N.; Marsland, A. On the concept of third occipital headache. J. Neurol. Neurosurg. Psychiatry 49:775–780; 1986.

Bogduk, N.; Lord, S. M.; Schwarzer, A. C. Post-traumatic cervical and lumbar zygapophyseal joint pain. In: Evans, R. W., ed. Neurology and trauma. Philadelphia: W. B. Saunders Co.; 1996: p. 363–372.

Bogduk, N. Cervical zygapophysial joint pain and percutaneous neurotomy. In: Gunzburg, R.; Szpalski, M., ed. Whiplash injuries: current concepts in prevention, diagnosis, and treatment of the cervical whiplash syndrome. Philadelphia: Lippincott-Raven; 1998: p. 211–219.

Borchgrevink, G.; Smevik, O.; Nordby, A.; et al. MR imaging and radiography of patients with cervical hyperextension-flexion injuries after car accidents. Acta Radiol. 36:425–428; 1995.

Brademann, G.; Reker, U. Paralysis of the superior laryngeal nerve after whiplash trauma. Laryngorhinootologie 77:3–6; 1998.

Brault, J. R.; Wheeler, J. B.; Siegmund, G. P.; Brault, E. J. Clinical response of human subjects to rear-end automobile collisions. Arch. Phys. Med. Rehabil. 79:72–80; 1998.

Brooke, R. I.; LaPointe, H. J. Temporomandibular joint disorders following whiplash. Spine 7:443–454; 1993.

Burke, J. P.; Orton, H. P.; West, J.; et al. Whiplash and its effect on the visual system. Graefes Arch. Clin. Exp. Ophthalmol. 230:335–339; 1992.

Byrn, C.; Bornstein, P.; Linder, L.-E. Treatment of neck and shoulder pain in whiplash syndrome patients with intracutaneous sterile water injections. Acta Anaesthesiol. Scand. 35:52–53; 1991.

Byrn, C.; Olsson, I.; Falkheden, L.; et al. Subcutaneous sterile water injections for chronic neck and shoulder pain following whiplash injuries. Lancet 341: 449–452; 1993.

Capistrant, T. D. Thoracic outlet syndrome in cervical strain injury. Minn. Med. 69:13–17; 1986.

Carette, S. Whiplash injury and chronic neck pain. N. Engl. J. Med. 330:1083–1084; 1994.

Castro, W. H. M.; Schilgen, M.; Meyer, S. Do "whiplash injuries" occur in low-speed rear impacts? Eur. Spine J. 6:366–375; 1997.

Chester, J. B. Whiplash, postural control, and the inner ear. Spine 16:716–720; 1991.

Conomy, J. P. Fender bender spine. Neurologist 4: 131–137; 1998.

Crowe, H. A new diagnostic sign in neck injuries. California Med. 100:12–13; 1964.

Davis, A. G. Injuries of the cervical spine. JAMA 127:149–156; 1945.

Davis, S. J.; Teresi, L. M.; Bradley, W. G.; Ziemba, M. A.; Bloze, A. E. Cervical spine hyperextension injuries: MR findings. Radiology 180:245–251; 1991.

Deans, G. T.; McGalliard, J. N.; Kerr, M.; Rutherford, W. H. Neck sprain—a major cause of disability following car accidents. Injury 18:10–12; 1987.

Deans, G. T.; McGalliard, J. N.; Rutherford, W. H. Incidence and duration of neck pain among patient's injured in car accidents. Br. Med. J. 292:94–95; 1986.

Di Stefano, G.; Radanov, B. P. Course of attention and memory after common whiplash: a two-year prospective study with age, education and gender pairmatched patients. Acta Neurol. Scand. 91:346–352; 1995.

Dolinis, J. Risk factors for 'whiplash' in drivers: a cohort study of rear-end traffic crashes. Injury 28:173–179; 1997.

Dougall, T. W.; Kay, N. R. M.; Turnbull, L. W. Acute cervical epidural haematoma after soft-tissue cervical spine injury. Injury 26:345–346; 1995.

Dukes, I. K.; Bannerjee, S. K. Hypoglossal nerve palsy following hyperextension neck injury. Injury 24: 133–134; 1993.

Dwyer, A.; Aprill, C.; Bogduk, N. Cervical zygapophyseal joint pain patterns. 1: a study in normal volunteers. Spine 15:453–457; 1990.

Eisenberg, D. M.; Davis, R. B.; Ettner, S. L.; et al. Trends in alternative medicine use in the United States, 1990–1997. Results of a follow-up national survey. JAMA 280:1569–1575; 1998.

Ellis, S. J. Tremor and other movement disorders after whiplash type injuries. J. Neurol. Neurosurg. Psychiatry 63:110–112; 1997.

Epstein, N.; Epstein, J. A.; Benjamin, V.; Ransohoff, J. Traumatic myelopathy in patients with cervical spinal stenosis without fractures or dislocation—methods of diagnosis, management, and prognosis. Spine 5:489–496; 1980.

Ettlin, T. M.; Kischka, U.; Reichmann, S.; et al. Cerebral symptoms after whiplash injury of the neck: a prospective clinical and neuropsychological study of whiplash injury. J. Neurol. Neurosurg. Psychiatry 55:943–948; 1992

Evans, R. W. The post-concussion syndrome: 130 years of controversy. Semin. Neurol. 14:32–39; 1994.

Evans, R. W. Whiplash around the world. Headache 35:262–263; 1995a.

Evans, R. W. Neurological manifestations of hyperventilation syndrome. Semin. Neurol. 15:115–125; 1995b.

Evans, R. W. Whiplash injuries. In: Evans, R. W., ed. Neurology and trauma. Philadelphia: W. B. Saunders; 1996: p. 439–457.

Evans, R. W.; Evans, R. I.; Sharp, M. J. The physician survey on the post-concussion and whiplash syndromes. Headache 35:268–274; 1994.

Ferrante, F. M.; Wilson, S. P.; Iacobo, C.; et al. Clinical classification as a predictor of therapeutic outcome after cervical epidural steroid injection. Spine 18:730–736; 1993.

Ferrari, R.; Russell, A. S. The whiplash syndrome—common sense revisited. J. Rheumatol. 24:618–622; 1997.

Fischer, A. J. E. M.; Verhagen, W. I. M.; Huygen, P. L. M. Whiplash injury. A clinical review with emphasis on neurootological aspects. Clin. Otolaryngol. 22:192–201; 1997.

Fisher, C. M. Whiplash amnesia. Neurology 32: 667–668; 1982.

Freeman, M. D.; Croft, A. C.; Rossignol, A. M.; et al. A review and methodologic critique of the literature refuting whiplash syndrome. Spine 24:86–98; 1999.

Friedenberg, Z. B.; Miller, W. T. Degenerative disc disease of the cervical spine. A comparative study of asymptomatic and symptomatic patients. J. Bone Joint Surg. 45A:1171–1178; 1963.

Gargan, M. F.; Bannister, G. C. Long term prognosis of soft tissue injuries of the neck. J. Bone Joint Surg. 72B:901–903; 1990.

Garvey, T. A.; Marks, M. R.; Wiesel, S. W. A prospective, randomized double-blind evaluation of trigger-point injection therapy for low-back pain. Spine 14: 962–964; 1989.

Gay, J. R.; Abbott, K. H. Common whiplash injuries of the neck. JAMA 152:1698–1704; 1953.

Gotten, N. Survey of 100 cases of whiplash injury after settlement of litigation. JAMA 162:865–867; 1956.

Graff-Radford, S. B.; Reeves, J. L.; Baker, R. L.; et al. Effects of transcutaneous electrical nerve stimulation on myofascial pain and trigger point sensitivity. Pain 37:1–5; 1989.

Greenfield, J.; Ilfeld, F. W. Acute cervical strain: evaluation and short term prognostic factors. Clin. Orthop. 122:196–200; 1977.

Griffiths, H. J.; Olson, P. N.; Everson, L. I.; Winemiller, M. Hyperextension strain or "whiplash" injuries to the cervical spine. Skeletal Radiol. 24: 263–266; 1995.

Hamer, A. J.; Gargan, M. F.; Bannister, G. C.; Nelson, R. J. Whiplash injury and surgically treated cervical disc disease. Injury 24:549–550; 1993.

Hildingsson, C.; Toolanen, G. Outcome after soft-tissue injury of the cervical spine. Acta Orthop. Scand. 61: 357–359; 1990.

Hinoki, M. Vertigo due to whiplash injury: a neurotological approach. Acta Otolaryngol. Suppl. (Stockh.) 419:9–29; 1985.

Hinse, P.; Thie, A.; Lachenmayer, L. Dissection of the extracranial vertebral artery: report of four cases and review of the literature. J. Neurol. Neurosurg. Psychiatry 54:863–869; 1991.

Hobson, D. E.; Gladish, D. F. Botulinum toxin injection for cervicogenic headache. Headache 37: 253–256; 1997.

Hohl, M. Soft tissue injuries of the neck in automobile accidents: factors influencing prognosis. J. Bone Joint Surg. 56A:1675–1682; 1974.

Hong, C. Z.; Simons, D. G. Response to treatment for pectoralis minor myofascial pain syndrome after whiplash. J. Musculoskel. Pain 1:89–129; 1993.

Irvine, D. H.; Fisher, J. B.; Newell, D. J.; Klukvin, B. N. Prevalence of cervical spondylosis in a general practice. Lancet 1:1089–1092; 1965.

Janjua, K. J.; Goswami, V.; Sagar, G. Whiplash injury associated with acute bilateral internal carotid arterial dissection. J. Trauma 40:456–458; 1996.

Jankovic, J. Post-traumatic movement disorders: central and peripheral mechanisms. Neurology 44: 2006–2014; 1994.

Jaspers, J. P. Whiplash and post-traumatic stress disorder. Disabil. Rehabil. 20:397–404; 1998.

Kahane, C. J. An evaluation of head restraints. U.S. Department of Transportation, National Highway Traffic Safety Administration Technical Report DOT HS-806-108, Springfield, Virginia, National Technical Information Service, February, 1982.

Karlsborg, M.; Smed, A.; Jespersen, H.; et al. A prospective study of 39 patients with whiplash injury. Acta Neurol. Scand. 95:65–72; 1997.

Keith, W. S. "Whiplash"—injury of the 2nd cervical ganglion and nerve. Can. J. Neurol. Sci. 13:133–137; 1986.

Kenna, C.; Murtagh. J. Whiplash. Aust. Fam. Physician 16:727,–729,733,736; 1987.

Kischka, U.; Ettlin Th.; Heim S; Schmid G. Cerebral symptoms following whiplash injury. Eur. Neurol.; 31:136–140; 1991.

Label, L. S. Carpal tunnel syndrome resulting from steering wheel impact. Muscle Nerve 14:904; 1991.

Livingston, M. Whiplash injury and peer copying. J. R. Soc. Med. 86:535–536; 1993.

Lord, S. M.; Barnsley, L.; Bogduk, N. Percutaneous radiofrequency neurotomy in the treatment of cervical zygapophyseal joint pain: a caution. Neurosurgery 36:732–739; 1995.

Lord, S. M.; Barnsley, L.; Wallis, B. J.; Bogduk, N. Third occipital headache: a prevalence study. J. Neurol. Neurosurg. Psychiatry 57:1187–1190; 1994.

Lord, S. M.; Barnsley, L.; Wallis, B. J.; Bogduk, N. Chronic cervical zygapophyseal joint pain after whiplash. A placebo-controlled prevalence study. Spine 21:1737–1745; 1996a.

Lord, S. M.; Barnsley, L.; Wallis, B. J.; et al. Percutaneous radio-frequency neurotomy for chronic cervical zygapophyseal-joint pain. N. Engl. J. Med. 335: 1721–1726; 1996b.

McKinney, L. A.; Dornan, J. O.; Ryan, M. The role of physiotherapy in the management of acute neck sprains following road-traffic accidents. Arch. Emerg. Med. 6:27–33; 1989.

MacNab, I. Acceleration injuries of the cervical spine. J. Bone Joint Surg. 46A:1797–1799; 1964.

Magnusson, T. Extracervical symptoms after whiplash trauma. Cephalalgia 14:223–2237; 1994.

Maimaris, C.; Barnes, M. R.; Allen, M. J. Whiplash injuries of the neck: a retrospective study. Injury 19:393–396; 1988.

Mayou, R.; Bryant, B. Outcome of 'whiplash' neck injury. Injury 27:617–623; 1996.

Mealy, K.; Brennan, H.; Fenelon, G. C. C. Early mobilization of acute whiplash injuries. Br. Med. J. 292: 656–657; 1986.

Mendelson, G. Not "cured by a verdict." Effect of legal settlement on compensation claimants. Med. J. Aust. 2:132–134; 1982.

Miles, K. A.; Maimaris, C.; Finlay, D.; Barnes, M. R. The incidence and prognostic significance of radiological abnormalities in soft tissue injuries to the cervical spine. Skeletal Radiol. 17:493–496; 1988.

Mills, H.; Horne, G. Whiplash—man-made disease? N. Z. Med. J. 99:373–374; 1986.

Morris, F. Do head-restraints protect the neck from whiplash injuries? Arch. Emerg. Med. 6:17–21; 1989.

Murray, R. H.; Rubel, A. J. Physicians and healers—unwitting partners in health care. N. Engl. J. Med. 326:61–64; 1992.

Neck injury and the mind (editorial). Lancet 338: 728–729; 1991.

Newman, P. K. Whiplash injury. Long term prospective studies are needed and, meanwhile, pragmatic treatment. BMJ 301:2–3; 1990.

Norris, S. H.; Watt, I. The prognosis of neck injuries resulting from rear-end vehicle collision. J. Bone Joint Surg. 65B:608–611; 1983.

Nygren, A. Injuries to car occupants: some aspects of the interior safety of cars. Acta Otolaryngol. Suppl. (Stockh.) 395:1–164; 1984.

Obelieniene, D.; Bovim, G.; Schrader, H.; et al. Headache after whiplash: a historical cohort study outside the medico-legal context. Cephalalgia 18: 559–564; 1998.

Obelieniene, D.; Schrader, H.; Bovim, G.; et al. Pain after whiplash: a prospective controlled inception cohort study. J. Neurol. Neurosurg. Psychiatry 66: 279–283; 1999.

Ommaya, A. K.; Faas, F.; Yarnell, P. Whiplash injury and brain damage—an experimental study. JAMA 204:285–289; 1968.

Oosterveld, W. J.; Kortschot, H. W.; Kingma, G. G.; et al. Electronystagmographic findings following cervical whiplash injuries. Acta Otolaryngol. (Stockh.) 111:201–205; 1991.

Otte, A.; Ettlin, T.; Fierz, L.; Mueller-Brand, J. Parieto-occipital hypoperfusion in late whiplash syndrome: first quantitative SPET study using technetium-99m bicisate (ECD). Eur. J. Nucl. Med. 23:72–74; 1996.

Otte, A.; Ettlin, T. M.; Nitzsche, E. U.; et al. PET and SPECT in whiplash syndrome: a new approach to a forgotten brain. J. Neurol. Neurosurg. Psychiatry 63:368–372; 1997.

Otte, A.; Mueller-Brand, J.; Fierz, L. Brain SPECT findings in late whiplash syndrome. Lancet 345: 1513–1514; 1995.

Parmar, H. V.; Raymakers, R. Neck injuries from rear impact road traffic accidents: prognosis in persons seeking compensation. Injury 24:75–78; 1993.

Pearce, J. M. S. Whiplash injury: a re-appraisal. J. Neurol. Neurosurg. Psychiatry 52:1329–1331; 1989.

Pearce, J. M. S. Polemics of chronic whiplash injury. Neurology 44:1993–1997; 1994.

Pennie, B. H.; Agambar, L. J. Whiplash injuries: a trial of early management. J. Bone Joint Surg. 72B: 277–279; 1990.

Peterson, D. I. A study of 249 patients with litigated claims of injury. Neurologist 4:131–137; 1998.

Pettersson, K.; Harrholm, J.; Toolanen, G.; Hildingsson, C. Decreased width of the spinal canal in patients with chronic symptoms after whiplash injury. Spine 20: 1664–1667; 1995.

Pettersson, K.; Hildingsson, C.; Toolanen, G.; et al. MRI and neurology in acute whiplash trauma. Acta Orthop. Scand. 65:525–528; 1994.

Pettersson, K.; Toolanen, G.; High-dose methylpred-nisolone prevents extensive sick leave after whiplash injury. A prospective, randomized, double-blind study. Spine 23:984–989; 1998.

Porter, K. M. Neck sprains after car accidents: a common cause of long term disability. BMJ 298:973–974;1989.

Quebec Task Force on Whiplash-Associated Disorders. Scientific monograph of the Quebec task force on whiplash-associated disorders. Spine 20(suppl. 8): 1S–73S; 1995.

Radanov, B. P. Common whiplash research findings revisited. J. Rheumatol. 24:623–625; 1997.

Radanov, B. P.; Di Stefano, G.; Schnidrig, A.; Ballinari, P. Role of psychosocial stress in recovery from common whiplash. Lancet 338:712–715; 1991.

Radanov, B. P.; Di Stefano, G.; Schnidrig, A.; Sturzenegger, M. Psychosocial stress, cognitive performance and disability after common whiplash. J. Psychosom. Res. 37:1–10; 1993.

Radanov, B. P.; Di Stefano, G.; Schnidrig, A.; Sturzenegger, M. Common whiplash: psychosomatic or somatopsychic? J. Neurol. Neurosurg. Psychiatry 57:486–90; 1994a.

Radanov, B. P.; Sturzenegger, M.; Di Stefano, G.; Schnidrig, A. Relationship between early somatic, radiological, cognitive and psychosocial findings and outcome during a one-year follow-up in 117 patients suffering from common whiplash. Br. J. Rheumatol. 33:442–448; 1994b.

Radanov, B. P.; Sturzenegger, M.; Di Stefano, G. Long-term outcome after whiplash injury. A 2-year follow-up considering features of injury mechanism and somatic, radiologic, and psychosocial findings. Medicine 74:281–297; 1995.

Radanov, B. P. Bicik, I.; Dvorak, J.; et al. Relation between neuropsychological and neuroimaging findings in patients with late whiplash syndrome. J. Neurol. Neurosurg. Psychiatry 66:485–489, 1999.

Rauschning, W.; Jónsson, H. Injuries of the cervical spine in automobile accidents: pathoanatomic and clinical aspects. In: Gunzburg, R.; Szpalski, M.; eds. Whiplash injuries: current concepts in prevention, diagnosis, and treatment of the cervical whiplash syndrome. Philadelphia: Lippincott-Raven; 1998: p. 33–52.

Robinson, D. D.; Cassar-Pullicino, V. N. Acute neck sprain after road traffic accident: a long-term clinical and radiological review. Injury 24:79–82; 1993.

Schmand, B.; Lindeboom, J.; Schagen, S.; et al. Cognitive complaints in patients after whiplash injury: the impact of malingering. J. Neurol. Neurosurg. Psychiatry 64:339–343; 1998.

Schofferman, J.; Wasserman, S. Successful treatment of low back pain and neck pain after a motor vehicle accident despite litigation. Spine 19:1007–1010; 1994.

Schrader, H.; Obelieniene, D.; Bovim, G.; et al. Natural evolution of late whiplash syndrome outside the medicolegal context. Lancet 347:1207–1211; 1996.

Schutt, C. H.; Dohan, F. C. Neck injury to women in auto accidents: a metropolitan plague. JAMA 206: 2689–2692; 1968.

Shapiro, A. P.; Roth, R. S. The effect of litigation on recovery from whiplash. Spine 7:531–556; 1993.

Sjaastad, O. The headache of challenge in our time: cervicogenic headache. Funct. Neurol. 5:155 1990.

Skovron, M. L. Epidemiology of whiplash. In: Gunzburg, R.; Szpalski, M., eds. Whiplash injuries: current concepts in prevention, diagnosis, and treatment of the cervical whiplash syndrome. Philadelphia: Lippincott-Raven; 1998; p. 61–67.

Smed, A. Cognitive function and distress after common whiplash injury. Acta Neurol. Scand. 95:73–80; 1997.

Stringer, W. L.; Kelly, D. L.; Johnston, F. R.; et al. Hyperextension injury of the cervical spine with esophageal perforation. J. Neurosurg. 53:541–543; 1980.

Sturzenegger, M.; DiStefano, G.; Radanov, B. P.; Schnidrig, A. Presenting symptoms and signs after whiplash injury: the influence of accident mechanisms. Neurology 44: 688–693; 1994.

Sturzenegger, M.; Radanov, B. P.; Di Stefano, G. The effect of accident mechanisms and initial findings on the long-term course of whiplash injury. J. Neurol. 242:443–449; 1995.

Swensen, R. S. The "double crush syndrome." Neurol. Chronicle 4(2):1–6; 1994.

Taylor, A. E.; Cox, C. A.; Mailis, A. Persistent neuropsychological deficits following whiplash: evidence for chronic mild traumatic brain injury? Arch. Phys. Med. Rehabil. 77:529–535; 1996.

Taylor, J. R.; Kakulas, B. A. Neck injuries. Lancet 338: 1343; 1991.

Taylor, J. R.; Twomey, L. T. Acute injuries to cervical joints. An autopsy study of neck sprain. Spine 18: 1115–1122; 1993.

Teresi, L. M.; Lufkin, R. B.; Reicher, M. A.; Moffit, B. J.; Vinuela, F. V.; Wilson, G. M.; Bentson, J. R.; Hanafee, W. N. Asymptomatic degenerative disk disease and spondylosis of the cervical spine: MR imaging. Radiology 164:83–88; 1987.

Totstein, O. D.; Rhame, F. S.; Molina, E.; et al. Mediastinitis after whiplash injury. Can. J. Surg. 29:54–56; 1986.

Trimble, M. R. Post-traumatic neurosis. Chichester: John Wiley & Sons; 1981.

Truong, D. D.; Dubinsky, R.; Hermanowicz, N.; et al. Posttraumatic torticollis. Arch. Neurol. 48:221–223; 1991.

Turner, J. A.; Deyo, R. A.; Loeser, J. D.; et al. The importance of placebo effects in pain treatment and research. JAMA 271:1609–1614; 1994.

Van Nechel, C.; Soeur, M.; Cordonnier, M.; Zanen, A. Eye movement disorders after whiplash injury.

In: Gunzburg, R.; Szpalski, M., eds. Whiplash injuries: current concepts in prevention, diagnosis, and treatment of the cervical whiplash syndrome. Philadelphia: Lippincott-Raven; 1998: p. 135–141.

Viktrup, L.; Knudsen, G. M.; Hansen, S. H. Delayed onset of fatal basilar thrombotic embolus after whiplash injury. Stroke 26:2194–2196; 1995.

Voyvodic, F.; Dolinis, J.; Moore, V. M. et al. MRI of car occupants with whiplash injury. Neuroradiology 39:35–40; 1997.

Wallis, B. J.; Lord, S. M.; Barnsley, L.; Bogduk, N. The psychological profiles of patients with whiplash-associated headache. Cephalalgia 18:101–105; 1998.

Wallis, B. J.; Lord, S. M.; Bogduk, N. Resolution of psychological distress of whiplash patients following treatment by radiofrequency neurotomy: a randomised, double-blind, placebo-controlled trial. Pain 73:15–22; 1997.

Weiss, H. D.; Stern, B. J.; Goldberg, J. Post-traumatic migraine: chronic migraine precipitated by minor head or neck trauma. Headache 31:451–456; 1991.

Wheeler, A. H. Botulinum toxin A, adjunctive therapy for refractory headaches associated with pericranial muscle tension. Headache 38:468–471; 1998.

Wickstrom, J.; Martinez, J.; Rodriguez, R. Cervical sprain syndrome and experimental acceleration injuries of the head and neck. In: Selzer, M. L.; Gikas, P. W.; Huelke, D. F., eds. Proc Prevention of Highway Accidents Symposium. University of Michigan; 1967: p. 182–187.

Winston, K. Whiplash and its relationship to migraine. Headache 27:452–457; 1987.

Yarnell, P. R., Rossie, G. V. Minor whiplash head injury with major debilitation. Brain Injury 2:255–258; 1988.

Yates, D. A. H.; Smith, M. A. Orthopaedic pain after trauma. In: Wall, P. D.; Melzack, R., eds. Textbook of pain. Edinburgh: Churchill Livingstone; 1994: p. 417.

# 11

# Reflex Sympathetic Dystrophy

ROBERT L. KNOBLER

Reflex sympathetic dystrophy (RSD) is a dreaded diagnosis in clinical medicine. At one end of the spectrum, it has an associated stigma of unrelenting pain, its principal clinical manifestation (Campbell and Raja 1995). Unfortunately, at the other end of the spectrum, there is the clinician's concern regarding reactive depression and drug-seeking behavior, as with any chronic pain sufferer, and even the possibility of malingering (Verdugo and Ochoa 1995). These issues, coupled with the inherent difficulties of treating what is incorrectly perceived by some as entirely a subjective disorder, because of poorly understood diagnostic criteria and lack of specific outcome measures of treatment, have led to difficulty in accepting RSD as a "real" condition. This has led to either subsequent reluctance in making this diagnosis, or its opposite, overdiagnosis.

The consequence of hesitation in the diagnosis of RSD is unfortunate, because early treatment for this disorder has the greatest chance of a good outcome. Therapy begins with the simple strategy of movement of the affected portions of the body. Delay in the diagnosis of RSD is not only tragic because early recognition and treatment of RSD can have a profoundly positive impact on this disorder, and thus the patient, but also because the lack of therapeutic intervention

may permit permanent sequelae to occur. Therefore, it is essential for all treating physicians, and especially neurologists, to have an appreciation of the full clinical picture of this disorder, its prognosis, and the impact of a delay in the initiation of effective treatment approaches (Kozin 1992; Schwartzman 1993).

The term RSD has become recognized through increased clinical usage in recent years, although this name is criticized as being inaccurate, since it does not properly describe the disorder, which is true. In reality, RSD is *not* characterized by an abnormal reflex action, nor is there uniform involvement of the sympathetic nervous system at all stages of this disorder, and there are not always dystrophic changes in the affected portions of the body. So, this criticism is justified. However, the term *RSD,* introduced by Evans (1947), when suggesting a hypothetical mechanism of its pathogenesis, does have some merit.

Many "different" diagnoses had previously been rendered by specific practitioners, dependent on their unique clinical perspectives of the causes of manifestations of this conditions including the following:

- Major causalgia
- Minor causalgia

- Shoulder–hand syndrome
- Sudeck's atrophy
- Traumatic angiospasm or vasospasm
- Post-traumatic osteoporosis

The eventual use of the term RSD to replace these other diagnoses, which were in some instances even more removed from an accurate description of the findings than the eponym RSD, came to have somewhat of a unifying effect.

Calling all of these disorders "RSD" meant recognizing and drawing attention to the reality that all of these "different" conditions were in fact manifestation variations of the same disorder, with a presumably common mechanism of causation and onset. Furthermore, the clinical features of RSD were identical to those described in the earlier characterization of causalgia, by S. Weir Mitchell, the father of American neurology and psychiatry at the time of the Civil War, but with an important distinction.

In causalgia, there was an underlying well-defined but incomplete lesion of a peripheral nerve that preceded the onset of the disorder. In contrast, although trauma often does precede the onset of RSD, a demonstrable peripheral nerve lesion is not usually evident. It is the absence of objective evidence, such as the demonstrable peripheral nerve lesion of causalgia, coupled with a potentially broad spectrum of clinical presentation, which may range from mild physical findings to a profoundly disfigured limb, occurring in the context of subjective complaints of pain that are often "out of proportion" to the precipitating injury, that makes RSD at once both so difficult to recognize and accept as a legitimate disorder.

In this chapter, the focus will be on the diagnosis and practical management of RSD as it relates to the prognosis of the disorder. These are not data based on the outcomes of controlled clinical trials, since there has not been a uniform code and method for staging RSD in place, and the outcome of any treatment is in significant part dependent both on the stage at which treatment is initiated and the participation of the patient in subsequent movement.

It is exceptional to find RSD as a primary disorder, without an obvious cause. Instead, RSD is almost always secondary, most often associated with a physical trauma of some sort, typically to an extremity. These may include, but are not limited to sprains, strains, crush injuries, or fractures with subsequent immobilization.

Simply stated, RSD is characterized by a collection of symptoms and signs as follows:

- Pain out of proportion to injury (burning or aching) in a regional distribution worse at the end of the limb (distally)
- Sensitivity to dependent posture, increased activity, and cold ambient temperature as is swelling and color change
- Swelling
- Sweating early, dryness later
- Temperature change: hot early, coldness later
- Color change: red-purple discoloration to blanched
- Altered growth: skin, hair and nails
- Movement disorder: spasm, cramping, tremor, decreased ability to initiate movements, altered posture (focal dystonia), increased reflexes
- Mirror image or unilateral spread of pain and secondary symptoms

Fluctuation of these symptoms with dependent posture, activity, and cold ambient temperatures, as well as spread of the pain to previously unaffected parts of the body, usually in a mirror image fashion at first, further adds to the difficulties in acceptance of RSD, since no other condition has such variability in its expression. Worsening with activity of the affected extremity also leads to difficulties in motivating and evaluating the success of the movement treatment strategies employed, since the patient invariably feels more pain by "movement" than by holding the affected limb immobile, like a "Napoleonic arm." Therefore, it is not unusual for the average qualified clinician to be skeptical when encountering such a presentation, especially if it is for their first time, even if previously aware that RSD exists as a clinical disorder.

The principal complaint of RSD pain is best characterized as a burning and/or aching pain, although other descriptors also apply, such as shooting, stabbing, squeezing, throbbing, and so on. It is not atypical to find that the pain of RSD is characterized as being "out of proportion" to the precipitating trauma, both by the patient and the clinician. However, the pain of the precipitating injury is separate and distinct, occurring immediately, from the pain that is secondary to the RSD.

The onset of RSD may be delayed by time periods of variable length, such as hours to a few weeks. Not infrequently, confusion arises regarding the time of onset of RSD, which may have implications in pinpointing events associated with its causation. This is most often because the time of onset is attributed to the time of recognition of the disorder, as opposed to the initial occurrence of its symptoms.

It has not yet been determined whether RSD is a primary consequence of the trauma, or as a secondary effect of either voluntary immobilization in attempt to reduce the pain and spasm that worsens upon movement, or involuntary immobilization because of the need for casting or splinting.

Certain features of RSD, such as its regional (global limb based), rather than neuroanatomical distribution (nerve root or peripheral nerve based), its mirror-image spread to a previously unaffected limb, its greatest severity distally, even if initiated by trauma to a more proximal location, and its potential for worsening even in the face of presumptively effective treatment, are contrary to general teachings in clinical neurology, and therefore, have fostered arguments over the validity of this painful condition.

These "validation" issues are further compounded by the addition of "reactive depression" subsequent to unanticipated problems with activities of daily living, including employment. This is because of pain and loss of sleep in the setting of clinical manifestations that are not always apparent to those unfamiliar with RSD. It can only be imagined how the admonition "it's all in your head," delivered by treating physicians, family and friends, and workers' compensation personnel, because of inadequate understanding of RSD, can impact the affected individual.

"Secondary gain" has also been emphasized as a potential explanation for the subjective symptom of pain of "out of proportion" to the injury in RSD. Thus, RSD victims are frequently accused of manifesting continuing pain symptoms for secondary gain because of several reasons. These include, but are not limited to, bias towards this diagnosis by some opinion leaders, restricted recognition of its physical manifestations by some clinicians, and limited knowledge of how applicable treatment strategies in the context of different stages of the natural history of RSD can influence the prognosis of this disorder.

This is not to say that there cannot be malingering in some of the individuals who carry the diagnosis of RSD, with or without the manifestations of RSD. Therefore, vigilance in searching for "objective" physical manifestations of RSD must be applied in rendering this diagnosis, to restrict the possibility of haphazardly and incorrectly labeling patients as having or not having this disorder.

Hopelessness associated with inadequate pain management and lack of psychosocial support in RSD has led to anger, despair, and even suicide in this patient population.

Movement therapy, however, has been recognized as the key to successful treatment, especially when it is initiated early. The application of additional therapeutic strategies, such as nerve blocks and adjunctive medications (Table 11-1), are essentially applied to reduce pain and thereby permit facilitation of movement.

Unfortunately, many still believe that a sympathetic nerve block should be done to establish the diagnosis of RSD, and that failure to respond suggests absence of the disorder. However, this is not true, and sympathetic nerve blocks performed specifically for the purpose of diagnosis can be misleading. In contrast, sympathetic nerve blocks can sometimes be therapeutically important, particularly early on. This is especially true if treating a precipitating injury requiring casting, which would of course impede the onset of movement therapy.

Amazingly, early mobilization and movement therapy, particularly in an aquatic environment,

**Table 11-1.** Recommended Treatment of RSD

First tier
    Identify and treat underlying disease: fracture, sprain, radiculopathies, spinal stenosis
    Symptomatic treatments: drugs (antidepressant, anticonvulsant, analgesic)
    Physical therapy: regular, repetitive as tolerated, self-directed, aquatherapy
    Counseling of patient and family in chronic pain management techniques
Second tier
    Blocks: chemical sympathectomy, depends on techniques and agents
    May include direct sympathetic blocks or regional intravenous blocks (Bier blocks)
Third tier
    Surgical sympathectomy: no longer regularly performed due to poor outcomes
    Dorsal column stimulator
    Morphine pump

which provides buoyancy and physical support while reducing the negative effects of both gravity and fluctuations in ambient temperature, is the treatment strategy associated with the best clinical outcome. Perhaps the importance of early mobilization can be best appreciated by recognizing that RSD is less common in professional athletes who are injured in games. Typically, they undergo a rapid evaluation to determine whether there is a contraindication to physical therapy (i.e., such as a fracture evident on x-ray or a torn ligament noted on a magnetic resonance imaging [MRI] scan). The diagnosis of RSD may never even have been considered in these individuals, but the appropriate treatment, of gradually escalated movement, is nevertheless initiated.

The major focus of treatment in professional players is the application of strategies employed to get the athlete back into action as rapidly as possible. There is the early and consistent application of gentle but regularly applied physical therapy measures and adjunctive medical therapies, if needed, to accomplish this goal. Since pain is expected to be a part of "playing the game," pain out of proportion to the injury, and other clinical features that might lead to the diagnosis of RSD, are rarely fully considered. Although there may be profound pain as the treatment regimen is initiated and continued, the early application of movement therapy typically results in rapid resolution of the painful symptoms, before there is the opportunity to recognize RSD as a secondary diagnosis.

In contrast, for the general public, the diagnosis of RSD may not be recognized either, but for entirely different reasons, and with a very different outcome. This is because consideration of this diagnosis in general practice is rarely made in the earliest stages of RSD. This is due in part to (1) general lack of awareness of the existence of this condition, or sometimes frank disbelief in its existence; (2) difficulty in differentiating between the pain, swelling, and color changes from the precipitating injury, as compared to their significance as early symptoms and signs of RSD; (3) failure to appreciate that RSD pain is commonly perceived as "out of proportion" to the injury, so that complaints of persistent severe pain get heeded when they occur rather than only receiving delayed attention; (4) limited understanding of the fact that RSD may develop very

early following an injury, without the more easily recognized severe manifestations that occur later in the course; and (5) lack of a definitive diagnostic test for this disorder, so there must be complete reliance only upon poorly understood clinical criteria to establish the diagnosis.

The diagnosis of RSD has also been delayed because of the common but incorrect perception that RSD is an oversubscribed "wastebasket" diagnosis for any form of chronic pain following an injury, rather than a specific disorder with its own diagnostic criteria. This wastebasket consideration unfortunately implies that the real cause of the pain must still be sought, further delaying proper diagnosis and treatment.

In contrast, reliance on clinical tests alone, such as the triple-phase bone scan, has also delayed the diagnosis of RSD. This is because this test is of diagnostic value when "positive," but not so when "negative." Therefore, a false-negative result on the triple-phase bone scan, or any other such laboratory test used to confirm the diagnosis, may erroneously lead to the conclusion that RSD is not present despite a corroborating history, symptom complex, and clinical signs indicating that it is present in the patient.

These perceptions must change, since RSD has proven to be most treatable when it first develops. Therefore, it must be properly diagnosed as soon after the injury as possible because of the importance of initiating movement therapy early. Therapy must be a gentle but sustained effort, not unlike the course pursued in the treatment of professional athletes.

It should be noted that in practice, physical therapy measures and adjunctive medical therapies, if applied at all after an injury to the average person, tend to be shortlived. This is particularly because pain that is already present will almost certainly intensify with movement. The perception of the patient is that they are doing worse with therapy, since they hurt more.

An important distinction is to be made, however, between the pain of RSD and the pain amplification with movement therapy, as opposed to pain associated with a persistent underlying orthopedic or soft tissue structural lesion such as a tear or fracture. The latter is evaluated by imaging studies, using x-rays or computed tomography (CT) for identifying orthopedic lesions and MRI for characterizing the soft tissue lesions. There is no permanent harm from the transient pain augmentation associated with gentle movement therapy. Nevertheless, it is in this clinical setting that the persistent pain of RSD is eventually first recognized, often weeks or months after the injury occurred, and the RSD has had its onset.

Although increased pain and spasm on movement is characteristic in RSD, only gradually increased movement will overcome this syndrome in its earliest phase. Since it is well recognized that RSD may progress in the face of immobilization, it is imperative that physical movement continues. Nerve blocks occasionally help to facilitate this course of treatment, as does the use of aquatic therapy, and, if needed, medications, sometimes in combination therapy to address the pain, the spasm, and the depression of RSD. Therefore, the prognosis regarding RSD is dependent on the ability to move the affected portion of the body, and the duration and severity of symptoms at the time such effective treatment is first initiated.

## Diagnostic Terminology

The International Association for the Study of Pain (IASP) has in recent years suggested a new nomenclature, proposing the name complex regional pain syndrome (CRPS) type I as the designation for RSD. This is to distinguish RSD from complex regional pain syndrome type II, causalgia (Table 11-2).

Causalgia, or CRPS type II, is the term applied to painful conditions with the identical clinical picture of RSD, but having an etiology secondary to an incomplete but definitive peripheral nerve lesion, such as a traumatic lesion to the femoral nerve. In contrast, RSD does not have a demonstrable partial nerve lesion. RSD (CRPS type I) most likely reflects local trauma to nerve endings in the skin, which are below the level of detection of present testing techniques. However, these pain syndromes are otherwise identical in their clinical features and approaches to treatment, although because of the presence of an incomplete

**Table 11-2.** Nomenclature for Complex Regional Pain Syndrome (CRPS)

Type I, RSD, no nerve injury demonstrated
Type II, causalgia, partial (incomplete) nerve injury

nerve lesion in causalgia (CRPS type II), it is more likely that there will be permanent sequelae.

In the past, there was even greater confusion regarding terminology, since there were many different diagnostic names (see above) that were being clinically used to describe essentially the same disorder. The reasons for this confusion were that (1) different specialists (i.e., orthopedic surgeons, rheumatologists, neurologists, anesthesiologists) used specific terms, unique to their specialties, to describe the painful conditions they observed in their own unique fashion; (2) different diagnoses were applied to painful conditions because they affected different regions of the body; and (3) different diagnoses were applied to painful conditions following a specific injury. The clinical features of RSD are all painted from the same palette, irrespective of the name applied to the diagnosis, so there is no difference in the spectrum of complaints and findings in any of these disorders. The unification of these varied conditions under the umbrella term of complex regional pain syndrome is, therefore, quite helpful from the perspective of focusing our interest on enhanced understanding of the pathogenesis of this condition and the development and administration of more targeted forms of treatment.

The IASP change in nomenclature to emphasize the "complex" and "regional" aspects of the pain is quite useful. The complexity of the CRPS disorders reflects the subtle features of autonomic dysfunction (which often go unrecognized until the condition progresses to a more severe form), its ability to spread to other limbs (often in a mirror-image fashion), and dissociation of the numerous symptoms found in CRPS from one another (i.e., pain, swelling, sweating, color change, temperature change) so that only a partial expression of the full spectrum of RSD may be manifest.

The regional distribution of the pain in the CRPS mirrors the network-like regional organization of the sympathetic fibers along blood vessels (i.e., all of the blood vessels supplying a limb). This regional pain pattern has been criticized by some physicians as nonanatomical, and has, therefore, been assumed to be nonphysiological, rather than the traditionally defined distribution of either a nerve root or peripheral nerve lesion which is emphasized on clinical grounds through anatomically based training focusing on locating the lesion.

In this regard, there are some who believe that the best way to establish a clinical diagnosis of

RSD is through demonstration of a positive response to a placebo-controlled, sympathetic nerve block, rather than on clinical features alone. This is based on the understanding that RSD, as a pain syndrome, is initially mediated through hyperactivity of the sympathetic nervous system. However, this too has its shortcomings.

When a patient responds to a properly performed sympathetic block (which blocks sympathetic activity, relieves pain, relieves swelling and warms the limb), their pain may be considered sympathetically mediated pain (SMP). However, failure to respond to a such a nerve block does not preclude the diagnosis of RSD, since the patient may have progressed to a state of sympathetically independent pain (SIP), yet still suffer from RSD. Pain syndromes other than RSD may also have elements of SMP or SIP, so the nature of the pain alone is not adequate to make the diagnosis of RSD.

The change from SMP to SIP is well recognized clinically (Table 11-3). It has no relation to the three stages of RSD (I through III) that have been recognized (Table 11-4), and described as the acute, dystrophic and atrophic stages. Instead, the progression from SMP to SIP is best conceptualized as "centralization" of the pain. This means the source of the pain has now been transferred from the point of injury origin in the periphery to within the central nervous system (CNS), with a concomitant resistance to previously effective treatment. The centralization of pain had been considered by some to be a learning phenomenon, but basic neuroscience research may give rise to a different perspective.

Experimentally obtained animal data in models of chronic neuropathic pain have demonstrated that there is a point in time, following the onset of pain, after which there are permanent degenerative changes localized within the relevant segments of the spinal cord dorsal root entry zone (DREZ). This is the region of the CNS where af-

**Table 11-3.** Classification of Pain

Sympathetically mediated pain (SMP)—responsive to sympathetic nerve blocks
Sympathetically independent pain (SIP)—unresponsive to sympathetic nerve blocks
Also referred to as "Centralization" of the pain of peripheral origin

**Table 11-4.** Stages of RSD*

Stage I, acute—variability of pain and other symptoms with activity, dependent posture, and cool ambient temperature
Stage II, dystrophic—consistency of pain and other symptoms from moment to moment, yet heightened by activity, dependent posture, and cool ambient temperature
Stage III, atrophic—unmistakable atrophy of a portion or all of an affected limb, with shiny, taut skin and tapered digits

*Previous literature had suggested that there was a "fixed" timecourse in each stage of RSD and, therefore, treatment must be instituted early to prevent progression. It has been empirically observed that individuals may stay in a particular stage (i.e., stage I) for a prolonged period, even years, without progressing into more advanced stages. For this reason, staging should refer to severity of disease, and not merely to its duration.

ferent sensory fibers, sympathetic fibers, and descending efferents for the affected segments converge, and is the first relay station of the CNS where sensory input and painful sensations can be modulated.

The dropout of neurons in the DREZ has been attributed to an uncontrolled aberrant release of excitatory neurotransmitters (i.e., glutamate) into this region as part of the triggered persistent pain response. Excitatory neurotransmitters do, in fact, have the potential for neurotoxicity when present in abundance, and trigger cell death of target field neurons. The loss of neurons renders the pain unresponsive to previously viable peripheral measures, such as nerve blocks and movement therapy, corresponding to the change from SMP to SIP. The anatomical and physiologic changes in the DREZ, secondary to persistence of the pain syndrome and release of excitatory neurotransmitters, now requires a different level of treatment to achieve pain relief and restore movement.

It should be noted that there are many links between the sensory and pain pathways and the control of movement. This should not be a surprising association in the context of recognizing that a primary goal of aversive movement is to avoid pain (i.e., the withdrawal reflex). While the goal of RSD treatment remains relief of pain and restoration of movement, the changes in the DREZ render further sympathetic blockade ineffective in the relief of pain symptoms. It is at this point in the clinical course, irrespective of the specific physical manifestations present, and thus staging, that narcotic medications, and possibly invasive procedures, such as the dorsal column stimulator (DCS) and morphine pump, become the only useful modalities to produce adequate pain relief and facilitate movement (Table 11-5).

Stated another way, when the clinical features of RSD are present, failure to respond to a technically well-performed sympathetic block, with a subsequent rise in skin temperature, does not rule out RSD. Instead, it provides supportive information indicating that there has been progression to the SIP state, rather than indicating SMP. Although RSD usually begins as SMP, this phase may go unrecognized, and thus the patient is first seen with SIP. Although the patient with SIP will no longer respond to a sympathetic block, it should be clear that the clinical diagnosis remains that of an advanced stage of RSD. This should help to now guide the clinician with certainty in the need for, and justification of the use of, pain-relieving medications in the treatment of this disorder.

Therefore, the diagnosis of RSD is best made on the basis of its clinical features. This diagnosis may or may not then be supported by laboratory studies where possible, and then further differentiated as either CRPS type I or type II.

## Clues to Pathogenesis

Initial involvement of the sympathetic nervous system, almost selectively, suggests two distinct possibilities that are not mutually exclusive. These are: (1) there is a sympathotrophic factor released as a result of trauma; and (2) there is activation of a sympathetic ganglionic inflammatory process, with potential systemic effects, as a result of trauma. Experimental studies support both of these notions.

Traumatic injury of peripheral nerves has experimentally been demonstrated to lead to the synthesis and release of nerve growth factor (NGF), which is normally only present during developmental stages, and then declines to low basal levels in the adult (Weskamp and Otten 1987). NGF is the most potent sympathotrophic factor recog-

nized, with equally dramatic impact on the dorsal root ganglion (DRG) sensory neurons as well.

The induction and release of NGF is accompanied by induction of the NGF receptor (Taniuchi et al. 1986). In addition to its trophic actions on the sympathetic and DRG cells, NGF has been recognized to have profound effects in stimulating inflammation. This includes activation of the complement system (Boyle and Young 1982), and promoting the expansion of antibody-producing B cells of the immune system (Otten et al. 1989). Of further interest, when NGF has been injected into humans, as part of a therapeutic clinical trial for the treatment of chemotherapy-induced peripheral neuropathy, it reproduces the burning pain characteristic of RSD at the site of the injection.

In this way trauma, whether to nerve endings alone, as in a sprain, or through an incomplete nerve injury, as in a gunshot or knife wound, would lead to the induction and release of NGF. The NGF signal would activate both the DRG and sympathetic ganglia. The activation of these neuronal cell populations (Table 11-6), would (1) heighten their sensitivity in all modalities; (2) lead to the release of excitatory neurotransmitters within the DREZ; and (3) produce potentially destructive lesions of these ganglionic or locally (limb) affected structures as a result of activation of inflammatory processes (specifically, the complement system and antibody-producing B cells). Opioids are able to counteract the immunological events to some degree (Morgan et al. 1990; Wybran et al. 1979).

Histopathologic investigation of sympathetic ganglia surgically removed in an effort to treat RSD has been performed. These ganglia were not previously traumatized by the performance of sympathetic nerve blocks at their location, since they were taken from sites remote from those at

**Table 11-5.** Long-Lasting Invasive Therapies*

---

Dorsal column stimulator—electrode placement and stimulation parameters are paramount

Morphine pump—intrathecal opioid is delivered continuously, with biweekly or monthly refill

---

*These modalities require a team approach in management. Not only must there be careful placement of the electrodes or the catheter for drug delivery, but trained personnel for readjustment of stimulator settings and pump refilling is mandatory for successful maintenance.

**Table 11-6.** Hypothetical Pathogenesis of RSD*

---

Trauma →
Release of NGF, SP, IL-2, etc. →
Activation of local peripheral neurogenic inflammation and stimulation of dorsal root ganglia (DRG) and sympathetic ganglia (SG) → RSD
Release of excitatory amino acid neurotransmitters in the dorsal root entry zone → stimulation of NMDA receptors →
Dorsal root entry zone degeneration → centralization of pain

---

*It must be emphasized that this is a hypothetical scheme for study of the pathogenesis of RSD, which incorporates elements of both animal and human studies, but complete evidence on the pathogenesis of this painful disorder is lacking at the present time.

which sympathetic nerve blocks had been administered to these patients. The ganglia analyzed demonstrated histopathological findings such as neuronal vacuolization and atrophy, axonal beading, endothelial cell damage with early thrombus formation, and perivascular lymphocytic infiltration. These findings are consistent with the interpretation of both "active" neurons and an active inflammatory process. Some investigators, such as Fields and Basbaum, have described similar findings experimentally as reflex neurogenic inflammation. Isolated findings in peripheral nerve of amputated limbs affected with RSD are consistent with small-fiber pathology (van der Laan et al. 1998).

Ultrastructural changes observed in the sympathetic ganglia removed corroborate the histopathological findings. These include the presence of intracytoplasmic vacuoles, secondary demyelination, onion bulb-like structures, dilated endoplasmic reticulum, and abnormal mitochondria within the neuronal cells of the sympathetic ganglia. These findings are also consistent with both NGF-activated neurons and an active inflammatory process.

Other candidate sympathotrophic and immunogenic molecules are also produced in response to local trauma. These include substance P (SP) and the lymphokine interleukin-2 (IL-2). SP is released from nerve terminals as an early post-traumatic event. SP functions as a potent vasoactive molecule that has profound actions during inflammatory events, but is a mediator of painful stimuli as well as having properties overlapping those of NGF. SP has also been shown to have direct stimulatory effects on sympathetic neurons and cells of the immune system, but may no longer play a role once the disease process becomes established, since it was not detected locally in skin from patients with long-established RSD (R. J. Schwartzman, personal communication).

IL-2 is an immune system signal normally associated with the expansion of reactive lymphocytes important in both cellular and humoral immunity. It may be derived from inflammatory cells specifically recruited and activated by the local release of cytokines in response to trauma. Alternatively, IL-2 may be released from non-specifically recruited cells trafficking through a traumatic lesion which become activated by the tissue factors present within the lesion. In either case,

IL-2 has been shown to selectively stimulate sympathetic neurons (Haugen and Letourneau 1990), in addition to its known immunologic effects.

Therefore, there is overlapping impact of three separate mediators (NGF, SP, and IL-2), which can each selectively stimulate sympathetic neurons in response to an injury. It is fairly straightforward to see how these molecules can be present in increased quantities following a local injury, as part of the local tissue response. Their impact on the sympathetic neurons associated with the affected region can be dramatic. From the perspective of survival, increased sensitivity to painful stimulation is advantageous because it contributes to a tendency toward protecting the affected limb from further trauma, as well as enhancing the withdrawal response from further painful, and perhaps dangerous, stimuli. However, movement of the affected limb is essential to overcome the downside of this protective mechanism, progresssion of the pain syndrome.

Potentially related painful phenomena, independent of the pain from the initial injury and that from the development of RSD, may contribute to further progression of the pain syndrome. This would occur through activation of latent herpesvirus infections known to commonly reside within the sympathetic and/or dorsal root ganglion cells as a direct consequence of local trauma (Price et al. 1975; Walz et al. 1974).

Activation of herpesvirus replication is followed both by direct herpes-associated damage, and immune attack due to an antiherpetic response. Experimentally, local trauma in the distribution of a neuron latently infected with herpesvirus has been demonstrated to reactivate the herpesvirus infection, leading to lytic replication in the neuron. In an immunologically intact individual an antiviral inflammatory response also follows in the distribution of sympathetic and dorsal root ganglion cells in the region of injury. Further studies are currently in progress to determine if herpesvirus antigens are detected in sympathetic ganglia removed at the time of surgical sympathectomy.

The documentation of a variety of localized skin reactions in RSD has been recognized and reflects the deposition of immune complexes in the skin (Webster et al. 1991, 1993). At present, these skin lesions are the most compelling observation of the involvement of cytokine, immune, and viral mechanisms in RSD.

Thus, at least two separate mechanisms of trauma-induced changes, sympathotrophic (NGF, SP, and IL-2) stimulation and herpesvirus reactivation, can occur and contribute to the histopathological features of RSD. These initiating events could then trigger subsequent events through humoral and inflammatory mechanisms.

In addition to the pain precipitated by trauma, RSD has also been observed to occur following lesions of the CNS, which have associated immobilization. Immobilization may affect multiple levels within the neuraxis, either independently or in concert. One such phenomenon is widening of the cortical receptive field, as in denervation supersensitivity, thus increasing the peripheral area of hypersensitivity. Therefore, multiple pathways, whether due to peripheral trauma or from CNS disease, can impact the pathogenesis of RSD. Furthermore, these mechanisms suggest interesting and testable hypotheses in the pathogenesis of this disorder, which must be better understood in order to provide more effective treatment.

## Clinical and Differential Diagnosis

RSD can occur in any age group but tends to be more common in women than in men for reasons that are not well understood, and usually follows injury to either a limb or another part of the body. The injury precipitating RSD need not be severe. The pain, however, persists beyond the anticipated time of recovery, and is described as worse than expected based on the scope of the injury. For example, injuries may range from minor traumas such as sprains and traction injuries, to more damaging crush injuries or fractures, which have an anticipated recovery time of 6 to 8 weeks. Therefore, the clinical suspicion of RSD should arise if traumatic pain persists, although not all sources of persistent pain are RSD. In addition to injury, RSD may also occur in the context of a paralyzed limb, associated with stroke, tumor, or other CNS lesions.

The distribution of the pain in RSD is not typically within the territory of peripheral nerves or nerve roots but is regional and primarily distal. This is consistent with the regional distribution and function of the sympathetic nervous system. During the initial phase of RSD, many symptoms and signs are attributable to overactivity of the sympathetic nervous system supplying affected area(s) of the body. However, burning or deep aching pain remains the cardinal feature of RSD.

The sometimes minimally traumatic origins, coupled with a regional pain distribution, often with subsequent spread to mirror-image regions of the opposite limb, in the context of limited familiarity of the full spectrum of symptoms and signs associated with even the earliest stages of this disorder, have allowed persistent skepticism regarding the validity of this diagnosis. Patients are often labeled as having a "psychogenic" source for their persistent pain rather than a physical disorder. It is not hard to see how reactive depression can develop under these circumstances, yet this is a secondary phenomenon to the persistent pain and consequent impairment of function.

Sympathetic hyperactivity is clinically recognized both by its interaction with somatic nerve fibers and direct involvement of sympathetic nerves that regulate blood flow and blood pressure. Interaction with somatic neurons and nerve fibers leads to altered sensation and altered movement.

Altered sensation includes such features as burning and/or deeply aching and throbbing pain, allodynia (altered perception of simple somatic sensations, such as light touch, as painful), hyperesthesia (increased sensitivity and lowered threshold to tactile and painful stimuli), and hyperpathia (increased pain perception, although with an elevated threshold to stimulation). All of these features are experienced as worse with movement, a dependent posture, and cold ambient temperature. This leads to patient resistance to mobilize the affected extremity.

In addition, there can be a variety of abnormalities of movement, which include difficulties in the initiation of movement, dystonic posturing, localized spasms with movement, increased muscle tone, brisk reflexes, and tremors as initially described by Schwartzman and Kerrigan (1990).

Direct involvement of the sympathetic nervous system includes tissue swelling (which is worst in a dependent posture, with increase in physical activity, and with cold ambient temperatures), color change (mottling of the skin, purple discoloration due to venous stasis), temperature changes (usually coolness, although increased skin temperature may variably be present in the earliest stages of the disorder), increased sweating, and trophic changes (shiny skin, early hair growth, and later hair loss, brittle nails).

It is at this stage that the disorder may be most responsive to sympathetic nerve blocks. Sometimes a positive response is used as a "diagnostic" sympathetic nerve block, and taken as proof of the presence of RSD because of pain relief by virtue of the block. However, as already discussed, there may be loss of responsiveness to sympathetic blocks due to progression of the condition to the phase of SIP. Therefore, lack of response to a nerve block does not prove that the individual does not have RSD, and it does not mean that RSD is ruled out.

Clinical worsening of the disease may involve spread to other extremities and other parts of the body, as well as the appearance of generalized symptoms including fevers and skin reactions suggestive of ongoing inflammation. The most advanced stage of RSD (stage III), is usually more readily recognized than the earlier stages because of its associated profound physical manifestations of atrophy and altered posturing of the affected extremity. Unfortunately, reversal of symptoms in stage III RSD is least likely, and only partial pain relief can commonly be achieved despite persistent treatment. Therefore, efforts to improve the awareness and recognition of RSD at earlier, more treatable stages coupled with intensively applied treatment strategies are warranted.

The pain and setting of the clinical presentation of RSD help to differentiate this condition from many other painful disorders (Table 11-7). However, it is imperative to note that there may be either confounding underlying or coexistent painful radiculopathies, nerve entrapment conditions, or other painful conditions that must be considered in the differential diagnosis of RSD pain. This list includes lumbar radiculopathy, sciatica, tarsal tunnel syndrome, Morton's neuroma, diabetes, and idiopathic painful polyneuropathy.

## Diagnostic Tests

Diagnostic tests of value in corroborating the clinical diagnosis of RSD include thermography, triple-phase bone scan, plain x-ray examination of bone, MRI with gadolinium, diagnostic nerve

**Table 11-7.** Differential Diagnosis of RSD

Deafferentation and phantom limb pain
Painful polyneuropathy
Neuralgia
Raynaud's disease
Cellulitis
Deep vein thrombosis

block, electromyography–nerve conduction velocity, and quantitative sensory testing, all of which are listed in Table 11-8.

Thermography can quantitatively reveal differences in limb temperatures in affected extremities, which is a function of C-fiber involvement in this disorder. However, these differences can also frequently be appreciated qualitatively by palpation and are not unique to RSD. Therefore, controversy his arisen regarding this form of evaluation, primarily because of interpretation of the results of this test with regard to a number of other disorders. Presently, this technique is claimed to be too imprecise to be relied on in the diagnosis of RSD because of the variability of the methods employed by different laboratories. However, it is the best functional test of C-fiber function.

Triple-phase bone scans can show increased uptake in the area affected by RSD, but are only of value when positive and cannot be used to rule out RSD if interpreted as negative. A plain x-ray film of bone in the affected limb often shows demineralization in the affected extremity. However, as with the triple-phase bone scan, it is of value when positive but cannot be used to rule out RSD if it is negative. In contrast, a recent advance in corroborating the diagnosis of early RSD (stage

**Table 11-8.** Diagnostic Tests in RSD

Thermography—quantitates limb temperature differences, reflecting C-fiber dysfunction, but is too nonspecific to be relied upon for diagnosis.

Triple-phase bone scan—may show increased uptake in the area affected by RSD. It is of value when positive, but cannot be used to rule out RSD if negative.

Plain x-ray film of bone—may show demineralization in the affected extremity. As with the triple-phase bone scan, it is of value when positive, but cannot be used to rule out RSD if negative.

MRI with gadolinium—shows skin thickening, subcutaneous contrast enhancement, and occasionally soft tissue edema in stage I RSD. Shows muscle atrophy in stage III RSD. It is not definitive for stage II RSD, which is an inconsistent transitional stage between I and II on MRI.

Diagnostic nerve block—pain relief when there is sympathetically maintained pain (SMP), but no relief when there is sympathetically independent pain (SIP). Pain relief, decreased swelling, and a rise in skin temperature are commonly transient even when the block is technically well performed.

Electromyography/nerve conduction velocity—C-fiber abnormalities characteristic of RSD are below the level of detection of this technique.

Quantitative sensory testing (QST)—identifies a raised threshold to sensory stimuli in severely affected extremities (stage III), but further testing of the technique is needed regarding specificity.

I) has been achieved through application of the MRI (Schweitzer et al. 1995).

An MRI with gadolinium can show skin thickening, subcutaneous contrast enhancement, and occasionally soft tissue edema in stage I RSD. At present, this appears to be the best technique for corroborating the diagnosis of stage I RSD. This is an important clinical adjunct in supporting consideration of the diagnosis of RSD at a time when there is a striking dichotomy between clinical signs that are often variable and quite subtle, and neurological symptoms of pain that are quite profound. In contrast, the MRI does not reveal anything definitive for stage II RSD, although the features of the disorder have become more constant. The reasons for the paucity of MRI findings characteristic of stage II RSD are not yet known, but this is a subject of intense investigation, specifically because it is a transitional stage into stage III RSD, characterized by dramatic findings of muscle atrophy.

The usefulness of sympathetic nerve blocks as a diagnostic tool in RSD are dependent on several conditions as follows: (1) sympathetic nerve blocks are only effective when there is SMP; (2) there is pain relief, albeit transiently, following the block; and (3) the blocks are properly performed. A technically satisfactory block is confirmed by a rise in peripheral skin temperature immediately following the sympathetic blockade. There will not be significant pain relief when the disorder has progressed to the stage of SIP. Failure to recognize the occurrence of a transition from SMP to SIP, and the impact of this change on the utility of a sympathetic nerve block in establishing the clinical diagnosis of RSD, can undermine the diagnostic process.

Electromyography–nerve conduction velocity (EMG/NCV) studies cannot demonstrate the small-fiber pathology mediating the effects of RSD, since C-fiber function is below the level of detection of standard EMG/NCV techniques. Quantitative sensory testing (QST) is a new technique currently under study that appears to identify a raised threshold to sensory stimuli in RSD-affected extremities. It remains to be determined if these are findings unique to RSD or are nonspecific.

## RSD Staging

Stage I RSD has been described as the "acute" stage (Table 11-4), because it occurs at the onset of the disorder and had initially been thought to be time limited to within the first 3 to 6 months. It is characterized by widespread variability in the nature of the symptoms present at any one time. The pain, however, is best described as being out of proportion to the precipitating insult and is quite intense. Autonomic signs of swelling and discoloration may be masked by traumatically induced inflammatory changes in the tissue.

The limb may be warmer or cooler to the touch at any given moment. The pain is described as a burning and/or deep aching pain and is worsened by movement, a dependent posture, and emotional distress. This leads toward a tendency to "guard" the limb and limit its movement or any degree of contact causing friction. The pain, swelling, and discoloration will often spread to the opposite limb in a mirror distribution and may still later become more generalized, even rarely throughout the entire body.

There is allodynia, hyperalgesia (increased areas of sensitivity to painful stimuli), and hyperpathia (an increased pain threshold with a disproportionate increase in perceived pain once the threshold is crossed). Edema is usually present in the affected area intermittently, along with increased hair growth (thicker and darker) and enhanced nail growth. The skin is initially hyperhidrotic. Bony changes (periarticular demineralization) are possible. This is the earliest stage of the disease. It is this stage that is most responsive to treatment and generally corresponds to the SMP phase.

There is no preset cadence at which all individuals will progress, and it is conceivable that a patient will remain in stage I indefinitely. However, when rapid progression occurs it tends to occur within the first 3 to 6 months after the onset of symptoms, although this is variable from person to person. Therapeutic mobilization of the limb at the patient's own pace, but with regularity, is associated with the best outcome.

Stage II RSD is the dystrophic stage (Table 11-4) and is marked by constancy of pain and "brawny" edema. There is sleep disruption, anxiety, and depression associated with this progression. The skin changes from moist (hyperhidrotic) to dry (hypohidrotic), shiny, cyanotic, and hypothermic, with a mottled meshwork pattern of the vessels described as livedo reticularis. There is now hair loss in the affected region with dulled, ridged, and cracked nails; x-ray films commonly show diffuse osteoporosis, as well as cystic changes and subchondral bone erosion. This stage is thought to be the most likely to correspond to the switch from SMP to SIP as has already been described.

Stage III is the atrophic stage (Table 11-4), and is not difficult to diagnose because of the often striking atrophy, coupled with tight, shiny skin and dramatically altered posture of the affected limb. The skin is thin, shiny, dry, and cold. Proximal migration of the pain occurs, if it has not already done so. This pattern is in sharp contrast to the distal spread of radicular pain. Irreversible skin, cartilaginous, muscle, and bone damage are evident. These include fascial thickening and limb contractures. The tips of the fingers and toes may appear tapered. Dupuytren's contracture is often seen; x-ray films show bony demineralization and ankylosis. There is atrophy of muscle groups in the affected limb. The patient may be wheelchair dependent. The movement disorder of RSD (difficulty initiating movements, tremor, weakness, spasm, increased reflexes, and dystonic posturing) is most dramatic at this stage.

Clinical worsening of the disease may also involve spread to other extremities and the appearance of generalized symptoms such as fevers and skin reactions suggestive of ongoing inflammation, as well as somatic changes such as decreased vision, hearing, and swallowing; broken teeth; and disrupted bladder and bowel functions. The latter are also further compromised by some of the medications used in an effort to provide symptomatic relief.

## RSD Symptom Complex

Sympathetic hyperactivity is clinically recognized as a constellation of variable symptoms that include burning or deep aching limb pain, which is maximal distally. The pain is regional and does not follow a nerve root, plexus, or peripheral nerve pattern, although secondary nerve entrapment (i.e., carpal tunnel syndrome) may occur as a consequence of local tissue swelling. Additional features include allodynia (mechanical sensation perceived as pain) and hyperesthesia, which leads the patient to "guard" the affected extremity, preferring to wrap the limb rather than risk exposure to contact with even a gentle breeze.

Other features are also often present, such as tissue swelling (worst in a dependent posture or with activity), color change (mottling of the skin, purple discoloration due to venous stasis), temperature change (initially variation between warmth and coolness and later only coolness), and increased sweating early and decreased sweating later, as well as trophic changes (shiny skin, altered hair growth, brittle nails). Bony demineralization in the affected extremity is commonplace and can be apparent on a plain x-ray film.

Abnormalities of movement are frequently present and include difficulty in the initiation of movements, weakness, dystonic posturing, a variety of tremors, spasms, and increased reflexes. These characteristics likely reflect the varied levels of interplay between the sympathetic nervous system and the somatic motor neurons in the anterior horn.

## Therapeutic Principles

It must be emphasized that RSD is extremely painful, and associated with severe spasms on even minor movements. These factors tend to combine to make the average patient quite reluctant to move an affected extremity without specific and persistent encouragement, for fear of worsening their situation. In contrast, the professional athlete benefits from sustained therapeutic efforts because of the need for their early mobilization. Working through pain is their motto. Athletes are not in fear of worsening their condition because of pain associated with their training regimen due to their level of motivation, and the observation that their consistent efforts lead to their improvement.

We must apply a similarly enthusiastic and supportive approach to the general public as regards treating RSD. This is especially important because common treatment strategies generally recommended for dealing with trauma to a limb, such as sprains, traction injuries, or broken bones, often utilize immobilization of the limb, including splinting or casting, further limiting the potential for movement necessary for remediating the painful condition of RSD.

Current treatments of RSD are based on decreasing the sympathetic activity in the affected extremity through the use of medications to limit the degree of pain associated with therapeutic programs of movement and physical therapy (Table 11-1). If there is a restriction to mobility (due to guarding or by virtue of a cast), rapid progression to more advanced stages of RSD, or severe edema in the affected limb, sympathetic nerve blocks should be attempted if initially effective. These are usually done as a series of five, with each block performed on alternate days.

Rarely, if RSD is diagnosed early and is not particularly responsive to physical therapy, but with limited yet definite responsiveness to sympathetic blocks, surgical sympathectomy may be considered. Caution should be used in performing surgical sympathectomies on more than one limb because of potential problems with the control of blood pressure, but this has not proven a major problem in practice. However, the actual use of therapeutic surgical sympathectomy has fallen into disfavor. This is because it is a challenging procedure after which there may be a postsympathectomy pain syndrome at the surgical site, as well as recurrence of the original pain. Crossed sympathetic nerve blocks are suggested as one way of handling this recurrent pain.

Many other treatments have been advocated over the years, but their effectiveness has not been established beyond anecdotal reports. Included among this group are systemic steroids, calcitonin, calcium-channel blockers, and $\alpha$-adrenergic blockers. An additional issue related to the use of the latter two groups of agents reflects the frequent occurrence of hypertension in the context of chronic pain syndromes, for which those and other antihypertensive therapies are appropriate. Similarly, diuretics have judiciously been used in an effort to control local edema, but this requires very close monitoring of the patient and should be reserved for only the most extreme circumstances.

Greater effectiveness has been achieved empirically through the early use of nonsteroidal antiinflammatory drugs (NSAIDs), antidepressants (Elavil, Prozac, Zoloft, and Effexor) and anticonvulsants (Dilantin, Tegretol, Neurontin, and Klonopin). Narcotic analgesics may frequently be required for adequate pain relief (Darvocet, Tylenol with codeine, Percocet, Lorcet 10/ 650, Norco, OxyContin, OxyIR, Methadone, MS Contin, MSIR, Dilaudid and Demerol). Attention to the combination of therapies used and the prospect that medication is provided by more than one source is necessary. A patient contract detailing the medications and sources is helpful in this regard.

If diagnosed early and treated with aggressive physical therapy (PT) early, RSD can be successfully treated. However, there is often a long lag between onset of symptoms and the initiation of a program of sustained aggressive therapy. The consequence of this delay is a more progressive phase of illness, such as SIP that is less responsive to analgesics, movement therapy, and sympathetic nerve blocks. This phase often requires more potent medications to reduce the pain to a more tolerable level and thus allow the individual to perform their activities of daily living.

Early involvement of the sympathetic nervous system in RSD, almost selectively, suggests release of a sympathotrophic factor as a result of trauma. NGF is one of the most potent sympathotrophic factors recognized. It is ordinarily present in highest concentrations during developmental stages and then declines in the adult. However, NGF is rapidly inducible following nerve injury, as is the NGF receptor. In addition to its trophic actions on the sympathetic and dorsal root ganglion cells, NGF has been recognized to have profound effects in mediating pain and stimulating inflammation.

Other candidate sympathotrophic molecules include SP and IL-2. SP is released from nerve terminals as an early post-traumatic event and may not only be a potent vasoactive molecule that has profound actions during inflammatory events but is a mediator of painful stimuli as well as having properties overlapping those of NGF. SP has also been shown to have direct stimulatory effects on sympathetic neurons, but may no longer play a role once the disease process is established, since it is not detected locally in skin from patients with established RSD. Capsaicin, derived from chili peppers, causes depletion of this molecule, and has been advocated by some in the treatment of RSD. However, the role of SP in the genesis of the pain of RSD may be a very early event, rendering capsaicin ineffective by the time it is used clinically.

### Specific Therapy

In determination of the specific course of treatment, the severity of the underlying primary clinical disorder, the severity and extent of the present pain complaint which presumably is the RSD, the overall duration of illness, previous treatments rendered along with their responses, side effects, and the continued need for retreatment are all important considerations. It is imperative to weigh the risk-ratio of the specific treatments chosen. This is especially true of the agents and modalities that are used in the treatment of RSD and their associated risks. A generalized approach is indicated in Table 11-1.

A hierarchical approach of progressively more involved treatment strategies is used in the treatment of RSD. A limited degree of pain control is first attempted with NSAID, tricyclic antidepressants, and anticonvulsants individually or in some combination that works best for the individual patient. A more potent analgesic may be needed to overcome severe pain and to help the patient sleep at night. However, these measures are usually ineffective alone in completely controlling the pain. The patient must be reassured that despite the pain, in the absence of an underlying structural abnormality (such as a fracture or torn ligaments), there is no harm done by movement of the painful limb, and that regular movement is the surest way to eventually combat the pain of early stage I RSD and overcome the disorder.

Patients are usually reluctant to accept PT as a treatment due to the intensity of the pain, but they must be motivated to move if there is no structural instability or immobilization, such as in the casting orthopedic injuries and some soft tissue injuries. In the event of the latter, one or more courses of five sympathetic nerve blocks per course, performed on alternate days, is administered to the affected region until movement can be resumed.

When patients attempt to reduce pain by "guarding" the limb, they are actually making the condition worse. PT is believed to lead to more rapid resolution of the underlying nerve injury. One particularly effective form of PT is aquatic therapy. Patients simply need to move around in a pool, in which the water supports the limb against gravity while simultaneously providing resistance to motion.

A self-directed PT program may be preferred, because some patients are inclined to stop treatment if the limb is manipulated too vigorously, and they work better at their own pace. However, some patients need the structure of a therapist-directed program. The addition of an aquatic component is very helpful. It does not need to be more complicated than getting into "tolerable" lukewarm water and moving around.

Throughout the self- or therapist-directed PT program, the author advocates the continued use of antidepressants such as Elavil (preferred over the generic amitriptyline, titrating up to 150 mg if that much is needed, at bedtime, in 10-mg intervals initially), anticonvulsants such as Neurontin (gabapentin, titrating up to as much as one or two 300-mg capsules three times daily, but beginning with 100 mg at bedtime), Klonopin (0.5 mg, one or two tablets at bedtime to aid sleep by helping to control myoclonic spasms) and the antispasm agent Zanaflex (tizanidine, 4 mg, starting with one-quarter of a tablet, 1 mg, as often as every 2 hours and titrating up to as many as eight full tablets per day if needed for the control of movement induced spasms and pain), and perhaps an NSAID with food.

If needed, a codeine-containing (Tylenol #3 one to two tablets at 4-hour intervals, limiting these to six tablets per day) or a hydrocodone-containing (Lorcet 10/650 or Norco 10/325, one to two tablets at 4-hour intervals, limiting these to six tablets per day) narcotic analgesic may be prescribed. These and other more potent narcotic analgesics may be added at any stage of treatment as a method of achieving better pain control, particularly for when patients are going to sleep.

The use of baclofen (Lioresal), titrating slowly up to 10 to 20 mg at a time, using one to two tablets three times daily, helps to overcome both dystonic posturing and falls from sudden "weakness and collapse" of the lower extremities. Such falls may be particularly profound in patients with RSD secondary to a brachial plexus traction injury (neurogenic thoracic outlet syndrome [TOS]), which is another primary condition that should also come under treatment if present to achieve better pain relief from the RSD. Surgery in the context of RSD is always a matter of concern, but it has successfully been performed by prearranging for epidural blocks to be performed prior to the procedure and then again afterward.

These initial steps may be followed by additional "chemical" sympathetic blockade using local anesthetic (the blocks at our center are performed by anesthesiologists), radiofrequency or surgical sympathectomy, dorsal column stimulation, and finally a morphine pump. Some form of counseling is of value if the pain persists to help both the individual and family members adjust to the alteration in lifestyle that often accompanies severe chronic pain.

More severe pain requires the use of a stronger narcotic analgesic. This may include methadone, used in 5- to 10-mg increments, with one to three tablets up to three times a day, oxycodone in the form of OxyContin (10-, 20-, 40-, and 80-mg tablets are available), which can be supplemented with immediate-release oxycodone in the form of OxyIR (5-mg tablets), or morphine in the form of Kadian (25, 50 or 100 mg daily) or MS Contin (15-, 30-, 60-, and 100-mg tablets are available), which can be supplemented with immediate-release morphine in the form of MSIR at 15 to 30 mg used up to four times daily for breakthrough pain. Severe limb swelling is often difficult to treat with oral medications alone, and has responded to intrathecal infusion of morphine.

Localized limb pain has also been successfully treated with a dorsal column stimulator. This technique can be quite helpful if there is truly isolated limb pain, but the downside is that the patient cannot have an MRI study with this paramagnetic device in place. More diffuse pain has been effectively treated with the intrathecal delivery of morphine through the use of a pump delivery system.

Finally, there are a variety of surgical ablative procedures that alter the patient's response to pain in the most severe circumstances and are truly last-resort measures for treatment. If these measures fail—whatever the reason—the only recourse is for medication and supportive counseling. Suicide has been a choice some patients have made because of difficulties in adjusting to their pain, so ongoing evaluation of how affected pain patients are coping is needed for comprehensive management, and a team approach is suggested to avoid "burnout" of both the patient and the caregiver.

Current treatments of RSD are based upon decreasing the sympathetic activity in the affected extremity through the use of physical therapy, sympathetic nerve blocks, surgical sympathectomy, and related treatments.

Therapeutic intervention is evolving along with our understanding of RSD. At the present time, early mobilization in an aquatic setting appears to be the best modality for treating the new onset of symptoms. Removing as many of the triggers of pain would appear to be the next modality. Finally, narcotic medications to address the chronic pain will be the last resort.

## References

Boyle, M. D. P.; Young, M. Nerve growth factor: activation of the classical complement pathway by specific substitution for component Cl. Proc. Natl. Acad. Sci. USA 79:2519–2522; 1992.

Campbell, J. N.; Raja, S. N. Reflex sympathetic dystrophy. Neurology 45:1235–1236; 1995.

Evans, J. A. Reflex sympathetic dystrophy: report on 57 cases. Ann. Intern. Med. 26:417–426; 1997.

Haugen, P. K.; Letourneau, P. C. Interleukin-2 enhances chick and rat sympathetic, but not sensory, neuritic outgrowth. J. Neurosci. Res. 25:443–452; 1990.

Kozin, F. Reflex sympathetic dystrophy syndrome: a review. Clin. Exp. Rheum. 10:401–409; 1992.

Morgan, E. L.; McClurg, M. R.; Janda, J. A. Suppression of human B lymphocyte activation by beta endorphin. J. Neuroimmunol. 28:209–217; 1990.

Otten, U.; Ehrhard, P.; Peck, R. Nerve growth factor induces growth and differentiation of human B lymphocytes. Proc. Natl. Acad. Sci. USA 86: 10059–10063; 1989.

Price, R. W.; Katz, B. J.; Notkins, A. L. Latent infection of the peripheral ANS with herpes simplex virus. Nature 257:686–688; 1975.

Schwartzman, R. J. Reflex sympathetic dystrophy. Curr. Opin. Neurol. Neurosurg. 6:531–536; 1993.

Schwartzman, R. J.; Kerrigan, J. The movement disorder of reflex sympathetic dystrophy. Neurology 40: 57–61; 1990.

Schweitzer, M. F.; Mandel, S.; Schwartzman, R. J.; et al. Reflex sympathetic dystrophy revisited: MR imaging findings before and after infusion of contrast material. Radiology 195:211–214; 1995.

Taniuchi, M.; Clark, H. B.; Johnson, E. M., Jr. Induction of nerve growth factor receptor in Schwann cells after axotomy. Proc. Natl. Acad. Sci. USA 83:4094–4098; 1986.

van der Laan, L.; ter Laak, H. J.; Gabreels-Festen, A.; Gabreels, F.; Goris, R. J. Complex regional pain syndrome type I (RSD): pathology of skeletal muscle and peripheral Nerve. Neurology 51:20–25; 1998.

Verdugo, R.; Ochoa, J. L. Reflex sympathetic dystrophy. Neurology 45:1236–1237; 1995.

Walz, M. A.; Price, R. W.; Notkins, A. L. Latent ganglionic infection with herpes simplex virus types 1 and 2: viral reactivation in vivo after neurectomy. Science 184:1185–1187; 1974.

Webster, G. F.; Schwartzman, R. J.; Jacoby, R. A.; Knobler R. L.; Uitto, J. J. Reflex sympathetic dystrophy. Occurrence of inflammatory skin lesions in patients with stages II and III disease. Arch. Dermatol. 127:1541–1544; 1991.

Webster, G. F.; Iozzo, R. V.; Schwartzman, R. J.; Tahmoush, A.; Knobler R. L.; Jacoby, R. A. Reflex sympathetic dystrophy: occurrence of chronic edema and non-immune bullous skin lesions. J. Am. Acad. Dermatol. 28:29–32; 1993.

Weskamp, G.; Otten, U. An enzyme-linked immunoassay for nerve growth factor (NGF): a tool for studying regulatory mechanisms involved in NGF production in brain and peripheral tissues. J. Neurochem. 48: 1779–1786; 1987.

Wybran, J.; Appelboom, T.; Famaey, J. P.; Govaerts, A. Suggestive evidence for receptors for morphine and methionine-enkephalin on normal human T lymphocytes. J. Immunol. 123:1068–1070; 1979.

# 12

# Primary Headache Disorders

TODD D. ROZEN AND STEPHEN D. SILBERSTEIN

Headache is a universal disorder. Most individuals experience at least one headache during their lifetime, and many have recurrent headaches (Rassmussen et al. 1991). The majority of these headaches are due to one of the primary headache disorders, such as migraine, cluster, or tension-type headache, and do not indicate an underlying pathologic process. These distinct, primary head pain syndromes, with stereotypic pain quality, location, and associated symptoms, afflict millions of individuals worldwide. Their natural history and prognosis are still not completely known, due, in part, to their episodic nature. Population-based epidemiologic studies are subject to recall bias, which makes it difficult to ascertain changes in attack frequency and quality over a period of time. Large-scale prospective studies in a representative population do not have this limitation.

In order to determine a disorder's prevalence and prognosis, it must be consistently diagnosed by different investigators in different regions at different times. The discrepancy in headache prevalence rates in early studies was due to lack of consistent case definitions and failure to account for influence of age and sex. The diagnostic guidelines for primary and secondary headache disorders that were created by the International Headache Society (IHS) (Headache Classification

Committee of the International Headache Society 1988) were designed, in part, to create uniform descriptive definitions of headache subtypes, and these have recently been used in headache epidemiologic studies. This chapter will discuss the epidemiology, treatment, natural history, and prognosis of the four main primary headache disorders: migraine, cluster, tension-type, and chronic daily headache. The influence of age and sex will be discussed.

## Migraine

### Epidemiology

Migraine afflicts 23 million Americans and has a major impact on both the individual and on society (Stewart et al. 1992). It has been postulated that migraine causes up to $17 billion of lost work productivity a year (Osterhaus et al. 1992). The true burden of migraine is not known, since 70% of migraineurs have not been diagnosed. Migraine prevalence and incidence are age- and gender-dependent (Silberstein and Lipton 1993). In childhood, boys and girls have the same migraine prevalence; with puberty, girls have a sharper rise in migraine prevalence and incidence than boys do. The gender ratio rises from puberty to age 40 and then declines, but never to the level of early child-hood (Silberstein and Lipton 1993).

According to the American Migraine Study (Stewart et al. 1992), 17.6% of women and 6% of men have one or more migraine attacks a year. Migraine incidence has been calculated in two population-based studies. Stang et al. (1992) reported an age-adjusted incidence of 137 per 100,000 person-years for men and 294 per 100,000 person-years for women in Olmsted County, Minnesota, from 1979 to 1981. Rozen et al. (1997), in the same population, calculated a 481 per 100,000 person-years age-adjusted inci-dence in women and 194 per 100,000 person-years in men from 1989 to 1990. These were the first migraine incidence studies across all age groups, based on clinic records, and suggest that migraine incidence is either increasing or is being increasingly ascertained.

Migraine was believed to be a disorder of the wealthy and educated, but this is not confirmed by recent epidemiologic studies. The American Migraine study (Stewart et al. 1992) found that migraine prevalence is inversely correlated with income, social class, and intelligence. It is only a disorder of the wealthy in the physician's office, not in the population. In fact, the peak 1-year mi-graine prevalence for women from low-income families has been reported to be as high as 40% (Silberstein and Lipton 1993).

The dawn of the 21st century is an exciting time for headache, and specifically for migraine re-search. We are beginning to understand the patho-genic mechanisms of migraine, and models based on these discoveries have led to new therapies. It is hoped that this trend will continue and have a marked impact on migraine-related disability.

## Natural History and Prognosis of Migraine in Adults

Migraine is a chronic, episodic headache syn-drome that often begins during childhood or ado-lescence and can last a lifetime (Table 12-1). Over the lifespan, migraine manifestations change. In children, migraine may present as episodic vertigo or abdominal pain without headache. These same children often develop typical migraine in their early teens. Migraine can also present as transient migraine accompaniments as described by Fisher (1980). Individuals of any age, but more commonly those over 40 (often with a history of migraine),

**Table 12-1.** IHS Features of Migraine With and Without Aura

---

Migraine Without Aura

---

Previously used terms: common migraine, hemicrania simplex
Diagnostic criteria:
A.  At least five attacks fulfilling B–D.
B.  Headache lasting 4 to 72 hours (untreated or unsuccess-fully treated).
C.  Headache has at least two of the following characteristics:
    1.  Unilateral location
    2.  Pulsating quality
    3.  Moderate or severe intensity (inhibits or prohibits daily activities)
    4.  Aggravation by walking stairs or similar routine physical activity
D.  During headache at least one of the following:
    1.  Nausea and/or vomiting
    2.  Photophobia and phonophobia

---

Migraine With Aura (Classic Migraine)

---

Diagnostic Criteria:
A.  At least two attacks fulfilling B
B.  At least three of the following four characteristics:
    1.  One or more fully *reversible* aura symptoms indicat-ing brain dysfunction
    2.  At least one aura symptom *develops gradually* over more than 4 minutes or 2 or more symptoms occur in succession
    3.  No single aura symptom *lasts more than 60 minutes*
    4.  *Headache follows aura* with a free interval of less than 60 minutes (it may also begin before or simulta-neously with the aura)
C.  History, physical examination and, where appropriate, diagnostic tests exclude a secondary cause

---

can develop attacks of episodic, transient neuro-logic dysfunction that last from 5 to 30 minutes. By definition, any underlying cerebrovascular etiology must be ruled out. The spells often come in clus-ters, may never recur, and about half the time are associated with a headache. These spells are prob-ably migrainous and have, in part, been classified by the IHS as migraine aura without headache.

Migraine may occur with or without aura, and most patients with aura also have attacks without aura. Migraine may be influenced by sex hor-mones. While the true prognosis of migraine is unknown, most believe that migraine attack fre-quency and severity decreases after age 40. Mi-graine attacks can stop, only to recur after many years of remission. Episodic migraine may also transform into a chronic daily headache (CDH) (transformed migraine) (see below).

Whitty and Hockaday (1968), in a clinic-based study, reported on 92 patients with a history of migraine for 16 to 69 years. After 15 to 20 years of follow-up, migraine remitted in one-third of patients, and attack frequency and intensity improved in the other two-thirds. In some patients, migraine remitted in young adulthood only to return later in life. Migraine persistence did not correlate with age of onset, age at the time of evaluation, or migraine duration.

Fry (1966), analyzing data from his general practice, found that migraine attack frequency and severity decreased with time. After 15 years, migraine remitted in 32% of men and 42% of women.

Migraine prevalence is age- and gender-dependent. Prevalence estimates range from 3.4% to 6.1% for men and from 12.9% to 17.6% for women (Silberstein and Lipton 1993). Migraine prevalence has been estimated in over 50 studies, but only 24 have looked at age- and gender-specific prevalence rates. Gender ratio appears to increase from the age of menarche to about age 40, declining thereafter. The American Migraine Study (Stewart et al. 1992), through regression analysis, found that age-specific prevalence rates increase up to about age 40 and then decrease for both men and women. As migraineurs age, headache prevalence decreases either from spontaneous remission or as a result of treatment. It is also possible that migraineurs have a higher mortality in their fifties and sixties, thus leading to a decline in prevalence. Leviton et al. (1974) found a 1.9-times increased mortality risk for migraineurs before the age of 70 compared to age-matched individuals without migraine. Waters et al. (1983), in contrast, found that women with one or more features of migraine had lower mortality than did women without migraine or with nonmigrainous headaches.

Migraine in the population decreases in prevalence after age 40, but it is not uncommon in the individual sufferer for it to continue, recur, or even begin in the elderly. Selby and Lance (1960), in a clinic-based sample of 500 migraineurs, found that 92% experienced their first attack in the first four decades of life, whereas only 2% had migraine onset after the age of 50 years. Long-term prospective studies are needed to assess the natural history of migraine and determine what factors contribute to cessation, recurrence, or continuance.

## Migraine and Hormones

Migraine incidence and prevalence is age- and sex-dependent. Migraine is as common in boys as it is in girls, with a prevalence of about 4% (Silberstein and Lipton 1993). In adults, migraine is two to three times as prevalent in women as in men. Migraine prevalence increases in women around the time of menarche (the first period). The trigger for menstrual migraine may be the decline in estrogen levels that are associated with menstruation. Migraine prevalence decreases in the elderly, often associated with menopause. In one clinic-based study, two-thirds of the women with natural menopause had headache relief compared to two-thirds of women whose headaches worsened following surgically induced menopause (Silberstein and Merriam 1997).

## Migraine and Pregnancy

Pregnancy has a profound influence on headache. Many women will have an increase in attacks during their first trimester and an improvement or cessation of attacks during the second and third trimesters (Silberstein 1997). Approximately two-thirds of women migraineurs improve during pregnancy, particularly if they had menstrually related migraine. Postpartum, migraine often returns. Stein (1981) found that women who develop postpartum headache usually have a history of migraine. Migraine can also occur for the first time during pregnancy. These patients may have a different prognosis than women who had migraine before becoming pregnant. This may be due to selection bias, as reported cases are often atypical or have prolonged aura. Chancellor et al. (1990) reported nine patients with migraine that occurred for the first time during pregnancy. None had a family history of migraine. Six patients were followed up to 4½ years and none had migraine attacks as severe as those that occurred during pregnancy. One patient had a single, milder attack, while another developed menstrually related migraine. Migraine that occurs for the first time with pregnancy may have a better prognosis than does migraine that initially occurs outside of pregnancy, but larger prospective studies are needed to confirm this observation.

In the Chancellor et al. (1990) study, the primiparous migraineurs developed many pregnancy-related complications. Two women developed pre-eclampsia that led to cesarian section, one had a threatened abortion, and two had premature deliveries. This study, with a small sample size, suggested that pregnancy outcome was worse in migraineurs than in the general population. Wain-scott and Volans (1978), in a much larger study, reviewed the pregnancy records of 777 female migraineurs and 182 nonheadache patients. The incidence of miscarriage, congenital anomalies, stillbirths, and toxemia were no different in migraineurs than in nonmigraineurs, suggesting that the outcome of pregnancy in migraine patients is no different than it is in the general population.

## Migraine in Children

It used to be believed that migraine was rare in children, but many retrospective studies suggest that migraine can begin before 3 years of age. Migraine prevalence ranges from 1.2% to 5.7% in children 7 years or younger (Sillanpää 1994). Prevalence increases in school aged children (ages 7 to 15 years) to 3.9% to 12% (Sillanpää 1994). Before puberty, migraine prevalence is equal in boys and girls; after puberty, migraine incidence and prevalence increase more rapidly in women than in men.

Migraine may have a different prognosis in children than in adults. This has been studied both retrospectively and prospectively. One-third of children will have a remission lasting for 10 years or more (Forsythe and Hockaday 1988). Hockaday (1988) studied 102 migraineurs who were diagnosed before the age of 20 years and followed them for 8 to 25 years. Migraine remitted in 26% and improved in 48% of the patients. Boys had a better prognosis than girls. Congdon and Forsythe (1979) found that 34% of 108 children had 10-year remissions, but only if the child was diagnosed before 18 years of age. Sillanpää (1983) looked at migraine prevalence longitudinally, in a cohort of Finnish children at age 7 and again at age 14. Migraine remitted in 22% and improved in 37%. Sillanpaa (1994), in another study, followed 2921 school children for 15 years. Migraine with onset before age 7 more commonly remitted in boys than in girls. By age 22, 51% of men and 62% of women still had migraine.

Metsahönkala et al. (1997) completed a migraine outcome study of 84 children from 8 to 12 years of age. After 3 years, 63.1% of the children still had migraine attacks, about half had increased attack frequency, and only four children (4.8%) had stopped having attacks. Boys had a worse prognosis than girls. Both sexes had the same intensity and duration of attacks, but boys more commonly used medication and had school absences. Children in households with parental problems (divorce/separation) had a worse prognosis; their migraine attack frequency was found to increase with time.

Bille (1997) conducted the largest childhood migraine prognosis study, following a subset of 9000 Swedish children, between the ages of 7 and 15, for up to 40 years. In the initial analysis, completed in 1955, migraine prevalence was 1.4% in children aged 7 years and increased to 5.3% in children age 15. Prior to age 11, boys and girls had equal prevalence, but after puberty girls had a higher prevalence than boys. Seventy-three children (32 men, 41 women) with severe migraine from the initial study group were followed for 40 years. After 6 years, 34% had a 1-year remission. After 16 years, 62% had been attack-free for longer than 2 years, but 22% relapsed. After 22 years, 40% were attack-free, and after 30 years 47% were attack-free. At the 40 year follow-up, final observations were made. By the age of 25, 23% of the initial cohort were attack-free, men twice as often as women. At 50 years of age, 51% of both men and women still had migraine attacks. Twenty-nine percent had at least one attack a year since onset, while another 22% had at least one remission of at least 2 years' duration. Over time, migraine attacks often decreased in frequency but pain intensity remained the same. Aura symptoms decreased over time: at the beginning, 70% had aura, this declined to 48% at the end of the study. Sixty-one of 73 study patients had children; 31 of the 61 parents (52%) had children with migraine.

Half of the children who develop severe migraine beginning between the ages of 7 and 15 will continue to have attacks into their fifties and sixties, although 20% become headache-free by 25 years of age. Whether less severely afflicted children have a better prognosis is uncertain.

## Migraine Therapy and Prognosis

Migraine therapy involves both drug and nondrug intervention. Acute treatment is used to abort an ongoing headache and its associated symptoms, whereas preventive treatment is designed to reduce migraine frequency or severity. Nondrug treatments include aerobic exercise, regular, balanced meals, and good sleep hygiene, all of which can help control headache. Drug therapy is patient specific and must take into account coexistent medical and psychiatric disorders, and the presence of migraine variants such as hemiplegic migraine or migraine with prolonged aura. In some individuals vasoactive drugs can be used with impunity, whereas in others they could possibly induce stroke or myocardial infarction. Good treatment outcomes depend on making the correct diagnosis. This requires obtaining a comprehensive headache history, performing a thorough neurologic examination, and eliminating underlying causes of secondary headache disorders if the history or examination suggests them. Coexistent and comorbid disorders must also be searched for. Once the correct diagnosis is made, most migraineurs can be helped.

## Migraine Abortive Medication

There has been an explosion in the development of specific acute migraine drugs designed to act at selected serotonin receptors. Sumatriptan, the first selective 5-HT$_1$ agonist, has revolutionized migraine treatment. Prospective studies attest to sumatriptan's long-term efficacy and tolerability. Gobel et al. (1996) reported on 2263 patients who used subcutaneous sumatriptan for 6 to 18 months. They had a total of 43,691 migraine attacks. Effective headache relief occurred 71% of the time, with 22.7% recurrence. This figure is probably low, due to selective dropout in this open study. Sumatriptan's effectiveness and tolerability did not change throughout the entire study. Leira et al. (1995) assessed the long-term efficacy and tolerability of subcutaneous sumatriptan in 32 patients with migraine with and without aura who were followed for 6 months. Headache severity and duration was reduced 71.8%; efficacy during the first and last month of treatment was identical. Sumatriptan maintains its effectiveness and tolerability over time.

One of the major problems with sumatriptan (and all the triptans) is the high headache recurrence rate. About 40% of all migraineurs treated with sumatriptan will have headache recurrence within 24 hours. Whether this is related to the short half-life of the drug is uncertain. Patients taking sumatriptan more than 3 to 4 days a week (mostly to abort headache recurrence) can also

develop rebound (drug-induced) headache. Visser et al. (1996) interviewed 366 migraine patients about headache recurrence on sumatriptan; individuals with menstrual migraine, severe headache intensity, longer untreated attack duration, and those experiencing a sensation of an ongoing migraine attack even after pain relief were most likely to develop headache recurrence. Recurrence was not related to the efficacy of sumatriptan, the timing of drug administration, or prior headache recurrence on ergotamine. Headache recurrence may reflect the inability of sumatriptan to shut off the hypothesized brain stem migraine generator. Weiller et al. (1995), using positron emission tomography (PET), demonstrated increased regional cerebral blood flow to medial brain stem structures (in addition to increased cortical blood flow) during a migraine attack. Sumatriptan eliminated the headache and reversed the cortical, but not the brain stem, increase in blood flow.

Newer antimigraine agents (triptans) have been specifically developed to have longer half-lives and greater central nervous system (CNS) penetration than sumatriptan. Rizatriptan and zolmitriptan have similar efficacy and recurrence and both have equal long-term efficacy and tolerability (Edmeads and Millson 1997; Gijsman et al. 1997). Naratriptan is less effective than other triptans at 2 hours, but may have a lower recurrence rate. It has very few adverse events (Mathew et al. 1997).

Dihydroergotamine (DHE) is an older established migraine-specific medication that is very effective in alleviating status migrainosus and helping patients with chronic daily headache. DHE has both a longer serum and biologic (sticks to the receptors) half-life than sumatriptan, which makes it more suitable for treating patients with recurrence. In addition, it can be used in patients with daily or near-daily headaches without the risk of medication-induced headache. DHE will be further discussed in the section on chronic daily headache. It is now available as a nasal spray with an efficacy similar to the triptans but a recurrence rate of less than 20%.

## Migraine Preventive Treatment

Individuals with migraine attacks that occur more often than twice a month or cause extreme disability are candidates for migraine prophylactic therapy. Since the average attack frequency of migraine is 1.5 attacks a month, most migraineurs do not need preventive treatment; however, many patients who do need it are not getting it. In fact, only 3% to 5% of migraineurs are on preventive drugs. Medications proven effective in migraine prevention include divalproex sodium/sodium valproate, amitriptyline, propranolol, timolol, nadolol, metoprolol, atenolol, flunarizine, methysergide, and riboflavin. Sacquegna et al. (1983) identified clinical factors that predicted better outcome on migraine preventives. Four hundred consecutive outpatients at an Italian headache center were placed on preventive drugs (either pizotifen, propranolol, methysergide, or amitriptyline) and followed from 3 to 12 months. Patients who did not respond to one medication could receive any of the other three drugs, alone or in combination. Patients treated for 1 year did better than those treated for 6 months, who did better than those treated for 3 months. The prognosis improved for patients who had more than three attacks a month and whose migraine duration was less than 10 years. Men did better than women. This study is subject to bias: Patients who were doing well would stay on the medication and have a better 1-year prognosis.

Most migraine treatments have not been vigorously studied in children. Many physicians choose alternate methods, such as behavioral therapy, to treat childhood headaches. Studies have examined behavioral therapy outcomes in childhood migraine and which psychosocial factors predict response to therapy. Osterhaus et al. (1993) reported 32 pediatric migraine patients who completed a 7-month follow-up study. After temperature biofeedback and relaxation training treatment (four sessions), 45% of patients had at least a 50% reduction in headache attack frequency. Almost all maintained their improvement at the 7-month follow-up. Female gender, shorter duration of migraine history, older age, and fewer somatic complaints predicted a favorable therapeutic response. A control group had no change in headache attack frequency over the same study period.

Hermann et al. (1997) looked at predictors of treatment outcome in 32 childhood migraineurs (aged 8 to 16 years) who received home-based biofeedback. No control groups were used in this study. Predictors of a good outcome included early age of headache onset, externalizing behavior (poor impulse control, acting out), and high levels of psychosomatic distress. Family functioning (ordered or chaotic) did not influence treatment outcome.

Larsson and Melin (1989) reported a 4-year follow-up on the effects of behavioral treatment (relaxation training) on adolescent migraine. Eighty-five percent of the patients who had achieved an initial 50% improvement in headache intensity after completing treatment continued to show improvement at 4 years. The only positive predictor of a favorable outcome was a high initial-pain-severity index.

## Quality of Life

Migraine is a lifelong disorder, but with appropriate therapy, migraineurs can live happy and successful lives. However, migraineurs even on medication are not as content with life as are non-headache patients. Dahlöf and Dimenäs (1995) compared the well-being of migraineurs between attacks with gender- and age-matched controls. One hundred thirty-eight migraineurs were administered three questionnaires: the Minor Symptoms Evaluation Profile, Subjective Symptoms Assessment Profile, and the Psychological General Well-Being Index. Compared with controls, migraineurs at baseline (outside of attacks) demonstrated less well-being, lower levels of contentment (happiness, self control, and tranquility), vitality (enthusiasm, endurance, and concentration), and sleep quality. Migraineurs had more subjective symptoms such as gastrointestinal distress, sex life disturbance, and dizziness than matched controls. The prognosis for migraineurs may improve if physicians concentrate not only on headache symptoms but on the general well-being of the individual.

Migraine therapy influences the quality of life of migraineurs. Solomon et al. (1995), in an open study, evaluated the impact of sumatriptan treatment on quality-of-life measurements in migraineurs. In this study, patients were given the SF-36 questionnaire and a pain questionnaire before treatment. These questionnaires were readministered following 6 to 9 months of sumatriptan therapy. Three SF-36 measurements (physical pain, bodily pain, and social functioning) showed statistically significant improvement. Four pain questionnaire parameters (enjoyment of life, pain interference with normal work, and ability to move and walk about) improved after sumatriptan therapy. Solomon et al.'s (1995) study suggests that migraineurs' quality of life and prognosis can be improved with therapy. Whether the improvement was to due the drug or to the care the patients received is uncertain.

## Cluster Headache

### Epidemiology and Clinical Characteristics

Cluster headache is a distinct primary headache disorder characterized by short-duration attacks of excruciating unilateral head pain and the presence of autonomic symptoms. Cluster affects about 0.07% of the population and occurs more commonly in men, with a male-female ratio of 5 to 6:1 (Kudrow 1997). The age-adjusted incidence of cluster headache in the population of Rochester, Minnesota, is 15.6 per 100,000 person-years for men and 4.0 per 100,000 person-years for women (Swanson et al. 1994).

Cluster is much less familial than migraine. The typical age of onset is between 20 and 40 years, although cluster can begin in children under the age of 10 and in individuals older than 70. The stereotypical cluster attack is characterized by severe unilateral pain, almost always without any side-shifting, in an orbital, supraorbital, or temporal distribution. Associated symptoms that reflect autonomic dysfunction include unilateral lacrimation, nasal congestion, ptosis, miosis, conjunctival injection, and eye tearing. Cluster patients are unable to get comfortable during an attack and will usually pace, rock, or take burning hot showers. Attacks last between 15 and 180 minutes, with a mean attack frequency of one to three headaches a day. The IHS criteria require at least five attacks during a lifetime, allow up to eight attacks in a day, and at least one of the associated autonomic symptoms (Table 12-2). Cluster can be episodic or chronic, based on the presence of remissions. Episodic cluster lasts from 7 days to 1 year, with at least one remission of 14 cluster-free days between bouts. Chronic cluster must last for more than 1 year, either without remissions or with less than 14 pain-free days.

There have been few prognostic studies of cluster headache, in part because of the rarity of the disorder and the fact that it is often misdiagnosed. Kudrow (1982) contacted 149 cluster patients who had been lost to follow-up for 3 to 8 years. Most of the dropout patients had episodic cluster

**Table 12-2.** Diagnostic Features of Cluster Headache (IHS)

A. At least five attacks fulfilling B–D
B. Severe unilateral orbital, supraorbital, and/or temporal pain lasting 15–180 minutes untreated
C. Headache associated with at least one of the following signs, which have to be present on the pain side:
   1. Conjunctival injection
   2. Lacrimation
   3. Nasal congestion
   4. Rhinorrhea
   5. Forehead and facial sweating
   6. Miosis
   7. Ptosis
   8. Eyelid edema
D. Frequency of attacks: from 1 every other day to 8 per day

headache (83.3%), while 25 patients (16.7%) had chronic cluster. Slightly over half of the episodic cluster patients (50.8%) had no change in attack pattern over time, while 5% developed chronic cluster. A prolonged remission (defined by the author as a remission longer than usual in duration) occurred in 38.7% of episodic cluster patients. Patients with more than a 20-year history of episodic cluster headache had more prolonged remissions, more conversion to chronic cluster, and higher mortality compared to patients who had shorter duration cluster, although none of these changes were statistically significant. Almost half of the chronic cluster patients (48%) had no change in headache pattern, while 20% converted to episodic cluster, 12% had a prolonged remission, and 25% died.

There was no significant difference in frequency of cluster conversion (episodic to chronic, chronic to episodic) or episodes of prolonged remission in men who experienced cluster for more or less than 20 years. Women with longer duration cluster had higher remission rates than did women with shorter duration cluster headache. In the dropout patient population, the longer a patient had cluster, the higher the frequency of remission and mortality. Individuals who had a remission of more than 1 year were much more likely to have periods of prolonged or even permanent remission. Overall, half of the studied cluster patients had no change in their cluster pattern, 7.4% switched patterns, and over 30% of patients had a prolonged remission. Seven patients died. Death, as expected, correlated with increasing age, although twice as many cluster patients died from cancer (two pulmonary) as opposed to a noncancer etiology (coronary artery disease). Cancer and noncancer mortality patients had almost equal cluster headache duration (about 26 years), although the age of cluster onset was much younger in the cancer group. Since cigarette smoking is common in cluster headache patients, and all of the cluster patients who died from cancer smoked, this may account for this association.

Sacquegna et al. (1987), in a clinic-based retrospective study, looked at the course of illness from onset to initial diagnosis in 72 episodic cluster headache patients. Most (86%) had a regular cluster cycle frequency, averaging one attack a year. Ten patients had a change in cluster frequency with the passage of time: the number of bouts of cluster headache decreased in six patients and increased in four. About 40% of patients had seasonally linked attacks (38% spring, 34% winter). Half of the episodic cluster patients had a fixed number of cluster episodes per year, a constant duration of individual attacks, and a near constant number of attacks per day. From this study, it appears that individual cluster patients have their own discrete cluster pattern, which usually remains unchanged over a lifetime.

Watson and Evans (1987) studied 60 chronic cluster headache patients using a retrospective record review. Each study patient had to have had at least one daily attack for 1 year. Mean cluster duration was 9.5 years. With therapy (lithium, methysergide, corticosteroids, indomethacin), 33% of patients were cluster free, and another 26% were satisfied with treatment. Eight patients did poorly or had no improvement.

Kunkel and Frame (1994) contacted 68 of 109 individuals who had been diagnosed with chronic cluster headache between 1970 and 1985. There was at least a 5-year interval between diagnosis and follow-up (study completed in 1990), with a mean follow-up time of 14 years. Of the 68 patients, 61% had chronic cluster from onset, while 39% had evolved from episodic cluster. Twenty of the contacted patients (29%) were poorly controlled on medications, while 22% were well controlled on preventive medication but were unable to discontinue their medication because of cluster recurrence. Twelve patients had a sustained remission that lasted from 2 to 18 years. About one-third of chronic patients converted into an episodic pattern. Equal numbers of primary and secondary chronic cluster patients went into remission or

converted to episodic cluster. Factors associated with prolonged remissions or conversion to an episodic pattern included surgery (9 of 33 patients), smoking cessation (3 of 33 patients), and preventive drug therapy (3 of 33 patients). In the Kunkel and Frame study, 70.5% of the contacted patients were either in prolonged remission, had converted to episodic cluster with headache-free time, or had stabilized on preventive medication. This study, as well as the Watson and Evans study, suggest that the prognosis of chronic cluster is not hopeless.

Pearce (1993) reported on 132 cluster patients (123 episodic, 9 chronic) who were diagnosed and followed from 1967 to 1982, with a mean follow-up of 14 years. The number of episodic cluster cycles, per year, decreased slightly over time (onset, 1.4 clusters per year; follow-up, 0.9 clusters per year), without a change in the cycle duration. Most episodic cluster patients (84%) had no change in cluster pattern, 3.96% converted to chronic cluster, and 11.8% had prolonged remissions (>4 years). Remissions typically occurred in patients who had had previous remissions lasting at least 1 year. Nine patients had chronic cluster: four had no change in cluster pattern, two converted to episodic cluster, and two had sustained remissions of 3 and 12 months but chronic cluster recurred in both. Medication controlled symptoms in 80% of episodic and 57% of chronic cluster patients. When medication was withdrawn during an active cluster cycle, symptoms quickly returned, suggesting that drugs do not change the natural history of the disorder, but just control the symptoms. Pearce concluded that episodic and chronic cluster patients continue to have attacks for at least 15 years after onset with little change in attack frequency or duration.

Krabbe (1991) did a long-term observation study of 226 cluster patients in Denmark seen from 1976 to 1989. Cluster duration was from 2 to 58 years. Conversion from chronic to episodic cluster occurred in 7.5% of patients; no information was given about the opposite conversion. Twenty-seven patients (12%) were cluster free (nothing mentioned about being on any treatment) from 1 to 9 years. Krabbe concluded that cluster is usually a lifelong illness, and that prolonged remissions do not mean a cure. One patient with a 15-year remission had a recurrence of episodic cluster.

Manzoni et al. (1991) followed 189 IHS-diagnosed cluster patients whose disease duration was over 10 years, in Parma and Pavia, Italy. The diagnosis of episodic or chronic cluster was based on the headache course in the first year of diagnosis: 140 patients (74%) had episodic cluster (118 men, 22 women) and 49 patients (25.9%) had chronic cluster (40 men, 9 women). Women had a younger age of onset for both cluster types. One patient developed new-onset cluster over the age of 60, while 15.3% continued to have cluster at this age. Approximately 81% of patients initially diagnosed with episodic cluster continued to have episodic cluster; 13% converted from episodic to chronic cluster. With longer disease duration, more cases of episodic cluster converted to chronic cluster. About one-quarter of patients with episodic cluster for longer than 20 years converted to chronic cluster; only 9% of patients whose cluster duration was less than 20 years converted. Men with episodic cluster had a nonstatistically significant higher conversion rate than women. Episodic cluster headache cycles occurred during the same months every year in 54% of patients; cluster cycle length increased in 48.2% of patients, and remained unchanged in 43.6%. Chronic cluster converted to episodic in one-third of patients, most of whom (56.2%) were on preventive therapy. Other factors influencing the conversion from chronic to episodic cluster included early age of disease onset, short disease duration, and (possibly) male gender (16 men, but no women switched). Prolonged remissions occurred in many patients (10%, 3 years; 4.8%, 5 years; 1.6%, 10 years). Patients who decreased or totally eliminated smoking did not have more remissions, but 4 of 19 patients who stopped drinking alcohol went into remission. Six patients died, half of them from cancer (one lung, one laryngeal, one pulmonary).

Episodic cluster headache does not change in most patients, but 20% of patients convert to chronic cluster. The conversion correlates to long disease duration (>20 years), older age of onset, and male gender. About 30% of chronic cluster patients convert to secondary episodic cluster; this correlated to an early age of onset, preventive therapy, and male gender, but not to duration of cluster or age of the patient.

## Cluster Therapy

There are no studies that look at the outcome of specific cluster therapies. Cluster is treated with acute medication (oxygen, corticosteroids, DHE, sumatriptan), preventive medication (verapamil, lithium, valproic acid, methysergide), and also with surgery (glycerol injection, radiofrequency gangliolysis, section of trigeminal nerve, gamma knife surgery). Many cluster sufferers require more than one drug to achieve control and 10% do not satisfactorily respond to medication.

### Acute Treatment

Oxygen via a nonrebreathing face mask is effective in 70% of cluster patients, normally within 10 minutes (Silberstein 1994). Short-term hyperbaric oxygen administration may have long-term benefit. Sumatriptan is effective in 74% of cluster patients (Silberstein 1994).

### Preventive Treatment

Methysergide appears to be effective in 65% to 69% of episodic cluster patients. In the Watson and Evans study (Watson and Evans 1987), methysergide gave sustained relief (>1 month) in 33% of chronic cluster patients and lithium carbonate gave sustained relief (3 months) in 39% of patients. Others have reported a 78% response to lithium carbonate in chronic cluster and a 63% response in episodic cluster (Ekbom and Sakai 1993). Approximately 20% of chronic cluster patients convert to an episodic cluster on lithium.

### Episodic Tension-Type Headache

Episodic tension type headache (ETTH) is defined as recurrent episodes of headache meeting the IHS diagnostic criteria (Table 12-3). TTH is the most common headache type, with a lifetime prevalence (in Denmark) of 69% in men and 88% in women and a 1-year prevalence of 63% in men and 86% in women (Rassmussen et al. 1991b).

TTH varies in frequency as well as in severity from rare, brief episodes to frequent, often-continuous, disabling headaches. TTH has no prodrome or aura. The pain is a dull, achy, nonpulsatile feeling of tightness, pressure, or constriction (vise-like or hatband-like), and is usually mild to moderate in severity, in contrast to the moderate to severe pain of migraine. Pain intensity increases with headache attack frequency (Rasmussen et al. 1992). Most patients have bilateral pain, but the location varies considerably within and between patients and can involve the frontal, temporal, occipital, or parietal regions,

**Table 12-3.** Tension-Type Headache (IHS)

2.1 Episodic tension-type headache
    Diagnostic criteria:
    A. At least 10 previous headache episodes fulfilling
       criteria B–D listed below. Number of days with
       such headache <180/yr (<15/mo)
    B. Headache lasting from 30 minutes to 7 days
    C. At least two of the following pain characteristics:
       1. Pressing/tightening (nonpulsating) quality
       2. Mild or moderate intensity (may inhibit, but
          does not prohibit activities
       3. Bilateral location
       4. No aggravation by walking stairs or similar
          routine physical activity
    D. Both of the following:
       1. No nausea or vomiting (anorexia may occur)
       2. Photophobia and phonophobia are absent, or
          one but not the other is present
2.1.1 Episodic tension-type headache associated with dis-
      order of pericranial muscles
      Diagnostic criteria:
      A. Fulfills criteria for 2.1
      B. At least one of the following:
         1. Increased tenderness of pericranial muscles
         2. Increased EMG level of pericranial muscles
2.1.2 Episodic tension-type headache unassociated with
      disorder of pericranial muscles
      Diagnostic criteria:
      A. Fulfills criteria for 2.1
      B. No increased tenderness or EMG activity of peri-
         cranial muscles.

EMG, electromyography.

alone or in combination, commonly changing locations during the attack.

Migraine and ETTH have traditionally been
considered distinct entities. However, some believe that migraine and TTH are related entities
that differ more in severity than kind (Rasmussen
et al. 1992). TTH may be two distinct disorders.
The first may be mild migraine attacks. The second may be a pure TTH that is not associated with
other features of migraine (sensitivity to movement, nausea, or photophobia) or with attacks of
severe migraine. What we call migraine may be
the upper end in a normal distribution of painful
episodic headaches. Whether TTH is a milder
form of migraine or is a distinct entity is still not
certain.

## Epidemiology

Tension-type headache is slightly more common
in women than in men (1.04 to 1.4:1), with peak
prevalence between the ages of 20 and 50 (Rasmussen et al. 1991b). Schwartz et al. (1998) recently published a prevalence study of ETTH uti-

lizing a telephone interview survey conducted in
Baltimore County, Maryland, from 1993 to 1994.
The overall 1-year period prevalence for ETTH
was 38.3%. Women had higher ETTH prevalence
rates than did men for all age, race, and education
subgroups. ETTH prevalence peaked between
30 to 37 years of age for both men and women.
ETTH prevalence also increased with educational
status. Over 71.8% of individuals with ETTH
experienced 30 or less headaches a year. ETTH
caused moderate disability, with 8.3% of patients
reporting lost workdays and 43.6% having had
decreased effectiveness at home, work, and school.
ETTH is very prevalent in society, causing moderate individual disability but substantial societal
impact.

Tension-type headache is a disorder of middle
life, striking individuals early in life and continuing to affect them through their peak productive
years. About 60% of tension-type headache patients have a diminished capacity for work or
other activities (Rasmussen et al. 1991b). Almost
one-half of TTH sufferers have to discontinue
normal activity and have some limitation of function. Most sufferers have less than one attack a
month, and about one-third have two or more attacks a month. Overall, the average frequency is
35 days per year.

Despite prominent disability, more than 80%
of tension-type headache patients have never consulted their general practitioner because of headache.

Frequent ETTH may be a risk factor for CTTH.
When migraine and TTH coexist, the TTH may
be more frequent and more severe. The process
whereby headache frequency increases and an
episodic disorder becomes chronic is sometimes
referred to as transformation. Overuse of ergotamine and/or analgesics is the most common factor leading to transformation (see below). If analgesics are not withdrawn, these patients may be
refractory to prophylactic therapy and have a very
poor prognosis.

## Treatment and Prognosis

The approach to the treatment of episodic headache, whether tension-type or migraine, is similar, and consists of psychophysiologic therapy,
physical therapy, and pharmacotherapy. Simple
analgesics and nonsteroidal anti-inflammatory

drugs (NSAIDs) are effective in TTH as demonstrated by the headache attack model for acute pain. Ibuprofen and naproxen are significantly more effective than placebo and may be more effective than aspirin or acetaminophen (Schoenen and Wang 1997). There is no evidence that muscle relaxants, such as the mephenesin-like compounds, baclofen, diazepam, tizanidine, cyclobenzaprine, or dantrolene sodium, are effective in the treatment of TTH (Schoenen and Wang 1997).

Prophylactic treatment, designed to reduce the frequency and severity of headache attacks, should be considered if the frequency (>2 per week), duration (>3 to 4 hours), and severity might lead to the overuse of abortive medication or significant disability. We prefer to begin treatment with antidepressants, but any of the "migraine" preventive drugs can be used empirically.

Relaxation and biofeedback are useful in the management of TTH. Relaxation training and/or electromyographic (EMG) biofeedback training can produce a 50% reduction in headache activity. Schoenen et al. (1985) found that relaxation training leading to a 50% or greater reduction in EMG activity by the fourth treatment session was predictive of a good outcome in TTH patients.

Cognitive behavioral interventions, such as stress management programs, may effectively reduce TTH activity when used alone, but they may be more useful in conjunction with biofeedback or relaxation therapies, particularly in patients with a high level of daily stress. Patients with continuous headache are less responsive to relaxation or biofeedback therapies, and patients with significant psychiatric comorbidity may do poorly with behavioral treatment that does not address the comorbid problem. Blanchard et al. (1982) found that patients with TTH who showed no improvement with biofeedback had the highest Beck Depression Inventory scores. The same investigators also found that positive depression scores on MMPIs correlated with poorer therapeutic success in TTH patients.

## Chronic Daily Headache

Chronic daily headache has a prevalence of 4.1% in the United States and 4.7% in Spain (Scher et al. 1998). Severe daily headache has a prevalence of 0.05% in the population and causes extreme economic and social disability (Newman et al. 1994).

Frequent headache sufferers most often have primary headache disorders aggravated by medication overuse, but an underlying pathologic condition must be excluded. Patients with chronic daily headache (CDH) are difficult to classify using the current IHS system. The major primary disorders to consider in individuals with near-daily headache include transformed migraine (TM), hemicrania continua (HC), chronic tension type headache (CTTH), and new daily persistent headache (NDPH).

### Transformed Migraine

TM is more common in the clinic (77%) but it is less common in the population, occuring in 1.3% in the United States and 2.2% in Spain. Patients with TM (Table 12-4) often have a past history of episodic migraine typically beginning in their teens or twenties (Silberstein et al. 1994). Most TM patients seen in subspecialty clinics are women; most (90%) have a history of migraine without aura (Silberstein and Lipton 1997). The TM patient often develops a daily or near-daily headache that resembles CTTH. Headache frequency increases over months to years and the associated symptoms of photophobia, phonophobia, and nausea become less severe and less frequent than they are in a typical migraine attack (Silberstein and Lipton 1997). About 80% of patients with TM overuse symptomatic medication (Mathew 1993).

**Table 12-4.** Proposed "1995" Criteria for Transformed Migraine

1.8 Transformed Migraine (TM)
  A. Daily or almost daily (>15 d/mo) head pain for >1 month
  B. Average headache duration of >4 h/d (if untreated)
  C. At least one of the following:
    1. History of episodic migraine meeting any IHS criteria 1.1 to 1.6
    2. History of increasing headache frequency with decreasing severity of migrainous features over at least 3 months
    3. Headache at some time meets IHS criteria for migraine 1.1 to 1.6 other than duration
  D. Does not meet criteria for New Daily Persistent Headache (4.7) or Hemicrania Continua (4.8)
  E. At least one of the following:
    1. There is no suggestion of one of the disorders listed in groups 5–11
    2. Such a disorder is suggested, but it is ruled out by appropriate investigations
    3. Such disorder is present, but first migraine attacks do not occur in close temporal relation to the disorder

Overuse has been defined as a regular intake of simple analgesics (aspirin, acetaminophen) or combination analgesics with additive barbiturates or caffeine more than 3 to 4 days a week for more than 1 to 2 months, or the use of opiates, ergots, or triptans more than twice a week. Headaches often increase in frequency when medication use is increased. Stopping the overused medication frequently results in distinct headache improvement, although improvement is not instantaneous and often takes days or weeks to develop. Many patients have significant long-term improvement after detoxification (see prognosis).

## Chronic Tension-Type Headache

Daily headaches may develop in patients with a history of ETTH. These headaches are often diffuse or bilateral and frequently involve the posterior aspect of the head and neck. In CTTH, in contrast to TM, most migraine features are absent, as is prior or coexistent episodic migraine.

CTTH requires head pain on at least 15 days a month for at least 6 months (Table 12-5); patients often have daily headaches. Although the pain criteria are identical to ETTH, the IHS classification allows nausea but not vomiting.

## New Daily Persistent Headache

NDPH (Table 12-6) is the abrupt development of a headache that does not remit. It often develops over less than 3 days, and some patients remember the exact day or time the headache started. NDPH is likely to be a heterogeneous disorder. Some cases may reflect a postviral syndrome (Vanast 1986). Patients with NDPH are generally younger than those with TM. There are no retrospective or prospective studies yet completed that offer insight into the prognosis of this unique headache syndrome.

## Hemicrania Continua

Hemicrania continua is a rare, indomethacin-responsive headache disorder characterized by a continuous, moderately severe, unilateral headache that varies in intensity, waxing and waning without disappearing completely (Table 12-7). It may rarely alternate sides (Bordini et al. 1991). It is frequently associated with jabs and jolt pains (idiopathic stabbing headache). Exacerbations of pain are often associated with autonomic disturbances, such as ptosis, miosis, tearing, and sweat-

**Table 12-5.** Proposed Criteria for Chronic Tension-Type Headache

2.2 Chronic tension-type headache
Diagnostic Criteria:
A. Average headache frequency more than 15 d/mo (180 d/yr) with average duration of ≥4 h/d (if untreated) for 6 months fulfilling criteria B–D listed below
B. At least two of the following pain characteristics:
   1. Pressing/tightening quality
   2. Mild or moderate severity (may inhibit, but does not prohibit activities)
   3. Bilateral location
   4. No aggravation by walking stairs or similar routine physical activity
C. History of episodic tension-type headache in the past (needs to be tested)
D. History of evolutive headaches which gradually increased in frequency over at least a 3-month period (needs to be tested)
E. Both of the following:
   1. No vomiting
   2. No more than one of nausea, photophobia, or phonophobia (needs to be tested)
F. Does not meet criteria for Hemicrania Continua (4.8), New Daily Persistent Headache (4.7), or transformed migraine (1.8)
G. At least one of the following:
   1. There is no suggestion of one of the disorders listed in groups 5–11
   2. Such a disorder is suggested, but it is ruled out by appropriate investigations
   3. Such disorder is present, but first headache attacks do not occur in close temporal relation to the disorder

**Table 12-6.** Proposed Criteria for New Daily Persistent Headache

4.7 New Daily Persistent Headache (NDPH)
A. Average headache frequency >15 d/mo for >1 month
B. Average headache duration >4 h/d (if untreated); frequently constant without medication but may fluctuate
C. No history of tension-type headache or migraine which increases in frequency and decreases in severity in association with the onset of NDPH (>3 months)
D. Acute onset (developing over <3 days) of constant unremitting headache
E. Headache is constant in location? (needs to be tested)
F. Does not meet criteria for Hemicrania Continua 4.8
G. At least one of the following:
   1. There is no suggestion of one of the disorders listed in groups 5–11
   2. Such a disorder is suggested, but it is ruled out by appropriate investigations
   3. Such disorder is present, but first headache attacks do not occur in close temporal relation to the disorder

**Table 12-7.** Proposed Criteria for Hemicrania Continua

4.8 Hemicrania Continua (HC)*
  A. Headache present for at least 1 month
  B. Strictly unilateral headache
  C. Pain has all three of the following present:
    1. Continuous but fluctuating
    2. Moderate severity, at least some of the time
    3. Lack of precipitating mechanisms
  D. 1. Absolute response to indomethacin or
    2. One of the following autonomic features with severe pain exacerbation
     (a) Conjunctival infection
     (b) Lacrimation
     (c) Nasal congestion
     (d) Rhinorrhea
     (e) Ptosis
     (f) Eyelid edema
  E. May have associated stabbing headaches
  F. At least one of the following
    1. There is no suggestion of one of the disorders listed in groups 5–11
    2. Such a disorder is suggested, but it is ruled out by appropriate investigations
    4. Such disorder is present, but first headache attacks do not occur in close temporal relation to the disorder

*HC is usually nonremitting, but rare cases of remission have been reported.

ing (Newman et al. 1993). Some patients may have photophobia, phonophobia, and nausea. Patients who respond to indomethacin demonstrate complete headache relief. If indomethacin is stopped, the headache usually returns within 2 to 3 days. The natural history of this disorder is not known. The prognosis is excellent if the patient can tolerate indomethacin. The prognosis is poor for individuals who have a contraindication to indomethacin (ulcer disease) because no other treatment has demonstrated the efficacy of indomethacin.

## Epidemiology of Chronic Daily Headache

The prevalence of daily headache has been estimated to be 2% in Denmark and 3% in the United States (Silberstein and Lipton 1997). Similar estimates come from Chile, but lower prevalence rates are reported from Asia and Africa (Scher et al. 1998). (Table 12-8). Schwartz et al. (1998) studied the prevalence of CTTH utilizing a telephone interview survey in Baltimore County, Maryland, from 1993 to 1994. The overall 1-year period prevalence for CTTH was 2.2%. CTTH declined with educational status and females had higher prevalence rates than males. CTTH patients demonstrated significant individual disability, but because of low prevalence rates, CTTH causes little societal impact.

    Frequent headache accounts for 30% to 75% of all subspecialty consults (Scher et al. in press). The largest and most complete study on the prevalence of frequent headache in the United States population came from Scher et al. (in press), using the same data base Schwartz et al. (1998) used. They completed a telephone interview survey in Baltimore County, Maryland, and calculated prevalence rates in individuals reporting 180 or more headaches a year. The headache types that were classified included frequent headache with migrainous features (Silberstein et al. 1994), CTTH, and unclassified frequent headache.

    The overall 1-year period prevalence of frequent headache was 4.1% (2.8% male, 5% fe-

**Table 12-8.** Summary of Population-Based Prevalence Estimates for Chronic Headache

| Author (Year of Publication) | Country | Method | Sample Size | Time Frame | Age | CTTH Prevalence | | |
|---|---|---|---|---|---|---|---|---|
| | | | | | | Total | Female | Male |
| Gobel et al. (1994) | Germany | Mail SAQ | 4061 | Lifetime | 18+ | 1.0% | 1.0% | 0.0% |
| Tekle Haimanot et al. (1995) | Ethiopia | Face-to-face/ clinic interview | 15,000 | 1 year | 20+ | 1.7% | 2.3% | 1.0% |
| Lavados and Tenham (1998) | Chile | Face-to-face | 1540 | 1 year | 14+ | 2.5% | 3.8% | 1.1% |
| Rasmussen (1995) | Denmark | Clinic interview | 740 | 1 year | 25–64 | 3.0% | 5.0% | 2.0% |
| Wong et al. (1995) | Hong Kong | Telephone | 7356 | 1 year | 15+ | 0.1% | | |
| Schwartz et al. (1998) | United States | Telephone | 13,343 | 1 year | 18–65 | 2.5% | 3.1% | 1.6% |
| Scher et al. (1998) | United States | Telephone | 13,343 | 1 year | 18–65 | 2.2% | | |
| Castillo et al. (1998) | Spain | Questionnaire/ face-to-face | 1883 | 1 year | | 2.4% | | |

SAQ, self-assessment questionaire.

male), with a 1.8:1 female-male ratio. About 50% of individuals met the criteria for CTTH (52% female, 56% male), with a 1-year period prevalence of 2.2%. One-third of patients had frequent headache with migrainous features with prevalence of 1.3% (33% female, 25% male), and the remainder were unclassified (15% female, 19% male) with prevalence of 0.6%. Prevalence was highest in Caucasians and those in the lowest educational group. Surprisingly, the Scher et al. (in press) study demonstrated a low prevalence of TM (frequent headache with migrainous features) in the general population. In specialty clinics, analgesic rebound headache can make up 80% of a referred population.

Castillo et al. (1998) reported on the epidemiology of CDH using the revised criteria of Silberstein et al. (1994). A questionnaire exploring headache frequency was distributed to 2252 unselected subjects. Those subjectively having headache 10 or more days a month were given a headache diary and seen by a neurologist, who classified them or not into CDH varieties.

One thousand eight hundred eighty-three subjects (83.5%) completed the questionnaire. One hundred thirty-five admitted to headache 10 or more days a month. Eighty-nine (4.7%) individuals fulfilled CDH criteria. Eighty were females. Forty-six (51.7% of CDH patients and 2.4% of all subjects in this work) had CTTH. Analgesic overuse was found in eight (17%). TM was diagnosed in 41 (46.1% of CDH patients and 2.2% of all subjects). Thirteen (31.7%) TM patients overused ergots or analgesics. The remaining two cases in this series met NDPH criteria. No patient was diagnosed as HC.

Almost 5% of the population (9% of women) suffers from CDH, the proportion of CTTH and TM being similar. Less than one-third overuse analgesics.

**Treatment and Prognosis**

Effective management requires excluding secondary headache disorders, diagnosing the specific primary CDH disorder, and identifying comorbid medical and psychiatric conditions, especially medication overuse.

If medication overuse is present, the goal of treatment is to safely detoxify the patient off rebounding medications. Overused medication is either tapered slowly or stopped abruptly, substituting neuroleptics, intravenous or intramuscular dihydroergotamine, a long-acting NSAID, or a short course of corticosteroids. Preventive medications are the primary therapy for CDH and should be instituted with the explicit understanding that they may not become fully effective until the overused medication has been eliminated. Antidepressants are attractive agents for use in CDH, since many patients have comorbid depression and anxiety. SSRIs, the new selective norepinephrine- and serotonin-reuptake inhibitors such as venlafaxine, and monoamine oxidase inhibitors, may have a therapeutic role, but this has not been proven to date. The anticonvulsant divalproex sodium is an important drug for use in CDH, even in patients who have failed other agents.

In some individuals, outpatient treatment will fail or be deemed unsafe (as, for example, the patient who is taking multiple narcotics daily and has a risk of withdrawal seizures), so inpatient treatment is instituted. Inpatient treatment modalities include detoxification, intravenous hydration, and combination therapy of intravenous dihydroergotamine and neuroleptics. Prophylactic medication is started concurrently.

No one knows the true natural history of medication-induced rebound headache; it is technically and perhaps ethically impossible to do this study. Retrospective studies suggest that the rebounder will experience episodes of stable drug consumption and spells of accelerated drug use, with eventual switching to different or more potent drugs to achieve equal therapeutic benefit. Without discontinuing the rebounding agent, spontaneous cessation of CDH probably will never occur. The prognosis for analyzing rebound headache is based on several studies (Table 12-9).

The prognosis of drug-induced analgesic rebound headache is good if the patient can successfully discontinue the offending agent and remain off the drug. The patient must also be given appropriate abortive and preventive therapy and, at times, nonmedicinal regimens, such as relaxation and biofeedback training. Between 1975 and 1996, 14 papers suggested a success rate of between 48% and 91% for treatment of CDH, with a 77% or higher success rate in seven of the papers. Saper and Lake (in press) have projected savings of greater than $100,000 for work-related disability by treating patients with analgesic rebound.

**Table 12-9.** Long-Term Outcome Studies for Analgesic Rebound Headache

| Study | No. of Patients | Drug E/A | Type of Therapy | Percentage Improved After Drug Withdrawal | Follow-up |
|---|---|---|---|---|---|
| Andersson (1975) | 44 | E | Outpatient | 91% | 6 months |
| Tfelt-Hansen et al. (1981) | 40 | E | Inpatient | 47.6% | 12 months |
| Ala-Hurula (1982) | 23 | E | Outpatient | 78% | 3–6 months |
| Mathew et al. (1982) | 200 | E/A | Outpatient | 86% | 3 months |
| Dichgans et al. (1984) | 52 | E/A | Inpatient | 77% | 16 months |
| Henry et al. (1984) | 22 | E/A | Outpatient | 78% | 4–24 months |
| Diener and Tfelt-Hansen (1993) | 85 | E/A | Inpatient | 69% | 10–75 months |
| Andersson (1988) | 32 | E | In/outpatient | 50% | 6 months |
| Baumgartner et al. (1989) | 54 | E/A | Inpatient | 60.5% | 17 months |
| Mathew et al. (1989) | 489 | E/A | In/outpatient | 69% | 18–72 months |
| Herring and Steiner (1991) | 46 | E/A | Outpatient | 80.4% | 6 months |
| Silberstein and Silberstein (1992) | 50 | E/A | Inpatient | 87% | 24 months |
| Lake et al. (1993) | 100 | E/A | Inpatient | 75% | 1 year |
| Schnider et al. (1996) | 36 | E/A | Inpatient | 50% (47.4% headache-free) | 5 years |

E, ergotamine tartrate; A, analgesics.

# References

Ala-Hurula, V.; Myllylä, V.; Hokkamen, E. Results of ergotamine discontinuation with special reference to plasma concentrations. Cephalalgia 2:187–195; 1982.

Andersson, P. G. Ergotamine headache. Headache 15: 118–121; 1975.

Andersson, P. G. Ergotism: the clinical picture. In: Diener, H. C.; Wilkinson, M. S., eds. Drug induced headache. Berlin: Springer; 1988: p.16.

Baumgartner, C.; Wessly, P.; Bingol, C.; Maly, J.; et al. Long-term prognosis of analgesic withdrawal in patients with drug-induced headaches. Headache 29:510; 1989.

Bille, B. A 40-year follow-up of school children with migraine. Cephalalgia 17:488–491; 1997.

Blanchard, E.; Andrasik, F.; Neff, D.; et al. Biofeedback and relaxation training with three kinds of headache: treatment effects and their predictions. J. Consul. Clin. Psychol. 50: 562–575; 1982.

Bordini, C.; Antonaci, F.; Stovner, L. J.; Schrader, H.; Sjaastad, O. "Hemicrania continua"—a clinical review. Headache 31: 20–26; 1991.

Castillo, J.; Munoz, P.; Guitera, V.; Pascual, J. Epidemiology of chronic daily headache in the general population. Headache 39:190–196;1999.

Chancellor, M. D.; Wroe, S. J. Migraine occurring for the first time in pregnancy. Headache 30: 224; 1990.

Congdon, P. G.; Forsythe, W. I. Migraine in childhood: a study of 300 children. Dev. Med. Child. Neurol. 21:209–216; 1979.

Dahlöf C. G. H.; Dimenäs migraine patients experience poorer subjective well-being/quality of life even between attacks. Cephalalgia 15:31–36; 1995.

Dichgans, J.; Diener, H. D.; Gerber, W. D.; et al. Analgetika-induzierter dauerkopfschmerz. Dtsch Med Wachanschr 109:369; 1984.

Diener, H. C.; Tfelt-Hansen, P. Headache associated with chronic use of substances. In: Olesen, J.; Tfelt-Hansen, P.; Welch, K. M. A., eds. The headaches. New York: Raven Press; 1993: p. 721.

Edmeads, J. G.; Millson, D. S. Tolerability profile of zolmitriptan (Zomig; 311C90), a novel dual central and peripherally acting 5HT1B/1D agonist. International clinical experience based on >3000 subjects treated with zolmitriptan. Cephalalgia 16:41–52; 1997.

Ekbom, K.; Sakai, F. Cluster headache: management. In: Olesen, J.; Tfelt-Hansen, P.; Welch, K. M. A., eds. The headaches. New York: Raven Press; 1993: p. 591–599.

Fisher, C. M. Late life migraine accompaniments as a cause of unexplained transient ischemic attacks. Can. J. Neurol. Sci. 7: 9–17; 1980.

Forsythe, I.; Hockaday, J. M. Management of childhood migraine. In: Hockaday, J. M., ed. Migraine in childhood. London: Butterworths; 1988: p. 63–74.

Fry, J. Profiles of disease. Edinburgh: Livingstone; 1966.

Gijsman, H.; Kramer, M. S.; Sargent, J.; Tuchman, M.; Matzura-Wolfe, D.; Polis, A.; Teall, J.; Block, G.; Ferrari, M. D. Double-blind, placebo-controlled, dose-finding study of rizatriptan (MK-462) in the acute treatment of migraine. Cephalalgia 17:647–651; 1997.

Gobel, H.; Petersen-Braun, M.; Soyka, D. The epidemiology of headache in Germany: a nationwide survey of a representative sample on the basis of the headache classification of the International Headache Society. Cephalalgia 14:97–106; 1994.

Gobel, H.; Stolz, H.; Heinze, A.; et al. Eighteen month long-term analysis of effectiveness, safety and tolerance of sumatriptan S.C. in acute therapy of migraine attacks. Nervenarzt 67:471–483; 1996.

Headache Classification Committee of the International Headache Society. Classification and diagnostic criteria for headache disorders, cranial neuralgia, and facial pain. Cephalalgia 8:1; 1988.

Henry, P.; Dartigues, J. F.; Benetier, M. P.; et al. Ergo-tamine- and analgesic-induced headache. In: Rose, F. C., ed. Migraine: proceedings from the fifth international migraine symposium. London; 1984: p. 197.

Hering, R.; Steiner, T. J. Abrupt outpatient withdrawal from medication in analgesic-abusing migraineurs. Lancet 337:1442; 1991.

Hermann, C.; Blanchard, E. B.; Flor, H. Biofeedback treatment for pediatric migraine: prediction of treatment outcome. J. Consul. Clin. Psychol. 65:611–616; 1997.

Hockaday, J. M. Definitions, clinical features, and diagnosis of childhood migraine. In: Hockaday, J. M., ed. Migraine in childhood. London: Butterworths; 1988: p. 5–24.

Krabbe, A. The prognosis of cluster headache. A long-term observation of 226 cluster headache patients. Cephalalgia Suppl. 11:250–291; 1991.

Kudrow, L. Natural history of cluster headache—part 1: outcome of dropout patients. Headache 22:203–206; 1982.

Kudrow, L. Cluster headache. In: Goadsby, P. J.; Silberstein, S. D., eds. Headache. Newton, MA: Butterworth-Heinemann; 1997: p. 227–242.

Kunkel, R. S.; Flame, J. R. Chronic cluster headache. In: Kunkel, R. S., ed. Headache classification and epidemiology. New York: Raven Press; 1994: p. 113–116.

Lake, A. E.; Saper, J. R.; Madden, S. F.; Kreeger, C. Comprehensive inpatient treatment for intractable migraine: a prospective long-term outcome study. Headache 33: 55–62; 1993.

Larsson, B.; Melin, L. Follow-up on behavioral treatment of recurrent headache in adolescents. Headache 29:249–253; 1989.

Lavados, P. M.; Tenham, E. Epidemiology of tension-type headache in Santiago, Chile: a prevalence study. Cephalalgia 18:552–558; 1998.

Leira, R.; Suarez, C.; Castillo, J.; Lema, M.; Noya, M. Subcutaneous sumatriptan in the treatment of migraine attacks. An analysis of its long-term efficaciousness and tolerance. Rev. Neurol. 23:752–755; 1995.

Leviton, A.; Malvea, B.; Graham, J. R. Vascular disease mortality and migraine in the parents of migraine patients. Neurology 24:669–672; 1974.

Manzoni, G. C.; Micieli, G.; Granella, F.; Tasorelli, C.; Zanferrari, C. Cluster headache—course over ten years in 189 patients. Cephalalgia 11:169–174; 1991.

Mathew, N. T. Transformed migraine. Cephalalgia 13:8–83; 1993.

Mathew, N. T.; Asgharnejad, M.; Peykamian, M.; Laurenza, A. Naratriptan is effective and well tolerated in the acute treatment of migraine. Results of a double-blind, placebo-controlled, crossover study. Naratriptan S2WA3001 Study Group. Neurology 49:1485–1490; 1997.

Mathew, N. T.; Kaiman, R.; Perez, F. Intractable chronic daily headache: a persistent neurobehavioral disorder. Cephalalgia 9:180–181; 1989.

Mathew, N. T.; Stubits, E.; Nigam, M. R. Transformation of episodic migraine into daily headache: analysis of factors. Headache 22:66–68; 1982.

Metsähonkala, L.; Sillanpää, M.; Tuominen, J. Outcome of early school-age migraine. Cephalalgia 17: 662–665; 1997.

Newman, L. C.; Lipton, R. B.; Solomon, S. Hemicrania continua: 7 new cases and a literature review. Headache 32:267; 1993.

Newman, L. D.; Lipton, R. B.; Solomon, S.; Stewart, W. F. Daily headache in a population sample: results from the American Migraine Study. Headache 34: 295; 1994.

Osterhaus, J.; Gutterman, D. L.; Pluchetka, J. R. Health-care resource and lost labor costs of migraine headache in the United States. Pharmacoeconomics 2: 67–76; 1992.

Osterhaus, S. O. L.; Passchier, J.; vanderHelm-Hylkema, H.; deJong, K. T.; Orlebeke, J. F. de Gauw.; Dekker, P. H. Effects of behavioral psychophysiological treatment on school children with migraine in a nonclinical setting: predictors and process variables. J. Pediatr. Psychol. 18:697–715; 1993.

Pearce, J. M. S. Natural history of cluster headache. Headache 33:253–256; 1993.

Rasmussen, B. K. Epidemiology of headache. Cephalalgia 15:45–68; 1995.

Rasmussen, B. K.; Jensen, R.; Olesen, J. A population-based analysis of the diagnostic criteria of the International Headache Society. Cephalalgia 11:129; 1991a.

Rasmussen, B. K.; Jensen, R.; Schroll, M.; Olesen, J. Epidemiology of headache in a general population-a prevalence study. J. Clin. Epidemiol. 44:1147–1157; 1991b.

Rasmussen, B. K.; Jensen, R.; Schroll, M.; Olesen, J. Interrelations between migraine and tension-type headache in the general population. Arch. Neurol. 49:914; 1992.

Rozen, T. D.; Swanson, J. W.; Stang, P. E.; McDonnell, S. K.; Rocca, W. A. Incidence of migraine headache: a 1989–1990 population-based study in Olmstead County, Minnesota. Neurology 3:122; 1997.

Sacquegna, T.; Baldrati, A.; D'Alessandro, P.; De-Carolis, P.; Santucci, M.; Lugaresi, E. Migraine prophylaxis: prognostic significance of clinical factors. Headache 23:34–36; 1983.

Sacquegna, T.; Curran, D. A.; Baldrati, A.; DeCarolis, P.; Tinuper, P. The natural history of episodic cluster headache. Minerva Med. 78:963–966; 1987.

Saper, J. R.; Lake, A. E. Tertiary care for headache: a six month outcome 1998 (in press).

Scher, A. I.; Stewart, W. F.; Liberman, J.; Lipton, R. B. Prevalence of frequent headache in a population sample. Headache 38:497–506; 1998.

Schnider, P.; Aull, S.; Baumgartner, C.; et al. Long-term outcome of patients with headache and drug abuse after inpatient withdrawal: five-year followup. Cephalalgia 16:481–485; 1996.

Schoenen, J.; Pholien, P.; Maertens deNoordhout, A. EMG biofeedback in tension-type headache: is the 4th session predictive of outcome? Cephalalgia 5: 132; 1985.

Schoenen, J.; Wang, W. Tension-type headache. In: Goadsby, P. J.; Silberstein, S. D., eds. Headache.

Newton, MA: Butterworth-Heinemann; 1997: p. 177–200.

Schwartz, B. S.; Stewart, W. F.; Simon, D.; Lipton, R. B. Epidemiology of tension-type headache. JAMA 279:381–383; 1998.

Selby, G.; Lance, J. W. Observation on 500 cases of migraine and allied vascular headaches. J. Neurol. Neurosurg. Psychiatry 23:23–32; 1960.

Silberstein, S. D. Pharmacological management of cluster headache. CNS Drugs 2:199–207; 1994.

Silberstein, S. D. Migraine and pregnancy. Neurol. Clin. 15:209–231; 1997.

Silberstein, S. D.; Lipton, R. B. Epidemiology of migraine. Neuroepidemiology 12:179–194; 1993.

Silberstein, S. D.; Lipton, R. B. Chronic daily headache. In: Goadsby, P. J.; Silberstein, S. D., eds. Headache. Newton, MA: Butterworth-Heinemann; 1997: p. 201–225.

Silberstein, S. D.; Lipton, R. B.; Solomon, S.; Mathew, N. T. Classification of daily and near daily headaches: proposed revisions to the IHS classification. Headache 34:1; 1994.

Silberstein, S. D.; Merriam, G. R. Sex hormones and headache. In: Goadsby, P. J.; Silberstein, S. D., eds. Headache. Newton, MA: Butterworth-Heinemann; 1997: p. 143–173.

Silberstein, S. D.; Silberstein, J. R. Chronic daily headache: prognosis following inpatient treatment with repetitive IV DHE. Headache 32:439; 1992.

Sillanpää, M. L. Changes in the prevalence of migraine and other headaches during the first seven school years. Headache 23:15–19; 1983.

Sillanpää, M. L. Headache in children. In: Olesen, J., ed. Headache classification and epidemiology. New York: Raven Press; 1994: 263–281.

Solomon, G. D.; Skobieranda, F. G.; Genzen, J. R. Quality of life assessment among migraine patients treated with sumatriptan. Headache 35:449–454; 1995.

Stang, P. E.; Yamagihara, T.; Swanson, J. W.; et al. Incidence of migraine headaches: a population-based study in Omstead County, Minnesota. Neurology 42: 1657–1662; 1992.

Stein, G. S. Headaches in the first postpartum week and their relationship to migraine. Headache 21:201; 1981.

Stewart, W. F.; Lipton, R. B.; Celentano, D. D.; Reed, M. L. Prevalence of migraine in the United States. JAMA 267:64–69; 1992.

Swanson, J. W.; Yamagihara, T.; Stang, P. E.; et al. Incidence of cluster headache: a population based study in Olmstead County, Minnesota. Neurology 44:433–437; 1994.

Tekle Haimanot, R.; Seraw, B.; Forsgren, L.; Ekbom, K.; Ekstedt, J. Migraine, chronic tension-type headache, and cluster headache in an Ethiopian rural community. Cephalalgia 15:482–488; 1995.

Tfelt-Hansen, P.; Aebelholt-Krabbe, A. Ergotamine abuse. Do patients benefit from withdrawal? Cephalalgia 1:27–32; 1981.

Vanast, W. J. New daily persistent headaches: definition of a benign syndrome. Headache 26:317; 1986.

Visser, W. H.; Jaspers, N. M.; deVriend, R. H.; Ferrari, M. D. Risk factors for headache recurrence after sumatriptan: a study in 366 migraine patients. Cephalalgia 16:264–269; 1996.

Wainscott, G.; Volans, G. N. The outcome of pregnancy in women suffering from migraine. Postgrad. Med. J. 54:98; 1978.

Waters, W. E.; Campbell, M. J.; Elwood, P. C. Migraine headache and survival in women. Br. Med. J. 287:1442–1443; 1983.

Watson, C. P.; Evans, R. J. Chronic cluster headache—a review of 60 patients. Headache 26:157–155; 1987.

Weiller, C.; May, A.; Limmroth, V.; et al. Brainstem activation in spontaneous human migraine attacks. Nat. Med. 1:658; 1995.

Whitty, C. W. M.; Hockaday, J. M. Migraine: a followup study of 92 patients. Br. Med. J. 1:735–736; 1968.

Wong, T. W.; Wong, K. S.; Yu, T. S.; Kay, R. Prevalence of migraine and other headaches in Hong Kong. Neuroepidemiology 14:82–91; 1995.

# 13

# Herpes Zoster and Postherpetic Neuralgia

C. PETER N. WATSON

I wish I could state anything more satisfactory as to the treatment of the after-pains,
which are sometimes so severe as to make the patient weary of existence.

William Bowman (1867)

When asked to revise a book chapter, one must address particularly the issue of what is new as well as retain what is of established substance in the previous work. New material, with regard to evaluating and changing the outlook with herpes zoster (HZ) and postherpetic neuralgia (PHN), includes the term zoster-associated pain (ZAP), the finding of racial differences in the incidence of HZ, and the view that the prognosis for many with HZ is for the development of an intractable, untreatable disorder (Watson 1998). This latter discouraging prospect may be avoided either by preventing HZ by vaccination or by aggressively treating the acute pain of HZ with antivirals, nerve blocks, antidepressants, and opioids. Whether these measures will attenuate the natural history of HZ and PHN is scientifically unknown at this time, but this approach appears reasonable and safe and may be of particular importance in high-risk populations.

A variety of therapies have been recommended to alter the course of HZ and PHN. Many of these studies have been of uncontrolled trials in populations of unknown age with postherpetic pain of unspecified duration. The chief difficulty is that the pain associated with HZ and PHN naturally improves with time and this gives a false impression of the efficacy of a remedy. This amelioration is most dramatic in the early weeks after the onset of the skin lesions but also is seen, to a lesser extent, in the ensuing months and years and even with PHN of long duration. This information about the pain's natural course is crucial for three reasons; first, it helps to reassure patients that improvement can occur even with pain of long duration; second, it becomes possible to interpret more knowledgeably the results of clinical trials and, finally, the researcher can more effectively design studies to assess the efficacy of a particular treatment. The clinical features, pathology and pathogenesis of PHN are not discussed in this chapter nor are prophylaxis and treatment discussed in any great detail.

## Definitions

A new term, zoster-associated pain (ZAP), has been introduced as a definition for postherpetic pain (Crooks et al. 1991). This definition has arisen because of problems occurring in studies of antiviral agents with HZ in order to remove the argument that occurs as to when HZ pain ceases and PHN begins. This term considers postherpetic pain as a continuum from its onset to its resolution. This appears, to the author, to be a good, novel idea for these studies of acute zoster pain. There is still, however, an important role for a uniform and separate definition of PHN for use in studies dealing particularly with populations of patients with established PHN.

A reasonable and general definition of PHN is neuropathic pain that persists in the area affected by HZ after the usual time for the skin lesions to heal (usually 4 weeks). As this chapter shows, resolution of pain continues to occur spontaneously in a considerable number of patients between 1 and 3 months. Therefore, to ensure a chronic, stable pain state for study design purposes, the author believes that it is preferable to choose patients with pain persisting for 3 months beyond the time of rash healing, which would be about 4 months after the onset of the rash or pain.

### What is the Natural History of Postherpetic Pain?

When PHN is defined as pain persisting more than 1 month after HZ, the incidence in all age groups has been found to be 9% (Ragozzino et al. 1982), 9.7% (Burgoon et al. 1957), and 14.3% (Hope-Simpson 1975) in different studies. Higher assessments have been made by DeMoragas and Kierland (1957) and Rogers and Tindall (1971). Perhaps differences are related to whether the inquiry was directed at any sort of discomfort or, rather, significant persistent pain. Edgar Hope-Simpson's graph of the incidence of HZ and PHN is illustrated (Fig. 13-1) because it is an original and singular study of a general practice population and pays tribute to the early work of this great scientist and family practitioner (Hope-Simpson 1975).

The number of patients suffering PHN for more than 1 year has been estimated to be 22% (Ragozzino et al. 1982) and 49% (DeMoragas and Kierland 1957) of the number affected at 1 month. Thus, of 100 patients of all ages with HZ, approximately ten will have pain at 1 month and between two and five at 1 year or more.

### What is the Natural Course of Established Postherpetic Neuralgia?

The author's data support continued improvement with established PHN even of long duration such as 1 year (Watson et al. 1992). A population of 132 patients with PHN was followed at intervals of 3 months, 6 months, and yearly thereafter for periods of up to 10 years after the initial pain clinic visit. At each interval, 35% to 50% of patients were doing well and having no pain or mild pain. Between 40% and 60% of patients doing well at each following assessment had the disorder for 1 year or more when first seen, so even long-lasting pain can improve with time. A disturbing group of 26 patients (20%) initially responded well to treatment but with time lost this effect and were repeatedly documented as having poor results despite retreatment with initially successful methods and others.

### Risk Factors for Postherpetic Neuralgia

Although the overall tendency for PHN is to improve, there is a strong relationship between age and the incidence and severity of this disorder.

**Figure 13-1.** Zoster—postherpetic neuralgia and age of patient.

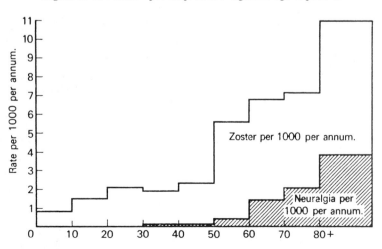

DeMoragas and Kierland (1957) found an increasing incidence of PHN lasting 1 month or more when patients were studied by age groups. The incidence was 33% between ages 40 and 49, increasing with each decade to 74% at age 70 and older. Also, the severity was increased (as measured by duration) with age, so that the prevalence of pain more than 1 year after HZ was 7% in the group aged 40 to 49, climbing to 47.5% in those older than 70 years. Other authors have also found this age-related increase in incidence (Burgoon et al. 1957; Glynn 1987; Rogers and Tindall 1971). Rogers and Tindall (1971) estimated the incidence of PHN lasting more than 4 weeks as 46.9% in a group older than 60 years and only 15.9% in those younger than 60 years.

A number of studies have indicated that women suffer PHN more commonly than men (Glynn 1987; Hope-Simpson 1975; Lewith et al. 1983; Russell et al. 1957; Watson et al. 1988). Although Hope-Simpson (1975) thought this was a true increase, Watson and colleagues (1988) and Glynn (1987) studied a larger number of patients and found that this female predominance simply reflected general population statistics.

There is good evidence from a number of studies that patients with greater pain with acute HZ are more likely to develop PHN (Molin 1969; Riopelle et al. 1984; Harding et al. 1987; Dworkin et al. 1992, 1995a, 1995b; Leijon et al. 1993; McKendrick et al. 1994; Whitley et al. 1995; Wood et al. 1996).

The greater severity of the rash is thought to influence the severity of PHN (Wilson 1986; Higa et al. 1988, 1992; Dworkin 1995a; Whitley et al. 1991). The presence of scarred skin and greater sensory dysfunction in the involved dermatome during HZ are also thought to be risk factors (Nurmikko et al. 1990; Leijon et al. 1993).

There is an increased tendency for PHN to affect the first division of the trigeminal nerve and thoracic, especially midthoracic, dermatomes (Glynn 1987; Watson et al. 1988). There is a corresponding lesser incidence in cervical and lumbosacral areas. This dermatomal distribution is similar to observations in HZ (Burgoon et al. 1957; Hope-Simpson 1975; Ragozzino et al. 1982) and also may reflect the centripetal distribution of varicella. PHN in the forehead area has also been reported to last longer (DeMoragas and

Kierland 1957; Hope-Simpson 1975; Watson et al. 1988). An increased incidence of this long-duration pain with trigeminal involvement has been found with increasing age (DeMoragas and Kierland 1957).

Although an increased risk of HZ has been associated with leukemia, lymphoma, and chemotherapy, no increased incidence of PHN has been reported with these conditions. Diabetes mellitus may predispose to HZ and increase the likelihood of PHN (Brown 1976; McCulloch et al. 1982).

Higa and associates (1988) have reported that the severity of HZ could be defined by the maximum antibody titer to varicella zoster virus and that, independently of age, this had the greatest influence on the duration of treatment of acute herpetic pain by sympathetic blockade. A greater magnitude and duration of cell-mediated immunity has been related to the severity of PHN as well (Dan et al. 1983; Higa et al. 1988, 1992).

A recent study by Schmader and colleagues (1995) has reported that blacks are less likely to develop herpes zoster than whites.

## Prevention of Postherpetic Neuralgia (Altering the Prognosis of HZ)

Data from clinical trials (Table 13-1) and the author's clinical experience indicate that at least 40% of patients with PHN are intractable or respond poorly to treatment. This may be because of irreversible damage to the nervous system (Watson 1998). Because of this it seems reasonable to try to prevent the disorder (Watson 1998). One approach is by vaccinating the older population and others at risk such as the immune-suppressed with varicella vaccine. Another approach to altering the prognosis is to aggressively treat herpes zoster pain to prevent virus-induced damage and/or the development of central (spinal) hyperexcitability resulting from continued and unrelieved nociceptive barrages. These measures might include treatment with antivirals such as valacyclovir or famciclovir within the first 72 hours, regional local anesthetic blockade, effective analgesia with opioids if necessary, and by the early use of antidepressant-analgesic therapy such as amitriptyline (Bowsher 1997). None of these approaches are scientifically proven except for the use of antivirals, but they appear reasonable and safe.

**Table 13-1.** Patients Responding Poorly or Not at All in Controlled Trials in Postherpetic Neuralgia

| Study | Efficacy Data With Number of Patients Unchanged and Poor Responses (%) | Placebo Controls Who Were Unchanged or Poor Responses | Agent |
|---|---|---|---|
| Watson et al. 1982 | 8/24 (33%) | 100% | Amitriptyline |
| Max et al. 1988 | 21/41 (53%) | 84% | Amitriptyline |
| Kishore-Kumar et al. 1990 | 14/26 (54%) | 89% | Desipramine |
| Watson et al. 1992 | 17/32 (53%) with MT and/or AT | No placebo | Amitriptyline (AT) vs. maprotiline (MT) |
| Watson et al. 1996 | 10/31 (32%) with NT and/or AT | No placebo | Amitriptyline vs. nortriptyline (NT) |
| Watson et al. 1997 | 17/38 (45%) | 82% | Oxycodone |

There is now support for a modest reduction in PHN by antiviral agents such as acyclovir, valacyclovir, and famciclovir. There is now a large literature on the use of opioids in nonmalignant pain indicating that the risk of psychological and physical dependency and tolerance is very low and that this is a reasonable approach without undue risk (Portenoy 1996). Possible side effects can be pre-empted by the use of stool softeners and antinauseants on a regular basis.

Many other approaches have been suggested for the prevention of PHN by treatment of HZ. Most have been studied with small numbers of patients and for short periods of follow-up. Controlled trials have appeared to support the use of oral corticosteroids in this fashion (Elliott 1964; Keczkes and Basheer 1980). Others (Esmann et al. 1987; Wood et al. 1996) have shown no benefit. Although there appears not to be a risk of the dissemination of the virus by this route, the author's view is that the evidence is not strong for using this approach and that the interventions above are more hopeful with the addition of steroids only adding to the risk of polypharmacy. There is a lack of good controlled trials of regional anesthesia with either somatic or sympathetic blocks. Nonetheless, in competent hands these procedures are of low risk and rational in the light of information about the prevention of windup and hyperexcitability in the nervous system. Other approaches, such as the use of amantadine (Galbraith 1983) levo-dopa (Kernbaum and Hauchecorne 1981), interferon-$\alpha$ (Merigan et al. 1978, 1981), vidarabine (Whitley et al. 1982), and adenosine monophosphate (Sklar et al. 1985) are either unsubstantiated, methodologically flawed, or too toxic and have never found general use.

## Treatment of Postherpetic Neuralgia

This chapter does not review exhaustively the treatment of PHN, and for this the reader is referred elsewhere (Kost and Strauss 1996). Because of the natural history of improvement with time, particularly soon after HZ onset, the definition of PHN and selection of a control population are important for evaluating any treatment approach. Only controlled trials with adequately defined study populations are considered here.

Randomized, double-blind, placebo-controlled trials support the analgesic effect of amitriptyline (AT) in PHN (Max et al. 1988; Watson et al. 1982). This effect was seen with mean doses of 65 mg (Max et al. 1988) and 75 mg (Watson et al. 1988) in approximately two-thirds of patients (Watson et al. 1982). The drug is thought to have an analgesic action independent of its antidepressant effect. After 12 months, 12 (55%) of 22 patients were maintaining a good response on AT (Watson et al. 1982). After 5 years, 10 (52%) of 19 were doing well, but only four were on AT. There is evidence also that the antidepressants desipramine and maprotiline also may be effective for PHN (Kishore-Kumar et al. 1990; Watson et al. 1992). Long-term data derived from 132 patients indicated that of patients doing well at follow-up, at least 50% continued to use antidepressants (AT, nortriptyline, maprotiline) at 3, 6, and 12 months and 2 and 3 years from the first pain clinic visit (Watson et al. 1992).

There is now some evidence that opioids can relieve some patients with PHN who are intractable to other measures (Watson and Babul 1998). As previously mentioned, there is now a significant literature concerning the use of opioids in nonmalignant pain of various sorts indicating that this approach is reasonable and safe and that psychological and physical dependency and tolerance are uncommon problems (Portenoy 1996). Side effects are to be expected and constipation and nausea, particularly, should be routinely treated, even pre-emptively. A single-dose opioid infusion study has demonstrated short-term reduction in pain in PHN (Rowbotham et al. 1991). A controlled trial of oxycodone versus placebo has shown at least moderate improvement in at least 58% of patients on drug versus 18% on placebo in cases of PHN (Watson and Babul 1998).

Topical agents, such as capsaicin, aspirin, and local anesthetics have shown some effectiveness in PHN but are generally disappointing for most patients in clinical practice.

The anticonvulsant gabapentin has recently been shown to be more effective than placebo in PHN by randomized trial (Rowbothan et al. 1991). It appears to have few serious side effects, and doses up to 3500 mg may be necessary.

Other medical approaches such as anticonvulsant therapy with carbamazepine or gabapentin do not currently have a good scientific basis and should be regarded as trial and error in nature. Regional anesthesia for PHN is unproven to relieve PHN and results have been discouraging (Colding 1969, 1973).

Although a number of surgical approaches to PHN have been suggested, results generally have been unsatisfactory. Dorsal root entry zone (DREZ) lesions have been reported to be of some use (Friedman et al. 1984; Friedman and Nashold 1984; Nashold et al. 1983) and report a beneficial effect of DREZ lesions in PHN in 50% to 66% of patients with follow-up of 6 to 25 months. Many of these patients had pain for at least 5 months and were refractory to many medical approaches. Significant complications can result from this operation including leg weakness; altered, disagreeable sensations below the lesion; and back discomfort at the level of surgery. Generally, surgical approaches have been abandoned for PHN and the current understanding is that this approach is currently rarely considered and only in refractory patients.

## Conclusions

In most patients, postherpetic pain improves with time. This occurs most dramatically soon after HZ onset but continues to occur during the ensuing months and years. A small number of patients initially may respond to therapy and then become intractable with time. Some remain so for years from the onset of the disorder. A direct relationship is present between advancing age and increasing risk of developing persistent pain. It may be possible to select patients at high risk for developing persistent pain as those over age 60 with severe pain and rash at onset and those with trigeminal involvement. It may be possible to alter the natural history by vaccination and by early, aggressive treatment with antivirals, opioids, nerve blocks, and early antidepressant therapy. For established PHN, the scientific literature supports the older generation antidepressants such as amitriptyline but not the newer agents such as fluoxetine. The anticonvulsant gabapentin has a scientific basis for efficacy with few serious side effects. Doses up to 3500 mg may be necessary. There is evidence that opioids are safe and effective in a proportion of patients with intractable disease refractory to all other measures.

## References

Bowman, W. Ophth. Hosp. Rep. 6:1–11; 1867.

Bowsher, D. The effects of pre-emptive treatment of postherpetic neuralgia with amitriptyline. J. Pain Symp. Manage. 13:327–331; 1997.

Brown, G. R. Herpes zoster. Correlation of age, sex, distribution, neuralgia, and associated disorders. South. Med. J. 69:576–578; 1976.

Burgoon, C. F.; Burgoon, J. S.; Baldridge, G. D. The natural history of herpes zoster. JAMA 164: 256–269; 1957.

Colding, A. The effect of sympathetic blocks on herpes zoster. Acta. Anaesthesiol. Scand. 13:113–141; 1969.

Colding, A. Treatment of pain: organization of a pain clinic, treatment of herpes zoster. Proc. R. Soc. Med. 66:541–543; 1973.

Crooks R. J.; Jones, D. A.; Fiddian A. P. Zoster-associated pain: overview of clinical trials with acyclovir. Scand. J. Infect. Dis. 80 (suppl. 6):62–68; 1991.

Dan, K.; Higa, K.; Noda, B. Nerve block for herpetic pain. In: Fields, H. L.; Dubner, R.;

Cervero, R., eds. Advances in pain research and therapy. Vol 9. New York: Raven Press; 1985: p. 831–838.

Dan, K.; Higa, K.; Tanaka, K.; Mori, R. Herpetic pain and cellular immunity. In: Yokota, T.; Dubner, R., eds. Current topics in pain research and therapy. Proceedings of the International Symposium on pain. Amsterdam: Excerpta Medica; 1983: p. 293–305.

DeMoragas, J. M.; Kierland, R. R. The outcome of patients with herpes zoster. Arch. Dermatol. 75: 193–196; 1957.

Dworkin, R. H.; Hartstein, G.; Rosner, H. L.; Walther, R. R.; Sweeney, E. W.; Brand, L. A. A high-risk method for studying psychosocial antecedents of chronic pain: the perspective investigation of herpes zoster. J. Abnorm. Psychol. 101:200–205; 1992.

Dworkin, R. H.; Boon, R. J.; Griffin, D. R. G. Covariates in herpes zoster and interpretation of clinical trial data. Antiviral Res. 26:A344; 1995a.

Dworkin, R. H.; Cooper, E. M.; Walther, R. R.; Sweeney, E. W. Predicting the development of postherpetic neuralgia in acute herpes zoster patients: a diathesis-stress model. Los Angeles: American Pain Society; 1995b.

Elliott, F. A. Treatment of herpes zoster with high doses of prednisone. Lancet 2:610–611; 1964.

Esmann, V.; Ipsen, J.; Peterslund, N. A.; Sayer-Hansen, K.; Schonheyder, H.; Juhl, H. Therapy of acute herpes zoster with acyclovir in the nonimmunocompromised host. Am. J. Med. 73:320–325; 1982.

Friedman, A. H.; Nashold, B. S.; Overmann-Levitt, J. DREZ lesions for postherpetic neuralgia. J. Neurol. 60:1258–1262; 1984.

Friedman, A. H.; Nashold, B. S. DREZ lesions for postherpetic neuralgia. Neurosurgery 15:969–970; 1984.

Galbraith, A. W. Treatment of acute herpes zoster with amantadine hydrochloride (Symmetrel). Br. Med. J. 4:693–695; 1983.

Glynn, C. A study of postherpetic neuralgia and its treatment. Pain Clin. 1(4):237–246; 1987.

Harding, S. P.; Lipton, J. R.; Wells, J. C. D. Natural history of herpes zoster ophthalmicus predictors of postherpetic neuralgia and ocular involvement. Br. J. Ophthalmol. 71:353–358; 1987.

Higa, K.; Dan, K.; Manabe, H.; Noba, D. Factors influencing the treatment of acute herpetic pain with sympathetic nerve block: importance of severity of herpes zoster assessed by the maximum antibody titres to varicella zoster virus in otherwise healthy patients. Pain 32:147–157; 1988.

Higa, K.; Noda, B.; Manabe, H.; Suto, S.; Dan, K. T-lymphocyte subsets in otherwise healthy patients with herpes zoster and relationships to the duration of acute herpetic pain. Pain 51:111–118; 1992.

Hope-Simpson, R. E. Postherpetic neuralgia. J. R. Coll. Gen. Pract. 25:571–575; 1975.

Keczkes, K.; Basheer, A. M. Do corticosteroids prevent postherpetic neuralgia? Br. J. Dermatol. 102:551–555; 1980.

Kernbaum, S.; Hauchecorne, J. Administration of levodopa for relief of herpes zoster pain. JAMA 246:132–134; 1981.

Kishore-Kumar, R.; Max, M. B.; Schafer, S. C.; et al. Desipramine relieves postherpetic neuralgia. Clin. Pharmacol. Ther. 47:305–312; 1990.

Kost, R. G.; Strauss, S. E. Drug therapy: postherpetic neuralgia. N. Engl. J. Med. 335:32–42; 1996.

Leijon, G.; Boivie, J.; Roberg, M.; Forsberg, P. Sensory abnormalities accompanying herpes zoster and postherpetic neuralgia. In: Abstracts, 7th World Congress on Pain. Seattle, WA: IASP Publications; 1993: p. 184–185.

Lewith, G. T.; Field, F.; Machin, D. Acupuncture versus placebo in postherpetic pain. Pain 17:361–368; 1983.

Max, M. B.; Schafer, R. N. C.; Culnane, M. Amitriptyline but not lorazepam relieves postherpetic neuralgia. Neurology 38:1427–1432; 1988.

McCulloch, D. K.; Fraser, D. M.; Duncan, L. P. J. Shingles in diabetes mellitus. Practitioner 226:531–532; 1982.

McKendrick, M. W.; Core, C. D.; Ogan, P.; Wood, M. J. A retrospective study of the epidemiology of zoster with particular reference to factors pertinent to the development of chronic pain. Second International Conference on the Varicella-Zoster Virus, Paris.

Merigan, T. C.; Gallagher, J. G.; Pollard, R. B. Short course human leukocyte interferon in treatment of herpes zoster in patients with cancer. Antimicrob. Agents Chemother. 19:193–195; 1981.

Merigan, T. C.; Rand, K. H.; Pollard, R. B.; et al. Human leukocyte interferon for the treatment of herpes zoster in patients with cancer. N. Engl. J. Med. 298:981–987; 1978.

Molin, L. Aspects of the natural history of herpes zoster. Acta. Dermatol. Venereol. 49:569–583; 1969.

Nashold, B. S., Jr.; Ostdahl, R. B.; Bullitt, E.; et al. Dorsal root entry zone lesions: a new neurosurgical therapy for deafferentation pain. In: Bonica, J. J.; Albefessard, D., eds. Advances in pain research and therapy. New York: Raven Press; 5:738–750; 1983.

Nurmikko, T. J.; Bowsher, D. Somatosensory findings in postherpetic neuralgia. J. Neurol. Neurosurg. Psychiatry 43:135–141; 1990.

Portenoy, R. K. Opioid therapy for chronic nonmalignant pain: a review of the critical issues. J. Pain Symptom Manag. 11:203–217; 1996.

Ragozzino, M. W.; Melton, I. J.; Kierland, L. T.; et al. Population based study of herpes zoster and its sequelae. Medicine 21:310–316; 1982.

Riopelle, J. M.; Naraghi, M.; Grush, K. P. Chronic neuralgia incidence following local anesthetic therapy for herpes zoster. Arch. Dermatol. 120:747–750; 1984.

Rogers, R. S.; Tindall, J. P: Geriatric herpes zoster. J. Am. Geriatr. Soc. 19:495–503; 1971.

Rowbothan, M. C.; Reisner-Keller, I. A.; Fields, H. L. Both intravenous lidocaine and morphine reduce the pain of postherpetic neuralgia. Neurology 41:1024–1028; 1991.

Russell, W. R.; Espir, M. L. E.; Morganstern, F. S. Treatment of postherpetic neuralgia. Lancet 1:242–245; 1957.

Schmader, K.; George, L. K.; Burchett, B. M.; Pieper, C. P.; Hamilton, J. D. Racial differences in the occurrence of herpes zoster. J. Infect. Dis. 171:701–704; 1995.

Sklar, S. H.; Blue, W. T.; Alexander, F. J.; et al. Herpes zoster, the treatment and prevention of neuralgia by adenosine monophosphate. JAMA 253:1427–430; 1985.

Watson, C. P. N. Postherpetic neuralgia: an end-stage untreatable disorder. J. Infect. Dis. 178 (suppl 1): S91–S94; 1998.

Watson, C. P. N.; Babul, N. Oxycodone relieves neuro-pathic pain: a randomized trial in postherpetic neu-ralgia. Neurology 50:1837–1841; 1998.

Watson, C. P. N.; Chipman, M.; Reed, K.; Evans, R. J.; Birkett, N. Amitriptyline versus maprotiline in post-herpetic neuralgia: a randomized, double-blind, crossover trial. Pain 48:29–36; 1992.

Watson, C. P. N.; Evans, R. J.; Reed, K.; et al. Amitriptyline versus placebo in postherpetic neural-gia. Neurology 32:670–673; 1982.

Watson, C. P. N.; Evans, R. J.; Watt, V. R.; Birkett, N. Postherpetic neuralgia: 208 cases. Pain 35:289–297; 1988.

Watson, C. P. N.; Watt, V. R.; Chipman, M.; Birkett, N.; Evans, R. J. The prognosis with postherpetic neuralgia. Pain 46:195–199; 1992.

Whitley, R. J.; Soong, S. J.; Dolin, R. Early vidarabine therapy to control the complications of herpes zoster in immunosuppressed patients. N. Engl. J. Med. 307:971–975; 1982.

Whitley, R. J.; Weiss, H.; Gnann, J.; Tyring, S.; Wolf, J.; Pollard, R.; Mertz, G.; Pappas, P.; Laughlin, C.; Sherrill, L.; Schlupner, C.; Soong, S. J.; and the NIAID Collaborative Antiviral Study Group. The efficacy of steroids and acyclovir therapy of herpes zoster in the elderly. Antiviral Res. 26:A303; 1991.

Wilson, J. B. Thirty-one years of herpes zoster in a rural practice. BMJ 293:1349–1351; 1986.

Wood, M. J.; Kay, R.; Dworkin, R. H.; Soong, S. J.; Whitley, R. J. Oral acyclovir accelerates pain resolu-tion in herpes zoster: a meta-analysis of placebo-controlled trials. Clin. Infect. Dis. 22:341–347; 1996.

PART V

# INFECTIOUS DISORDERS

# 14

# Acute Meningitis

KAREN L. ROOS

Before sulfonamide therapy and the discovery of penicillin in 1931, bacterial meningitis was almost always a fatal disease. Despite the availability of a number of effective antimicrobial agents that penetrate into the cerebrospinal fluid (CSF) in adequate concentrations to eradicate the infection, meningitis remains a devastating neurologic disease of infancy, childhood, and adulthood. The mortality rate for acute bacterial meningitis has not changed significantly over the last several decades. The mortality rate for community-acquired bacterial meningitis is 10% to 30% (Durand et al. 1993; Berg et al. 1996), with a slightly higher mortality rate of 30% to 40% for pneumococcal meningitis (Pfister et al. 1993). The neurological complications of bacterial meningitis are a major cause of the morbidity and mortality. The major neurological complications of this infection include cerebrovascular disease, cerebral edema, communicating and obstructive hydrocephalus, cerebral herniation, seizure activity and status epilepticus, focal neurological deficits, cranial nerve palsies, and subdural effusions and empyemas. The recent emphasis has been on understanding the pathophysiology of the neurological complications in order to develop effective therapies to decrease the host's inflammatory response and thus minimize the neurological complica-

tions. The pathophysiology of bacterial meningitis will be reviewed in order to discuss how present therapies can be used to alter the pathophysiology and improve outcome. The prognostic factors for specific etiological organisms in childhood and adulthood bacterial meningitis will be described with an emphasis on how management can affect outcome. The management of each of the major neurological complications of bacterial meningitis will be discussed. The rationale for the use of dexamethasone and the results of clinical trials to date using adjunctive agents will be reviewed. The major systemic complications of bacterial meningitis, which include septic shock, disseminated intravascular coagulation, the syndrome of inappropriate secretion of antidiuretic hormone, the adult respiratory distress syndrome, and deep vein thrombosis also contribute significantly to outcome, but a discussion of these will not be included in this chapter, except to describe the effect of fluid restriction on outcome of acute bacterial meningitis in childhood. The impact of the emergence of penicillin- and cephalosporin-resistant pneumococcal isolates on clinical disease will be described.

The majority of this chapter will be dedicated to a discussion of the prognosis of acute bacterial meningitis. Viruses, specifically enteroviruses, herpes simplex virus, and the human immuno-deficiency virus (HIV), are also the causative organisms of acute meningitis, but acute viral meningitis is typically a self-limited illness with an excellent prognosis. A discussion of viral meningitis is included with an emphasis on short-term morbidity.

## Bacterial Meningitis

### Pathophysiology

The most common bacteria that cause meningitis, *Neisseria meningitidis* and *Streptococcus pneumoniae* initially colonize the nasopharynx by attaching to the nasopharyngeal epithelial cells. They are then carried across the cell in membrane-bound vacuoles to the intravascular space (Quagliarello and Scheld 1992). Once the bacteria gain access to the bloodstream, they are successful in avoiding phagocytosis by neutrophils because of the presence of a polysaccharide capsule. Bacteria that are able to survive in the bloodstream then enter the CSF through the choroid plexus of the lateral ventricles and through other areas of altered blood-brain barrier permeability. The CSF is an area of impaired host defense. Once meningeal pathogens gain access to the CSF, there are insufficient complement components and immunoglobulins for the opsonization of bacteria, an essential step for phagocytosis by neutrophils. Normal uninfected CSF contains no phagocytic cells, has a low protein concentration, contains no IgM, and has low concentrations of complement components (Zwahlen et al. 1982). The multiplication of bacteria proceeds rapidly. From observations in a rabbit model of pneumococcal meningitis, it appears that once the bacterial concentration in the subarachnoid space reaches a threshold range (approximately $10^6$ colony-forming units [cfu] per milliliter), the inflammatory response commences (Pfister et al. 1994).

The release of bacterial cell-wall components by the lysis of bacteria in the subarachnoid space due to their multiplication and due to bactericidal antibiotic therapy is the initial step in the induction of the inflammatory process and the formation of a purulent exudate in the subarachnoid space. It is not simply the presence of bacteria in the subarachnoid space that induces the inflammatory response, but rather the presence of bacterial cell-wall components due to lysis of bacteria that induces the inflammatory response. The lipopolysaccharide molecules (endotoxin) attached to the outer membranes of gram-negative bacteria and the teichoic acid and peptidoglycan components of the pneumococcal cell wall have been demonstrated in experimental models of meningitis to induce meningeal inflammation by stimulating the production of the proinflammatory cytokines, tumor necrosis factor (TNF) and interleukin-1 (IL-1), by brain astrocytes and microglia (central nervous system [CNS] macrophage-equivalent cells). In experimental models of meningitis, within 1 to 3 hours after the intracisternal inoculation of lipopolysaccharide, TNF and IL-1 are present in CSF followed by the onset of increased concentrations of protein and leukocytes in the CSF. One of the major contributors to the purulent exudate in the subarachnoid space is the increased number of neutrophils in the CSF. The inflammatory cytokines recruit polymorphonuclear leukocytes from the bloodstream and upregulate the expression of selectins on cerebral capillary endothelial cells and leukocytes, which allows for leukocytes to adhere to vascular endothelial cells, and to subsequently migrate into the CSF. Large numbers of leukocytes in the subarachnoid space contribute to the purulent exudate, and obstruct the flow of CSF. The adherence of leukocytes to cerebral capillary endothelial cells increases the permeability of blood vessels, allowing for the leakage of plasma proteins through open intercellular junctions leading to vasogenic brain edema. The results of experimental models of meningitis suggest that bacterial eradication from the CSF is not a leukocyte-dependent phenomenon. The fluid medium of the CSF impairs the phagocytosis of bacteria by neutrophils (Simberkoff et al. 1980; Zwahlen et al. 1982). Neutrophils in the subarachnoid space degranulate and release cytotoxic molecules. The presence of an inflammatory exudate in the subarachnoid space obstructs the flow and resorption of CSF resulting in a transependymal movement of fluid from the ventricular system into the brain parenchyma and interstitial edema. The combination of vasogenic, interstitial, and cytotoxic edema leads to increased intracranial pressure (ICP) and coma.

In both experimental models of meningitis and in clinical studies, it has been shown that during the very early stages of meningitis there is an increase in cerebral blood flow followed soon thereafter by a decrease in cerebral blood flow and a loss of cerebrovascular autoregulation. Cerebral perfusion pressure (CPP) is defined as the difference between the mean arterial pressure (MAP) and the intracranial pressure (CPP = MAP − ICP). Cerebral perfusion pressure is protected by cerebrovascular autoregulation, which dilates or constricts cerebral resistance vessels in response to alterations in cerebral perfusion pressure, due to either changes in the mean arterial blood pressure or changes in intracranial pressure. A loss of cerebrovascular autoregulation means that cerebral blood flow increases when the systemic blood pressure is raised and decreases when systemic blood pressure is lowered. An increase in systemic blood pressure leads to an increase in cerebral blood flow and an increase in ICP. A decrease in mean systemic arterial pressure due to septic shock results in a decrease in cerebral blood flow and cerebral ischemia and infarction. The cerebrovascular complications of bacterial meningitis include not only a loss of cerebrovascular autoregulation, but also narrowing of the large arteries at the base of the brain due to encroachment on the vessel by the purulent exudate in the subarachnoid space and infiltration of the arterial wall by inflammatory cells with intimal thickening, vessel wall irregularities and obstructions of branches of the middle cerebral artery, and thrombosis of the major sinuses and thrombophlebitis of the cerebral cortical veins (Pfister et al. 1992).

There are a number of possible mediators of neuronal injury during bacterial meningitis, including nitric oxide and superoxide produced by activated inflammatory cells, reactive nitrogen species, endogenous excitatory amino acids, and macrophages, all of which are presently under investigation (Pfister et al. 1994).

## Prognostic Factors

### Mortality

In a review of 296 episodes of community-acquired meningitis, in which *Streptococcus pneumoniae* accounted for 37%, *Neisseria meningitidis* for 13%, and *Listeria monocytogenes* for 10% of cases, risk factors for death included older age (≥60 years of age), obtundation on admission, and seizures within the first 24 hours (Durand

et al. 1993). Autopsy records were available for review on 27 of the 40 patients who died within 7 days of presentation. There was evidence of temporal lobe herniation in eight cases; four also had cerebellar herniation. In five, clinical signs of herniation developed within a period ranging from several minutes to several hours after a lumbar puncture; opening pressures were recorded for four patients and were greater than 500 mm of $H_2O$ (Durand et al. 1993).

Older individuals have an increased risk of mortality from pneumococcal meningitis. In a review of 77 cases of pneumococcal meningitis, those patients over 60 years of age had a significantly greater mortality than younger patients ($p < .05$) (Kirkpatrick et al. 1994). In 31 adult patients with pneumococcal meningitis, there was a case fatality rate of 9% for individuals less than 70 years of age, and a case fatality rate of 33% for those older than 70 years of age (Kragsbjerg et al. 1994). The mortality rate of pneumococcal meningitis is lower among children than among adults. An increased rate of mortality from pneumococcal meningitis in children is associated with an altered level of consciousness at the time of admission especially if the child is comatose, the presence of shock, and the need for mechanical ventilation (Kornelisse et al. 1995). The laboratory values associated with a poor outcome from bacterial meningitis in childhood are the following: a decreased CSF glucose concentration, an elevated CSF protein concentration (≥2.5 g/L), and a low serum sodium level (<135 mmol/L) (Kornelisse et al. 1995).

Meningococcal meningitis has a 10% mortality rate. Major risk factors significantly associated with death include the following: (1) age—the case fatality rate is highest in infants less than 5 months of age, individuals over 50 years of age, and children and adolescents between 10 and 19 years of age (Scholten et al. 1994; Olivares et al. 1993); (2) a decreased level of consciousness (Anderson et al. 1997); (3) the presence of purpura fulminans (Olivares et al. 1993); (4) the presence of septicemia (Olivares et al. 1993); and (5) a history of convulsions (Anderson et al. 1997). The serogroup of *Neisseria meningitidis* has been significantly associated with death in some series but not in others. Serogroup A has been associated with a higher risk of death than serogoup B (Olivares et al. 1993).

*Streptococcus agalactiae,* or group B streptococcus (GBS), is a leading causative organism of bacterial meningitis in neonates and is increasingly reported as the etiologic organism of severe infection in adults. The mortality rate from meningitis due to this organism in adults is high, with most series reporting mortality rates of 24% to 50% (Dunne and Quagliarello 1993; Domingo et al. 1997), a case fatality rate comparable to that associated with pneumococcal, gram-negative bacillary and staphylococcal meningitis, all of which tend to occur in debilitated severely ill patients (Domingo et al. 1997; Jensen et al. 1993). Mortality is significantly increased in those patients with a comorbid condition, including diabetes, malignancy, renal failure, cardiac disease, collagen-vascular disease, and concomitant steroid therapy (Dunne and Quagliarello 1993). The mortality rate from bacterial meningitis in infants is also high, ranging from 15% to 30% depending on the etiological organism, immaturity of the infant, and experience of the medical staff with this disease (Trujillo and McCracken 1997).

Mortality rates of 50% are reported in series of *Staphylococcus aureus* meningitis, particularly when *S. aureus* meningitis results from hematogenous spread of infection from a distant extracranial focus, such as endocarditis, and in association with older age and the presence of septic shock (Jensen et al. 1993).

In general, the risk of death from bacterial meningitis is significantly associated with the following: a decreased level of consciousness on admission, the onset of seizures within 24 hours of admission (Durand et al. 1993), signs of increased intracranial pressure, young age (infancy) and age over 50, the presence of a comorbid condition, the presence of shock and/or the need for mechanical ventilation, and delay in the initiation of treatment. Abnormal CSF values, specifically decreased glucose concentration (<40 mg/dl) and increased protein concentration (≥300 mg/dl) reach statistical significance as factors predictive of increased mortality rate in some series but not in others (Durand et al. 1993; Kornelisse et al. 1995).

### Neurological Complications

Most series that look at prognostic indicators and outcome of bacterial meningitis do not separate those prognostic factors that are associated with acute neurological complications, such as increased intracranial pressure, seizure activity, hydrocephalus, stroke, transient sensorineural hearing impairment, from those prognostic factors that are associated with neurological sequelae, such as permanent sensorineural hearing impairment, chronic seizure disorder, mental retardation, and spastic quadriplegia. The importance of making such a distinction is suggested by the observations of a number of investigators that a higher percentage of children with bacterial meningitis have neurological abnormalities at the time of discharge than have neurological abnormalities 5 years later (Feigin 1992; Pikis et al. 1996). On the other hand, many of the same prognostic factors that are associated with acute neurological complications would be expected to be associated with neurologic sequelae. In a series that looked at outcome of bacterial meningitis in school-age survivors, children with acute neurological complications were at increaed risk for neurological sequelae (Grimwood et al. 1995). In general, the presence of coma and/or shock on admission, hypotension within the first 24 hours after pediatric intensive care unit (ICU) admission, and a CSF glucose concentration of less than 0.6 mmol/L are associated with sequelae in children (Kornelisse et al. 1995; Madagame et al. 1995). The presence of coma on admission appears to be the strongest predictor of increased morbidity (Pikis et al. 1996). Neurological sequelae, including hearing loss, hydrocephalus, seizure activity, and mental retardation have been reported in 29% to 56% of children with pneumococcal meningitis (Kornelisse et al. 1995). The causative organism of the meningitis appears to be significantly associated with outcome in children. Pneumococcal meningitis is reported to have the highest frequency of later sequelae followed by *Haemophilus influenzae* and meningococcal meningitis (Kaaresen and Flaegstad 1995; Baraff et al. 1993). Overall, 25% of children with bacterial meningitis have functionally important disabilities years later, including mild to moderate hearing loss, learning disabilities, and behavior problems (Grimwood et al. 1995). Approximately 10% of children who survive bacterial meningitis have major neurological sequelae, including seizures, hydrocephalus, spasticity, blindness, or severe to profound hearing loss (Grimwood et al. 1995). The risk of permanent neurological sequelae in gram-negative bacillary meningitis in the newborn period is high. In a series of 98 newborns and infants ranging in age from 1 day to 2 years with gram-negative enteric bacillary meningitis, 34 of 59 (58%) survivors had permanent neurological sequelae, including hydrocephalus in 16 (27%), seizure disorder in 21 (36%), permanent spastic paralysis in 18 (31%), and. severe neurological deficits requiring constant care in 13 (22%). Thirty-seven percent of the patients had developmental delay, of whom 59% had severe mental retardation. A hearing deficit was documented in 17% of the patients. Factors associated significantly with sequelae included a platelet count less than 100,000/mm$^3$, a CSF leukocyte count greater than 2000/mm$^3$, a CSF to serum glucose ratio less than 0.5, a CSF protein concentration greater than or equal to 200 mg/dl, and a positive CSF culture for 48 hours or more after the start of treatment (Unhanand et al. 1993).

In adults, the major neurological complications of bacterial meningitis include seizure activity, cerebral edema, hydrocephalus, arterial and venous cerebrovascular disease, cerebral herniation, cranial nerve palsies, subdural effusion, and brain abscess. There were abnormalities on cranial computed tomography (CT) scan in 34 of 87 (39%) adult patients with community-acquired bacterial meningitis, including ventriculomegaly or hydrocephalus (13 patients), cerebral edema (five), meningeal enhancement (four), cerebral infarction (four), subdural effusion (two), abscess (two), lesions consistent with septic emboli (two), cavernous sinus thrombosis (one), and subdural empyema (one). Cerebral infarctions that were not apparent on the admission CT scan were seen on later CT scans (>72 hours after admission) in four patients (Durand et al. 1993). *Streptococcus pneumoniae* accounted for 37% of the cases of community-acquired bacterial meningitis, *Neisseria meningitidis* for 13%, and *Listeria monocytogenes* for 10%. Cerebrovascular disease and brain edema were the most important and most severe neurological complications in 86 adult patients (between the ages of 15 and 87 years) with bacterial meningitis (Pfister et al. 1993). In this series, *Streptococcus pneumoniae* was the causative organism in 30 patients (34.9%), *Neisseria meningitidis* in five (5.8%), *Haemophilus influenzae* in six (7%), *Staphylococcus aureus* in 5 (5.8%), and other organisms, including *Listeria*

*monocytogenes, Escherichia coli,* and *Streptococcus viridans* in the remainder. Cerebrovascular complications were identified in 13 patients who underwent angiography, including (1) arterial narrowing of the supraclinoid portion of the internal carotid artery; (2) vessel wall irregularities, focal dilatations, and occlusions of distal branches of the middle cerebral artery; (3) focal abnormal parenchymal blush; and (4) thrombosis of the superior sagittal sinus and cortical veins. Cerebral herniation occured in seven patients during the first 5 days of illness, and was caused by edema in four patients, by angiographically documented sinus venous thrombosis in two, and by hydrocephalus in one. Communicating hydrocephalus developed in eight patients and obstructive hydrocephalus in two. Of the 70 survivors of bacterial meningitis in this series, two (2.3%) remained in a vegetative state, seven (8.1%) had severe disability, five (5.8%) had moderate or slight disability, and 56 (65.1%) recovered completely. Patients with pneumococcal meningitis had the worst prognosis.

## Improving Outcome

The prevention and management of the neurological complications of bacterial meningitis is the best means to improve outcome. Each of the neurological complications and their management will be discussed. Fluid management in children is also reviewed.

### Coma

Raised intracranial pressure as a result of vasogenic, interstitial, and cytotoxic edema is the major cause of coma in this disease. Vasogenic edema is due to altered blood-brain permeability, interstitial edema is due to obstruction of CSF flow and altered CSF resorption resulting in acute hydrocephalus, and cytotoxic edema is due to ischemia from arterial and venous infarction and also the degranulation of polymorphonuclear leukocytes. As described above, coma is a poor prognostic indicator. Patients that are obtunded or comatose should have an ICP measurement and monitoring device. Normal ICP, as measured by an ICP monitoring device, is less than 10 mm Hg. Sustained elevations in ICP above 15 mm Hg should be treated. The treatment of raised intracranial pressure is as outlined below (Chang and Bleck 1997):

1. Elevate the head of the bed 30 degrees and keep the head in the midline position.
2. Hyperventilation to maintain $PaCO_2$ between 25 and 33 mm Hg. Do not decrease below 25 mm Hg, as this may cause cerebral ischemia.
3. Mannitol: 1.0 g/kg bolus injection and then 0.25 to 0.5 g/kg every 4 to 6 hours based on ICP measurements. The effect of mannitol reaches its peak between 30 and 60 minutes after it is administered and lasts for 4 to 6 hours. Keep serum osmolarity between 295 and 320 mOsm/L.
4. Dexamethasone 0.15 mg/kg every 6 hours.
5. Pentobarbital coma:
   Loading dose: 10 to 15 mg/kg intravenously given at a rate of 1 mg/kg/min.
   Maintenance dose: 1 to 3 mg/kg/h. Therapy can be titrated to achieve a therapeutic serum level of 25 to 40 mg/L or a burst-suppression pattern on electroencephalography (EEG).
6. Thiopental: The dose is 1 to 5 mg/kg bolus. Thiopental is shorter acting than pentobarbital in bolus doses and can be used to treat brief increases in intracranial pressure such as occurs with endotracheal intubation. When continuous infusion is necessary, tissue accumulation of thiopental occurs. Pentobarbital should be used for continuous infusion.

### Cerebral Herniation

Cerebral edema, either focal or generalized, can lead to cerebral herniation. In a review of autopsy records of 27 patients who died within 7 days of presentation of bacterial meningitis, there was evidence of temporal lobe herniation in eight cases; four also had cerebellar herniation. All had cerebral edema; two also had dural sinus or cortical vein thrombosis (Durand et al. 1993). In a series of acute bacterial meningitis in 302 infants and children, cerebral herniation occurred in 18 cases (6%). In all 18 patients, cerebral herniation happened within 8 hours of admission, and in eight cases cerebral herniation occurred within 30 minutes of admission. Three of the patients with this complication died, and 4 of the 15 patients who survived had severe neurologic deficits at the time of discharge from the hospital. In the eight patients who developed clinical signs of cerebral herniation within 30 minutes of admission to the hospital, a possible relationship to lumbar puncture was suggested. In each case the amount of CSF removed

was approximately 2 to 3 ml. One of the patients developed respiratory arrest and fixed and dilated pupils immediately following lumbar puncture (Horwitz et al. 1980). In Durand's series, clinical signs of herniation developed within a period ranging from several minutes to several hours after lumbar puncture in five patients. In their classic paper on bacterial meningitis, Dodge and Swartz addressed the issue of the relationship of cerebral herniation to lumbar puncture. In this series of 29 patients dying with acute bacterial meningitis, there were three cases of temporal lobe herniation, and seven cases of cerebellar herniation. Death from herniation followed lumbar puncture immediately or within 2 hours in three cases. The difficulty in attributing these episodes of cerebral herniation to lumbar puncture is emphasized by the patient with meningococcal meningitis in this series who died of medullary compression from a cerebellar pressure cone before lumbar puncture (Dodge and Swartz 1965). In a prospective study of 86 patients with bacterial meningitis between the ages of 15 and 87, cerebral herniation occurred in seven patients during the acute phase of the illness. This was due to cerebral edema in four patients, angiographically documented sinus venous thrombosis in two patients, and hydrocephalus in one patient (Pfister et al. 1993).

In a retrospective study to determine whether the incidence of cerebral herniation was increased immediately after lumbar puncture, the medical records of 445 children (aged 1 month and older) with bacterial meningitis were reviewed. Cerebral herniation occurred in 19 (4%) of the 445 children. Herniation occurred within 3 hours of lumbar puncture in eight children. Of these children, three had signs suggesting impending herniation at the time of the procedure (these children were comatose and unresponsive to pain at the time of the lumbar puncture), cerebral herniation had occurred previously in one child (this child had had dilatation of one pupil before being paralyzed and mechanically ventilated), one child with cerebral palsy was hard to assess, and one child had decerebrate posturing at the time of lumbar puncture. Six of the 19 episodes of herniation occurred before lumbar puncture or in a child that did not undergo lumbar puncture (Rennick et al. 1993; Jones and Webb 1993).

The risk of cerebral herniation from acute bacterial meningitis is approximately 6% to 8%. Focal

ability to live outside of an institution. Moderate impairment was defined as requiring institutional care, while severe impairment was essentially a vegetative state. This study looked at the prognostic significance of lesions on magnetic resonance imaging (MRI), electrolyte abnormalities, and degree of CSF pleocytosis. On the MRIs, 13 out of 14 patients had abnormalities and all comatose patients had abnormal MRIs. The MRI appearance did not, however, have prognostic significance. Most commonly, lesions on MRI were found in the thalamus and basal ganglia in 70% of patients. Brain stem lesions were found in 43% of patients. CSF pleocytosis was common and was neutrophilic (median white blood cell [WBC] count was 370 cells/mm$^3$ with a median of 70% neutrophils). There was only a moderate increase of CSF protein (median, 92 mg/dl) and no hypoglycorrhachia was noted. The two main prognostic factors at initial presentation were degree of pleocytosis and hyponatremia. If normal and mild impairment are labeled as favorable outcomes and moderate and severe impairment are denoted unfavorable, it was found that 10 of 13 (77%) patients with a CSF pleocytosis of greater than 500 cells/mm$^3$ had unfavorable outcomes, while only 6 of 21 (29%) of those with a pleocytosis less than 500 cells/mm$^3$ had unfavorable outcomes. Of patients with a serum sodium of less than 130 mmol/L, 12 of 14 (86%) had an unfavorable outcome, while of those with a sodium greater than 130 mmol/L only 4 of 16 (25%) did so.

The prognosis of EEE is therefore rather poor, both for survival and meaningful neurological recovery. The mortality rate in the older series was about 70%, while more recent series showed mortality rates of 30% to 40%, possibly reflecting improved support of patients in the acute phase of the disease. Evolution of the host-virus interaction may also have led to the lower level of mortality of more recently described cases. Extremes of age, high pleocytosis, hyponatremia, and rapid onset of disease are negative prognostic factors.

### Western Equine Encephalitis

Western equine encephalitis (WEE) is seen in the western United States and Canada. It is caused by an alphavirus, as is EEE, which is maintained in birds and transmitted by the mosquito *Culex tarsalis*. It is rare and usually seen in epidemics. There is less known about WEE than EEE, per-

haps because of the lack of proximity of large academic medical centers to areas where epidemics occur, but it appears to have a somewhat less grim prognosis (Herzon et al. 1957). Of 636 cases summarized from a review of the literature, only about 13.5% had major sequelae, which included quadriplegia, paraplegia, rigidity, and mental retardation (Herzon et al. 1957). Infants were particularly vulnerable, and 30% of those less than 1 year of age, and especially less than 3 months, were left with severe residua. About 30% of those beyond infancy developed a parkinsonian-like state (Herzon et al. 1957). While dementia can improve over the year following the acute illness, personality changes can persist. In some autopsies, exclusively in patients with severe residua, active inflammatory changes can be seen years after the acute illness, and this has been interpreted as a chronic encephalitis (Herzon et al. 1957). In a more recent study of 35 patients with WEE, 12 (34 %) had significant sequelae (Earnest et al. 1971). Of the 14 children aged less than 1 year when the illness occurred, nine (64%) had significant sequelae (mental retardation, spasticity, and recurrent seizures). Of the five patients who were between 1 and 2 years of age when the illness occurred, three (60%) had mild cognitive deficits. Of the 16 patients over 2 years of age when the illness occurred, none had unequivocal sequelae. The degree of severity of the residua correlated with the severity of the initial illness. The fatality rate of WEE is low. In a series of 39 patients with WEE acquired during the 1975 epidemic in North Dakota and western Minnesota, the case fatality rate was 7.7% (Leech et al. 1981).

The prognosis is guarded, especially in those with severe illness, and in very young children. Older children have a much better prognosis.

### Japanese B Encephalitis

Japanese B encephalitis (JBE) is endemic in Southeast Asia and is caused by a mosquito-borne flavivirus of the West Nile complex, with a single-stranded, positive-sense RNA genome. The virus occurs in birds and pigs and is transmitted by *Culex tritaeniorhyncus* mosquitoes. Most human infections are inapparent, but a variable (1:50 to 1:1000) proportion of infections result in encephalitis.

Much of the initial information about JBE was obtained from illness occurring in U.S. servicemen stationed in various areas of Southeast Asia, as well as the civilians living there. An epidemic of JBE occurred in Okinawa in 1945, and 66 patients, civilians living in the area, were reported on (Table 16-3) (Lewis et al. 1947). There were 22 patients between the ages of 12 and 16 years and 28 between 5 and 9 years of age. The two patients over 30 years of age were 36 and 51. Seventeen (26%) patients recovered completely, nine (14%) patients died, and 39 patients had a long, protracted illness. Eighteen of these patients (46%) had good recoveries, 17 (44%) had neurological residua, and four (10%) died. Thus, overall, 53% of JBE patients had good recoveries, 26% had residual neurological deficits, and 20% died. Of the patients who survived, recovery began within 3 to 41 days.

A large epidemic occurred in Korea in 1950, and approximately 300 servicemen were affected. Two hundred of these cases were seen at an evacuation hospital in Pusan, and were summarized and reported in 1952 (Lincoln and Sivertson 1952). All patients were men aged between 18 and 24 years of age. The acute mortality rate was 8.5%. All patients had high fever. Continual rise in temperature and the appearance of diaphoresis, tachypnea, and accumulation of bronchial secretions were grave prognostic signs, usually followed by death in a day or so. Long-term follow-up data were not given in this report. Another series reported 299 servicemen who developed JBE between July and October 1950 while serving in Korea (Dickerson et al. 1920). The immediate mortality rate was 10%. Follow-up was reported for 110 patients, all of whom had a uniform clinical picture, but only 65 of whom had serological confirmation of the diagnosis. Ten weeks after onset of the illness, only 12 of the 65 (18%) were significantly impaired, mostly intel-

lectually and behaviorally. In those that recovered, resolution of the neurological deficits was often astonishingly sudden and rapid. Poor prognostic indicators included positive Babinski's signs, prolonged fever (>10 days), albuminuria, and very high pleocytosis (>1000 cells/mm³).

Fifty-seven U.S. servicemen developed JBE during an epidemic in Vietnam in 1969 (Ketel and Ognibene 1971). Only one patient died. This unusually low mortality was attributed by the authors to the rapid provision of intensive supportive care. Residual difficulties in mentation, memory and attention deficits, and dementia reportedly occurred in 95% of patients, but further details were not given, and it is impossible to know what proportions of these were mild, moderate, or severe.

In a series of 49 patients in Thailand seen at a major medical center between June and August 1983, the mortality rate was 33% (Burke et al. 1985). Patients with JBE virus (JBEV) isolatable from the CSF, low levels of JBEV IgG and IgM in the CSF, and semicoma or coma had the worst prognosis. Age, gender, days ill before admission, distance of home to hospital, CSF protein, and degree of CSF pleocytosis were not significant prognostic factors.

Children appear to have a worse prognosis than adults, in some studies. In one series of 132 child patients, ages 6 months to 12 years, from India, the acute mortality rate was 36.9%. Rapid onset of the disease, deep coma, respiratory abnormalities, and decerebrate posturing were significantly predictive of mortality (Kumar et al. 1990). In a follow-up study of 55 survivors in this series, only 29.2% were completely normal, and only 25.4% were felt to have minor residua (Kumar et al. 1993).

In a clinical trial of the effect of dexamethasone on outcome in JBE, 65 patients were randomized

**Table 16-3.** Reports of Epidemics of Japanese B Encephalitis

| Year | Location | Number and Type of Patients | Mortality (%) | Recovery with Residual Deficits (%) | Mild to No Deficits | Reference |
|------|----------|-----------------------------|---------------|-------------------------------------|---------------------|-----------|
| 1945 | Okinawa | 66 (civilians) | 20 | 26 | 53 | Lewis et al. |
| 1950 | Korea | 200 (military) | 8.5 | | | Lincoln and Sivertson |
| 1950 | Korea | 110 (military) | 10 | 18 | | Dickerson |
| 1969 | Vietnam | 57 (military) | 2 | 95 | | Ketel and Ognibene |
| 1983 | Thailand | 49 (civilians) | 33 | | | Burke et al. |
| 1991 | China | 70 (civilians) | 4 | 47% | | Dapeng et al. |
| 1985–88 | Lucknow, India | 93 (civilians) | 36.9 | | | Kumar et al. |

to either dexamethasone 0.6 mg/kg loading dose, and 0.2 mg/kg intravenously every 6 hours for 5 days, or to identical-appearing placebo (Hoke et al. 1992). There was no benefit to dexamethasone administration, since survival (mortality rate was 24% in the treatment group and 27% in the control group) and neurological status 3 months after discharge from hospital (45% abnormal in each group) were the same in the two groups.

Japanese B encephalitis is a severe disease, with a mortality rate between 2% and 40%, and a variable frequency of residual deficits. The reason for the highly variable mortality and morbidity rates between different epidemics is not clear, and may involve the availability of medical care, different patient populations, or different strains of the virus. The overall prognosis is guarded.

### Tick-Borne Encephalitis

Tick-borne encephalitis (TBE) consists of several diseases, Powassan encephalitis in North America, and Western (WTBE) and Far Eastern tick-borne encephalitis, also known as Russian spring-summer encephalitis (RSSE) in Central Europe and the easternmost part of the former Soviet Union, respectively. Powassan encephalitis is extremely rare. These viruses are related flaviviruses, consisting of a single-stranded, positive-sense RNA genome. The literature on WTBE and RSSE in English is sparse.

The Far Eastern form of TBE is a typical acute encephalitis, with mortality rates between 5% and 30% (Smorodintsev 1958). A variable proportion of patients are left with lower motor weakness in the neck and shoulders, and it is said that in parts of the former Soviet Union, flaccidity of shoulder muscles and weakness of the neck (often requiring the patient to prop up his head manually), with a compatible history, is virtually pathognomonic of a previous episode of RSSE (Smorodintsev 1958). A small proportion of patients with RSSE develop a chronic progressive encephalitis 6 months to many years after the initial illness. This is stated to occur in 1% to 20% of RSSE patients (Asher 1979). One well-documented case occurred in a Japanese man who had RSSE while in a prisoner-of-war camp, and who recovered with shoulder atrophy. Thirteen years later, he developed headache, memory problems, tinnitus, dysarthria, and gait ataxia, which progressed to death over a course of 10 years (Ogawa et al. 1973). Another characteristic sequela of RSSE is that of a focal continuous partial epilepsy, epilepsia partialis continua, or Kozhevnikov's epilepsy. Approximately 1% to 2% of RSSE patients are said to develop Kozhevnikov's epilepsy (Brody 1964).

The Western form of TBE is also clinically a typical acute encephalitis, but the prognosis appears to be better than in the Far Eastern form of the disease. About half the cases have a biphasic course, with an acute febrile illness that resolves after a few days and is then followed by the encephalitis phase. In 20 children with the disease, 19 were said to have a benign course (Kaiser 1995). The overall mortality rate is about 1%, and about 10% of patients appear to have residual neurological deficits (Valdueza et al. 1996).

Powassan encephalitis is a tick-borne encephalitis transmitted by *Ixodes* ticks (which also transmit Lyme disease) in North America. It is quite rare, but has been reported to occur in New York State, New Jersey, Ontario, and Quebec. Of 16 cases in the literature, outcomes were reported in 14. Two patients (14%) died, seven (50%) had severe motor deficits, one had recurrent severe headaches (7%), and four (29%) had no residua (Wilson et al. 1979; Jackson 1989).

## Parainfectious Encephalitides

### Acute Disseminated Encephalomyelitis

Acute disseminated encephalomyelitis (ADEM) is an acute, usually monophasic, diffuse or multifocal inflammatory, usually demyelinating disease of the CNS, characterized by a febrile encephalopathy with variable focal abnormalities (Tselis and Lisak 1997). It generally begins a few days to a few weeks after a nonspecific viral syndrome, with the abrupt onset of confusion, fever, and focal weakness, and may progress to stupor or coma. The disease can be difficult to differentiate from a viral encephalitis clinically, but MRI of the brain shows extensive white matter lesions, in contrast to the gray matter lesions of lytic viral encephalitis. The disease may, rarely, be confused with the heralding manifestation of multiple sclerosis. Focal, restricted presentations, which include optic neuritis, transverse myelitis, and brain stem leukoencephalitis, are more often the initial presentations of multiple sclerosis.

In the past, the most frequent inciting illness has been measles, but most cases of ADEM now follow upper respiratory infections, the etiology of which is usually undiagnosed. Vaccination with rabies vaccine prepared in neural tissues is a common trigger of the disease in the Third World. The pathogenesis is uncertain but involves a cell-mediated autoimmune attack on CNS myelin. The pathology consists of perivenular infiltrates of inflammatory cells and variable degrees of demyelination. No virus (or other agent) is isolated from brain. Various treatments have been attempted, the most common being high-dose intravenous methylprednisolone, but none has been subject to a proper clinical trial. Most patients survive, with varying degrees of deficit but, astonishingly, complete recoveries can occur (Tselis and Lisak 1997). Case series of ADEM are rarely published nowadays, since the main recognizable triggers of the disease—measles, mumps, rubella, and varicella—have been almost completely eradicated by modern vaccine strategies, and so ADEM following these diseases is quite rare. It is to older, or Third World, series that we must turn to learn the natural history of the disease.

For ADEM following measles, a mortality of 22.1% is quoted in a review of parainfectious encephalomyelitides published in 1956 (Miller et al. 1956). For ADEM following rubella, varicella, and mumps, the mortality rates were 20%, 10%, and 22.2%, respectively. Significant sequelae were common (Miller et al. 1956). More recent data suggest a much more benign prognosis. In a more recent series of 121 children (some of whom had restricted forms of ADEM, such as transverse myelitis), however, none died and 82% had complete recoveries (Rust et al. 1997). Seventeen of these patients (14%) eventually had further episodes that satisfied the criteria of multiple sclerosis. It is likely that the better outcome of the more recent series illustrates the advances in the intensive care of these patients. It is also possible that ADEM triggered by a more modern spectrum of viruses has a different natural history than that due to the measles, rubella, and varicella infections that were much more common before the modern era of vaccination.

## Subacute and Chronic Encephalitides

### Human Immunodeficiency Virus Encephalitis

This is the most common form of chronic viral encephalitis in North America and is discussed in a separate chapter.

## Subacute Sclerosing Panencephalitis

Subacute sclerosing panencephalitis (SSPE) is a chronic progressive infection of the brain with a defective measles virus (single-stranded, positive-sense RNA genome). SSPE occurred after a several-month to several-year latent period in about 1 per 1 million patients with preceding measles infection before vaccination was widespread. It was essentially no longer seen in North America, once measles vaccination became widespread (Modlin et al. 1979). Typically, patients are in late childhood or early adolescence at the onset of disease. The disease often occurs in those patients who had natural measles at an age of less than 2 years.

The first case of SSPE was reported by Dawson in 1933 (Dawson 1933). This was a 16-year-old boy who presented with personality changes, poor memory, and slowness of behavior that progressed to lethargy, increasing myoclonic jerks, high fever, and death. At autopsy, perivascular infiltrates, neuronal dropout and necrosis, and intraneuronal cytoplasmic inclusion bodies were seen. This course illustrates the stereotyped progression of the disease, which begins with behavioral changes and progresses to a vegetative state (Freeman 1969). The course is usually steadily progressive, leading to death about 9 months after onset (Freeman 1969). Very rapid progression, with death 5 and 6 weeks after onset, has been reported (Gilden et al. 1975). Long survivals of 8 years (Landau and Luse 1958) and 14 years with a remitting-relapsing course (Cobb et al. 1984) have also been reported. It has been estimated that about 5% of patients with SSPE have spontaneous long-term improvement (Risk et al. 1978). However, even these patients are severely impaired, even though they may be able to carry out activities of daily living (Risk et al. 1978).

Therapy for SSPE has not been conspicuously successful. Only modest therapeutic responses have been achieved (Huttenlocher and Mattson 1979; Huttenlocher et al. 1986). The prognosis of SSPE is therefore poor.

### Progressive Rubella Panencephalitis

This is an exceedingly rare disease, of which there are very few reports. It is a chronic progressive degenerative disease due to infection of the brain with rubella virus. The virus is a member of the rubivirus genus of the *Togaviridae* family, and consists of a single-stranded, positive-sense RNA genome. The disease occurs almost exclusively in those with congenital rubella syndrome, and is characterized by progressive dementia, myoclonus, and cerebellar ataxia in children and young adults, with high titers of antibody to rubella virus in serum and CSF. No treatment has been described, and the disease progresses steadily over several years (Townsend et al. 1975). It may resemble SSPE (Weil et al. 1975). The prognosis appears to be very poor.

### Progressive Multifocal Leukoencephalopathy

Progressive multifocal leukoencephalopathy (PML) is due to a papovavirus infection of oligodendrocytes and astrocytes in patients with moderate to severe cell-mediated immune dysfunction, most commonly in patients with AIDS. Before the AIDS epidemic, the disease was seen in patients with lymphoma, Hodgkin's disease, cancer, sarcoidosis, and tuberculosis, and very rarely in those without obvious immune deficiency. Papovaviruses consist of a circular, double-stranded DNA genome, and the virus that causes PML is known as JC papovavirus. The disease causes multifocal areas of myelin destruction in the CNS and is progressive. Clinically, it is characterized by a progressive dulling of behavior, weakness, central visual loss, ocular motor dysfunction, spastic hemiparesis, gait ataxia, and death. In a review of 22 cases of PML published before the AIDS epidemic, Richardson noted a survival of 3 to 4 months from onset of neurological signs (Richardson 1961). Twenty-two cases of PML in AIDS patients had a similar survival (Berger et al. 1987). A recent trial of cytosine arabinoside in AIDS-associated PML, diagnosed by biopsy in patients with a compatible clinical presentation and MRI findings, showed no benefit (Hall et al. 1998).

### Prion diseases

#### Creutzfeldt-Jakob Disease, Gerstmann-Straussler-Scheinker Syndrome, and Fatal Familial Insomnia

Prion diseases are a fascinating group of degenerative brain diseases in which there is accumulation of an abnormal isoform (PrP-sc) of a normal cellular protein (PrP-c) in the brain. This leads to neuronal dropout, status spongiosus, a few amyloid plaques, and astrocytosis. The clinical presentation consists of forgetfulness, and unsteadiness of gait, progressing to dementia, spasticity, ataxia, and myoclonus, leading eventually to a vegetative state. In most patients, the electroencephalogram (EEG) shows periodic discharges that evolve into a burst-suppression pattern. The disease usually occurs in late middle age, being very rare before the age of 40 years. The diseases are also known as transmissible spongiform encephalopathies, because of their transmissibility to laboratory primates and characteristic neuropathology. There are several forms of prion disease: Creutzfeldt-Jakob disease (CJD), which presents with dementia; Gerstmann-Straussler-Scheinker syndrome, which presents with gait ataxia; and fatal familial insomnia, which presents with insomnia and autonomic instability. The progression of all of these leads to a final common state of unresponsiveness and inanition and to death within 6 months of onset (Brown et al. 1994). However, a case of Creutzfeldt-Jakob disease of 14 years' duration has been reported (Cutler et al. 1984). There is no effective treatment for prion diseases.

There are three basic modes of prion disease occurrence: sporadic, familial, and iatrogenic. The disease occurs sporadically in about 1 case per 1 million people per year. About 10% of prion diseases display an autosomal dominant transmission. The disease can be transmitted by corneal (Duffy et al. 1974) and dural grafts (Clavel and Clavel 1996), and pituitary extracts (Brown et al. 1985). For this reason, transplant organs are no longer obtained from patients dying of undiagnosed neurological disease and pituitaries are not harvested from autopsies.

#### New Variant Creutzfeldt-Jakob Disease and Bovine Spongiform Encephalopathy

Recently, a new form of prion disease has been described. Ten cases of an unusual illness in young people, all less than 40 years of age at onset, was reported in which the patients had emotional disturbances, leading to dementia, myoclonus, ataxia, and death (Will et al. 1996). The EEG did not show the typical pattern of periodic sharp wave complexes in these patients, and prion disease was diagnosed generally at autopsy. The duration of illness has been between 7.5 and 22.5

months, with a median of 12 months. The disease was different from most cases of Creutzfeldt-Jakob disease in that patients were young, less than 40 years of age, and there was a very much greater quantity of disseminated amyloid (or kuru) plaques than is usually seen in CJD. This new form of prion disease has been labeled new variant Creutzfeldt-Jakob disease (nvCJD).

Although rare, nvCJD is of great importance, since it has been linked to contamination of the food supply by infected beef. It was noted in 1986 that some cattle in England were disoriented, ataxic, and abnormally aggressive. The disease was variously called mad cow disease and bovine spongiform encephalopathy (BSE). On neuropathological examination, the affected animals were found to have a spongiform encephalopathy (Wells et al. 1986). Epidemiological studies showed that the onset of the disease followed several years after changes in the manufacturing process of meat and bone meal (MBM), which was used as a protein supplement in cattle feed (Wilesmith 1996). It is probable that the previous manufacturing process inactivated the infectivity of the BSE agent. Banning of supplementation of cattle feed with MBM was followed by a progressive reduction in BSE, which has been projected to be essentially eliminated by the year 2000 (Nathanson et al. 1997). There is evidence that nvCJD occurs in humans who have ingested BSE-contaminated beef in England. Indeed, the pathology of nvCJD is reminiscent of kuru, which was likely to have been orally transmitted. Furthermore, the neuropathological and incubation time spectra of BSE and nvCJD transmitted to various strains of mice were very similar to each other, and different from the patterns seen from transmission from sporadic CJD and from scrapie (Bruce et al. 1997; Hill et al. 1997). This is strong evidence that nvCJD is the human form of BSE. It is unclear how far the disease has penetrated the human population, although the recent observation of prion immunoreactivity in the appendix prior to the onset of nvCJD may allow that to be assessed (Hilton et al. 1998).

## Conclusion

Viral encephalitis is usually a severe, devastating disease, with variable prognosis, depending on the causative virus and host factors such as age. In some viral encephalitides, the prognosis is uniformly good (La Crosse encephalitis) or grim (rabies, SSPE, PRP, prion disease). In others, it is guarded (EEE, WEE, Japanese encephalitis, SLE). Generally, patients with greater severity of symptoms tend to have more adverse outcomes. Those at the extremes of age are usually at greater risk of mortality or, if they survive, of residual morbidity. Encephalitis patients with a deepening coma and autonomic signs have a very poor prognosis for survival. In some viral encephalitides (Japanese B encephalitis and eastern equine encephalitis), a high pleocytosis is indicative of a poor prognosis.

There are many cases in which the causative virus is never discovered. The prognosis in such cases is highly uncertain, but impressive recoveries can occur after a very long convalescence, and it is reasonable to treat patients aggressively.

## References

Alvarez, L.; Fajardo, R.; Lopez, E.; Pedroza, R.; Hemachudha, T.; Kamolvarin, N.; et al. Partial recovery from rabies in a nine year old boy. Pediatr. Infect. Dis. J. 13:1154–1155; 1994.

Arribas, J. R.; Storch, G. A.; Clifford, D. B.; Tselis, A. C. Cytomegalovirus encephalitis. Ann. Intern. Med. 125:577–587; 1996.

Artenstein, A. W.; Hicks, C. B.; Goodwin, B. S., Jr.; Hilliard, J. K. Human infection with B virus following a needlestick injury. Rev. Infect. Dis. 13:288–291; 1991.

Asher, D. M. Persistent tick-borne encephalitis infection in man and monkeys: relation to chronic neurologic disease. In: Arctic and tropical arboviruses. New York: Academic Press; 1979.

Ayres, J. C.; Feemster, R. F. The sequelae of eastern equine encephalitis. N. Engl. J. Med. 240: 960–962; 1957.

Balfour, H. H., Jr.; Siem, R. A.; Bauer, H.; Quie, P. G. California arbovirus (La Crosse) infections. 1. Clinical and laboratory findings in 66 children with meningoencephalitis. Pediatrics 52:680–691; 1973.

Berger, J. R.; Kaszovitz, B.; Post, M. J. D.; Dickinson, G. Progressive multifocal leukoencephalopathy associated with human immunodeficiency virus infection. A review of the literature with a report of sixteen cases. Ann. Intern. Med. 107:78–87; 1987.

Bernstein, T. C.; Wolff, H. G. Involvement of the nervous system in infectious mononucleosis. Ann. Intern. Med. 35:1120–1138; 1950.

Bistrian, B.; Phillips, C. A.; Kaye, I. S. Fatal mumps meningoencephalitis. Isolation of virus premortem and postmortem. JAMA 222:478–479; 1972.

Bodensteiner, J. B.; Morris, H. H.; Howell, J. T.; Schochet, S. S. Chronic echo type 5 virus meningoencephalitis in X-linked hypogammaglobulinemia: treatment with immune plasma. Neurology 29:815–819; 1979.

Bray, P. F.; Culp, K. W.; McFarlin, D. E.; Panitch, H. S.; Torkelson, R. D.; Schlight, J. P. Demyelinating disease after neurologically complicated primary Epstein-Barr virus infection. Neurology 42:278–282; 1992.

Brody, J. A. Chronic sequelae of tick-borne encephalitis and Vilyuisk encephalitis. National Institute of Neurological Disorders and Blindness Institute Monograph No.2. Slow, latent and temperate virus infections. U.S. Government Printing Office; 1964: p. 111–113.

Brown, P.; Gajdusek, D. C.; Gibbs, C. J., Jr.; Asher, D. M. Potential epidemic of Creutzfeldt-Jakob disease from human growth hormone therapy. N. Engl. J. Med. 313:728–731; 1985.

Brown, P.; Gibbs, C. J.; Rodgers-Johnson, P.; Asher, D. M.; Sulima, M.; et al. Human spongiform encephalopathy: the National Institutes of Health series of 300 cases of experimentally transmitted disease. Ann. Neurol. 35:513–529; 1994.

Bruce, M. E.; Will, R. G.; Ironside, J. W.; McConnell, I.; Drummond, D.; Suttie, A.; McCardle, L.; Chree, A.; Hope, J.; et al. Transmission to mice indicate that 'new variant' CJD is caused by the BSE agent. Nature 389:498–501; 1997.

Burke, D. S.; Lorsomrudee, W.; Leake, C. J.; Hoke, C. H.; Nisalak, A.; Chongswasdi, V.; Laorakpongse, T. Fatal outcome in Japanese encephalitis. Am. J. Trop. Med. Hyg. 34:1203–1210; 1985.

Centers for Disease Control. Rabies in a laboratory worker. MMWR Morb. Mortal. Wkly. Rep. 26: 183–184; 1977.

Centers for Disease Control. MMWR update: progress toward global eradication of poliomyelitis. MMWR Morb. Mortal. Wkly. Rep. 45:565–568; 1996.

Centers for Disease Control and Prevention. Outbreak of Hendra-like virus—Malaysia and Singapore, 1989–1999. MWRR Morb. Mortal. Wkly. Rep. 48: 265–269; 1999.

Chopra, J. S.; Banerjee, A. K.; Murthy, J. M. K.; Pal, S. R. Paralytic rabies. A clinico-pathological study. Brain 103:789–802; 1980.

Chou, S. M.; Roos, R.; Burrell, R.; Gutmann, L.; Harley, J. B. Subacute focal adenovirus encephalitis. J. Neuropathol. Exp. Neurol. 32:34–50; 1973.

Cinque, P.; Cleator, G. M.; Weber, T.; Montayne, P.; Sindic, C. J.; van Loon, A. M.; the EU Concerted Action on Virus Meningitis and Encephalitis. The role of laboratory investigation in the diagnosis and management of patients with suspected herpes encephalitis: a consensus report. J. Neurol. Neurosurg. Psychiatry 61:339–345; 1996.

Clavel, M.; Clavel, P. Creutzfeldt-Jakob disease transmitted by dura mater graft. Eur. Neurol. 36:239–240; 1996.

Cobb, W. A.; Marshall, J.; Scaravilli, F. Long survival in subacute sclerosing panencephalitis. J. Neurol. Neurosurg. Psychiatry 47:176–183; 1984.

Counsell, C. E.; Taylor, R.; Whittle, I. R. Focal necrotising herpes simplex encephalitis: a report of two cases with good clinical and neuropsychological outcomes. J. Neurol. Neurosurg. Psychiatry 57: 1115–1117; 1994.

Cramblett, H. G.; Stegmiller, F.; Spencer, C. California encephalitis virus infection in children. Clinical and laboratory studies. JAMA 198:128–132; 1966.

Cutler, N. R.; Brown, P. W.; Narayan, T.; Parisi, J. E.; Janotta, J.; Baron, H. Creutzfeldt-Jakob disease: a case of 16 years' duration. Ann. Neurol. 15:107–110; 1984.

Davenport, D. S.; Johnson, D. R.; Holmes, G. P.; Jewett, D. A.; Ross, S. C.; Hilliard, J. K. Diagnosis and management of human B virus (Herpesvirus simiae) infections in Michigan. Clin. Infect. Dis. 19:33–41; 1994.

Dawson, J. R., Jr. Cellular inclusions in cerebral lesions of lethargic encephalitis. Arch. Pathol. 9:7–15; 1933.

Deresiewicz, R. L.; Thaler, S. J.; Hsu, L.; Zamani, A. A. Clinical and neuroradiographic manifestations of eastern equine encephalitis. N. Engl. J. Med. 336:1867–1874; 1997.

Dickerson, R. B.; Newton, J. R.; Hansen, J. E. Diagnosis and immediate prognosis of Japanese encephalitis. Observations based on more than 200 patients with detailed analysis of 65 serologically confirmed cases. Am. J. Med. 12:277–279; 1952.

Donat, J. F.; Rhodes, K. H.; Groover, R. V.; Smith, T. F. Etiology and outcome in 42 children with acute nonbacterial meningoencephalitis. Mayo Clin. Proc. 55:156–160; 1980.

Duffy, P.; Wolf, J.; Collins, G.; DeVoe, A. G.; Streeten, B.; Cowen, D. Possible person-to-person transmission of Creutzfeldt-Jakob disease. N. Engl. J. Med. 290:692; 1974.

Dupont, J. R.; Earle, K. M. Human rabies encephalitis. A study of forty-nine fatal cases with a review of the literature. Neurology 15:1023–1034; 1966.

Dwyer, J. M.; Erlendsson, K. Intraventricular gammaglobulin for the management of enterovirus encephalitis. Pediatr. Infect. Dis. J. 7:S30–S33; 1986.

Earnest, M. P.; Goolishian, H. A.; Calverley, J. R.; Hayes, R. G.; Hill, H. R. Neurologic, intellectual and psychologic sequelae following western encephalitis. A followup study of 35 cases. Neurology 21:969–974; 1971.

Erlendsson, K.; Swartz, T.; Dwyer, J. M. Successful reversal of echovirus meningoencephalitis in X-linked hypogammaglobulinemia by intraventricular administration by immunoglobulin. N. Engl. J. Med. 312: 351–353; 1997.

Farber, S.; Hill, A.; Connelly, M. L.; Dingle, J. H. Encephalitis in infants and children. Caused by the virus of the eastern variety of equine encephalitis. JAMA 114:1725–1731; 1940.

Freeman, J. M. The clinical spectrum and early diagnosis of Dawson's encephalitis. With preliminary notes on treatment. J. Pediatr. 75:590–603; 1969.

Fujimoto, S.; Kobayashi, M.; Uemura, O.; Iwasa, M.; Ando, T.; Katoh, T.; et al. PCR on cerebrospinal fluid to show influenza-associated acute encephalopathy or encephalitis. Lancet 352:873–875; 1998.

Gilden, D. H.; Rorke, L. B.; Tanaka, R. Acute SSPE. Arch. Neurol. 32:644–646; 1975.

Goldfield, M.; Sussman, O. The 1959 outbreak of Eastern encephalitis in New Jersey. I. Introduction and description of the outbreak. Am. J. Epidemiol. 87:1–10; 1968.

Gordon, B.; Selnes, O. A.; Hart, J., Jr.; Hanley, D. F.; Whitley, R. J. Long-term cognitive sequelae of acyclovir-treated herpes simplex encephalitis. Arch. Neurol. 47:646–647; 1990.

Hall, C. B.; Hall, C. B.; Dafhi, U.; Simpson, D.; Clifford, D.; Wetherill, P. E.; Cohen, B.; McArthur, J.; Hollander, H; et al. Failure of cytarabine in progressive multifocal leukoencephalopathy associated with human immunodeficiency virus infection. N. Engl. J. Med. 338:1345–1351; 1998.

Hattwick, M. A. W.; Weis, T. T.; Stechschulte, J.; Baer, G. M.; Gregg, M. B. Recovery from rabies. A case report. Ann. Intern. Med. 76:931–942; 1972.

Herzon, H.; Shelton, J. T.; Bruyn, H. B. Sequelae of western equine and other arthropod-borne encephalitides. Neurology 7:535–548; 1957.

Hill, A. E.; Desbruslais, M.; Joiner, S.; Sidle, K. C. L.; Gowland, I.; Collinge, J.; Doey, L.; Lantos, P. The same prion strain causes vCJD and BSE. Nature 389:448–450; 1997.

Hilton, D. A.; Fathers, E.; Edwards, P.; Ironside, J. W.; Zajicek, J. Prion immunoreactivity in appendix before clinical onset of variant Creutzfeldt-Jakob disease. Lancet 352:703–704; 1988.

Hilty, M. D.; Haynes, R. E.; Azimi, P. H.; Cramblett, H. G. California encephalitis in children. Am. J. Dis. Child. 124:530–533; 1972.

Hoke, C. H.; Vaughn, D. W.; Nisalak, A.; Intralawan, P.; Poolsuppasit, S.; et al. Effect of high dose dexamethasone on the outcome of acute encephalitis due to Japanese encephalitis virus. J. Infect. Dis. 165: 631–637; 1992.

Hokkanen, L.; Launes, J. Cognitive recovery instead of decline after acute encephalitis: a prospective followup study. J. Neurol. Neurosurg. Psychology 63:222–227; 1997.

Holmes, G. P.; Chapman, L. E.; Stuart, J. A.; Straus, S. E.; Hilliard, J. K.; Davenport, D. S.; and the B Virus Working Group. Guidelines for the prevention and treatment of B virus infections in exposed persons. Clin. Infect. Dis. 20:421–439; 1995.

Holmes, G. P.; Hilliard, J. K.; Klontz, K. C.; Rupert, A. H.; Schindler, C. M.; et al. B virus (herpesvirus simiae) infection in humans: epidemiologic investigation of a cluster. Ann. Intern. Med. 112:833–839; 1990.

Houff, S. A.; Burton, R. C.; Wilson, R. W.; et al. Human-to-human transmission of rabies virus by a corneal transplant. N. Engl. J. Med. 300:603–604; 1979.

Huttenlocher, P. R.; Mattson, R. H. Isoprinosine in subacute sclerosing panencephalitis. Neurology 29: 763–771; 1979.

Huttenlocher, P. R.; Pichietti, D. L.; Roos, R. P.; Cashman, N. R.; et al. Intrathecal interferon in subacute sclerosing panencephalitis. Ann. Neurol. 19:303–305; 1986.

Jackson, A. C. Leg weakness associated with Powassan virus infection—Ontario. Can. Dis. Week. Rep. 14:123–124; 1989.

Johnson, P. R., Jr.; Edwards, K. M.; Wright, P. F. Failure of intraventricular gamma globulin to eradicate echovirus encephalitis in a patient with X-linked agammaglobulinemia. N. Engl. J. Med. 313: 1546–1547; 1985.

Kaiser, R. Tick-borne encephalitis in southern Germany. Lancet 345:463; 1995.

Kennard, C.; Swash, M. Acute viral encephalitis. Its diagnosis and outcome. Brain 104:29–148; 1981.

Kennedy, C. R.; Duffy, S. W.; Smith, R.; Robinson, R. O. Clinical predictors of outcome in encephalitis. Arch. Dis. Child. 62:1156–1162; 1987.

Ketel, W. B.; Ognibene, A. J. Japanese B encephalitis in Vietnam. Am. J. Med. Sci. 261:271–279; 1971.

Kilham, L. Mumps meningoencephalitis with and without parotitis. Am. J. Dis. Child. 78:324–333; 1949.

Klapper, P. E.; Cleator, G. M.; Longson, M. Mild forms of herpes encephalitis. J. Neurol. Neurosurg. Psychiatry 47:1247–1250; 1984.

Koskiniemi, M.; Donner, M.; Pettay, O. Clinical appearance and outcome in mumps encephalitis in children. Acta Pediatr. Scand. 72:603–609; 1983.

Kumar, R.; Mathur, A.; Kumar, A.; Sharma, S.; Chakraborty, S.; Chaturvedi, U. C. Clinical features and prognostic indicators of Japanese encephalitis in children in Lucknow (India). Indian J. Med. Res. 91:321–327; 1990.

Kumar, R.; Mathur, A.; Singh, K. B.; Sitholey, P.; Prasad, M.; Shukla, R.; Agarwal, S. P.; Arockiasamy, J. Clinical sequelae of Japanese encephalitis in children. Indian J. Med. Res. 97:9–13; 1993.

Landau, W. M.; Luse, S. A. Relapsing inclusion encephalitis (Dawson type) of eight years duration. Neurology 8:669–676; 1958.

Lange, B. J.; Berman, P. H.; Bender, J.; Henle, W.; Hewetson, J. F. Encephalitis in infectious mononucleosis: diagnostic considerations. Pediatrics 58: 877–880; 1976.

Launes, J.; Siren, J.; Valanne, L.; Salonen, O.; Nikkinen, P.; Seppalainen, A. -M.; Liewendahl, K. Unilateral hyperperfusion in brain-perfusion SPECT predicts poor prognosis in acute encephalitis. Neurology 48:1347–1351; 1997.

Leech, R. W.; Harris, J. C.; Johnson, R. M. 1975 encephalitis epidemic in North Dakota and western Minnesota. Minn. Med. September 545–548; 1981.

Lewis, L.; Taylor, H. G.; Sorem, M. B.; Norcross, J. W.; Kindsvatter, V. H. Japanese B encephalitis.

Clinical observations in an outbreak on Okinawa Shima. Arch. Neurol. Psychiatry 57:430–463; 1947.

Levitt, L. P.; Rich, T. A.; Kinde, S. W.; Lewis, A. L.; Gates, E. H.; Bond, J. O. Central nervous system mumps. A review of 64 cases. Neurology 20:829–834; 1970.

Lincoln, A. F.; Sivertson, S. E. Acute phase of Japanese B encephalitis. Two hundred and one cases in American soldiers, Korea, 1950. JAMA 150:268–273; 1952.

Linneman, C. C., Jr.; May, D. B.; Schubert, W. K.; Caraway, C. F.; Schiff, G. M. Fatal viral encephalitis in children with X-linked hypogammaglobulinemia. Am. J. Dis. Child. 126:100–103; 1973.

McGrath, N.; Anderson, N. E.; Croxson, M. C.; Powell, K. F. Herpes simplex encephalitis treated with acyclovir: diagnosis and long-term outcome. J. Neurol. Neurosurg. Psychiatr. 63:321–326; 1997.

McKinney, R. E., Jr.; Katz, S. L.; Wilfert, C. M. Chronic enteroviral encephalitis in agammaglobulinemic patients. Rev. Infect. Dis. 9:334–356; 1987.

McLean, D. M.; Bach, R. D.; Larke, R. P. B.; McNaughton, G. A. Mumps meningoencephalitis, Toronto, 1963. Can. Med. Assoc. J. 90:458–462; 1964.

Mease, P. J.; Ochs, H. D.; Wedgwood, R. J. Successful treatment of echovirus meningoencephalitis and myositis-fasciitis with intravenous immune globulin therapy in a patient with X-linked agammaglobulinemia. N. Engl. J. Med. 304:1279–1281; 1981.

Miller, H. G.; Stanton, J. B.; Gibbons, J. L. Parainfectious encephalomyelitis and related syndromes. A critical review of the neurological complications of certain specific fevers. Q. J. Med. 25:428–505; 1956.

Miller, J. D.; Ross, C. A. C. Encephalitis. A four year survey. Lancet i:1121–1126; 1968.

Modlin, J. F.; Halsey, N. A.; Eddins, D. L.; Conrad, J. L.; Johnson, J. T.; Jabbour, J. T.; Chien, L.; Robinson, H. Epidemiology of subacute sclerosing panencephalitis. J. Pediatr. 94:231–236; 1979.

Nathanson, N.; Wilesmith, J.; Griot, C. Bovine spongiform encephalopathy (BSE): causes and consequences of a common source epidemic. Am. J. Epidemiol. 145:959–969; 1997.

Ogawa, M.; Okubo, H.; Tsuji, Y.; Yasui, N.; Someda, K. Chronic progressive encephalitis occurring 13 years after Russian spring-summer encephalitis. J. Neurol. Sci. 19:363–373; 1973.

O'Sullivan, J. D.; Allworth, A. M.; Paterson, D. L.; Snow, T. M.; Boots, R.; et al. Fatal encephalitis due to novel paramyxovirus transmitted from horses. Lancet 349:93–95; 1997.

Palmer, A. E. B virus, herpes simiae: historical perspective. J. Med. Primatol. 16:99–130; 1987.

Porras, C.; Barboza, J. J.; Fuenzalida, E.; Lopez Adaros, H.; Oviedo de Diaz, M.; Furst, J. Recovery from rabies in man. Ann. Intern. Med. 85:44–48; 1976.

Powell, K. E.; Blakey, K. L. St Louis encephalitis. The 1975 epidemic in Mississippi. JAMA 237:2294–2298; 1977.

Powell, K. E.; Kappus, K. D. Epidemiology of St Louis encephalitis and other acute encephalitides. In: Shoen-

berg, B. S., ed. Advances in neurology. Vol. 19. New York: Raven Press; 1978.

Przelomski, M. M.; O'Rourke, E.; Grady, G. F.; Berardi, V. P.; Markley, H. G. Eastern equine encephalitis in Massachusetts: a report of 16 cases, 1970–1984. N. Engl. J. Med. 38:736–739; 1988.

Quick, D. T.; Thompson, J. M.; Bond, J. O. The 1962 epidemic of St Louis encephalitis in Florida. IV. Clinical features of cases occurring in the Tampa Bay Area. Am. J. Epidemiol. 81:415–427; 1965.

Rautonen, J.; Koskiniemi, M.; Vaheri, A. Prognostic factors in childhood acute encephalitis. Pediatr. Infect. Dis. J. 10:441–446; 1991.

Richardson, E. P., Jr. Progressive multifocal leukoencephalopathy. N. Engl. J. Med. 265:815–823; 1961.

Rie, H. E.; Hilty, M. D.; Cramblett, H. G. Intelligence and coordination following California encephalitis. Am. J. Dis. Child. 125:824–827; 1973.

Risk, W. S.; Haddad, F. S.; Chemali, R. Substantial spontaneous long-term improvement in subacute sclerosing panencephalitis. Six cases from the Middle East and a review of the literature. Arch. Neurol. 35:494–502; 1978.

Rose, E.; Prabhakar, P. Influenza A virus associated neurological disorders in Jamaica. West Indian Med. J. 31:29–33; 1982.

Rotbart, H. A. Enteroviral infections of the nervous system. Clin. Infect. Dis. 20:971–981; 1995.

Rust, R. S.; Dodson, W.; Prensky, A.; Chun, R.; Devivo, D.; Dodge, P.; Fishman, M.; Noetzel, M.; Trosser, J.; Volpe, J.; Zupanc, M. Classification and outcome of acute disseminated encephalomyelitis. Ann. Neurol. 38:491; 1997.

Sabin, A. B.; Wright, A. M. Acute ascending myelitis following a monkey bite, with the isolation of a virus capable of reproducing the disease. J. Exp. Med. 59:115–136; 1934.

Sage, J. I.; Weinstein, M. P.; Miller, D. C. Chronic encephalitis possibly due to herpes simplex virus: two cases. Neurology 35:1470–1472; 1985.

Schnell, R. G.; Dyck, P. J.; Walter Bowie, E. J.; Klass, D. W.; Taswell, H. F. Infectious mononucleosis: neurologic and EEG findings. Medicine 45:51–63; 1966.

Sells, C. J.; Carpenter, R. L.; Ray, C. G. Sequelae of central nervous system enterovirus infections. N. Engl. J. Med. 293:1–4; 1975.

Shill, M.; Baynes, R. D.; Miller, S. D. Fatal rabies encephalitis despite appropriate post-exposure prophylaxis. N. Engl. J. Med. 316:1257–1258; 1987.

Silcott, W. L.; Neuberger, K. Acute lymphocytic choriomeningitis. Report of three cases with neuropathological findings. Am. J. Med. Sci. 200:253–259; 1940.

Silverstein, A.; Steinberg, G.; Nathanson, M. Nervous system involvement in infectious mononucleosis. Arch. Neurol. 26:353–358; 1972.

Skoldenberg, B.; Forsgren, M.; Alestig, K.; Bergstrom, T.; et al. Acyclovir versus vidarabine in herpes simplex encephalitis. Randomized multicentre study in consecutive Swedish patients. Lancet 2:707–711; 1984.

Smorodintsev, A. A. Tick-borne spring-summer encephalitis. Prog. Med. Virol. 1:210–248; 1958.

Sworn, M. J.; Urich, H. Acute encephalitis in infectious mononucleosis. J. Pathol. 100:201–205; 1970.

Taylor, F. B.; Toreson, W. E. Primary mumps meningoencephalitis. Arch. Intern. Med. 112:114–119; 1963.

Thompson, W. H.; Kalfayan, B.; Anslow, R. O. Isolation of a California encephalitis group virus from a fatal human illness. Am. J. Epidemiol. 81:245–253; 1966.

Townsend, J. J.; Baringer, J. R.; Wolinsky, J. S.; Malamud, N.; Mednick, J. P.; et al. Progressive rubella panencephalitis. Late onset after congenital rubella. N. Engl. J. Med. 292:990–993; 1975.

Tselis, A.; Lisak, R. P. Acute disseminated encephalomyelitis. In: Antel, J.; Birnbaum, G.; Hartung, H. -P., eds. Clinical neuroimmunology. London: Blackwell Scientific; 1997.

Tyler, K. L.; Tedder, D. G.; Yamamoto, L. J.; Klapper, J. A.; et al. Recurrent brainstem encephalitis associated with herpes simplex virus type 1 DNA in cerebrospinal fluid. Neurology 45:2246–2250; 1995.

Valdueza, J. M.; Weber, J. R.; Harms, L.; Bock, A. Severe tick-borne encephalomyelitis after tick bite and passive immunization. J. Neurol. Neurosurg. Psychiatr. 60: 593–594; 1996.

von Economo, C. Encephalitis lethargica. Its sequelae and treatment. Translated by Newman, K. O. London; Oxford University Press, 1931.

Warkel, R. L.; Rinaldi, C. F.; Bancroft, W. H.; Cardiff, W. D.; Holmes, G. E.; Wilsnack, R. E. Fatal meningencephalitis due to lymphocytic choriomeningitis virus. Neurology 23:198–203; 1973.

Warrell, D. A. The clinical picture of rabies in man. Trans. R. Soc. Trop. Med. Hyg. 70:188–195; 1976.

Webster, A. D. B.; Tripp, J. H.; Hayward, A. R.; Dayan, A. D.; Doshi, R.; MacIntyre, E. H.; Tyrrell, D. A. J. Echovirus encephalitis and myositis in primary immunoglobulin deficiency. Arch. Dis. Child. 53: 33–37; 1978.

Weigler, B. J. Biology of B virus in macacque and human hosts: a review. Clin. Infect. Dis. 14:555–567; 1992.

Weil, M. L.; Itabashi, H. H.; Cremer, N. E.; Oshiro, L. S.; Lennette, E. H.; Carnay, L. Chronic progressive panencephalitis due to rubella virus simulating subacute sclerosis panencephalitis. N. Engl. J. Med. 292:994–998; 1975.

Wells, G. A.; Scott, A. C.; Johnson, C. T.; et al. A novel progressive spongiform encephalopathy in cattle. Vet. Rec. 121:419–420; 1987.

Whitley, R. J.; Alford, C. A.; Hirsch, M. S.; et al. Vidarabine versus acyclovir therapy in herpes simplex encephalitis. N. Engl. J. Med. 314:144–149; 1986.

Whitley, R. J.; Soong, S. J.; Dolin, R.; et al. Adenine arabinoside therapy of biopsy-proved herpes simplex encephalitis. National Institute of Allergy and Infectious Diseases Collaborative Antiviral Study. N. Engl. J. Med. 297:289–294; 1977.

Whitley, R. J.; Soong, S. J.; Hirsch, M. D.; Karchner, A. W.; Dolin, R.; Galasso, G.; et al. Herpes simplex encephalitis. vidarabine therapy and diagnostic problems. N. Engl. J. Med. 304:313–318; 1981.

Wildemann, B.; Ehrhart, E.; Storch-Hagenlocher, B.; Meyding-Lamade, U.; et al. Quantitation of herpes simplex virus type 1 DNA in cells of cerebrospinal fluid of patients with herpes simplex encephalitis. Neurology 48:1341–1346; 1997.

Wilesmith, J. W. Bovine spongiform encephalopathy: methods of analyzing the epidemic in the United Kingdom. In: Baker, H. F.; Ridley, R. M., eds. Prion diseases. New York: Humana Press; 1996

Wilfert, C. M.; Buckley, R. H.; Mohanakumar, T.; Griffith, J. F.; Katz, S. L.; Whisnant, J. K.; Eggleston, P. A.; et al. Persistent and fatal central nervous system echovirus infections in patients with agammaglobulinemia. N. Engl. J. Med. 296:1485–1489; 1977.

Will, R. G.; Ironside, J. W.; Zeidler, M.; Cousons, S. N.; Estibeiro, K.; Alperovitch, A.; et al. A new variant of Creutzfeldt-Jakob disease in the UK. Lancet 347:921–925; 1996.

Wilson, M. S.; Wherrett, B. A.; Mahdy, M. S. Powassan virus meningoencephalitis: a case report. Can. Med. Assoc. J. 121:320–323; 1979.

Winter, W. D., Jr. Eastern equine encephalomyelitis in Massachusetts in 1955. N. Engl. J. Med. 255: 262–267; 1956.

Young, D. J. California encephalitis virus. Report of three cases and a review of the literature. Ann. Int. Med. 65:419–428; 1966.

# 17

# HIV-1 and Associated Infections

AFSHAN M. KHAN, NADA G. ABOU-FAYSSAL,
AND DAVID M. SIMPSON

Neurological involvement in the acquired immunodeficiency syndrome (AIDS) is a common clinical problem. The spectrum of neurological disorders associated with human immunodeficiency virus type 1 (HIV-1) has expanded widely since the initial recognition of AIDS in 1982 (Britton et al. 1982; Horowitz et al. 1982; Miller et al. 1982). Such disorders may result from direct or indirect injury to the nervous system by the HIV virus itself or be a result of the vulnerability of the nervous system to the complications of immunosuppression (Snider et al. 1983; Shaw et al. 1985; Petito et al. 1986; Gray et al. 1988). Table 17-1 lists the spectrum of neurological disorders that occur in association with HIV-1 infection.

Neurological complications of HIV-1 infection can occur at any level of the neuraxis, and multiple levels can be affected simultaneously (Snider et al. 1983; Levy et al. 1985). Involvement of the nervous system is very common in all stages of the disease. It has been estimated that neurological manifestations are present during HIV seroconversion in approximately 16% of patients (Clark et al. 1991). In the AIDS population, the prevalence of neurological disease is 39% to 63% and in 10% to 20%, neurological disease is the presenting manifestation of AIDS (Levy et al. 1985; Berger et al. 1986b). Postmortem studies

demonstrate an even higher prevalence of central nervous system (CNS) disease approximating 80% (Petito et al. 1986; Anders et al. 1986).

Neurological complications add considerably to the morbidity and mortality of HIV infection. For example, the presence of HIV dementia is an independent predictor of survival (McArthur 1987; Navia and Price 1987). The type of neurological disease correlates strongly with the stage of HIV infection and particularly reflects the degree of immunosuppression. A thorough knowledge of these neurological disorders helps in their early diagnosis and treatment, hence improving patients' survival and quality of life. Figure 17-1 outlines the relationship between the degree of immunocompromise and major neurological disease.

## Diffuse Brain Lesions

### HIV Leukoencephalopathy

One of the most common and enigmatic of the neurological complications of HIV infection is progressive dementia. This disorder has a number of names including AIDS dementia complex and HIV-associated cognitive motor complex. Neuropathological nomenclature includes HIV encephalitis and HIV leukoencephalopathy. This is a

**Table 17-1.** Major Neurological Disorders
Associated With HIV-1 Infection

**Cerebral disorders**
  Diffuse brain lesions
    HIV-1 encephalopathy
    CMV encephalitis
    VZV encephalitis
  Focal brain lesions
    Primary and metastatic lymphoma
    Metastatic Kaposi's sarcoma
    Infectious (i.e., toxoplasmosis, tuberculoma, cryptococ-
      coma, gumma)
    Progressive multifocal leukoencephalopathy
    Cerebrovascular disease
**Spinal cord disorders**
  Vacuolar myelopathy
  VZV, CMV myelitis
  Focal lesions (i.e., toxoplasmosis, tuberculoma, lymphoma)
**Meningeal disorders**
  Acute aseptic meningitis
  Chronic aseptic meningitis
  Cryptococcal meningitis
  Tuberculous meningitis
  Neurosyphilis
  Lymphomatous meningitis
**Neuromuscular disorders**
  Peripheral neuropathy
    Distal symmetrical polyneuropathy
    Mononeuropathy multiplex
    Acute demyelinating polyneuropathy
    Chronic idiopathic demyelinatng polyneuropathy
    Progressive polyradiculopathy
    Autonomic neuropathy
  Myopathy
    HIV myositis
    Zidovudine myopathy
    HIV wasting syndrome

HIV-1, human immunodeficiency virus type 1; CMV, cytomegalovirus; VZV, varicella zoster virus.

complex progressive neuropsychiatric disorder
seen in about 15% to 20% of patients with AIDS
(McArthur et al. 1993; Price et al. 1988; Navia
et al. 1986b) usually in late stages of the disease.
However, about 4% to 10% of HIV-infected patients may develop ADC as their primary or AIDS
defining illness (Navia et al. 1987).

The likelihood that an HIV-infected individual
develops neurological disease, and the stage of infection in which the clinical signs become apparent, is related to a combination of host and viral
factors. Host factors include the competency of
immune responses and cellular expression of viral
coreceptors. Viral factors include cell tropism and
sequences that determine neurovirulence.

HIV dementia (HIVD) is distinguished from
other viral diseases of the CNS by its chronic
course, paucity of infected cells, and minimal evidence of neuronal infection despite widespread

cognitive and motor decline. HIV remains con-
centrated in microglia and macrophages and is
present to a lesser extent in astrocytes and endothelial cells (Gabuzda et al. 1986; Wiley et al.
1986; Brew et al. 1995). The events leading to dementia are not clearly understood and despite
considerable research there is no clear consensus
on a unifying theory of its mechanism.

### Pathogenesis

The cause of CNS injury in HIV-1 infection is not
well understood. Many gaps remain in our knowledge of the pathogenesis of AIDS dementia.
HIVD occurs in only a subset of AIDS patients.
The reason for this is not well understood. HIV is
thought to enter the nervous system via the
macrophages and probably enters the brain at the
time of seroconversion. However, clinical dementia usually appears when there is marked immunodeficiency. HIV mainly infects microglia
and only rarely neurons. Despite the severe cognitive deficits the number of macrophages and microglia infected by HIV is small. These findings
support the view that both direct and indirect effects of brain HIV infection contribute to the development of dementia.

Various factors that have been implicated include HIV itself, cytokine dysregulation, release
of toxic substances from macrophages (i.e., nitric
oxide), toxic effect of viral proteins (i.e., gp120,
gp141, tat, nef), and secretory products (i.e.,
tumor necrosis factor α [TNF-α] and platelet-
activating factor [PAF]) (Giulian et al. 1993, 1996;
Genis et al. 1992).

Several HIV-1 gene products including HIV-1
nef and HIV-1 tat have been identified as neurotoxins. Synthetic tat is neurotoxic in mice (Sabatier
et al. 1991) and gp120 envelope glycoprotein of
HIV-1 has been shown to be toxic to rodent neurons (Dreyer et al. 1990), whose neurotoxicity is
mediated via factors released by activated macrophages, microglia, and astrocytes. Neuronal death
occurs as a consequence of excessive calcium
influx via overactivation of neuronal N-methyl-
D-aspartate (NMDA) receptors. This in turn leads
to hyperactivity of a variety of enzyme systems
and release of the neurotransmitter glutamate,
which stimulates the neighboring neuronal NMDA
receptors causing further damage. It is postulated
that NMDA receptor antagonists such as memantine may ameliorate the damage.

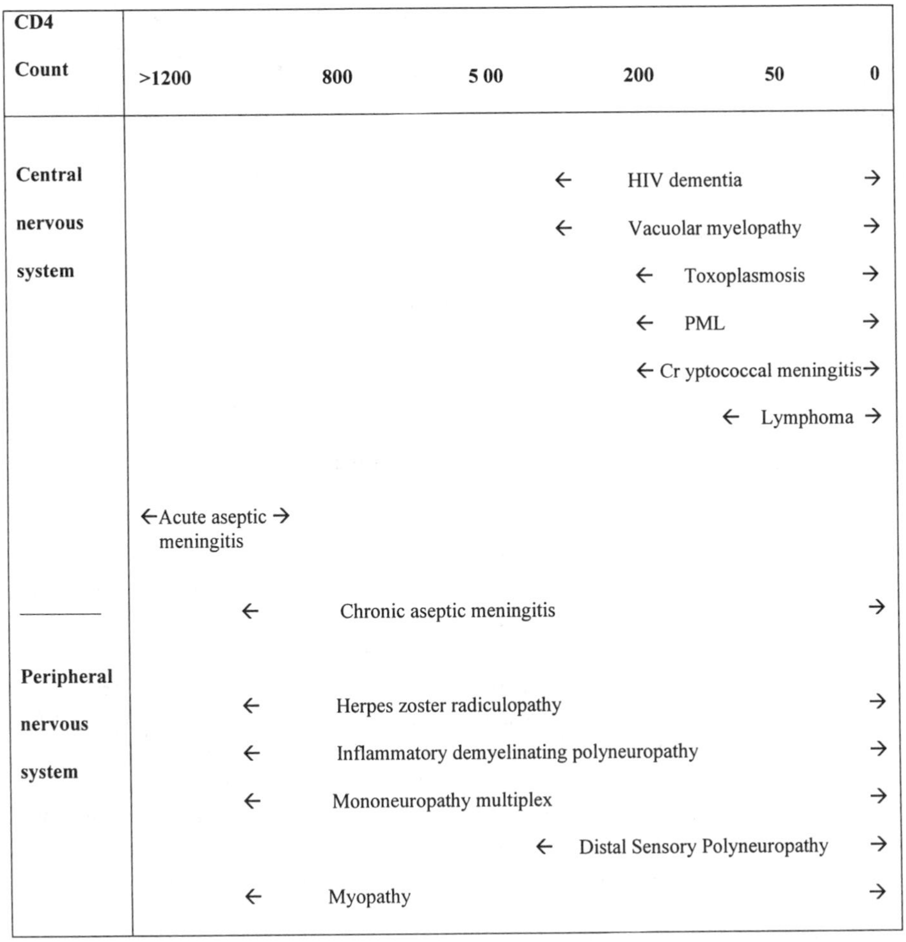

| CD4 Count | >1200 | 800 | 5 00 | 200 | 50 | 0 |
|---|---|---|---|---|---|---|
| **Central nervous system** | | | | ← HIV dementia | → | |
| | | | | ← Vacuolar myelopathy | → | |
| | | | | ← Toxoplasmosis | → | |
| | | | | ← PML | → | |
| | | | | ← Cr yptococcal meningitis → | | |
| | | | | ← Lymphoma | → | |
| | ←Acute aseptic → meningitis | | | | | |
| ——— | ← | Chronic aseptic meningitis | | | | → |
| **Peripheral nervous system** | ← | Herpes zoster radiculopathy | | | | → |
| | ← | Inflammatory demyelinating polyneuropathy | | | | → |
| | ← | Mononeuropathy multiplex | | | | → |
| | | | ← Distal Sensory Polyneuropathy | | | → |
| | ← | Myopathy | | | | → |

**Figure 17-1.** Correlation of CD4 count with major HIV-1–related neurological diseases. (Adapted from Johnson et al. 1988.)

HIV-1 gp120 induces arachidonic acid metabolites, interleukin-1β (IL-1β), and TNF-α in monocytes. In turn TNF amplifies production of arachidonic acid metabolites in response to IL-1. As a result there is overproduction of cytokines that act as direct neurotoxins, or in synergy with excitotoxic agents like glutamate.

In recent years, it has been possible to assay HIV viral RNA levels directly in the cerebrospinal fluid (CSF). The magnitude of CSF viral load correlates with the clinical severity of dementia, supporting a direct role for HIV in the mechanism of dementia (Ellis et al. 1997; McArthur et al. 1997).

In summary a complex interaction occurs between HIV-infected macrophages, microglia, and astrocytes resulting in the production of proinflammatory cytokines, arachidonic acid metabolites, and PAF, which are thought to mediate damage.

The ultimate result is apoptosis of neurons and astrocytes caused by HIV-1 infection; however, all the apoptotic stimuli have not yet been identified.

*Pathology*

The hallmark of HIV-1 infection of the CNS is the multinucleated giant cell (MGC), which is characterized as a macrophage-derived cell (Gabuzda et al. 1986). The formation of MGC is thought to be due to syncytia formation between infected macrophages and microglia (Sharer 1992; Wiley and Achim 1994). This results from an interaction between the viral envelope proteins gp120 and gp41 and cellular receptors for the virus. Viral particles can be demonstrated by electron microscopy in the cytoplasm of these cells, which contain large amounts of HIV-1 protein. However, the MGC is not unique to HIV-1 and has also been seen in other forms of viral encephalitis (Genis et al. 1992). They can be found anywhere in the CNS and the spinal cord but are most commonly seen in the deep white matter of the cerebral hemispheres, basal ganglia, and brain stem.

Another pathological feature of HIVD is diffuse white matter pallor (HIV leukoencephalopathy). These changes may be seen with or without MGC together with pronounced astrogliosis. The axons are usually spared, although there may be focal axonal loss (Giulian et al. 1993). Additionally, minor alterations of neocortical dendritic processes have been seen.

### Clinical Features

Neurobehavioral features of HIVD include both cognitive and affective changes. A small group of asymptomatic seropositive persons show subtle changes in mentation without affective changes. HIVD is generally considered to be a subcortical dementia even though neuropathological and neuroradiological data show cortical and subcortical involvement. Memory impairment is the earliest and most prominent abnormality, followed by frontal and executive dysfunction (Tross et al. 1988). Other symptoms include loss of libido and gait difficulty. Brain MRI in HIV dementia characteristically reveals global cerebral atrophy associated with bilateral symmetrical white matter abnormalities (leukoencephalopathy). Newer functional imaging procedures such as proton magnetic resonance spectroscopy show promise as a surrogate marker of brain function in these patients (Yiannoutsos et al. 1999).

### Treatment

There is evidence that HIV dementia is ameliorated by zidovudine (AZT) treatment with improvement in neuropsychological test performance (Sidtis et al. 1992; Simpson 1999). The optimal dosage of AZT has not been established. However, the maximal efficacy found in placebo-controlled studies has been obtained with high-dose AZT (1000 to 2000 mg/d).

A controlled study of approximately 100 patients with HIV dementia did not reveal that abacavir was superior to placebo in improving neuropsychological performance (Brew et al. 1998). Most other antiretroviral agents (ARVs) have not been assessed in the treatment of HIVD. However, if one considers that antiretroviral penetration into the brain is important in this setting, the ability of ARVs to penetrate the blood brain barrier (BBB) is important. The agents with maximal BBB penetration include the nucleoside analogues AZT, stavudine (d4T), abacavir (1592u89), and the non-nucleoside reverse transcriptase inhibitor nevirapine. Notably, the protease inhibitors do not penetrate the BBB well.

Nimodipine, a calcium channel antagonist has shown promise in a preliminary trial of HIVD although further studies are needed to evaluate this agent more fully (Navia et al. 1998). A number of other agents under investigation in the treatment of HIVD include memantine, deprenyl, and lexipiphant.

### Prognosis

HIVD often develops in conjunction with progressive systemic disease. It is usually seen in patients with CD4 counts of less than 200 cells/mm$^3$ (Giulian et al. 1996). Cross-sectional studies have found a correlation between CSF HIV RNA levels and the severity of neurocognitive impairment (discussed above). A prospective longitudinal study revealed that the level of CSF HIV RNA at baseline predicts later neurocognitive decline (Ellis et al. 1999). The severity of dementia is linked to immune activation within the CSF and brain parenchyma as noted by increased levels of IL-1, IL-6, and $\beta_2$-microglobulin. Alcohol and other substances that might be implicated in neurocognitive impairment do not contribute materially to the mental decline. Additionally, intravenous drug abuse has not been shown to be an adverse prognostic factor (Davis et al. 1992). Aging does not increase vulnerability to HIV dementia. For unclear reasons, the progression of HIV dementia can be variable. Once diagnosed with HIVD, most patients die within 6 months or less (McArthur et al. 1993), with a small subset showing prolonged survival. Factors contributing to prolonged survival are not known, but higher CD4 cell counts probably play a role. The advent of highly active antiretroviral therapy has resulted in an improved lifespan of HIV-infected patients, and appears to have reduced the frequency of HIVD. Data from the multicenter AIDS Cohort Study indicate that the incidence of HIV dementia has declined in recent years (1990–92: 21.1/1000 person years; 1993–95:17.4/1000 person years; 1996–97: 14.7/1000 person years) (Sacktor et al. 1999).

## Focal Brain Lesions

### Primary CNS Lymphoma

Primary lymphoma of the central nervous system (PCNSL) is the most common brain neoplasm that occurs in association with HIV infection. About 0.6% to 5% of AIDS patients present with PCNSL (Levy et al. 1988a, 1988b) and 2% to 5% patients ultimately develop it (Eikin et al. 1986). PCNSL in an HIV-seropositive individual is considered an AIDS-defining illness. Its incidence is rising in both AIDS and non-AIDS populations (DeAngelis 1995). PCNSL is the second most common cause of CNS mass lesions in HIV-infected adults and the most common cause of CNS mass lesions in HIV-infected children. It usually presents as a brain tumor, but may also involve the leptomeninges, eyes, or spinal cord (DeAngelis 1992).

#### Pathology

Immunohistochemical studies of PCNL identify this neoplasm to be of B-cell origin. In AIDS patients PCNSL usually contains Epstein-Barr virus (EBV) and runs an aggressive course (Morgello et al. 1997). The prevalence of EBV in AIDS-associated PCNSL ranges from 94% to 100%. This consistent association supports a pathogenetic role for EBV in AIDS-related PCNSL (Hochberg et al. 1983). In addition, human herpes virus-8 DNA has been found in a significant number of patients with PCNSL with and without AIDS (Corboy et al. 1998).

In most cases of PCNSL the lesions are multiple and supratentorial. They may be superficial (corticomedullary junction) or deep (basal ganglia, thalamus, and corpus callosum). The posterior fossa may also be involved. Grossly, the tumor is bulky with indistinct borders, and often contiguous with meningeal or ventricular surfaces. The lesions have high mitotic rates and varying degrees of microglial reaction and necrosis. AIDS-related PCNSL has a tendency to be more hemorrhagic and necrotic than non–AIDS-related PCNSL (Remick et al. 1990).

#### Clinical Features

PCNSL usually occurs in the profoundly immunocompromised patient with CD4 lymphocyte counts below 50 cells/mm$^3$. The presenting symptoms are varied and nonspecific and include focal neurological deficits (38% to 78%), altered level of consciousness (57%), seizures (23%), cranial nerve deficits (13%), and increased intracranial pressure (5%). Systemic signs include fever, night sweats, and weight loss. It is difficult to clinically differentiate between PCNSL and other intracranial masses, especially *Toxoplasma* encephalitis. Patients with AIDS-related lymphoma tend to be younger (34 years old vs. 59 years old), predominantly male, and have more constitutional symptoms as compared to patients with non–AIDS-related lymphoma (Remick et al. 1990).

#### Diagnosis

PCNSL has a variable MRI appearance that correlates with the severity of intratumoral necrosis. Most lesions enhance in a diffuse and homogeneous pattern. A contrast-enhancing ring lesion may occur in 5% to 10% of cases (Remick et al. 1990). Varying degrees of edema and mass effect may be seen. Lesions may be single or multiple. They may be present as homogenous masses or be nodular in configuration (Hochberg and Miller 1988). About 50 % of the lesions are located in the cortical grey matter or adjacent white matter, and about 25% of the lesions are found in the basal ganglia, thalamus, and corpus callosum. The presence of a solitary lesion does not necessarily favor lymphoma over toxoplasmosis (Porter and Sande 1993). About 14% of patients with *Toxoplasma* encephalitis have a single lesion on magnetic resonance imaging (MRI) (Porter and Sande 1993). Involvement of the spinal cord is extremely rare (Hochberg and Miller 1988).

Radiographically, it is difficult to distinguish PCSNL from other CNS infectious processes such as toxoplasmosis. Toxoplasmosis resembles PCSNL radiographically in about 50% to 80% of cases. Findings suggestive of PCSNL in AIDS patients with intracranial pathology are callosal involvement, periventricular location, ependymal enhancement, and presence of lesions with irregular enhancing margins. Additionally, these lesions are usually isointense or hypointense to parenchyma on all MRI sequences (Zimmerman 1990) unlike many other neoplastic lesions. This may be due to the dense cellularity of the lesions. Rapid progression of the lesions on serial imaging studies also favors lymphoma.

Thallium-201 brain single photon emission computed tomography (SPECT) is a valuable method for the differential diagnosis of PCNSL and toxoplasmosis in patients with AIDS with lesions of at least 6 to 8 mm (Mordechai et al. 1996), with a high sensitivity and specificity. Neoplasm shows increased uptake of thallium due to metabolic activity while infection does not. With lesions less than 6 mm to 8 mm, increased uptake may not be seen. A positive thallium-201 brain SPECT study is strongly suggestive of lymphoma or another neoplasm in AIDS patients. Fluorodeoxyglucose positron emission tomography (FDG-PET) has also shown promise in differentiating lymphoma from infectious lesions in the CNS of patients with HIV infection. Larger prospective studies are needed to confirm this impression.

Stereotactic brain biopsy yields a specific diagnosis in more than 95% of cases of PCNSL (Levy et al. 1991). CSF cytology is diagnostic in only 10% to 30% of patients. Increased CSF protein, mild pleocytosis, and decreased glucose levels may be observed (Case Records of the Massachusetts General Hospital 1983). EBV may be detected in the CSF in almost 100% of patients with AIDS-associated lymphoma, although this assay is predominantly relegated to research uses, rather than routine clinical diagnosis.

### Treatment

The primary treatment modality for AIDS-associated PCNSL is radiation therapy (Sagerman et al. 1967). Adjunctive therapy in the form of chemotherapy may also be used, but has limited usefulness in view of the underlying immunodeficiency (Remick et al. 1990). Curative surgical treatment is not feasible in view of the multicentric nature of the lymphoma. Corticosteroids may reduce enhancement on CT or MRI studies, and provide misleading diagnostic information.

Since there is a strong histological association between PCNSL and EBV, it has been suggested that systemic prophylaxis against EBV may prevent development of lymphoma. Valaciclovir, a proform of acyclovir, has in vitro activity against EBV and shows promise in demonstrating a protective effect on developing cerebral lymphoma. Chemotherapy has been added to radiotherapy in a small number of patients in an effort to improve response duration (Cinque et al. 1993). This combination has resulted in a median survival of about 4 months.

### Prognosis

Whole-brain irradiation results in improvement of neurological status and prolongs median survival to 3 to 4 months (Remick et al. 1990) as opposed to 1 to 2 months in untreated patients (Gills et al. 1985). Patients with AIDS-related PCNSL have a worse outcome from radiation treatment as compared to patients with non–AIDS-related PCNSL. Median survival is 12 to 18 months in the non-AIDS patient (Formenti et al. 1989). The poor outcome for patients with AIDS-related PCNSL might be due to the fact that the tumor may be relatively radioresistant and biologically different from non–AIDS-related PCNSL (Jellinger et al. 1975). Survival following irradiation is correlated with younger age, high Karnofsky performance status, CD4 count greater than 200 cells/mm$^3$ and a biologically effective dose of cranial radiotherapy (Jellinger et al. 1975). Additionally, patients with AIDS-associated PCNSL have advanced immunosuppression and are susceptible to opportunistic infections, making the use of potent chemotherapeutic agents difficult.

### Kaposi's Sarcoma

Rarely, Kaposi's sarcoma (KS) may metastasize to the brain and involve the cerebrum and cerebellum with hemorrhagic lesions (Kelly et al. 1983). Radiographic findings are similar to lymphoma and toxoplasmosis (Levy et al. 1986). Survival is extremely short due to rapid progression of widespread KS. AIDS-related CNS KS is generally viewed as a terminal event for these patients even though the tumor is radiosensitive (Ariza et al. 1988).

### Toxoplasmosis

The most common cause of an intracerebral mass lesion in AIDS patients is toxoplasmosis. *Toxoplasma gondii* is an obligate intracellular protozoan acquired by ingestion of undercooked meat. More than 95% of toxoplasma encephalitis (TE) is secondary to reactivation of latent infection (Luft and Remington 1992). About 30% of AIDS patients develop TE. The prevalence of toxoplasmosis is higher in Hispanics, African Americans, and heterosexual males. There is a geographical distribution, with the disease being three times more prevalent in Florida than in other states, probably secondary to ethnic distribution (Luft and Catro 1991; Levy et al. 1988b). More than 80% of patients who are seropositive for *Toxoplasma gondii* develop TE when CD4 counts drop below 100 cells/mm$^3$ The pathogenesis of TE is related to factors including host immune status and timing of infection. The presence of CNS involvement in the absence of systemic symptomatology is due to containment of infection by host immunity.

### Pathology

*Toxoplasma* produces hemorrhagic or coagulative necrosis in the CNS, leading to abscess formation. Ventricular ependymitis and vasculitis may occasionally be seen (Farkesh et al. 1986; Navia et al. 1986c). Lesions may be multiple or single and vary in size. All parts of the CNS may be affected including gray and white matter, but the leptomeninges are usually spared. Areas such as the thalamus, basal ganglia, and corticomedullary junction are more frequently involved.

### Clinical Features

Toxoplasmosis usually presents subacutely with focal neurologic signs (50% to 90%). In later stages there may be diffuse cerebral dysfunction. Seizures may be the presenting manifestation in about 15% to 25% of patients. The most frequent focal abnormalities are hemiparesis and aphasia. Generalized dysfunction manifests as altered mental status in the form of lethargy and confusion (Farkash et al. 1986). Neuropsychiatric manifestations include personality changes and psychosis.

### Diagnosis

The diagnosis of TE is usually presumptive, initially based on the presence of multiple or single enhancing lesions on neuroimaging studies in the appropriate clinical setting. Serological evidence of prior exposure to *Toxoplasma* is present in almost 100% of cases. The absence of *Toxoplasma* antibodies casts doubt on the diagnosis and suggests an alternate diagnosis.

MRI is the imaging modality of choice (Porter and Sande 1993). Solitary lesions occur in about 15% cases of TE (Porter and Sande 1993). The solitary enhancing lesions must be differentiated from cerebral lymphoma. As discussed earlier,

SPECT or PET scan may help in separating these etiologies, with increased uptake favoring lymphoma (Ruiz et al. 1994). Stereotactic brain biopsy confirms the diagnosis of lymphoma.

### Treatment

In current practice, presumptive TE is treated empirically with pyrimethamine and sulfadiazine (P/S) with a therapeutic response generally occurring in 10 to 14 days. Treatment is administered for at least 3 weeks and often extended to 6 weeks before excluding the possibility of response. The response rate varies from 68% to 95% (Luft and Remington 1985). Duration of treatment in confirmed cases of TE is lifelong. Clindamycin is an alternative agent for the treatment of TE, particularly when there are adverse reactions to P/S. Other substitute agents include atovaquone, azithromycin, and clarithromycin.

### Prognosis

Despite initial successful treatment, about 30% to 60% of patients will relapse if they discontinue medication (Porter and Sande 1993). Factors that increase the risk of recurrence include persistence of radiographic abnormalities despite adequate treatment (Laissey et al. 1994). Some patients with TE demonstrate no response to suitable treatment due to presence of another coexisting infection, or secondary to the simultaneous presence of lymphoma. Current recommendations mandate prophylactic treatment for TE with P/S for HIV-infected patients with CD4 counts of 100 cells/mm$^3$ or less.

## Progressive Multifocal Leukoencephalopathy

Progressive multifocal leukoencephalopathy (PML) is a progressive and usually fatal demyelinating disease of the CNS that is associated with infection of the oligodendrocytes by the papovavirus JC (JCV). JCV is ubiquitous; about 80% of adults are infected by middle age and 50% of children by 10 years of age (Walker and Padgett 1993). The incidence of PML in HIV infection is about 4% to 5% based on autopsy series (Berger et al. 1987a). JCV is the primary cause of PML. In three cases, another papovavirus, the SV40 virus has been implicated. Another papovavirus, the BK virus, is probably not neuropathogenic. The greatest incidence of PML occurs in the age range of 20 to 50 years (Holman et al.

1991). PML is rarely observed in the immuno-suppressed child, since only a very small number of children have been exposed to JCV. The frequency of PML as an indicator disease of AIDS ranges from 0.8% to 1.6% (Casabona et al. 1991). At autopsy, 2% to 7% of AIDS cases have PML (Anders et al. 1986).

## Pathogenesis

PML results from systemic or CNS reactivation of JC virus triggered by immunodeficiency associated with HIV infection. JC virus replication in oligodendrocyte nuclei causes cell dysfunction and death. JC virus shed from infected cells spreads to adjacent cells and thus extension of infection occurs along myelin tracts. Since most patients develop PML following reactivation of a latent JCV infection, JCV latency and reactivation are integral in the emergence of PML in immunosuppressed patients. Sites of latency include brain, kidney, and certain lymphoid cells (B cells). Investigation of the effects of different cytokines and chemokines on JCV replication in immune cells may provide clues as to the mechanism of viral reactivation.

Although the molecular control of JCV gene expression and DNA replication is well studied in glial cells, transcription factors affecting JCV have only recently been studied. The molecular pathogenesis of this fatal CNS disease requires further study.

## Pathology

Macroscopically the hallmark of PML is demyelination. Typically this occurs as a multifocal process. A predilection for the parieto-occipital region has been noted. PML may involve the gray matter, cerebellum, brain stem, and rarely the spinal cord. Lesions range in size from 1 mm to several centimeters. Large lesions are normally the result of coalescence of multiple smaller ones.

The diagnostic features of PML are enlarged oligodendroglial nuclei, multifocal demyelination, and enlarged bizarre astrocytes. By electron microscopy the JC virions can be seen singly or in dense crystalline arrays and measure 28 to 45 nm in diameter. Virions are not generally seen in the large astrocytes. Macrophage infiltration of demyelinating lesions represent the predominant immune response to JCV infection of neuroglial cells.

## Clinical Features

The presentation of the AIDS patient with PML is not significantly different from that of patients with PML complicating other immunosuppressive conditions such as Hodgkin's lymphoma and other myeloproliferative diseases. The symptoms and signs of PML are the result of multifocal demyelination in the CNS white matter. PML usually begins subacutely with focal neurological deficits. Common presenting manifestations are cognitive abnormalities, visual disturbances (cortical blindness, hemianopia, alexia without agraphia), and hemiparesis (Brooks and Walker 1984). About 80% of patients have weakness at the time of diagnosis. Visual symptoms occur in 50% of patients. Cerebellar dysfunction may also be seen. Sensory deficits occur less frequently and are present in about 10% to 20% of patients (Brooks and Walker 1984). Seizures are very rare. Most patients eventually develop multiple neurological signs as multifocal areas undergo demyelination.

## Diagnosis

Radiographically, PML lesions appear on MRI scan as hypointense on $T_1$-weighted scans and hyperintense on $T_2$-weighted scans without mass effect or enhancement with gadolinium. In 5% to 10% of patients, faint peripheral enhancement may be seen (Whiteman et al. 1993). The lesions of PML in AIDS preferentially affect frontal and parieto-occipital lobes but may occur anywhere in the brain. Demyelination associated with HIV dementia (i.e., leukoencephalopathy) resembles PML and may have overlapping clinical and radiographic features. Serum JCV antibodies are not helpful diagnostically, since about 80% of the population is seropositive by adulthood. Routine CSF studies reveals no diagnostic abnormalities. CSF analysis for JCV polymerase chain reaction (PCR) is about 82% sensitive and 100% specific for the diagnosis of PML (Weber et al. 1990). Stereotactic brain biopsy remains the "gold standard" for the definitive diagnosis of PML.

## Treatment and Prognosis

The mean survival in HIV-infected patients with PML is between 3 and 5 months (Berger et al. 1987a). Long-term survival is seen in about 7% to 15% of the total number of patients with PML complicating AIDS. The explanation of this phenomenon is unknown (Berger and Mucke 1998).

When compared with patients with the typical course of PML, the patients with prolonged survival or neurological improvement had higher CD4 counts, PML as the initial manifestation of AIDS, and were systemically healthier. Of note is the fact that cerebellar and brain stem disease was not observed in this group. Additionally, enhancement of lesions on neuroimaging studies was more often present. Histopathological study often reveals inflammatory infiltrates. However, in general more than 80% of patients with AIDS-associated PML die within 3 to 4 months from the time of diagnosis (Berger et al. 1987a; Brooks et al. 1984).

Antiretroviral therapy may improve the course of PML. A recent study of the natural history of PML in the post-HAART (highly active anti-retroviral therapy) era has been conducted within the Neurologic AIDS Research Consortium (Clifford 1999). This study of 37 subjects indicated that patients with well-controlled plasma HIV viral load have a significantly prolonged survival. An open-label, retrospective study by Huang et al. (1988) suggest that treatment with interferon-$\alpha$ (IFN-$\alpha$) may significantly increase the survival of HIV-positive PML patients as compared to untreated controls. Median survival of deceased treated patients was 127.5 days longer than that of untreated patients who died. However, a controlled clinical trial is warranted for confirmation of this observational study. AIDS Clinical Trials Group Study 243 demonstrated that treatment with cytarabine either intravenously or intrathecally did not improve the prognosis of PML complicating AIDS (Hall et al. 1998). Novel treatments under investigation for the treatment of AIDS-associated PML include cidofovir, topotecan, IFN-$\alpha$ and peptide-T.

## Spinal Cord Lesions

### Vacuolar Myelopathy

HIV-1–associated vacuolar myelopathy (VM) is a common neurological disorder associated with AIDS. Pathological studies indicate a prevalence of 22% to 25% (Petito et al. 1986; Navia et al. 1986; Artigas et al. 1990), although its clinical frequency is unknown. Vacuolar myelopathy has been identified in nearly 50% of autopsies of unselected patients who died of AIDS (Dal-Pan et al. 1994). VM generally occurs during advanced immunosuppression (Petito et al. 1985). However, there are reports of VM occurring at the time of seroconversion (McArthur et al. 1987). Subclinical myelopathy may also be detected (Jakobsen et al. 1989) with somatosensory evoked potentials.

Other kinds of myelopathy related to HIV-1 have also been described. A relapsing and remitting myelopathy with optic neuritis has been noted in patients with HIV-1 infection, resembling multiple sclerosis, and occurring during the early stages of HIV-1 infection. Dal Pan et al. presented three cases of cervical myelopathy presenting with spastic quadriparesis (Dal-Pan et al. 1994). No patient had characteristic features of VM on spinal cord biopsy. Infectious or neoplastic causes were not identified. Vitamin $B_{12}$ deficiency has clinical and pathological findings that resemble VM. However, cervical cord abnormalities predominate in $B_{12}$ deficiency, while the thoracic cord is primarily affected in HIV VM.

HIV-1 VM has certain similarities with HTLV-1–associated myelopathy but unlike HIV-1 VM, patients with HTLV-1 myelopathy may rarely show a sensory level. Coinfection of HIV with HTLV-1 is correlated with higher frequency of myelopathy than single infection with HIV.

Additionally, coinfection confers a higher likelihood of developing peripheral neuropathy (40%). Rarely, progressive myelopathy has been seen with severe immunosuppression with herpes simplex virus (HSV). Other etiologies of myelopathy reported in association with HIV infection include syphilis (Berger 1992), mycobacteria (Woolsey et al. 1988), herpes virus, *Toxoplasma,* and lymphoma (Klein et al. 1990).

### *Clinical Features*

VM presents in an insidious fashion with progressive spastic paraparesis and less often as monoparesis, with impairment of position sense and vibration (Ho et al. 1985). Dal-Pan et al. reported that among 56 patients with pathologically proven VM, only 15 had clinical evidence of myelopathy antemortem (Dal-Pan et al. 1994). Mild to moderate limb weakness was present in all cases. Lower limb spasticity was noted in 53%, spastic gait in 60%, and knee hyperreflexia in 93%. Sphincter dysfunction was described in only one patient, although in our experience, sphincter and erectile symptoms are frequently present early in the course of HIV-associated VM (Di Rocco and Simpson et al. 1998). A sensory level is usually absent. In late stages of the disease the patient is usually wheelchair bound.

### Diagnosis

Serological blood studies should be performed to exclude HTLV-1, syphilis, and vitamin $B_{12}$ and folate deficiencies. CSF analysis in VM occasionally reveals a mild nonspecific pleocytosis ranging from 5 to 10 cells/mm$^3$ (Dal-Pan et al. 1994). CSF protein is usually mildly elevated. Other CSF abnormalities include increased $\beta_2$-microglobulin, neopterin, and TNF-$\alpha$ (Tyor et al. 1993). Imaging studies of the spine reveal nonspecific changes including spinal cord atrophy and white matter changes. Somatosensory evoked potentials, particularly of lower extremity nerves, reveals abnormalities consistent with myelopathy, although coexisting peripheral neuropathy may complicate their interpretation. VM is a diagnosis of exclusion and should be considered when other potentially treatable causes have been considered.

### Pathology

The spinal cord in VM is characterized by the presence of intramyelinic and periaxonal vacuoles. These changes are most prominent in the dorsal and lateral columns. Most of the pathology occurs at the midthoracic level (Goldstick et al. 1985). The vacuoles are produced due to the presence of lipid-laden macrophages. The posterior columns are most affected rostrally, while the lateral columns are most affected caudally (Goldstick et al. 1985). Varying degrees of astrogliosis is also present (Artigas et al. 1990). TNF-$\alpha$ is present in significant amounts within the affected areas of the spinal cord within the macrophages and the microglia (Tan et al. 1996) as demonstrated by immunostaining. The presence of large amounts of TNF-$\alpha$ in early stages of the disease suggests that it might play a role in causing myelin vacuolation in VM. Multinucleated giant cells and microglial nodules are infrequently seen and lymphocytic infiltrates are absent. A grading system has been developed by Petito et al. (1986) from grade 1 to 3 based on the degree of vacuolization.

### Pathogenesis

The pathogenesis of AIDS-associated VM is unknown. Although HIV-1 virus is present in the spinal cord of patients with VM (Weiser et al. 1990), its direct role in the development of VM is questionable. It is possible that HIV indirectly causes myelin damage via macrophage-derived toxins or cytokines, such as TNF-$\alpha$. The prominence of activated macrophages in mild to moderate VM suggests that they may be involved in the early phases of disease activation.

Macrophage infiltration usually precedes the development of vacuoles and is closely involved in their pathogenesis. Macrophage-derived TNF-$\alpha$ is neurotoxic with myelinotoxic properties (Selmaj et al. 1988), and is also involved in the pathogenesis of multiple sclerosis (Hofman et al. 1989). Increased macrophage activity occurs in late HIV infection due to decreased production of cytokines such as interleukin-4 (IL-4) and IL-10 by CD4 cells, which are macrophage inhibitors. It is unclear why myelin changes occur in such a characteristic distribution in the spinal cord in VM.

Since there is a similarity between VM and subacute combined degeneration (SACD) of the spinal cord, it is postulated that abnormalities involving the $B_{12}$ and folate pathways may contribute to the myelin damage. However, this has not been confirmed. Persistent myelin damage could lead to increased requirement for metabolic products for repair mechanisms. One such agent is the universal methyl donor (S-adenosylmethionine), which is involved in the methylation of fatty acids, polysaccharides, and myelin basic protein. This is a product of the methyl transfer pathway involving folate and $B_{12}$ metabolism (Tan et al. 1996). When consumption of the methyl groups becomes excessive, a secondary methyl group deficiency develops that is similar to that of SACD of the cord without decreased $B_{12}$ and folate levels. This may partially explain the similarity between VM and SACD.

### Treatment

The treatment of VM is mainly symptomatic with physical therapy. Spasticity may be treated with baclofen or botulinum toxin. Di Rocco and colleagues are conducting an experimental placebo-controlled study of methionine in the treatment of

HIV VM. The authors are also conducting an open-label pilot trial of intravenous immunoglobulin in the treatment of HIV VM.

### Prognosis

There is a paucity of data concerning prognostic factors in VM. Once VM develops, it generally pursues a relentlessly progressive course, although a longitudinal natural history study has not been performed. The effects of specific therapeutic interventions remain a matter of conjecture. Thus, results of current therapeutic trials are eagerly awaited.

## Meningeal Disorders

### Systemic Lymphoma With CNS Involvement

One of the most common systemic malignancies associated with HIV infection is non-Hodgkin's lymphoma, present in 7% to 10% of patients (Levine 1987). CNS spread occurs in about 30% of patients (Levine et al. 1991a), usually in the form of leptomeningeal involvement. Presenting signs include headache, fever, night sweats, weight loss, and lymphadenopathy. Such patients may also develop cranial nerve palsies and meningismus. However, 17% of patients with leptomeningeal involvement are asymptomatic (Levine et al. 1991a).

### Cryptococcal Meningitis

*Cryptococcus neoformans* (CN) is a common fungus found throughout the world and commonly isolated from soil and pigeon droppings. It enters the human body through the respiratory tract and in immunocompromised hosts behaves as a pathogen, disseminates widely, and causes a life-threatening infection (Diamond 1995). CN is the fourth most common cause of life-threatening infection among patients with AIDS after *cytomegalovirus, Pneumocystis carinii,* and *Mycobacterium avium-intracellulare* (Kovacs et al. 1985). Cryptococcosis is estimated to occur in 5% to 8% of the AIDS population, mostly as a meningoencephalitic involvement, although extrameningeal sites including lungs, genitourinary tract, and bone marrow are frequently involved (Kovacs et al. 1985; Eng et al. 1986; Zuger et al. 1986; Chuck and Sande 1989). It is also noted that cryptococcal infection in AIDS patients is usually associated with profound immunosuppression (Crowe et al. 1991; Larsen et al. 1994).

Cryptococcal meningoencephalitis (CME), the most common manifestation of CN in HIV infection, occurs in 5% of AIDS patients. It has a racial and geographic tendency with a higher prevalence in African Americans, Haitians, and in intravenous drug abusers. It also has a particularly high frequency in New Jersey, with a prevalence of 7.8% (Levy et al. 1988b).

### Pathology

The pathological features of CME are different in HIV-infected and -uninfected patients. While HIV-uninfected patients exhibit a classical granulomatous inflammation, the CNS in HIV-infected patients often shows little inflammatory response consisting mainly of macrophage and microglial infiltration. Patients with HIV infection also exhibit multifocal invasion, more widespread tissue cryptococcal antigen deposit, and a prominent encephalitic component when compared to HIV-seronegative patients. A dysregulation in microglia/macrophage defense mechanisms against CN in HIV patients may explain these pathological findings (Lee et al. 1996).

### Clinical Features

The clinical course of CME in AIDS patients is indolent, with a mean duration from onset of symptoms to diagnosis of 1 month (Zuger et al. 1986). Symptoms are nonspecific, including fever, headache, and general malaise (Chuck and Sande 1989; Zuger et al. 1986; Kovacs et al. 1985). Altered mental status and focal neurological deficits are seen in only 15% to 19% of patients, and meningismus is present in 27% to 31% of patients. Half of AIDS patients with *Cryptococcus* meningitis have extrameningeal involvement as compared to 12% in non-AIDS patients (Eng et al. 1986).

### Diagnosis

Routine blood and CSF studies are often of little help in diagnosing CME. The CSF usually exhibits a mild lymphocytosis. Glucose levels may vary from normal to low, and protein from normal to mildly high. The diagnosis of CME does not necessarily require a positive CSF culture. Identifying the organism by India ink staining is a rapid means of establishing the diagnosis with a sensitivity of 85% and a specificity of 53% (Gal et al. 1987).

An assay of cryptococcal antigen (CRAG) in serum and CSF is both sensitive and specific. Chuck et al. reported that serum CRAG is more sensitive in diagnosing CME than CSF CRAG (99% vs. 91%) (Chuck and Sande 1989). Increased CSF opening pressure of greater than or equal to 200 mm Hg at the time of the lumbar puncture was noted in 62% to 66% of patients (Chuck and Sande 1989; Zuger et al. 1986).

### Treatment and Prognosis

Cryptococcal meningitis is fatal if untreated. The mortality during initial therapy is 10% to 40% (Diamond and Bennett 1974; Kovacs et al. 1985; Zuger et al. 1986; Eng et al. 1986; Saag et al. 1992). Pretreatment factors predictive of high mortality include an abnormal mental status at presentation, a CSF white blood cell (WBC) count less than or equal to 20 cells/mm$^3$, a positive CSF India ink, and a CSF CRAG greater than or equal to 1:1024 dilution (Saag et al. 1992; Dismukes et al. 1987).

Amphotericin B with or without flucytosine for 4 to 6 weeks was considered to be the standard treatment of CME in the pre-AIDS era with a success rate of 75% to 85% (Bennett et al. 1979; Dismukes et al. 1987). In AIDS patients, several retrospective studies have evaluated the response to treatment, which included amphotericin B at a dosage of 0.3 to 0.5 mg/kg/d with or without flucytosine. The success rate defined by negative cultures and clinical improvement at the completion of therapy did not exceed 50%. Flucytosine improved the overall success rate when added to amphotericin B but was associated with a high toxicity rate, particularly granulocytopenia (Kovacs et al. 1985; Zuger et al. 1986; Chuck and Sande 1989).

When compared to amphotericin B at 0.3 mg/kg/d, fluconazole at 400 mg/d showed an identical response rate, although both regimens were suboptimal for high-risk patients (Saag et al. 1992). Higher doses of amphotericin B may have a better success rate (Van Der Horst et al. 1997).

Without any suppressive treatment, the relapse rate of CME is as high as 50% to 60% (Zuger et al. 1986; Chuck and Sande 1989; Kovacks et al. 1985), thus maintenance therapy is required. The two primary agents for maintenance therapy are weekly intravenous injection of amphotericin B or oral fluconazole. Stern et al. reported an open trial of fluconazole as maintenance therapy with encouraging results (Stern et al. 1988). In a prospective study conducted by Powderly et al. in 1992, fluconazole at 200 mg/d orally was superior to placebo and weekly injections of amphotericin B in preventing relapse (97% vs. 78%, respectively).

The primary prophylaxis of cryptococcosis in severely immunocompromised AIDS patients is under investigation. Several studies showed promising results with fluconazole. The dosage and frequency is yet to be defined (Quagliarello et al. 1995; Singh et al. 1996).

### Neurosyphilis

There is evidence that concurrent HIV-1 infection alters the natural history of syphilis and its response to treatment. In the pre-AIDS era and after the introduction of penicillin, neurosyphilis had become rare (Niedelman 1956; Perdrup et al. 1981; Jaffe and Kabins 1982). With the advent of HIV-1 infection, the prevalence of symptomatic and asymptomatic neurosyphilis has risen to 5.7% to 12.5% and 2% to 54%, respectively (Berger 1991; Holtom et al. 1992; Brandon et al. 1993; Zisfein et al. 1993). HIV-1–infected patients, despite adequate treatment for early syphilis, were noted to develop neurosyphilis, an unusual occurrence prior to the 1980s (Bayne et al. 1986; Berry et al. 1987; Musher et al. 1990; Telzak et al. 1991). Symptomatic neurosyphilis in HIV-1 infection is reported to present early in the course of coinfection, with a spectrum of manifestations that include meningitis, meningovascular syphilis, polyradiculopathy, transverse myelitis, and optic neuritis.

The course of neurosyphilis in HIV-1–infected patients appears to be more aggressive (Lanska et al. 1988; Feraru et al. 1990; Berger 1992), although several studies have failed to support these findings (Fiumara et al. 1989; Gourevitch et al. 1993). The diagnosis of neurosyphilis should be pursued in all HIV-1 patients with a reactive serum rapid plasma reagin (RPR) and fluorescent treponemal antibody absorption (FTA-ABS). Such diagnoses are based on clinical findings and supported by CSF pleocytosis, elevated protein, and a reactive Venereal Disease Research Laboratories (VDRL) test. Caution should be taken in interpreting CSF serology in the HIV-infected patient, as pleocytosis could be due to HIV alone and CSF-VDRL may show a delayed seroconversion or remain nonreactive in proven cases of neurosyphilis (Johns et al. 1987; Feraru et al. 1990).

Since treatment of neurosyphilis in HIV-1–infected patients may have a high relapse rate (Malone et al. 1995), such patients should be treated aggressively and followed closely. The Centers for Disease Control (CDC) has recommended treating neurosyphilis in HIV-1 subjects with either aqueous crystalline penicillin G, 2 to 4 million U intravenous every 4 hours for 10 to 14 days or procaine penicillin 2.4 million U intramuscularly once a day, plus probenecid 500 mg by mouth four times a day, both for a total of 10 to 14 days (CDC 1993). Some authors recommend obtaining serum nontreponemal tests monthly for the first 3 months after treatment and every 3 to 6 months thereafter until titers are nonreactive or reactive at a titer of less than or equal to 1 : 8. Similarly, The CSF should be examined at 3 months after therapy and every 6 months thereafter until normal (Berger and Levy 1997).

## Neuromuscular Disorders

### Peripheral Neuropathy

Early retrospective studies showed that peripheral involvement occurs in 5% to 8% of HIV patients (Snider et al. 1983; Levy et al. 1985; Parry 1988) and represents 15% to 20% of all neurological complications related to HIV infection (Dalakas and Pezeshkpour 1988). Subclinical evidence of peripheral neuropathy has been found in 50% to 90% of AIDS patients (Comi et al. 1986; De la Monte et al. 1988; Barohn et al. 1989; Gastaut et al. 1989). Peripheral neuropathies that may present early in HIV-1 infection include inflammatory demyelinating polyneuropathy and cranial neuropathy (Piette et al. 1986; Berger et al. 1987b; Cornblath et al. 1987; Vendrell et al. 1987). With advanced immunosuppression, distal symmetrical polyneuropathy and polyradiculopathy are more common (Ghika-Schmid et al. 1994). It is critical to distinguish among the various forms of neuropathy because their pathogenesis, prognosis, and treatment vary. We will review in this section the most common peripheral neuropathies in HIV.

### Distal Symmetrical Polyneuropathy

Distal symmetrical polyneuropathy (DSP) is the most common form of neuropathy in HIV infection (Miller et al. 1988; Simpson and Wolfe 1991; Ghika-Schmid et al. 1994). DSP is present in 35% of AIDS patients (So et al. 1988), particularly in later stages of the disease when immunosuppression is advanced (Barohn et al. 1993; Simpson et al. 1994). DSP presents predominantly as a sensory polyneuropathy with burning and painful paresthesias involving the feet more than the hands. Distal weakness develops only late in its course. Physical examination reveals distal symmetrical loss of sensory function with diminished distal reflexes (Lange et al. 1988; So et al. 1988). Electrophysiological studies show that sural nerve amplitude is significantly reduced (Fuller et al. 1991; Simpson et al. 1994). Needle electromyography (EMG) may demonstrate signs of active or chronic denervation in distal leg muscles (Bailey et al. 1988; Lange et al. 1988). Nerve biopsy demonstrates axonal degeneration and loss of large myelinated fibers with occasional perivascular mononuclear inflammation (Mah et al. 1988; De la Monte et al. 1988).

The pathogenesis of HIV-associated DSP is uncertain. Direct viral infection is unlikely to be the primary cause of DSP (De la Monte et al. 1988). Indirect immune mechanisms such as cytokine toxicity may be pathogenetic (Wesselingh et al. 1993). DSP may also result from vitamin $B_{12}$ deficiency, although this is not a common cause in HIV-infected subjects (Kieburtz et al. 1991). DSP is also a well-defined side effect of the antiretroviral nucleoside analogue didanosine (ddI), zalcitabine (ddC), and stavudine (d4T) (Kieburtz et al. 1992; Dubinsky et al. 1989; Berger et al. 1993b; Browne et al. 1993; Simpson and Tagliati 1995). Patients with a history of subclinical neuropathy prior to initiation of such antiretroviral regimens are more susceptible to developing symptomatic neuropathy after the drug is started.

Nucleoside-related DSP tends to evolve more rapidly (Simpson and Tagliati 1994) and usually responds to withdrawal of the neurotoxin, although a coasting period of sympton intensification may occur for 4 to 8 weeks before improvement is seen (Berger et al. 1993b). The treatment of DSP is essentially symptomatic and includes analgesics, tricyclic antidepressants, anticonvulsants, and topical agents (Cornblath et al. 1988). Recent controlled clinical trials have demonstrated the efficacy of recombinant human nerve growth factor (McArthur et al. 1998) and the novel anticonvulsant lamotrigine. (Simpson et al. 1998). We are currently investigating the efficacy of topical lidocaine in DSP (Khan et al. 1998).

### Inflammatory Demyelinating Polyneuropathy

Inflammatory demyelinating polyneuropathy (IDP) occurs in HIV infection either as an acute (AIDP) or chronic, relapsing form (CIDP). It is more commonly found in asymptomatic stages of HIV infection, can be the initial manifestation of the disease (Cornblath et al. 1987; Lange et al. 1988), and may coincide with seroconversion (Piette et al. 1986).

Clinically, histologically, and electrophysiologically, IDP does not differ in HIV-negative and HIV-positive patients (Cornblath et al. 1987). Patients present with acute or subacute, relapsing or progressive weakness with minimal sensory signs. Electrophysiological studies show evidence of conduction block, prolonged distal latencies, prolonged or absent late responses, and reduced motor nerve compound action potential amplitudes (Miller et al. 1988). CSF reveals a lymphocytic pleocytosis in HIV-seropositive patients as compared to acellular CSF found in HIV-seronegative patients (Dalakas 1986; Cornblath et al. 1987). Nerve biopsy shows segmental demyelination and perivascular lymphocytic infiltrates (Cornblath et al. 1987).

The etiology of IDP in HIV patients is thought to be autoimmune with mechanisms similar to those proposed in HIV-seronegative patients (Dalakas and Pezeshkpour 1988; Simpson and Wolfe 1991). While controlled studies have not been done, observations have shown that the clinical course and the response to treatment is similar in HIV-infected and HIV-uninfected patients. Case reports have indicated that prednisone, plasmapheresis, and intravenous immunoglobulin (IVIG) may be effective in the treatment of IDP in HIV-induced patients (Cornblath et al. 1988; Miller et al. 1988; Leger et al. 1989).

### Mononeuropathy Multiplex

Mononeuropathy multiplex (MM) may occur in association with HIV infection (Lipkin et al. 1985). MM is multifocal and typically involves multiple spinal, cranial or peripheral nerves resulting in sensory or motor deficits in the distribution of involved nerves. MM occurs at different stages of HIV disease. In the early stages it generally involves a few nerves (especially the facial nerve) and usually resolves spontaneously, while in later stages MM has a rapidly progressive course and carries a poor prognosis (Lange et al. 1988; So et al. 1991).

Pathological studies have revealed several patterns associated with MM. Axonal degeneration is seen early in HIV infection, and cytomegalic inclusion bodies in advanced stages of HIV. Necrotizing arteritis is a less common pathological feature (Dalakas and Pezeshkpour 1988). An autoimmune mechanism has been postulated for early MM (Dalakas and Pezeshkpour 1988), while CMV is a primary pathogenetic agent in late stages, particularly when CD4 lymphocyte counts are below 50 cells/mm$^3$ (So 1992). Varicella-zoster virus (VZV) and lymphoma should also be considered in the differential diagnosis of MM (Engstrom et al. 1991; Berger et al. 1993a). CSF may show elevated protein and pleocytosis. Assay of the CSF for CMV by PCR may provide helpful diagnostic information, particularly in patients with advanced immunosuppression (Roullet et al. 1994). Electrodiagnostic studies in MM indicate a multifocal process with axonal degeneration.

The treatment of MM depends on the etiology and stage of the disease. Early in HIV infection MM tends to have a benign course and resolves spontaneously, requiring no treatment or immunomodulatory therapy such as prednisone or IVIG. In advanced AIDS, MM is mainly due to CMV and requires rapid diagnosis and treatment with ganciclovir, foscarnet, or cidofivir in order to prevent a poor outcome (Said et al. 1991; So 1992).

### Progressive Polyradiculopathy

Progressive polyradiculopathy (PP) generally occurs with advanced immunosuppression and usually coexists with systemic CMV infection (Eidelberg et al. 1986; Miller et al. 1990). CMV has been implicated in the pathogenesis of this syndrome, since CMV infiltration of nerve roots has been identified (Behar et al. 1987; Grafe and Wiley 1989; Said et al. 1991). PP presents as a rapidly progressive paraparesis, sensory loss mainly in the sacral distribution, and early sphincter dysfunction (Eidelberg et al. 1986). CSF usually demonstrates increased protein and polymorphonuclear pleocytosis. CMV can occasionally be detected in CSF by culture, but PCR is the assay of choice in establishing the diagnosis (Roullet et al. 1994; Cinque et al. 1993). EMG reveals widespread denervation in lower extremity muscles and lumbar paraspinal muscles while nerve conduction velocities are only mildly affected (Miller et al. 1990; Said et al. 1991). Since PP has a specific treatment, early diagnosis and treatment is critical in achieving a good outcome (Glass et al. 1993). Although no controlled studies have been done, anti-CMV therapy as discussed above is often effective in stabilizing the clinical course (de Gans et al. 1990; Kim and Hollander 1993; So and Olney 1994). If therapy is delayed by more than several days, irreversible nerve root necrosis may occur predicting a poor clinical outcome.

### Autonomic Neuropathy

Anecdotal reports of autonomic nervous system (ANS) dysfunction in HIV infection were recorded as early as 1987 (Lin-Greenberg and Taneja-Uppal 1987; Craddock et al. 1987; Evenhouse et al. 1987; Villa et al. 1987). While autonomic studies indicate dysfunction occurs in 60% to 75% of AIDS patients, it is frequently subclinical or overlooked (Welby et al. 1991; Ruttimann et al. 1991; Villa et al. 1992).

Autonomic dysfunction involves both parasympathetic and sympathetic divisions (Cohen and Laudenslager 1989; Freeman et al. 1990) and may be the result of CNS or peripheral nervous system involvement (Cohen and Laudenslager 1989). Batman et al. showed the presence of abnormal and depleted autonomic axons in small bowel mucosa (Griffin et al. 1988; Batman et al. 1991). Purba et al. demonstrated the existence of a decreased number of oxytocin neurons in the periventricular nucleus of the hypothalamus (Purba et al. 1993). Despite these pathological observations, the pathogenesis of HIV-associated ANS dysfunction is unknown. HIV has been postulated as a causative agent in ANS dysfunction (Freeman et al. 1990; Scott et al. 1990). Villa et al. proposed an immune theory underlying autonomic impairment in HIV infection (Villa et al. 1992).

Pentamidine and other drugs used in HIV infection have been associated with autonomic dysfunction (Hemlick and Green 1985). Autonomic dysfunction is more commonly seen later in the course of HIV (Welby et al. 1991) but subclinical forms have been detected early by autonomic nervous system tests (Villa et al. 1992; Mulhall and Jennens 1987). The severity of autonomic dysfunction correlates with the extent of immunosuppression (Ruttimann et al. 1991). Clinical manifestations include impotence, diarrhea, bladder dysfunction, decreased sweating, and cardiovascular dysregulation (Lin-Greenberg and Taneja-Uppal 1987; Craddock et al. 1987; Evenhouse et al. 1987; Batman et al. 1991). Progressive involvement of the autonomic nervous system during the course of HIV infection has been suggested (Ruttimann et al. 1991; Becker et al. 1997). Cardiac dysregulation due to autonomic dysfunction has been associated with high mortality (Craddock et al. 1987).

## Myopathy

### HIV-Associated Myopathy

Myopathy in HIV-1 infection is infrequent as compared to other HIV-related neurological complications. It occurs at all stages of HIV infection and occasionally constitutes the presenting manifestation of disease (Snider et al. 1983; Stern et al. 1987; Simpson and Bender 1988; Lange et al. 1988; Dalakas and Pezeshkpour 1988). The histopathological spectrum of HIV-associated myopathy can be broadly divided into two groups: inflammatory and noninflammatory (Dalakas et al. 1986; Dalakas et al. 1987; Illa et al. 1991; Dwyer et al. 1992).

The inflammatory myopathies in HIV disease are indistinguishable from those occurring in seronegative patients. Muscle biopsy usually shows necrotic fibers and inflammatory infiltrates, although the extent of inflammation is generally less in HIV-infected patients (Dalakas et al. 1986; Lange et al. 1988; Simpson and Bender 1988; Illa et al. 1991). The noninflammatory myopathies, which include nemaline (rod) myopathy, are still a poorly understood group. Muscle biopsy may exhibit intracytoplasmic rod bodies in atrophic type 1 myofibers, selective loss of thick fibers, and cytoplasmic microvesiculation (Dalakas and Pezeshkpour 1988; Gonzales et al. 1988; Wrzoleck et al. 1990; Simpson and Bender 1988). The pathogenesis of HIV-associated myopathy is hypothetically based on an immune mechanism involving cytokines (Illa et al. 1991; Gherardi et al. 1994). HIV antigens have not been reliably isolated from muscle fibers (Illa et al. 1991; Leon-Monzon et al. 1993).

The primary clinical symptom of myopathy is slowly progressive proximal muscle weakness with occasional myalgia and mild to moderate elevation in creatine kinase (CK) (Lange et al. 1988; Simpson and Bender 1988; Masanes et al. 1995). Myopathy is one of the causes of HIV wasting syndrome (Simpson et al. 1990; Belec et al. 1993; Masanes et al. 1995). HIV-myopathy tends to respond to immunomodulatory therapy, including corticosteroids. The authors are conducting a pilot study of IVIG in the treatment of HIV myopathy.

### Zidovudine Myopathy

Since the introduction of AZT in the treatment of HIV infection, several authors have associated myopathy with this medication (Dalakas et al. 1990; Mhiri et al. 1991; Grau et al. 1993). Zidovudine is thought to cause a reversible myopathy through inhibition of mitochondrial DNA polymerase gamma and mitochondrial depletion (Simpson et al. 1989; Arnaudo et al. 1993). The frequency of AZT myopathy is unclear, since study designs vary among different investigators.

Dalakas et al. reported an AZT-associated myopathy associated with ragged red fibers. This group later demonstrated the presence of abnormal mitochondria and depletion of mtDNA on electron microscopy (Dalakas et al. 1990; Pezeshkpour and Dalakas et al. 1991). Chariot and Gherardi measured mitochondrial dysfunction in AZT-treated patients by demonstrating partial deficiency in cytochrome-c oxidase activity and a high lactate/pyruvate ratio in blood (Chariot et al. 1993, 1994). Nonetheless, the notion that AZT myopathy is distinguishable from HIV myopathy is not universally accepted. Simpson et al. and Morgello et al. have noted that similar mitochondrial abnormalities are present in patients with HIV myopathy whether or not they have been treated with zidovudine (Simpson et al. 1993; Morgello et al. 1995). Clinically and electrophysiologically, AZT myopathy is similar to HIV-associated myopathy, with progressive proximal weakness. The extent to which withdrawal of AZT improves muscular weakness varies among series (Mhiri et al. 1991; Manji et al. 1993), although in our experience the majority of patients do not improve with AZT withdrawal (Simpson et al. 1993).

Immunomodulatory therapy including prednisone may have a role in refractory cases of AZT myopathy (Manji et al. 1993; Simpson et al. 1993). Dalakas et al. demonstrated that AZT-induced mitochondrial toxicity results in decreased carnitine levels in the muscle, suggesting that L-carnitine supplementation might have a role in improving AZT myopathy (Dalakas et al. 1994).

## References

Anders, K. H.; Guerra, W. F.; Tomiyasu, U.; et al. The neuropathology of AIDS: UCLA experience and review. Am. J. Pathol. 124:537–558; 1986.

Anders, P.; Munoz, A.; Vlahov, D.; Friendland, G. H. The incubation period of human immunodefiency virus. Epidemiol. Rev. 15:305–318; 1993.

Ariza, A.; Kim, J. H. Kaposi's sarcoma of the dura mater. Hum. Pathol. 19:1461–1462; 1988.

Arnaudo, E.; Dalakas, M. C.; Shanske, S.; et al. Depletion of muscle mitochondrial DNA in AIDS patients with ZDV-induced myopathy. Lancet 337:508–510; 1993.

Artigas, J.; Grosse, G.; Niedobitek, F. Vacuolar myelopathy in AIDS. A morphological analysis. Pathol. Res. Pract. 186:228–237; 1990.

Artigas, J.; Grosse, G.; Niedobitek, F.; et al. Severe toxoplasmic ventriculomeningoencephalomyelitis in two AIDS patients following treatment of cerebral toxoplasmic granuloma. Clin. Neuropathol. 13:120–126; 1994.

Bailey, R. O.; Baltch, A. L.; Miller, E. N.; et al. Sensory motor neuropathy associated with AIDS. Neurology 38:886–891; 1988.

Barohn, R. J.; Gronseth, G. S.; Leforce, B. R.; et al. Peripheral nervous system involvement in a large cohort of human imunodeficiency virus-infected individuals. Arch. Neurol. 50:167–171; 1993.

Barhon, R. J.; LeForce, B. R.; McVey, A. L.; et al. Peripheral nervous system involvement in human immunodeficiency virus (HIV) infection: a prospective study of a large cohort of HIV-seropositive individuals. Muscle Nerve 9:762; 1989.

Batman, P. A.; Miller, A.; Sedgwick, P. M.; et al. Autonomic denervation in jejunal mucosa of homosexual men infected with HIV. AIDS 5:1247–1252; 1991.

Bayne, L. L.; Schmidely, J. W.; Goodin, D. S. Acute syphilitic meningitis. Its occurrence after clinical and serological cure of secondary syphilis with penicillin G. Arch. Neurol. 43:137–138; 1986.

Becker, K.; Gorlach, I.; Frieling, T.; et al. Characterization and natural course of cardiac autonomic nervous system dysfunction in HIV-infected patients. AIDS 11:751–757; 1997.

Behar, R.; Wiley, C.; McCutchan, J. A. Cytomegalovirus polyradiculopathy in acquired immunodeficiency syndrome. Neurology 37:557–561; 1987.

Belec, L.; Mhiri, C. H.; Constanzo, B.; Gherardi, R. The HIV wasting syndrome. Muscle Nerve 15:856–857; 1993.

Bennett, J. E.; Dismukes, W. E.; Duma, R. J.; et al. A comparison of amphotericin B alone and combined with flucytosine in the treatment of cryptococcal meningitis. N. Engl. J. Med. 301:126–131; 1979.

Berger, A. R.; Arezzo, J. C.; Schaumburg, H. H.; et al. 2′,3′-dideoxycitidine (ddC) toxic neuropathy: a study of 52 patients. Neurology 43: 358–362; 1993.

Berger, J. R. Neurosyphilis in human immunodeficiency virus type 1-seropositive individuals. A prospective study. Arch. Neurol. 48:700–702; 1991.

Berger, J. R. Spinal cord syphilis associated with human immunodeficiency virus infection: a treatable myelopathy. Am. J. Med. 92:101–103; 1992.

Berger, J. R.; Flaster, M.; Schatz, N.; et al. Cranial neuropathy heralding otherwise occult AIDS-related large cell lymphoma. J. Clin. Neurophysiol. 13: 113–118; 1993.

Berger, J. R.; Kaszovitz, B.; Post, M. J.; Dickinson, G. Progressive multifocal leukoencephalopathy associated with human immunodeficiency virus infection: a review of the literature with a report of sixteen cases. Ann. Intern. Med. 107:78–87; 1987a.

Berger, J. R.; and Levy, R. M., eds. AIDS and the nervous system. 2nd ed. Philadelphia: Lippincott-Raven; 1997: p. 687–688.

Berger, J. R.; Moskowitz, L.; Fischl, M.; et al. Neurologic disease as the presenting manifestation of acquired immunodeficiency syndrome. South. Med. J. 80:683–686; 1987b.

Berger, J. R.; Mucke, L. Prolonged survival and partial recovery in AIDS-associated progressive multifocal leukoencephalopathy. Neurology 38:1060–1065; 1988.

Berry, C. D.; Hooton, T. M.; Collier, A. C.; Lukehart, S. A. Neurological relapse after benzathine penicillin therapy for secondary syphilis in a patient with HIV infection. N. Engl. J. Med. 316:1587–1589; 1987.

Brandon, W. R.; Boulos, L. M.; Morse, A. Determining the prevalence of neurosyphilis in a cohort co-infected with HIV. Int. J. STD AIDS 4:99–101; 1993.

Brew, B. J.; Rosenblum, M.; Cronin, K.; Price, R. W. AIDS demetia complex and HIV-1 brain infection: clinical-virological correlations. Ann. Neurol. 38: 563–570; 1995.

Brew, B.; Brown, S.; Catalan, J.; Simpson, D.; and the CNA3001 International Study Team: Phase III, randomized, double blind, placebo controlled, multicentre study to evaluate the safety and efficacy of abacavir (ABC, 1592) in HIV-1 infected patients with AIDS dementia complex (abstract). Proceedings of the 12th World AIDS Conference, Geneva, Switzerland, 1998.

Britton, C. B.; Marquardt, M. D.; Garvey, G.; Miller, J. R. Neurological complications of the gay immuno-

suppressed syndrome: clinical and pathological features. Ann. Neurol. 12:80; 1982.

Brooks, B. R.; Walker, D. L. Progressive multifocal leukoencephalopathy. Neurol. Clin. 2:229–313; 1984.

Browne, M. J.; Mayer, K. H.; Chafee, S. B.; et al. 2′,3′-dideoxyhydro-3′-deoxythymidine (d4T) in patients with AIDS or AIDS-related complex: a phase I trial. J. Infect. Dis. 166:21–29; 1993.

Casabona, J.; Sanchez, E.; Graus, F.; et al. Trends and survival for AIDS patients presenting with indicative neurologic diseases. Acta Neurol. Scand. 84:51–55; 1991.

Case Records of the Massachusetts General Hospital. N. Engl. J. Med. 309:359–369; 1983.

Centers for Disease Control and Prevention. 1993 Sexually transmitted diseases treatment guidelines. MMWR Morb. Mortal. Wkly. Rep. 42:27–46; 1993.

Chariot, P.; Benbrik, E.; Schaeffer, A.; Gheraldi, R. Tubular aggregates and partial cytochrome C oxidase deficiency in skeletal muscle in patients with AIDS treated with zidovudine. Acta Neuropathol. 85: 431–436; 1993.

Chariot, P.; Monnet, I.; Mouchet, M.; Gheraldi, L.; et al. Determinant of the blood lactate:pyruvate ratio as a noninvasive tool for the diagnosis of zidovudine myopathy. Arthritis Rheum. 37:583–586; 1994

Chuck, S. L.; Sande, M. A. Infections with cryptococcus neoformans in the acquired immunodeficiency syndrome. N. Engl. J. Med. 321:794–799; 1989.

Clark, S. J.; Saag, M. S.; Becker, W. D.; et al. Hightiters of cytopathic virus in plasma of patients with symptomatic primary HIV-1 infection. N. Engl. J. Med. 324:1954–1960; 1991.

Cinque, P., Bryting, M.; Vago, L.; et al. Epstein Barr virus DNA in cerebrospinal fluid from patients with AIDS-related primary lymphoma of the central nervous system. Lancet 342:398–401; 1993.

Clifford, D.; Yiannoutsos, C.; Glicksman, M.; et al. HAART improves prognosis in HIV-associated progressive multifocal leukoencephalopathy. Neurology 52:623–625; 1999.

Cohen, J. A.; Laudenslager, M. Autonomic nervous system involvement in patients with human immunodeficiency virus infection. Neurology 39:1111–1112; 1989.

Comi, G.; Medaglini, S.; Galardi, G.; et al. Subclinical neuromuscular involvement in acquired immune deficiency syndrome (abstract). Muscle Nerve 9: 65; 1986.

Corboy, J. R.; Garl, P. J.; Kleinschmidt-Demasters, B. K. Human herpesvirus 8 DNA in CNS lymphomas from patients with and without AIDS. Neurology 50: 335–340; 1998.

Cornblath, D. R. Treatment of the neuromuscular complications of human immunodeficiency virus infection. Ann. Neurol. 23(suppl.):S88–S91; 1988.

Cornblath, D. R.; McArthur, J. C.; Kennedy, P. G. E.; et al. Inflammatory demyelinating peripheral neuropathies associated with human T-cell lymphotrophic virus type III infection. Ann. Neurol. 2:32–40; 1987.

Craddock, C.; Pasvol, J.; Bull, R.; et al. Cardiorespiratory arrest and autonomic neuropathy in AIDS. Lancet 2:16–18; 1987.

Crowe, S. M.; Carlin, J. B.; Stewart, K. I.; et al. Predictive value of CD4 lymphocyte numbers for the development of opportunistic infections and malignancies in HIV-infected persons. J. Acquir. Immune. Defic. Syndr. 4:770–776; 1991.

Dalakas, M. C. Neuromuscular complications of AIDS. Muscle Nerve 9:92; 1986.

Dalakas, M. C.; Illa, I.; Pezeshkpour, G. H.; et al. Mitochondrial myopathy caused by long term zidovudine therapy. N. Engl. J. Med. 322:1098–1105; 1990.

Dalakas, M. C.; Leon-Monzon, M.; Bernardini, I.; et al. Zidovudine-induced mitochondrial myopathy is associated with muscle carnitine deficiency and lipid storage. Ann. Neurol. 35:482–487; 1994.

Dalakas, M. C.; Pezeshkpour, G. H. Neuromuscular diseases associated with human immunodeficinecy virus infection. Ann. Neurol. 23(suppl.):S38–S48; 1988.

Dalakas, M. C.; Pezeshkpour, G. H.; Flaherty, M. Progressive nemaline (rod) myopathy associated with HIV infection. N. Engl. J. Med. 317:1602–1603; 1987.

Dalakas, M. C.; Pezeshkpour G. H.; Gravell, M.; Server, J. L. Polymyositis associated with AIDS retrovirus. JAMA 256:2381–2383; 1986.

Dal-Pan, G. J.; Glass, J. D.; McArthur, J. C. Clinicopathologic correlations of HIV-associated vacuolar myelopathy: an autopsy-based case-control study. Neurology 44:2159–2164; 1994.

Davis, L. E., Hjelle, B. L.; Miller, V. E.; et al. Early viral brain invasion in iatrogenic human immunodefiency virus infection. Neurology 42:1736–1739; 1992.

De Gans, J.; Portegies, P.; Tiessens, G.; et al. Therapy for cytomegalovirus polyradiculopathy in patients with AIDS. Treatment with ganciclovir. AIDS 4:421–425; 1990.

De la Monte, S. M.; Gabuzda, D. H.; Ho, D. D.; et al. Peripheral neuropathy in the acquired immune deficiency syndrome. Ann. Neurol. 23:485–492; 1988.

DeAngelis, L. M. Primary CNS lymphoma. In DeVita, V. T. Jr.; Hellman, S.; Rosenberg, S. A., eds. Principles and practice of oncology updates. Philadelphia: J. B. Lippincott; 1992.

DeAngelis, L. M. Current management of primary central nervous system lymphoma. Oncology 9:63–78; 1995.

Di Rocco, A.; Simpson, D. AIDS-associated vacuolar myelopathy, AIDS Patients Care STDs 12:457–460; 1998.

Diamond R. D. Cryptococcus neoformans. In Mandel, G. L.; Douglas, R. G.; Bennett, J. E., eds. Principles and practice of infectious diseases. New York: Churchill Livingstone; 1995: p. 2331–2332.

Diamond, R. D.; Bennett, J. E. Prognostic factors in cryptococcal meningitis: a study of 111 cases. Ann. Intern. Med. 80:176–81; 1974.

Dismukes, W. E.; Cloud G.; Gallis, H. A.; et al. Treatment of cryptococcal meningitis with combination of amphotericin B and flucytosine for four as compared with six weeks. N. Engl. J. Med. 317:334–341; 1987.

Dreyer, E. B.; Kaiser, P. K.; Offermann, J. T.; Lipton, S. A. HIV-1 coat protein neurotoxicity prevented by calcium channel antagonists. Science 248:364–367; 1990.

Dubinsky, R. M.; Yarchoan, R.; Dalakas, M.; et al. Reversible axonal neuropathy from the treatment of AIDS and related disorders with 2′,3′-dideoxycytidine (ddC). Muscle Nerve 12:856–860; 1989.

Dwyer, B. A.; Mayer, R. F.; Lee, S. C. Progressive nemalin (rod) myopathy as a presentation of human immunodeficiency virus. Arch. Neurol. 49:440; 1992.

Eidelberg, D.; Sotrel, A.; Vogel, A. T.; et al. Progressive polyradiculopathy in acquired immune deficiency syndrome. Neurology 36:912–916; 1986.

Eikin, C. M.; Leon, E.; Grenell, S. L.; Leeds, N. E. Intracranial lesions in the acquired immunodeficiency large cell lymphoma (abstract). Blood 68:124; 1986.

Ellis, R.; Hsia, K.; Spector S.; et al. CSF HIV-1 RNA levels are elevated in neurocognitively impaired individuals. Ann. Neurol. 42:679–688; 1997.

Ellis, R. J.; McCutchan, J. A. Heaton, R. K.; et al. Elevated HIV RNA levels in cerebrospinal fluids predict increased subsequent risk for the development of neurocognitive disorders (abstract). Neurology 52 (suppl. 2):S253, 1999.

Eng, R. H. K.; Bishburg, E.; Smith, S. M.; Kapila, R. Cryptococcal meningitis in patients with acquired immunodeficiency syndrome. Am. J. Med. 81:19–23; 1986.

Engstrom, J. W.; Lewis, E.; McGuire, D. Cranial neuropathy and the acquired immunodeficiency syndrome. Neurology 41(suppl 1):S374; 1991.

Evenhouse, M.; Haas, E.; Snell, E.; et al. Hypotension in infection with the human immunodeficiency virus. Ann. Intern. Med. 107:598–599; 1987.

Farkash, A. E.; Maccabee, P. J.; Sher, J. H. CNS toxoplasmosis in acquired immunodeficiency syndrome: a clinical-pathology-radiological review of 12 cases. J. Neurol. Neurosurg. Psychiatry 49:744–748; 1986.

Feraru, E. R.; Aronow, H. A.; Lipton, R. B. Neurosyphilis in AIDS patients: initial CSF VDRL may be negative. Neurology 40:541–543; 1990.

Fiumara, N. Human immunodeficiency virus infection and syphilis. J. Am. Acad. Dermatol. 21:141–142; 1989.

Formenti, S. C.; Gill, P. S.; Lean, E.; et al. Primary central nervous system lymphoma in AIDS: results of radiation therapy. Cancer 63:1101–1107; 1989.

Freeman, R.; Roberts, M. S.; Friedman, L. S.; Broadbridge, C. Autonomic function and human immunodeficiency virus infection. Neurology 40:575–578; 1990.

Fuller, G. N.; Jacobs, J. M.; Guiloff, R. J. Subclinical peripheral nerve involvement in AIDS. An electrophysiological and pathological study. J. Neurol. Neurosurg. Psychiatry 54:318–324; 1991.

Gabuzda, D. H.; Ho, D. D.; de la Monte, S. M.; et al. Immunohistochemical identification of HTLV-III antigen in brains of patients with AIDS. Ann. Neurol. 20:289–295; 1986.

Gal, A. A.; Evans, S.; Meyer, P. R. The clinical laboratory evaluation of cryptococcal infections in the acquired immunoeficiency syndrome. Diagn. Microbiol. Infect. Dis. 7:249–254; 1987.

Gastaut, J. L.; Gastaut, J. A.; Pellissier, J. F.; et al. Neuropathies périphériques au cours de l'infection par le virus de l'immunodéficience humaine. Rev. Neurol. (Paris) 145:451–459 1989.

Genis, P.; Jett, M.; Bernton, E. W.; et al. Cytokines and arachidonic metabolites produced during human immunodeficiency virus (HIV)-infected macrophage astroglia interactions: implications for the neuropathogenesis of HIV disease. J. Exp. Med. 176:170–178; 1992.

Gherardi, R. K.; Florea-Strat, A.; Fromont, G.; et al. Cytokine expression in the muscle of HIV-infected patients: evidence for interleukin-1a accumulation in mitochondria of AZT fibers. Ann. Neurol. 36: 752–758; 1994.

Ghika-Schmid, F.; Kuntzer, T.; Chave, J. P.; et al. Diversite de l'atteinte neuromusculaire de 47 patients infectes par le virus de l'immunodeficience humaine. Schweiz. Med. Wochenschr. 124:791–800; 1994.

Gills, P. S.; Levine, A. M.; Meyer, P. R.; et al. Primary central nervous system lymphoma in homosexual men. Clinical, immunological and pathological features. Am. J. Med. 78:742–748; 1985.

Giulian, D.; Wendt, E.; Vaca, K.; Noonan, C. A. The envelope glycoprotein of neurotoxins from monocytes. Proc. Natl. Acad. Sci. USA 90:2769–2773; 1993.

Giulian, D.; Yu, J.; Li, X.; et al. Study of receptor-mediated neurotoxins released by HIV-1 infected mononuclear phagocytes found in human brain. J. Neurosci. 16:3139–3153; 1996.

Glass, J. D.; Erozan, Y. S. Rapid diagnosis of cytomegalovirus polyradiculitis in a patient with acquired immunodeficiency syndrome (letter). Ann. Neurol. 34:239; 1993.

Glass, J. D.; Wesselingh, S. L.; Seines, O. A.; McAuthur, J. C. Clinical-neuropathologic correlation in HIV-associated dementia. Neurology 43:2230–2237; 1993.

Goldstick, L.; Mandybur, T. I.; Bode, R. Spinal cord degeneration in AIDS. Neurology 35:103–106; 1985.

Gonzalez, M. F.; Olney, R. K.; So, Y. T.; et al. Subacute structural myopathy associated with human immunodeficiencxy virus infection. Arch. Neurol. 45: 585–587; 1988.

Gourevitch, M. N.; Selwyn. P. A.; Daverny, K.; et al. Effects of HIV infection on the serologic manifestations and response to treatment of syphilis in intravenous drug users. Ann. Intern. Med. 18:350–355; 1993.

Grafe, M. R.; Wiley, C. A.: Spinal cord and peripheral nerve pathology in AIDS: the role of cytomegalo-

virus and human immunodeficiency virus. Ann. Neurol. 25:561–566; 1989.

Grau, J. M.; Masanes, F.; Casademont, J.; et al. Human immunodeficiency virus type 1 infection and myopathy: clinical relevance of zidovudine therapy in AIDS. Ann. Neurol. 34:206–211; 1993.

Gray, F.; Gherardi, R.; Keohane, C.; et al. Pathology of the central nervous system in 40 cases of acquired immune deficiency syndrome (AIDS). Neuropathol. Appl. Neurobiol. 14: 365–380; 1988.

Griffin, G. E.; Miller, A.; Batman, P.; et al. Damage to jejunal intrinsic autonomic nerves in HIV infection. AIDS 2:379–382; 1988.

Hall, C. D.; Urania, D.; Simpson, D.; et al. Failure of cytarabine in progressive multifocal leukoencephalopathy associated with human immunodeficiency virus infection. N. Engl. J. Med. 338: 1345–1351; 1998.

Hemlick, C. G.; Green, J. K. Pentamidine-associated hypotension and route of administration. Ann. Intern. Med. 103:480; 1985.

Ho, D. D.; Rota, T. R.; Schooley, R. T.; et al. Isolation of patients with neurologic syndromes related to the acquired immunodeficiency syndrome. N. Engl. J. Med. 313:1493–1497; 1985.

Hochberg, F. H.; Miller, D. C. Primary central nervous system lymphoma. J. Neurosurg. 68:835–853; 1988.

Hochberg, F. H.; Miller, G.; Schooley, R. T.; et al. Central nervous system lymphoma related to Epstein-Barr virus. N. Engl. J. Med. 309:813–881; 1983.

Hofman, F. M.; Hinton, D. R.; Johnson, K.; Merrill, J. E. Tumor necrosis factor identified in multiple sclerosis brain J. Exp. Med. 170:607–612; 1989.

Holman, R. C.; Janssen, R. S.; Buehler, J. W.; Zelasky, M. T.; Hooper, W. C. Epidemiology of PML in the US: analysis of national mortality and AIDS surveillance data. Neurology 41:1733–1736; 1991.

Holtom, P. D.; Larsen, R. A.; Leal, M. E.; Leedom, J. M. Prevalence of neurosyphilis in human immunodeficiency virus-infected patients with latent syphilis. Am. J. Med. 93:9–12; 1992.

Horowitz, S. L.; Benson, D. F.; Gottlieb, M. S.; et al. Neurological complications of gay-related immunodeficiency disorder. Ann. Neurol. 12:80; 1982.

Huang, S. S.; Skolasky, R. L.; Dal Pan, G. L.; et al. Survival prolongation in HIV-associated progressive multifocal leucoencephalopathy treated with alpha-interferon: an observational study. J Neurovirol. 4:324–332; 1988.

Illa, I.; Nath, A.; Dalakas, M. Immunocytochemical and virological characteristics of HIV-associated inflammatory myopathy: similarities with seronegative polymyositis. Ann. Neurol. 29:474–481; 1991.

Jaffe, H. W.; Kabins, S. A. Examination of cerebrospinal fluid in patients with syphilis. Rev. Infect. Dis. 4(suppl.):S842–S847; 1982.

Jakobsen, J.; Smith, T.; Gaub. J.; et al. Progressive neurological dysfunction during latent HIV infection. BMJ 299:225–228; 1989.

Jellinger, K.; Raskiewicz, T. H.; Slowik, F. Primary malignant lymphoma of the central nervous system in man. Acta Neuropathol. (Berl.) 6(suppl.):S95–102; 1975.

Johns, D. R.; Tierney, M.; Parker, S. W. Pure motor hemiplegia due to meningovascular neurosyphilis. Arch. Neurol. 44:1062–1065; 1987.

Kelly, W. M.; Brant-Zawadzki, M. Acquired immunodeficiency syndrome: neuroradiological findings. Radiology 149:485–491; 1983.

Khan, A.; Dorfman, D.; Dalton, A.; et al. 5% Lidoderm in the treatment of painful peripheral HIV-neuropathy (abstract). J Neurovirol. 4:355; 1998.

Kieburtz, K. D.; Ciang, D. W.; Schiffer, R. B.; et al. Abnormal vitamin B12 metabolism in human immunodeficiency virus infection: association with neurological dysfunction. Arch. Neurol. 48:312–314; 1991.

Kieburtz, K. D.; Siedlin, M.; Lambert, J. S.; et al. Extended follow up of peripheral neuropathy in patients with AIDS and AIDS-related complex treated with dideoxyinosine. J. Acquir. Immune Defic. Syndr. 5: 60–64; 1992.

Kim, Y. S.; Hollander, H. Polyradiculopathy due to cytomegalovirus: report of two cases in which improvement occurred after prolonged therapy and review of the literature. Clin. Infect. Dis. 176:32–37; 1993.

Klein, P.; Zientek, G.; Vandenberg, S. R.; Lothman, E. Primary CNS lymphoma: lymphomatous meningitis presenting as a cauda equina lesion in an AIDS patient. Can. J. Neurol. Sci. 17:329–331; 1990.

Kovacs, J. A.; Kovacs, A. A.; Poli, M.; et al. Cryptococcosis in the acquired immunodeficiency syndrome. Ann. Intern. Med. 103:533–538; 1985.

Laissy, J. P.; Soyer, P.; Parlier, C.; et al. Persistent enhancement after treatment for cerebral toxoplasmosis in patients with AIDS: predictive value for subsequent recurrence. Am. J. Neuroradiol. 15:1773–1778; 1994.

Lange, D. J.; Britton, C. B.; Youger, D. S.; et al. The neuromuscular manifestations of human immunodeficiency virus infections. Arch. Neurol. 45: 1084–1088; 1988.

Lanska, M. J.; Lanska, D. J.; Schmidley, J. W. Syphilitic polyradiculopathy in an HIV-positive man. Neurology 38:1297–1301; 1988.

Larsen, R. A.; Bozette, S. A.; Jones, B. E.; et al. Fluconazole combined with flucytosine for treatment of cryptococcal meningitis in patients with AIDS. Clin. Infect. Dis. 19:741–745; 1994.

Lee, S. C.; Dickson, D. W.; Casadevall, A. Pathology of cryptococcal meningoencephalitis: analysis of 27 patients with pathogenic implications. Hum. Pathol. 27:839–847; 1996.

Leger, J. M.; Bouche, P.; Bolgert, F.; et al. The spectrum of polyneuropathies in patients infected with HIV. J. Neurol. Neurosurg. Psychiatry 52:1369–1374; 1989.

Leon-Monzon, M.; Lamphert, L.; Dalakas, M. C. Search for HIV proviral DNA and amplified sequences in the muscle biopsies of patients with HIV polymyositis. Muscle Nerve 16:408–413; 1993.

Levine, A. M. Non-Hodgkin's lymphoma and other malignancies in the acquired immune deficiency syndrome. Semin. Oncol. 14(suppl.):S34–S39; 1987.

Levine, A. M.; Sullivan-Halley, J.; Pike, M. C.; et al. HIV-related lymphoma: prognostic factors predictive of survival. Cancer 68:2466–2472; 1991a.

Levine, A. M.; Wernz, J. C.; Kaplan, L.; et al. Low dose chemotherapy with CNS prophylaxis and zidovudine maintenace for AIDS-related lymphoma: a prospective multi-institutional trial. JAMA 266: 84–88; 1991b.

Levy, R. M.; Bredesen, D. E.; Rosenblum, M. L. Neurological manifestations of the acquired immunodeficiency syndrome (AIDS): experience at the UCSF and review of the literature. J. Neurosurg. 62: 475–495; 1985.

Levy, R. M.; Janssen, R. S.; Bush, T. J.; et al. Neuroepidemiology of acquired immunodeficiency syndrome. In: Rosenblum, M. L.; Levy, R. M.; Bredesen, D. E.; eds. AIDS and the nervous system. New York: Raven Press; 1988a: p. 13–27.

Levy, R. M.; Jansen, R. S.; Bush, T. J.; Rosenblum, M. L. Neuroepidemiology of acquired immunodefiency syndrome. J. Acquir. Immune Defic. Syndr. 1: 31–40; 1988b.

Levy, R. M., Rosenblum, M. L. Neurosurgical aspects of HIV-1 infection. In: Wilkins, R. H.; Rengachary, S. S., eds. Neurosurgery update II. New York: McGraw-Hill, 1991: p. 257–268.

Levy, R. M.; Rosenblom, S.; Perrett, L. V. Neuroradiological findings in the acquired immunodeficiency syndrome (AIDS): a review of 200 cases AJNR Am. J. Neuroradiol. 7:833–839; 1986.

Lin-Greenberg, A.; Taneja-Uppal, N. Dysautonomia and infection with the human immunodeficiency virus . Ann. Intern. Med. 106:167; 1987.

Lipkin, W. I.; Parry, G.; Kiprov, D.; et al. Inflammatory neuropathy in homosexual men with lymphadenopathy. Neurology 35:1479–1483; 1985.

Lorberboym, M.; Estok, L.; Machac, J.; et al. Rapid differential diagnosis of cerebral toxoplasmosis and primary central nervous system lymphoma by thallium - 201 SPECT. J. Nucl. Med. 37:1150–1154; 1996.

Luft, B. J.; Catro, K. G. An overview of the problem of toxoplasmosis and pneumocystosis in AIDS in the USA: implication from future therapeutic trials. Eur. J. Clin. Microbiol. Infect. Dis. 10:178–181; 1991.

Luft, B. J.; Remington, J. S. Toxoplasmosis of the central nervous system. In: Remington, J. S.; Swartz, W. M., eds. Current clinical topics in infectious diseases. New York: McGraw-Hill; 1985: p. 315.

Luft, B. J.; Remington, J. S. Toxoplasmic encephalitis in AIDS. Clin. Infect. Dis. 15:177–187; 1992.

Mah, V.; Vartavarian, L. M.; Akers, M. A.; et al. Abnormalities of peripheral nerve in patients with human immunodeficiency virus infection. Ann. Neurol. 24:713–717; 1988.

Major, E. O.; Ault, G. S. Progressive multifocal leukoencephalopathy: clinical and laboratory observation on a viral induced demyelinating disease in the immunodeficient patient. Curr. Opin. Neurol. 8: 184–190; 1995.

Malone, J. L.; Wallace, M. R.; Hendrick, B. B. Syphilis and neurosyphilis in a human immunodeficiency virus type-1 seropositive population: evidence for frequent serologic relapse after treatment. Am. J. Med. 99:55–63; 1995.

Manji, H.; Harrison, M. J. G.; Round, J. M.; et al. Muscle disease, HIV and zidovudine: the spectrum of muscle disease in HIV-infected individuals treated with zidovudine. J. Neurol. 240:479–488; 1993.

Masanes, F.; Pedrol, E.; Grau, J. M.; et al. Symptomatic myopathies in HIV-1 infected patients untreated with antiretroviral agents—a clinico-pathological study of 30 consecutive patients. Clin. Neuropathol. 15: 221–225; 1995.

McArthur, J. C. Neurologic manifestations of AIDS. Medicine (Baltimore) 66:407–437; 1987.

McArthur, J. C.; Cohen, B. A.; Farzedegan, H.; et al. Cerebrospinal fluid abnormalities in homosexual men with and without neuropsychiatric findings. Ann. Neurol. 23(suppl.):34–37; 1988.

McArthur, J. C.; Hoover, D. R.; Bacellar, H.; et al. Dementia in AIDS patients: incidence and risk factors. Neurology 43: 2245–2252; 1993.

McArthur, J. C.; McClernon, D. R.; Cronin, M. F.; et al. Relationship between human immunodeficiency virus associated dementia and viral load in cerebrospinal fluid and brain. Ann. Neurol. 42:689–698; 1997.

McArthur, J.; Yiannoutsos, C.; Simpson, D.; and the ACIG 291 Study Team. Trial of recombinant human nerve growth factor for HIV-associated sensory neuropathy (abstract). J. Neurovirol. 4:359;1998.

Mhiri, C.; Baudrimont, M.; Bonne, G.; et al. Zidovuine myopathy: a distinctive disorder associated with mitochondrial dysfunction. Ann. Neurol. 29:606–614; 1991.

Miller, J. R.; Barrett, R. E.; Britton, B. C.; Bruno, M. S.; et al. Progressive multifocal leukencephalopathy in a male homosexual with T-cell immune deficiency. N. Engl. J. Med. 307:1436–1438; 1982.

Miller, R. G.; Parry, G.; Lang, W.; et al. The spectrum of peripheral neuropathy associated with ARC and AIDS. Muscle Nerve 11:857–863; 1988.

Miller, R. G., Storey, J. R.; Greco, C. M. Ganciclovir in the treatment of progressive AIDS-related polyradiculopathy. Neurology 40:569–574; 1990.

Morgello, S.; Tagliati, M.; Ewart, M. R. HHV-8 and AIDS-related CNS lymphoma. Neurology 48: 1333–1335; 1997.

Morgello, S.; Wolfe, D.; Simpson, D., et al. Mitochondrial abnormalities in human deficiency virus-associated myopathy. Acta Neuropathol. 90: 366–374; 1995.

Mulhall, B. P.; Jennens, I. Testing for neurological involvement in HIV infection. Lancet 26:1531–1532; 1987.

Musher, D. M.; Hamill, R. J. Baughn, R. E. Effect of human immunodeficiency virus infection in the course of syphilis and the response to treatment. Ann. Intern. Med. 113:872–881; 1990.

Navia, B. A.; Cho, E.; Petito, C.; Price, R. W. The AIDS dementia complex: II. Neuropathology. Ann. Neurol. 19:525–535; 1986a.

Navia, B. A.; Petito, C. K.; Gold, J. W. M.; Cho, E.-S.; Jordan, B. D.; Price, R. W. Cerebral toxoplamosis complicating the acquired immune deficiency syndrome: clinical and neuropathological findings in 27 patients. Ann. Neurol. 6:224–238; 1986b.

Navia, B. A.; Price, R. W. The acquired immunodeficiency syndrome dementia complex as the presenting sole manifestation of human immunodeficiency virus infection. Arch. Neurol. 44:65–69; 1987.

Parry, G. J. Peripheral neuropathies associated with human immunodeficiency virus. Ann. Neurol. 23 (suppl.):S49–S53; 1988.

Perdrup, A.; Jorgensen, B. B.; Pederson, N. S. The profile of neurosyphilis in Denmark. A clinical and serological study of all patients in Denmark with neurosyphilis disclosed in the years 1971–1979 inclusive by Wasserman reaction (CWRM) in the cerebrospinal fluid. Acta Derm. Venereol. Suppl. (Stokh.) 96:1F–14; 1981.

Petito, C. K.; Cho, E. S.; Lemann, W.; Navia, B. A.; Price, R. W. Neuropathology of acquired immunodeficiency syndrome (AIDS): an autopsy review. J. Neuropathol. Exp. Neurol. 45:635–646; 1986.

Petito, C. K.; Navia, B. A.; Cho, E. S.; et al. Vacuolar myelopathy pathologically resembling subacute combined degeneration in patients with the acquired immunodeficiency syndrome. N. Engl. J. Med. 312:874–879; 1985.

Pezeshkpour, G.; Illa, I.; Dalakas, M. C. Ultrastructural characteristics and DNA immunocytochemistry in human immunodeficiency virus and zidovudine-associated myopathies. Hum. Pathol. 22:1281–1289; 1991.

Piette, A. M.; Tusseau, F.; Vignon, D.; et al. Acute neuropathy coincident with seroconversion for anti-LAV/HTL-III. Lancet 1:852; 1986.

Porter, S. B.; Sande, M. A. Toxoplasmosis of the central nervous system in the acquired immunodeficiency syndrome. N. Engl. J. Med. 327: 1643–1648; 1993.

Powderly, W. G.; Saag, M. S.; Cloud, G. A.; et al. A controlled trial of fluconazole versus amphotericin B to prevent relapse of cryptococcal meningitis in patients with the acquired immunodeficiency syndrome. N. Engl. J. Med. 326:793–798; 1992.

Price, R. W.; Brew, B.; Sidtis, J. J.; et al. The brain in AIDS: central nervous system HIV-1 infection and AIDS dementia complex. Science 239:586–592; 1988.

Purba, J. S.; Hofman, M. A.; Portegies, P.; et al. Decreased number of oxytocin neurons in the paraventricular nucleus of the human hypothalamus in AIDS. Brain 116:795–809; 1993.

Quagliarello, V. J.; Viscoli, C.; Horwitz, R. I. Primary prevention of cryptococcal meningitis by fluconazole in HIV-infected patients. Lancet 345:548–552; 1995.

Remick, S. C.; Diamond. C.; Migiozz, J. A.; et al. Primary central nervous system lymphoma in patients with and without the acquired immune deficiency syndrome. Medicine 69;345–360; 1990.

Roullet, E,; Assuerus, V.; Gozlan, J.; et al. Cytomegalovirus multifocal neuropathy in AIDS: analysis of 15 consecutive cases. Neurology 44: 2174–2182; 1994.

Ruiz, A.; Ganz, W. I.; Post, J. D.; et al. Use of thallium-201 SPECT to differentiate cerebral lymphoma from toxoplasma encephalitis in AIDS patients. Am. J. Neuroradiol. 15:1885–1894; 1994.

Ruttimann, S.; Hilti, P.; Spinas, G. A.; et al. High frequency of human immunodeficiency virus-associated autonomic neuropathy and more severe involvement in advanced stages of human immunodeficiency virus disease. Arch. Intern. Med. 151:2441–2443; 1991.

Saag, M. S.; Powderly, W. G.; Cloud. G. A.; et al. Comparison of amphotericin B with fluconazole in the treatment of acute AIDS-associated cryptococcal meningitis. The NIAD Mycoses Study Group and the AIDS Clinical Trials Group. N. Engl. J. Med. 326:83–89; 1992.

Sabatier, J. M.; Vives, E.; Mabrouk, K.; et al. Evidence for neurotoxic activity of tat from human immunodeficiency virus type 1. J. Virol. 65:961–967; 1991.

Sacktor, N.; Lyles, R. H.; McFarlane G.; et al. HIV-1 related neurological dosage incidence changes in the era of highly active antiretroviral therapy (abstract). Neurology 52(suppl. 2):S252, 1999.

Sagerman, R. H.; Cassady, J. R.; Chang, C. H. Radiation therapy for intracranial lymphoma. Radiology 88: 552–554; 1967.

Said, G.; Lacroix, C.; Chemoulli, P.; et al. Cytomegalovirus neuropathy in acquired immunodeficiency syndrome: a clinical and pathological study. Ann. Neurol. 29:139–146; 1991.

Scott, G.; Piagessi, A.; Ewing, D. Sequential autonomic function tests in HIV infection. AIDS 4:1279–1282; 1990.

Selmaj, K. W.; Raine, C. S. Tumor necrosis factor mediates myelin and oligodendrocyte damage in vitro. Ann. Neurol 23:339–346; 1988.

Sharer, L. R. Pathology of HIV-1 infection of the central nervous system. J. Neuropathol. Exp. Neurol. 51: 3–11; 1992.

Shaw, G. M., Harper, M. E.; Hahn, B. H.; et al. HTLV-III infection in brain of children and adults with AIDS encephalopathy. Science 227:177–182; 1985.

Sidtis, J. J.; Gatsonis, C.; Price, R. W.; et al. Zidovudine treatment of the AIDS dementia complex: result of a placebo controlled trial. Ann. Neurol. 33:343–349; 1992.

Simpson, D. M. Human immunodeficiency virus-associated dementia: review of pathogenesis, prophylaxis, and treatment studies of zidovudine therapy. Clin. Infect. Dis. 29:19–34; 1999.

Simpson, D. M.; Bender, A. N. Human immunodeficiency virus-associated myopathy: analysis of 11 patients. Ann. Neurol. 24:79–84; 1988.

Simpson D. M.; Bender, A. N.; Farraye, J.; et al. Human immunodeficiency virus wasting syndrome

may represent a treatable myopathy. Neurology 40:535–538; 1990.

Simpson, D. M.; Citak, K. A.; Godfrey, E.; et al. Myopathies associated with human immunodeficiency virus and zidovudine: can their effect be distinguished? Neurology 43:971–976; 1993.

Simpson, D. M.; Olney, R. K.; McArthur, J. C.; et al. A placebo controlled study of lamotrigine in the treatment of painful sensory polyneuropathy associated with HIV infection (abstract). J. Neurovirol. 4:366; 1998.

Simpson, D. M.; Tagliati, M. Neurologic manifestation of HIV infection. Ann. Intern. Med. 121:769–785; 1994.

Simpson, D. M.; Tagliati, M. Nucleoside analogue-associated peripheral neuropathy in human immunodeficiency virus infection. J. AIDS 9:153–161; 1995.

Simpson, D. M.; Tagliati, M.; Grinnell, J.; et al. Electrophysiological findings in HIV infection: association with distal symmetrical polyneuropathy and CD4 level. Muscle Nerve 17:1113–1114; 1994.

Simpson, D. M.; Wolfe, D. Neuromuscular complications of HIV infection and its treatment. AIDS 5: 917–927; 1991.

Simpson, M. V.; Chin, C. D.; Keilbough, S. A.; et al. Studies on the inhibition of mitochondrial DNA replication of 3-azido-3'-deoxythymidine and other dideoxynucleoside analogs which inhibit HIV-1 replication. Biochem. Pharmacol. 38:1033–1036; 1989.

Singh, N.; Barnish, M. J.; Berman, S.; et al. Low dose fluconazole as primary prophylaxis for cryptococcal infection in AIDS patients with CD4 cell counts of < or = $100/mm^3$: demonstration of efficacy in a positive, multicenter trial. Clin. Infect. Dis. 23: 1282–1286; 1996.

Snider, W. D.; Simpson, D. M.; Nielson, S.; et al. Neurological complications of acquired immune deficiency syndrome: analysis of 50 patients. Ann. Neurol. 14: 403–418; 1983.

So, Y. T. Clinical subdivision of mononeuropathy multiplex in patients with HIV infection. Neurology 429(suppl. 3):409; 1992.

So, Y. T.; Holtzman, D. M.; Abrams, D. I.; et al. Peripheral neuropathy associated with AIDS. Arch. Neurol. 45:945–948; 1988.

So, Y. T.; Olney, R. K. The natural course of mononeuritis multiplex and simplex in HIV infection. Neurology 41(suppl. 1):375; 1991.

So, Y. T.; Olney, R. K. Acute lumbosacral polyradiculopathy in acquired immunodeficiency syndrome: experience in 23 patients. Ann. Neurol. 35:53–58; 1994.

Stern, J. J.; Hartman, B. J.; Sharkey, P.; et al. Oral fluconazole therapy for patients with acquired immunodeficiency syndrome and cryptococcosis: experience with 22 patients. Am. J. Med. 85: 477–480; 1988.

Stern, R.; Gold, J.; DiCarlo, F. Myopathy complicating the acquired immune deficiency. Muscle Nerve 10: 318–322; 1987.

Tan, S. V.; Guiloff, R. J.; Henderson, D. C.; Gazzard, B. G. Aids-associated vacuolar myelopathy and tumor necrosis factor alpha. J. Neurol. Sci. 138: 134–144; 1996.

Telzak, E. E.; Zweig Greenberg, M. S.; Harrison, J.; et al. Syphilis treatment response in HIV-infected individuals. AIDS 5:591–595; 1991.

Tross, S.; Price, R. W.; Navia, B.; Thaler, H. T.; Gold, J.; Sidtis, J. J. Neuropsychological characterization of the AIDS dementia complex: a preliminary report. AIDS 2:81–88; 1988.

Tyor, W. R.; Glass, J. D.; Bauring, N.; et al. Cytokine expression of macrophages in HIV-1 associated vacuolar myelopathy. Neurology 43:1002–1009; 1993.

Van Der Horst, C. M.; Saag, M. S.; Cloud, G. A.; et al. Treatment of cryptococcal meningitis associated with the acquired immunodeficiency syndrome. N. Engl. J. Med. 337:15–20; 1997.

Vendrell, J.; Heredia, C.; Pujol, M.; et al. Guillain-Barre syndrome associated with seroconversion for anti-HTLV-III. Neurology 37:544; 1987.

Villa, A.; Foresti, V.; Confalonieri, F. Autonomic neuropathy and HIV infection. Lancet 2:915; 1987.

Villa, A.; Foresti, V.; Confalonieri, F. Autonomic nervous system dysfunction associated with HIV infection in intravenous heroin users. AIDS 6:85–89; 1992.

Walker, D. L.; Padgett, B. L. The epidemiology of human polyomaviruses. In: Polyomaviruses and human neurological diseases. New York: Alan R. Liss; 1993: p. 99–106.

Weber, T.; Tuner, R. W.; Ruf, B.; et al. JC virus detected by polymerase chain reaction in cerebrospinal fluid of AIDS patients with PML. In: Berger, J. R.; Levy, R. L., eds. Neurological and neuropsychological complications of HIV infection. Proceedings from the Satellite Meeting of the International Conference on AIDS; 1990: p. 100.

Weiser, B.; Press, N.; LaNeve, D.; et al. Human immunodeficiency virus type 1 expression in the central nervous system correlates directly with extent of disease. Proc. Natl. Acad. Sci. USA 3997:4001; 1990.

Wesselingh, S. L.; Power, C.; Fox, R.; et al. Cytokine mRNA expression in HIV-associated neurological disease. Neurology 43(suppl. 2):291; 1993.

Welby, S. B.; Rogerson, S. J.; Beeching, N. J. Autonomic neuropathy is common in human immunodeficiency virus infection. J. Infect. 23:123–128; 1991.

Whiteman, M.; Post, M. J.; Berger, J. R.; et al. Progressive multifocal leucoencephalopathy in 47 HIV-patients. Radiology 187:233–240; 1993.

Wiley, C. A.; Achim, C. A. Human immunodeficiency virus encephalitis is the pathological correlation of dementia in acquired immunodeficiency syndrome. Ann. Neurol. 36:673–676; 1994.

Wiley, C. A.; Schrier, R. D.; Nelson, J. A.; et al. Cellular localization of human immunodeficiency virus infection within the brains of acquired immune deficiency syndrome patients. Proc. Natl. Acad. Sci. USA 83:7089–7093; 1986.

Woolsey, R. M.; Chambers, T. J.; Chung, H. D.; McGarry, J. D. Mycobacterial meningomyelitis associated with human immunodeficiency virus infections. Arch Neurol 45:691–693; 1988.

Wrzolek, M. A.; Sher, J. H.; Kozlowski, P. B.; et al. Skeletal muscle pathology in AIDS: an autopsy study. Muscle Nerve 13:508–515; 1990.

Yianoutsos, C.; Miller, E.; Chang, L.; et al. Proton MRS and neuropsychological assessments in AIDS dementia complex (abstract). Neurology 52(suppl. 2):S253; 1999.

Zimmerman, R. A. Central nervous system lymphoma. Radiol. Clin. North. Am. 28:697–721; 1990.

Zisfein, J.; DiPietro, D.; Lugo-Torres, O. CSF venereal disease research laboratory in neurologically asymptomatic HIV-infected patients with serological evidence for syphilis. Ann Neurol 34:283; 1993.

Zuger, A.; Louie, E.; Holzman, R. S.; et al. Cryptococcal disease in patients with the acquired immunodeficiency syndrome: diagnostic features and outcome of treatment. Ann. Intern. Med. 104:234–240; 1986.

# 18

# Brain Abscesses

MAX KOLE, THOMAS J. MAMPALAM, AND MARK L. ROSENBLUM

Focal suppurative infections of the brain parenchyma have been recognized since the time of Hippocrates in 460 BC. In 1893, Sir William Macewen described the etiology and pathogenesis of brain abscesses in his monograph *Pyogenic Infective Diseases of the Brain and Spinal Cord* and is considered the first physician to diagnose, localize, and surgically treat brain abscesses. Historically, the prognosis of a patient with a brain abscess has been poor, with high mortality rates and neurological sequelae. In recent years, however, the advent of computed tomography (CT) and magnetic resonance imaging (MRI), advances in surgical techniques (i.e., the operating microscope, stereotaxy, and real-time ultrasonography), improved microbiological identification, and more effective antibiotic regimens have improved the prognosis of brain abscess. This chapter briefly reviews the incidence, etiology, and treatment of brain abscesses, emphasizing the prognosis of this disorder.

## Incidence

The incidence of brain abscess has remained relatively stable in the antibiotic era (Wispelwey et al. 1997). Bacterial brain abscesses occur in approximately 1500 to 2500 patients each year in

the United States (Mamelak et al. 1995). Brain abscess accounts for approximately 1 in 10,000 general hospital admissions, with four to ten cases seen annually at major neurosurgical centers in developed countries (Wispelwey et al. 1997). However, with the increasing prevalence of immunocompromised states, the incidence of focal central nervous system (CNS) infections may be on the rise.

## Etiology

The formation of a cerebral abscess occurs in association with the following predisposing states: (1) a contiguous suppurative focus, (2) hematogenous or metastatic dissemination, (3) after penetrating craniocerebral trauma, (4) after neurosurgery, (5) in immunocompromised states, and (6) cryptogenic. Approximately 80% of patients with a brain abscess have a known predisposing factor that has contributed to the development of the intracranial infection. The remaining 20% are cryptogenic (Rosenblum et al. 1986).

Suppurative processes of the paranasal sinuses, middle ear, and mastoid are the most common sources of underlying infection in most clinical series (Loftus and Biller 1996). Paranasal sinus infection can spread intracranially to the frontal or temporal lobe via retrograde thrombophlebitis of the diploic veins. Osteomyelitis and dehiscence of the posterior table of the frontal sinus may also result in direct extension of infection to the anterior and basal regions of the frontal lobe. Middle ear infections can lead to temporal lobe abscess. Direct extension of mastoiditis can lead to temporal or cerebellar abscesses. The frequency of brain abscess as a result of sinusitic and otic origin may be declining because of earlier and more effective treatment of sinus, middle ear, and mastoid infections.

Metastatic abscesses occur through hematogenous dissemination of micro-organisms from a remote site of infection. Common primary foci include skin pustules, pulmonary infections, dental abscess, bacterial endocarditis, cyanotic congenital heart disease, and pulmonary arteriovenous fistulas. Metastatic abscesses tend to be multiple and located at the corticomedullary junction proportionate to the regional cerebral blood flow. However, they can also occur in the thalamus, brain stem, and cerebellum.

Penetrating craniocerebral trauma is another well-recognized cause of brain abscess. Skull fractures with dural tear, contaminated bone fragments, and debris provide a nidus of infection that may evolve into a brain abscess. Most cases are a sequel to compound injury, with a reported incidence ranging from 3% to 16% (Patir et al. 1995). Brain abscess rarely complicates neurosurgical procedures; only 0.06% to 0.17% of clean neurosurgical procedures result in brain abscess formation (Wispelwey et al. 1997).

Interestingly, transient bacteremia by itself is unlikely to result in brain abscess formation because of the inherent resistance of the blood-brain barrier to infection. In addition, brain abscess rarely complicates meningitis with the exception of gram-negative meningitis in the neonate. Abscess formation has been associated with more than 70% of cases of *Citrobacter diversus* meningitis in the infant (Wispelwey et al. 1997).

Brain abscesses are caused by a wide variety of bacteria, fungi, and parasites. The bacteriological profile found within an abscess is closely related to the etiology of the infection. Overall, the organisms most frequently isolated from cerebral abscesses are streptococci, both anaerobic and aerobic, and staphylococci. Gram-negative organisms are an increasing cause of cerebral abscesses.

Mixed infections can occur in up to one-third of cases. An understanding of the predisposing condition has important implications to the likely microbacterial agent, location of abscess, the solitary nature or multiplicity of abscesses, and the prognosis.

## Treatment

The goals in treating brain abscesses are to reduce mass effect, decrease intracranial pressure, prevent herniation or intraventricular rupture and ventriculitis, identify the causative micro-organism, and establish antibiotic sensitivities. There are no randomized, prospective trials on the treatment of brain abscess and its management remains a subject of controversy. The various treatment modalities include surgical excision, surgical aspiration (stereotactic vs. free-hand), and empiric antibiotics. Surgery is considered the treatment of choice for most cases, although favorable outcomes have been reported with antibiotics alone. Modern-day treatment of brain abscesses generally includes a combined surgical and medical approach.

The authors advocate the following treatment algorithm: All patients suspected of harboring a brain abscess should receive a contrast CT or MRI immediately to confirm this suspicion. If multiple ring-enhancing lesions are found, the patient is taken urgently to surgery and all abscesses larger than 2.5 cm in diameter or that are causing significant mass effect are either excised or preferably stereotactically aspirated. Exceptions include abscesses in an early cerebritis phase, which are therefore more likely to respond to antibiotic therapy alone. An abscess diameter of 2.5 cm is the conservative cutoff used in cases of multiple lesions, based on a previous report demonstrating that solitary abscesses 3 cm or less in diameter could be treated nonsurgically, whereas larger abscesses were more likely to require surgery for cure. If all abscesses are smaller than 2.5 cm in size or not causing mass effect, the largest and/or most accessible abscess should be aspirated for diagnostic purposes and antibiotic selection. If another source of infection has been clearly identified, therapy for the brain lesions may be started empirically based on those culture results. If the patient neurologically deteriorates or shows an increase in abscess size at any time or if 2 weeks of antibiotic therapy fails to shrink these lesions, aspiration for diagnostic purposes should be ascertained. Antibiotics are not started until appropriate cultures are sent. Antibiotics are continued for a minimum of 6 to 8 weeks and in immunocompromised patients often for 1 year or longer (Mamelak et al. 1995). In the case of nocardial abscesses, the drainage of the cavity may prove inadequate. The excision of the entire abscess cavity may be the only means to ensure complete response (Mamelak et al. 1994). Similarly, posttraumatic abscesses tend to be multiloculated and neither antibiotics nor aspiration can prevent recurrence resulting from indriven bone or external debris necessitating craniotomy with surgical excision (Patrir et al. 1995).

## Prognosis

The prognosis of patients with brain abscesses may be considered in terms of mortality statistics and neurological sequelae. The most important determinants of morbidity and mortality are the condition of the patient at the start of treatment and the rapidity of disease progression. Early diagnosis and prompt initiation of appropriate therapy are necessary to ensure a satisfactory therapeutic outcome.

No evidence suggests that standard demographic characteristics, such as sex or ethnic origin, influence the mortality rate among patients with brain abscess. Although age at diagnosis is an important determinant of long-term neurological status, it has no consistent relationship with the mortality rate (Bhatia et al. 1973; Britt et al. 1981; Carey et al. 1971, 1972; Garfield 1969; Jooma et al. 1951; Joubert and Stephanov 1977; Loeser and Scheinberg 1957; Mampalam and Rosenblum 1988; Morgan et al. 1973), except among neonates with gram-negative abscesses (Reiner et al. 1988). The high mortality rate in such patients may be related to immaturity, the virulence of the gram-negative organisms, and coexistent systemic disease. Abscesses in this population are most frequently caused by *Proteus* or *Citrobacter* species, organisms notorious for inducing a fulminant necrotizing reaction with destruction of large amounts of brain parenchyma (Osenbach and Loftus 1992). In the University of California, San Francisco (UCSF) series, which included patients aged 6 weeks to 78 years (mean,

34.9 years), the mortality rate did not correlate with age (Mampalam and Rosenblum 1988).

The risk of death from brain abscess depends on the neurological condition at diagnosis (Table 18-1) (Alderson et al. 1981; Carey et al. 1971, 1972; Garfield 1969; Jooma et al. 1951; Joubert and Stephanov 1977; Karandanis and Shulman 1975; Loeser and Scheinberg 1957; Mampalam and Rosenblum 1988; Morgan et al. 1973). The mortality rate exceeds 60% if signs of brain herniation are present (Yang 1981) and is approximately 90% among comatose patients (Alderson et al. 1981; Bhatia et al. 1973; Garfield 1969; Karandanis and Shulman 1975). Among alert patients, however, the mortality rate is less than 20%, even in older studies (Alderson et al. 1981; Karandanis and Shulman 1975; Mampalam and Rosenblum 1988; Svanteson et al. 1988). Misdiagnosis was the main reason for the high mortality rate from brain abscess in previous decades (Bhatia et al. 1973; Garfield 1969; Loeser and Scheinberg 1957; Rosenblum et al. 1986; Samson and Clark, 1973).

The advent of CT has been the most important factor in reducing the mortality rate among patients with brain abscess (Joubert and Stephanov 1977; Renier et al. 1988; Rosenblum et al. 1978; Svanteson et al. 1988). The prompt and accurate localization of the lesions by CT has reduced the previous mortality rate of 30% to 50% to less than 15% in most series (Alderson et al. 1981; Bhatia et al. 1973; Britt et al. 1981; Carey et al. 1971, 1972; Garfield 1969; Jooma et al. 1951; Joubert and

**Table 18-1.** Factors Affecting the Prognosis of Patients With Brain Abscess

| Factor | Mortality Rate (%) |
|---|---|
| Before advent of CT | 30–50 |
| After advent of CT | 0–15 |
| Neurological condition at diagnosis | |
|   Alert, no deficit | 0–20 |
|   Comatose | 25–90 |
| Etiology | |
|   Local infection | 6–50 |
|   Metastatic | 12–100 |
| Number of abscesses | |
|   Solitary | 0–45 |
|   Multiple | 8–100 |
| Type of treatment | |
|   Aspiration | 0–45 |
|   Excision | 0–30 |
|   Nonoperative | 0–13 |

From Mampalam and Rosenblum (1988).

Stephanov 1977; Karandanis and Shulman 1975; Mampalam and Rosenblum 1988; Rosenblum et al. 1978, 1986; Samson and Clark 1973; Stephanov 1988; Svanteson et al. 1988; Van Alphen and Dreissen 1976; Yang 1981). Since CT scanning became a routine diagnostic test at one major neurosurgical center, the diagnosis of brain abscess has not been missed in any patient, and the mortality rate has decreased from 40.9% to 4.3% (Mampalam and Rosenblum 1988). During this period there were no significant changes in the culture identification of organisms or in antibiotic regimens to account for the remarkable drop in mortality rate.

Certain characteristics of brain abscesses have been associated with higher mortality rates. In patients with post-traumatic brain abscesses without signs of herniation the mortality rate was 12.5% in one series (Patir et al. 1995). Abscesses arising from adjacent otogenous infections or previous craniotomy seem to carry lower mortality rates than those caused by metastatic spread (Bhatia et al. 1973; Carey et al. 1972; Karandanis and Shulman 1975; Loeser and Scheinberg 1957; Van Alphen and Dreissen 1976). Metastatic abscesses tend to be deep and multiple and occur more often in patients with serious systemic disease, such as endocarditis or pulmonary infections. In addition, the diagnosis of metastatic abscess may be delayed because the index of suspicion for abscess is higher when a patient has an adjacent infection than when the source is remote from the brain.

Multiple abscesses also have been associated with high mortality rates, up to 100% in older studies (Garfield 1969; Karandanis and Shulman 1975). Liske and Weikers (1964) found a 70% mortality rate in patients with multiple abscesses, compared to only 45% in those with solitary abscesses. CT scanning, more effective antibiotic regimens, and stereotactic surgical procedures have markedly diminished the difficulty of managing multiple lesions. In several series all patients with multiple abscesses were treated successfully (Mampalam and Rosenblum 1988; Rosenblum et al. 1978, 1986). In 1988, Dyste et al. reported on eight patients with multiple brain abscesses and achieved results similar to those with solitary lesions. In 1995, Mamelak et al. demonstrated a mortality rate of only 6% in their series of 16 patients with multiple brain abscesses.

In the series by Mampalam and Rosenblum (1988), the size of the abscess was the only factor other than the initial neurological grade that influenced the mortality rate. Patients who died tended to have larger abscesses than those who survived. Rupture of an abscess into the ventricle is associated with an unfavorable outcome, causing ventriculitis, acute hydrocephalus, and death if a large volume of purulent material enters the ventricle. If only a small amount of pus reaches the ventricle and if a ventriculostomy is performed without delay, the prognosis is better. Immunocompromised patients and those with coexisting septicemia or cardiac disease have higher mortality rates than other patients (Britt et al. 1981; Kagawa et al. 1983; Rosenblum et al. 1986).

Although most observe no important influence of bacteriology, an increased mortality has been occasionally reported with anaerobic and gram-negative rods. Fungal, mycobacterial, and parasitic brain abscesses are predominantly seen in the immunocompromised state and have a different prognosis than the typical pyogenic brain abscess.

No prospective, randomized trial comparing the different treatment modalities for brain abscesses has been performed. Rosenblum et al. (1986) analyzed the five largest series concerning nonoperative management of brain abscesses and found an overall collective success rate of 74%, with a mortality rate of 4% among 50 patients. In the series of medically treated brain abscesses, the mean diameter of abscesses that were cured with antibiotics alone was 1.7 cm compared to 4 cm for those that required aspiration (Rosenblum et al. 1980). In fact, no abscess larger than 2.5 cm resolved without surgical intervention. Although some patients may respond favorably to empirical antibiotics alone, most require surgery for optimal management.

Differences in perioperative mortality rates between aspiration and excision procedures seem to be related to patient selection criteria rather than to the safety of the respective treatments. Stephanov (1988) reviewed the literature on surgical treatment of brain abscesses and found mortality rates of 38% (356 of 941) after aspiration and 19% (283 of 1505) after excision. Most of these patients, however, were treated before CT became available, and in most series the initial neurological or general medical condition was worse among patients whose lesions were aspirated than among those who underwent excision. Given similar initial conditions, the results of aspiration and excision appear to be comparable. Series published during the CT era have shown an 11% mortality rate for aspiration compared to 8% for excision (Dyste et al. 1988). In the UCSF series, the perioperative mortality rate was 6.1% after aspiration and 8.7% after excision ($p = $ NS) (Mampalam and Rosenblum 1988). Seydoux and Francioli (1992) analyzed 39 cases of brain abscess diagnosed since the advent of CT and found an overall mortality rate of 13% and severe sequelae in 22% of the survivors. There was no apparent correlation between the outcome and the presence of predisposing factors; radiological, biological, and microbiological findings; or the treatment modalities. No detectable difference in outcome occurred between the patients who underwent excision versus those who underwent stereotactic aspiration. In a recent review of the surgical management of brain abscesses, Ng et al. (1995) reported that 86% who underwent aspiration alone made a good recovery compared with 81% of the group who underwent excision. One prominent finding of this study was that repeat operations were often necessary especially for the aspiration group (73% vs. 25%), although the overall outcome was similar. In reviewing results from 17 reported series from 1979 to 1996 that employed CT-guided stereotactic aspiration of brain abscesses, the mortality rate was approximately 10%

(Table 18-2). Konziolka et al. (1994) defined adverse conditions that affected outcome in reference to the stereotactic aspiration of brain abscesses. Long-term immunosuppression, concomitant antineoplastic chemotherapy, chronic steroid use, retained foreign body, and insufficient initial drainage or antibiotic course were factors that decreased the likelihood of successful treatment. The literature lacks conclusive evidence to suggest superiority of one surgical treatment modality over another in terms of mortality or neurological sequelae.

## Neurological Sequelae

Despite successful eradication of the infection, many patients with brain abscess in early series suffered persistent neurological sequelae, most likely due to delayed diagnosis, poor initial neurological condition, and larger abscesses. The surgical technique might have also contributed to the higher morbidity rate. Before CT was introduced, there was no way to localize the lesions precisely before and during the operation. With modern imaging capabilities, earlier diagnosis will lead to lower long-term morbidity. The morbidity from brain abscess has already decreased markedly; at one university center, for example, none of 43 patients treated successfully between 1981 and 1986 had significant neurological deficits when discharged from the hospital (Mampalam and Rosenblum 1988).

**Table 18-2.** Reported Case Series (1979–1996) of CT-Guided Stereotactic Aspiration of Brain Abscess

| Authors | Year | Cases | Death | Severe | Moderate | Good |
|---|---|---|---|---|---|---|
| Wise and Gleason | 1979 | 1 | | | | 1 |
| Walsh et al. | 1980 | 2 | | | 1 | 1 |
| Lunsford and Nelson | 1982 | 1 | | | | 1 |
| Hollander et al. | 1987 | 1 | | | | 1 |
| Itakura et al. | 1987 | 14 | 1 | | | 13 |
| Hall et al. | 1987 | 3 | 1 | | | 2 |
| Apuzzo et al. | 1987 | 89 | | No information given | | |
| Nauta et al. | 1987 | 4 | | No information given | | |
| Dyste et al. | 1988 | 8 | 1 | 1 | 1 | 5 |
| Goodman and Coffey | 1989 | 1 | | | | 1 |
| Stapleton et al. | 1993 | 11 | 3 | 1 | | 7 |
| Laborde et al. | 1993 | 2 | | | | 2 |
| Hasdemir and Ebeling | 1993 | 24 | 1 | | 5 | 18 |
| Konziolka | 1994 | 29 | 6 | 3 | 1 | 19 |
| Rajshekhar and Chandy | 1994 | 1 | | | 1 | |
| Shahzadi et al. | 1996 | 20 | | | 4 | 16 |
| Skrap et al. | 1996 | 9 | 1 | | | 8 |
| Total | | 220 | 14 | 5 | 13 | 95 |

The most common neurological sequelae of brain abscesses are cognitive deficits, hemiparesis, and seizures. Earlier studies reported permanent neurological deficits, such as hemiparesis and dysphasia in 27% of 505 patients with brain abscesses (Carey et al. 1971, 1972; Nielsen et al. 1983). Infants and children have a worse outcome than adults. Most neonates with brain abscess subsequently have IQs lower than 80 (Renier et al. 1988). In one study, 70% of the children had difficulties with school performance and 38% had severe hemiparesis, whereas 87% of the adults were able to continue their normal work and none had severe hemiparesis (Carey et al. 1971).

Seizure disorders occur in about 50% of patients with brain abscess (range, 15% to 92%) (Jooma et al. 1951; Legg et al. 1973; Nielsen et al. 1983; Northcraft and Wyke 1957; Shaw 1990), usually within 3 to 4 years after treatment (Legg et al. 1973). Children are more likely than adults to develop epilepsy after brain abscess (Carey et al. 1971). Seizures are most common in patients with lesions of the frontal and temporal lobes; seizures after occipital lobe abscesses are unusual, and cerebellar abscesses do not predispose to seizures (Carey et al. 1971; Northcraft and Wyke 1957). Empiric administration of anticonvulsant drugs is recommended for all patients with brain abscess.

Deficiencies in cell-mediated immunity stemming from immunosuppressive therapy for organ transplantation and from acquired immunodeficiency syndrome (AIDS) have resulted in an increasing incidence of brain abscesses. Brain abscesses were responsible for 33% of all CNS infections in patients with cancer and in 35% to 44% of those after heart and heart-lung transplantation in one large series (Hall 1992). Intracerebral brain abscess is the most common CNS infection in patients with leukemia, and 4% of bone marrow transplant recipients develop brain abscess (Hall 1992). In the series by Mampalam and Rosenblum (1988), approximately 6% of the brain abscesses reviewed were associated with non-AIDS immunodeficiency. In addition, AIDS has become one of the most important risk factors for the development of CNS infection. It is estimated that up to 40% to 70% of all persons infected with HIV will develop symptomatic neurological disease (Berger and Simpson 1997). For example, estimates of the prevalence of cerebral toxoplasmosis alone in patients with AIDS range from 2.6% to 30.8% (Wispelwey et al. 1997).

The clinical presentation of brain abscesses in the immunocompromised patient is different than that of the typical pyogenic abscesses. Immunocompromised patients have a poor inflammatory response and are less likely to complain of constitutional symptoms such as headache or meningismus. Lesions detected on CT or MRI scans are less likely to show enhancement and surrounding vasogenic edema than are similar lesions in the nonimmunocompromised patient. This lack of ring enhancement is believed to be an indication of inadequate inflammatory response and a poor prognostic factor (Mathisen and Johnson 1997).

Numerous pathogens causing brain abscess in the immunocompromised patient have been described including *Toxoplasma gondii,* mycobacterial species, *Nocardia asteroides, Listeria monocytogenes, Cryptococcus neoformans, Candida albicans, Aspergillus* species, and many others.

Cerebral toxoplasmosis is the most common cerebral mass lesion in patients with AIDS. Central nervous system toxoplasmosis usually occurs in advanced HIV infection when CD4 counts are lower than 200 cells/mm$^3$. Toxoplasmic lesions begin as a foci of encephalitis that progress rapidly to parenchymal abscesses with central necrosis and surrounding inflammation. Most patients with cerebral toxoplasmosis respond favorably to empiric antibiotics, pyrimethamine and sulfadiazine. However, adverse side effects such as rash nephrotoxicity and hematological toxicity complicate this regimen. If no radiological or clinical response is obtained within 1 to 2 weeks, stereotactic biopsy is recommended for definitive diagnosis. The mean survival for patients with *Toxoplasma* encephalitis was $265 \pm 212$ days in one study (Porter and Sande 1992). Although survival of 1 to 2 years is not uncommon, early death appears to correlate directly with mental function at the time treatment is instituted (Levy and Berger 1992).

Fungal brain abscesses are mostly seen in immunocompromised patients. Although *Candida* species are the most common fungi found within the CNS and *Cryptococcus* is the most common cause of fungal meningitis, *Aspergillus* is the most common fungal source of brain abscess. *Aspergillus* brain abscesses are usually characterized by rapid progression of disease and high mortality rates despite aggressive surgical and antifungal therapy (Mathisen and Johnson 1997). An aggressive surgical approach in nonimmunocompromised patients helped reduce the mortality from 64% to 39% in one series (Young et al. 1985). However, mortality rates remain disturbingly high in the immunocompromised, with 80% to 97% of patients dying regardless of the treatment modality (Wispelwey et al. 1997; Artico et al. 1997).

The mortality rate for nocardial brain abscess has dropped almost 50% since the advent of CT. However, the rate has remained virtually unchanged in immunocompromised patients (55%), and is three times higher than that of other bacterial brain abscesses (30% vs. 10%) (Mamelak et al. 1994).

Extrapulmonary tuberculosis, including CNS tuberculosis, occurs in more than 70% of those with tuberculosis and pre-existing AIDS (Zuger and Lowry 1997). Most commonly this manifests as tuberculous meningitis and tuberculomas. In cases of intracranial tuberculomas, neurosurgical intervention is recommended only if there is no sign of clinical improvement within 3 or 4 weeks of antituberculous triple or quadruple treatment. However, the treatment of true tuberculous brain abscesses warrants a more aggressive surgical approach. When the caseous core of a tuberculoma liquefies, a tuberculous brain abscess will result. True tuberculous brain abscesses, an encapsulated collection of pus containing viable tubercle bacilli, are rare. In the pre-AIDS era (up to 1978), there were only 17 reported cases of tuberculous brain abscess. There have been 12 documented cases of tuberculous brain abscess in patients with AIDS (Farrar et al. 1997). Pathologically, tuberculous brain abscesses differ from tuberculomas in that they lack the giant cell and epithelioid granulomatous reaction in the central necrotic area. Tuberculous brain abscesses have vascular granulation tissue with acute and chronic inflammatory cells similar to pyogenic brain abscesses, but they have much thicker walls (Ildan et al. 1994). This characteristic makes tuberculous brain abscess less amenable to aspiration techniques (Ildan et al. 1994). The mortality rate of CNS tuberculosis is high and the treatment of tuberculous brain abscess mandates an aggressive combined surgical and medical approach (Farrar et al. 1997).

Immunosuppression secondary to HIV has become an important risk factor in the development of brain abscess. The prognosis is generally worse than that of the nonimmunocompromised and is most often dictated by the concomitant systemic illnesses. Rapid diagnosis and effective medical and surgical treatments are essential to preserve neurological function.

## References

Alderson, D.; Strong, A. J.; Ingham, H. R.; Selkon, J. B. Fifteen-year review of the mortality of brain abscess. Neurosurgery 8:1–5; 1981.
Apuzzo, M. L. J.; Chandrasoma, P. T.; Cohen, D.; Zee, C.; Zelman, V. Computed imaging stereotaxy: experience and perspective related to 500 procedures applied to brain masses. Neurosurgery 20:930–937; 1987.
Artico, M.; Pastore, F. S.; Polosa, M.; Sherat, S.; Neroni, M. Intracerebral aspergillus abscess: case report and review of the literature. Neurosurg. Rev. 20:135–138; 1997.
Berger, J. R.; Simpson, D. M. Neurologic complications of AIDS. In: Scheld, W. M.; Whitly, R. J.; Durack, D. T. (eds). Infections of the central nervous system. 2nd ed. Philadelphia, Lippincott-Raven; 1997: p. 255–271.
Bhatia, R.; Tandon, P. N.; Baneji, A. K. Brain abscess—an analysis of 55 cases. Int. J. Surg. 58:565–568; 1973.
Britt, R. H.; Enzmann, D. R.; Remington, J. S. Intracranial infection in cardiac transplant recipients. Ann. Neurol. 9:107–119; 1981.
Carey, M. E.; Chou, S. N.; French, L. A. Long-term neurological residua in patients surviving brain abscess with surgery. J. Neurosurg. 34:652–656; 1971.
Carey, M. E.; Chou, S. N.; French, L. A. Experience with brain abscesses. J. Neurosurg. 36:1–9; 1972.
Dyste, G. N.; Hitchon, P. W.; Menezes, A. H.; Van-Gilder, J. C.; Greene, G. M. Stereotaxic surgery in the treatment of multiple brain abscesses. J. Neurosurg. 69:188–194; 1988.
Farrar, D. J.; Flanigan, T. P.; Gordan, N. M.; Gold, R. L.; Rich, J. D. Tuberculous brain abscess in a patient with HIV infection: case report and review. Am. J. Med. 102:297–301; 1997.
Garfield, J. Management of supratentorial intracranial abscess: a review of 200 cases. Br. Med. J. 2:7–11; 1969.
Goodman, M. L.; Coffey, R. J. Stereotactic drainage of Aspergillus brain abscess with long term survival: a case report and review. Neurosurgery 24:96–99; 1989.
Hall, W. A. Neurosurgical infections in the compromised host. Neurosurg. Clin. N. Am. 3:435–442; 1992.
Hall, W. A.; Martinez, A. J.; Dummer, J. S.; Lunsford, L. D. Nocardial brain abscess: diagnostic and therapeutic use of stereotactic aspiration. Surg. Neurol. 28:114–118; 1987.
Hasdemir, M. G.; Ebeling, V. CT-guided stereotactic aspiration and treatment of brain abscesses. An ex-

perience with 24 cases. Acta Neurochir. (Wien) 125:58–63; 1993.

Hollander, D.; Villemore, J. G.; Leblanc, R. Thalamic abscess: a stereotactically treatable lesion. J. Appl. Neurophysiol. 50:168–171; 1987.

Ildan, F.; Gursoy, F.; Gul, B.; Boyar, B.; Kilic, C. Intracranial tuberculous abscess mimicking malignant glioma. Neurosurg. Rev. 17:317–320; 1994.

Itakura, T.; Yokote, H.; Ozaki, F.; et al. Stereotactic operation for brain abscess. Surg. Neurol. 28:196–200; 1987.

Jooma, O. V.; Pennybacker, J. B.; Tutton, G. K. Brain abscess: aspiration, drainage, or excision? J. Neurol. Neurosurg. Psychiatry 14:308–313; 1951.

Joubert, M. J.; Stephanov, S. Computerized tomography and surgical treatment in intracranial suppuration. Report of 30 consecutive unselected cases of brain abscess and subdural empyema. J. Neurosurg. 47:73–78; 1977.

Kagawa, M.; Takeshita, M.; Yato, S.; Kitamura, K. Brain abscess in congenital cyanotic heart disease. J. Neurosurg. 58:913–917; 1983.

Karandanis, D.; Shulman, J. A. Factors associated with mortality in brain abscess. Arch. Intern. Med. 135:1145–1150; 1975.

Konziolka, D.; Duma, Ch. M.; Lunsford, L. D. Factors that enhance the likelihood of successful stereotactic treatment of brain abscesses. Acta Neurochir. 127:85–90; 1994.

Laborde, G.; Klimek, L.; Harders, A.; Gilsbach, J. Frame-less stereotactic drainage of intracranial abscesses. Surg. Neurol. 40:16–21; 1993.

Legg, N. J.; Gupta, P. C.; Scott, D. F. Epilepsy following cerebral abscess: a clinical and EEG study of 70 patients. Brain 96:259–268; 1973.

Levy, R. M.; Berger, J. R. Neurosurgical aspects of human immunodeficiency virus infection. Neurosurg. Clin. N. Am. 3:443–465; 1992.

Liske, E.; Weikers, N. J. Changing aspects of brain abscesses. Review of cases in Wisconsin 1940 through 1962. Neurology 14:294–300; 1964.

Loeser, E., Jr.; Scheinberg, L. Brain abscess: a review of ninety-nine cases. Neurology 7:601–609; 1957.

Loftus, C. M.; Biller, J. Brain Abscess. In: Rengachary, S. S.; Wilkins, R. H. (eds). Principles of Neurosurgery. London: McGraw-Hill Publishing; 1996: p. 3285–3296.

Lunsford, L. D.; Nelson, P. B. Stereotactic aspiration of a brain abscess using the "therapeutic" CT scanner: a case report. Acta Neurochir. (Wien) 62:25–29; 1982.

Mamelak, A. N.; Mampalam, T. J.; Obana W. G.; Rosenblum, M. L. Improved management of multiple brain abscesses: a combined medical and surgical approach. Neurosurgery 36:75–86; 1995.

Mamelak, A. N.; Obana, W. G.; Flaherty, J. F.; Rosenblum, M. L. Nocardial brain abscesses: treatment strategies and factors influencing outcome. Neurosurgery 35:622–631; 1994.

Mampalam, T. J.; Rosenblum, M. L. Trends in the management of bacterial brain abscesses: a review of 102 cases over 17 years. Neurosurgery 23:451–458; 1988.

Mathisen, G. E.; Johnson, J. P. Brain abscess. Clin. Infect. Dis. 25:763–781; 1997.

Morgan, H.; Wood, M. W.; Murphey, F. Experience with 88 consecutive cases of brain abscess. J. Neurosurg. 38:698–704; 1973.

Nauta, H. J.; Contreras, W. F. L.; Weiner, R. L.; Crofford, M. J. Brain stem abscess managed with computed tomography-guided stereotactic aspiration. Neurosurgery 20:476–480; 1987.

Ng, P. Y.; Seow, W. T.; Ong, P. L. Brain abscesses: review of 30 cases treated with surgery. Aust. N. Z. J. Surg. 65:664–666; 1995.

Nielsen, H.; Harmsen, A.; Gyldensted, C. Cerebral abscess: a long term follow-up. Acta Neurol. Scand. 67:330–337; 1983.

Northcraft, G. B.; Wyke, B. D. Seizures folowing surgical treatment of intracranial abscesses: a clinical and electroencephalographic study. J. Neurosurg. 14:249–263; 1957.

Osenbach, R. K.; Loftus, C. M. Diagnosis and management of brain abscess. Neurosurg. Clin. N. Am. 3:403–420; 1992.

Patir, R.; Sood, S.; Bhatia, R. Post-traumatic brain abscess: experience of 36 patients. Br. J. Neurosurg. 19:29–35; 1995.

Porter, S. B.; Sande, M. A. Toxoplasmosis of the central nervous system in the acquired immunodeficiency syndrome. N. Engl. J. Med. 327:1643–1648; 1992.

Rajshekhar, V.; Chandy, M. J. Successful stereotactic management of a large cardiogenic brain stem abscess. J. Neurosurg. 34:368–371; 1994.

Renier, D.; Flandin, C.; Hirsch, E.; Hirsch, J. F. Brain abscesses in neonates. A study of 30 cases. J. Neurosurg. 69:877–882; 1988.

Rosenblum, M. L.; Hoff, J. T.; Norman, D.; Edward, M. S.; Berg, B. O. Nonoperative treatment of brain abscesses in selected high-risk patients. J. Neurosurg. 52:217–225; 1980.

Rosenblum, M. L.; Hoff, J. T.; Norman, D.; Weinstein, P. R.; Pitts, L. Decreased mortality from brain abscesses since the advent of computerized tomography. J. Neurosurg. 49:658–668; 1978.

Rosenblum, M. L.; Mampalam, T. J.; Pons, V. Controversies in the management of brain abscesses. Clin. Neurosurg. 33:603–632; 1986.

Samson, D. S.; Clark, K. A current review of brain abscess. Am. J. Med. 54:201–210; 1973.

Seydoux, C. H.; Francioli, P. Bacterial brain abscesses: factors influencing mortality and sequelae. Clin. Infect. Dis. 15:394–401; 1992.

Shahzadi, S.; Lozano, A. M.; Bernstein, M.; Guha, A.; Tasker, R. R. Stereotactic management of bacterial brain abscesses. Can. J. Neurol. Sci. 23:34–39; 1996.

Shaw, M. Post-operative epilepsy and the efficacy of anticonvulsant therapy. Acta Neurochir. Suppl. 50:55–57; 1990.

Skrap, M.; Melatini, A.; Vassallo, A.; Sidoti, C. Stereotactic aspiration and drainage of brain abscesses.

Experience with 9 cases. Minim. Invasive Neuro-surg. 39: 108–112; 1996.

Stapleton, S. R.; Bell, B. A.; Uttley, D. Stereotactic aspiration of brain abscesses is the treatment of choice? Acta Neurochir. 121:15–19; 1993.

Stephanov, S. Surgical treatment of brain abscess. Neurosurgery 22:724–730; 1988.

Svanteson, B.; Nordstrom, C. H.; Rausing, A. Non-traumatic brain abscess. Acta Neurochir. (Wien) 94: 57–65; 1988.

Van Alphen, H. A. M.; Dreissen, J. J. R. Brain abscess and subdural empyema: factors influencing mortality and results of various surgical techniques. J. Neurol. Neurosurg. Psychiatry 39:481–490; 1976.

Walot, I.; Miller B. L.; Chang, L; Mehringer, C. M. Neuroimaging findings in patients with AIDS. Clin. Infect. Dis. 22:906–919; 1996.

Walsh, P. R.; Larson, S. J.; Rytel, M. W.; Maiman, D. J. Stereotactic aspiration of deep cerebral ab-scesses after CT-directed labeling. Appl. Neuro-physiol. 43:205–209; 1980.

Wise, B. L.; Gleason, C. A. CT-directed stereotactic surgery in the management of brain abscess. Ann. Neurol. 6:457; 1979.

Wispelwey, B.; Dacey, R.; Scheld, W. Brain Abscess. In: Scheld, W. M.; Whitley, R. J.; Durack, D. T., eds. Infections of the central nervous system. 2nd ed. Philadelphia: Lippincott-Raven; 24:463–493; 1997.

Yang, S. Y. Brain abscess: a review of 400 cases. J. Neurosurg. 55:794–799; 1981.

Young, R. F.; Gade, G.; Grinnell, V. Surgical treatment for fungal infections in the central nervous system. J. Neurosurg. 63:371–381; 1985.

Zuger, A.; Lowry, F. Tuberculosis. In: Scheld, W. M.; Scheld, R. J.; Durack, D. T., eds. Infections of the cen-tral nervous system. 2nd ed. Philadelphia: Lippincott-Raven; 23:417–443; 1997.

# PART VI

# INFLAMMATORY DISORDERS

# 19

# Multiple Sclerosis

EMMANUELLE L. WAUBANT AND DONALD E. GOODKIN

Multiple sclerosis (MS) is a demyelinating disease of the central nervous system (CNS) that affects between 1 and 1.25 million persons worldwide (Dean 1994). Prevalence rates in the United States and Europe range from 15 to 145 per 100,000 and disease susceptibility appears to be influenced by genetic determinants, one's distance of residence from the equator, and possibly to age of exposure to certain infectious agents (National Center for Health Statistics 1989; Kurtzke 1993). Persons with MS often experience a variety of neurological symptoms including disturbances of vision, co-ordination; sensation; gait; endurance; and bowel, bladder, and sexual function. The diagnosis is traditionally clinically based and made only after excluding other medical conditions known to mimic MS (Natowicz and Bejjani 1994). To meet criteria for the diagnosis of *clinically definite* MS (Schumacher et al. 1965), patients must experience two or more episodes of symptoms, referred to as bouts or exacerbations, or continuous progression of abnormal neurological signs for 6 or more months. Exacerbations must last more than 24 hours, be separated by 4 or more weeks, and be accompanied by abnormal neurological signs attributable to involvement of separate anatomical locations in the brain or spinal cord. The diagnostic criteria for MS were revised in 1983 to incorporate magnetic resonance imaging (MRI) and other paraclinical tests that are frequently abnormal in patients with clinically definite MS (Poser et al. 1983). These criteria permit an abnormal MRI scan or paraclinical test such as a visual evoked response to be used in place of a second neurological sign. A diagnosis of *laboratory supported definite* MS may be established when there is one bout, one abnormal neurological sign, an abnormal paraclinical test, and intrathecal synthesis of immunoglobulin.

The brains and spinal cords of patients with MS evidence well-defined perivenular "plaques" of demyelination accompanied by variable amounts of leukocytic infiltrate and axonal transection (Allen and McKeown 1979; McDonald et al. 1992; Ferguson et al. 1997; Trapp et al. 1998). There is accumulating evidence that edema and inflammatory infiltrates produce disability that is transient, whereas disability resulting from demyelination and axonal transection is relatively irreversible (McDonald et al. 1992; Trapp et al. 1998). The earliest event in the formation of new lesions appears to be a breakdown in the blood-brain barrier that can be detected on serial gadolinium-enhanced MRI scans (Kermode et al. 1990). These histopathological and imaging observations as well as convergent lines of immunological, genetic, and epidemiological evidence suggest that tissue injury results from an immune response that is misdirected to one or more antigens of myelin in the CNS. The results of therapeutic trials with immunomodulatory agents support this concept, since treatments that augment proinflammatory immune function have exacerbated disease activity, while immunosuppressive and immunomodulating treatments have produced modest clinical benefits (Goodkin 1992).

In this chapter we review (1) the natural history of MS; (2) monosymptomatic demyelinating optic neuritis (ON), brain stem syndromes (BSS), and myelopathy (MYE) and their prognosis for spontaneous recovery and conversion to MS; (3) prognosis for recovery from acute exacerbations, progression of disability and survival from MS; (4) the effect of treatment for monosymptomatic ON, BSS, and MYE; and (5) the effect of treatment for exacerbations, sustained progression of disability, and MRI activity of MS.

## Natural History of MS

The natural history of MS has been defined in terms of clinical activity and activity detected by MRI scans (Fig. 19-1).

## Clinical Patterns of MS

The clinical course of MS evolves in one of four patterns (Lublin and Reingold 1996) (Fig. 19-2). Relapsing remitting (RR) MS is seen at the onset of disease in approximately 85% of patients. This clinical course is characterized by recurrent exacerbations with or without complete recovery of neurological impairment (Fig. 19-2A and B). Patients with RRMS are clinically stable between exacerbations. Within 10 years of disease onset, more than 50% of patients with RRMS transition to a secondary progressive (SP) clinical course that is characterized by gradual progression of disability between relapses or gradual progression of disability without superimposed relapses (Fig. 19-2C and D). Approximately 10% of all MS patients experience gradual progression of disability from disease onset unaccompanied by abrupt exacerbations. This clinical pattern is called primary progressive (PP) MS (Fig. 19-2E and F). Less than 5% of MS patients experience a primary progressive onset that is subsequently accompanied by one or more exacerbations. This clinical pattern is called progressive relapsing MS (Fig. 19-2G). The appearance of gadolinium-enhanced MRI lesions correlates to a limited extent with clinical exacerbations and, like exacer-

**Figure 19-1.** Natural history of MS: MRI and clinical patterns. MS natural history can be defined by progression of disability (*solid line*) or serial MRI scans as the appearance of new lesions that enhance transiently on $T_1$-weighted MRI sequences (*arrows*) and by increase of total $T_2$-weighted lesion burden (*dotted line*). (Adapted from Wolinsky 1993.)

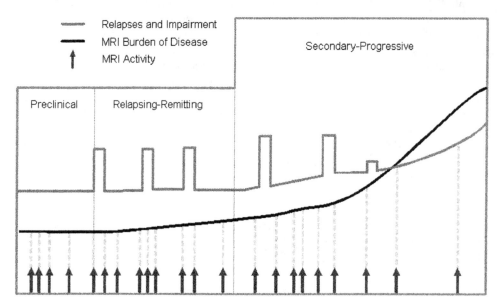

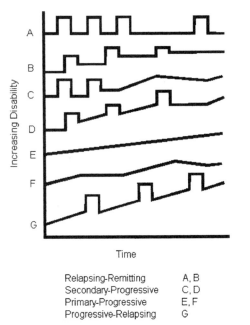

Time

| Relapsing-Remitting | A, B |
| Secondary-Progressive | C, D |
| Primary-Progressive | E, F |
| Progressive-Relapsing | G |

**Figure 19-2.** Clinical patterns of MS. Each line corresponds to different patterns of occurrence of MS symptoms over time (see text for further description).

bations, the appearance of new MRI lesions tends to be most frequent during the early or relapsing-remitting phase of the disease (Fig. 19-1).

## MRI Activity in MS

Focal $T_2$-weighted (T2W) MRI lesions correspond anatomically to MS plaques observed in fresh brain specimens (Grossman 1996). Studies of monthly MRI scans show the appearance of new focal T2W lesions that enhance on $T_1$-weighted (T1W) sequences following injection of intravenous gadolinium contrast agents. Gadolinium enhancement provides an imaging marker for disruption to the normal vascular endothelial barrier that limits movement of large molecules from the intravascular space into the brain parenchyma. Since most new focal lesions are unaccompanied by clinical symptoms (Miller et al. 1993), and disruption of the blood-brain barrier is considered to be an early event in the formation of new MS lesions, gadolinium-enhanced MRI lesions provide a useful surrogate measure for clinical disease activity.

Gadolinium enhancement of new MS lesions generally lasts for less than 2 months. Thereafter, each new lesion persists on T2W imaging sequences. On average, T2W lesion load increases

by 5% to 10% every year. One might expect change in total T2W lesion volume to correlate robustly with change in disability. Unfortunately, this is not the case (Paty et al. 1993). The lack of robust correlation between change in MRI T2W lesion load and change in disability may be explained by (1) the relative importance of lesion location, (2) the poor histopathological specificity of T2W lesions, and (3) the inability to image microscopic disease in normal appearing white matter. Progressive atrophy of the cervical spinal cord, third and lateral ventricles, and total T1W lesion area appear to provide more robust imaging correlates with change in measures of disability (Lossef et al. 1996b; Simon et al. 1998a). These findings suggest measures of atrophy and $T_1$ hypointensity provide more specific markers of irreversible tissue damage. Preliminary data suggest that change in measures of atrophy and T1W focal hypointense areas may be eventually used as surrogate markers for progression of disability in natural history studies and controlled clinical trials.

## Monosymptomatic Demyelinating Optic Neuritis, Brain Stem Syndromes, and Myelopathy

The probability of developing additional demyelinating episodes after an initial episode of monosymptomatic demyelinating ON, BSS, or MYE is of interest because patients who experience a second event of symptoms referable to dysfunction in the brain or spinal cord generally meet criteria for the diagnosis of clinically definite MS. This has prognostic implications and affects the ability of individuals to secure medical and life insurance. In this section we consider the prognosis for spontaneous recovery from each of these entities and their rates of conversion to multiple sclerosis.

### Prognosis for Spontaneous Recovery from ON, BSS, and MYE

#### Recovery from ON

The prognosis for spontaneous recovery from ON is favorable. Recovery of visual acuity equal to or better than 20/40 occurs in at least 85% of patients who experience an isolated episode of monosymptomatic ON (Bradley and Whitty 1967; Cohen et al. 1979; Beck et al. 1992). Of those who recover to this level, 50% do so within 1 month and 60% to 75% at 6 months. One year after onset of a first bout of ON fewer than 6% experience a recovery of visual acuity that is worse than 20/50 (Bradley and Whitty 1967; Beck et al. 1992). Prognosis appears to be related to the severity of visual impairment soon after the onset of ON. Of those who experience impairment of visual acuity worse than 20/200, 37% ($n = 24$) experience no recovery and 58% had improved to 20/20 when re-examined 5 years later (Cohen et al. 1979).

### Recovery from BSS

In contrast to ON, reliable data for rates of spontaneous recovery from BSS are not available.

### Recovery from MYE

Patients with complete acute myelopathies are less likely to recover than those with partial acute myelopathies (Lipton and Teasdall 1973; Ford et al. 1992). Likewise, patients with acute transverse myelitis in the context of Devic's syndrome usually recover poorly (O'Riordan et al. 1996).

## Prognosis for Conversion from ON, BSS, and MYE to Multiple Sclerosis

### Conversion from ON to MS

Approximately 17% of patients who meet diagnostic criteria for clinically definite MS have experienced ON as a presenting symptom (Weinshenker et al. 1989a). Between 35% and 68% of patients with an initial episode of ON will convert to MS within 12 to 15 years (Francis et al. 1987; Rizzo and Lessell 1988; Sandberg-Wollheim et al. 1990) and the rate appears to increase with time.

Conclusions regarding which clinical variables increase the probability of converting from ON to MS are based on limited data and should be considered tentative. Young adults age 21 to 40 years (Rizzo and Lessell 1988; Sandberg-Wollheim et al. 1990) are reported to be at increased risk to develop MS when compared to older patients. It has been suggested that the risk of developing MS is lowest if ON is experienced before age 16. A retrospective study (Lucchinetti et al. 1997) reports that 13% of patients under age 16 ($n = 79$) with isolated ON progressed to clinically or laboratory supported definite MS by 10 years of follow-up. The rate for children increases to 19% by 20 years. It is unknown why the risk to convert to

MS after an ON seems lower in childhood than in adults. There are no convincing data that gender is related to probability of converting to MS (Beck et al. 1993). Patients who experience an infection 2 weeks prior to ON (Lucchinetti et al. 1997), no retrobulbar pain, the presence of optic disc swelling, and mild visual acuity loss (Beck et al. 1993) appear to be at low risk to convert to MS. Patients who experience simultaneous bilateral ON may have a lower risk to develop MS than patients with unilateral or sequential bilateral ON (Parkin et al. 1984).

There is general agreement that MRI scans can discriminate which patients with ON are most likely to convert to MS (Table 19-1). The risk of conversion from ON to MS is related to the number of MRI lesions and total T2W lesion load. In the ON treatment trial, the 5-year risk of converting to MS ranges from 16% in patients with no brain MRI lesion to 51% in patients with three or more lesions (Optic Neuritis Study Group 1997). Similarly, 5 years after onset of ON, BSS, or MYE, 85% of the patients with four or more lesions ($n = 33$) convert to MS compared with 54% of the patients who have less than four lesions ($n = 24$) ($\chi^2 = 6.48$; $p < .02$) (Morrissey et al. 1993). Eighty-six percent of these patients with a lesion load greater than 1.23 cm$^3$ and 25% of patients with a lesion load less than 1.23 cm$^3$ convert to MS within 5 years (Filippi, 1994). Although larger initial T2W lesion load correlates with decreasing time to convert to MS, more than three-quarters of patients who develop MS do so

**Table 19-1.** Risk to Convert from ON, MYE, and BSS to MS According to MRI Status: 5-Year Follow-up

|  | Number of Patients Converting MS/Total Number Patients | |
| --- | --- | --- |
|  | Abnormal MRI | Normal MRI |
| Monosymptomatic demyelinating ON | | |
| Morrissey et al. 1993 | 23/28 (82%) | 1/16 (6%) |
| ONTT 1997 | 88/149 (59%) | 49/202 (24%) |
| Monosymptomatic demyelinating MYE | | |
| Morrissey et al. 1993 | 10/17 (59%) | 1/11 (9%) |
| Monosymptomatic demyelinating BSS | | |
| Morrissey et al. 1993 | 8/12 (67%) | 0/5 (0%) |

ON, optic neuritis; MYE, myelopathy; BSS, brain stem syndromes; MRI, magnetic resonance imaging; MS; multiple sclerosis; ONTT, Optic Neuritis Treatment Trial.

within the first 2 years of follow-up. In patients with abnormal MRI shortly after onset of ON, BSS, or MYE, conversion to MS over 5 years is highest in those who develop new lesions ($n = 48$) (81%), compared those who do not (22%) ($n = 9$) (Morrissey et al. 1993). T2W lesion load soon after onset of ON is correlated with lesion load 5 years after ON (Spearman's rank correlation coefficient [SRCC] = 0.862; $p < .0001$) and the severity of disability at 5 years is significantly correlated to increase in lesion load over the same time frame (SRCC = 0.62; $p < .0001$) (Filippi et al. 1994).

The presence of intrathecal oligoclonal bands (OB) that are not observed in the systemic circulation or increased intrathecal synthesis of immunoglobulin G (IgG) increases the risk of conversion from ON, BSS, and MYE to MS (Moulin et al. 1983; Miller et al. 1989; Lee et al. 1991; Sharief and Thompson 1991). Table 19-2 summarizes these data for ON, BSS, and MYE.

MRI appears to better discriminate which patients with ON, BSS, or MYE are most likely to convert to MS than IgG or OB (Morrissey et al. 1993; Lee et al. 1991). For example, in acute partial transverse myelopathy, 93% of patients with abnormal MRI convert to MS compared with 78% of patients with OB and 30% of patients with abnormal evoked potentials (Ford et al. 1992). The risk of conversion to MS is greater than 93% for patients with MYE who evidence three or more lesions on MRI and who additionally evidence abnormal OB or IgG (Soderstrom et al. 1994). By contrast, fewer than 5% of patients who experience an episode of ON, BSS, MYE who have normal MRI and cerebrospinal fluid (CSF) will over 2 years convert to MS (Miller et al.

1989; Lee et al. 1991; Morrissey et al. 1993). This observation has led to the notion that examination of CSF IgG and OB may be most useful in monosymptomatic patients who evidence normal brain MRI. Preliminary data suggest that CSF IgM may better discriminate which patients with ON are most likely to convert to MS than CSF IgG (Sharief and Hentges 1991).

Conversion from ON, BSS, and MYE to MS is associated with the DRB1*1501, DQA1*0102, DQB1*0602 haplotype, but this effect is only significant in patients with disseminated T2W abnormalities on brain MRI (Kelly et al. 1993). It is not yet established whether HLA type independently influences the prognosis for conversion from ON, BSS, and MYE to MS.

### Conversion from BSS to MS

In contrast to patients who experience ON, there are no clinical data that indicate which patients with BSS are most likely to convert to MS.

Although data from imaging studies are limited, the ability of MRI to predict which patients with BSS are most likely to convert to MS are similar to those that discriminate which patients with ON are most likely to convert to MS (Table 19-1). Forty-seven percent of patients ($n = 17$) with monosymptomatic demyelinating BSS who evidence abnormal MRI scans convert to MS on average over 5 years (Filippi, 1994). None of the patients with BSS and normal brain MRI converted to MS within the same follow-up period. Data regarding the ability of IgG, IgM, and OB to discriminate which patients with monosymptomatic BSS are most likely to convert to MS are presented in the preceding section, Conversion from ON to MS.

**Table 19-2.** Percent of Patients With Abnormal CSF Who Develop MS

|  |  | Follow-up | CSF at Onset | Number of Patients | Progression to MS (%) | Relative Risk | $p$ Value |
|---|---|---|---|---|---|---|---|
| Miller et al. 1989 | Spinal cord | 14 mo | OB+ | 14 | 10 (71%) | 25 | <.005 |
|  |  |  | OB− | 11 | 1 (9%) |  |  |
|  | Brain stem | 14 mo | OB+ | 8 | 7 (87%) | 19 | <.01 |
|  |  |  | OB− | 11 | 3 (27%) |  |  |
| Lee et al. 1991 | Monosymptomatic | 2 yr | OB+ | 91 | 38 (42%) | 3.2 | .0005 |
|  |  |  | OB− | 93 | 17 (18%) |  |  |
| Soderstrom et al. 1994 | ON | 2 yr | OB+ | 41 | 16 (39%) | 10.8 | .009 |
|  |  |  | OB− | 18 | 1 (5%) |  |  |

CSF, cerebrospinal fluid; MS, multiple sclerosis; OB+, oligoclonal band positive; OB−, oligoclonal band negative; ON, optic neuritis

## Conversion from MYE to MS

Data for clinical variables that discriminate patients with MYE who are most likely to convert to MS are limited. Five years after MYE, only 1 of 31 patients with *complete* transverse myelitis convert to MS (Lipton and Teasdell 1973; Morrissey et al. 1993). Patients with monosymptomatic *partial* transverse myelitis are more likely to convert to MS. Thirty-nine percent of the patients with partial MYE (*n* = 28) convert to MS during a mean follow-up of approximately 5 years (Morrissey et al. 1993).

Imaging data that discriminate patients with MYE who are most likely to convert to MS are also limited. Eighty percent of patients with partial MYE who have normal MRI (*n* = 18) and 93% (*n* = 12) of patients who have abnormal MRI convert to MS after a mean follow-up of 3 years (Ford et al. 1992). Data regarding the ability of CSF IgG, IgM, and OB to discriminate which patients with monosymptomatic BSS are most likely to convert to MS are presented in the preceding section, Conversion from ON to MS.

## Multiple Sclerosis: Prognosis for Acute Exacerbations, Progression of Disability, and Survival

Although the natural history of MS is highly variable between and within patients, data from large cohorts of patients with MS indicate trends where demographic, clinical, imaging, and laboratory variables appear to be related to the extent of recovery from exacerbations, sustained progression of disability, and survival.

### Prognosis for Acute Exacerbations

Approximately 85% of patients with MS experience an acute event at disease onset and approximately 85% of those initial exacerbations improve spontaneously (McAlpine 1961). Recovery rates from initial exacerbations are inversely related to the duration of symptoms produced by the bout (Muller 1949) (Table 19-3).

Rates for improvement of impairment and disability resulting from acute exacerbations have been most rigorously studied in hospitalized male World War II veterans (Kurtzke 1956). Change in impairment and disability in that study was defined as change of at least 1 DSS point (see Ap-

**Table 19-3.** Patients Experiencing Complete Symptomatic Recovery from Initial Exacerbations

| Initial Symptom | Percent Recovery by Duration of Symptoms | |
|---|---|---|
| | < 2 mo | ≥2 mo |
| Diplopia | 94 | 16 |
| "Giddiness" | 86 | Not available |
| Paresthesia | 83 | 25 |
| Hemiparesis | 57 | Not available |
| Optic neuritis | 56 | 12 |
| Monoparesis | 45 | 33 |

Adapted from Muller (1999) and Goodkin (1992).

pendix A). Rates for complete recovery to pre-exacerbation DSS score were not provided. Of those patients who improved spontaneously, 80% did so within 2 months of the onset of exacerbation. The probability of spontaneous improvement declined markedly 1 month after the onset of an exacerbation (Fig. 19-3).

### Prognosis for the Frequency of MS Exacerbations

Acute exacerbations are the most obvious clinical manifestation of disease activity. Exacerbation rates in most cross-sectional studies range from of 0.4 to 1 per year (Weinshenker and Ebers 1987). The frequency of exacerbations in untreated patients spontaneously decreases as disease duration increases (Muller 1949; McAlpine and Compston 1952; Leibowitz et al. 1964; Weinshenker and Ebers 1987) even over short periods of time (Goodkin et al. 1991; INFB Multiple Sclerosis Study Group 1995; Johnson et al. 1995; Jacobs et al. 1996). Since cases of MS tend to come to medical attention shortly after an exacerbation, the relationship between exacerbation frequency and disease duration to some extent reflects case ascertainment bias. Thus, the tendency for exacerbation frequency to decline after case ascertainment may result in part from "spontaneous regression to the mean" exacerbation rate of larger populations. However, a decline in exacerbation rate also probably reflects spontaneous conversion to gradual progression of disability without superimposed relapses. It is assumed that the progressive phase of MS results from irreversible demyelination and axonal loss, which become more prominent as the parenchymal burden of disease increases.

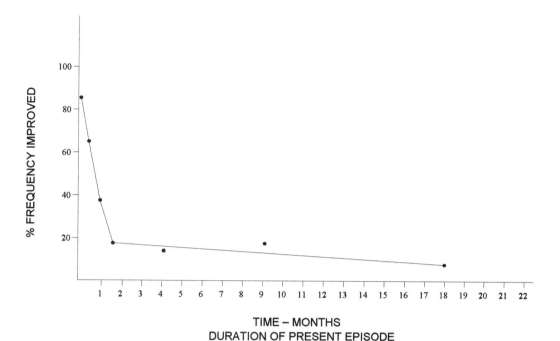

**Figure 19-3.** Recovery from exacerbations. The percentage of patients who improve following a relapse declines as a function of time. The probability of spontaneous improvement declines markedly 1 month after the onset of an exacerbation (Adapted from Kutzke 1956.)

## Prognosis for Sustained Progression of Disability Resulting from MS

Retrospective studies indicate that 34% to 44% of untreated patients lose the ability to ambulate independently 5 years after experiencing the onset of initial symptom. The proportion of patients who lose the ability to ambulate independently is related to disease duration—47% to 58% lose that ability after 10 years and 56% to 66% after 15 years (Muller 1949, McAlpine 1961; Leibowitz et al. 1964). Similar trends for rates of sustained progression of disability as measured by the Disability Status Scale (DSS) and Expanded Disability Status Scale (EDSS) (Kurtzke 1983) are seen in prospective natural history studies. These scales range from 0 (no disability) to 10 (death due to MS) (see Appendix A for the EDSS). DSS and EDSS scores of 6.0 mark the transition from independent ambulation to ambulation with a unilateral assistance such as a cane. In these studies, 25% to 55% of patients reach DSS 6.0 10 years after disease onset (Confavreux et al. 1980; Weinshenker et al. 1989a). Ten years after disease onset, between 15% and 40% of patients retain an EDSS score less than 3.5 (Kurtzke et al. 1977;

McAlpine 1961; Confavreux et al. 1980; Thompson et al. 1986; Miller et al. 1992). This score indicates a moderate disability involving not more than two of the following functional systems: pyramidal, cerebellar, brain stem, sensory, visual, bowel, or bladder function (Kurtzke 1983). Table 19-4 summarizes rates of progression of disability reported in large retrospective and prospective natural history studies.

There is evidence that clinical, demographic, MRI, and biological markers may in large MS cohorts be related to the risk of exacerbation and sustained progression of disability. These variables include (1) age at onset of disease, (2) gender, (3) initial symptoms, (4) relapse rate during the first 2 years of the disease, (5) level of disability 5 years after the onset of disease, (6) clinical pattern of disease, (7) stress, (8) pregnancy, (9) infection, (10) vaccination, (11) MRI, (12) intrathecal synthesis of immunoglobulin, (13) genetic factors, and (14) adhesion molecules and cytokines. Attempts to incorporate some of these clinical and demographic variables into mathematical models that can predict the prognosis for sustained progression of disability in individual

**Table 19-4.** Percentage of Patients Ambulatory After 5, 10, and 15 Years (EDSS of 6.0 or Less)

| | Number of Patients | % of Patients Ambulatory Without Assistance (EDSS ≤ 6.0) | | |
| --- | --- | --- | --- | --- |
| | | After 5 yr | After 10 yr | After 15 yr |
| Muller 1949 | 793 | 56% | 44% | 34% |
| McAlpine 1961 | 241 | | 42% | 34% |
| Leibowitz et al. 1964 | 266 | 66% | 53% | 44% |
| Kurtzke et al. 1977 | 403 | | 56% | 50% |
| Confavreux et al. 1980 | 349 | 92% | 75% | 60% |
| Weinshenker et al. 1989a, 1989b | 1099 | 86% | 68% | 50% |
| Runmaker and Andersen 1993 | 308 | 85% | 65% | 50% |

EDSS, Expanded Disability Status Scale.

patients have been disappointing (Wolfson and Confavreux 1987; Weinshenker et al. 1991; Runmarker et al. 1994).

### Age at Onset of Disease

Several investigators have reported that patients whose age at onset of disease is less than 40 years are less likely to experience sustained progression of disability (Muller 1949; McAlpine and Compston 1952; Panelius 1969; Visscher et al. 1984; Thompson 1986; Wolfson and Confavreux 1987; Weinshenker 1989a; Phadke 1990; Miller et al. 1992; Trojano et al. 1995) (Table 19-5). Data for 15-year follow-up indicate that 76% of children are still ambulatory (Duquette et al. 1987). In contrast, 32% to 76% of adults require assistance to walk within 15 years of disease onset (Weinshenker and Ebers 1987; Weinshenker et al. 1989b).

### Gender

Most investigators report that after controlling for disease duration and age, male patients are more likely to experience sustained progression of disability (Muller 1949; Panelius 1969; Wolfson and Confavreux 1987; Weinshenker et al. 1989b; Runmarker and Andersen 1993) (Table 19-5).

### Symptoms at Onset

Patients who experience monosymptomatic sensory symptoms or optic neuritis are less likely to experience sustained progression of disability as long as 25 years after disease onset (Muller 1949; McAlpine and Compston 1952; Minderhoud et al. 1988; Weinshenker et al. 1989b; Phadke 1990; Runmarker and Andersen 1993) (Table 19-5). In contrast, patients who experience cerebellar or pyramidal dysfunction at disease onset are more likely to experience sustained progression of disability (Muller 1949, McAlpine and Compston 1952; Kurtzke et al. 1977; Miller et al. 1992; Visscher et al. 1984; Thompson et al. 1986; Riise et al. 1992; Runmarker and Andersen 1993; Trojano et al. 1995). On average, data indicate that patients who fail to experience recovery after an initial bout are more likely to convert to secondary progressive MS (Weinshenker 1989b; Phadke 1990; Runmarker and Andersen 1993). Furthermore, these patients convert to the progressive phase of the illness at an earlier time than patients who experience some improvement from their initial bout (Trojano et al. 1995).

### Relapse Rate During the First 2 Years of the Disease

Some investigators report that relapse rate during the first 2 years of the disease is related to probability of sustained progression of disability (Table 19-5) The risk to progress to DSS 3.0 to 6.0 is reported to be greater for patients who experience two or more attacks during the first 2 years of their illness (Confavreux et al. 1980; Weinshenker et al. 1989b). Similarly, a long interval between the first two bouts appears to be associated with a more favorable prognosis (Thompson et al. 1986; Phadke 1990; Weinshenker et al. 1989b). On average, 50% of patients reach DSS 6.0 within 7 years if during the first 2 years of their illness they experience five or more attacks ($n = 34$), 13 years if they experience two to four attacks ($n = 244$), and within 18 years if they experience fewer than two attacks ($n = 452$) (Weinshenker 1995). However, other investigators fail to detect any relationship between attack frequency during the first 2 years of the disease and probability of experiencing sustained progression of disability (Runmarker et al. 1994). Thus the relationship between attack rate during the first 2 years of the illness and probability of experiencing sustained progression of disability remains uncertain.

**Table 19-5.** Potential Prognostic Markers of Later Severity of Disability from Selected Natural History Studies

| | Female | Young Age of Onset | ON | Sensory Symptoms | Motor Symptoms | Cerebellar Symptoms | Number of relapses in first years | Long First Remission | Recuperation of First Relapse | Mono-sypmtomatic Onset | Relapsing-Remitting | Chronic Progressions | Low Level of Disability at 5 Years |
|---|---|---|---|---|---|---|---|---|---|---|---|---|---|
| Muller 1949 | + | + | | +− | − | | | | | | + | | + |
| McAlpine and Compston 1952 | 0 | + | + | + | − | − | − | | | | + | − | + |
| Kurtzke 1956 | | 0 | | 0 | 0 | 0 | 0 | | | | + | − | |
| McAlpine 1961 | | 0 | + | 0 | − | 0 | 0 | | | | + | − | + |
| Leibowitz et al. 1964 | − | | 0 | 0 | 0 | 0 | | | | | + | − | |
| Panelius 1969 | + | + | | | | | | | | | | | |
| Fog and Linnemann 1970 | | | | | | | | | | | | | |
| Kurtzke et al. 1977 | 0 | 0 | + | 0 | − | 0 | 0 | | | | + | 0 | + |
| Wolfson and Confavreux 1987 | 0 | 0 | 0 | 0 | − | − | 0 | | | | 0 | 0 | |
| Minderhoud et al. 1988 | + | 0 | + | 0 | 0 | 0 | − | | | − | + | − | |
| Goodkin et al. 1989 | − | 0 | + | | − | 0 | 0 | | | 0 | + | − | |
| Phadke 1990 | 0 | + | + | + | − | 0 | | | | + | + | − | |
| Weinshenker 1989b | 0 | + | + | 0 | 0 | − | | + | + | | + | − | +++ |
| Miller et al. 1992 | + | + | 0 | 0 | − | − | − | | + | | + | − | + |
| Riise et al. 1992 | 0 | + | 0 | 0 | − | − | 0 | | | | + | − | |
| Runmarker and Andersen 1993 | 0 | + | + | + | − | − | 0 | + | + | + | + | − | + |
| Trojano et al. 1995 | + | + | + | | − | − | − | | + | + | + | − | + |
| Weinshenker 1995 | + | + | | | | | | | ++ | ++ | | | |

U, no effect on prognosis; +, positive effect on prognosis; −, negative effect on prognosis; ON, optic neuritis;

## Level of Disability 5 Years
## After the Onset of Disease

Most investigators report that level of disability 5 years after onset of disease is predictive of level of disability 10 and 15 years after disease onset (Muller 1949; McAlpine and Compston 1952; Kurtzke et al. 1977; Miller et al. 1992; Weinshenker et al. 1989b; Runmarker and Andersen 1993). This relationship is illustrated in Table 19-6.

### Clinical Pattern of Disease

Although the definitions for clinical patterns of disease have changed to reflect the broad consensus of MS investigators (Lublin and Reingold 1996), most agree that patients who experience any definition of progressive MS are more likely to experience sustained progression of disability than patients with relapsing forms of MS (Muller 1949; McAlpine and Compston 1952; McAlpine 1961; Kurtzke 1956; Leibowitz et al. 1964; Fog and Linnemann 1970; Wolfson and Confavruex 1987; Minderhoud et al. 1988, Goodkin et al. 1989; Miller et al. 1992; Riise et al. 1992; Weinshenker and Ebers 1987; Trojano et al. 1995). For example, it has been reported that 10 years after onset of disease 46% of patients who meet the definition for secondary progressive MS ($n = 69$) and 53% of patients who meet the definition for primary progressive MS ($n = 60$) lose ability to ambulate independently. This stands in sharp contrast to a report that only 2% of patients who meet the definition for relapsing remitting disease experience this level of disability over a similar time frame (Trojano et al. 1995).

### Stress

The relationship between stress and MS clinical activity remains poorly defined. One rigorously controlled study found patients who experienced extremely stressful life events were 3.7 times as

**Table 19-6.** Predicting DSS Score at 15 Years from DSS Score at 5 Years

| DSS at Year 5 | DSS at Year 15 | |
| --- | --- | --- |
| | 0–2 | >6 |
| 0–2 | 66% | 11% |
| 3–5 | 14% | 40% |
| >6 | 1% | 99% |

From Goodkin (1992), adapted from Kurtzke et al. (1977).
DSS, Disability Status Scale.

likely to exacerbate as those not exposed to such events (Franklin 1988). Studies investigating the relationship between stress and MRI activity are ongoing (Mohr et al. 1997).

### Pregnancy

It is reported that annualized relapse rate decreases during pregnancy (Sadovnick et al. 1994), particularly during the third trimester thereof (Korn-Lubetzki et al. 1984; Confavreux et al. 1998). In a single study of two patients who were monitored with brain MRIs during and after pregnancy, new MRI lesions were not found during the third trimester but reappeared after delivery (van Walderveen et al. 1994). However, these clinical observations have not been confirmed in a rigorously controlled prospective study in which no decline in exacerbation rate was observed after conception (Roullet et al. 1993). On the other hand, there is general agreement that 20% to 53% of female patients experience a relapse during the 3 months following delivery. Thus the annualized exacerbation rates increase approximately twenty-threefold during the first 3 months after delivery and thereafter return to baseline (Birk et al. 1990; Sadovnick et al. 1994; Roullet et al. 1993; Confavreux et al. 1998). Anecdotal experience suggests that relapses may be milder during pregnancy, and those during the 3 months following delivery may be more severe (Roullet et al. 1993; Worthington and Crawford 1994).

There is consensus that the long-term prognosis for sustained progression of disability following pregnancy is probably similar to that for women who do not become pregnant (Roullet et al. 1993). However, some reports suggest pregnancy before and after onset of MS may be protective. Although prone to case ascertainment bias, two studies suggest the relative risk for developing MS may be lower in women with more than two children than in those with fewer than two children (Villard-Mackintosh and Vessey 1993; Runmarker and Andersen 1995). Others report that pregnancy after onset of MS is associated with a longer time to sustained progression of disability (Verdru et al. 1994), reduced probability of conversion from relapsing to progressive MS (Runmarker and Andersen 1995), and a lower annualized relapse rate when compared with patients who do not become pregnant after the onset of MS (Roullet et al. 1993). There is no evidence that MS has a deleterious effect on pregnancy (Damek and Shuster 1997).

## Infections

Preliminary evidence suggests that viral infections may increase the risk of developing a subsequent relapse (Sibley et al. 1985, Panitch 1994). Rigorously controlled studies are needed to confirm these provocative findings.

## Vaccinations

A possible relationship between hepatitis B vaccination and MS exacerbations is reported (Nadler 1993). Reassuringly, there is no increase in relapse rate following vaccination during a multicenter, randomized, double-blind, placebo-controlled trial of influenza immunization in patients with MS (Miller et al. 1997). Similarly, preliminary data suggest there is no evidence of any increase in MRI activity following vaccination for influenza (Salvetti et al. 1995).

## Magnetic Resonance Imaging

In cross-sectional studies, T2W and to a greater extent T1W total lesion area correlate significantly with level of disability (Grossman 1996). Furthermore, patients with relapsing-remitting MS who evidence gadolinium-enhanced lesions are more likely to experience future exacerbations during the next 2 to 3 years (Smith et al. 1993; Koudriavtseva et al. 1997). The presence of at least one enhancing lesion also predicts the appearance of new gadolinium-enhancing lesions over the next 6 months (Koudriavtseva et al. 1997). Although total T2W lesion number and area are useful for identifying which patients with ON, BSS, and MYE are more likely to develop severe disability resulting from MS, imaging data from patients with established MS do not reliably identify those who are most likely to progress. Perhaps this should not be surprising, since (1) focal T2W lesions do not discriminate reversible edema from relatively irreversible demyelination and axonal transection, (2) disability may correlate more robustly with lesion location than lesion number or lesion area, and (3) T2W imaging sequences do not provide a measure of microscopic disease within normal appearing white matter. Currently, no measure of MRI activity whether it be T2W, T1W lesions, gadolinium enhancement, magnetic transfer imaging, or proton magnetic resonance spectroscopic imaging has

been shown to reliably predict which patients are most likely to experience sustained progression of disability (Losseff et al. 1996a).

## Intrathecal Synthesis of Immunoglobulins

Once the diagnosis of MS is established, measures of intrathecal synthesis of immunoglobulins do not correlate reliably with disease activity or sustained progression of disability.

## Genetic Factors

Evidence for genetic susceptibility to MS has been reported in studies of ethnic groups and in family, adoption, and twin studies (Oksenberg and Hauser 1997). Siblings of affected individuals have a lifetime risk for MS of 2% to 5%, whereas the risk for parents or for children of affected individuals is somewhat lower. Recent adoption and half-sibling studies from Canada (Ebers et al. 1995) support the concept that familial aggregation in MS is determined by genetics rather than environment. Twin studies demonstrate concordance rates of 25% to 30% in monozygotic and of only 2% to 5% in dizygotic twins. In Caucasians, MS is four times more likely to occur with haplotype HLA-DRB1*1501-DQA1*0102-DQB1*0602. In Asians, disseminated but not a more restricted disease is associated with DRB1*1501 and DRB5*0101 alleles (Kira et al. 1996). There is but a single study that reports an association of HLA type with clinical disease course: relapsing-remitting MS with DRw15, DQw6 and DRw17, and Dqw2 and primary progressive MS with DR4, and Dqw8 (Olerup et al. 1989). These findings have not been replicated in other populations and there is as yet no convincing evidence that HLA type is related to overall prognosis.

## Adhesion Molecules, Cytokines, Matrix Metalloproteinases (MMP) and their Inhibitors

High levels of soluble intercellular adhesion molecule 1 (ICAM-1) and vascular cell adhesion molecule 1 (VCAM-1) are detected in patients exhibiting clinical exacerbations and gadolinium-enhanced MRI lesions (Giovannoni et al. 1997; Hartung et al. 1995). Although circulating ICAM levels may correlate with exacerbations (Rieckman et al. 1994), high levels of serum ICAM-1 (sICAM-1) do not correlate with nor do they predict progression of disability (Giovannoni et al.

1997). Increased serum interferon-γ, tumor necrosis factor (TNF) production, and TNF mRNA expression in blood mononuclear cells appear to precede clinical relapses and new MRI activity (Beck et al. 1988; Rieckmann et al. 1995). Serum levels of soluble TNF receptor are also raised in patients with active disease (Hartung et al. 1995). Thus far, only one study suggests any correlation between level of TNF-α in the CSF and rate of neurological deterioration ($r = .74$; $p < .001$) (Sharief and Hentges 1991). High serum levels of MMP-9, an enzyme likely involved in cell migration through the blood-brain barrier, and low serum levels of its inhibitor, tissue inhibitor of MMP-type 1 (TIMP-1) appear to precede clinical and MRI activity (Lee et al. 1999; Waubant et al. 1999).

## MS: Prognosis for Survival

It is important to know what percentage of MS patients will die from MS or related problems and to be able to predict those patients who are at high risk to do so. A significant reduction in survival time is frequently reported in earlier studies. These data are difficult to interpret because of retrospective data acquisition (Muller 1949), small sample size (Allison 1950), or hospital- rather than clinic-based data collection (McAlpine 1961). Additionally, these studies were performed during the preantibiotic era.

Kurtzke et al. estimated a mean survival period exceeding 30 years in U.S. male armed service veterans (Kurtzke et al. 1977). Weinshenker et al. reported a median survival time of 15.1 years for their total population of 1099 patients (Weinshenker et al. 1989a). A subgroup of their total population followed since onset of the disease sustained only 1 death in 197 patients followed for a mean of 4.2 years.

Phadke et al. (1987) presented data on 1055 patients who had been followed for more than 10 years as part of an epidemiological investigation. A centralized record-keeping system of death certificates for the region enabled continuous monitoring of the entire population for recorded death. Between 1970 and 1980, 216 deaths occurred and the mean survival time was 24.5 years. Information recorded included sex, age at onset, initial symptoms, course of the disease, and survival calculated from the year of first symptoms. Initial symptoms and course of the disease were clearly defined. There was no difference in time of

survival between sexes. The life expectancy of the patients compared to the Scottish general population using life table analysis demonstrated only a slight reduction in short-term (<10 years) survival in all age groups with the exception of those with onset age above 50 years. A 44% reduction in survival for males and 22% for females was observed in the latter group. Long-term (≥10 years) life expectancy was markedly reduced in all age groups compared with controls. In the 40- to 49-year-old disease onset group, only 26% of females and 5% of males were alive at 30 years after onset compared to 70% of females and 60% of males for age-matched general population controls. Survival time also correlated with level of disability at the time of the initial examination. A mean of 94% of those without significant disability survived 10 years compared to 28% of those who were no longer functional ambulators. Similar results have been reported by others (Hyllested 1961; Gudmendsson 1971). Survival was significantly shorter for those patients in all age groups who sustained a relapse within 6 months of disease onset, compared to those whose relapse occurred later than 6 months, and for those who had a progressive course since onset as opposed to a relapsing course. Patients with cerebellar symptoms at onset had a significantly shorter survival, and those with optic neuritis or isolated brain stem initial symptoms had longer survival than those with other presentations. Sixty-two percent died of causes directly related to MS (pneumonia, sepsis), 12% from hematological or malignant disease, and 19% from coronary artery disease.

The possibility that additional illnesses might contribute to death rates in MS patients has also been considered. Zimmerman et al. reported an uncontrolled series of 41 autopsied MS cases in which an insignificant increase in the prevalence of coexistent malignant disease was noted (Zimmerman and Netsky 1950). This trend has not been seen by others (Kurtzke et al. 1970; Allen et al. 1978).

In summary, survival is reduced in MS patients compared to age-matched population controls. Data suggest that survival is predominantly influenced by older age of onset, male sex, and advanced level of disability at initial examination.

The risk for suicide among MS patients is reported to be approximately 7.5 times greater than that for the age-matched general population

(Sadovnick et al. 1991). Risk factors for suicide include (1) patients with mild to moderate disability (average EDSS, 4.5) (Sadovnick et al. 1991), (2) first 5 years following diagnosis (Stenager et al. 1992), (3) absence of social support systems, (4) hopelessness, and (5) self-perceived religiosity (Long and Miller 1991). Unemployed males experiencing financial stress may be more likely to commit suicide (Berman and Samuel 1993).

## Effect of Disease-Modifying Therapies for Monosymptomatic ON, BSS, MYE, and MS

### Monosymptomatic Episodes of Demyelinating ON, BSS, and MYE

#### Effect of Treatment Compared to Spontaneous Recovery from ON

Most of the data regarding recovery from acute ON have been generated from the Optic Neuritis Treatment Trial (ONTT) (Beck et al. 1992). In that trial, patients were treated with placebo, oral prednisone, or intravenous methylprednisolone. Compared with placebo, methylprednisolone administered intravenously 250 mg every 6 hours for 3 days followed by oral prednisone 1 mg/kg/d for 11 days improved short-term recovery of visual acuity. Most of the difference in the rate of recovery of vision between these treatment arms was seen during the first 2 weeks. Thereafter, differences in visual function were small and after 1 year of follow-up there were no significant differences between treatment arms in visual acuity, contrast sensitivity, color vision, or visual fields. Patients treated with oral prednisone administered 1 mg/kg/d for 14 days appeared to experience more new attacks of optic neuritis in both the initially affected and fellow eyes. Within 2 years of follow-up, new attacks of optic neuritis in either eye occurred in 30% of the patients in the oral prednisone group, compared with 16% in the placebo group and 14% in the intravenous group.

#### Effect of Treatment on the Probability of Conversion from ON to MS

Two-year data from the ONTT indicate that intravenous methylprednisolone (IVMP) recipients were less likely to convert to MS than the placebo or oral prednisone recipients (Beck et al. 1993). At 2 years, 7.5% of the IVMP recipients converted to

MS compared with 16.7% of the placebo and 14.7% of the oral prednisone recipients. Most of the treatment effect occurred in the patients with abnormal brain MRI scans at baseline. Five-year rates for conversion from ON to MS were again greater for patients with abnormal MRI scans at baseline; 51% versus 16%. However, the treatment effect observed at 2 years was no longer evident after 5 years (Optic Neuritis Study Group 1997): 27% of the IVMP, 32% of the oral prednisone, and 31% of the placebo recipients converted to MS. These data raise the possibility that the treatment effect observed with IVMP at 2 years was due to chance. Since the significance of the 2-year survival data remains unclear to several investigators, we believe there is no treatment that convincingly delays the conversion of monosymptomatic demyelinating ON to MS. Trials are currently in progress to determine if a combination of interferon-β and IVMP is more efficacious than IVMP in delaying the conversion of ON to MS.

#### Effect of Treatment on Recovery from Monosymptomatic Demyelinating BSS and MYE

Although patients who experience monosymptomatic episodes of demyelinating BSS and MYE are routinely treated with corticosteroids and there is a notion that IVMP shortens the duration of disability resulting from these syndromes, there have been no rigorous controlled clinical trials to clarify whether treatment is actually efficacious.

#### Effect of Treatment on Conversion from BSS and MYE to MS

There have been no rigorous clinical trials to determine whether IVMP or any other disease-modifying intervention reduces the probability of converting from a first episode of BSS or MYE to MS.

## Multiple Sclerosis: The Effect of Treatment for Acute Exacerbations, Sustained Progression of Disability, and MRI Activity

### Effect of Treatment on Recovery from Acute Exacerbations of MS

The effect of placebo-controlled treatments on the recovery of acute exacerbations of MS is confined to corticotropin (ACTH) and glucocorticosteroids (Andersson and Goodkin 1996). Patients in the

Cooperative Study in the Evaluation of Therapy in Multiple Sclerosis (Rose et al. 1970) were randomized to receive ACTH gel (40 U intramuscularly [IM] twice daily for 7 days, 20 U IM twice daily for 4 days, and 20 U IM each day for 3 days) or matched placebo within 8 weeks of an exacerbation. Significantly more ACTH- than placebo-treated patients (65% vs. 47%) exhibited improvement in DSS score 4 weeks after initiating therapy. The duration of these benefits was not determined, since the patients were not followed for longer than 4 weeks.

In 1985, Barnes et al. reported that patients treated with 1 g of IVMP for 7 days were clinically more improved than patients treated with 60 U IM ACTH tapered by 20 U each week for 3 weeks (Barnes et al. 1985). However, the treatment benefit was no longer evident 3 months after initiating therapy. Other investigators observed similar clinical improvements for 4 to 12 weeks with either a shorter course of IVMP (1 g IV daily for 3 days) or the ACTH protocol used in the Cooperative Study (80 U for 7 days, 40 U for 4 days, and 20 U for 3 days) (Thompson et al. 1989). Although clinical benefits appeared to be equal across treatment groups, fewer adverse effects were observed with IVMP. Similar benefits have resulted from alternative protocols of IVMP administered in other double-blind, placebo-controlled, randomized clinical trials (Durelli et al. 1986; Milligan et al. 1987). The doses used in these treatment protocols ranged from 15 mg/kg/d for 3 days tapered over 15 days, to 500 mg daily for 5 days. It is claimed that the benefits of methylprednisolone 500 mg each day for 5 days are demonstrable if administered intravenously or orally (Alam et al. 1993). A second study comparing high-dose IVMP and oral prednisone (Barnes et al. 1997) has reached similar conclusions. Support for glucocorticosteroid treatment is provided by the observation that high-dose IV MP reduced intrathecal immunoglobulin production (Trotter and Garvey 1980; Troiano et al. 1984), plaque edema, and gadolinium enhancement evidenced by serial computed tomography (CT) and MRI scans (Troiano et al. 1985; Barkhof et al. 1991; Oliveri et al. 1998). These effects may be less evident with lower doses of corticosteroids (Troiano et al. 1985; Oliveri et al. 1998). Although there is presently no agreement regarding the optimal dose, duration, or route of administration for glucocorticosteroid therapy for MS exacerbations, experience suggests that most neurologists administer 500 to 1000 mg of IVMP daily for 3 to 7 days followed by a tapering course of oral prednisone over 10 to 21 days. This dose range of IV MP is generally well tolerated, but insomnia, restlessness, euphoria, hypomania, and weight gain can be problematic (Myers 1992).

## Effect of Treatment on Annualized MS Exacerbation Rates

Annualized MS exacerbation rates are significantly reduced by interferon beta-1b (Betaseron), interferon beta-1a (Avonex and Rebof), glatiramer acetate (Copaxone), azathioprine, intravenous immunoglobulin G (IVIG) and mitoxantrone. A comparison of the reduction in annualized exacerbation rates achieved with selected treatments is illustrated in Figure 19-4. The details of the design and results of these clinical trials have been published (Goodkin et al. 1991; INFB Multiple Sclerosis Study Group 1995; Johnson et al. 1995; Jacobs et al. 1996; Fazekas et al. 1997; Achiron et al. 1998).

## Effect of Treatment on Sustained Progression of Disability Resulting from MS

The most clinically relevant outcome in controlled clinical trials is *sustained* progression of disability. This outcome is most appealing because confirmation of progression of disability helps to distinguish *transient* changes in disability due to exacerbations or pseudoexacerbations from sustained progression of disability resulting from irreversible demyelination and axonal transection. Interferon beta-1a is the only disease-modifying treatment that during a Phase III trial convincingly delayed the onset of sustained progression of disability in patients with relapsing forms of MS. Interferon beta-1b and mitoxantrone have a similar effect in SPMS (European Study Group of Interferon beta-1b in Secondary Progressive MS 1998; Hartung et al. 1999). These results provide strong support for the notion that disease-modifying treatment should be initiated early in the course of the disease before irreversible tissue damage has occurred. Similar effects in Phase II trials have been reported for methotrexate and intravenous methylprednisolone (Goodkin et al. 1996, 1998) (Table 19–7).

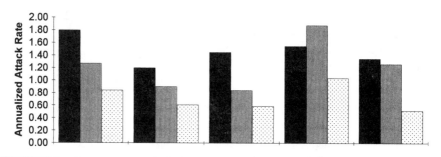

| | | 1) IFNβ1b | 2) IFNβ1a | 3) Copolymer | 4) Azathioprine | 5) IVIG |
|---|---|---|---|---|---|---|
| Pre-Entry | ■■■ | 1.80 | 1.20 | 1.45 | 1.55 | 1.35 |
| Placebo | ▨▨▨ | 1.27 | 0.90 | 0.84 | 1.88 | 1.26 |
| Active Drug | ▦▦▦ | 0.84 | 0.61 | 0.59 | 1.04 | 0.52 |

1) IFNB Multiple Sclerosis Study Group, 1993.
2) Jacobs 1996.
3) Johnson, 1995.
4) Goodkin, 1991.
5) Fazekas, 1997.

**Figure 19-4.** Annualized attack rates in various clinical trials. The reduction in relapse rate is compared before study entry, during placebo, and active treatment for five different trials.

## The Effect of Treatment on MRI Activity

### Gadolinium Enhancement

Glucocorticosteroids reduce the intensity and duration of enhancement of new gadolinium-enhancing lesions (Barkhof et al. 1991). The benefits are transient and persist for less than 1 week. It has been suggested that IVMP reduces the appearance of new gadolinium-enhancing lesions for up to 3 months (Smith et al. 1993; Oliveri et al. 1998). These results provide imaging correlates for the short-term benefits observed when glucocorticosteroids are administered for acute relapses of MS. The long-term effects of cyclical pulses of IVMP on new gadolinium-enhancing lesions are not known.

Interferon beta-1b and interferon beta-1a convincingly reduce the number of new gadolinium-enhancing lesions observed on monthly brain MRI scans (Stone et al. 1995; Pozzilli et al. 1996; Edan 1997; Millefiorini et al. 1997; European Study Group 1998; Mancardi, et al. 1998; Oliveri et al. 1998; PRIMS 1998; Simon et al. 1998b; Comi and Filippi 1999; Hartung et al. 1999; Waubant el al. in press). For interferons on average, the percent reduction in new gadolinium-enhancing lesions (50% to 70%) is greater than the percent reduction in clinical relapses (30% to 35%). However, not all patients experience a reduction in the number of new gadolinium-enhancing lesions and the effects of dose and route of administration of interferon beta-1a and -1b have not been rigorously evaluated. Preliminary evidence also indicates that the number of new gadolinium-enhancing lesions is also reduced by other off-label treatments for patients with re-

**Table 19-7.** FDA-Approved and Off-Label Disease-Modifying Treatments in MS

| Relapsing-Remitting MS | Secondary Progressive MS | | Primary Progressive MS |
|---|---|---|---|
| | With Relapses | Without Relapses | |
| Interferon beta-1a | Interferon beta-1a | Oral methotrexate* | No effective treatment available |
| Interferon beta-1b | Interferon beta-1b | IVMP* | |
| Copolymer | Cytoxan* | | |
| IVIG* | Mitoxantrone* | | |
| Cytoxan* | Cladribine* | | |
| Mitoxantrone* | | | |
| Cladribine* | | | |

*Off-label use.

FDA, Food and Drug Administration; MS, multiple sclerosis; IVIG, intravenous immunoglobulin; IVMP, intravenous methylprednisolone.

lapsing forms of MS. These include IVIG (Soel-berg Sørensen et al. 1997 Sorenson et al. 1998), 2-chlorodeoxyadenosine (Cladribine) (Sipe 1992; Sipe et al. 1997), and azathioprine (Cavazzuti et al. 1995).

### Number and Area of T2W Lesions

Interferon beta-1b, interferon beta-1a mitrox-antrone and Copaxone reduce the progression of total T2W lesion number and area in patients with relapsing-remitting MS and SPMS (INFB Multi-ple Sclerosis Study Group 1995; Jacobs et al. 1996; PRIMS 1998; Comi and Filippi 1999; Har-tung et al. 1999). These benefits measured by annual MRI scans are observed for at least 1 year with interferon beta-1a and for at least 2 years for interferon beta-1b. Similar benefits are ob-served for up to 2 years with methotrexate in patients with chronic progressive forms of MS (Goodkin 1996). These studies provide imaging correlates that support the clinical treatment ef-fects observed with those interventions. Prelimi-nary reports also suggest that treatment effect with interferon beta-1a (AVONEX) correlates with measures of progression of brain atrophy (Rudick et al. 1999).

## References

Achiron, A.; Gabbay, U.; Gilad, R.; Hassin-Baer, S.; Barak, Y.; Gornish, M.; Elizur, A.; Goldhammer, Y.; Sarova-Pinhas, I. Intravenous immunoglobulin treat-ment in multiple sclerosis. Effect on relapses. Neu-rology 50:398–402; 1998.

Alam, S. M.; Kyriakides, T.; Lawden, M.; Newman, P. K. Methylprednisolone in multiple sclerosis: a comparison of oral with intravenous therapy at equivalent high dose. J. Neurol. Neurosurg. Psychi-atry 56:1219–1220; 1993.

Allen, I. V.; Millar, J. H. D.; Hutchinson, M. J. General disease in 120 necropsy-proven cases of multiple sclerosis. Neuropathol. Appl. Neurobiol. 4:279–284; 1978.

Allen, I. V.; McKeown, S. R. A histological, histo-chemical and biochemical study of the macroscopi-cally normal white matter in multiple sclerosis. J. Neurol. Sci. 41:81–91; 1979.

Allison, R. S. Survival in disseminated sclerosis: a clin-ical study of a series of cases first seen twenty years ago. Brain 73:103–120; 1950.

Andersson, P.-B.; Goodkin, D. Current pharmacologic treatments of multiple sclerosis. West. J. Med. 165: 313–317; 1996.

Barnes, M. P.; Bateman, D. E.; Cleland, P. G.; Dick, D. J.; Walls, T. J., Newman; P. K., Saunders, M.; Tilley, P. J. B. Intravenous methylprednisolone for multiple sclerosis in relapse. J. Neurol. Neurosurg. Psychiatry 48:157–159; 1985.

Barnes, D.; Hughes, R. A. C.; Morris, R.; et al. Ran-domised trial of oral and intravenous methylpred-nisolone in acute relapses of multiple sclerosis. Lancet 349:902–906; 1997.

Barkhof, F.; Hommes, O. R.; Scheltens, P.; Valk, J. Quantitative MRI changes in gadolinium-DPTA enhancement after high-dose intravenous methyl-prednisolone in multiple sclerosis. Neurology 41: 1219–1222; 1991.

Beck, J.; Rondot, P.; Catinot, L.; et al. Increased pro-duction of interferon gamma and tumor necrosis fac-tor precedes clinical manifestation in multiple scle-rosis: do cytokines trigger off exacerbations? Acta Neurol. Scand. 78:318–323; 1988.

Beck, R. W.; Cleary, P. A.; Anderson, M. M.; Keltner, J. L.; Shults, W. T.; Kaufman, D. I.; Buckley, E. G.; Corbett, J. J.; Kupersmith, M. J.; Miller, N. R.; Savino, P. J.; Guy, J. R.; Trobe, J. D.; McCrary, J. A.; Smith, C. H.; Chrousos, G. A.; Thompson, H. S.; Katz, B. J.; Brodsky, M. C.; Goodwin, J. A.; Atwell, C. W.; and the Optic Neuritis Study Group. A ran-domized, controlled trial of corticosteroids in the treatment of acute optic neuritis. N. Engl. J. Med. 326:581–588; 1992.

Beck, R. W.; Cleary, P. A.; Trobe, J. D.; Kaufman, D. I.; Kupersmith, M. J.; Paty, D. W.; Brown, C. H.; and the Optic Neuritis Study Group. The effect of corticosteroids for acute optic neuritis on the subse-quent development of multiple sclerosis. N. Engl. J. Med. 329:1764–1769; 1993.

Berman, A. L.; Samuel, L. Suicide among people with multiple sclerosis. J. Neurol. Rehabil. 7:53–62; 1993.

Birk, K.; Ford, C.; Smeltzer, S.; Ryan, D.; Miller, R.; Rudick, R. A. The clinical course of multiple sclero-sis during pregnancy and the puerperium. Arch. Neurol. 47:738–742; 1990.

Bradley, W. G.; Whitty, C. W. M. Acute optic neuritis: its clinical features and their relation to prognosis for recovery of vision. J. Neurol. Neurosurg. Psychiatry 30:531–538; 1967.

Cavazzuti, M.; Tassone, G.; Canafoglia, L.; Merelli, E. Lesion load quantification in serial MRI of MS pa-tients under azathioprine treatment: a retrospective analysis (abstract). J. Neuroimmunol. Suppl. 1:16; 1995.

Cohen, M. M.; Lessell, S.; Wolf, P. A. A prospective study of the risk of developing multiple sclerosis in uncomplicated optic neuritis. Neurology 29: 208–213; 1979.

Comi, G. Filippi, M.; for the Copaxone MRI Study Group. The effect of glatiramer acetate (Copaxone) on disease activity as measured by cerebral MRI in patients with relapsing-remitting multiple sclerosis (RRMS): a multi-center, randomized, double-blind, placebo-controlled study extended by open-label treatment. Neurology 52(suppl. 2):A289; 1999.

Confavreux, C.; Aimard, G.; Devic, M. Course and prognosis of multiple sclerosis assessed by the com-puterized data processing of 349 patients. Brain 103:281–300; 1980.

Confavreux, C.; Hutchinson, M.; Hours M. M.; Cortinovis-Tourniaire P.; Moreau T.; and the Pregnancy in Multiple Sclerosis Group. Rate of pregnancy-related relapse in multiple sclerosis. N. Engl. J. Med. 339:285–291; 1998.

Damek, D. M.; Shuster, E. A. Pregnancy and multiple sclerosis. Mayo Clin. Proc. 72:977–989; 1997.

Dean, G. How many people in the world have multiple sclerosis? Neuroepidemiology 13:1–7; 1994.

Duquette, P.; Murray, T. J.; Pleines, J.; Ebers, G. C.; Sadovnick, D.; Weldon, P.; Warren, S.; Paty, D. W.; Upton, A.; Hader, W.; Nelson, R.; Auty, A.; Neufeld, B. ; Meltzer, C. Multiple sclerosis in childhood: clinical profile in 125 patients. J. Pediatr. 111:359–363; 1987.

Durelli, L.; Cocito, D.; Riccio, A.; et al. High-dose intravenous methylprednisolone in the treatment of multiple sclerosis: clinical-immunologic correlations. Neurology 36:238–243; 1986.

Ebers, G. C.; Sadovnick, A. D.; Risch, N. J. A genetic basis for familial agregation in MS. Nature 377: 150–151; 1995.

Edan, G.; Miller, D.; Clanet, M.; Confavreux, C.; Lyon-Caen, O.; Lubetzki, C.; Brochet, B.; Berry, I.; et al. Therapeutic effect of mitoxantrone combined with methylprednisolone in multiple sclerosis: a randomised multicentre study of active disease using MRI and clinical criteria. J. Neurol. Neurosurg. Psychiatry 62:112–118; 1997.

European Study Group on Interferon β-1b in Secondary Progressive MS. Placebo-controlled multicentre randomised trial of interferon β-1b in treatment of secondary progressive multiple sclerosis. Lancet 352:1491–1497; 1998.

Fazekas, F.; Deisenhammer, F.; Strasser-Fuchs, S.; Nahler, G.; Mamoli, B. Randomised placebo-controlled trial of monthly intravenous immunoglobulin therapy in relapsing-remitting multiple sclerosis. Lancet 349:589–593; 1997.

Ferguson, B.; Matyszak, M. K.; Esiri, M. M.; Perry, V. H. Axonal damage in acute multiple sclerosis lesions. Brain 120:393–399; 1997.

Filippi, M.; Horsfield, M. A.; Morrissey, S. P.; MacManus, D. G.; Rudge, P.; McDonald, W. I.; Miller, D. H. Quantitative brain MRI lesion load predicts the course of clinically isolated syndromes suggestive of multiple sclerosis. Neurology 44:635–641; 1994.

Fog, T.; Linnemann, F. The course of multiple sclerosis in 73 cases with computer-designed curves. Acta Neurol. Scand. 47:11–175; 1970.

Ford, B.; Tampieri, D.; Francis, G. Long-term follow-up of acute partial transverse myelopathy. Neurology 42:250–252; 1992.

Francis, D. A.; Compston, D. A. S.; Batchelor, J. R.; McDonald, W. I. A reassessment of the risk of multiple sclerosis developing in patients with optic neuritis after extended follow-up. J. Neurol. Neurosurg. Psychiatry 50:758–765; 1987.

Franklin, G. M.; Nelson L. M.; Heaton, R. K.; Burks, J. S.; Thompson, D. S. Stress and its relationship to acute exacerbations in multiple sclerosis. J. Neurol. Rehabil. 2:7–11, 1988.

Giovannoni, G.; Lai, M.; Thorpe, J.; Kidd, D.; Chamoun, V.; Thompson, A. J.; Miller, D. H.; Feldmann, M.; Thompson, E. J. Longitudinal study of soluble adhesion molecules in multiple sclerosis: correlation with gadolinium enhanced magnetic resonance imaging. Neurology 48:1557–1565; 1997.

Goodkin, D. E.; Hertsgaard, D.; Rudick, R. A. Exacerbation rates and adherence to disease type in a prospectively followed-up population with multiple sclerosis: implications for clinical trials. Arch. Neurol. 46:1107–1112; 1989.

Goodkin, D. E.; Baily, R. C.; Teetzen, M. L.; Hertsgaard, D.; Beatty, W. W. The efficacy of azathioprine in relapsing-remitting multiple sclerosis. Neurology 41:20–25; 1991.

Goodkin, D. E. The natural history of multiple sclerosis. In: Rudick, R. A.; Goodkin, D. E., eds. Treatment of multiple sclerosis: trial design, results and future perspectives. London: Springer-Verlag; 1992: p. 17–45.

Goodkin, D. E.; Rudick, R. A.; VanderBrug Medendorp, S.; Daughtry, M. M.; Van Dyke, C. D. Low-dose oral methotrexate in chronic progressive multiple sclerosis: analyses of serial MRI's. Neurology 47:1153–1157; 1996.

Goodkin, D. E.; Kinkel, R. P.; Weinstock-Guttman, B.; VenderBrug Medendorp S.; Secic M.; Gogol, D.; Perryman J. E.; Uccelli, M. M.; Neilley, L. A phase II study of IV methylprednisolone in secondary progressive multiple sclerosis. Neurology 51:239–245; 1998.

Grossman, R. I. Magnetic resonance imaging: current status and strategies for improving multiple sclerosis clinical trial design. In: Rudick, R. A.; Goodkin, D. E., eds. Multiple sclerosis: advances in clinical trial design, treatment and future perspectives. London: Springer; 1996: p. 161–186.

Gudmendsson, K. R. Clinical studies of multiple sclerosis in Iceland—a follow-up of previous survey and reappraisal. Acta Neurol. Scand. 48:1–78; 1971.

Hartung, H.; Reiners, K.; Archelos, J. J.; Michels, M.; Seeldrayers, P.; Heidenreich, F.; Pflughaupt, K. W.; Toyka, K. V. Circulating adhesion molecules and tumor necrosis factor receptor in multiple sclerosis: correlation with magnetic resonance imaging. Ann. Neurol. 38:186–193; 1995.

Hartung, H. P.; Gonsette, R.; and the MIMS-Study Group. Mitoxantrone in progressive multiple sclerosis: a placebo-controlled, randomized, observer-blind phase III trial: clinical results and three-year follow-up. Neurology 52(suppl. 2) A290; 1999.

Hyllested, K. Lethality, duration and mortality of disseminated sclerosis in Denmark. Acta Psychiatr. Scand. 36:553–564; 1961.

IFNB Multiple Sclerosis Study Group. Interferon beta-1b is effective in relapsing-remitting multiple sclerosis: I. Clinical results of a multicenter, randomized, double-blind, placebo-controlled trial. Neurology 43:655–661; 1993.

IFNB Multiple Sclerosis Study Group. Interferon beta-1b in the treatment of multiple sclerosis: initial outcome of the randomized controlled trial. Neurology 45:1277–1285; 1995.

Jacobs, L. D.; Cookfair, D. L.; Rudick, R. A.; Herndon, R. M.; Richert, J. R.; Salazar, A. M.; Fischer, J. S.; Goodkin, D. E.; Granger, C. V.; Simon, J. H.; Alam, J. J.; Bartoszak, D. M.; Bourdette, D. N.; Braiman, J.; Brownscheidle, C. M.; Coats, M. E.; Cohan, S. L.; Dougherty, D. S.; Kinkel, R. P.; Mass, M. K.; Munschauer, F. E.; Priore, R. L.; Pullicino, P. M.; Scherokman, B. J.; Weinstock-Guttman, B.; Whitham, R. H.; and the Multiple Sclerosis Collaborative Research Group. Intramuscular interferon beta-1a for disease progression in relapsing multiple sclerosis. Ann. Neurol. 39:285– 294; 1996.

Johnson, K. P.; Brooks, B. R.; Cohen, J. A.; Ford, C. C.; Goldstein, J.; Lisak, R. P.; Myers, L. W.; Panitch, H. S; Rose, J. W.; Schiffer, R. B.; Vollmer, T.; Weiner, L. P.; Wolinsky, J. S.; and the Copolymer 1 Multiple Sclerosis Study Group. Copolymer 1 reduces relapse rate and improves disability in relapsing-remitting multiple sclerosis: results of a phase III multicenter, double-blind, placebo-controlled trial. Neurology 45:1268–1276; 1995.

Kelly, M. A.; Cavan, D. A.; Penny, M. A.; Mijovic, C. H.; Jenkins, D.; Morrissey, S.; Miller, D. H.; Barnett, A. H.; Francis, D. A. The influence of HLA-DR and -DQ alleles on progression to multiple sclerosis following a clinically isolated syndrome. Hum. Immunol. 37:185–191; 1993.

Kermode, A. G.; Thompson, A. J.; Tofts, P.; et al. Breakdown of the blood-brain barrier precedes symptoms and other MRI signs of new lesions in multiple sclerosis. Brain 113:1477–1489; 1990.

Kira, J.; Kanai, T.; Nishhimura, S.; Yamasaki, K.; Matsushita, S.; Kawano, S.; Hasuo, K.; Tobimatsu, S.; Kobayashi, T. Western versus Asian types of multiple sclerosis: immunogenetically and clinically distinct disorders. Ann. Neurol. 40:569–574; 1996.

Korn-Lubetzki, I.; Kahana, E.; Cooper, G.; Abramsky, O. Activity of multiple sclerosis during pregnancy and puerperium. Ann. Neurol. 16:229–231; 1984.

Koudriavtseva, T.; Thompson, A. J.; Fiorelli, M.; Gasperini, C.; Bastianello, S.; Bozzao, A.; Paolillo, A.; Pisani, A.; Galgani, S.; Pozzilli, C. Gadolinium enhanced MRI predicts clinical and MRI disease activity in relapsing remitting multiple sclerosis. J. Neurol. Neurosurg. Psychiatry 62:285–287; 1997.

Kurtzke, J. F. Course of exacerbations of multiple sclerosis in hospitalized patients. Arch. Neurol. 76: 175–184; 1956.

Kurtzke, J. F.; Beebe, G. W.; Nagler, B.; Nefziger, M. D.; Auth, T. L.; Kurland, L. T. Studies on the natural history of multiple sclerosis. V. Longterm survival in young men. Arch. Neurol. 22:215–225; 1970.

Kurtzke, J. F.; Beebe, G. W.; Nagler, B.; Kurlands, L. T.; Auth, T. L. Studies on the natural history of multiple sclerosis—8: early prognostic features of the later course of the illness. J. Chron. Dis. 30: 819–830; 1977.

Kurtzke, J. F. Rating neurologic impairment in multiple sclerosis: an expanded disability status scale (EDSS). Neurology 33:1444–1452; 1983.

Kurtzke, J. F. Epidemiologic evidence for multiple sclerosis as an infection. Clin. Microbiol. Rev. 6: 382–427; 1993.

Lee, K. H.; Hashimoto, S. A.; Hooge, J. P.; Kastrukoff, L. F.; Oger, J. J. F.; Li, D. K. B.; Paty, D. W. Magnetic resonance imaging of the head in the diagnosis of multiple sclerosis: a prospective 2-year follow-up with comparison of clinical evaluation, evoked potentials, oligoclonal banding, and CT. Neurology 41:657–660; 1991.

Lee, M. A.; Palace, J.; Stabler, G.; Ford, J.; Gearing, A.; Miller, K. Serum gelatinase B, TIMP-1 and TIMP-2 levels in multiple sclerosis: a longitudinal clinical and MRI study. Brain 122:191–197; 1999.

Leibowitz, U.; Alter, M.; Halpern, L. Clinical studies of multiple sclerosis in Israel. 3. Clinical course and prognosis related to age at onset. Neurology 14: 926–932; 1964.

Lipton, H. L.; Teasdall, R. D. Acute transverse myelopathy in adults: a follow-up study. Arch. Neurol. 28:252–257; 1973.

Long, D. D.; Miller, B. J. Suicidal tendancy and MS. Health Soc. Work 16:104–109; 1991.

Lossef, N. A.; Kingsley, D. P. E.; McDonald, W. I.; Miller, D. H.; Thompson, A. J.. Clinical and magnetic resonance imaging predictors of disability in primary and secondary progressive multiple sclerosis. Multiple Sclerosis 1;218–222; 1996a.

Lossef, N. A.; Webb, S. L.; O'Riordan, J. I.; Page, R.; Wang, L.; Barker, G. J.; Tofts, P. S.; McDonald, W. I.; Millar, D. H.; Thompson, A. J. Spinal cord atrophy and disability in multiple sclerosis: a new reproducible and sensitive MRI method with potential to monitor disease progression. Brain 119: 701–709; 1996b.

Lublin, F. D.; Reingold, S. C. Defining the clinical course of multiple sclerosis: results of an international survey. Neurology 46:907–911; 1996.

Lucchinetti, C. F.; Kiers, L.; O'Duffy, A.; Gomez, M. R.; Cross, S.; Leavitt, J. A.; O'Brien, P.; Rodriquez, M. Risk factors for developing multiple sclerosis after childhood optic neuritis. Neurology 49: 1413–1418; 1997.

Mancardi, G. L.; Sardanelli, F.; Parodi, R. C.; Melani, E.; Capello, E.; Inglese, M.; Ferrari, A.; Sormani, M. P.; Ottonello, C.; Levrero, F.; Ucelli, A.; Bruzzi, P. Effect of copolymer-1 on serial gadolinium-enhanced MRI in relapsing remitting multiple sclerosis. Neurology 50:1127–1133; 1998.

McAlpine, D.; Compston, N. Some aspects of the natural history of disseminated sclerosis. 1. The incidence, course, and prognosis. 2. Factors affecting the onset and course. Q. J. Med. 21:135–160; 1952.

McAlpine, D. The benign form of multiple sclerosis: a study based on 241 cases seen within three years of onset and followed up until the tenth year or more of the disease. Brain 84:186–203; 1961.

McDonald, W. I.; Miller, D. H.; Barnes, D. Annotation: the pathological evolution of multiple sclerosis. Neuropathol. Appl. Neurobiol. 18:319–334; 1992.

Millefiorini, E.; Gasperini, C.; Pozzilli, C.; D'Andrea, F.; Bastianello, S.; Trojano, M; Morino, S.; Morra,

V. B.; Bozzao, A.; Calo', A.; et al. Randomized placebo-controlled trial of mitoxantrone in relapsing-remitting multiple sclerosis: 24-month clinical and MRI outcome. J. Neurol. 244:153–159; 1997.

Miller, D. H.; Ormerod, E. C.; Rudge, P. L.; Kendall, B. E.; Moseley, I. F.; McDonald, W. I. The early risk of multiple sclerosis following isolated acute syndromes of the brainstem and spinal cord. Ann. Neurol. 26:635–639; 1989.

Miller, D. H.; Hornabrook, R. W.; Purdie, G. The natural history of multiple sclerosis: a regional study with some longitudinal data. J. Neurol. Neurosurg. Psychiatry 55:341–346; 1992.

Miller, D. H.; Barkhof, F.; Nauta, J. J. Gadolinium enhancement increases the sensitivity of MRI in detecting disease activity in multiple sclerosis. Brain 116:1077–1094; 1993.

Miller, A. E.; Morgante, L. A.; Buchwald, L. Y.; Nutile, S. M.; Coyle, P. K.; Krupp, L. B.; Doscher, C. A.; Lublin, F. D.; Knobler, R. L.; Trantas, F.; Kelley, L.; Smith, C. R.; La Rocca, N.; Lopez, S. A multicenter, randomized, double-blind, placebo-controlled trial of influenza immunization in multiple sclerosis. Neurology 48:312–314; 1997.

Milligan, N. M.; Newcombe, R.; Compston, D. A. A double-blind controlled trial of high dose methylprednisolone in patients with multiple sclerosis. 1. Clinical effects. J. Neurol. Neurosurg. Psychiatry 50:511–516; 1987.

Minderhoud, J. M.; van der Hoeven, J. H.; Prange, A. J. A. Course and prognosis of chronic progressive multiple sclerosis. Acta Neurol. Scand. 78:10–15; 1988.

Mohr, D.; Russo, D.; Reiss, M.; Chang, J.; Goodkin, D. E. Relationship of stress, psychological distress, and disease activity in multiple sclerosis (abstract). Ann. Neurol. 42:443; 1997.

Morrissey, S. P.; Miller, D. H.; Kendall, B. E.; Kingsley, D. P. E.; Kelly, M. A.; Francis, D. A.; MacManus, D. G.; McDonald, W. I. The significance of brain magnetic resonance imaging abnormalities at presentation with clinically isolated syndromes suggestive of multiple sclerosis. Brain 116:135–146; 1993.

Moulin, D.; Paty, D. W.; Ebers, G. C. The predictive value of cerebrospinal fluid electrophoresis in 'possible' multiple sclerosis. Brain 106:809–816; 1983.

Muller, R. Studies on disseminated sclerosis with special reference to symptomatology, course and prognosis. Acta Neurol. Scand. 222:1–214; 1949.

Myers, L. Treatment of multiple sclerosis with ACTH and corticosteroids. In: Rudick, R. A.; Goodkin, D. E., eds. Treatment of multiple sclerosis: trial design, results and future perspectives. New York: Springer-Verlag: 1992.

Nadler, J. P. Multiple sclerosis and hepatitis B vaccination. Clin. Infect. Dis. 17:928–929; 1993.

National Center for Health Statistics: Current estimates from the Health Interview Survey, United States, 1989. Vital and health statistics, series 10, No. 176. DHHS Pub. No. (PHS) 90-1504. Public Health Service. Washington, DC: U.S. Government Printing Office, 1990.

Natowicz, M. R.; Bejjani, B. Genetic disorders that masquerade as multiple sclerosis. Am. J. Med. Genet. 49:149–169; 1994.

Oksenberg, J. R.; Hauser, S. L. New insights into the immunogenetics of multiple sclerosis. Curr. Opin. Neurol. 10:181–185, 1997.

Olerup, O.; Hillert, J.; Fredrikson, S.; Olsson, T.; Kam-Hansen, S.; Moller, E.; Carlsson, B.; Wallin, J. Primarily chronic progressive and relapsing/remitting multiple sclerosis: two immunogenetically distinct disease entities. Proc. Natl. Acad. Sci. USA 86: 7113–7117; 1989.

Oliveri, R. L.; Valentino, P.; Russo, C.; Sibilia, G.; Aguglia, U.; Bono, F.; Fera, F.; Gambardella, A.; Zappia, M.; Pardatscher, K.; Quattrone, A. Randomized trial comparing two different high doses of methylprednisolone in MS. A clinical and MRI study. Neurology 1833–1836; 1998.

Optic Neuritis Study Group. The 5-year risk of MS after optic neuritis: experience of the Optic Neuritis Treatment Trial. Neurology 49:1404–1413; 1997.

O'Riordan, J. I.; Gallagher, H. L.; Thompson, A. J.; Howard, R. S.; Kingsley, D. P. E.; Thompson, E. J.; McDonald, W. I.; Miller, D. H. Clinical, CSF, and MRI findings in Devic's neuromyelitis optica. J. Neurol. Neurosurg. Psychiatry 60:382–387; 1996.

Panelius, M. Studies on epidemiological, clinical and etiological aspects of multiple sclerosis. Acta Neurol. Scand. 45:1–82; 1969.

Panitch, H. S. Influence of infection on exacerbations of multiple sclerosis. Ann. Neurol. 36:S25–S28; 1994.

Parkin, P. J.; Hierons, R.; McDonald, W. I. Bilateral optic neuritis: a long-term follow-up. Brain 107: 951–964; 1984.

Paty, D. W.; Li, D. K. B.; UBC MS/MRI Study Group; IFNB Multiple Sclerosis Study Group. Interferon beta-1b is effective in relapsing-remitting multiple sclerosis: II. MRI analysis results of a multicenter, randomized double-blind, placebo-controlled trial. Neurology 43:662–667; 1993.

Phadke, J. G. Survival pattern and cause of death in patients with multiple sclerosis: results from an epidemiological survey in north east Scotland. J. Neurol. Neurosurg. Psychiatry 50:523–531; 1987.

Phadke, J. G. Clinical aspects of multiple sclerosis in north-east Scotland with particular reference to its course and prognosis. Brain 113:1597–1628; 1990.

Poser, C. M.; Paty, D. W.; Scheinberg, L.; et al. New diagnostic criteria for multiple sclerosis: guidelines for research protocols. Ann. Neurol. 13:227–231; 1983.

Pozzilli, C.; Bastianello, S.; Koudriavtseva, T.; et al. Magnetic resonance imaging changes with recombinant human interferon-beta-1a : a short term study in relapsing-remitting multiple sclerosis. J. Neurol. Neurosurg. Psychiatry 61:251–258; 1996.

PRIMS Study Group. Randomised double-blind placebo-controlled study of interferon beta-1a in relapsing/ remitting multiple sclerosis. Lancet 352: 1498–1504; 1998.

Rieckmann, P.; Martin, S.; Weichselbraun, I.; Albrecht, M.; Kitze, B.; Weber, T.; Tumani, H.; Broocks, A.; Luer, W.; Helwig, A.; Poser, S. Serial analysis of circulating adhesion molecules and TNF receptor in serum from patients with multiple sclerosis: cICAM-1 is an indicator for relapses. Neurology 44:2367–2372; 1994.

Rieckmann, P.; Albrecht, M.; Kitze, B.; Weber, T.; Tumani, H.; Broocks, A.; Luer, W.; Helwig, A.; Poser, S. Tumor necrosis factor-α messenger RNA expression in patients with relapsing-remitting multiple sclerosis is associated with disease activity. Ann. Neurol. 37:82–88; 1995.

Riise, T.; Gronning, M; Fernandez, O.; et al. Early prognostic factors for disability in multiple sclerosis, a European multicenter study. Acta Neurol. Scand. 85:212–218; 1992.

Rizzo, J. F.; Lessell, S. Risk of developing multiple sclerosis after uncomplicated optic neuritis: a long-term prospective study. Neurology 38:185–190; 1988.

Rose, A. S.; Kuzma, J. W.; Kurtzke, J. F.; et al. Cooperative study in the evaluation of therapy in multiple sclerosis: ACTH vs placebo. Neurology 20(part II): 1–59, 1970.

Roullet, E.; Verdier-Taillefer, M.; Amarenco, P.; Gharbi, G.; Alperovitch, A.; Marteau, R. Pregnancy and multiple sclerosis: a longitudinal study of 125 remittent patients. J. Neurol. Neurosurg. Psychiatry 56: 1062–1065; 1993.

Rudick, R.; Fisher, E.; Lee, J. C.; Simon, J.; Miller, D.; Jacobs, L.; and MSCRG. The effect of AVONEX (IFNβ-1a) on cerebral atrophy in relapsing multiple sclerosis. Neurology 52(suppl. 2):A289; 1999.

Runmarker, B.; Andersen, O. Prognostic factors in a multiple sclerosis incidence cohort with twenty-five years of follow-up. Brain 116:117–134; 1993.

Runmarker, B.; Andersson, C.; Oden, A.; Andersen, O. Prediction of outcome in multiple sclerosis based on multivariate models. J. Neurol. 241: 597–604; 1994.

Runmarker, B.; Andersen, O. Pregnancy is associated with a lower risk of onset and a better prognosis in multiple sclerosis. Brain 118:253–261; 1995.

Sadovnick, A. D.; Eisen, K.; Ebers, G. C.; Paty, D. W. Cause of death in patients attending multiple sclerosis clinics. Neurology 41:1193–1196; 1991.

Sadovnick, A. D.; Eisen, K.; Hashimoto, S. A.; Farquhar, R.; Yee, I. M. L.; Hooge, J.; Kastrukoff, L.; Oger, J. J. F.; Paty, D. W. Pregnancy and multiple sclerosis: a prospective study. Arch. Neurol. 51: 1120–1124; 1994.

Salvetti, M.; Pisani, A.; Bastianello, S.; Millefiorini, E.; Buttinelli, C.; Pozzilli, C. Clinical and MRI assessment of disease activity in patients with multiple sclerosis after influenza vaccination. J. Neurol. 242: 143–146; 1995.

Sandberg-Wollheim, M.; Bynke, H.; Cronqvist, S.; Holtas, S.; Platz, P.; Ryder, L. P. A long-term prospective study of optic neuritis: evaluation of risk factors. Ann. Neurol. 27:386–393; 1990.

Schumacher, G. A.; Beebe, G.; Kibler, R. E., et al. Problems of experimental trials of therapy in multiple sclerosis: report by the panel on evaluation of experimental trials of therapy in multiple sclerosis. Ann. N. Y. Acad. Sci. 122: 552–568, 1965.

Sharief, M. K.; Thompson, E. J. The predictive value of intrathecal immunoglobulin synthesis and magnetic resonance imaging in acute isolated syndromes for subsequent development of multiple sclerosis. Ann. Neurol. 29:147–151; 1991.

Sharief, M. K.; Hentges, R. Association between tumor necrosis factor-α and disease progression in patients with multiple sclerosis. N. Engl. J. Med. 325: 467–472; 1991.

Sibley, W. A.; Bamford, C. R.; Clark, K. Clinical viral infections and multiple schlerosis. Lancet 1 (8441): 1313–1315; 1985.

Simon, J. H.; Jacobs, L. D.; Campion, M.; Wende, K.; Simonian, N.; Cookfair, D.; Rudick, R.; Herndon, R. M.; Richert, J.; Salazar, A. M.; Alam, J. J.; Fisher J. S.; Goodkin, D. E.; Granger, C. V.; Lajeunie, M.; Martens-Davidson, A. L.; Meyer, M. J.; Sheeder. J.; Choi, K.; Scherzinger, A. L.; Bartoszak, D. M.; Bourdette, D. N.; Braiman, J.; Brownscheidle, C. M.; Coats, M. E.; Cohan, S. L.; Dougherty, D. S.; Kinkel, R.; Mass M. K.; Munschaure, F. E.; Priore, R. L.; Pullicino, P. M.; Scherokman, B. J.; Weinstock-Guttman, B.; Whitham, R. H.; and The Multiple Sclerosis Collaborative Research Group. Magnetic resonance studies of intramuscular interferon beta-1a for relapsing multiple sclerosis. Ann. Neurol. 43:79–87; 1998.

Simon, J. H.; Jacobs, L. D.; Campion, M.; Wende, K.; Simonian, N.; Cookfair, D. L.; Rudick, R. A. Magnetic resonance studies of intramuscular interferon β-1a for relapsing multiple sclerosis. Ann. Neurol. 43:79–87; 1998b.

Sipe, J. C. Treatment of multiple sclerosis with Cladribine. In: Rudick, R. A.; Goodkin, D. E., eds. Treatment of multiple sclerosis: trial design, results and future perspectives (clinical medicine and the nervous system series). London: Springer-Verlag, 1992: p. 313–334.

Sipe, J. C.; Romine, J. S.; Koziol, J; Zyroff, J.; McMillan R.; Beutler, E. Cladribine improves relapsing-remitting multiple sclerosis : a double blind, placebo controlled study (abstract). Neurology 48:A340; 1997.

Smith, M. E.; Stone, L. A.; Albert, P. S.; Frank, J. A.; Martin, R.; Armstrong, M.; Maloni, H.; McFarlin, D. E.; McFarland, H. F. Clinical worsening in multiple sclerosis is associated with increased frequency and area of gadopentetate dimeglumine-enhancing magnetic resonance imaging lesions. Ann. Neurol. 33:480–489; 1993.

Soderstrom, M.; Lindqvist, M.; Hillert, J.; Kall, T.; Link, H. Optic neuritis; findings on MRI, CSF examination and HLA class II typing in 60 patients and results of a short-term follow-up. J. Neurol. 241: 391–397; 1994.

Soelberg Sørensen, P.; Wanscher, B.; Schreiber, K.; Blinkenberg, M.; Jensen, C. V.; Ravnnborg, M. Effect of intravenous immunoglobulin (IVIG) on gadolinium enhancing lesions on MRI in multiple sclerosis (MS): final results of a double-blind cross-over trial. Multiple Sclerosis. 3:268; 1997.

Sorensen, P. S.; Wanscher, B.; Jensen, C. V.; Schreiber, K.; Blinkenberg, M.; Ravnborg, M.; Kirsmeier, H.; Larsen, V. A.; Lee, M. L. Intravenous immunoglobulin G reduces MRI activity in relapsing multiple sclerosis. Neurology 50:1273–1281; 1998.

Stone, L. A.; Frank, J. A.; Albert, P. S.; Bash, C. N.; Smith, M. E.; Maloni, H.; McFarland, H. F. The effect of interferon beta on blood-brain-barrier disruptions demonstrated by contrast-enhanced magnetic resonance imaging in relpasing-remitting multiple sclerosis. Ann. Neurol. 37:611–619, 1995.

Stenager, E. N.; Stenager, E.; Koch-Henriksen, N.; et al: Suicide and MS: an epidemiological investigation. J. Neurol. Neurosurg. Psychiatry 55:542–545; 1992.

Thompson, A. J.; Hutchinson, M.; Brazil, J.; Feighery, C.; Martin, E. A. A clinical and laboratory study of benign multiple sclerosis. Q. J. Med. 58:69–80; 1986.

Thompson, A. J.; Kennard, C.; Swash, M.; et al. Relative efficacy of IV methylprednisolone and ACTH in the treatment of acute relapses in multiple sclerosis. Neurology 39:969–971, 1989.

Trapp, B. D.; Peterson, J.; Ransohoff, R. M.; Rudick, R.; Mork, S.; Bo, L. Axonal transection in the lesions of multiple sclerosis. N. Engl. J. Med. 338:278–285; 1998.

Troiano, R.; Hafstein, M.; Ruderman, M.; et al. Effect of high dose intravenous steroid administration on contrast-enhancing computed tomographic scan lesion in multiple sclerosis. Ann. Neurol. 15:257–263; 1984.

Troiano, R.; Hafstein, M.; Zito, G.; et al. The effect of oral corticosteroid dosage on CT-enhancing multiple sclerosis plaques. J. Neurol. Sci. 70:67–72; 1985.

Trojano, M.; Avolio, C.; Manzari, C.; Calo, A.; De Robertis F.; Serio, G.; Livrea, R. Multivariate analysis of predictive factors of multiple sclerosis course with a validated method to assess clinical events. J. Neurol. Neurosurg. Psychiatry 58:300–306; 1995.

Trotter, J. L.; Garvey, W. F. Prolonged effects of large-dose methylprednisolone infusion in multiple sclerosis. Neurology 30:702–708, 1980.

Van Walderveen, M. A.; Tas, M. W.; Barkhof, F.; Polman, C. H.; Frequin, S. T.; Hommes, O. R.; Valk, J. Magnetic resonance evaluation of disease activity during pregnancy in multiple sclerosis. Neurology 44:327–329; 1994.

Verdru, P.; Theys, P.; D'Hooghe, M. B.; Carton, H. Pregnancy and multiple sclerosis: the influence on long term disability. Clin. Neurol. Neurosurg. 96: 38–41; 1994.

Villard-Mackintosh, L.; Vessey, M. P. Oral contraceptives and reproductive factors in multiple sclerosis incidence. Contraception 47:161–168; 1993.

Visscher, B. R.; Liu, K.; Clark, V. A.; Detels, R.; Malmgren, R. M.; Dudley, J. P. Onset symptoms as predictors of mortality and disability in multiple sclerosis. Acta Neurol. Scand. 70:321–328; 1984.

Waubant, E.; Gee, L.; Sloan, R.; Stewart, T.; Andersson, P-B.; Miller, K.; Stabler, G.; Goodkin, D. Serum levels of matrix metalloprotease-9 (MMP-9) and natural tissue inhibitor of matrix metalloprotease-type 1 (TIMP-1) predict MRI activity in relapsing-remitting patients. Neurology 52 (suppl. 2):A567; 1999.

Waubant, E.; Goodkin, D.; Sloan, R.; Andersson, P. B. A pilot study of the effect of MRI activity before and during interferon beta-1a (AVONEX) therapy. Neurology (in press).

Weinshenker, B. G.; Ebers, G. C. The natural history of multiple sclerosis. J. Can. Sci. Neurol. 14:255–261; 1987.

Weinshenker, B. G.; Bass, B.; Rice, G. P. A.; Noseworthy, J.; Carriere, W.; Baskerville, J.; Ebers, G. C. The natural history of multiple sclerosis: a geographically based study. 1. Clinical course and disability. Brain 112:133–146; 1989a.

Weinshenker, B. G.; Bass, B.; Rice, G. P. A.; Noseworthy, J.; Carriere, W.; Baskerville, J.; Ebers, G. C. The natural history of multiple sclerosis: a geographically based study. II. Predictive value of the early clinical course. Brain 112:1419–1428; 1989b.

Weinshenker, B. G.; Rice, G. P. A.; Noseworthy, J. H.; Carriere, W.; Baskerville, J.; Ebers, G. C. The natural history of multiple sclerosis: a geographically based study. 3. Multivariate analysis of predictive factors and models of outcome. Brain 114:1045–1056; 1991.

Weinshenker, B. G. The natural history of multiple sclerosis. Neurol. Clin. 13:119–146; 1995.

Wolfson, C.; Confavreux, C. Improvements to a simple Markov model of the natural history of multiple sclerosis. Neuroepidemiology 6:101–115; 1987.

Wolinsky, J. Multiple sclerosis. In: Appel, S. H., ed. Current neurology. St. Louis: Mosby Yearbook Inc., 1993:p.167–207.

Worthington, J. J. R.; Crawford, M. F. A. Pregnancy and multiple sclerosis: a 3-year prospective study. J. Neurol. 241:228–233; 1994.

Zimmerman, H. M.; Netsky, M. G. The pathology of multiple sclerosis. Research publications—Association for Research in Nervous and Mental Disease 28:271–312;1950.

**Appendix A**  Kurtzke Expanded Disability Status Scale (Kurtzke 1983)

| | |
|---|---|
| 0.0 | Normal neurological examination. |
| 1.0 | No disability, minimal signs in one FS (i.e., grade 1). |
| 1.5 | No disability, minimal signs in more than one FS (more than 1 grade 1). |
| 2.0 | Minimal disability in one FS (one FS grade 2, others 0 or 1). |
| 2.5 | Minimal disability in two FS (two FS grade 2, others 0 or 1). |
| 3.0 | Moderate disability in one FS (one FS grade 3, others 0 or 1) or mild disability in 3 or 4 FS (3 or 4 FS grade 2, others 0 or 1) though fully ambulatory. |
| 3.5 | Fully ambulatory but with moderate disability in one FS (one grade 3) and 1 or 2 FS grade 2 or 2 grade 3 (others 0 or 1) or 5 grade 2 (others 0 or 1). |
| 4.0 | Fully ambulatory without aid (usual FS equivalents are 1 FS grade 4, others 0 or 1, or combination of lesser grades); the patient would be able to walk at least 500 m without assist or rest. |
| 4.5 | Fully ambulatory without aid (usual FS equivalents are one FS grade 4 or combinations of lesser grades exceeding limits of previous steps) and walks at least 300 m without assist or rest. |
| 5.0 | Ambulatory without aid (usual FS equivalents are one grade 5 alone, others 0 or 1 or combinations of lesser grades) and walks at least 200 m without aid or rest. |
| 5.5 | Ambulatory without aid (usual FS equivalents are one grade 5 alone, others 0 or 1; or combinations of lesser grades) and walks at least 100 m without aid or rest. |
| 6.0 | Intermittent or unilateral constant assistance required to walk at least 100 m without rest (usual FS equivalents are combinations with more than one FS grade 3). |
| 6.5 | Constant bilateral assistance required to walk at least 20 m without resting (usual FS equivalents are combinations with more than one FS grade 3). |
| 7.0 | Unable to walk beyond 5 m even with aid, essentially restricted to wheelchair; wheels self and transfers alone (usual FS equivalents are combinations with more than one FS grade 4; very rarely pyramidal grade 5 alone). |
| 7.5 | Unable to take more than a few steps, restricted to wheelchair, wheels self but may need aid in transfers (usual FS equivalents are combinations with more than 1 grade 4; very rarely grade 5 pyramidal alone). |
| 8.0 | Essentially restricted to chair or perambulated in wheelchair but out of bed most of day, retains many self-care functions, generally has effective use of arms (usual FS equivalents are combinations generally grade 4+ in several FS). |
| 8.5 | Essentially restricted to bed most of day, has some effective use of arm(s), retains some self-care functions (usual FS equivalents are combinations generally 4+ in several systems). |
| 9.0 | Helpless bed patient, can communicate and eat (usual FS equivalents are combinations mostly grade 4+). |
| 9.5 | Totally helpless bed patient, unable to communicate effectively or eat or swallow (usual FS equivalents are combinations almost all grade 4+). |
| 10. | Death due to MS. |

**Functional Systems Scores** (Kurtzke 1983; Goodkin et al. 1996)
**Pyramidal Functions**

| | |
|---|---|
| 0. | Normal. |
| 1. | Abnormal signs without weakness. |
| 2. | Mild weakness (4/5 in one extremity or 4+/5 in more than one extremity). |
| 3. | Moderate paraparesis or hemiparesis (4/5 or 4–/5); or severe monoparesis (≤3/5). |
| 4. | Severe triparesis, paraparesis or hemiparesis (≤3/5); moderate quadriparesis (4/5 or 4–/5); or monoplegia. |
| 5. | Paraplegia, hemiplegia, or severe quadriparesis (≤3/5). |
| 6. | Quadriplegia. |
| 7. | Untestable. |
| 8. | Unknown. |

**Cerebellar Functions**
Note: Test finger to nose, heel/knee/shin, rapid alternating movements, and gait. This is a test of cerebellar function and not of weakness. If one or more limbs cannot be tested for any reason, score only the remaining limbs.

| | |
|---|---|
| 0. | Normal. No evidence of cerebellar dysfunction. This score may be used if one or more limbs are uncoordinated due to weakness, apraxia, or sensory loss. |
| 1. | Abnormal signs without interference in routine function. |
| 2. | Mild ataxia. Limb ataxia in any or all limbs or gait ataxia that is adequate to interfere with routine function. |
| 3. | Moderate ataxia. Moderate ataxia of one or more limbs or gait that requires some physical or mechanical adaptation to complete a targeted activity. Examples include the requirement to hold a wall or a companion's arm to hop or tandem walk, or to use a buttonhole device to fasten buttons. The adaptation permits the activity to be completed. |
| 4. | Severe ataxia. This score is applied when there is ataxia of 1 or more limbs or gait. Patients with a severe ataxia cannot complete a targeted activity even with mechanical or human assistance even though the activity may be initiated. |
| 5. | Unable to perform coordinated limb movements or gait. This score is only used when routine activities in one or more limbs or gait cannot even be initiated because ataxia is so severe that injury will result. |
| 6. | Untestable. This score will be applied most commonly when motor strength is 3/5 or less in all four limbs. |
| 7. | Unknown. |

**Brain Stem Functions**

| | |
|---|---|
| 0. | Normal. |
| 1. | Signs only. There is no interference with function. Use this score for unsustained nystagmus. |

2.      Mild impairment. Use this score for sustained conjugate nystagmus, dysconjugate eye movements without associated nystagmus (incomplete INO), or paresis of one or more extraocular muscles innervated by neurons originating in the brain stem.

3.      Moderate impairment. Use this score for dysconjugate nystagmus (complete INO), paralysis of one or more extraocular muscles innervated by neurons originating in the brain stem, or when speech is affected due to brain stem dysfunction but remains intelligible.

4.      Severe impairment. Use this score when speech is impaired by brain stem dysfunction and is marginally intelligible.

5.      Inability to swallow or speak due to brain stem dysfunction.

6.      Untestable.

7.      Unknown.

## Sensory Function

0.      Normal.

1.      Mild impairment. There is a loss of vibration, pain or temperature, or position sense involving the toes or fingers of one or more limb.

2.      Moderate impairment. There is a loss of vibration, pain or temperature, or position sense up to the ankle or wrist in one or more limbs.

3.      Severe impairment. There is a loss of vibration, pain or temperature, or position sense up to the knee or elbow in one or more limbs.

4.      Loss of above-described sensory function(s) proximal to the knee or elbow in one limb.

5.      Loss of above-described sensory function(s) in more than one limb.

6.      Untestable.

7.      Unknown.

## Bowel and Bladder Function.

Ask about both bladder and bowel function during the past 2 weeks. Score the worst as follows. Place an "X" after bladder score if the patient performs intermittent self-catheterization.

### Bladder

0.      Normal.

1.      Bladder symptoms but not incontinence.

2.      Incontinence less than twice per week.

3.      Incontinence two or more times per week but not daily.

4.      Daily incontinence.

5.      Indwelling catheter.

6.      Grade 5 bladder function plus grade 5 bowel function.

7.      Untestable. Use this score if change in function is due to change in medication or presence of infection.

8.      Unknown.

### Bowel

0.      Normal.

1.      Mild or intermittent constipation but no incontinence.

2.      Severe and continuous constipation but no incontinence.

3.      Incontinence less than twice per week.

4.      Incontinence two or more times per week but not daily.

5.      Daily incontinence.

6.      Grade 5 bowel function plus grade 5 bladder function.

7.      Untestable. Use this score if change in function appears to be due to change in medication or presence of infection.

8.      Undetermined.

## Visual Function

Note: All visual acuities (VA) are best corrected.

0.      VA equal to or better than 20/30 and no sign of optic nerve disease.

1.      VA equal to or better than 20/30 with signs of optic nerve disease (e.g., afferent pupil defect).

2.      Worst eye with maximal corrected VA 20/40–20/50.

3.      Worst eye with maximal corrected VA 20/70.

4.      Worst eye with maximal corrected VA 20/100– 20/200.

5.      Worst eye with maximal corrected VA worse than 20/200 and maximal VA of better eye better than 20/60.

6.      Grade 5 plus maximal VA in better eye worse than 20/60.

7.      Untestable.

8.      Unknown.

## Mental Functions

Note: This score is not used in calculation of EDSS scores when neuropsychological testing is performed as part of a controlled clinical trial.

0.      Normal.

1.      Mood alteration only.

2.      Mild decrease in mentation.

3.      Moderate decrease in mentation.

4.      Marked decrease in mentation.

5.      Dementia or chronic brain syndrome.

6.      Untestable.

7.      Unknown.

# 20

# NEUROSARCOIDOSIS

BARNEY J. STERN

Neurological disease occurs in 5% of patients with sarcoidosis (Stern et al. 1985). Central (CNS) or peripheral nervous system (PNS) dysfunction is the presenting feature of sarcoidosis in one-half or more of the patients with neurosarcoidosis (Oksanen 1986; Pentland et al. 1985; Stern et al. 1985). Furthermore, approximately three-fourths of sarcoidosis patients who are destined to develop neurological disease do so within the first 2 years of their systemic illness (Stern et al. 1985). Unfortunately, it is not known why only a small proportion of patients with sarcoidosis have neurological problems or how to predict which patients will encounter neurological difficulties (Newman et al. 1997).

Therefore, neurosarcoidosis is a diagnostic consideration in patients with sarcoidosis who develop neurological signs or symptoms and in patients without known sarcoidosis who develop an illness consistent with neurosarcoidosis. Sarcoidosis presents with a variety of neurological problems, as outlined in Table 20-1.

Two-thirds of patients with neurosarcoidosis have a monophasic illness with minimal residual neurological deficits (Luke et al. 1987; Oksanen 1986; Pentland et al. 1985). These patients typically have a cranial mononeuropathy. Approximately one-third of patients have a remitting-

relapsing or chronically progressive illness that is associated with substantial morbidity and a mortality approximating 10% (James and Sharma 1967; Luke et al. 1987). These patients often have CNS mass lesions, hydrocephalus, or a relatively diffuse encephalopathy/vasculopathy (Luke et al. 1987; Oksanen 1986; Pentland et al. 1985). Patients with recurrent aseptic meningitis, cranial polyneuropathies, myopathy, or neuropathy can have a protracted course but usually survive their illness albeit with considerable morbidity at times (Ando1985; Luke et al. 1987). It is not possible to confidently identify which patients will have a relapsing course (Chen and McLeod 1989), but those who are destined to do so tend to have recurrent disease presenting with similar neurological manifestations (Luke et al. 1987). Although controversial (Sharma 1997), patients with either an acute or more chronic neurological presentation do not differ in their prognosis (Chapelon et al. 1990).

The true natural history of neurosarcoidosis is not well known. Therefore, it is difficult to report specific numbers from large clinical series regarding the prognosis of the various neurological manifestations of sarcoidosis. Also, reports from referral centers probably reflect a skewed patient population. Most patients with neurological com-

**Table 20-1.** Manifestations of Neurosarcoidosis

Cranial neuropathy
Meningeal disease
   Aseptic meningitis
   Dural mass
Myopathy
Neuropathy
Hydrocephalus
Parenchymatous disease
   Endocrinopathy
   Mass lesion(s)
   Encephalopathy/vasculopathy
   Seizures

plications of sarcoidosis are treated with corticosteroids (Newman et al. 1997) or rarely with other therapies, such as radiation or immunosuppressive agents. Published observations of treated patients may, however, approximate the natural history of the disease; Zaki and associates (1987) have noted no significant differences in the outcome of 183 patients with pulmonary sarcoidosis randomized to either corticosteroid therapy or placebo. Corticosteroids are effective treatments for the *symptoms* of sarcoidosis (Israel 1987), but whether corticosteroids affect the ultimate prognosis of sarcoidosis or neurosarcoidosis remains to be determined (Chapelon et al. 1990; Hunninghake et al. 1994). Other therapeutic modalities are needed to alter the outcome of patients with refractory disease.

Sharma (1997) reports an 18% (6 of 37 patients) mortality rate in his series of neurosarcoidosis patients. Patients with CNS sarcoidosis who die tend to do so at a young age. In the pathological series reviewed by Manz (1983), the mean age at death of patients with CNS sarcoidosis ranged from 24 to 38.2 years. The mean duration of neurological disease ranged from 2.3 to 4.7 years before death. Even allowing for the bias inherent in a pathological analysis, these data reinforce the potentially fulminant course of CNS sarcoidosis.

## Cranial Neuropathy

Peripheral facial palsy, the most common neurological complication of sarcoidosis, has a good prognosis (Colover 1948; James and Sharma 1967; Silverstein et al. 1965; Wiederholt and Siekert 1965), with improvement in more than 80% of patients (Stern et al. 1985; Oksanen 1886).

Patients typically recover over several weeks, although residual weakness may remain (Matthews 1979).

Eighth nerve dysfunction, whether auditory or vestibular, can recover or have a less fortunate outcome, characterized by sudden deafness, fluctuating or progressive symptomatology with persistent hearing loss, tinnitus, or vestibular dysfunction (O'Reilly et al. 1995).

Unilateral or bilateral optic neuropathy, often accompanied by chiasmatic infiltration, can lead to progressive visual loss (Gelwan et al. 1988). Optic atrophy can develop insidiously and serial neuro-ophthalmological assessments are necessary to monitor the clinical course.

Any of the other cranial nerves can be involved in CNS sarcoidosis. The clinical outcome typically is benign (Chapelon et al. 1990), especially if only one or two nerves are involved and disease is limited to the cranial nerves. If CNS parenchymal disease or hydrocephalus is present, the prognosis seems to parallel the course of these problems, rather than the cranial neuropathy.

Patients with a single cranial neuropathy have been treated with corticosteroids, although it is unclear whether this alters the generally benign clinical course. Patients with optic or eighth nerve disease often require protracted corticosteroid therapy to maintain function. Progressive optic neuropathy may warrant more aggressive immunotherapy (Abgobu et al. 1995).

## Meningeal Disease

Symptomatic acute aseptic meningitis usually is a self-limited problem (Chapelon et al. 1990), but it may be recurrent. Typically, patients are offered corticosteroid therapy. A chronic cerebrospinal fluid (CSF) pleocytosis is not usually symptomatic, but a persistent pleocytosis, hypoglycorrachia, elevated immunoglobulin G (IgG) index, oligoclonal bands, and elevated CSF angiotensin converting enzyme (ACE) level suggest continuing CNS inflammation. The relevance of these findings to the clinical outcome is unclear. If a patient is clinically stable or asymptomatic, the author has not tried to normalize the CSF with immunosuppressive therapy, but has titrated therapy to the development of new signs or symptoms. Rigorous data to support this approach are lacking.

A dural granulomatous mass requires a more cautious prognosis. These lesions may respond to therapy and not recur following withdrawal of corticosteroid therapy, or they may develop into a chronic problem and exhibit a chronic remitting-relapsing or progressive course. In the latter case, the patient's outcome is similar to that of patients with CNS parenchymatous disease.

## Myopathy

Patients with myopathy have a guarded prognosis (Chapelon et al. 1990). An acute myositis can resolve after several months of corticosteroid therapy. More commonly, there is a chronic, indolent myopathy that can be remitting-relapsing or chronically progressive and debilitating (Matthews 1979; Wolfe et al. 1987). Long-term corticosteroid treatment is routinely used and can be helpful.

## Neuropathy

A mononeuropathy implies a good prognosis, whereas the outcome of patients with a mononeuritis multiplex or generalized sensory, motor, or sensorimotor neuropathy is guarded (Zuniga et al. 1991). A Guillain-Barre syndrome can occur with good recovery (Zuniga et al. 1991; Miller et al. 1991). A trial of corticosteroid therapy is indicated (Scott et al. 1993).

## Hydrocephalus

The prognosis of hydrocephalus is related to the underlying cause. Hydrocephalus can be due to active granulomatous inflammation involving the choroid plexus or ependymal lining of the ventricles or causing a periventricular parenchymal mass or meningitis. Hydrocephalus can result from an end-stage fibrotic process obstructing CSF flow. Patients can develop acute life-threatening increased intracranial pressure (Maisel and Lynam 1996), or they may have a subacute or even asymptomatic presentation.

Patients with an active inflammatory component to their hydrocephalus may improve, at least temporarily, with corticosteroid therapy (Lundh and Wikkelso 1987). However, concurrent parenchymal disease and the hydrocephalus typically require continuing therapy (Foley et al. 1989).

Often a ventriculoperitoneal shunt is required because the patient becomes intolerant of the high-dose corticosteroid needed to maintain CSF flow or the hydrocephalus is progressive in spite of high corticosteroid doses. A patient with symptomatic hydrocephalus due to end-stage fibrosis would not be expected to respond to medical management with corticosteroids and therefore requires a ventriculoperitoneal shunt.

Once a shunt is placed, the patient is at risk not only from the underlying inflammatory disease and the concurrent medication needed to keep this under control, but also from shunt complications, such as infection and obstruction. Blockage of the shunt can be related to a high CSF protein or spread of granulomatous inflammation onto and within the shunt tubing (B. J. Stern, unpublished data, 1985).

With all the complications associated with hydrocephalus due to sarcoidosis, it is clear why these patients constitute a particularly high-risk group (Chapelon et al. 1990).

## CNS Parenchymatous Disease

The most common CNS parenchymal lesions involve the hypothalamus and cause neuroendocrinological dysfunction and vegetative symptoms. Once altered, it is unusual for hormonal function to normalize (Scott et al. 1987). However, hyperprolactinemia can resolve (Nakao 1978), and rarely normal gonadotropin function can return (Hidaka et al. 1987). Altered sleep patterns may improve with corticosteroid therapy.

Patients with one or more CNS granulomatous mass lesions have a guarded prognosis. Untreated, these patients usually progressively deteriorate. However, although resolution of the disease can be achieved in some patients (Chapelon et al. 1990), many patients have continuing disease characterized by remissions and exacerbations that are linked to their corticosteroid dose. Other patients exhibit a progressive deterioration in spite of "optimal" therapy. Surgical intervention is best reserved for diagnostic purposes or for patients who deteriorate in spite of aggressive medical management (Peeples et al. 1991). Radiation therapy and immunosuppressive agents other than corticosteroids occasionally are used in refractory patients and may improve neurological function (Agbogu et al. 1995).

A sarcoidosis-related diffuse encephalopathy/ vasculopathy can present as a monophasic illness and resolve, but more commonly, it exhibits a remitting-relapsing or chronically progressive course in spite of intense medical management (Agbogu et al. 1995).

Convulsions suggest the presence of parenchymal brain disease if there is no obvious metabolic perturbation accounting for the seizures. Typically the seizures are not difficult to treat, but the underlying parenchymal disease often is the limiting factor regarding patient outcome (Krumholz et al. 1988). Therefore, seizures are a potential marker for cerebral sarcoidosis and are poor prognostic indicators (Delaney 1980).

Spinal sarcoidosis manifests as extradural and intradural extramedullary disease, intramedullary lesions, the cauda equina syndrome, and arachnoiditis (Junger et al. 1993). Dural extramedullary disease evolves in an analogous manner to cranial dural lesions, as previously discussed. Intramedullary spinal cord disease typically presents as focal or diffuse inflammation that may be responsive to immunosuppressive therapy (Junger et al. 1993). Spinal cord atrophy suggests that treatment may not be beneficial (Junger et al. 1993). Radiculopathies can respond to immunosuppressive therapy as can a cauda equina syndrome (Ku et al. 1996).

As previously mentioned, patients with CNS parenchymatous disease involving the brain or spinal cord account for much of the morbidity and mortality attributed to neurosarcoidosis, especially if there is associated hydrocephalus (Agbogu et al. 1995). Patients are at risk not only for progressive neurological deterioration, but also therapy can pose significant hazards. Complications of prolonged corticosteroid administration, such as infection and osteoporosis (Rizzato et al. 1987), are particular problems.

## Conclusion

Neurosarcoidosis can exhibit a broad spectrum of manifestations. In an analogous manner, the prognosis is varied and linked not only to the extent of neurological disease, but also to the complications that arise from therapeutic interventions. Fortunately, most patients with sarcoidosis do well, but 1% to 2% of all patients with sarcoidosis encounter considerable neurological difficulties that challenge their fortitude and the skills of their physician.

## References

Agbogu, B. N.; Stern, B. J.; Sewell, C.; Yang, G. Therapeutic considerations in patients with refractory neurosarcoidosis. Arch. Neurol. 52:875–879; 1995.

Ando, D. G.; Lynch, J. P.; Fantone, J. C. Sarcoid myopathy with elevated creatine phosphokinase. Am. Rev. Respir. Dis. 131:298–300; 1985.

Chapelon, C.; Ziza, J. M.; Piette, J. C.; Levy, Y.; Raguin, G.; Wechsler, B.; Bitker, M. O.; Blétry, O.; Laplane, D.; Bousser, M. G.; Godeau, P. Neurosarcoidosis: signs, course and treatment in 35 confirmed cases. Medicine 69:261–276; 1990.

Chen, R. C. Y.; McLeod, J. G. Neurological complications of sarcoidosis. Clin. Exp. Neurol. 26:99–112; 1989.

Colover, J. Sarcoidosis with involvement of the nervous system. Brain 71:451–475; 1948.

Delaney, P. Seizures in sarcoidosis: a poor prognosis. Ann. Neurol. 7:494; 1980.

Foley, K. T.; Howell, J. D.; Junck, L. Progression of hydrocephalus during corticosteroid therapy for neurosarcoidosis. Postgrad. Med. J. 65:481–484; 1989.

Gelwan, M. J.; Kellen, R. I.; Burde, R. M.; Kupersmith, M. J. Sarcoidosis of the anterior visual pathway: successes and failures. J. Neurol. Neurosurg. Psychiatry 51:1473–1480; 1988.

Hidaka, N.; Takizawa, H.; Miyachi, S.; Hisatomi, T.; Kosuda, T.; Sato, T. Case report: a case of hypothalamic sarcoidosis with hypopituitarism and prolonged remission of hypogonadism. Am. J. Med. Sci. 294:357–363; 1987.

Hunninghake, G. W.; Gilbert, S.; Pueringer, R.; Dayton, C.; Floerchinger, C.; Helmers, R.; Merchant, R.; Wilson, J.; Galvin, J.; Schwartz, D. Outcome of the treatment for sarcoidosis. Am. J. Respir. Crit. Care. Med. 149:893–898; 1994.

Israel, H. L. Corticosteroid treatment of sarcoidosis—who needs it? N. Y. State J. Med. 87:490; 1987.

James, D. G.; Sharma, O. P. Neurological complications of sarcoidosis. Proc. R. Soc. Med. 60: 1169–1170; 1967.

Junger, S. S.; Stern, B. J.; Levine, S. R.; Sipos, E.; Marti-Masso, J. F. Intramedullary spinal sarcoidosis: clinical and magnetic resonance imaging characteristics. Neurology 43:333–337; 1993.

Krumholz, A.; Stern, B. J.; Stern, E. G. Clinical implications of seizures in neurosarcoidosis. Arch. Neurol. 48:842–844; 1991.

Ku, A.; Lachmann, E.; Tunkel, R.; Nagler, W. Neurosarcoidosis of the conus medullaris and cauda equina presenting as paraparesis: case report and literature review. Paraplegia 34:116–120; 1996.

Luke, R. A.; Stern, B. J.; Krumholz, A.; Johns, C. J. Neurosarcoidosis: the long-term clinical course. Neurology 37:461–463; 1987.

Lundh, T.; Wikkelso, C. Sarcoidosis with hydro-cephalus: report of a case successfully treated with a ventriculo-peritoneal shunt and methylprednisolone pulse therapy. Acta. Neurol. Scand. 76:365–368; 1987.

Maisel, J. A.; Lynam, T. Unexpected sudden death in a young pregnant woman: unusual presentation of neurosarcoidosis. Ann. Emerg. Med. 28:94–97; 1996.

Manz, H. J. Pathobiology of neurosarcoidosis and clinicopathologic correlation. Can. J. Neurol. Sci. 10:50–55; 1983.

Matthews, W. B. Neurosarcoidosis. Handbook of clinical neurology. New York: Elsevier-North Holland, Inc., 1979.

Miller, R.; Sheron, N.; Semple, S. Sarcoidosis presenting with an acute Guillain-Barré syndrome. Postgrad. Med. J. 65:765–767; 1989.

Nakao, K.; Noma, K.; Sato, B.; Yano, S.; Yamamura, Y.; Hibano, T. Serum prolactin levels in eighty patients with sarcoidosis. Eur. J. Clin. Invest. 8:37–40; 1978.

Newman, L. S.; Rose, C. S.; Maier, L. A. Sarcoidosis. N. Engl. J. Med. 336:1224–1234; 1997.

Oksanen, V. Neurosarcoidosis: clinical presentations and course in 50 patients. Acta Neurol. Scand. 73:283–290; 1986.

O'Reilly, B. J.; Burrows, E. H. VIIIth cranial nerve involvement in sarcoidosis. J. Laryngol. Otol. 109: 1089–1093; 1995.

Peeples, D. M.; Stern, B. J.; Violet, J.; Sahni, K. S. Germ cell tumors masquerading as central nervous system sarcoidosis. Arch. Neurol. 48:554–556; 1991.

Pentland, B.; Mitchell, J. D.; Cull, R. E.; Ford, M. J. Central nervous system sarcoidosis. Q. J. Med. 56: 457–465; 1985.

Rizzato, G.; Fraioli, P. Natural and corticosteroid-induced osteoporosis in sarcoidosis: prevention, treatment, follow up, and reversibility. Sarcoidosis 7: 89–92; 1990.

Scott, I. A.; Stocks, A. E.; Saines, N. Hypothalamic/pituitary sarcoidosis. Aust. N. Z. J. Med. 17:243–245; 1987.

Scott, T. S.; Brillman, J.; Gross, J. A. Sarcoidosis of the peripheral nervous system. Neurol. Res. 15:389–390; 1993.

Sharma, O. P. Neurosarcoidosis. A personal perspective based on the study of 37 patients. Chest 112: 220–228;1997.

Silverstein, A.; Feuer, M. M.; Siltzbach, L. E. Neurologic sarcoidosis. Arch. Neurol. 12:1–11; 1965.

Stern, B. J.; Krumholz, A.; Johns, C.; Scott, P.; Nissim, J. Sarcoidosis and its neurological manifestations. Arch. Neurol. 42:909–917; 1985.

Wiederholt, W. C.; Siekert, R. G. Neurologic manifestations of sarcoidosis. Neurology 15:1147–1154; 1965.

Wolfe, S. M.; Pinals, R. S.; Aelion, J. A.; Goodman, R. E. Myopathy in sarcoidosis: clinical and pathologic study of four cases and review of the literature. Semin. Arthritis Rheum. 16:300–306; 1987.

Zaki, M. H.; Lyons, H. A.; Leilop, L.; Huang, C. T. Corticosteroid therapy in sarcoidosis. A five-year, controlled follow-up study. N. Y. State J. Med. 87:496–499; 1987.

Zuniga, G.; Ropper, A. H.; Frank, J. Sarcoid peripheral neuropathy. Neurology 41:1558–1561; 1991.

# 21

# Vasculitis and Immune-Mediated Vascular Diseases

PATRICIA M. MOORE

The vasculitides are a diverse group of diseases characterized by inflammation in the blood vessel wall with attendant tissue damage usually from ischemia. Despite their relative rarity, many types of vasculitis are increasingly recognized and treated in modern medicine. Neurological manifestations of vasculitis range from frequent in temporal (giant cell) arteritis and the systemic vasculitides to exclusive in isolated angiitis of the central nervous system (CNS) to infrequent or rare in many of the cutaneous vasculitides. The prognoses, both in terms of sequelae and recurrence of disease, improved dramatically with refined diagnosis, identification and treatment of underlying causes, and therapy with immunosuppressive agents. However, given the side effects of medications and the still imprecise estimates of prevalence, vigilance in the diagnoses and recognition of the natural history of disease remain critical.

## Classification and Epidemiology

The term *idiopathic vasculitides* encompasses a variety of diseases. Classification and epidemiology of these unusual and pleomorphic vascular disorders remain a topic of active discussion and study. Although precise diagnosis could provide general prognostic information and guide initial therapy, a widely accepted and validated nomenclature has proved elusive. Despite several recent attempts at classification, there is debate about both the specificity and the sensitivity of criteria used in individual diagnostic categories (Bruce and Bell 1997; Hunder et al. 1990; Wu et al. 1994). The sensitivity and specificity of the classification rules in one schema of seven major vasculitides vary from 70% to over 99%. Clinically well-defined diseases such as temporal (giant cell) arteritis, Churg-Strauss syndrome, and Takayasu's arteritis have high indices, while hypersensitivity vasculitis, a pleomorphic cutaneous vasculitis, has the lowest values (Sherman et al. 1990). Diagnosis is also confounded by the reclassification that now distinguishes polyarteritis nodosa from microscopic polyarteritis on the basis of features including the size of affected vessels and biological measures such as circulating antineutrophilic cytoplasmic antibodies (cANCA) (Carruthers et al. 1996). The overlap of histopathological features among the vasculitides further hinders precise categories. (Tables 21–1 and 21–2).

Another concern is early recognition of vasculitis and features that distinguish it from other inflammatory, nonvasculitic diseases. The current classifications only address features that distin-

**Table 21-1.** The Vasculitides Affecting the Nervous System

Polyarteritis nodosa
Microscopic polyarteritis
Churg-Strauss syndrome
Wegener's granulomatosis
Temporal (giant cell) arteritis
Takayasu's arteritis
Behçet's disease
Isolated angiitis of the CNS
Secondary vasculitides
   Vasculitis secondary to infections
   Vasculitis secondary to toxins
   Vasculitis secondary to neoplasia
   Vasculitis associated with connective tissue diseases

guish one type of vasculitis from another; these criteria are not appropriate to use for diagnosis of individual patients. Because little information is available on the early features and subsequent course of patients with possible vasculitis, longitudinal studies comparing patients with vasculitis with other inflammatory or autoimmune conditions are needed.

There are some epidemiological data. Recent epidemiological studies indicate that in addition to improved recognition, the incidence of some vasculitides is rising (Cotch and Rao 1996; Scott and Watts 1994; Watts et al. 1995; Watts and Scott 1997). Furthermore, seasonal (Guillevin and Lhote 1997; Salvarani et al. 1995) or geographical factors (Numano 1997) influence certain diseases.

**Table 21-2.** Current Estimates of Incidence/ Prevalence Rates

| Disease/Syndrome | Incidence per 1 Million Persons | Prevalence per 1 Million Persons |
|---|---|---|
| Polyarteritis nodosa | 2.4 | |
| | 9 | |
| | 77 | |
| Microscopic polyarteritis | 2.4 (3.6) | |
| Wegener's granulomatosis | 8.5 | 30 |
| Churg-Strauss angiitis | 2.4 | |
| Temporal arteritis | 178 | |
| Takayasu's arteritis | 0.8 (2.6) | |
| Behçet's disease | | |
| Rheumatoid vasculitis | 12.5 | |
| Isolated angiitis of the CNS | | |

## Pathophysiology

Inflammation in and around blood vessels is central to numerous physiological and pathological processes. Communications between immune cells and the blood vessel wall pivot around the temporal and spatial expression of cell surface molecules on leukocytes and endothelial cells. These molecules, which include the selectins, integrins, immunoglobulin superfamily, and chemokines, mediate the spectrum, location, and duration of infiltrating immune cells in the vessel wall and tissue parenchyma (Lawrence and Springer 1991; Weyand and Goronzy 1997). The physiological processes provide rapid response and delivery of cells to regions where the integrity of the tissue is threatened. Delivery of cells to the tissue through the vasculature is critical to eradication of infections and for healing. However, in some circumstances, tissue damage may also result from inflammation of the blood vessel wall either acutely or over a longer term. The pathophysiological mechanisms in these diseases are multiple, and are well defined in only a few of the disorders. Notably, many of the observed pathological processes differ from physiological inflammation only in the extent, duration, or location of the inflammation. Tissue injury from intense, excessive, or prolonged vascular inflammation is usually due to ischemia. Tissue ischemia may develop because cells that indurate the vessel wall mechanically narrow or obstruct the lumen. In addition, soluble mediators released by immune, vascular, and parenchymal cells influence coagulation and vasomotor tone. The combination of physical obstruction of blood flow, increased coagulation, and contraction of vessel diameter impedes the flow of blood and delivery to tissue. Given the enigma surrounding the etiology of inflammation in most of the autoimmune diseases, treatment is directed at diminishing inflammatory signals and local leukocyte expansion.

Recovery of the vessel wall appears to depend largely on the stimulus for inflammation and type of cell in the infiltrate. In general, vessel wall damage is more pronounced with neutrophilic infiltrates than with mononuclear cell infiltrates. Degranulation of neutrophils releases lysosomes, reactive oxygen species, and collagenases (Bruce et al. 1997; Harlan et al. 1981; Sacks et al. 1978).

The etiological stimulus is a major determinant of the infiltrate. For example, many infectious agents prominently recruit neutrophils. The subsequent scarring of the vessel wall renders it vulnerable to additional damage by hypertension, hyperlipidemia, and potentially adverse effects of corticosteroid therapy. Although the details are less well delineated, granulomatous processes associated with activated macrophages also appear to be associated with cicatrized vessels. In contrast, lymphocyte-mediated vascular inflammation results in less long-term injury to the vessel. At least in animal models of vasculitis, viral infections and associated infiltrating lymphocytes may result in transiently denuded endothelial cell linings that heal without sequelae (Henson and Crawford 1974). The extent to which this is true in humans is unknown. Other cells that may play prominent roles in vasculitis include eosinophils (Tai et al. 1984). Eosinophilic infiltrates are notable in idiopathic vasculitides such as Churg-Strauss angiitis and the parasitic diseases.

## Factors Affecting Prognosis

The prognoses of the vasculitides vary greatly among the individual disorders. Among the numerous groups, primarily cutaneous vasculitis is largely benign while the systemic vasculitides may be fatal or recurrent and chronic. In those vasculitides that affect vital visceral organs and the nervous systems, the clinical manifestations and short-term outcome depend on (1) the location and extent of damage from the initial event, (2) identification of underlying causes of the inflammation, and (3) side effects from medications. Over the longer term, outcome of the vasculitides depends on the (1) extent of scarring in the blood vessel wall and (2) recurrence of vascular inflammation.

The dramatic increase in survival with the advent of cytotoxic therapy has reduced the mortality; however, deaths in the systemic or CNS vasculitides are not rare. Currently, the most prominent factor contributing to short-term mortality is the presence of organ failure. Modern treatments allowing longer term follow-up reveal that many vasculitides are chronic relapsing diseases with high morbidity (Exley and Bacon 1996). Because the long-term prognosis depends on occurrences of relapses (requiring repeat im-

munosuppressive therapy) and the development of consequences of vascular damage (requiring prevention and rehabilitation), newer outcome measures are being developed. Measures of outcome such as disease activity, disease-related damage, and functional outcome are increasingly important. Furthermore, there is a significant morbidity due to drug toxicity despite remission of active disease. In the systemic vasculitides, disease-related damage as measured by the Vasculitis Damage Index (64 items in 11 organ-based systems) has proved a useful prognostic tool showing that damage occurs early in systemic vasculitis and that the type and extent of damage predicts outcome (Exley et al. 1997). Similarly, persistent subclinical disease and early recognition of relapse direct treatment. Also, the Birmingham Assessment of disease severity in systemic vasculitis is a measure of mortality, which is now uncommon, and morbidity, which is increasing in significance. Morbidity includes permanent scars or damage, an evolving concept that may be particularly valuable in chronic disease. A close relationship between damage and disease severity in Wegener's granulomatosis and systemic rheumatoid vasculitis is described. Finally, the relapse rate is important in assessing the prognosis of many types of vasculitis. Relapses studied in 150 consecutive patients with an idiopathic necrotizing vasculitis reveal a considerable nonfatal relapse rate in these diseases that contributes to chronic morbidity. Examples of relapse rates (and median time to relapse) were 41.7% (and 33 months) in classical polyarteritis, 25.4% (and 24 months) in microscopic polyarteritis, and 44% (and 42 months) in Wegener's granulomatosis. Laboratory tests were not helpful in predicting relapse (Gordon et al. 1993).

## Specific Diseases

### Polyarteritis Nodosa

Polyarteritis nodosa (PAN) affects medium- and small-sized vessels throughout the body, has various clinical manifestations, a spectrum of severity and, probably, numerous causes. A distinction between PAN and microscopic PAN, which is based on the presence in the latter of microvascular disease, glomerulonephritis, and an association with antineutrophilic cytoplasmic antibodies

(ANCAs), has regrouped current classifications. Recently, hepatitis B–associated PAN is separated from other forms of PAN to emphasize that the addition of antiviral agents in association with immunosuppressive and anti-inflammatory therapy improves the outcome. The increased incidence of hepatitis C also reveals the likelihood of another chronic viral infection as a cause of recurrent vascular inflammation (Nityanand et al. 1997).

*Systemic*

The 5-year survival of patients with PAN rose from 18% untreated to 55% with corticosteroid therapy alone to about 79% with the current combination prednisone/cyclophosphamide therapy (Cohen et al. 1980; Langford 1997). Mortality is greatest in the first year of disease. A recent prospective study of 326 patients confirms that organ failure, particularly of the gastrointestinal tract, remains the predominant feature determining survival over the 3-year course of the study. Gastrointestinal tract failure is largely irreversible. Although early proteinuria is associated with increased mortality, overt renal failure is reversible in many patients. CNS disease and cardiomyopathy did appear as overall risk factors for death but did not individually increase early mortality (Guillevin et al. 1996). Degenerative and hypertensive vascular disease as well as the effects of hypertension affect the heart, CNS, and kidneys. It is not clear whether the pathophysiology of the degenerative changes results from a subclinical vasculitis in the coronary and cerebral vasculature healing with fibrosis and scarring or the vasculopathy is primarily a degenerative process and exacerbated by hypertension and medications such as prednisone (Fortin et al. 1995).

*Neurological*

Peripheral neuropathies are one of the defining features of disease (Hawke et al. 1991; Moore 1995; Moore and Fauci 1981). Except for seizures and subarachnoid hemorrhage that may occur early, CNS abnormalities, such as stroke, usually occur later in the course of disease. The frequent ischemic neuropathies heal well albeit slowly (months to years) and, when recurrence of the PAN is controlled, the neuropathies are not quantitatively prominent in the mortality of disease, although in individual patients the morbidity may be considerable. Similarly, seizures are seldom recurrent and are easily controlled with current medications. Visual abnormalities develop from vasculitis in regions spanning the orbits, the optic nerve and tracts, and the visual cortex as well as the cranial nerves and brain regions controlling ocular motility. We anticipate, although it is not yet studied, that addition to the medical regimen of therapeutic agents that minimize platelet aggregation and vasoconstriction, as well as using the lowest clinically effective dosages of corticosteroids will reduce the longer-term complications of disease. For patients who have been refractory to therapy, several maneuvers including plasmapheresis or humanized monoclonal antibodies such as anti-CD4 and anti-CDw52 antibodies have had anecdotal success not confirmed in controlled studies (Lockwood 1994a, 1994b).

## Microscopic Polyarteritis

Microscopic polyarteritis has been recently individualized from classical polyarteritis nodosa. Microscopic polyangiitis (MPA) is a systemic necrotizing vasculitis clinically and histologically affecting small-sized vessels without granulomata and is associated with focal segmental glomerulonephritis. Renal disease is the major feature but pulmonary involvement, particularly hemorrhage, is also prominent. The presence of ANCAs is an additional feature distinguishing MPA from PAN. Clinical features of systemic inflammation are common. The distinction between MPA and PAN has changed the reported incidence of these diseases (Watts et al. 1996). Neurological features of MPA are not yet well defined, but the incidence of peripheral neuropathies, reported at 14% to 36% of patients, is considerably less than PAN (Lhote et al. 1996)

## Churg-Strauss Syndrome

Churg-Strauss syndrome (CSS) was first described in 1951, on the basis of distinctive features in the autopsies of 13 patients who died after an illness characterized by fever, asthma, eosinophilia, and a systemic illness. This disease was initially included with polyarteritis nodosa but is increasingly regarded as a distinct entity, although a recognized overlap exists. Histologically, medium and small vessels are affected. The two diagnostically essential lesions are angiitis and extravascular necrotizing granulomas usually with eosinophilic infiltrates In any single biopsy specimen, however, the changes may appear very similar to PAN. The disease is often heralded by rhinitis and then increasingly severe asthma. This prodrome may precede the development of eosinophilia and systemic vasculitis by 2 to 20 years. Clinical and hematological features distinguish it from PAN. Early features may include anemia, weight loss, heart failure, recurrent pneumonia, and bloody diarrhea. Pulmonary involvement is typical in CSS and rare in PAN. Similarly, the eosinophilia that is characteristic in CSS is not a feature of PAN. Cutaneous manifestations include palpable purpura, erythema, and subcutaneous nodules.

### Systemic

The mortality of the disease reflects the distribution of the systemic vasculitis, with visceral organ failure the prominent determining feature. Notably, the asthma plays little role in the outcome. Recent studies on the prognosis of Churg-Strauss syndrome suggest that sequelae of early episodes and recurrences are less than with the other systemic vasculitides (Abu-Shakra et al. 1994). The roles of infection and other side effects of immunosuppression are similar to those discussed in PAN.

### Neurological

Clinically, neuropathies occur in over 60% of patients and, as in PAN, are often part of the defining features of the disease (Sehgal et al. 1995). Mononeuropathy multiplex is the predominant pattern, but distal symmetrical and occasional asymmetrical polyneuropathies and radiculopathies occur (Ng et al. 1997). Of the cranial nerve abnormalities, ischemic optic neuropathy and trigeminal neuropathy predominate (Giorgi et al. 1997). CNS manifestations vary, but 10% to 15% of patients develop subarachnoid hemorrhage, visual loss, or stroke (Liou et al. 1997a; 1997b). Encephalopathies, abnormalities in cognition with or without changes in level of arousal, appear to be more frequent than in the other systemic necrotizing vasculitides, but whether this reflects increased incidence or increased recognition is not known. Despite their frequency, the role of the neurological abnormalities in the morbidity and mortality of Churg-Strauss syndrome is not clearly defined.

## Wegener's Granulomatosis

Wegener's granulomatosis may be the most frequently encountered of the idiopathic systemic necrotizing vasculitides, with a recently estimated incidence of 8.5 per 1 million (Cotch et al. 1996; Watts et al. 1995). Characteristic features of upper and lower respiratory tract involvement, glomerulonephritis, and systemic vasculitis define the disease. The strong association of Wegener's and ANCA is an aid in diagnosis. The more specific association of disease is with cANCAs (with a target epitope of proteinase C) (Bini et al. 1992). The role of ANCA in the pathogenesis of disease remains undefined. In vitro studies reveal activation of both neutrophils and endothelial cells that could result in vascular injury and inflammation (Gross et al. 1993; Jennette and Falk 1995). Clinically, none of the forms of ANCAs are currently useful in determining overall relapse rate, type of relapse, morbidity, or longevity (Cohen et al. 1995; Kerr et al. 1993).

### Systemic

The early mortality results from progressive disease resulting in organ failure despite therapy. Because of a higher relapse rate in Wegener's granulomatosus than PAN or CSS, acute complications of disease extend beyond 1 year (Gordon et al. 1993; Jayne and Rasmussen 1997). Patients with Wegener's granulomatosis have benefited from a dramatic improvement in survival with the advent of cyclophosphamide therapy. Previously, the disease was fatal over 4 to 6 months in untreated patients and 11 months with prednisone therapy alone. Long-term survivals are now routine in patients treated with prednisone/cyclophosphamide therapy. Recurrences do occur and particular features of disease may be relatively refractory to therapy (Gordon et al. 1993; Matteson et al. 1996). To reduce the long-term features of diseases and the side effects of medication, recent trials have examined the effects of the antimicrobial trimethoprim-sulfamethoxazole with reported success (Stegeman et al. 1996). Other therapies based on anatomical features and maintenance of remission, or refractory disease include monoclonal antibodies to lymphocyte antigens, methotrexate, and varying protocols for cytotoxic therapy (Jayne and Rasmussen 1997; Kallenberg 1996).

### Neurological

Overall, neurological abnormalities have declined since the advent of combination therapy, but peripheral neuropathies, meningeal inflammation, and cranial neuropathies occur and may appear early in the disease (Nishino et al. 1993). The very erosive nature of the upper respiratory tract lesions involves contiguous structures such as the optic and cranial nerves (Bajema et al. 1997; Cruz and Segal 1997; Jinnah et al. 1997; Shiotani et al. 1997; Spranger et al. 1997; Yokote et al. 1997). Nonetheless, the frequency of neurological abnormalities is not a prominent contributor to the overall prognosis of the disease (Exley et al. 1998).

## Giant Cell Arteritis

Giant cell arteritis (temporal arteritis), the most frequent inflammatory vasculopathy, preferentially affects medium- and large-sized arteries, especially those branching from the proximal aorta (Hunder et al. 1990). It typically affects persons over the age of 50 years and is more prevalent among women of northern European background. Several studies reveal both a seasonal and cyclic (over 5 to 7 years) variation in incidence (Machado et al. 1988). The systemic nature of the disease is apparent in its close relation to polymyalgia rheumatica, a syndrome of proximal muscle aching and stiffness. Although there is some overlap with polymyalgia rheumatica, rigorous attention to diagnostic criteria will facilitate correct diagnosis and therapy. Although this is a systemic arteritis, clinical features, except for malaise and arthralgias, seldom occur below the neck. When systemic features are prominent the diagnosis is more likely to be PAN or CSS. Temporal arteritis is suggested by the pattern of clinical manifestations and confirmed on temporal artery biopsy. Advances in the understanding of the formation of inflammatory infiltrates may improve diagnosis and provide new strategies for therapy. Histological evidence for persistence of the transforming growth factor-$\beta$1 (TGF-$\beta$ -1)– transcribing macrophages in temporal arteries despite paralysis of T-cell function during corticosteroid therapy provides an explanation for the chronicity of the disease (Achkar et al. 1994; Weyand et al. 1997).

In a recent clinical study, follow-up for 205 patients in the 1990 American College of Rheumatology vasculitis classification study revealed that life expectancy of patients with giant cell arteritis is the same as that of the general population (Matteson et al. 1996). Corticosteroids diminish the feared complication of tissue ischemia, particularly blindness, but do not alter the course of disease. The complication rate of corticosteroid therapy is, however, high. Tissue biopsy is recommended to accurately distinguish between temporal arteritis and other inflammatory diseases of the elderly that would respond to lower dosages of prednisone or alternative therapies.

### Systemic

Feared complications include blindness, stroke, aortic arch syndrome, and rupture of aortic aneurysms (Machado et al. 1988; Michel et al. 1996; Swannell 1997).

### Neurological

Headaches, tender temporal arteries, and jaw claudication predominate, although ischemic optic neuropathies remain the feared complication. Occasionally, intracranial disease referable to the posterior circulation occurs (Achkar et al. 1995; Caselli and Hunder 1994; Rivest et al. 1995). When blindness arises, recovery of vision is infrequent, occurring in less than 15% of patients (Aiello et al. 1993). The less frequent ophthalmoplegias share a better prognosis with substantial improvement or resolution in most patients (Barricks et al. 1977; Mehler and Rainowich 1988).

## Takayasu's Arteritis

Takayasu's arteritis is a chronic vasculitis, heterogeneous in presentation, evolution, and response to therapy (Numano 1997). This condition involves primarily the aorta, its main branches, and the coronary and pulmonary arteries. Part of the difficulty in determining the prognosis and therapy is the disease stems from its apparent biphasic nature. The early inflammatory phase may be clinically silent; the chronic vaso-occlusive stage usually initiates the organ damage and medical investigations. It is the only vasculitis for which angiography is usually sufficient for diagnosis. An epidemiological characteristic of this condition is the geographical distribution. Almost all patients come from Asian and South American countries, which has led to searches in the role of genetic factors in its pathogenesis (Vanoli et al. 1995).

A recent study using life-table methods and Cox regression analyses applied to clinical data on 120 patients followed for a median of 13 years provides prognostic information. The overall survival rate at 15 years after the diagnosis was 82.9% and remained the same for the remainder of the follow-up period. Of six variables evaluated at diagnosis, four complications (retinopathy, hypertension, aortic regurgitation, and aneurysm), progressive course, older age at onset, and year of onset were statistically significant predictors of a poorer prognosis. The 15-year survival was 66.3% versus 96.4% for patients with and without a major complication, 67.9% versus 92.9% for patients with and without a progressive course, 58.3% versus 92.7% for age greater than 35 years and less than or equal to 35 years, and 79.9% versus 96.5% for patients diagnosed from 1957 through 1975 and from 1976 through 1990, respectively. In contrast to other vasculitides, a delay in diagnosis and the erythrocyte sedimentation rate (ESR) were of marginal significance. The presence of both major complication and progressive course (stage 3) was the worst prognostic indicator (43% survival at 15 years). Aggressive medical and surgical treatment may be considered for patients with a major complication and a progressive course (stage 3) (Ishikawa and Maetani 1994).

Neurological complications of Takayasu's arteritis result largely from hypertensive and occlusive cerebrovascular disease (Edwards et al. 1989; Numano 1997; Pariser 1994).

## Isolated Angiitis of the CNS

Isolated angiitis of the CNS (IAC) is an idiopathic vasculitis affecting blood vessels of the CNS within the dural reflections. Originally described as fatal, treatment with cyclophosphamide dramatically decreases the morbidity and mortality of the disease. The name for this disease, isolated angiitis of the CNS, reflects the major feature, a recurrent vasculitis clinically confined to the CNS. It does not comment on granulomata, which may or may not be present Current issues focus more on the prevalence rather than therapy for the disease. The apparent increase in frequency of diagnosis of CNS vasculitis (e.g., granulomatous angiitis, primary angiitis), particularly those reports in which there are no histological data, likely results from a lack of widely accepted criteria (Calabrese and Mallek 1988; Scolding et al. 1997; Stubgen and Lotz 1991). The author uses criteria published previously: (1) clinical features consistent with recurrent, multifocal vascular disease; (2) exclusion of an underlying systemic inflammatory process or infection; (3) neuroradiographic studies, usually a cerebral angiogram, supporting diagnosis of vasculopathy; and (4) brain biopsy to establish the presence of vascular inflammation and exclude infection, neoplasia, or alternate causes of vasculopathy (Moore 1989).

### Systemic

Systemic features are absent from this disease, which targets the CNS vasculature. Any evidence of systemic disease should be used to initiate a search for alternative diagnoses.

### Neurological

Neurological features are protean, although typically headaches, encephalopathy, and multifocal signs suggest the diagnosis. Untreated, recurrent ischemia leads to coma and death, although the time frame is not clearly established. Early studies described the mortality in untreated patients as 9 months to a year. More recently, we observe that untreated disease may smolder over several years, although recurrent disease is the rule. Patients treated with prednisone alone have a high relapse rate, probably greater than 80%. Therapy with cyclophosphamide usually in combination with a low dosage of prednisone results in a cure in many patients. Although we cannot determine accurately the relapse rate, given the rarity of the disease, it appears to be below 10% (manuscript in preparation). To some extent this depends on the duration of cyclophosphamide therapy. An early series of patients treated for 6 months after clinical remission of symptoms developed a relapse in 30% of patients. The current protocol of 12 months of therapy corresponds to a relapse rate lower than 10%. The outcome of individual neurological episodes is fairly good, with many patients returning to normal function. As with other types of vascular injury, the occipital cortex heals poorly and hemianopsias are usually persistent. The radiculopathies/myelopathy features encountered in some patients do heal albeit slowly. Episodes of mania or psychoses may be recurrent and difficult to treat but do subside with therapy.

As discussed before, the side effects of therapy remains a concern (Alhalabi and Moore 1994; Calabrese et al. 1993; Moore 1992). Multicenter studies using appropriately defined criteria for disease would be extremely useful.

### Behçet's Disease

Behçet's disease is a multisystem disorder of unknown etiology with prominent mucocutaneous and ocular manifestations. Although any organ system may be involved, the classic clinical triad is that of recurrent oral and genital aphthae with uveitis. The natural history of the disease varies but, although recurrent painful skin lesions and occasionally blindness are sources of morbidity, the disease is seldom fatal.

Diagnostic criteria remain somewhat controversial. The International Study Group (ISG) for Behçet's disease proposed new international criteria for Behçet's disease in 1990. More recently, studies assessing the utility of these criteria in new patient groups in 300 patients in seven countries determined that sensitivity still exceeds specificity (O'Neill et al. 1994). Earlier criteria emphasized the presence of several criteria and specific exclusions of inflammatory bowel disease, systemic lupus erythematosus (SLE), Reiter's syndrome, and orogenital herpesvirus infection (O'Duffy 1990).

In many patients, symptoms are relieved with chlorambucil, azathioprine, or dapsone. A study of 10-year mortality among 152 patients who had registered at a Behçet's syndrome outpatient clinic indicated an increased mortality compared with the general population, particularly in the young male patients (Yazici et al. 1996). The two prominent systemic arterial lesions in patients with Behçet's are occlusive and aneurysmal. In a study of 25 patients with arteriographically proven arterial lesions, occlusive lesions were present in seven patients, aneurysms in three, and both occlusive and aneurysmal lesions in 15. High-dose corticosteroids were not effective in isolated occlusive lesions and probably contributed to one fatal infection. Death was related to aneurysms in five patients. A high postoperative morbidity was associated with vascular surgery to address thromboses but was considered life saving in patients with aneurysms (Le Thi Huong et al. 1995).

Neurological manifestations occur in about 25% of patients with Behçet's disease. Meningo-encephalitis (headaches, fever, confusion, meningismus, cerebrospinal fluid [CSF] pleocytosis), the most frequent manifestation, requires careful exclusion of infection with each episode. Brain stem abnormalities and cranial neuropathies are the second group of neurological changes and an obvious source of morbidity. Other reported neurological abnormalities include benign intracranial hypertension, extrapyramidal dysfunction, and peripheral neuropathies (Fenwick et al. 1997; Serdaroglu et al. 1989a, 1989b). A recent examination of the effects of neurological manifestations on prognosis showed neurological abnormalities in 24 of 41 patients. Eleven patients showed evidence of increased intracranial pressure, and ten of these had radiologically confirmed dural sinus thrombosis. Five patients presented with a meningoencephalitic or meningomyelitic picture, three with a stroke-like picture, and three with primarily brain stem signs. One patient developed trigeminal neuritis, and five patients exhibited (along with other features) variable degrees of psychological manifestations. Of the patients treated with steroids and/or other immunosuppressant drugs and colchicine, only one patient died of the disease. Although this suggests a more favorable prognosis, the short term of follow-up and the prominent morbidity remain high (Farah et al. 1998). Another study re-examined 46 patients after 7 years who were the subjects of a previous report with short-term follow-up. Twenty-seven patients had had headaches without any neurological symptoms or signs previously. Two of these developed an acute neurological event, and a further seven patients showed minor abnormalities on neurological examination. Among the previous neuro-Behçet's group ($n = 15$), as defined by the presence of neurological signs or symptoms, other than headache, seven had a stationary course, while eight had been progressive. Three of the latter group had died The long-term prognosis in neuro-Behçet's syndrome does not seem to be as favorable as the earlier observation, (Akman-Demir et al. 1996).

Loss of vision in Behçet's disease due to an occlusive vasculitis is one of the most common, as well as one of the most serious, of its varied manifestations. Both iridocyclitis and retinovascular lesions, especially necrotizing retinitis, are prominent. Blindness, which occurs in up to 25% of patients, is one of the major causes of permanent disability (Kim 1997).

## SECONDARY VASCULITIDES

It is important to recognize and correctly diagnosies the secondary vasculitides:

- Vasculitis secondary to infections
- Vasculitis secondary to toxins
- Vasculitis secondary to neoplasia

They occur more frequently than the idiopathic vasculitides. Prompt diagnosis and appropriate therapy greatly improve prognosis; tissue is often the sole test that will distinguish between the secondary and idiopathic disorders. It appears that the secondary vasculitides involve the central nervous system more than the peripheral nervous system, although this may be an artifact of recognition.

The author groups the secondary vasculitides together, not because there is no difference in the prognoses between vasculitis secondary to infections and vasculitis secondary to toxins, but because the prognoses depend so much on the specific underlying etiology that differences between the groups are less critical (Fortin 1996; Giang 1994). In general, as would be anticipated, the more virulent the underlying process the worse the outcome for the vasculitic components of disease. Thus, the vasculitis associated with a bacterial meningitis has a higher mortality and morbidity (strokes, cranial neuropathies) than vasculitis associated with treponemal infections. With the indolent infections, an important variable in prognosis is duration of disease prior to diagnosis and treatment. In these cases, treatment of the acute inflammation does not diminish the damage from the chronic cicatrization of the blood vessel wall. The ischemia from scarring is as devastating as that from the acute inflammatory process. Clinical manifestations are often similar to those observed in polyarteritis nodosa or cryoglobulinemia. Identification of viral infection is a cause of vasculitis directs therapy. Treatment with combination of antiviral agents and symptomatic or immunomodulating therapies improves virus clearance and seroconversion to specific antibodies. Both steroids and cytotoxic agents stimulate virus replication and favor disease chronicity and deleterious effects due to the presence of the virus. Hepatitis B virus–related polyarteritis nodosa can be cured

with the combination of antiviral agents (mainly interferon alfa) and plasma exchanges. Hepatitis C virus–related cryoglobulinemia responds to interferon alfa and sometimes to plasma exchanges, but responses are usually partial and relapses occur in the majority of cases (Guillevin et al. 1997)

Vasculitides associated with malignancy occur infrequently, although Hodgkin's disease is a striking example of a secondary vasculitis that may improve dramatically with successful treatment of the underlying disease (Somer and Finegold 1995). However, in the central nervous system the well-documented mimicry of isolated angiitis of the CNS and lymphoma illustrates the necessity of tissue for accurate diagnosis of vasculitis.

The vascular diseases associated with toxins reveal that vascular inflammation occurs in only a small percentage of toxin-mediated vascular injury. However, the frequency of drug abuse does lead to cerebral vascular inflammation and degeneration, particularly in sympathomimetic types of drugs such as amphetamines and cocaine (Citron et al. 1970; Krendel et al. 1990; Wiggins and Cochrane 1981). Although the disease improves with discontinuation of the underlying substance, there are cases with a recurrent course.

### Vacsulopathies Associated with Immune-Mediated Injury

Vascular inflammation is often a dramatic manifestation of an illness and directs the patient and physician to early diagnosis and intervention. Inflammation is, however, only part of the spectrum of immune-mediated vascular disease. Evident in certain disorders such as SLE, yet, undoubtedly underdiagnosed, degenerative vasculopathies illustrate alternate results of immune injury. Vasculitis of the CNS is rare in SLE, although vascular abnormalities, particularly of small vessels, are frequent. Histopathological features of the vasculature on postmortem are scanty, usually revealing a bland vasculopathy (Hanly et al. 1992; Tsokos et al. 1986). Studies in animal models of autoimmunity indicate that persistent, albeit low-level, immune complexes are associated with a degenerative vasculopathy rather than the inflammatory disorder associated with induced immune complex disease. The numerous contributing features to the CNS vascular abnormalities are not yet definable yet do profoundly influence the prognosis of SLE (Moore 1997; Welch et al. 1997). The vascular disease, when clinically manifest, is not treatable with anti-inflammatory medications; in fact, these may deteriorate the histological picture. Further studies and the prevention of vascular disease are more likely to impact prognosis.

Similarly, the role of antiphospholipid antibodies in inflammatory or immune-mediated vasculopathies is yet to be defined. To date, therapies aimed at reducing the titer of antiphospholipid antibodies have not altered the recurrence or sequelae of vascular disease. Other antibodies, such as antiendothelial antibodies, are even more difficult to associate with specific clinical features. These statements are not to dismiss the role of antibodies in vascular injury. Numerous factors associated with systemic inflammation do influence vascular tone and coagulation. The dynamic interaction of lymphocytes, adhesion molecules, and cytokines as well as antibodies and complement induce short-term and long-lived changes in the vasculature. How these affect the prognosis of vascular disease is awaiting discovery.

## Therapy-Effects on Prognosis

With the improvement in the mortality of vasculitis, the side effects of medications make a greater relative contribution to mortality. Vasculitis treatment should be chosen according to etiology, classification, pathogenic mechanisms, severity, and predicted outcome. Treatment of vasculitis ranges from the simple measures of removing the cause of the chronic inflammation to the corticosteroid/cyclophosphamide immunosuppressive mainstays of some diseases to experimental measures in refractory vasculitis. As information on the mechanisms of vascular inflammation increases, more specific, less toxic therapies can be developed. Treatment of patients with vasculitis requires expertise with a spectrum of vasculitides and autoimmune diseases so that there will be an appreciation for the potential of overlap syndromes or evolution of a specific diagnosis over time. Experience in the use of immunosuppressant medications is also important because of the wide range of potential and actual side effects. Side effects occur with any of these agents and the physician should be thoroughly acquainted with all potential side effects before initiating treatment. Most patients do well on the standard regimens. More difficult are those patients who only partially respond to treatment. The physician must determine whether the clinical effects are from persistent inflammation or other causes. Excluding infection should remain a high priority. Ischemia may result not only from the inflammation but also from chronic changes in the vessel wall accompanied by thrombosis and/or hemorrhage.

## Antiplatelet Agents and Anticoagulation

In certain of the vasculitides, there is evidence of a coagulopathy. Active Takayasu's disease is associated with hyperfibrinogenemia and hypofibrinolytic activity. Studies in patients with Kawasaki disease reveal thrombocytosis, diminished fibrinolytic activity, and increased platelet-derived β-thromboglobulin. Fewer data exist for other vasculitides, but thrombosis is a common clinical and histological feature. A potentially simple solution with minimal side effects would be to continue low-dose aspirin during immunosuppressive therapy. This, however, has not been rigorously studied. Anticoagulation with heparin or Coumadin therapy has both theoretical and practical limitations. First, parts of the coagulation in the vessels may be a physiological effect to protect the vessel and tissue. In addition, many of the vasculitides demonstrate histological evidence of perivascular hemorrhage. The risk of intracranial hemorrhage with these medications is potentially high.

Another prominent feature determining survival and morbidity centers on the complication rate of corticosteroid and immunosuppressive therapy. Of appropriate concern is the occurrence of infections. A wide gamut of identified organisms and variable clinical tempo, from indolent to fulminant, emphasizes the need for clinical vigilance. Among the numerous observable complications of prednisone including cognitive abnormalities, mood changes, cataracts, osteoporosis, hyperlipidemia, glucose intolerance, osteoporosis, and hypertension indicate the wide array of short- and long-term conditions that result from corticosteroid therapy. Concerns about cyclophosphamide focus on the neutropenia (that can be ameliorated by monitoring dosage), hemorrhagic cystitis (that can be reduced by maintaining adequate hydration and minimizing contact of the metabolites with the bladder wall), and bladder and systemic malignancies. The incidence of malignancy developing years after therapy with cyclophosphamide is low (<1%) and depends upon total dosage of medication and the underlying disease (Bradley et al. 1989; Langford 1997; Martin et al. 1997).

## References

Abu-Shakra, M.; Smythe, H.; Lewtas, J.; Badley, E.; Weber, D.; Keystone, E. Outcome of polyarteritis nodosa and Churg-Strauss syndrome. An analysis of twenty-five patients. Arthritis Rheum. 37:1798–1803; 1994.

Achkar, A. A.; Lie, J. T.; Gabriel, S. E.; Hunder, G. G. Giant cell arteritis involving the facial artery. J. Rheumatol. 22:360–362; 1995.

Achkar, A. A.; Lie, J. T.; Hunder, G. G.; O'Fallon, W. M.; Gabriel, S. E. How does previous corticosteroid treatment affect the biopsy findings in giant cell (temporal) arteritis? Ann. Intern. Med. 120:987–992; 1994.

Aiello, P. D.; Trautmann, J. C.; McPhee, T. J.; Kunselman, A. R.; Hunder, G. G. Visual prognosis in giant cell arteritis. Ophthalmology 100:550–555; 1993.

Akman-Demir, G.; Baykan-Kurt, B.; Serdaroglu, P.; Gurvit, H.; Yurdakul, S.; Yazici, H.; Bahar, S.; Aktin, E. Seven-year follow-up of neurologic involvement in Behcet syndrome. Arch. Neurol. 53:691–694; 1996.

Alhalabi, M.; Moore, P. M. Serial angiography in isolated angiitis of the central nervous system. Neurology 44:1221–1226; 1994.

Bajema, I. M.; Hagen, E. C.; Weverling-Rijnsburger, A. W.; van der Pijl, H.; van Dorp, W. T.; van Ravenswaay Claasen, H. H.; Bruijn, J. A. Cerebral involvement in two patients with Wegener's granulomatosis. Clin. Nephrol. 47:401–406; 1997.

Barricks, M. E.; Traviesa, D. B.; Glaser, J. S.; Levy, I. S. Ophthalmoplegia in cranial arteritis. Brain 100:209–221; 1977.

Bini, P.; Gabay, J. E.; Teitel, A.; Melchior, M.; Zhou, J.; Elkon, K. B. Antineutrophil cytoplasmic autoantibodies in Wegener's granulomatosis recognized confirmational epitope(s) on proteinase 3. J. Immunol. 149:1409–1415; 1992.

Bradley, J. D.; Brandt, K. D.; Katz, B. P. Infectious complications of cyclophosphamide treatment for vasculitis. Arthritis Rheum. 32:45–53; 1989.

Bruce, I.; McNally, J.; Bell, A. Enhanced monocyte generation of reactive oxygen species in primary systemic vasculitis. J. Rheumatol. 24:2364–2370; 1997.

Bruce, I. N.; Bell, A. L. A comparison of two nomenclature systems for primary systemic vasculitis. Br. J. Rheumatol. 36:453–458; 1997.

Calabrese, L. H.; Gragg, L. A.; Furlan, A. J. Benign angiopathy: a distinct subset of angiographically defined primary angiitis of the central nervous system. J. Rheumatol. 20:2046–2050; 1993.

Calabrese, L. H.; Mallek, J. A. Primary angiitis of the central nervous system. Report of 8 new cases, review of the literature, and proposal for diagnostic criteria. Medicine 67:20–39; 1988.

Carruthers, D. M.; Watts, R. A.; Symmons, D. P.; Scott, D. G. Wegener's granulomatosis—increased incidence or increased recognition? Br. J. Rheumatol. 35:142–145; 1996.

Caselli, R. J.; Hunder, G. G. Neurologic complications of giant cell (temporal) arteritis. Semin. Neurol. 14:349–353; 1994.

Citron, B. P.; Halpern, M.; McCarron, M.; Lundberg, G. D.; McCormick, R.; Pincus, I. J.; Tatter, D.; Haverback, B. J. Necrotizing angiitis with drug abuse. N. Engl. J. Med. 283:1003–1011; 1970.

Cohen, P.; Guillevin, L.; Baril, L.; Lhote, F.; Noel, L. H.; Lesavre, P. Persistence of antineutrophil cytoplasmic antibodies (ANCA) in asymptomatic patients with systemic polyarteritis nodosa or Churg-Strauss syndrome: follow-up of 53 patients. Clin. Exp. Rheumatol. 13:193–198; 1995.

Cohen, R. D.; Conn, D. L.; Ilstrup, D. M. Clinical features, prognosis, and response to treatment in polyarteritis. Mayo Clin. Proc. 55:146–155; 1980.

Cotch, M. F.; Hoffman, G. S.; Yerg, D. E.; Kaufman, G. I.; Targonski, P.; Kaslow, R. A. The epidemiology of Wegener's granulomatosis. Estimates of the five-year period prevalence, annual mortality, and geographic disease distribution from population-based data sources. Arthritis Rheum. 39:87–92; 1996.

Cotch, M. F.; Rao, J. K. New insights into the epidemiology of systemic vasculitis. Curr. Opin. Rheumatol. 8:19–25; 1996.

Cruz, D. N.; Segal, A. S. A patient with Wegener's granulomatosis presenting with a subarachnoid hemorrhage: case report and review of CNS disease associated with Wegener's granulomatosis (review). Am. J. Nephrol. 17:181–186; 1997.

Edwards, K. K.; Lindsley, H. B.; Lai, C.; Van Veldhuizen, P. J. Takayasu arteritis presenting as retinal and vertebrobasilar ischemia. J. Rheumatol. 16:1000–1002; 1989.

Exley, A. R.; Bacon, P. A. Clinical disease activity in systemic vasculitis. Curr. Opin. Rheumatol. 8:12–18; 1996.

Exley, A. R.; Bacon, P. A.; Luqmani, R. A.; Kitas, G. D.; Carruthers, D. M.; Moots, R. Examination of disease severity in systemic vasculitis from the novel perspective of damage using the vasculitis damage index (VDI). Br. J. Rheumatol. 37:57–63; 1998.

Exley, A. R.; Bacon, P. A.; Luqmani, R. A.; Kitas, G. D.; Gordon, C.; Savage, C. O.; Adu, D. Development and initial validation of the Vasculitis Damage Index for the standardized clinical assessment of damage in the systemic vasculitides. Arthritis Rheum. 40:371–380; 1997.

Exley, A. R.; Carruthers, D. M.; Luqmani, R. A.; Kitas, G. D.; Gordon, C.; Janssen, B. A.; Savage, C. O.;

Bacon, P. A. Damage occurs early in systemic vasculitis and is an index of outcome. Q. J. Med. 90:391–399; 1997.

Farah, S.; Al-Shubaili, A.; Montaser, A.; Hussein, J. M.; Malaviya, A. N.; Mukhtar, M.; Al-Shayeb, A.; Khuraibet, A. J.; Khan, R.; Trontelj, J. V. Behcet's syndrome: a report of 41 patients with emphasis on neurological manifestations. J. Neurol. Neurosurg. Psychiatry 64:382–384; 1998.

Fenwick, S.; Goonetilleke, A.; Santosh, C. G.; Newman, P. K. Cerebral venous thrombosis in Behcet's disease. J. Neurol. Neurosurg. Psychiatry 63:419; 1997.

Fortin, P. R. Vasculitides associated with malignancy (review). Curr. Opin. Rheumatol. 8:30–33; 1996.

Fortin, P. R.; Larson, M. G.; Watters, A. K.; Yeadon, C. A.; Choquette, D.; Esdaile, J. M. Prognostic factors in systemic necrotizing vasculitis of the polyarteritis nodosa group—a review of 45 cases. J. Rheumatol. 22:78–84; 1995.

Giang, D. W. Central nervous system vasculitis secondary to infections, toxins, and neoplasms. Semin. Neurol. 14:313–319; 1994.

Giorgi, D.; Lagana, B.; Giorgi, A.; Verrastro, G.; Grandinetti, F.; Grandinetti, P. P.; Gabrieli, C. B. Ischemic optic neuritis in Churg-Strauss syndrome. Recenti Prog. Med. 88:273–275; 1997.

Gordon, M.; Luqmani, R. A.; Adu, D.; Greaves, I.; Richards, N.; Michael, J.; Emery, P.; Howie, A. J.; Bacon, P. A. Relapses in patients with a systemic vasculitis. Q. J. Med. 86:779–789; 1993.

Gross, W. L.; Schmitt, W. H.; Csernok, E. ANCA and associated diseases: immunodiagnostic and pathogenetic aspects. Clin. Exp. Immunol. 91:1–12; 1993.

Guillevin, L.; Lhote, F. Classification and management of necrotising vasculitides. Drugs 53:805–816; 1997.

Guillevin, L.; Lhote, F.; Gayroud, M.; Cohen, P.; Jarrousse, B.; Lortholary, O.; Thibult, N.; Casassus, P. Prognostic factors in polyarteritis nodosa and Churg-Straus syndrome. A prospective study in 342 patients. Medicine 75:17–28; 1996.

Guillevin, L.; Lhote, F.; Gherardi, R. The spectrum and treatment of virus-associated vasculitides. Curr. Opin. Rheumatol. 9:31–36; 1997.

Hanly, J. G.; Walsh, N. M. G.; Sangalang, V. Brain pathology in systemic lupus erythematosus. J. Rheumatol. 19:732–741; 1992.

Harlan, J. M.; Killen, P. D.; Harker, L. A. Neutrophil mediated endothelial injury in vitro. J. Clin. Invest. 68:1394–1403; 1981.

Hawke, S. H.; Davies, L.; Pamphlett, R.; Guo, Y. P.; Pollard, J. D.; McLeod, J. G. Vasculitis neuropathy. A clinical and pathologic study. Brain 114:2175–2190; 1991.

Henson, J. B.; Crawford, T. B. The pathogenesis of virus-induced arterial disease—Aleutian disease and Equine viral arteritis. Adv. Cardiol. 13:183–191. 1974.

Hunder, G. G.; Arend, W. P.; Bloch, D. A.; Calabrese, L. H.; Fauci, A. S.; Fries, J. F.; Leavitt, R. Y.; Lie, J. T.; Lightfoot, R. W., Jr.; Masi, A. T. The American College of Rheumatology 1990 criteria for the classification of vasculitis. Introduction. Arthritis Rheum. 33:1065–1067; 1990.

Hunder, G. G.; Bloch, D. A.; Michel, B. A.; et al. The American College of Rheumatology 1990 criteria for the classification of giant cell arteritis. Arthritis Rheum. 33:1122–1128; 1990.

Ishikawa, K.; Maetani, S. Long-term outcome for 120 Japanese patients with Takayasu's disease. Clinical and statistical analyses of related prognostic factors. Circulation 90:1855–1860; 1994.

Jayne, D. R.; Rasmussen, N. Treatment of antineutrophil cytoplasm autoantibody-associated systemic vasculitis: initiatives of the European Community Systemic Vasculitis Clinical Trials Study Group. Mayo Clin. Proc. 72:737–747; 1997.

Jennette, J. C.; Falk, R. J. Clinical and pathological classification of ANCA-associated vasculitis: what are the controversies? Clin. Exp. Immunol. 101:18–22; 1995.

Jinnah, H. A.; Dixon, A.; Brat, D. J.; Hellmann, D. B. Chronic meningitis with cranial neuropathies in Wegener's granulomatosis. Case report and review of the literature (review). Arthritis Rheum. 40:573–577; 1997.

Kallenberg, C. G. Treatment of Wegener's granulomatosis: new horizons? Clin. Exp. Rheumatol. 14:1–4; 1996.

Kerr, G. S.; Fleisher, T. A.; Hallahan, C. W.; Leavitt, R. Y.; Fauci, A. S.; Hoffman, G. S. Limited prognostic value of changes in antineutrophil cytoplasmic antibody titer in patients with Wegener's granulomatosis. Arthritis Rheum. 36:336–371; 1993.

Kim, H. B. Ophthalmologic manifestation of Behcet's disease. Yonsei. Med. J. 38:390–394; 1997.

Krendel, D. A.; Ditter, S. M.; Frankel, M. R.; Ross, W. K. Biopsy-proven cerebral vasculitis associated with cocaine abuse. Neurology 40:1092–1094; 1990.

Langford, C. A. Chronic immunosuppressive therapy for systemic vasculitis (review). Curr. Opin. Rheumatol. 9:41–47; 1997.

Lawrence, M. B.; Springer, T. A. Leukocytes roll on a selectin at physiological flow rates: distinction from and prerequisite for adhesion through integrins. Cell 65:859–873; 1991.

Le Thi Huong, D.; Wechsler, B.; Papo, T.; Piette, J. C.; Bletry, O.; Vitoux, J. M.; Kieffer, E.; Godeau, P. Arterial lesions in Behcet's disease. A study in 25 patients. J. Rheumatol. 22:2103–2113; 1995.

Lhote, F.; Cohen, P.; Genereau, T.; Gayraud, M.; Guillevin, L. Microscopic polyangiitis: clinical aspects and treatment (review). Ann. Med. Interne (Paris) 147:165–177; 1996.

Liou, H. H.; Liu, H. M.; Chiang, I. P.; Yeh, T. S.; Chen, R. C. Churg-Strauss syndrome presented as multiple intracerebral hemorrhage. Lupus 6:279–282; 1997a.

Liou, H. H.; Liu, H. M.; Chiang, I. P.; Yeh, T. S.; Chen, R. C. Churg-Strauss syndrome presented as multiple intracerebral hemorrhage. Lupus 6:279–282; 1997b.

Lockwood, C. M. Approaches to specific immunotherapy for systemic vasculitis. Semin. Neurol. 14:387–392; 1994a.

Lockwood, C. M. Approaches to specific immunotherapy for systemic vasculitis (review). Semin. Neurol. 14:387–392; 1994b.

Machado, E. B.; Michet, C. J.; Ballard, D. J.; Hunder, G. G.; Beard, C. M.; Chu, C. P.; O'Fallon, W. M. Trends in incidence and clinical presentation of temporal arteritis in Olmsted County, Minnesota, 1950–1985. Arthritis Rheum. 31:745–749; 1988.

Martin, F.; Lauwerys, B.; Lefebvre, C.; Devogelaer, J. P.; Houssiau, F. A. Side-effects of intravenous cyclophosphamide pulse therapy. Lupus 6:254–257; 1997.

Matteson, E. L.; Gold, K. N.; Bloch, D. A.; Hunder, G. G. Long-term survival of patients with giant cell arteritis in the American College of Rheumatology giant cell arteritis classification criteria cohort. Am. J. Med. 100:193–196; 1996.

Matteson, E. L.; Gold, K. N.; Bloch, D. A.; Hunder, G. G. Long-term survival of patients with Wegener's granulomatosis from the American College of Rheumatology Wegener's Granulomatosis Classification Criteria Cohort. Am. J. Med. 101:129–134; 1996.

Mehler, M. F.; Rainowich, L. The clinical neuro-ophthalmologic spectrum of temporal arteritis. Am. J. Med. 85:839–844; 1988.

Michel, B. A.; Arend, W. P.; Hunder, G. G. Clinical differentiation between giant cell (temporal) arteritis and Takayasu's arteritis. J. Rheumatol. 23:106–111; 1996.

Moore, P. M. Diagnosis and management of isolated angiitis of the central nervous system. Neurology 39:167–173; 1989.

Moore, P. M. Isolated angiitis of the central nervous system. In: Berlit, P.; Moore, P. M., eds. Vasculitis, rheumatic disease and the nervous system. New York: Springer-Verlag; 1992.

Moore, P. M. Neurological manifestation of vasculitis: update on immunopathogenic mechanisms and clinical features. Ann. Neurol. 37 (suppl 1):S131–S141; 1995.

Moore, P. M. Neuropsychiatric systemic lupus erythematosus. Stress, stroke, and seizures. Ann. N. Y. Acad. Sci. 823:1–17; 1997.

Moore, P. M.; Fauci, A. S. Neurologic manifestations of systemic vasculitis. A retrospective and prospective study of the clinicopathologic features and responses to therapy in 25 patients. Am. J. Med. Sci. 71:517–524; 1981.

Ng, K. K.; Yeung, H. M.; Loo, K. T.; Chan, H. M.; Wong, C. K.; Li, P. C. Acute fulminant neuropathy in a patient with Churg-Strauss syndrome. Postgrad. Med. J. 73:236–238; 1997.

Nishino, H.; Rubino, F. A.; DeRemee, R. A.; Swanson, J. W.; Parisi, J. E. Neurological involvement in Wegener's granulomatosis: an analysis of 324 consecutive patients at the Mayo Clin. Ann. Neurol. 33:4–9; 1993.

Nityanand, S.; Holm, G.; Lefvert, A. K. Immune complex mediated vasculitis in hepatitis B and C infections and the effect of antiviral therapy. Clin. Immunol. Immunopathol. 82:250–257; 1997.

Numano, F. Differences in clinical presentation and outcome in different countries for Takayasu's arteritis. Curr. Opin. Rheumatol. 9:12–15; 1997.

O'Duffy, J. D. Behcet's syndrome. N. Engl. J. Med. 322:326–328; 1990.

O'Neill, T. W.; Rigby, A. S.; Silman, A. J.; Barnes, C. Validation of the International Study Group criteria for Behcet's disease. Br. J. Rheumatol. 33:115–117; 1994.

Pariser, K. M. Takayasu's arteritis. Curr. Opin. Cardiol. 9:575–580; 1994.

Rivest, D.; Brunet, D.; Desbiens, R.; Bouchard, J. P. C-5 radiculopathy as a manifestation of giant cell arteritis. Neurology 45:1222–1224; 1995.

Sacks, T.; Moldow, C.; Craddock, P.; Bowers, T.; Jacob, H. Oxygen radicals mediate endothelial cell damage by complement-stimulated granulocytes. An in vitro model of immune vascular damage. J. Clin. Invest. 61:1161–1167; 1978.

Salvarani, C.; Gabriel, S. E.; O'Fallon, W. M.; Hunder, G. G. The incidence of giant cell arteritis in Olmsted County, Minnesota: apparent fluctuations in a cyclic pattern [see comments]. Ann. Intern. Med. 123:192–194; 1995.

Scolding, N. J.; Jayne, D. R.; Zajicek, J. P.; Meyer, P. A.; Wraight, E. P.; Lockwood, C. M. Cerebral vasculitis—recognition, diagnosis and management. Q. J. Med. 90:61–73; 1997.

Scott, D. G.; Watts, R. A. Classification and epidemiology of systemic vasculitis. Br. J. Rheumatol. 33:897–899; 1994.

Sehgal, M.; Swanson, J. W.; DeRemee, R. A.; Colby, T. V. Neurologic manifestations of Churg-Strauss syndrome. Mayo Clin. Proc. 70:337–341; 1995.

Serdaroglu, P.; Yazici, H.; Ozdemir, C.; Yurdakul, S.; Bahar, S.; Akin, E. Nerologic involvement in Behcet's syndrome: a prospective study. Arch. Neurol. 46:270–273; 1989a.

Serdaroglu, P.; Yazici, H.; Ozdemir, C.; Yurdakul, S.; Bahar, S.; Aktin, E. Neurologic involvement in Behcet's syndrome. A prospective study. Arch. Neurol. 46:265–269; 1989b.

Sherman, G.; Morrison, L.; Rosen, G.; Behan, P.; Galaburda, A. Brain abnormalities in immune defective mice. Brain Res. 532:25–33; 1990.

Shiotani, A.; Mukobayashi, C.; Oohata, H.; Yamanishi, T.; Hara, T.; Itoh, H.; Nishioka, S. Wegener's granulomatosis with dural involvement as the initial clinical manifestation. Intern. Med. 36:514–518; 1997.

Somer T.; Finegold S. M. Vasculitides associated with infections, immunization, and antimicrobial drugs. Clin. Infect. Dis. 20:1010–1036; 1995.

Spranger, M.; Schwab, S.; Meinck, H. M.; Tischendorf, M.; Sis, J.; Breitbart, A.; Andrassy, K. Meningeal involvement in Wegener's granulomatosis confirmed and monitored by positive circulating antineutrophil cytoplasm in cerebrospinal fluid. Neurology 48:263–265; 1997.

Stegeman, C. A.; Cohen Tervaert, J. W.; de Jong, P. E.; Kallenberg, C. G. Trimethoprim-sulfamethoxazole (co-trimoxazole) for the prevention of relapses of Wegener's granulomatosis. Dutch Co- Trimoxazole Wegener Study Group. N. Engl. J. Med. 335:16–20; 1996.

Stubgen, P.; Lotz, B. P. Isolated angiitis of the central nervous system: involvement of penetrating vessels at the base of the brain. J. Neurol. 238:235–238; 1991.

Swannell, A. J. Polymyalgia rheumatica and temporal arteritis: diagnosis and management. BMJ 314:1329–1332; 1997.

Tai, P. C.; Holt, M. E.; Denny, P.; Gibbs, A. R.; Williams, B. D.; Spry, C. J. F. Deposition of eosinophil cationic protein in granulomas in allergic granulomatosis and vasculitis: the Churg-Strauss syndrome. Br. Med. J. 289:400–402; 1984.

Tsokos, G. C.; Tsokos, M.; le Riche, N. G. H.; Klippel, J.H. A clinical and pathologic study of cerebrovascular disease in patients with systemic lupus erythematosus. Semin. Arthritis Rheum. 16:70–78; 1986.

Vanoli, M.; Miani, S.; Amft, N.; Bacchiani, G.; Radelli, L.; Scorza, R. Takayasu's arteritis in Italian patients. Clin. Exp. Rheumatol. 13:45–50; 1995.

Watts, R. A.; Carruthers, D. M.; Scott, D. G. Epidemiology of systemic vasculitis: changing incidence or definition? Semin. Arthritis Rheum. 25:28–34; 1995.

Watts, R. A.; Jolliffe, V. A.; Carruthers, D. M.; Lockwood, M.; Scott, D. G. Effect of classification on the incidence of polyarteritis nodosa and microscopic polyangiitis. Arthritis Rheum. 39:1208–1212; 1996.

Watts, R. A.; Scott, D. G. Classification and epidemiology of the vasculitides (review). Baillieres Clin. Rheumatol. 11:191–217; 1997.

Welch, K. M.; Nagesh, V.; Boska, M.; Moore, P. M. Detection of cerebral ischemia in systemic lupus erythematosus by magnetic resonance techniques. Ann. N. Y. Acad. Sci. 823:120–131; 1997.

Weyand, C. M.; Goronzy, J. J. Multisystem interactions in the pathogenesis of vasculitis. Curr. Opin. Rheumatol. 9:3–11; 1997.

Weyand, C. M.; Tetzlaff, N.; Bjornsson, J.; Brack, A.; Younge, B.; Goronzy, J. J. Disease patterns and tissue cytokine profiles in giant cell arteritis. Arthritis Rheum. 40:19–26; 1997.

Wiggins, R. C.; Cochrane, C. G. Current concepts in immunology—immune-complex-mediated biologic effects. N. Engl. J. Med. 304:518–519; 1981.

Wu, J.; Zhou, T.; Zhang, J.; He, J.; Gause, W. C.; Mountz, J. D. Correction of accelerated autoimmune disease by early replacement of the mutated lpr gene with the normal Fas apoptosis gene in the T cells of transgenic MRL-lpr/lpr mice. Proc. Natl. Acad. Sci. USA 91:2344–2348; 1994.

Yazici, H.; Basaran, G.; Hamuryudan, V.; Hizli, N.; Yurdakul, S.; Mat, C.; Tuzun, Y.; Ozyazgan, Y.; Dimitriyadis, I. The ten-year mortality in Behcet's syndrome. Br. J. Rheumatol. 35:139–141; 1996.

Yokote, H.; Terada, T.; Nakai, K.; Itakura, T. Subdural and meaningful involvement related to Wegener's granulomatosis: case report. Neurosurgery 40:1071–1073; 1997.

PART VII

# TRAUMA

# 22

# Traumatic Brain Injury

LORI A. SHUTTER, JACK I. JALLO, AND RAJ K. NARAYAN

The ability to predict outcome from traumatic brain injury (TBI) is of obvious importance, but remains complicated by the diversity of clinical presentations and the variability of clinical course. Some of the factors affecting outcome, such as age, are unchangeable, but others, such as blood pressure and intracranial pressure, can be modified by medical interventions. As physicians we must use the prognostic information available to us to not only answer questions for the patient and family but also to make appropriate management decisions. The luxury of postponing outcome predictions for weeks into the course of treatment is slipping away as pressures mount to make determinations regarding long-term care earlier and earlier. Many health care providers are involved in the care of a TBI patient, and each provider places an emphasis on different aspects of prognostic information. Thus, the focus of prognostication can differ considerably depending on whether one is contemplating the withdrawal of care, placement in an appropriate rehabilitation setting, or the effect of the long-term sequelae of head trauma.

It should be emphasized at the very onset that almost any variable could be shown to correlate with outcome (Table 22-1). However, when these various prognostic factors are subjected to a logistic regression analysis, most factors are found to be insignificant. Some of the more robust factors that hold up after detailed analysis include the Glasgow coma scale (GCS) score, age, pupillary reactivity, and blood pressure. This chapter will review a large number of these factors, although much of the literature falls into class III evidence, along with some class II data.

In its simplest form, prognosis is often described in terms of survival. As aggressive early management of the TBI patient has resulted in decreased mortality, the focus of outcome predictions is increasingly being directed to residual disability and quality-of-life issues. Thus, prognosis after TBI is increasingly being referred to in terms of functional outcome.

## Measuring Outcome

The terms *outcome* and *prognosis* after TBI may mean different things to the medical care providers, the hospital administrator, the HMO/insurance caseworker, the patient, and the family. In addition, outcome prediction measures vary among physicians of different specialties. Thus, the neurosurgical and trauma literature emphasizes different "outcome measures" than the rehabilitation literature. A survey of neurosurgeons found that the majority felt prognostic factors

**Table 22-1.** Preinjury Prognostic Factors and Demographic Variables Affecting Outcome from TBI

| Variable | Finding | Authors |
|---|---|---|
| Age | Increased mortality<br>Elderly<br>Very young (≤4) | Kilaru et al. 1996; Luerssen et al. 1988; Pennings et al.<br>1993; Vollmer et al. 1991<br>Levin et al. 1992; Luerssen et al. 1988 |
|  | Increased morbidity<br>Elderly<br>Young (<8) | Cifu et al. 1996; Goldstein et al. 1994; Katz and Alexander<br>1994; Kilaru et al. 1996; Pennings et al. 1993<br>Asikainen et al. 1996; Thompson et al. 1994 |
| Gender | Mortality ratio 3:1 M:F<br>Predicts length of stay<br>Female hormones may improve<br>recovery—animal studies | Sosin et al. 1989<br>Spettell et al. 1991<br>Garcia-Estrada et al. 1993; Emerson et al. 1993; Roof,<br>1993; Roof et al. 1996 |
| Genetics | APOE-ε4 predicts outcome | Jordan et al. 1997; Teasdale et al. 1997 |
| Psychosocial factors | Median income inversely<br>related to TBI incidence<br>and mortality | Kraus et al. 1986; Whitman et al. 1984 |
| Education | Better outcome with<br>higher education | Asikainen et al. 1996; Dikmen et al. 1989; Girard et al.<br>1996; Mayes et al. 1989 |
| Recurrent head trauma | Additive damage | Gronwall and Wrightson 1975; Jordan and Zimmerman<br>1990; Salcido and Costrich 1992 |
| Substance abuse | Increased mortality and morbidity | Corrigan 1995; Girard et al. 1996; Kelly M et al. 1997 |

would allow decisions to be made within 3 days following injury (Barlow and Teasdale 1986). In comparison, rehabilitation specialists remain skeptical about outcome predictions even months following injury. These variations may be due to different priorities and perceptions, the use of different outcome measures, span of time frames reviewed, and population sizes (Sandel 1994).

Prognostic outcome measures must be selected in response to what questions are being asked. The model of disease impact established by the World Health Organization (WHO) can provide guidance regarding this selection (WHO 1980). This model identifies four areas in which an injury can be assessed: pathology, impairment, disability, and handicap. *Pathology* is determined by the lesion characteristics, such as location, hemorrhage, focal contusions, diffuse axonal injury, hypoxia, hypotension, intracranial pressure, and the like. These parameters are assessed in the acute care

setting by use of the neurological examination, physiological monitoring, anatomic and metabolic imaging, and laboratory testing. Mortality and disability are correlated with this information, and the prognostic data provided by these parameters will be discussed later in this chapter.

Pathology may result in *impairment,* which in the TBI patient refers primarily to neurological deficits. Neurological impairment can be measured with tools such as the GCS (Table 22-2) (Teasdale and Jennett 1974), Rancho Los Amigos Coma Score, Galveston Orientation & Amnesia Test (GOAT) (Levin et al. 1979), neurological exam, and neuropsychological testing. This information has a role in predicting long-term outcome and will be addressed in more detail.

The realm of *disability* is often discussed in terms of what level of assistance is needed to perform the necessary activities of daily living (ADL). Evaluations are made regarding things such as

**Table 22-2.** Glasgow Coma Scale*

| Eye Opening (E) | | Verbal Response (V) | | Best Motor Response (M) | |
|---|---|---|---|---|---|
| Spontaneous | 4 | Oriented | 5 | Follows commands | 6 |
| To command | 3 | Confused | 4 | Localizes to pain | 5 |
| To pain | 2 | Inappropriate | 3 | Withdraws to pain | 4 |
| No response | 1 | Incomprehensible | 2 | Flexor posturing | 3 |
|  |  | No response | 1 | Extensor posturing | 2 |
|  |  |  |  | No response | 1 |

* Scores from each category are added for the total coma score, with a range from 3 to 15. Lower scores indicate greater severity of injury.

self-care, continence, walking, and household management skills. *Handicap* is defined in terms of how the disability impacts on a person's life. Can a person continue working in a chosen profession, participating in their prior leisure activities, or living in their previous environment? These two areas can be assessed by a number of measurement tools; examples include the Glasgow Outcome Scale (GOS) (Jennett and Bond 1975), the Disability Rating Scale (DRS) (Rappaport et al. 1982) and Functional Independence Measure (FIM) (Hamilton et al. 1987), socioeconomic measures, quality of life measures, and caregiver burden measures.

The GOS was designed by the developers of the GCS and is frequently used as an assessment of disability in the neurosurgical literature (Table 22-3) (Jennett and Bond 1975). The GOS is made up of five categories: good recovery, moderate disability, severe disability, vegetative state, and death. Favorable outcomes are defined as good recovery or moderate disability; the remaining categories are considered unfavorable. The GOS has proven reliability, but the broad categories of outcome result in a lack of sensitivity for changes seen in patients over time. This can lead to erroneous assumptions regarding the prognosis for recovery. In an effort to address this concern, Jennett et al. proposed a modification of the GOS that subdivided patients with good recovery, moderate disability, or severe disability into "better or worse" outcomes within each category (Jennett et al. 1981). This modified version of the GOS has not gained widespread usage.

The DRS is frequently reported in the rehabilitation literature as a measure of disability. It is a reliable, easily performed test that assesses eight items in four categories consisting of alertness, cognition for self-care, dependence, and psychosocial adaptability (Table 22-4). In a direct comparison of these two measures, the DRS was found to be more sensitive to change than the GOS over the first year after injury (Hall et al. 1985).

The FIM (Table 22-5) is the most widely used general disability measure among rehabilitation specialists. It consists of a seven-point scale that grades the level of assistance needed by a patient on 18 different tasks and can document functional change during inpatient rehabilitation better than the DRS (Bowers et al. 1989). The FIM has validity as a TBI outcome measure (Corrigan et al. 1997), but it must be supplemented with neuropsychological evaluations, since it does not adequately address the cognitive, behavioral, and psychosocial issues that occur after TBI. Many different tools may be used to assess TBI patients during the course of their recovery. Combining the unique pieces of information provided by each individual measure may yield the most comprehensive and sensitive assessment of a patient's outcome.

## The Cost of Brain Injury

TBI has been called the silent epidemic, and young men between the ages of 15 and 24 are the most frequent victims. The incidence of brain injury varies depending on the definition of severity used, the means of injury identification, and the geographical and social group being studied. It has been reported that 80% of all injuries are in the mild category, with moderate and severe injuries being approximately 10% each (Kraus and McArthur 1996; Jennett 1996). A recent literature review of TBI epidemiology studies estimated that in a typical Unites States community the annual incidence of all new brain injuries was approximately 200 per 100,000 (Sorenson and Kraus 1991). There is a wide variation in the severity of these injuries, as these figures include immediate fatalities in addition to hospital admis-

**Table 22-3.** Glasgow Outcome Scale

| Unfavorable Outcomes | | | Favorable Outcomes | |
|---|---|---|---|---|
| 1 | 2 | 3 | 4 | 5 |
| Death | Persistent vegetative state | Severe disability | Moderate disability | Good recovery |
| Loss of life due to head injury | Unresponsive, + sleep cycles, + eye opening | Conscious but disabled, dependent for daily care | Disabled but independent, able to care for self | Resumes normal life, minor residual deficits |

**Table 22-4.** Disability Rating Scale

| Category | Item | Scoring |
|---|---|---|
| Arousability, awareness, and responsibility | Eye opening | Spontaneous = 0, To speech = 1, To pain = 2, None = 3 |
| | Verbalization | Oriented = 0<br>Confused = 1<br>Inappropriate = 2<br>Incomprehensible = 3<br>None = 4 |
| | Motor response | Obey = 0<br>Localizes = 1<br>Withdraws = 2<br>Flexor = 3<br>Extensor = 4<br>None = 5 |
| Cognitive ability for self-care activities | Feeding | Ignore motor disability |
| | Toileting | Complete = 0<br>Partial = 1 |
| | Grooming | Minimal = 2<br>None = 3 |
| Dependence on others | Level of functioning | Independent = 0<br>Independent in special setting = 1<br>Mildly dependent = 2<br>Markedly dependent = 3<br>Totally dependent = 4 |
| Psychosocial adaptability | Employability | Not restricted = 0<br>Selective jobs, competitive = 1<br>Sheltered workshop = 2<br>Nonemployable = 3 |

DRS Disability Scores

| 0 | 1 | 2–3 | 4–6 | 7–11 | 12–16 | 17–21 | 22–24 | 25–29 | 30 |
|---|---|---|---|---|---|---|---|---|---|
| No disability | Mild | Partial | Moderate | Moderately severe | Severe | Extremely severe | Vegetative state | Extreme vegetative state | Death |

**Table 22-5.** Functional Independence Measure

Categories

| Self-care | Mobility | Cognition |
|---|---|---|
| Eating | | |
| Grooming | Transfers—bed, chair | Comprehension |
| Bathing | Transfers—toilet | Expression |
| Dressing—upper body | Transfers—tub, shower | Social interaction |
| Dressing—lower body | Locomotion—walk, wheelchair | Problem solving |
| Toileting | Locomotion—stairs | Memory |
| Bladder management | | |
| Bowel management | | |

Scoring

| Independent<br>—No Helper | | Dependent—Requires Helper | | | | |
|---|---|---|---|---|---|---|
| | | Modified Dependence | | | Complete Dependence | |
| Complete independence | Modified independence | Supervision or setup | Minimal assistance | Moderate Assistance | Maximal assistance | Total assistance |
| 7 | 6 | 5 | 4 | 3 | 2 | 1 |

\* Each of the 18 categories are scored on a 7-point scale. Total scores can range from 18 to 126.

sions. The prehospital TBI mortality rate has been calculated to range from 14 to 30 per 100,000 per year, with a mean rate of 22 per 100,000 (Kraus and McArthur 1996).

The majority of moderate and severe brain injuries that survive, as well as some of the mild injuries, will have a residual neurological disability. It has been estimated that some degree of impairment will remain in 10% of all new mild TBI patients, 67% of those with moderate TBI, and 100% of severe injuries that survive hospitalization. After excluding early and in-hospital fatalities from the yearly incidence rate, this results in a calculated disability rate of just under 35 per 100,000 people (Sorenson and Kraus 1991). This figure may underestimate the full scope of this problem. A recent study estimates that only 75% of patients sustaining mild to moderate head injury seek medical assistance (Sosin et al. 1996). In addition, many patients with mild TBI are sent home from the emergency room and found on follow-up to have residual problems. Some of these patients may never return to seek further medical attention.

The health care cost of brain injury is high. In 1988 dollars the calculated direct and indirect costs of TBI annually was $44 billion (Max et al. 1991). Acute care costs were found by Brooks et al. to range from $10,990 for mild injuries up to $81,152 for severe injuries (Brooks et al. 1995). The average cost of rehabilitation of the TBI population ranges from $35,000 to $110,000 per case (Bryant et al. 1993; Whitlock and Hamilton 1995; Ashley et al. 1997). This has increasing significance in the changing medical climate, as long-term and follow-up services must be justified. Data on the effectiveness of various treatments with regards to prognosis and long-term outcome need to be collected.

## Prognostic Factors

Many factors have been evaluated for their prognostic abilities after TBI. We have attempted to briefly review the available data, but certain caveats must be emphasized. The clinician has to remain aware that numbers derived from groups of patients give only a general sense of the prognostic correlations. However, in daily practice each patient must be considered as an individual with unique characteristics that can affect outcome differently.

Prognostic factors are merely associations between a clinical finding and outcome, they do not provide a definitive answer in each individual case. As stated earlier, one must remember that almost any variable can be shown to correlate with outcome. However, when these various prognostic factors are subjected to a logistic regression analysis, most factors are found to be insignificant. In addition, head injury initiates a dynamic process in brain tissues with changes that occur over variable time spans. Thus, ongoing assessments are required to reflect a patient's current status. Decisions regarding the level of medical care must be based on firm clinical and diagnostic data, especially when considering the withdrawal of support. Finally, the field of neuroscience is in a state of rapid growth and the advances in our knowledge may have implications for the TBI patient.

## Preinjury Factors

There are some demographic factors that have been shown to have an impact on recovery from TBI (Table 22-1).

### Age

Age has been found to be a strong independent predictor of mortality (Luerssen et al. 1988). Higher mortality rates are seen in children under the age of 5 and in individuals over 65 (Levin et al. 1992; Kilaru et al. 1996; Vollmer et al. 1991). Age also has an impact on the level of residual disability with effects reported on both functional and cognitive outcomes (Katz and Alexander 1994; Kilaru et al. 1996; Vollmer et al. 1991; Pennings et al. 1993; Cifu et al. 1996; Goldstein et al. 1994; Thompson et al. 1994; Asikainen, 1996). A study of 40 elderly patients with severe TBI found no functional improvement after 3 years (Kilaru, 1996). Another study found that functional change did occur in the patients over 55, but they required longer rehabilitation programs and had a lower rate of change when compared to patients under 55 (Cifu et al. 1996). Goldstein et al. found that patients over 50 with only mild to moderate injuries had marked problems with memory and executive function tasks on neurobehavioral studies (Goldstein et al. 1994). Brain injuries prior to the age of 8 result in a greater likelihood of severe disability on the GOS, as well as evidence of impaired motor and visuomotor development (Asikainen et al. 1996; Thompson et al. 1994).

## Gender

A significant difference between genders is seen in both incidence and mortality TBI data. TBI occurs much more frequently in males, with a 3:1 male-female mortality rate that may simply represent differences in the severity of injury (Sosin et al. 1989). The effect of gender on recovery after TBI remains unclear. Animal studies imply that gonadal hormones can influence outcome from brain injury, but only a few human studies have suggested a gender effect. Garcia-Estrada et al. found that rats treated with progesterone, estradiol, or testosterone after an induced brain injury had a significant decrease in the number of reactive astrocytes near the lesion (Garcia-Estrada et al. 1993). Studies by Roof et al. have shown that progesterone significantly decreases the amount of cerebral edema following TBI in rats, thus suggesting that this hormone may have a protective effect on the brain (Roof et al. 1993, 1996). Another group of researchers found that estrogen exacerbated brain injury in female rats, but was beneficial in male rats (Emerson et al. 1993). The influence of gender has not been widely investigated in the human literature on brain injury. One study of penetrating brain injury in children and adolescents found that sex did correlate with outcome (Levy et al. 1993a). Gender was also found to be a predictor of the length of rehabilitation stay in a recent study (Spettell et al. 1991).

## Genetics

The influence of genetics on recovery from brain injury has received recent attention. The increased risk of Alzheimer's disease with the presence of an apolipoprotein ε-4 (APOE-ε4) genotype is well known. Recent studies are suggesting that TBI patients with this same genotype may have a greater risk of persistent deficits due to the possibility of histopathological changes in response to the injury. Boxers with the APOE-ε4 genotype and 12 or more professional bouts have shown significantly higher impairments on a scale specifically designed to test for the traumatic encephalopathy associated with boxing (Jordan et al. 1997). Teasdale et al. recently reported on the results of a prospective study assessing the APOE genotype in 93 TBI patients. A higher proportion of the patients with the APOE-ε4 genotype had a GCS score of less than 13. In addition, the 6-month GOS determination found that 57% of the patients with APOE-ε4 had a poor outcome compared to 27% of the patients without APOE-ε4 ($p = .006$) (Teasdale et al. 1997). Further studies are needed on the long-term predictive value provided by this information.

## Race

Race and socioeconomic factors do correlate with the incidence of TBI by placing people in an environment with higher risks for head injury. Sosin et al. recently reported that the TBI mortality rates for black males has risen since 1984, whereas the rate has fallen for white males. This was attributed to a significant increase in black male firearm-related deaths, with an associated decrease in motor-vehicle-related deaths in white males (Sosin et al. 1995). Median family income has shown an inverse relationship to both the incidence and mortality rate of TBI (Kraus et al. 1986; Whitman et al. 1984). Patients with a higher premorbid level of education and intelligence carry a better prognosis for recovery from TBI (Asikainen et al. 1996; Dikmen et al. 1989; Girard et al. 1996; Mayes et al. 1989). Neuropsychological testing of intelligence in the acute phase after TBI has also shown a positive correlation with outcome (Klonoff et al. 1993). This may relate in some way to the neural reserve available to a person after TBI. Recurrent head injuries have been shown to result in cumulative damage over time, and even mild trauma may result in significant deficits if there is a prior history of TBI (Gronwall and Wrightson 1975; Jordan and Zimmerman 1990; Salcido and Costrich 1992).

## Substance Abuse

A review of recent research on this topic by Corrigan found that alcohol intoxication was present in one-third to one-half of all TBI hospitalizations. A history of some form of substance abuse is present in approximately two-thirds of TBI patients going on to rehabilitation. Higher mortality rates, increased acute complications with longer hospitalizations, worse discharge status, and a greater likelihood of repeat injuries were all associated with a history of substance abuse (Corrigan, 1995). A history of substance abuse also has a negative influence on cognitive performance after TBI (Girard et al. 1996). This association was confirmed recently; Kelly et al. found lower scores on multiple neuropsychological test parameters in TBI patients with a positive toxicology screen on admission (Kelly M et al. 1997).

## Nature of the Injury

### Type of Injury

As previously mentioned, the pathology of TBI has a bearing on the outcome. Brain injury can be described in terms of the mechanism and morphology of injury. Mechanism of injury refers to blunt versus penetrating trauma, whereas morphology describes the presence of focal or diffuse intracranial injury. The mechanism of injury carries implications regarding outcome. Penetrating trauma occurs less frequently than blunt trauma in most series, but the mortality rate is significantly higher (Aldrich et al. 1992b; Shaffrey et al. 1992; Siccardi et al. 1991; Kaufman 1993). Outcome after penetrating head injury follows a strongly bimodal pattern (i.e., either patients do quite well or they die). In closed head injury, the intermediate outcomes are much better represented. An overall mortality rate of 55% was seen at 1 week after penetrating brain injury in a retrospective study of 62 patients with severe TBI (Shaffrey et al. 1992). A prospective study found that patients with penetrating head injuries with a GCS score of 6 to 8 had a 70% mortality rate, this rate jumped to 94% when the initial GCS score was 3 to 5 (Aldrich et al. 1992b). The presence of a traumatic subarachnoid hemorrhage (tSAH) is a poor prognostic sign after penetrating head injury (Levy et al. 1993b, 1994). Although there is a greater likelihood of death after a penetrating head injury, survival does not necessarily imply a poor long-term outcome. A recent study comparing the functional outcome of 25 cases of penetrating TBI survivors with the same number of blunt TBI survivors found no significant differences in the outcome variables 1 year following injury (Zafonte et al. 1997b).

As the name implies, diffuse axonal injury (DAI) represents a form of diffuse trauma and may occur either in isolation, or with coexisting focal hematomas. Neuroimaging studies are generally not diagnostic and DAI remains a histological diagnosis. Recent data suggest that a form of apoptotic cellular death in response to trauma may compound the effect of DAI (Clark et al. 1997). Clinically, the syndrome of DAI has three separate stages: first is immediate unconsciousness, followed by a longer period of confusion and associated post-traumatic amnesia (PTA), and finally a prolonged recovery period. The amount and density of DAI determine the clinical course; and the factors that are most predictive of outcome include the length of PTA, duration of coma, and the GCS score (Blumbergs et al. 1989; Gennarelli et al. 1982; Katz and Alexander 1994). Secondary injuries, most notably due to hypotension and hypoxia, are often associated with brain injury. Furthermore, metabolic and neurochemical disturbances can contribute to the cellular injury and influence the clinical course. Subarachnoid hemorrhage is another form of diffuse injury seen in TBI. Greene et al. compared differences in the clinical course of TBI patients with tSAH to patients of similar GCS scores without tSAH. The tSAH patients were found to have more medical complications, as well as an increased number of days in both the intensive care unit (ICU) and in the hospital. The clinical outcome for tSAH was also worse; these patients had higher mortality rates, lower GOS scores on discharge, and a smaller number were discharged to home (Greene et al. 1997). However, all of these studies are based on relatively few patients, thus precluding valid statistical analyses.

Cortical contusions, subdural, extradural, and intracranial hematomas comprise the majority of focal pathologies. The recovery from these types of injury is variable and depends on the location, size, and depth of the lesion. At one time it was suggested that lesions in the left hemisphere were associated with an increased duration of unresponsiveness. Further studies found that the length of time to develop localized pain responses was similar regardless of the hemispheric localization of injury. The interpretation of this result was that impaired language skills provided the explanation for any delayed responsiveness seen with left hemisphere lesions (Levin et al. 1989).

The presence of subdural hematoma (SDH) and epidural hematoma can affect outcome and often require neurosurgical intervention. Seelig et al. found that outcome from SDH is related to the length of time between injury and surgical decompression. Patients had a 30% mortality rate if decompression was accomplished within 4 hours, whereas delays of more than 4 hours increased the mortality rate to 90% (Seelig et al. 1981). The presence of a greater than 15-mm midline shift on computed tomography (CT) due to an SDH has also been associated with late deterioration and death (Marshall et al. 1983b). An outcome study focusing on patients with epidural hematomas suggests that 23% have a poor outcome and 77% have good recovery or moderate disability by GOS. These results were found to have an association with GCS scores, other intracerebral injuries, and intracranial pressure (ICP) management (Heinzelmann et al. 1996). Levin et al. related the depth of a lesion with both injury severity and the duration of altered consciousness. A brain magnetic resonance imaging (MRI) scan was done at 3-months after TBI to determine lesion depth and they found that this factor was predictive of the 6-month GOS (Levin et al. 1988).

*Severity of Injury*

Traumatic brain injury is the single largest contributor to trauma center deaths, with a higher mortality rate than other forms of trauma. A review of 95 trauma centers found an overall trauma mortality rate of 6.1%, but this rate increased to 18.2% in the TBI patients (Gennarelli et al. 1989). One of the strongest predictors of mortality is severity of injury, and this is usually determined by assessing the level of consciousness. This information can also provide some guidance regarding the possibility and amount of any residual disability. The most widely used scale to assess the level of consciousness is the GCS, which was developed by Teasdale and Jennett in 1974 (Teasdale and Jennett 1974). Scores are assigned after a simple assessment of the patient's ocular, verbal, and motor response to stimulation (see Table 22-2). A score of 13 to 15 places a patient in the mild category, 9 to 12 is considered a moderate injury, and 8 or less defines a severe injury. As a measure of injury severity, the GCS has shown a strong relationship to outcome in numerous studies (Zafonte et al. 1996a; Siegel, 1995; Litofsky et al. 1994; Levin et al. 1990; Diringer and Edwards 1997). Another scale to assess the severity of injuries frequently used in trauma centers is the Revised Trauma Score (RTS) (Boyd et al. 1987). It is arrived at by adding the GCS, systolic blood pressure, and respiratory rate. Although it has been shown to have good predictive value regarding mortality, it has limited usefulness in predicting disability (Champion et al. 1989; Cooke et al. 1995; Zafonte et al. 1996b).

One must remain aware of the fact that the GCS score can change rapidly in response to medical interventions in the early stages after TBI. For this reason, the scale's developers have recommended that a standardized postresuscitation time be identified for assessment of the GCS score (Teasdale and Jennett 1976). Other researchers have found that both the first GCS score obtained and the worst postresuscitation GCS score could be highly predictive of neurobehavioral functioning 1 year after injury (Levin et al. 1990). An isolated GCS may actually have a somewhat limited value as a predictor of functional outcome (Zafonte, 1996a; Diringer and Edwards 1997). Alternative scales have been proposed but, although these other scales may provide more specific information, the GCS remains the most widely used and has a reasonably good interobserver reliability (Benzer et al. 1991). However, significant variations have been noted depending on who is assessing the GCS (Marion and Carlier 1994).

Although recent advances in emergent and acute care have resulted in improved outcomes, severe TBI (GCS score ≤8) continues to have a significant mortality and disability rate. The NIH Traumatic Coma Data Bank (TCDB) was a cooperative effort of six clinical head injury centers to collect data regarding acute and long-term prognosis after severe TBI (Marshall et al. 1983a). This study reported a decrease in TBI mortality from 50% in the 1970s to approximately 30% in a 1991 review. It also found that moderate disability or good recovery occurred in only 16% of patients with a GCS score less than 6 (Marshall et al. 1991). Poor or substantially limited reintegration in the community has been found in 76% of severe TBI patients for up to 6 years after injury. The subgroup of patients with good recovery or moderate disability by the GOS showed only a 50% rate of good community reintegration (Tate et al. 1989). Moderate TBI carries a much better prognosis, with one study finding that patients with a GCS score of 9 to 13 had a mortality rate of 0.9%. The 6-month outcome analysis found 86% with moderate disability or good recovery, 7% with severe disability, and only 7% in the vegetative/dead category (Stein and Ross 1992). Overall, mild head injury (GCS score ≥14) has a good prognosis, although some recommend classifying it into uncomplicated versus complicated (or high-risk) categories. Complicated mild TBI patients are those with a GCS score of 13 to 14, or 15 with radiographic abnormalities. This group demonstrates worse outcomes when compared to patients with a GCS score of 15 without radiographic findings (Hsiang et al. 1997). Postconcussion syndrome (PCS) can follow a mild head injury. The symptoms are diverse, but commonly include headache, irritability, dizziness, and cognitive impairments. Levin reports that there is consistent evidence for the recovery of the cognitive deficits within 1 to 3 months after injury (Levin, 1996). The majority of patients will experience substantial or complete recovery of symptoms by 3 months after injury. Unfortunately, 1 year after injury residual symptoms are still reported in 7% of mild TBI patients (Rutherford et al. 1979). The persistence of PCS 6 months after injury raises concerns that psychological factors may be contributing to the symptoms (Alexander, 1992). Researchers have reported on the high prevalence of PCS-like symptoms in the general population, as well as in patients with either medical or psychiatric problems (Dikmen and McLean 1986; Fox et al. 1995; Iverson and McCracken 1997; Gouvier et al. 1992; Mittenberg et al. 1992; Wong et al. 1994). TBI patients may underestimate the prevalence of these symptoms in the general population, thus causing them to associate these symptoms directly to their injury (Mittenberg, 1992).

Prognosis from TBI may be better determined by looking at more than one variable, especially in the severe head-injured patient. Many researchers have proposed the need for multidimensional analysis tools (Table 22-6). Choi et al. reported that the combination of patient's age, best GCS motor response, and pupillary response at admission provided the most accurate prediction of outcome (Choi et al. 1988). He, with other colleagues, went on to propose using these variables in a decision tree algorithm (Figure 22-1). Clinical use of this tool found it to have an accuracy rate of 77.7%. The prediction accuracy was highest for patients at the GOS extremes (i.e., death vs. good recovery) compared to those in the intermediate categories (Choi et al. 1991). Levin found that the 1-year GOS could be predicted by using the lowest postresuscitation GCS and pupil reactivity (Levin et al. 1990). Others have found that the combination of age, depth and duration of coma (as measured by the GCS), pupil reactivity to light, and spontaneous and reflex eye movements could predict outcome with a high level of accuracy (Braakman et al. 1980). Narayan et al. found that the combination of clinical data (i.e., age, GCS score, pupillary response, extraocular motility) predicted outcome with considerable accuracy. ICP data and multimodal evoked potentials could add somewhat to the confidence of the prediction (Narayan et al. 1981). In the pediatric population brain injury severity, extracranial injury severity, and pupillary response in the emergency department (ED) have been shown to be predictive of mortality. The most prognostic factors for disability in the same cohort were 72-hour postinjury GCS motor response and early oxygenation status (Michaud et al. 1992).

**Table 22-6.** Multidimensional Assessments for Outcome Prediction after TBI

| Author | Variables Affecting Outcome | Outcome Measurement |
|---|---|---|
| Braakman et al. 1980 | Age, GCS, pupil reactivity, spontaneous & reflex eye movements, length of coma | 6-month GOS |
| Narayan et al. 1981 | GCS, pupillary response, ICP, EPs, age | 2-category GOS (D+VS+SD; MD+GR) |
| Born et al. 1985) | GCS motor response, brain stem reflexes, age | 3-category GOS (D; VS+SD; MD+GR) |
| Choi et al. 1988 | Best motor response by GCS, admission pupillary response, age | 4-category GOS (D+VS; SD; MD; GR) |
| Levin et al. 1990 | Lowest postresuscitation GCS, pupil reactivity | 1-year GOS |
| Michaud et al. 1992 (pediatric) | Brain and extracranial injury severity, pupil response | Survival |
| | 72-hour GCS motor response, early oxygenation status | Disability |
| Ong et al. 1996 (pediatric) | 24-hour GCS, admission hypoxia, CT findings | 2-category GOS (D+VS+SD; MD+GR) |

GCS, Glasgow Coma Scale; GOS, Glasgow Outcome Scale; ICP, intracranial pressure; EPs, evoked potentials; VS, vegetative state; D, death; CT, computed tomography; SD, severe disability; MD, moderate disability; GR, good recovery.

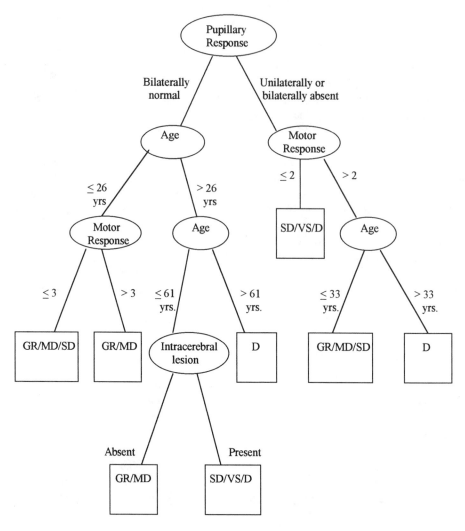

**Figure 22-1.** TBI outcome prediction tree based on pupillary response, motor response, and age. (From Choi et al. 1991.)

Present information supports efforts to make mortality predictions by using a limited number of variables in the acute phase after injury, with the primary focus on age, injury severity (especially the GCS motor component), and pupillary reactions. Although this is the trend, it must be emphasized that life is inherently unpredictable. A falsely optimistic prediction suggests a favorable outcome when the patient actually does poorly, and a falsely pessimistic one suggests an unfavorable outcome when the patient actually does well. These inaccurate predictions can have serious and devastating implications. The recently described Leeds scale reported a 100% accuracy rate for predicting mortality in severe

brain injury (Gibson and Stephenson 1989), but the reliability of this scale has been questioned. When the Leeds scale was applied to a different patient population, Feldman et al. found only a 60% to 70% fatality accuracy rate (Feldman et al. 1991). A wrongful prediction of death (falsely pessimistic) in more than 30% is unacceptable when making decisions about early termination of care. Quigley and colleaques recently reported a "3-4-5" rule after evaluating the use of age and admission GCS score for predicting survival (Quigley et al. 1997). They found only nonfunctional survival (death or vegetative) in those patients whose age was beyond the 30s with a GCS score of 3, beyond the 40s with a GCS score of 4, or beyond the 50s with a GCS score of 5. In their discussion they stressed that any "rule" will have exceptions. Thus, prognostic factors should not be used for definitive decisions to treat or not treat, but instead should act as guides for treatment decisions and expectations. The prediction of long-term disability poses even greater challenges and requires a broader base of information gathered over a longer time frame.

### Associated Injuries

The presence of extracranial traumatic injuries can have a significant effect on recovery after TBI. Of the 1709 TBI patients reviewed by Siegel et al, 60% had associated systemic injuries and 40% had an isolated TBI. The patients with systemic injuries had a mortality rate of 21.8% compared to an 11% rate in the isolated TBI group. The subgroup of patients with systemic injuries involving the spine, lung, viscera, pelvis, or extremities showed an even higher mortality rate of greater than 25% (Siegel et al. 1991). Associated systemic injuries can also impact on the average total cost of care over the first year after injury. These costs increase from $59,000 in isolated severe TBI to $90,000 when additional systemic injuries are present (Siegel et al. 1991; Siegel, 1995). The patient's long-term level of recovery may be affected by the presence of associated injuries. A longer duration of coma has been reported in TBI patients with multiple injuries, as well as greater problems with long-term psychosocial functioning, memory, attention, and learning (Woischneck et al. 1997; Moore et al. 1990). Masson et al. looked at a group of 149 patients 5 years after a mild to moderate TBI and found that the majority of disabilities reported were related to their systemic injuries (Masson et al. 1996). Similar findings have been reported in the pediatric population. A study of 95 pediatric patients found that those with TBI plus multiple trauma had a 2 1/2 times greater frequency of poor outcome even though the severity of head injury was greater in the patients with isolated TBI (Mayer et al. 1981).

## Postinjury Factors

### ED/ICU Management

Recent advances in urgent and acute medical care of TBI have been associated with a decrease in mortality rates (Marshall et al. 1991; Warme et al. 1991). In particular, the ability of emergency medical service (EMS) teams to accurately assess the TBI patient at the accident scene has improved triage. A delay in care or transportation to a facility that is not prepared to manage a trauma patient can have a negative long-term effect (Morgan, 1994). A prospective study evaluating the effects of prehospital and acute clinical management on the 6-month GOS is being undertaken by Lehr et al. (1997). The primary injury after TBI is the biomechanical damage that occurs directly to the central nervous system (CNS). Commonly, trauma-related secondary insults of hypotension, hypoxia, hypovolemia, and elevated ICP also occur. These entities can result in the secondary injuries of ischemia and diffuse cerebral edema. The focus of early TBI management should include minimizing any secondary insults. Wald et al. grouped patients by the presence or absence of secondary brain injury and found no significant differences in the mortality rates between a rural setting and an urban community with access to trauma centers (Wald et al. 1993). In a comparative analysis of TBI survival in New Delhi, India, and Charlottesville, Virginia, Colohan et al. found that early management might affect outcome. The availability of better critical care improved the mortality rate of the Virginia patients who localized to painful stimuli (GCS motor score = 5) (Colohan et al. 1989). The combination of prehospital variables with clinical and radiographic findings has shown predictive power on mortality and outcome (Fearnside et al. 1993). Systemic complications after injury can also influence TBI recovery; postinjury pulmonary, cardiovascular, hematological, or infectious problems are associated with poor outcomes (Bratton and Davis 1997; Piek et al. 1992). Increased efforts by ED and ICU staff to prevent secondary insults and systemic complications may result in improved survival with less disability.

There is an emphasis in the neurosciences to develop multidisciplinary approaches to patient care. The TBI population is a patient group that may benefit from this treatment approach. Trauma teams, neurosurgeons, and ED staff work closely together to coordinate the initial care. After the acute stabilization, the treatment team expands to include orthopedic surgery, neurology, rehabilitation services (including the physiatrist, physical and occupational therapist, and speech-language pathologist), respiratory therapy, nursing, nutrition, and social services. The use of a formalized team approach of aggressive early intervention has recently been compared to a traditional, nonformalized program. Patients in the formalized program had a significant decrease in both coma duration and length of stay in the inpatient rehabilitation setting. Improvements were also seen in discharge impairment scores, motor, sensory, and cognitive function. This resulted in 94% of the formalized program patients being discharged to their home compared to only 57% of those patients in the nonformalized program (Mackay et al. 1992). Specialized "acute TBI units" may actually provide an optimal treatment setting with cost-effective medical care resulting in improved outcomes. However, data to date are nonrandomized, noncontrolled, and generally with limited numbers of patients; therefore, any conclusions regarding efficacy need to be made with great caution.

### Hemodynamic Factors

The physiological effects of hypotension and hypoxia can result in secondary brain injuries and thus worsen the prognosis for recovery. They are extremely detrimental after TBI, and every effort should be made to avoid their development. Increased mortality and morbidity have been associated with early postinjury episodes of systolic blood pressure below 90 mm Hg or respiratory compromise (apnea, cyanosis, or $PaO_2 < 60$ mm Hg). One or both of these parameters have been reported at some time after injury and through resuscitation in 57% of comatose TBI patients (Chestnut et al. 1993b). Another study found that only 23% of the patients with a history of hypotension or hypoxia had a good recovery versus 56% of the patients without either factor. In addition, the presence of either one doubled the mortality rate (Wald et al. 1993). These physiological parameters have a negative impact on outcome and can be modified by therapeutic interventions; therefore, an emphasis must be placed on their management in any TBI-related treatment protocol.

Many researchers have confirmed that hypotension has a negative impact on TBI survival and recovery (Fearnside et al. 1993; Piek et al. 1992; Chestnut et al. 1993a; Klauber et al. 1989; Winchell et al. 1996; Chestnut et al. 1993b; Pietropaoli et al. 1992; Pigula et al. 1993). Mortality rates are doubled (55% vs. 27%) in the patients

that are hypotensive on admission, and they have shown a significant increase in morbidity compared to normotensive patients (Chestnut et al. 1993a). Transient episodes of hypotension may commonly occur in the ICU after TBI. The total number of these episodes has been associated with increased mortality and a decrease in the number of patients' discharged to their home, with the most detrimental effects occurring in patients having an initial GCS score greater than 8 (Winchell et al. 1996). The TCDB review found that 32% of 493 patients developed late hypotension, and 24% had hypotensive episodes only in the ICU. This group showed a very poor outcome, 66% were in a vegetative state or dead compared to only 17% of the group without late hypotension falling into these categories (Chestnut et al. 1993a). Hypotension that occurs intraoperatively during the first 72 hours after injury has been associated with a higher mortality rate compared to normotensive TBI patient (82% vs. 25%). The same study also reported an inverse relationship between hypotension and GOS scores (Pietropaoli et al. 1992). In the pediatric TBI population the development of hypotension resulted in a fourfold increase in mortality (Pigula et al. 1993). Recent studies suggest that the use of small-volume hypertonic saline solutions for blood pressure resuscitation provide a therapeutic effect that may help to improve outcome from severe TBI (Vassar et al. 1993; Wade et al. 1997).

The detrimental effects of hypoxemia after TBI are recognized in both animal models of injury and humans. In animal models, mild to moderate hypoxemia augments neuronal death and functional motor deficits even though there is no increase in the lesion volume (Clark et al. 1997). The monitoring of hypoxia in the clinical setting has been aided with recent technological advances, and knowledge of cerebral oxygen utilization may provide some insight regarding cerebral perfusion in the early stages after TBI. Information regarding the balance between cerebral oxygen delivery and consumption may be obtained by monitoring jugular venous oxyhemoglobin saturation ($SjvO_2$) (Prough and Lang 1997; Robertson et al. 1995). Desaturation ($SjvO_2 < 50\%$) has been reported to occur at least once in 39% of TBI patients, and was related to both intracranial hypertension and systemic causes (Robertson et al. 1995). Episodes of desaturation have been correlated with poor outcomes, which supports the thought that reductions in oxygen delivery contribute to secondary neurological injury (Robertson et al. 1995; Cruz, 1996). Other tools for detecting early ischemic secondary injury include brain tissue partial pressure of oxygen (ti-$P_{O_2}$) and cerebral arteriovenous oxygen difference ($AVDO_2$). Falls of ti-$P_{O_2}$ below 10 mm Hg for more than 15 minutes is consistent with ischemia and has been associated with unfavorable outcomes (Kiening et al. 1997). Late cerebral infarction and poor outcome can also be predicted by the failure of $AVDO_2$ to fall in response to treatment interventions (LeRoux et al. 1997). A constant, noninvasive means of monitoring cerebral oxygenation may be provided by near-infrared spectroscopy (NIRS), but the validity of this tool has not been proven (Prough and Lang 1997). A multimodality recording system has allowed the comparison of NIRS with other monitoring parameters. NIRS was found to correlate with 97% of the cerebral hemodynamic changes; this was compared to only a 53% correlation provided by $SjvO_2$ measures. At this time NIRS should not be used in isolation, but can supply information regarding clinical trends (Kirkpatrick et al. 1995). Hyperbaric oxygen therapy has been used in efforts to improve oxygenation after TBI. A benefit in mortality was seen, with only 17% of the treatment group dying compared to 32% of the control group. Unfortunately, this benefit did not carry through to long-term results, as there was no increase in the number of survivors with favorable outcomes (Rockswold et al. 1992).

Cerebral vasculature and cerebral blood flow (CBF) are altered after TBI, and this can lead to changes in cerebral oxygen metabolism ($CMRO_2$). Failure to maintain adequate CBF increases the risk of secondary ischemia. Cerebral ischemia (CBF <18 ml/100 g/min) occurs in up to 30% of TBI patients in the first hours after injury (Bouma and Muizelaar 1995). Hypovolemic shock associated with TBI has a mortality rate of 62%, and there is a direct relationship between mortality and the volume of blood required for resuscitation in the first 24 hours (Siegel, 1995). In severe TBI there may be an association between low CBF and 3-month mortality; patients with CBF values of 29 ml/100 g/min had a mortality rate of 32% versus 20% for CBF values of 62 ml/100 g/min (Robertson et al. 1992). In addition, an increased need for inpatient rehabilitation has been shown when hypovolemic shock occurs after TBI (Siegel, 1991).

The relationship between blood flow changes and outcome following TBI has been assessed with [133]Xe-CBF studies. CBF is lowest on the day of injury; subsequently there is an increase in flow over the next 1 to 5 days. Favorable outcome at 6-months after injury has been reported in 58.8% of the patients that consistently maintained a CBF greater than or equal to 33 ml/100 g/min, but favorable recovery occurred in none of those patients whose rate fell below that level. This suggests that a phasic elevation in CBF after TBI is necessary for functional recovery (Kelly D et al. 1997). The combination of increased CBF with an elevated ICP may indicate the loss of cerebral autoregulation, whereas increased CBF with a normal ICP suggests an appropriate relationship between metabolism and CBF, thus improving the chance for a favorable outcome (Kelly et al. 1996; Kelly D et al. 1997). Although the early changes in postinjury CBF are uncertain in the pediatric patient, the contribution of hypovolemia and CBF to mortality and morbidity has been established in this population (Mayer et al. 1981; Sharples et al. 1995).

It has been suggested that $CMRO_2$ is a stronger predictor of outcome than CBF. A significant association was seen between low $CMRO_2$ values and death or persistent vegetative state at 6 months after injury (Jaggi et al. 1990). In most children the cerebral metabolism is initially normal. However, at 1 to 3 days after injury a fall in both $CMRO_2$ and $AVDO_2$ can be observed. The likelihood of an unfavorable GOS outcome was greater in those children with a lower mean $CMRO_2$ over the first 24 hours (Sharples et al. 1995). Diaspirin crosslinked hemoglobin (DCLHb) has been used in efforts to increase the mean arterial pressure (MAP) and improve CBF. In animals, this agent also raises the cerebral perfusion pressure (CPP) and results in lower fluid loads for MAP maintenance. The effects on long-term outcome have not been assessed, but DCLHb may prove to be beneficial in the early treatment of hypovolemia and CBF (Chappell et al. 1996). The physiological effects of alterations in CBF after TBI remain unclear, as one study suggests a better outcome when isolated focal hyperemia is seen near intraparenchymal or extracerebral lesions. This information is confounded by the possibility that these patients may have initially sustained a less severe injury (Sakas et al. 1995). The variations in CBF and $CMRO_2$ following a brain injury may actually represent a continuum of hemodynamic responses to injury; mild changes could be part of the normal recovery process, but extreme fluctuations may result in secondary insults to the brain that further injury and worsen outcome.

### Intracranial Pressure

The normal ICP is between 0 and 10 mm Hg, and most centers involved in TBI management define an elevated ICP as any value above 20 mm Hg. In order to meet metabolic demands and prevent secondary complications the brain must have adequate tissue perfusion. Severe TBI patients are at great risk for developing intracranial hypertension, which can result in impaired cerebral perfusion. Sustained episodes of an ICP above 25 mm Hg have been associated with increased mortality and poor outcome by many researchers (Marshall et al. 1991; Aldrich et al. 1992a; Fearnside et al. 1993; Marmarou et al. 1991; Gopinath et al. 1993; Resnick et al. 1997). Although ICP elevations can have a negative influence, a prognosis should not be made on this information alone. Favorable GOS outcomes have been reported in 38% of severe TBI patients with prolonged (>96 hours) ICP elevations. This percentage increased to 60% in the younger patients, and rose even further when the GCS score was greater than 5 (Resnick et al. 1997).

A parameter that may be more important than absolute ICP is CPP, which is calculated by subtracting the ICP from the MAP (CPP = MAP − ICP). A low CPP can lead to cerebral ischemia and contribute to further neurological injury. One of the most important stategies in providing adequate cerebral oxygenation is maintenance of the CPP above 50 mm Hg (Prough and Lang 1997; Kiening et al. 1997). Rosner et al. have reported on the benefits of keeping the CPP at a minimum of 70 mm Hg. Patients treated to maintain this CPP parameter had a 29% mortality rate, and favorable GOS outcomes ranged from 35% in those patients with an initial GCS of 3 up to 75% for patients with a GCS score of 7. Volume expansion, ventriculostomy drainage, vasopressors, and mannitol were used to maintain the CPP (Rosner et al. 1995). Another study has shown the adverse effect of a CPP below 60 mm Hg (Gopinath et al. 1993). However, a recently completed study at Baylor College of Medicine showed that while maintaining a higher CPP resulted in a 20% reduction in the incidence of jugular oxygen desaturation, there was also a substantial increase in the incidence of adult respiratory distress syndrome (ARDS), which cancelled out any positive effect on outcome (C. S. Robertson, personal communication).

### Morphological Variables

CT and MRI can provide information regarding injury morphology and severity. Researchers have identified specific findings on imaging studies that are correlated with outcome (Table 22-7). Abnormalities that are predictive of mortality and disability include midline shift, compression or obliteration of the mesencephalic cisterns, subarachnoid blood (SAH), intraventricular hemorrhage (IVH), large-volume mass lesions, and diffuse edema or bilateral swelling (Aldrich et al. 1992a, 1992b; Eisenberg et al. 1990; Fearnside

**Table 22-7.** CT Findings and Clinical Effects

| Authors | Patient Population | CT Findings | Effects |
|---|---|---|---|
| Narayan et al. 1981 | Adults | High-density mass lesion | Unfavorable outcome by GOS |
| Marshall et al. 1983b | Adults | Midline shift, SDH | Clinical deterioration, mortality |
| Toutant et al. 1984 | Adults | Compressed cisterns | Increased mortality, severe disability |
| Eisenberg et al. 1990 | Adults | Midline shift, mass lesion, compressed cisterns, SAH | Increased mortality, elevated ICP |
| Marshall et al. 1991 | Adults | Midline shift, mass lesion, brain stem lesion | Increased mortality |
| Kido et al. 1992 | Adults | High-volume lesion | Unfavorable outcome by GOS |
| Fearnside et al. 1993 | Adults | Midline shift, cerebral edema, IVH, compressed cisterns | Increased mortality |
| | | Intracerebral contusion, SAH, hematoma | Unfavorable outcome by GOS |
| Aldrich et al. 1992b | Adults, penetrating injury | Midline shift, compressed cistern, SAH, IVH, hyperdense lesion | Unfavorable outcome by GOS |
| Levin et al. 1992 | ≤15 years | Diffuse swelling, mass lesion | Unfavorable outcome by GOS |
| Aldrich et al. 1992a | ≤16 years | Diffuse swelling | Increased mortality |

et al. 1993; Kido et al. 1992; Levin et al. 1992; Marshall et al. 1991, 1983b; Narayan et al. 1981; Toutant et al. 1984). The use of CT findings combined with prehospital and clinical variables can predict mortality with 84.4% accuracy; the same information can differentiate good versus poor outcome with an accuracy of 72.5% (Fearnside et al. 1993). The appearance of the basal cisterns on the initial CT can provide significant prognostic information. The mortality rate has been reported at 77% if the perimesencephalic cisterns are obliterated, 39% if they are compressed, and 22% if they are normal. In addition, patients with a GCS score of 6 to 8 and obliterated cisterns had a much higher risk of unfavorable outcome compared to those with normal cisterns (Toutant et al. 1984). Diffuse hemispheric edema on CT has been associated with early hypoxia and hypotension (Eisenberg et al. 1990). In children age 16 or younger, diffuse edema carries a high mortality rate of 53% compared to a rate of 16% in children without this finding (Aldrich et al. 1992a). CT imaging can also be beneficial in the chronic stage following TBI. Enlargement of the width of the third ventricle suggests diencephalic atrophy and has been correlated with persistent cognitive deficits, behavioral problems, and vocational outcome (Reider-Groswasser et al. 1993). Widening of the septum-caudate distance indicates loss of the deep gray nuclei and catastrophic injury; it has been correlated with the overall prognosis for recovery from a vegetative state after severe TBI (Reider-Groswasser et al. 1997).

MRI provides greater imaging detail and may reveal lesions not seen on CT. One study found that MRI detected a greater number of lesions when compared with CT studies in 85% of mild or moderate TBI patients (Levin et al. 1987). Decreases in brain volume and expansion of cerebrospinal fluid (CSF) spaces as measured by MRI volumetric studies have been correlated with neuropsychological outcome. This suggests that MRI volumetrics may be a useful tool in efforts to predict long-term cognitive outcome (Blatter et al. 1997). Single photon emission computed tomography (SPECT) and positron emission tomography (PET) can provide information on the functional state and metabolic activity of brain tissue. These tools are beginning to have a role in evaluations of TBI patients. SPECT shows promise in the assessment of mild to moderate TBI. Alterations identified on SPECT images in this population have correlated well with injury severity, and a negative early study is thought to be predictive of a good outcome. SPECT may become a useful tool in attempts to objectify sequelae in those patients with persistent postconcussive complaints (Jacobs et al. 1994). PET can show focal uptake in regions beyond those identified by MRI and CT, which may allow for diagnostic localization of both structural and functional lesions (Jansen et al. 1996). Dynamic and functional neuroimaging may have a future role in TBI management by providing information about cerebral function.

### Duration of Coma or Post-traumatic Amnesia

After a severe brain injury patients can have a variable amount of time in a nonresponsive and confusional state. The importance of this period has been recognized since 1932, when Russell proposed that the sum of the comatose and confusional periods would be the most useful predictor of outcome (Russell, 1932). The duration of coma provides useful information regarding injury severity, and the significant prognostic implications of this measure were first described by Symonds in 1928 (Symonds, 1928). When DAI is the primary injury there is almost a linear relationship between the duration of coma and recovery time (Katz, 1992). The length of coma has also been correlated with the presence of residual impairments (Hall et al. 1993; Spettell et al. 1991; Wilson et al. 1991; Woischneck et al. 1997; Katz and Alexander 1994). One study found that none of the patients remaining comatose for more than 2 weeks had a good outcome. It was suggested that increasing periods of coma might have a proportional relationship to functional outcome (Katz and Alexander 1994). Another study suggests that the GOS is a direct reflection of whatever process determines the length of coma (Spettell et al. 1991). Cognitive function after TBI (including memory, attention, and learning skills) has been associated with coma duration (Wilson et al. 1991; Woischneck et al. 1997). The length of coma also relates to the ability for returning to work or school (Katz, 1992; Ruff et al. 1993). In addition, the recovery of motor function after TBI has been correlated with the duration of coma (MacPherson et al. 1992). The adequate assessment and documentation of coma length should be emphasized in TBI management to provide assistance with long-term decision making and prognostic efforts.

The recovery of consciousness also proceeds along a different time-line for each patient. During this process the TBI patient will demonstrate a period of PTA, which is defined as the time from injury until the patient shows continuous memory for ongoing events. Since 1961, PTA has been identified as "the best yardstick" to measure the severity of a head injury (Editorial, 1961). The presence of PTA is often assessed prospectively by using the GOAT scale (Appendix B), with a score of greater than 75 marking the end of PTA. It can also be estimated retrospectively with good validity (McMillan et al. 1996). Many researchers have reported on the powerful prognostic value of PTA duration as a measure of injury severity (Katz and Alexander 1994; Hall et al. 1993; Bishara et al. 1992; Zafonte et al. 1997b). Patients with prolonged PTA have shown more extensive tissue damage on MRI, with lesions present in both central structures and hemispheric areas (Wilson et al. 1993). Katz and Alexander found that PTA has a strong predictive relationship to GOS in those patients with DAI, with a direct correlation between longer duration of PTA and worse outcomes. No patients having a PTA longer than 12 weeks had a good recovery, whereas 80% of patients with PTA less than 2 weeks had a good recovery (Katz and Alexander 1994). Another study found that the duration of PTA was predictive of acute rehabilitation FIM scores, as well as both admission and discharge DRS results (Zafonte et al. 1997b). Monitoring of PTA can provide a global measurement of brain damage and is a key element in prognostic efforts after TBI.

### Neurophysiological Variables

Evoked potentials can be used in the assessment of the TBI patient to evaluate the responsiveness of the CNS to external stimuli. They also provide information that can assist in outcome predictions. However, they require some expertise and are not widely used for outcome prediction. Evoked potentials that have been assessed after TBI include the somatosensory (SSEP), visual (VEP), auditory (BAEP), and P300 responses. One study found that the combined multimodality evoked potentials (MEP) test was the single best prognostic indicator when compared to the clinical exam, CT, and ICP. Combining the MEP with the clinical exam provided the maximum predictive accuracy (Narayan et al. 1981). Many researchers have found a high predictive accuracy for poor progno-

sis when there is bilateral loss of the SSEP due to diffuse injury (Pohlmann-Eden et al. 1997; Moulton et al. 1994; Gutling et al. 1993; Beca et al. 1995). The reliability of SSEP data increases with serial recordings. During hourly ICU monitoring one study has found that deterioration in the SSEPs would often occur prior to elevations of ICP, and the final summed SSEP correlated with the GOS (Konasiewicz et al. 1994). VEPs are easy to perform and interpret, but they do not have the predictive accuracy of SSEPs. Prolongation of the VEP has shown a linear relationship with changes in ICP, and thus may have some relationship to outcome (Kane et al. 1996; York et al. 1981). Although generally less reliable than SSEP findings, BAEP may be a useful monitoring tool in the acute phase after injury, as these responses are the least likely to be affected by barbiturates (Newlon et al. 1983). A potential problem in their clinical effectiveness is that they rely on an intact peripheral auditory system. Serial BAEPs can potentially give an early warning of uncal herniation, since changes in the responses have been seen prior to pupillary changes (Barelli et al. 1991). Often, early after injury the TBI patient cannot undergo direct cognitive testing at that time, these modalities can help provide information regarding cognitive function. In this setting evoked responses are best used in a serial fashion to monitor for change and assist in rehabilitation planning. In the chronic phase the SSEP and BAEP can continue to provide predictive information, but SSEPs maintain a higher predictive value for functional recovery (Shin et al. 1989; Goldberg and Karazim 1998). Long-latency somatosensory (LL-SEP) and cortical auditory (CAER) evoked potentials may give better prognostic information in the chronic phase after TBI (Rappaport et al. 1990b, 1991). The combination of testing all three sensory modalities has demonstrated a high correlation with the patient's clinical condition in the rehabilitation setting and outcome at 1 year after injury (Rappaport et al. 1981).

Recently, an evoked potential paradigm has been used to assess cognition and neuropsychological activity. Long-latency event-related potentials (ERP) are obtained in response to the infrequent presentation of a novel, brief stimulus within a background of brief, frequently repeating stimuli. The modality for the stimuli may be the same (i.e., two different auditory tones) or different (i.e., visual or auditory). The ERP is a positive deflection that occurs approximately 300 ms (P300) after presentation of the novel stimuli, and can be seen both passively or with the patient actively counting the stimuli. The passive response can be enhanced by the use of different sensory stimuli in the testing paradigm (Rappaport et al. 1990a). This testing technique provides a means for cognitive assessment in nonresponsive patients; it is thought to reflect the cortical processing of information and can be used as a measure of cognitive recovery (Clark et al. 1992). A prolonged latency of this response has been shown with both PTA and severe TBI (Papanicolaou et al. 1984; Rappaport and Clifford 1994). The ERP may also provide prognostic information for severe injuries. It has shown a very significant correlation with 3-month outcome (Kane et al. 1996), and absence of this response suggests that a patient will not regain consciousness (Rappaport and Clifford 1994).

A conventional electroencephalogram (EEG) has limited value in predicting acute events or outcome from TBI. In the early postinjury phase there are a few EEG findings that can provide some clinical information. The presence of normal sleep spindles 48 hours or beyond after injury has been associated with a favorable outcome (Rumpl et al. 1983). In addition, death has been associated with the presence of an isoelectric study or repeated isoelectric intervals, nonreactive alpha, or a theta pattern of EEG activity (Hutchison et al. 1991; Synek, 1988). Late in the clinical course a low-voltage, nonreactive EEG suggests a poor outcome (Bricolo and Turella 1990). The combination of EEG reactivity with SSEP data has been able to predict a good versus bad outcome with 98% accuracy (Gutling et al. 1995). Recently, a variation of the conventional EEG called compressed spectral array (CSA) has shown good prognostic accuracy for brain injury. The combination of CSA-EEG with the GCS at the time of the EEG has reportedly been able to discriminate between death and good outcome at 1 year with 95.8% accuracy (Thatcher et al. 1991). In general, these neurophysiological studies are most useful for predicting survival in the acute unresponsive period after severe TBI.

## Management Issues

There are several aspects of the management of patients with head injury that can impact on the ultimate outcome. These are briefly reviewed here, since they directly or indirectly alter prognosis.

## ICP Management

### Hyperventilation

Hypothermia has been used for more than 2 decades in the treatment of TBI for its effects on ICP. A survey in 1995 found that hyperventilation was still a common method of ICP control (Ghajar et al. 1995). This common practice needs to be modified in response to more recent data demonstrating its potentially adverse effects in the TBI patient. CBF is decreased during the first 24 hours after TBI. The vasoconstrictive effects of severe hyperventilation ($PCO_2$ <25) can further decrease CBF thus causing secondary ischemia (Kiening et al. 1997). Thus, hyperventilation clearly can reduce ICP, but it has a negative influence on many other parameters including ti-$PO_2$, $SjvO_2$, cerebral autoregulation, $CMRO_2$, and $AVDO_2$ (Obrist et al. 1984; 1987; Unterberg et al. 1997). In addition, recent animal studies found that hippocampal CA3 neurons have a selective vulnerability to hyperventilation (Forbes et al. 1998). Prophylactic prolonged hyperventilation has been shown to result in worse outcomes at 6 months when compared to patients that remained normocapneic (Muizelaar et al. 1991). Short-term hyperventilation therapy can be helpful in patients who are herniating, but at this time long-term prophylactic hyperventilation is not indicated in severe TBI due to the potential for secondary ischemia (AANS, 1995).

### Pharmacological Agents

Sedation and neuromuscular blockade is often used during transportation and in the ED for severe TBI patients. One study looked at the role of early, prophylactic neuromuscular blockade on outcome and found there was no clear beneficial effect. In fact, results suggested that the use of neuromuscular was detrimental due to increases in the length of ICU stays, pneumonia, and sepsis. This study recommended that only sedation be used in early ICU care after brain injury, and neuromuscular blockade be reserved for refractory ICP elevations (Hsiang et al. 1994). If sedation and chemical paralysis are necessary, then short-acting agents are recommended in order to minimize the effects these agents have on the ability to obtain a proper neurological evaluation.

Mannitol has been used for over 20 years as an agent to manage ICP. Although there have been no placebo-controlled trials to assess the effects of mannitol on functional outcome, it has shown beneficial effects on CPP, CBF, and metabolism. The effects of mannitol and hyperventilation on ICP control have been compared. Both agents improved CPP and lowered ICP, but mannitol accomplished the task without affecting cerebral oxygenation, whereas hyperventilation resulted in decreased oxygenation (Unterberg et al. 1997). Another study compared the effects of mannitol versus barbiturates for ICP management. Mannitol was found to maintain the desired CPP range better than barbiturates. In addition, the mannitol group had a 41% mortality rate compared to a 77% rate in the barbiturate group (Schwartz et al. 1984).

Barbiturates have been used for managing ICP since the 1930s; these agents have been used for both preventing and treating ICP elevations. One proposed mechanism of action is by lowering cerebral metabolic requirements, which should result in less demand for CBF with subsequent reduction in cerebral blood volume and ICP. One study suggested that barbiturates should not be used as a prophylactic treatment due to the possible development of hypotension and secondary ischemia. Additionally, the group receiving prophylactic treatment showed no benefit on the GOS at 1 year (Ward et al. 1985). Barbiturate therapy may have a role in treating refractory ICP elevations when other interventions have failed. Lower mortality rates have been reported for patients that achieve ICP control with barbiturate therapy compared to nonresponding patients (Rea and Rockswold 1983; Eisenberg et al. 1988). Outcome assessments of patients with an ICP greater than 40 mm Hg also suggest that 50% of those patients who respond to barbiturates have a good recovery (Marshall et al. 1979). Unfortunately, barbiturates may have adverse effects on other parameters that can also influence outcome. In some patients, barbiturate therapy leads to a fall in $SjvO_2$ below 45%; these patients had a significantly worse outcome even though the two groups showed no differences in ICP or CPP after treatment (Cruz, 1996). A literature review of barbiturate use in pediatric TBI patients found that there was no clear-cut benefit from this therapy, and it was associated with significant complications. It was therefore recommended that barbiturates should not be used routinely for ICP control in this population (Trauner, 1986). Although mortality data suggest that barbiturate therapy may have a role in management of refractory ICP elevations, there is a paucity of information regarding the morbidity in survivors. Barbiturate therapy increases the risk of hypotension and hypoxia, both of which have known adverse effects on TBI outcome. Barbiturates should therefore not be used indiscriminately in the TBI patient. In patients who are hypotensive, the use of barbiturate coma is contraindicated (Eisenberg et al. 1988).

## Surgery

The importance of neurosurgical intervention for a hematoma or contusion with significant mass effect has already been mentioned. Early surgery is generally warranted for a traumatic subdural, epidural, or intracerebral hematoma causing a midline shift of greater than 5 mm on CT (Seelig, 1981; Marshall et al. 1983b). Surgery may also play a role in management of ICP. A small study on the use of decompressive bifrontal craniectomy to treat post-traumatic refractory cerebral edema found benefit from this intervention, with a mortality rate of 23% and a favorable recovery seen in 37% of the survivors. The patients undergoing surgery within 48 hours of injury and before the ICP was greater than 40 mm Hg for any sustained period of time had the best results, and this group had a favorable recovery rate of 60% (Polin et al. 1997). In certain patients, neurological deterioration or intractable ICP may also respond to a lobectomy. A small study reported a favorable recovery in over 50% of patients receiving this treatment. Younger age, higher initial GCS, and better pupillary reactivity were associated with a better outcome (Litofsky et al. 1994).

## Steroids

Glucocorticoids have been used in the treatment of brain edema since the early 1960s. Their role in the management of cerebral edema secondary to trauma is unclear. A review of the randomized, controlled clinical trials evaluating steroids in the management of TBI could prove neither benefit nor harm from their use (Alderson and Roberts 1997). The 1995 Guidelines for the Management of Severe Head Injury published by the AANS state that the use of glucocorticoids is not recommended for improving outcome or ICP control in severe TBI (AANS, 1995). Use of these agents may actually result in hyperglycemia and lead to other complications (Kelly, 1995; Lam et al. 1991).

Inflammatory responses may contribute to the pathophysiology of TBI, which has led researchers to investigate the role of anti-inflammatory agents in the care of brain injury. Indomethacin is one such agent, and its role in the management of ICP has been recently reviewed (Harrigan et al. 1997). It is a cyclo-oxygenase inhibitor, and acts similar to hyperventilation through vasoconstriction and CBF reduction with the benefit of not affecting $CMRO_2$ (Jensen et al. 1991). In animals, it has been shown to lower ICP by decreasing cerebral edema (Deluga et al. 1991) and CSF production (Schalk et al. 1992). Indomethacin has recently been used in severe TBI patients for treatment of elevated ICP; a 50-mg bolus was found to significantly reduce ICP and improve CPP (Biestro et al. 1995). In addition, the antipyretic properties of indomethacin may provide some neuroprotective tissue effects through the lowering of body temperature (Jensen et al. 1991; Benedek et al. 1987). The advantages of indomethacin use include easy administration, a lack of systemic adaptation, and beneficial effects on cerebral edema and metabolism that help decrease the risk of secondary ischemia (Harrigan et al. 1997). Large, randomized controlled trials will be needed to assess the role of indomethacin in acute TBI management.

## Hypothermia

Moderate hypothermia as a therapeutic intervention following TBI has been the focus of many recent studies. The results of a Phase II trial of moderate hypothermia in severe TBI were published in 1993. Cooling blankets were placed on patients in the treatment group within 6 hours of injury. The goal was to achieve an intravascular temperature of 32° to 33°C, maintain this range for 48 hours, and then gradually rewarm the patient. The follow-up analysis found that there was a 16% increase in the number of patients with a favorable GOS recovery at 3 months as compared to those with an unfavorable GOS (Clifton et al. 1993a). These promising early results led to a pilot randomized, controlled trial assessing moderate hypothermia for 24 hours in severe TBI patients. In this study a favorable outcome by GOS was seen in 62% of the hypothermic group at the 12-month follow-up compared to 38% of the normothermic group. Hypothermia was associated with significantly improved 3- and 6-month outcomes in those patients with an initial GCS of 5 to 7, but this

difference was not maintained at 12 months, suggesting that it hastened the recovery process of the treatment group. Unfortunately, hypothermia was not beneficial for patients with an admission GCS of 3 to 4 (Marion et al. 1997). The mechanism of action through which hypothermia provides neuroprotection is unclear. It has been reported to decrease cerebral oxygen metabolism, lower ICP, and attenuate the negative neurochemical cascade effects initiated after TBI (Busto et al. 1989; Marion et al. 1996). A larger prospective, randomized, multicenter trial of hypothermia in severe head injury has prematurely closed patient accrual and the trial results are to be announced soon (G. L. Clifton, personal communication, 1998).

## Hyperglycemia and Nutrition

Metabolic alterations after brain injury may contribute to the neuronal injury and neurological impairment. Hyperglycemia is a component of the stress response after TBI, and serum glucose levels above 200 mg/dl have shown significant correlation with unfavorable recovery in all age groups (Lam 1991; Young et al. 1989, Michaud et al. 1992). In animals, the use of 5% dextrose solution for fluid resuscitation after cerebral injury resulted in hyperglycemia and significantly higher mortality rates (Feldman et al. 1995).

The alterations in energy metabolism following TBI have prompted investigations into the role of nutrition on recovery. Metabolic expenditures of comatose patients vary from 120% to 250% of expected levels. Increased mortality was seen in patients unable to receive complete nutritional support for 2 weeks after injury compared to patients that tolerated full feeding by day 7 (Rapp et al. 1983). In small studies, early nutritional support appeared to be associated with a better rate of neurological recovery (Young et al. 1987).

## Post-traumatic Seizures and Anticonvulsants

Post-traumatic epilepsy (PTE) has been reported in up to 53% of the patients sustaining a penetrating brain injury in a military combat setting (Salazar et al. 1985). An extensive study on the incidence of unprovoked post-traumatic seizures in civilians has recently been published (Annengers et al. 1998). It reviewed 30 years of data and reported that there was a significant relation between the severity of injury and the risk of post-traumatic seizures. The 5- and 30-year cumulative seizure probabilities for patients with a mild head injury were 0.7% and 2.1%, respectively. These rates increased in those patients with moderate injuries to 1.2% and 4.2%. Severe TBI patients had the highest cumulative probability, with 10% at 5 years and an increase to 16.7% over 30 years. The first year after injury showed the greatest incidence of seizure occurrence among all levels of severity. The incidence remained fairly stable after 1 year in those patients with mild injuries. Patients with moderate injuries showed an increase in the risk of seizures for up to 10 years before they stabilized. Severe TBI patients demonstrated a significantly elevated seizure risk throughout the follow-up period. After a patient has their first post-traumatic seizure there are often questions raised as to whether it represents an isolated event or implies the start of a chronic problem. A study addressing this issue found that recurrent seizures occurred in 86% of the patients who had an unprovoked late post-traumatic seizure. The majority of recurrent seizures were seen in the first year after the initial event (Haltiner et al. 1997). Risk factors associated with the development of post-traumatic seizures include intracerebral contusion, SDH, prolonged coma or PTA, and skull fracture (Annengers et al. 1998; Haltiner et al. 1997). The mechanism or event that initiates post-traumatic seizures is still unknown. It has been suggested that the biochemical reactions to the release of blood products into brain tissue may be the inciting process (Willmore, 1990).

The high incidence of recurrence after an initial late post-traumatic seizure argues for aggressive treatment with anticonvulsants in an effort to prevent further events. Unfortunately, the data regarding the effectiveness of therapy are not very promising. A well-designed study investigating the use of phenytoin for prevention of post-traumatic seizures found that it was only useful during the first week after TBI. There was a 73% decrease in seizure risk for the phenytoin group in that time period. Beyond 1 week there was no benefit to phenytoin therapy. During the first year, seizures occurred in 22% of the treatment group and 16% of the placebo group, by the second year these numbers were 28% and 21%, respectively (Temkin et al. 1990). Although there was not a statistically significant difference between the two groups, a larger percentage of patients in the phenytoin group developed late seizures. Phenytoin therapy has also shown negative cognitive effects on

neurobehavioral assessments at 1 month after injury when compared to a placebo group (Dikmen et al. 1991). The apparent lack of efficacy and potential for adverse effects with phenytoin use has led researchers to consider other anticonvulsants. Carbamazepine may provide effective early seizure control, but it also did not show any benefit for preventing late seizures (Schierhout and Roberts 1998). A recent study using valproic acid for post-traumatic seizure prophylaxis found no benefit for either early or late seizure control (N. R. Temkin, personal communication, 1998). Carbamazepine and valproic acid are thought to have fewer adverse effects on cognition and be less sedating than phenytoin; thus they are the preferred anticonvulsants for seizure management in the rehabilitation setting. Unfortunately, recent studies are raising doubts about these assumptions. All three agents have been shown to impair cognitive function, especially with higher plasma levels (Kirschner et al. 1991; Massagli, 1991). It is hoped that one of the newly introduced anticonvulsants will provide effective post-traumatic seizure prophylaxis with limited cognitive effects.

## Neuroprotective Agents

A cascade of biochemical events is initiated following a traumatic injury to the brain, and can result in secondary injury. The cascade starts with a release of primarily excitatory neurotransmitters (glutamate and acetylcholine). Alterations in cellular receptor channels follow, leading to changes of ionic concentrations, increased arachidonic acid metabolism, and free oxygen radical formation. A full discussion of this process is beyond the scope of this chapter. Readers interested in further information are directed to the extensive reviews on neurochemical changes and potential pharmacological interventions after TBI by McIntosh (McIntosh 1993, 1994). Modulation of this cascade at different levels is being attempted through the use of neuroprotective pharmacological agents. Although there have been some promising preliminary data, clinical studies have not been positive to date (Doppenberg and Bullock 1997). A number of factors may contribute to the differences between animal data, early human data, and final large clinical studies. These include heterogeneous patient populations, variations in the mechanism of experimental and clinical injury, time differences in the "therapeutic window" for neurochemical responses between animal and human injury, changes in the neurochemical balances due to alterations in the blood-brain barrier, measurement techniques and limitations, and outcome assessment parameters (Bullock 1993).

## Rehabilitation Issues

The intensity of rehabilitation services required after brain injury is primarily determined by the severity of injury. Mild head injury usually does not require inpatient rehabilitation services; instead, education regarding the clinical course and potential sequelae from this type of injury is helpful in facilitating the natural recovery process. Inpatient rehabilitation for moderate and severe injury appears to have a positive effect on functional outcome, but this has not been subjected to a prospective randomized trial.

Thus, although it is generally believed that early rehabilitative efforts help maximize ultimate recovery from TBI, there are very limited data that prove this. A recent study evaluating the functional outcomes after rehabilitation for severe TBI reported that over 73% of patients had a significant increase in FIM scores during their inpatient rehabilitation admission, with 53% of the patients being discharged to their homes (Whitlock and Hamilton 1995). How much of this improvement was due to the rehabilitative efforts as opposed to the natural course of recovery is difficult to discern. A review of the literature on long-term effects of rehabilitation was published in 1995. Although a direct comparison of the studies could not be accomplished due to the variations in outcome measures used, overall each study reported that rehabilitation was beneficial following TBI (Hall and Cope 1995). The time frame for initiation of rehabilitation services has changed in the present managed care environment. It is currently believed that rehabilitation should start immediately after medical stabilization in the ICU setting. One study has found that an early transfer to the inpatient rehabilitation setting (i.e., <35 days following injury) can result in an overall decrease in the length of hospitalization. These patients had been matched for age, severity of injury, neuroimaging results, and neurosurgical procedures (Cope and Hall 1982). However, many insurance companies will not pay for inpatient rehabilitation unless a patient can participate in at least 3 hours of therapy a day. Further-

more, most patients have a limited number of inpatient rehabilitation days allowed on their coverage. These factors often require a patient to first go to subacute rehabilitation units or to a long-term nursing facility until their level of consciousness improves and they are capable of more fully cooperating with their therapists.

Strength, sitting, and standing balance on admission to the rehabilitation setting, (in addition to age and initial GCS score) have shown predictive value for the functional outcome at discharge (Black et al. 1997). The length of acute hospitalization and gender can also be used to help predict the rehabilitation length of stay (Spettell et al. 1991). Recently, a tool has been designed that uses disability measures to predict what length of stay will be necessary in the rehabilitation setting to achieve specific functional gains (Davis et al. 1997). In the present era of cost-effective medical care this type of information is vital to the clinical decision-making process regarding the appropriate levels of long-term care following TBI.

Although it is commonly believed that the majority of recovery following any brain injury occurs in the first 6 months following injury, the length of rehabilitation and time course of recovery can be difficult to predict. A recent study of recovery following a severe brain injury found that many patients progress for 6 months and then improvement levels off (Choi et al. 1994). In addition, the 3-month GOS was predictive of the 6-month outcome. A favorable recovery was seen at 6 months in 56% of the patients discharged with severe disability, and by 12 months further progress was seen with 76% having a favorable outcome. The most striking finding was seen in those patients discharged in a vegetative state: at 12 months only 28% remained vegetative, 44% were severely disabled, and 28% had achieved a favorable outcome. Another study assessing the recovery of patients discharged in a vegetative state found that 58% had regained consciousness by 3 years after injury. Unfortunately, they were unable to identify variables that could be used to predict which patients would emerge from the vegetative state (Levin et al. 1991). These data suggest that decisions regarding continuation of supportive care for the vegetative patient should best be deferred to beyond 6 months, especially in young patients. One study found that 90% of severe TBI patients had returned to a home environment by 1 year after rehabilitation. Of these, 16% required supervision, 82% were independent most of the day, and 25% had returned to some level of work (Hawkins et al. 1996). A long-term follow-up study found that, although visual difficulties, headaches, and fatigue often persist, many improvements in functional outcome can occur far beyond 6 months after injury. They reported increases in independence for personal, domestic, and community activities, as well as cognitive, behavioral, and emotional changes during years 2 to 5 following injury (Olver et al. 1996). This information suggests that intermittent rehabilitation interventions may be beneficial for years after the original injury. The gains achieved in functional recovery through rehabilitation are stable for up to 14 years following TBI, with younger patients showing the maximum stability and best outcomes (Ashley et al. 1997). Rehabilitation should not be viewed as a static event following a severe brain injury, but instead should be considered a lifelong continuum of recovery and progress.

Recent advances in understanding the biomechanical and neurochemical events of brain injury have led to a greater role for pharmacological interventions in the rehabilitation process. Targeted neurotransmitter pathways include the dopaminergic, cholinergic, γ-aminobutyric acid, serotonergic, and noradrenergic systems (Boyeson and Harmon 1994). Arousal, motivation, and responsiveness have been shown to increase with the use of dopamine agonists, psychostimulants, and tricyclic antidepressants. These agents, as well as certain anticonvulsants (valproic acid, carbamazepine), β-adrenergic antagonists, antipsychotics, buspirone, and lithium may be beneficial in treating agitation and aggression (Mysiw and Sandel 1997). The use of any pharmacological agent must be tempered by an awareness of the potential for adverse effects. The sedation caused by benzodiazepines may slow the emergence from coma; motor recovery can be impaired by the use of antipsychotics and carbamazepine. Readers interested in further information on this topic are directed to the extensive subject reviews that have recently been published (Mysiw and Sandel 1997; Boyeson and Harmon 1994).

### Cognitive and Vocational Outcome

The cognitive deficits after TBI are commonly assessed through neuropsychological tests. Unfortunately, a complete neuropsychological battery

is a challenging and often overwhelming endeavor for many TBI survivors. Efforts have been made to identify the least number of tests done in the acute period that can provide the greatest amount of relevant, prognostic information for 3- and 6-month outcomes. Four tests have been identified: Controlled Oral Word Association, Grooved Pegboard, Trailmaking Part B, and the Rey-Osterrieth Complex Figure Delayed Recall. The Grooved Pegboard test assesses fine motor coordination and can account for 80% of the GOS variance. Only 15% of the study patients with severe TBI could not complete this battery of tests (Clifton et al. 1993b). Serial neuropsychological test data have found that information processing speed, memory skills, and simultaneous processing abilities are related to the level of functional outcome (Girard et al. 1996). Levin et al. report that impairment in memory and slowness of information processing are common 1 year after severe TBI, but language and visuospatial ability often recover to a normal range (Levin et al. 1990). Five years after injury 50% of severe, 14.3% of moderate, and 3.1% of mild injuries still demonstrate cognitive impairments (slow speech or reaction time) and attention and comprehension problems. The prevalence of post injury headaches, dizziness, and anxiety may be similar among all three TBI groups, but long-term memory impairments and depressed mood tend to increase with injury severity (Masson et al. 1996).

Cognitive screening finds that memory, followed by attention and reasoning abilities, are the areas most frequently affected in the mild TBI patient. Patients with a GCS score of 13 or 14 had more problems identified on the screening tests when compared to the patients with a GCS score of 15 (Blostein et al. 1997). Cognitive screening provides data that can assist in the early planning of appropriate rehabilitation programs, and subsequent follow-up studies can contribute further information to help with predicting functional recovery and long-term prognosis.

A greater emphasis is being placed on community re-entry and vocational rehabilitation after TBI, with specialized postacute rehabilitation programs being developed to help patients achieve their maximum potential. These programs have reported that 56% of the patients gain independence in work, school, or homemaking compared to 43% of the patients that were not participating in a specialized re-entry program (Malec and Basford 1996). Formalized case-management systems have been suggested as a way to facilitate the start of vocational and rehabilitation services after a brain injury (Malec et al. 1995). Factors that can help predict a return to work or school include the patient's age, verbal intellectual power, information processing speed, performance IQ, emotional disturbances, and the presence of vocational services (Ruff et al. 1993; Ip et al. 1995; Crepeau and Schevzer 1993; Dikmen et al. 1994).

A recent South Australian study assessed the 5-year outcome of TBI patients, 73% of whom had severe injuries: 40% were employed full-time, 6% maintained part-time employment, and 50% of the patients were reliant on welfare (Hillier et al. 1997). A study based out of Seattle, Washington, looked at the probability of previously employed patients returning to work following a brain injury. At 1 year after injury, 80% of the patients with mild head injuries had returned to work compared to only 25% of those with severe TBI. In contrast, a 48% employment rate was found in the patients that had sustained severe trauma without an associated brain injury. Patients that returned to work usually did so within the first 6 months after injury. The amount of time necessary prior to returning to work was related to the patient's age, severity of injury, duration of coma, level of education, and preinjury work stability patterns. A coma duration of 29 days or greater was strongly predictive of a failure to return to work, with only 8% of these patients being employed by 2 years after injury. This can be compared to the 96% employment rate found for patients that showed excellent cognitive functioning on their 1-month postinjury testing (Dikmen et al. 1994).

Community activities are an essential part of our daily lives, and program development emphasizing vocational and community re-entry for TBI survivors needs to become an integral part of rehabilitation services. It should be emphasized that in assessing outcome in any patient group, the preinjury or baseline performance is a critical factor. A poorly educated and unemployed patient is unlikely to become a high-performing individual after the injury, regardless of the acute or post-acute interventions. While this may seem self-evident, correcting for such issues is difficult due to the limited amount of population-specific neuropsychological data.

## Conclusions

Much has been learned over the past 2 decades about the factors that predict outcome after traumatic brain injury. While the initial and serial neurological exams form the primary basis for prognostication, the confidence of such predictions can be enhanced modestly with additional data derived from CT, ICP, EPs, and other such tests. However, no prognostic system can be unfailingly accurate because of the inherent unpredictability of biological systems. Thus, predictions may be falsely optimistic or falsely pessimistic. Earlier in the course, most errors tend to be in the falsely optimistic category due to subsequent complications. However, falsely pessimistic predictions are perhaps more dangerous, since they foster therapeutic nihilism. One must be very wary about throwing in the proverbial towel, especially in young patients early in the postinjury period. Unless patients are virtually brain dead when seen, we tend to treat them aggressively. While several systems have been reported for predicting outcome after severe brain injury, caution should be exercised in applying one center's statistics to another because of differences in populations, management techniques, and a host of other variables.

## References

AANS, Foundation TBT. Guidelines for the management of severe head injury, 1995.

Alderson, P.; Roberts, I. Corticosteroids in acute traumatic brain injury: systemic review of randomized controlled trials. BMJ 314:1855–1859; 1997.

Aldrich, E.; Eisenberg, E.; Saydjari, C.; et al. Diffuse brain swelling in severely head-injured children. A report from the NIH Traumatic Coma Data Bank. J. Neurosurg. 76:450–454; 1992a.

Aldrich, E.; Eisenberg, H.; Saydjari, C.; et al. Predictors of mortality in severely head-injured patients with civilian gunshot wounds: a report from the NIH Traumatic Coma Data Bank. Surg. Neurol. 38:418–423; 1992b.

Alexander, M. Neuropsychiatric correlates of persistent postconcussive syndrome. J. Head Trauma Rehabil. 7:60–69; 1992.

Annengers, J.; Hauser, W.; Coan, S.; et al. A population-based study of seizures after traumatic brain injuries. N. Engl. J. Med. 338:20–24; 1998.

Ashley, M.; Persel, C.; Clark, M.; et al. Long-term follow-up of post acute traumatic brain injury rehabilitation: a statistical analysis to test for stability and predictability of outcome. Brain Injury 11:677–690; 1997.

Asikainen, I.; Kaste, M.; Sarna, S. Patients with traumatic brain injury referred to a rehabilitation and re-employment programme: social and professional outcome for 508 Finnish patients 5 or more years after injury. Brain Injury 10:883–899; 1996.

Barelli, A.; Valente, M.; Clemente, A.; et al. Serial multi-modality evoked potentials in severely head injured patients: diagnostic and prognostic implications. Crit. Care Med. 19:1374–1381; 1991.

Barlow, P.; Teasdale, G. Prediction of outcome and the management of severe head injuries: the attitude of neurosurgeons. Neurosurgery 19:989–991; 1986.

Beca, J.; Cox, P.; Taylor, M.; et al. Somatosensory evoked potentials for prediction of outcome in acute severe brain injury. J. Pediatr. 126:44–49; 1995.

Benedek, G.; Toth-Daru, P.; Janaky, J.; et al. Indomethacin is effective against neurogenic hyperthermia following cranial trauma or brain surgery. Can. J. Neurol. Sci. 14:145–148; 1987.

Benzer, A.; Mitterschiffthaler, G.; Marosi, M.; et al. Prediction of non-survival after trauma: Innsbruck Coma Scale. Lancet 338:977–978; 1991.

Biestro, A.; Alberti, R.; Soca, A.; et al. Use of indomethacin in brain-injured patients with cerebral perfusion impairment: a preliminary report. J. Neurosurg. 83:627–630; 1995.

Bishara, S.; Partidge, F.; Godfrey, H.; et al. Post-traumatic amnesia and Glasgow Coma Scale related to outcome in survivors in a consecutive series of patients with severe closed head injury. Brain Injury 6:373–380; 1992.

Black, K.; Mann, N.; Zafonte, R.; et al. Sitting balance following brain injury: does it predict outcome? (poster presentation). Atlanta, GA: American Academy of Physical Medicine & Rehabilitation Annual Meeting; 1997.

Blatter, D.; Bigler, E.; Gale, S.; et al. MR-based brain and cerebrospinal fluid measurement after traumatic brain injury: correlation with neuropsychological outcome. Am. J. Neuroradiol. 18:1–10; 1997.

Blostein, P.; Jones, S.; Buechler, C.; et al. Cognitive screening in mild traumatic brain injuries: analysis of the neurobehavioral cognitive status examination when utilized during initial trauma hospitalization. J. Neurotrauma 14:171–177; 1997.

Blumbergs, P.; Jones, N.; North, J. Diffuse axonal injury in head trauma. J. Neurol. Neurosurg. Psychiatry 52:838–841; 1989.

Born, J.; Albert, A.; Hans, P.; et al. Relative prognostive value of best motor response and brain stem reflexes in patients with severe brain injury. Neurosurgery 16:595–601; 1985.

Bouma, G.; Muizelaar, J. Cerebral blood flow in severe clinical head injury. New Horizons 3:384–394; 1995.

Bowers, D.; Kofroth, L. Comparisons of Disability Rating Scale and Functional Independence Measures during recovery from traumatic brain injury (abstract). Arch. Phys. Med. Rehabil. 70:A58; 1989.

Boyd, C.; Tolson, M.; Copes, W. Evaluating trauma care: the TRISS method. Trauma Score and the Injury Severity Score. J. Trauma 27:370–378; 1987.

Boyeson, M.; Harmon, R. Acute and postacute drug-induced effects on rate of behavioral recovery after brain injury. J. Head Trauma Rehabil. 9:78–90; 1994.

Braakman, R.; Gelpke, G.; Habbema, J.; et al. Systemic selection of prognostic features in patients with severe head injury. Neurosurgery 6:362–370; 1980.

Bratton, S.; Davis, R. Acute lung injury in isolated traumatic brain injury. Neurosurgery 40:707–712; 1997.

Bricolo, A.; Turella, G. Electrophysiology of head injury. In: Vinken, P.; Bruyn, G.; Klawans, H., eds. Handbook of clinical neurology. New York: Elsevier; 1990.

Brooks, C.; Lindstrom, J.; McCray, J.; et al. Cost of medical care for a population-based sample of persons surviving traumatic brain injury. J. Head Trauma Rehabil. 10:1–13; 1995.

Bryant, E.; Sundance, P.; Hobbs, A.; et al. Managing costs and outcome of patients with traumatic brain injury in the HMO setting. J. Head Trauma Rehabil. 8:15–29; 1993.

Bullock, R. Opportunities for neuroprotective drugs in clinical management of head injury. J. Emerg. Med. 11:23–30; 1993.

Busto, R.; Globus, M.; Dietrich, D.; et al. Effect of mild hypothermia on ischemia-induced release of neurotransmitters and free fatty acids in the rat brain. Stroke 20:904–910; 1989.

Champion, H.; Sacco, W.; Copes, W.; et al. A revision of the trauma score. J. Trauma 29:623–629; 1989.

Chappell, J.; McBride, W.; Shackford, S. Diaspirin cross-linked hemoglobin resuscitation improves cerebral perfusion after head injury and shock. J. Trauma 41:781–788; 1996.

Chestnut, R.; Marshall, L.; Klauber, M.; et al. The role of secondary brain injury in determining outcome from severe head injury. J. Trauma 34:216–222; 1993a.

Chestnut, R.; Marshall, S.; Piek, J.; et al. Early and late hypotension as a frequent and fundamental source of cerebral ischemia following severe brain injury in the Traumatic Coma Data Bank. Acta Neurochir. Suppl. (Wien) 59:121–125; 1993b.

Choi, S.; Barnes, T.; Bullock, R.; et al. Temporal profiles of outcome in severe head injury. J. Neurosurg. 81:169–173; 1994.

Choi, S.; Muizelaar, J.; Barnes, T.; et al. Prediction tree for severely head-injured patients. J. Neurosurg. 75:251–255; 1991.

Choi, S.; Narayan, R.; Anderson, R.; et al. Enhanced specificity of prognosis in severe head injury. J. Neurosurg. 69:381–385; 1988.

Cifu, D.; Kreutzer, J.; Marwitz, J.; et al. Functional outcomes of older adults with traumatic brain injury: a prospective, multicenter analysis. Arch. Phys. Med. Rehabil. 77:883–888; 1996.

Clark, C.; O'Hanlon, A.; Wright, M.; et al. Event-related potential measurement of deficits in information processing following moderate to severe closed head injury. Brain Injury 6:509–520; 1992.

Clark, R.; Kochanek, P.; Dixon, C.; et al. Early neuropathologic effects of mild or moderate hypoxemia after controlled cortical impact injury in rats. J. Neurotrauma 14:179–189; 1997.

Clifton, G.; Allen, S.; Barrodale, P.; et al. A phase II study of moderate hypothermia in severe brain injury. J. Neurotrauma 10:263–271; 1993a.

Clifton, G.; Kreutzer, J.; Choi, S.; et al. Relationship between Glasgow Outcome Scale and neuropsychological measures after brain injury. Neurosurgery 33:34–38; 1993b.

Colohan, A.; Alves, W.; Gross, C.; et al. Head injury mortality in two centers with different emergency medical services and intensive care. J. Neurosurg. 71:202–207; 1989.

Cooke, R.; McNicholl, B.; Brynes, D. Use of the Injury Severity Score in head injury. Injury 26:399–400; 1995.

Cope, D.; Hall, K. Head injury rehabilitation: benefit of early intervention. Arch. Phys. Med. Rehabil. 63:433–437; 1982.

Corrigan, J. Substance abuse as a mediating factor in outcome from traumatic brain injury. Arch. Phys. Med. Rehabil. 76:302–309; 1995.

Corrigan, J.; Smith-Knapp, K.; Granger, C. Validity of the functional independence measure for persons with traumatic brain injury. Arch. Phys. Med. Rehabil. 78:828–834; 1997.

Crepeau, F.; Scherzer, P. Predictors and indicators of work status after traumatic brain injury: a meta-analysis. Neuropsych. Rehabil. 3:5–35; 1993.

Cruz, J. Adverse effects of pentobarbital on cerebral venous oxygenation of comatose patients with acute traumatic brain swelling: relationship to outcome. J. Neurosurg. 85:758–761; 1996.

Davis, C.; Fardanesh, L.; Rubner, D.; et al. Profiles of functional recovery in fifty traumatically brain-injured patients after acute rehabilitation. Am. J. Phys. Med. Rehabil. 76:213–218; 1997.

Deluga, K.; Plotz, F.; Betz, A. Effect of indomethacin on edema following single and repetitive cerebral ischemia in the gerbil. Stroke 22:1259–1264; 1991.

Dikmen, S.; McLean, A.; Temkin, N. Neuropsychological and psychosocial consequences of minor head injury. J. Neurol. 49:1227–1232; 1986.

Dikmen, S.; Temkin, N.; Armsden, G. Neuropsychological recovery: relationship to psychosocial functions and postconcussional complaints. In: Levin, H.; Eisenberg, H.; Benton, A.; eds. Mild head injury. New York: Oxford University Press; 1989.

Dikmen, S.; Temkin, N.; Machamer, J.; et al. Employment following traumatic head injuries. Arch. Neurol. 51:177–186; 1994.

Dikmen, S.; Temkin, N.; Miller, B.; et al. Neurobehavioral effects of phenytoin prophylaxis of posttraumatic seizures. JAMA 265:1271–1277; 1991.

Diringer, M.; Edwards, D. Does modification of the Innsbruck and the Glasgow Coma Scales improve their ability to predict functional outcome? Arch. Neurol. 54:606–611; 1997.

Doppenberg, E.; Bullock, R. Clinical neuro-protection trials in severe traumatic brain injury: lessons from previous studies. J. Neurotrauma 14:71–80; 1997.

Editorial. The best yardstick we have. Lancet ii: 1445–1446; 1961.

Eisenberg, H.; Frankowski, R.; Contant, C.; et al. High-dose barbiturate control of elevated intracranial pressure in patients with severe head injury. J. Neurosurg. 69:15–23; 1988.

Eisenberg, H.; Gary, H.; Aldrich, E.; et al. Initial CT findings in 753 patients with severe head injury. A report from the NIH Traumatic Coma Data Bank. J. Neurosurg. 73:688–698; 1990.

Emerson, C.; Headrick, J.; Vink, R. Estrogen improves biochemical and neurological outcome following traumatic brain injury in male rats, but not in females. Brain Res. 608:95–100; 1993.

Fearnside, M.; Cook, R.; McDougall, P.; et al. The Westmead Head Injury Project outcome in severe head injury. A comparative analysis of pre-hospital, clinical and CT variables. Br. J. Neurosurg. 7:267–279; 1993.

Feldman, Z.; Contant, C.; Robertson, C.; et al. Evaluation of the Leeds prognostic score for severe head injury. Lancet 337:1451–1453; 1991.

Feldman, Z.; Zachari, S.; Reichenthal, E.; et al. Brain edema and neurological status with rapid infusion of lactated Ringer's or 5% dextrose solution following head trauma. J. Neurosurg. 83:1060–1066; 1995.

Forbes, M.; Clark, R.; Dixon, C.; et al. Augmented neuronal death in CA3 hippocampus following hyperventilation early after cortical impact. J. Neurosurg. 88:549–556; 1998.

Fox, D.; Lees-Haley, P.; Earnest, K.; et al. Post-concussive symptoms: base rates and etiology in psychiatric patients. Clin. Neuropsychol. 9:89–92; 1995.

Garcia-Estrada, J.; Del Rio, J.; Luquin, S.; et al. Gonadal hormones down-regulate reactive gliosis and astrocyte proliferation after a penetrating brain injury. Brain Res. 628:271–278; 1993.

Gennarelli, T.; Champion, H.; Sacco, W.; et al. Mortality of patients with head injury and extracranial injury treated in trauma centers. J. Trauma 29:1193–1201; 1989.

Gennarelli, T.; Thibault, L.; Adams, J.; et al. Diffuse axonal injury and traumatic coma in the primate. Ann. Neurol. 12:564–574; 1982.

Ghajar, J.; Hairiri, R.; Narayan, R.; et al. Survey of critical care management of comatose, head-injured patients in the United States. Crit. Care Med. 23: 560–567; 1995.

Gibson, R.; Stephenson, G. Aggressive management of severe closed head trauma: time for reappraisal. Lancet 2:369–371; 1989.

Girard, D.; Brown, J.; Burnett-Stolnack, M.; et al. The relationship of neuropsychological status and productive outcomes following traumatic brain injury. Brain Injury 10:663–676; 1996.

Goldberg, G.; Karazim, E. Application of evoked potentials to the prediction of discharge status in minimally responsive patients: a pilot study. J. Head Trauma Rehabil. 13:51–68; 1998.

Goldstein, F.; Levin, H.; Presley, R.; et al. Neurobehavioral consequences of closed head injury in older adults. J. Neurol. Neurosurg. Psychiatry 57:961–966; 1994.

Gopinath, S.; Contant, C.; Robertson, C.; et al. Critical thresholds for physiological parameters in patients with severe head injury. Vancouver, British Columbia; Congress of Neurological Surgeons Annual Meeting; 1993.

Gouvier, W.; Cubic, B.; Jones, G.; et al. Postconcussion symptoms and daily stress in normal and head-injured college populations. Arch. Clin. Neuropsychol. 7:193–211; 1992.

Greene, K.; Jacobowitz, R.; Marciano, F.; et al. Impact of traumatic subarachnoid hemorrhage on outcome in non-penetrating head injury. Part II: relationship to clinical course and outcome variables during acute hospitalization. J. Trauma 42:964–971; 1997.

Gronwall, D.; Wrightson, P. Cumulative effect of concussion. Lancet 2:995–997; 1975.

Gutling, E.; Gonser, A.; Imhof, H.; et al. EEG reactivity in the prognosis of severe head injury. Neurology 45:915–918; 1995.

Gutling, E.; Gonser, A.; Regard, M.; et al. Dissociation of frontal and parietal components of somatosensory evoked potentials in severe head injury. Electroencephalogr. Clin. Neurophysiol. 88:369–376; 1993.

Hall, K.; Cope, D. The benefit of rehabilitation in traumatic brain injury: a literature review. J. Head Trauma Rehabil. 10:1–13; 1995.

Hall, K.; Cope, D.; Rappaport, M. Glasgow Coma Scale and Disability Rating Scale: comparative usefulness in following recovery in traumatic head injury. Arch. Phys. Med. Rehabil. 66:35–37; 1985.

Hall, K.; Hamilton, B.; Gordon, W.; et al. Characteristics and comparisons of functional assessment indices: Disability Rating Scale, Functional Independence Measure and Functional Assessment Measure. J. Head Trauma Rehabil. 8:60–74; 1993.

Haltiner, A.; Temkin, N.; Dikmen, S. Risk of seizure recurrence after the first late posttraumatic seizure. Arch. Phys. Med. Rehabil. 78:835–840; 1997.

Hamilton, B.; Granger, C.; Sherwin, F.; et al. A uniform national data system for medical rehabilitation. In: Fuhrer, M., ed. Rehabilitation outcomes: analysis and measurement. Baltimore: Paul H. Brooks; 1987.

Harrigan, M.; Tuteja, S.; Neudeck, B. Indomethacin in the management of elevated intracranial pressure: a review. J. Neurotrauma 14:637–650; 1997.

Hawkins, M.; Lewis, F.; Medeiros, R. Serious traumatic brain injury: an evaluation of functional outcomes. J. Trauma 41:257–263; 1996.

Heinzelmann, M.; Platz, A.; Imhof, H. Outcome after acute extradural haematoma, influence of additional injuries and neurological complications in the ICU. Injury 27:345–349; 1996.

Hillier, S.; Sharpe, M.; Metzer, J. Outcomes 5 years post-traumatic brain injury with further reference to neurophysical impairment and disability. Brain Injury 11:661–675; 1997.

Hsiang, J.; Chestnut, R.; Crisp, C.; et al. Early routine paralysis for intracranial pressure control in severe head injury: is it necessary? Crit. Care Med. 22:1471–1476; 1994.

Hsiang, J.; Yeung, T.; Yu, A.; et al. High risk mild head injury. J. Neurosurg. 87:234–238; 1997.

Hutchison, D.; Frith, R.; Shae, N.; et al. A comparison between electroencephalography and somatosensory evoked potentials for outcome prediction following severe head injury. Electroencephalogr. Clin. Neurophysiol. 78:228–233; 1991.

Ip, R.; Dornan, J.; Schentag, C. Traumatic brain injury: factors predicting return to work or school. Brain Injury 9:517–532; 1995.

Iverson, G.; McCracken, L. 'Postconcussive' symptoms in persons with chronic pain. Brain Injury 11:783–790; 1997.

Jacobs, A.; Put, E.; Ingels, M.; et al. Prospective evaluation of technetium-99m-HMPAO SPECT in mild and moderate traumatic brain injury. J. Nucl. Med. 35:942–947; 1994.

Jaggi, J.; Obrist, W.; Gennarelli, T.; et al. Relationship of early cerebral blood flow and metabolism to outcome in acute head injury. J. Neurosurg. 72:176–182; 1990.

Jansen, H.; van der Naalt, J.; van Zomeran, A.; et al. Cobalt-55 positron emission tomography in traumatic brain injury: a pilot study. J. Neurol. Neurosurg. Psychiatry 60:221–224; 1996.

Jennett, B. Epedemiology of head injuries. J. Neurol. Neurosurg. Psychiatry 60:362–369; 1996.

Jennett, B.; Bond, M. Assessment of outcome after severe brain damage: a practical scale. Lancet 7905:480–484; 1975.

Jennett, B.; Snoek, J.; Bond, M.; et al. Disability after severe head injury: observations on the use of the Glasgow Outcome Scale. J. Neurol. Neurosurg. Psychiatry 44:285–293; 1981.

Jensen, K.; Ohrstrom, J.; Cold, G.; et al. The effects of indomethacin on intracranial pressure, cerebral blood flow and cerebral metabolism in patients with severe head injury and intracranial hypertension. Acta Neurochir. (Wien) 108:116–121; 1991.

Jordan, B.; Relkin, N.; Ravdin, L.; et al. Apolipoprotein E episolon4 associated with chronic traumatic brain injury in boxing. JAMA 278:136–140; 1997.

Jordan, B.; Zimmerman, R. Computed tomography and magnetic resonance imaging comparisons in boxers. JAMA 263:1670–1674; 1990.

Kane, N.; Curry, S.; Rowlands, C.; et al. Event-related potentials—neurophysiological tools for predicting emergence and early outcome from traumatic coma. Intensive Care Med. 22:39–46; 1996.

Katz, D. Neuropathology and neurobehavioral recovery from closed head injury. J. Head Trauma Rehabil. 7:1–15; 1992.

Katz, D.; Alexander, M. Traumatic brain injury: predicting course of recovery and outcome for patients admitted to rehabilitation. Arch. Neurol. 51:661–670; 1994.

Kaufman, H. Civilian gunshot wounds to the head. Neurosurgery 32:962–964; 1993.

Kelly, D. Steroids in head injury. New Horizons 3:453–455; 1995.

Kelly, D.; Kordestani, R.; Martin, N.; et al. Hyperemia following traumatic brain injury: relationship to intracranial hypertension and outcome. J. Neurosurg. 85:762–771; 1996.

Kelly, D.; Martin, N.; Kordestani, R.; et al. Cerebral blood flow as a predictor of outcome following traumatic brain injury. J. Neurosurg. 86:633–641; 1997.

Kelly, M.; Johnson, C.; Knoller, N.; et al. Substance abuse, traumatic brain injury and neuropsychological outcome. Brain Injury 11:391–402; 1997.

Kido, D.; Cox, C.; Hamill, R.; et al. Traumatic brain injuries: predictive usefulness of CT. Radiology 182:777–781; 1992.

Kiening, K.; Hartl, R.; Unterberg, A.; et al. Brain tissue po2-monitoring in comatose patients: implications for therapy. Neurol. Res. 19:233–240; 1997.

Kilaru, S.; Garb, J.; Emhoff, T.; et al. Long term functional status and mortality of elderly patients with severe closed head injury. J. Trauma 41:957–963; 1996.

Kirkpatrick, P.; Smielewski, P.; Czosnyka, M.; et al. Near-infrared spectroscopy use in patients with head injury. J. Neurosurg. 83:963–970; 1995.

Kirschner, K.; Sahgal, V.; Armstrong, K.; et al. A comparative study of the cognitve effects of phenytoin and carbamazepine in patients with blunt head injury. J. Neurol. Rehabil. 5:169–174; 1991.

Klauber, M.; Marshall, L.; Luerssen, T.; et al. Determinants of head injury mortality: importance of the low risk patient. Neurosurgery 24:31–36; 1989.

Klonoff, H.; Clark, C.; Klonoff, P. Long-term outcome of head injuries: a 23 year follow up study of children with head injuries. J. Neurol. Neurosurg. Psychiatry 56:410–415; 1993.

Konasiewicz, S.; Moulton, R.; Shedden, P. Somatosensory evoked potentials and intracranial pressure in severe head injury. Can. J. Neurol. Sci. 21:219–226; 1994.

Kraus, J.; Fife, D.; Ramstein, K.; et al. The relationship of family income to the incidence, external causes, and outcomes of serious brain injury, San Diego County, California. Am. J. Public Health 6:1345–1347; 1986.

Kraus, J.; McArthur D. Epidemiology of brain injury. In: Evans, R., ed. Neurology and trauma. Philadelphia: W. B. Saunders Co.; 1996.

Lam, A.; Winn, H.; Cullen, B.; et al. Hyperglycemia and neurologic outcome in patients with head injury. J. Neurosurg. 75:545–551; 1991.

Lehr, D.; Baethmann, A.; Reulen, H.; et al. Management of patients with severe head injury in the preclinical phase: a prospective analysis. J. Trauma 42(suppl):S71–S75; 1997.

LeRoux, P.; Newell, D.; Lam, A.; et al. Cerebral arteriovenous oxygen difference: a predictor of cerebral infarction and outcome in patients with severe head injury. J. Neurosurg. 87:1–8; 1997.

Levin, H. Outcome from mild head injury. In: Narayan, R.; Wilberger, J.; Povlishock, J., eds. Neurotrauma. New York: McGraw-Hill; 1996.

Levin, H.; Aldrich, E.; Saydjari, C.; et al. Severe head injury in children: experience of the Traumatic Coma Data Bank. Neurosurgery 31:435–443; 1992.

Levin, H.; Amparo, E.; Eisenberg, H.; et al. Magnetic resonance imaging and computerized tomography in relation to the neurobehavioral sequelae of mild and moderate injuries. J. Neurosurg. 66:706–713; 1987.

Levin, H.; Gary H., Eisenberg, H. Duration of impaired consciousness in relation to side of lesion after severe head injury. NIH Traumatic Coma Data Bank Research Group. Lancet 1:1001–1003; 1989.

Levin, H.; Gary, H., Eisenberg, H.; et al. Neurobehavioral outcome 1 year after severe head injury: experience of the Traumatic Coma Data Bank. J. Neurosurg. 73:699–709; 1990.

Levin, H.; O'Donnell, V.; Grossman, R. The Galveston orientation and amnesia test: a practical scale to assess cognition after head injury. J. Nerv. Ment. Dis. 167:675–684; 1979.

Levin, H.; Saydjari, C.; Eisenberg, H.; et al. Vegetative state after closed head injury. A Traumatic Coma Data Bank Report. Arch. Neurol. 48:580–585; 1991.

Levin, H.; Williams, D.; Crofford, M.; et al. Relationship of depth of brain lesions to consciousness and outcome after closed head injury. J. Neurosurg. 69:861–866; 1988.

Levy, M.; Masri, L.; Lavine, S.; et al. Outcome prediction after penetrating craniocerebral injury in a civilian population: aggressive surgical management in patients with admission Glasgow Coma Scores of 3, 4, or 5. Neurosurgery 35:77–84; 1994.

Levy, M.; Masri, L.; Levy, K.; et al. Prenetrating craniocerebral injury resultant from gunshot wounds: gang-related injury in children and adolescents. Neurosurgery 33:1018–1024; 1993a.

Levy, M.; Rezai, A.; Masri, L.; et al. The significance of subarachnoid hemorrhage after penetrating craniocerebral injury: correlation with angiography and outcome in a civilian population. Neurosurgury 32:532–540; 1993b.

Litofsky, N.; Chin, L.; Tang, G.; et al. The use of lobectomy in the management of severe closed-head trauma. Neurosurgery 34:628–632; 1994.

Luerssen, T.; Klauber, M.; Marshall, L. Outcome from head injury related to patient's age. A longitudinal prospective study of adult and pediatric head injury. J. Neurosurg. 68:409–416; 1988.

Mackay, L.; Bernstein, B.; Chapman, P.; et al. Early intervention in severe head injury: long-term benefits of a formalized program. Arch. Phys. Med. Rehabil. 73:635–641; 1992.

MacPherson, V.; Sullivan, S.; Lambert, J. Prediction of motor status 3 and 6 months post severe traumatic brain injury: a preliminary study. Brain Injury 6:489–498; 1992.

Malec, J.; Basford, J. Postacute brain injury rehabilitation. Arch. Phys. Med. Rehabil. 77:198–207; 1996.

Malec, J.; Buffington, A.; Moessner, A.; et al. Maximizing vocational outcome after brain injury: integration of medical and vocational hospital-based services. Mayo Clin. Proc. 70:1165–1171; 1995.

Marion, D.; Carlier, P. Problems with initial Glasgow Coma Scale assessment caused by prehospital treatment of patients with head injuries: results of a national survey. J. Trauma 36:89–95; 1994.

Marion, D.; Leonov, Y.; Ginsberg, M.; et al. Resuscitative hypothermia. Crit. Care Med. 24(suppl): S81–S89; 1996.

Marion, D.; Penrod, L.; Kelsey, S.; et al. Treatment of traumatic brain injury with moderate hypothermia. N. Engl. J. Med. 336:540–546; 1997.

Marmarou, A.; Anderson, R.; Ward, J.; et al. Impact of ICP instability and hypotension on outcome in patients with severe head trauma. J. Neurosurg. 75: S59–S66; 1991.

Marshall, L.; D. P. B.; S. A. B.; et al. The National Traumatic Coma Data Bank. Part 1: Design, purpose, goals, and results. J. Neurosurg. 59:276–284; 1983a.

Marshall, L.; Gautille, T.; Klauber, M.; et al. The outcome of severe closed head injury. J. Neurosurg. 71(suppl.):S28–S36; 1991.

Marshall, L.; Smith, R.; Shapiro, H. The outcome with aggressive treatment in severe head injuries. J. Neurosurg. 50:26–30; 1979.

Marshall, L.; Toole, B.; Bowers, S. The National Traumatic Coma Data Bank. Part 2: patients who talk and deteriorate: implications for treatment. J. Neurosurg. 59:285–288; 1983b.

Massagli, T. Neurobehavioral effects of phenytoin, carbamazepine, and valproic acid: implications for use in traumatic brain injury. Arch. Phys. Med. Rehabil. 72:219–226; 1991.

Masson, F.; Maurette, P.; Salmi, L.; et al. Prevalence of impairments 5 years after a head injury, and their relationship with disabilities and outcome. Brain Injury 10:487–497; 1996.

Max, W.; MacKenzie, E.; Rice, D.; Hicac, J. H. T. R.-P. Head injuries: cost and consequences. J. Head Trauma Rehabil. 6:76–91; 1991.

Mayer, T.; Walker, M.; Sasha, I.; et al. Effect of multiple trauma on outcome of pediatric patients with neurologic injuries. Childs Brain 8:189–197; 1981.

Mayes, S.; Pelco, L.; Campbell, C. Relationships among pre- and post-injury intelligence, length of coma and age in individuals with severe closed-head injuries. Brain Injury 3:301–313; 1989.

McIntosh, T. Neurochemical sequelae of traumatic brain injury: therapeutic implications. Cerebrovasc. Brain Metab. Rev. 6:109–164; 1994.

McIntosh, T. Novel pharmacologic therapies in the treatment of experimental traumatic brain injury: a review. J. Neurotrauma 10:215–261; 1993.

McMillan, T.; Jongen, E.; Greenwood, R. Assessment of post-traumatic amnesia after severe closed head injury: retrospective or prospective. J. Neurol. Neurosurg. Psychiatry 60:422–427; 1996.

Michaud, L.; Rivara, F.; Grady, M.; et al. Predictors of survival and severity of disability after severe brain injury in children. Neurosurgery 31:254–264; 1992.

Mittenberg, W.; DiGiulio, D.; Perrin S.; et al. Symptoms following mild head injury: expectation as etiology. J. Neurol. Neurosurg. Psychiatry 55:200–204; 1992.

Moore, A.; Stambrook, M.; Peters, L.; et al. Long-term multi-dimensional outcome following isolated traumatic brain injuries and traumatic brain injuries associated with multiple trauma. Brain Injury 4: 379–389; 1990.

Morgan, A. The trauma center as a continuum of care for persons with severe brain injury. J. Head Trauma Rehabil. 9:1–10; 1994.

Moulton, R.; Sheddon, P.; Tucker, W.; et al. Somatosensory evoked potential monitoring following severe closed head injury. Clin. Invest. Med. 17:187– 195; 1994.

Muizelaar, J.; Marmarou, A.; Ward, J.; et al. Adverse effects of prolonged hyperventilation in patients with severe head injury: a randomized clinical trial. J. Neurosurg. 75:731–739; 1991.

Mysiw, W.; Sandel, M. The agitated brain injured patient. Part 2: pathophysiology and treatment. Arch. Phys. Med. Rehabil. 78:213–220; 1997.

Narayan, R.; Greenberg, R.; Miller, J.; et al. Improved confidence of outcome prediction in severe head injury. A comparative analysis of the clinical examination, multimodality evoked potentials, CT scanning and intracranial pressure. J. Neurosurg. 54:751–762; 1981.

Newlon, P.; Greenberg, R.; Enas, G.; et al. Effects of therapeutic pentobarbital coma on multimodality evoked potentials recorded from severely head-injured patients. Neurosurgery 12:613–619; 1983.

Obrist, W.; Clifton, G.; Robertson, C.; et al. Cerebral metabolic changes induced by hyperventilation in acute head injury. Cerebral Vascular Disease: Proceedings of the World Federation of Neurology, 13th International Salzburg Conference. Salzburg, Austria; 1987: p. 251–255.

Obrist, W.; Langfitt, T.; Jaggi, J.; et al. Cerebral blood flow and metabolism in comatose patients with acute head injury. Relationship to intracranial hypertension. J. Neurosurg. 61:241–253; 1984.

Olver, J.; Ponsford, J.; Curran, C. Outcome following traumatic brain injury: a comparison between 2 and 5 years after injury. Brain Injury 10:841–848; 1996.

Ong, L.; Selladurai, B.; Dhilion, M.; et al. The prognostic value of the Glasgow Coma Scale, hypoxia and computerized tomography in outcome prediction of pediatric head injury. Pediatr. Neurosurg. 24:285–291; 1996.

Papanicolaou, A.; Levin, H.; Eisenberg H.; et al. Evoked potential correlates of posttraumatic amnesia after closed head injury. Neurosurgery 14:676–678; 1984.

Pennings, J.; Bachulis, B.; Simons, C.; et al. Survival after severe brain injury in the aged. Arch. Surg. 128:787–793; 1993.

Piek, J.; Chestnut, R.; Marshall, L.; et al. Extracranial complications of severe head injury. J. Neurosurg. 77:901–907; 1992.

Pietropaoli, J.; Rogers, F.; Shackford, S.; et al. The deleterious effects of intraoperative hypotension on outcome in patients with severe head injury. J. Trauma 33:403–407; 1992.

Pigula, F.; Wald, S.; Shackford, S.; et al. The effect of hypotension and hypoxia on children with severe head injuries. J. Pediatr. Surg. 28:310–314; 1993.

Pohlmann-Eden, B.; Dingethal, K.; Bender, H.; et al. How reliable is the predictive value of SEP (somatosensory evoked potentials) patterns in severe brain damage with special regard to the bilateral loss of cortical responses? Intensive Care Med. 23:301–308; 1997.

Polin, R.; Shaffrey, M.; Bogaev, C.; et al. Decompressive bifrontal craniectomy in the treatment of severe refractory posttraumatic cerebral edema. Neurosurgery 41:84–92; 1997.

Prough, D.; Lang, J. Therapy of patients with head injuries: key parameters for management. J. Trauma 42:S10–S18; 1997.

Quigley, M.; Vidovich, D.; Cantella, D.; et al. Defining the limits of survivorship after very severe head injury. J. Trauma 42:7–10; 1997.

Rapp, R.; Young, B.; Twyman, D.; et al. The favorable effect of early parenteral feeding on survival in head injured patients. J. Neurosurg. 58:906–912; 1983.

Rappaport, M.; Clifford, J. Comparison of passive P300 brain evoked potentials in normal and severely traumatically brain injured patients. J. Head Trauma Rehabil. 9:94–104; 1994.

Rappaport, M.; Clifford, J. J.; Winterfield, K. P300 response under active and passive attentional states and uni- and bimodality stimulus presentation conditions. J. Neuropsychiatry Clin. Neurosci. 2:399–407; 1990a.

Rappaport, M.; Hall, K.; Hopkin, K.; et al. Disability rating scale for severe head trauma: coma to community. Arch. Phys. Med. Rehabil. 63:118–123; 1982.

Rappaport, M.; Hemmerle, A.; Rappaport, M. Intermediate and long latency SEPs in relation to clinical disability in traumatic brain injury patients. Clin. Electroencephalogr. 21:188–191; 1990b.

Rappaport, M.; Hemmerle, A.; Rappaport, M. Short and long latency auditory evoked potentials in traumatic brain injuy patients. Clin. Electroencephalogr. 22:199–202; 1991.

Rappaport, M.; Hopkins, H.; Hall, K.; et al. Evoked potentials and head injury: 2. Clinical applications. Clin. Electroencephalogr. 12:167–176; 1981.

Rea, G.; Rockswold, G. Barbiturate therapy in uncontrolled intracranial hypertension. Neurosurgery 12:401–405; 1983.

Reider-Groswasser, I.; Cohen, M.; Costeff, H.; et al. Late CT findings in brain trauma: relationship to cognitive and behavioral sequelae and to vocational outcome. AJR Am. J. Roentgenol. 160:147–152; 1993.

Reider-Groswasser, I.; Costeff, H.; Sazbon, L.; et al. CT findings in persistent vegetative state following blunt traumatic brain injury. Brain Injury 11:865–870; 1997.

Resnick, D.; Marion, D.; Carlier, P. Outcome analysis of patients with severe head injuries and prolonged intercranial hypertension. J. Trauma 42:1108–1111; 1997.

Robertson, C.; Contant, C.; Gokaslan, Z.; et al. Cerebral blood flow, arteriovenous oxygen difference, and outcome in head injured patients. J. Neurol. Neurosurg. Psychiatry 55:594–603; 1992.

Robertson, C.; Gopinath, S.; Goodman, J.; et al. Sjvo2 monitoring in head-injured patients. J. Neurotrauma 12:891–896; 1995.

Rockswold, G.; Ford, S.; Anderson, D.; et al. Results of a prospective randomized trial for treatment of severely brain-injured patients with hyperbaric oxygen. J. Neurosurg. 76:29–34; 1992.

Roof, R.; Duvdevani, R.; Heyburn, J.; et al. Progesterone rapidly decreases brain edema: treatment delayed up to 24 hours is still effective. Exp. Neurol. 138:246–251; 1996.

Roof, R.; Duvdevani, R.; Stein, D. Gender influences outcome of brain injury: progesterone plays a protective role. Brain Res. 607:333–336; 1993.

Rosner, M.; Rosner, S.; Johnson, A. Cerebral perfusion pressure: management protocol and clinical results. J. Neurosurg. 83:949–962; 1995.

Ruff, R.; Marshall, L.; Crouch, J.; et al. Predictors of outcome following severe head trauma: follow-up data from the Traumatic Coma Data Bank. Brain Injury 7:101–111; 1993.

Rumpl, E.; Prugger, M.; Bauer, G.; et al. Incidence and prognostic value of sleep spindles in post-traumatic coma. Electroencephalogr. Clin. Neurophysiol. 56:420–429; 1983.

Russell, W. Cerebral involvement in head injury. Brain 55:549–603; 1932.

Rutherford, W.; Merrett, J.; McDonald, J. Symptoms at one year following concussion from mild head injuries. Injury 10:225–230; 1979.

Sakas, D.; Bullock, M.; Patterson, J.; et al. Focal cerebral hyperemia after focal head injury in humans: a benign phenomenon? J. Neurosurg. 83:277–284; 1995.

Salazar, A.; Jabbari, B.; Vance, S.; et al. Epilepsy after penetrating head injury. I. Clinical correlates: a report of the Vietnam Head Injury Study. Neurology 35:1406–1414; 1985.

Salcido, R.; Costrich, J. Recurrent traumatic brain injury. Brain Injury 6:293–298; 1992.

Sandel, M. Outcome measures and prognosis in traumatic brain injury. Washington, DC: American Academy of Neurology Annual Meeting; 1994.

Schalk, K.; Faraci, F.; Heistad, D. Effect of endothelin on production of cerebrospinal fluid in rabbits. Stroke 23:560–563; 1992.

Schierhout, G.; Roberts, I. Prophylactic antiepileptic agents after head injury: a systemic review. J. Neurol. Neurosurg. Psychiatry 64:108–112; 1998.

Schwartz, M.; Tator, C.; Rowed, D. The University of Toronto Head Injury Treatment Study: a prospective randomized comparison of pento-barbital and mannitol. Can. J. Neurol. Sci. 11:434–440; 1984.

Seelig, J.; Becker, D.; Miller, J.; et al. Traumatic acute subdural hematoma: major mortality reduction in comatose patients treated within four hours. N. Engl. J. Med. 304:1511–1518; 1981.

Shaffrey, M.; Polin, R.; Phillips, C.; et al. Classification of civilian craniocerebral gunshot wounds: a multivariate analysis predictive of mortality. J. Neurotrauma 9:S279–S285; 1992.

Sharples, P.; Stuart, A.; Matthews, D.; et al. Cerebral blood flow and metabolism in children with severe head injury. Part I: relation to age, Glasgow coma score, outcome, intracranial pressure, and time after injury. J. Neurol. Neurosurg. Psychiatry 58:145–152; 1995.

Shin, D.; Ehrenberg, B.; Whyte, J.; et al. Evoked potential assessment: utility in prognosis of chronic head injury. Arch. Phys. Med. Rehabil. 70:189–193; 1989.

Siccardi, D.; Cavaliere, R.; Pau, A.; et al. Penetrating craniocerebral missile injuries in civilians: a retrospective analysis of 314 cases. Surg. Neurol. 35: 455–460; 1991.

Siegel, J. The effect of associated injuries, blood loss, and oxygen debt on death and disability in blunt traumatic brain injury: the need for early physiologic predictors of severity. J. Neurotrauma 12:579–590; 1995.

Siegel, J.; Gens, D.; Mamantov, T.; et al. Effect of associated injuries and blood volume replacement on death, rehabilitation needs, and disability in blunt traumatic brain injury. Crit. Care Med. 19:1252–1265; 1991.

Sorenson, S.; Kraus, J. Occurrence, severity, and outcomes of brain injury. J. Head Trauma Rehabil. 6:1–10; 1991.

Sosin, D.; Sacks, J.; Smith, S. Head injury-associated deaths in the United States from 1979 to 1986. JAMA 262:2251–2255; 1989.

Sosin, D.; Sniezek, J.; Thurman, D. Incidence of mild and moderate brain injury in the United States, 1991. Brain Injury 10:47–54; 1996.

Sosin, D.; Sniezek, J.; Waxweiler, R. Trends in death associated with traumatic brain injury, 1979 through 1992. Success and failure. JAMA 273:1778–1780; 1995.

Spettell, C.; Ellis, D.; Ross, S.; et al. Time of rehabilitation admission and severity of trauma: effect on brain injury outcome. Arch. Phys. Med. Rehabil. 72:320–325; 1991.

Stein, S.; Ross, S. Moderate head injury: a guide to initial management. J. Neurosurg. 77:562–564; 1992.

Symonds, C. Observations on the differential diagnosis and treatment of cerebral states consequent upon head injuries. Br. Med. J. 2:828–832; 1928.

Synek, V. Prognostically important EEG coma patterns in diffuse anoxic and traumatic encephalopathies in adults. J. Clin. Neurophysiol. 5:161–174; 1988.

Tate, R.; Lulham, J.; Broe, G.; et al. Psychosocial outcome for the survivors of severe blunt head injury: the results from a consecutive series of 100 patients. J. Neurol. Neurosurg Psychiatry 52:1128–1134; 1989.

Teasdale, G.; Jennett, B. Assessment and prognosis of coma after head injury. Acta. Neurochir. 34:45–55; 1976.

Teasdale, G.; Jennett, B. Assessment of coma and impaired consciousness. A practical scale. Lancet 2: 81–84; 1974.

Teasdale, G.; Nicoll, J.; Murray, G.; et al. Association of apolipoprotein E polymorphism with outcome after head injury. Lancet 350:1069–1071; 1997.

Temkin, N.; Dikmen, S.; Wilensky, A.; et al. A randomized, double-blind study of phenytoin for the prevention of post-traumatic seizures. N. Engl. J. Med. 323:497–502; 1990.

Thatcher, R.; Cantor, D.; McAlaster, R.; et al. Comprehensive predictions of outcome in closed head-injured patients. The development of prognostic equations. Ann. N.Y. Acad. Sci. 620:82–101;

Thompson, N.; Francis, D.; Steubing, K.; et al. Motor, visual-spatial, and somatosensory skills after traumatic brain injury in children and adolescents: a study of change. Neuropyschologia 8:333–342; 1994.

Toutant, S.; Klauber, M.; Marshal, L.; et al. Absent or compressed basal cisterns on first CT scan: ominous predictors of outcome in severe head injury. J. Neurosurg. 61:691–694; 1984.

Trauner, D. Barbiturate therapy in acute brain injury. J. Pediatr. 109:742–746; 1986.

Unterberg, A.; Kiening, K.; Hartl, R.; et al. Multimodal monitoring in patients with head injury: evaluation of the effects of treatment on cerebral oxygenation. J. Trauma 42(suppl):S32–S40; 1997.

Vassar, M.; Fischer, R.; O'Brien, P.; et al. A multicenter trial for resuscitation of injured patients with 7.5% sodium chloride. The effect of added dextran 70. The Multicenter Group for the Study of Hypertonic Saline in Trauma Patients. Arch. Surg. 128:1003–1011; 1993.

Vollmer, D.; Torner, J.; Jane, J.; et al. Age and outcome following traumatic coma: why do older patients fare worse? J. Neurosurg. 75(suppl):S37–S49.

Wade, C.; Grady, J.; Kramer, G.; et al. Individual patient cohort analysis of efficacy of hypertonic saline/dextran in patients with traumatic brain injury and hypotension. J. Trauma 42(suppl):S61–S65; 1997.

Wald, S.; Shackford, S.; Fenwick, J. The effect of secondary insults on mortality and long-term disability after severe head injury in a rural region without a trauma system. J. Trauma 34:377–381; 1993.

Ward, J.; Becker, D.; Miller, J.; et al. Failure of prophylactic barbiturate coma in the treatment of severe head injury. J. Neurosurg. 62:383–388; 1985.

Warme, P.; Bergstrom, R.; Persson, L. Neurosurgical intensive care improves outcome after severe head injury. Acta Neurochir. (Wien) 110:57–64; 1991.

Whitlock, J.; Hamilton, B. Functional outcome after rehabilitation for severe traumatic brain injury. Arch. Phys. Med. Rehabil. 76:1103–1112; 1995.

Whitman, S.; Coonley-Hoganson, R.; Desai, B. Comparative head trauma experiences in two socioeconomically different Chicago-area communities: a population study. Am. J. Epidemiol. 119:570–580; 1984.

WHO. The International Classification of Impairments, Disabilities, and Handicaps. Geneva: World Health Organization; 1980.

Willmore, L. Post-traumatic epilepsy: cellular mechanisms and implications for treatment. Epilepsia 31(suppl):S67–S73; 1990.

Wilson, B.; Vizor, A.; Bryant, T. Predicting severity of cognitive impairment after severe head injury. Brain

Injury 5:189–197; 1991.

Wilson, J.; Teasdale, G.; Hadley, D.; et al. Post-traumatic amnesia: still a valuable yardstick. J. Neurol. Neurosurg. Psychiatry 56:198–201; 1993.

Winchell, R.; Simons, R.; Hoyt, D. Transient systolic hypotension. A serious problem in the management of head injury. Arch. Surg. 131:533–539; 1996.

Woischneck, D.; Firsching, R.; Ruckert, M.; et al. Clinical predictors of the psychosocial long-term outcome after brain injury. Neurol. Res. 19:305–310; 1997.

Wong, J.; Regennitter, R.; Barrios, F. Base rate and simulated symptoms of mild head injury among normals. Arch. Clin. Neuropsychol. 9:411–425; 1994.

York, D.; Pulliam, M.; Rosenfield, J.; et al. Relationship between visual evoked potentials and intracranial pressure. J. Neurosurg. 55:909–916; 1981.

Young, B.; Ott, L.; Dempsey, R.; et al. Relationship between admission hyperglycemia and neurologic outcome in severely brain-injured patients. Ann. Surg. 210:466–473; 1989.

Young, B.; Ott, L.; Twyman, D.; et al. The effect of nutritional support on outcome from severe head injury. J. Neurosurg. 67:668–676; 1987.

Zafonte, R.; Hammond, F.; Mann, N.; et al. Relationship between Glasgow Coma Scale and functional outcome. Am. J. Phys. Med. Rehabil. 75:364–369; 1996a.

Zafonte, R.; Hammond, F.; Mann, N.; et al. Revised Trauma Score: an additive predictor of disability afollowing brain injury? Am. J. Phys. Med. Rehabil. 75:456–460; 1996b.

Zafonte, R.; Mann, N.; Millis, S.; et al. Functional outcome after violence related traumatic brain injury. Brain Injury 11:403–407; 1997a.

Zafonte, R.; Mann, N.; Mills, S.; et al. Posttraumatic amnesia: it's relation to functional outcome. Arch. Phys. Med. Rehabil. 78:1103–1106; 1997b.

**Appendix B.** Galveston Orientation and Amnesia Test (GOAT)

Include documentation of the patient's name, age, sex, injury date, and date/day/time of test

| | Error Point Value | Error Points |
|---|---|---|
| 1. What is your name? | 2 | _____ |
| When were you born? | 4 | _____ |
| Where do you live? | 4 | _____ |
| 2. Where are you now? City | 5 | _____ |
| Hospital (unnecessary to state name of hospital) | 5 | _____ |
| 3. On what date were you admitted to this hospital? | 5 | _____ |
| How did you get here? | 5 | _____ |
| 4. What is the first event you can remember after the injury? | 5 | _____ |
| Can you describe in detail (e.g., date, time, companions) the first event you can recall after injury. | 5 | _____ |
| 5. What is the last event you can remember before the injury? | 5 | _____ |
| Can you describe in detail (e.g., date, time, companions) the last event you can recall before injury? | 5 | _____ |
| 6. What time is it now? (1 point for each 1/2 hour removed from correct time to maximum of 5) | 5 (maximum) | _____ |
| 7. What day of the week is it? (1 point for each day removed from correct day) | 3 (maximum) | _____ |
| 8. What day of the month is it? (1 point for each day removed from correct date to maximum of 5) | 5 (maximum) | _____ |
| 9. What is the month? (5 points for each month removed from correct month to maximum of 15) | 15 (maximum) | _____ |
| 10. What is the year? (10 points for each year removed from correct year to maximum of 30) | 30 (maximum) | _____ |
| Total Error Points | | _____ |
| Total Goat Score (100 - total error points) | | _____ |
| Range: normal, 76–100; borderline, 66–75; impaired, ≤ 65 | | |

# 23

# Postconcussion Syndrome

RANDOLPH W. EVANS

The postconcussion syndrome refers to a large number of symptoms and signs that may occur alone or in combination, usually following mild head trauma (Evans 1992, 1996a). Concussion is a trauma-induced alteration in mental status that may or may not involve loss of consciousness (Kelly and Rosenberg 1997; Practice parameter, 1997). Loss of consciousness does not have to occur for the postconcussion syndrome to develop. The following symptoms and signs are associated with the syndrome which develops in over 50% of those who have mild head injuries (Bazarian et al. 1999): headaches, dizziness, vertigo, tinnitus, hearing loss, blurred vision, diplopia, convergence insufficiency, light and noise sensitivity, diminished taste and smell, irritability, anxiety, depression, personality change, fatigue, sleep disturbance, decreased libido, decreased appetite, post-traumatic stress disorder, memory dysfunction, impaired concentration and attention, slowing of reaction time, and slowing of information processing speed. Rare sequelae of mild head injury include subdural and epidural hematomas, cerebral venous thrombosis, second impact syndrome, seizures, nonepileptic post-traumatic seizures, transient global amnesia, tremor, and dystonia (Table 23-1). Headaches, dizziness, fatigue, irritability, anxiety, insomnia, loss of concentration and memory, and noise sensitivity are the most common complaints (Rutherford et al. 1977; Minderhoud et al. 1980; Dikmen et al. 1986; Edna 1987).

## Epidemiology

Head trauma is a cause of significant morbidity and mortality in all societies. Mild head injury accounts for 75% or more of all brain injuries (Krause and Nourjah 1988). The annual incidence of mild head injury per 100,000 population has been estimated to be 149 for Olmsted County, Minnesota (Annegers et al. 1980), 131 for San Diego County, California (Kraus et al. 1984), and 511 for Auckland, New Zealand (Wrightson 1989). However, the incidence of mild head injury may be as high as 640 persons per 100,000 population, as many cases go unreported (Bernstein 1999). In addition, some patients may have "hidden" traumatic brain injury where they develop a postconcussion syndrome but do not make the causal connection between the injury and its consequences (Gordon et al. 1998).

In an industrialized country such as the United States, the relative causes of head trauma are approximately as follows: motor vehicle accidents, 45%; falls, 30%; occupational accidents, 10%; recreational accidents, 10%; and assaults, 5%

**Table 23-1.** Sequelae of Mild Head Injury

**Headaches**
  Muscle contraction or tension type
  Cranial myofascial injury
  Secondary to neck injury (cervicogenic)
    Myofascial injury
    Intervertebral discs
    Cervical spondylosis
    C2–3 facet joint (third occipital headache)
  Secondary to temporomandibular joint injury
  Greater and lesser occipital neuralgia
  Migraine with and without aura
  Footballer's migraine
  Medication rebound
  Cluster
  Supraorbital and infraorbital neuralgia
  Due to scalp lacerations or local trauma
  Dysautonomic cephalgia
  Orgasmic cephalgia
  Carotid or vertebral artery dissection
  Subdural or epidural hematomas
  Hemorrhagic cortical contusions
  Mixed
**Cranial nerve symptoms and signs**
  Dizziness
  Vertigo
  Tinnitus
  Hearing loss
  Blurred vision
  Diplopia
  Convergence insufficiency
  Light and noise sensitivity
  Diminished taste and smell
**Psychological and somatic complaints**
  Irritability
  Anxiety
  Depression
  Personality change
  Post-traumatic stress disorder
  Fatigue
  Sleep disturbance
  Decreased libido
  Decreased appetite
  Initial nausea/vomiting
**Cognitive impairment**
  Memory dysfunction
  Impaired concentration and attention
  Slowing of reaction time
  Slowing of information processing speed
**Rare sequelae**
Subdural and epidural hematomas
Cerebral venous thrombosis
Second impact syndrome
Seizures
Nonepileptic post-traumatic seizures
Transient global amnesia
Tremor
Dystonia

(Jennett and Frankowski 1990). About one-half of all patients with mild head injury are between the ages of 15 and 34. Motor vehicle accidents are more common in the young and falls more common in the elderly (Roy et al. 1986).

## Historical Aspects

The postconcussion syndrome has been controversial for over a century (Strauss and Savitsky 1934; Trimble 1981; Evans 1994a). One interesting historical case involved a 26-year old maid servant who had been hit over the head with a stick and reported symptoms of retrograde amnesia. Six months later she still complained of headaches, dizziness, tinnitus, and tiredness. In 1694, a judge requested a specialists' report of the Swiss physician J. J. Wepfer and two other surgeons who stated, "We can't say anything definite, but it is certain that there has been a grave contusion of the head and that this will leave its mark in the form of an impediment (De Morsier 1943).

Rigler raised the issue of "postcompensation neurosis" in 1879 (Rigler 1879). He described the increased incidence of post-traumatic invalidism after a system for financial compensation was established for accidental injuries on the Prussian railways in 1871. The London surgeon John Erichsen (1882) took an opposing viewpoint. He argued that minor injuries to the head and spine could result in severe disability due to "molecular disarrangement" and/or anemia of the spinal cord.

In more recent times, Henry Miller (1961) summarized the viewpoint of those who believe that the postconcussion syndrome is really a compensation neurosis: "The most consistent clinical feature is the subject's unshakable conviction of unfitness for work. . . ." Sir Charles Symonds (1962) took an equally strong opposing viewpoint when he wrote, "It is, I think, questionable whether the effects of concussion, however slight, are ever completely reversible."

## The Hollywood Head Injury Myth

Many physicians, lay persons, defense attorneys, and agents of insurance companies have serious doubts about the existence of the postconcussion syndrome (McMordie 1988; Evans et al. 1994b). A group of Canadian college students did not find the symptoms of postconcussion syndrome credible (Aubrey et al. 1989). Among their doubts were that the patients had sustained only minor head injuries, they appeared normal, and they had multiple vague complaints. The group suspected that they wanted to get out of school or work responsibilities or enhance a compensation claim.

Other than not being familiar with the literature, another explanation for these doubts is the Hollywood head-injury myth, which Robertson (1988) has called the "Three Stooges model."

Most people's knowledge of the sequelae of mild head injuries is largely the product of movie magic. Some of the funniest scenes in slapstick comedies and cartoons depict the character sustaining single or multiple head injuries, looking dazed, and then recovering immediately. In cowboy movies, detective and action stories, and boxing and Kung Fu films, seemingly serious head trauma is often inflicted by blows from guns and heavy objects, falls, motor vehicle injuries, fists, and kicks, all without lasting sequelae. Our experience is minuscule compared to the thousands of simulated head injuries witnessed in the movies and on television. Because of this compelling mythology, the physician has a difficult job educating patients, their families, and others in the realities of mild head injuries.

In addition to summarizing the literature on mild head injury, the physician can counter the myths by the use of vivid examples from sports. The public is quite familiar with the punch-drunk syndrome of cumulative head trauma in boxers (Martland 1928). The examples of two successful boxers, Joe Louis and Muhammad Ali, are well-known. Many have witnessed powerful punches resulting in dazed, disoriented boxers or knock-outs. There is also growing awareness of the effect of cumulative concussions in other sports including professional football (e.g., quarterbacks Steve Young, Troy Aikman, and Stan Humphries) and hockey (Pat Lafontaine) (Kelly and Rosenberg 1997). Finally, there is recent evidence of cumulative brain injury from collisions and repetitive heading of the ball in professional soccer players resulting in abnormal cognitive functioning (Matser et al. 1998). Considering the common incidence of head injuries, the example of family members, friends, or acquaintances with sequelae from mild head injuries sometimes can be used as well.

## Evidence for Organicity

In 1835 Gama wrote, "Fibers as delicate as those of which the organ of mind is composed are liable to break as a result of violence to the head" (Gama 1835). Over the last 30 years, a growing body of evidence strongly supports the organic theory. Diffuse axonal injury has been documented with mild head injury in neuropathological studies of humans and animals (Oppenheimer 1968; Blumbergs et al. 1989; Povlishock and Coburn 1989). A neurochemical substrate for mild head injury has also been suggested (Graham and McIntosh 1996). Neuroimaging studies including magnetic resonance imaging (MRI), single photon emission computed tomography (SPECT), and positron emission tomography (PET) can show structural and functional deficits (Packard and Ham 1994; Ruff et al. 1994).

Other testing also demonstrates abnormalities. Although not prognostically helpful, in some cases auditory brain stem responses have been reported as abnormal in mild head injury (Schoenhuber et al. 1988; Drake et al. 1996). Neuropsychological studies have revealed deficits in information processing, memory, reaction time, and attention (Levin 1989; Levin et al. 1992; Capruso and Levin 1996). Prognostic studies have shown the persistence of symptoms over time as compared to controls.

## Symptoms and Signs

### Headaches

Headaches have been estimated to occur in about 30% to 90% of patients who are symptomatic after mild head injury (Minderhoud et al. 1980; Evans 1996a). Headaches may occur more often and with longer duration in those with mild head injury compared to others with more severe degrees of trauma (Couch and Bearss 1994). Post-traumatic headaches are more common in those with a history of headache (Jensen and Nielsen 1990; Russell and Olesen 1996). According to the International Headache Society criteria (Headache Classification Committee 1988), the headache should occur less than 14 days after the injury, although Haas (1996) suggests within 3 months. Tension headaches, often associated with occipital neuralgia, account for about 85% (Packard 1994). Episodic migraine with and without aura de novo can also be a consequence of mild head injury (Weiss et al. 1991; Russell and Olesen 1996). In addition, impact can trigger acute migraine with and without aura, "footballer's headache" (Matthews 1972). Migraine triggered by mild head injury in sports often occurs in athletes, especially adolescents (Weinstock and Rothner 1995) with a family history of migraine. (The most famous example is the acute migraine with aura of Terrell Davis, who had pre-existing migraine, after a ding on the head in the 1998 Super Bowl.) Rarely, cluster headaches can develop after mild head injury. In patients with chronic post-traumatic headaches, medication rebound should also be considered (Evans 1996b; Haas 1996). Other headache types can also follow mild head injury (Table 23–1).

## Cranial Nerve Symptoms and Signs

Various cranial nerve symptoms and signs can occur after mild head injury. Dizziness is reported by 53% of patients within 1 week of injury (Levin et al. 1987). Central and peripheral pathologies including labyrinthine concussion, perilymph fistula, and benign positional nystagmus can result (Keane and Baloh 1996). Blurred vision is reported by 14% of patients (Minderhoud et al. 1980) with convergence insufficiency the most common cause. Optic nerve contusions can result in decreased visual acuity and hue discrimination. Mild head injury can also cause diplopia due to cranial nerve III, IV, and VI palsies (Keane and Baloh 1996). Decreased smell and taste are reported by more than 5% of patients following mild head injury (Minderhoud et al. 1980). Light and noise sensitivity are rather common complaints after mild head injury (Bohnen et al. 1991).

## Psychological and Somatic Complaints

Psychological and somatic complaints are common following mild head injury. Within 3 months of injury, between 51% and 84% of patients have post-traumatic psychological symptoms (Rimel et al. 1981; Rutherford et al. 1977). The prevalence of depression is at least 35% (Busch and Alpern 1998). In a study of patients who sustained a mild head injury in a motor vehicle accident, post-traumatic stress disorder was diagnosed in 14% within 1 month and 24% at 6 months after the injury (Bryant and Harvey 1998). Fatigue is a common complaint reported by 29% of patients at 4 weeks after the trauma and by 23% at 6 months (Minderhoud et al. 1980). Sleep disturbance is common (Perlis et al. 1997), with difficulty falling asleep and arousals reported by

15% at 6 weeks following injury (Rutherford et al. 1977)

## Rare Sequelae

A variety of rare sequelae have been reported. For adults after mild injury, the incidence of subdural hematomas is 1% or less (Jeret et al. 1993) and for epidural hematomas also 1% or less (Stein and Ross 1992). Both subdural and epidural hematomas can later appear after an initial computed tomography (CT) scan is normal. Diffuse cerebral swelling is a rare complication of mild head injury usually occurring in children and adolescents resulting in death or a persistent vegetative state (Bruce 1984). When diffuse cerebral swelling occurs after a second concussion when an athlete is still symptomatic from an earlier concussion, the term "second impact syndrome" is used. Although the second impact syndrome is a rare complication and somewhat controversial (McCrory and Berkovic 1998), guidelines have been suggested for return to play after concussions (Practice parameter 1997). Seizures can occasionally result from mild head injury. Lee and Lui (1992) reported an incidence of 2.36% of patients who developed seizures within 1 week. Annegers et al. (1998) found a standardized incidence ratio of 1.5 after mild head injuries but with no increase over the expected number after 5 years. Nonepileptic post-traumatic seizures usually follow mild rather than more severe degrees of head injury and typically present during the first year after the injury (Barry et al. 1998). Mild head injury can rarely trigger transient global amnesia, which in children may actually be confusional migraine (Sheth et al. 1995). Rarely, cerebral venous thrombosis may result in cerebral venous thrombosis (Couban and Maxner 1991; Ochagavia et al. 1996). Finally, mild head injury can result in an essential type tremor (Biary et al. 1989); multiple episodes of mild head injury can result in Parkinson's syndrome (Jankovic 1994).

## Variables in Prognosis

Although many prognostic studies have been reported during the last 70 years, comparison among the studies is difficult. There are significant differences including the definition of mild head injury, use of testing, study design, and subject variables (Table 23-2) (Levin et al. 1987a; Berstein 1999).

**Table 23-2.** Variables in Prognostic Studies

**Definition of mild head injury**
    Loss of consciousness and if so, duration
    Duration, if present, of post-traumatic amnesia
    Glasgow Coma Scale score
    Inclusion of skull fractures and/or cerebral contusions
    Radiological
    Neurophysiological
    Neuropsychological
    Use of testing
**Study design**
    Prospective vs. retrospective
    Length of follow-up
    Spontaneous volunteering of symptoms vs. responding
    to a checklist
    Face-to-face interview vs. a mailed questionnaire
    Use of matched controls
    Number of subjects
    Symptoms assessed
**Subject variables**
    Cause of head injury
    Hospital vs. outpatient presentation
    Geographic and cultural differences
    Age and gender
    Socioeconomic and educational level
    Premorbid personality and psychopathology
    Prior head trauma
    Use of alcohol and drugs
    Multiple trauma
    Pending or completed litigation
    Attrition rate of subjects

## Definition of Mild Head Injury

Although the terms mild and minor head injury are often used interchangeably, "mild head injury" is preferred in delineating the continuum of mild, moderate, and severe. Mild head injury is nonuniformly defined in different studies by different criteria including loss of consciousness and, if present, duration of the loss; duration of post-traumatic amnesia, if present; and a Glasgow coma scale (GCS) score of 13 to 15. In some studies, patients with skull fractures and/or cerebral contusions are included. Strict criteria used in recent studies (Dikmen et al. 1986; Levin et al. 1987b) are crucial to ensure studying similar types of injuries without confounding variables. For future studies, the author proposes the following criteria for mild head injury: loss of consciousness does not have to occur; if it does occur, a duration of 30 minutes or less; an initial GCS score rating of 13 to 15 without subsequent deterioration; and absence of focal neurological deficits without evidence of depressed skull fracture, intracranial hematomas, or other neurosurgical disease. However, heterogeneity may exist even with

this definition. Culotta et al. (1996) suggest segregating those with GCS scores of 15 from those with 13 and 14.

The persistence and severity of symptoms and neuropsychological deficits are not predicted by a loss of consciousness of less than 1 hour as compared to a patient being just dazed (Denker 1944; Leininger et al. 1990). The consideration of post-traumatic amnesia is problematic as a criteria for mild head injury, since the duration is frequently not reliably reported by the patient or observers. In addition, the duration of post-traumatic amnesia has been variably reported as being predictive (Minderhoud 1980; Vander Naalt et al. 1999) and not predictive (Edna 1987) of postconcussion sequelae. Wrightson and Gronwall (1981) found no correlation between duration of post-traumatic amnesia and time off work following the injury.

## Diagnostic Testing

Imaging studies, as well as neurophysiological and neuropsychological testing have been used to variable degrees in prognostic studies. Electroencephaographic (EEG) studies have frequently been used to assess patients with mild head injury. Since there is a significant incidence of premorbidly abnormal EEGs (Lorenzoni 1970), an abnormal EEG cannot be stated unequivocally to be caused by mild head injury without a preinjury study to compare. For the specific patient, EEG results do not have predictive value. Dow et al. (1944) found that an EEG taken immediately following head injury was borderline or abnormal in 43% of patients compared to 38% of controls. An abnormal EEG study was less predictive than clinical judgment in predicting time lost from work. However, for certain population groups, there may be some predictive information. For example, an increased incidence of abnormal EEGs has been found in former soccer players with chronic postconcussion symptoms (Tysvaer et al. 1989). A significant correlation has also been reported between EEG abnormalities and the number of bouts fought by ex-boxers (Ross et al. 1983). Abnormalities in EEG power spectral analyses have been reported after mild head injury (Thatcher et al. 1989). However, the results of brain mapping may not be sensitive, specific, and reproducible (Nuwer 1997) and can contain a high frequency of serious errors when presented as evidence in U.S. courtrooms (Nuwer and Hauser 1994). The American Academy of Neurology and the American Clinical Neurophysiology Society do not recommend the routine use of EEG brain mapping for evaluation of mild head injury and the postconcussion syndrome (Nuwer 1997). Although auditory brain stem responses have been reported as being abnormal in mild head injury, there is no correlation between abnormal results and postconcussion symptoms (Schoenhuber et al. 1988; Drake et al. 1996).

MRI of the brain is more sensitive than CT scan in evaluating mild head injury. Levin et al. (1992), in a comparison study between MRI and CT scan in evaluating mild to moderate head injury, found that MRI detected lesions in 85% of patients that were not detected by CT scan. Most of the lesions detected were in the frontal and temporal regions. Lesions present on the MRI scan had prognostic value for deficits of frontal lobe functioning and memory. Follow-up scans at 1 and 3 months showed marked reduction of lesion size with improvement in cognition and memory. Subsequent MRI studies have demonstrated clinically occult contusions and white matter changes (Hesselink et al. 1988; Yokota et al. 1991; Mittl et al. 1994), primarily in the frontotemporal region (Levin et al. 1992). Fluid-attenuated inversion-recovery (FLAIR) MRI is equal or superior to conventional spin-echo sequences for demonstrating traumatic lesions (Ashikaga et al. 1997).

Although SPECT scans are more sensitive than MRI and CT scans in detecting lesions (Kant et al. 1997; Abdel-Dayem et al. 1998), the findings may not have prognostic significance (Mitchener et al. 1997). SPECT scan abnormalities are also nonspecific. Depression and polydrug abuse can produce deficits similar to those seen after mild head injury (Juni 1994; Lesser et al. 1994). The scientific literature does not support the routine use of SPECT for the evaluation of patients with mild head injuries or the postconcussion syndrome (Report of the Therapeutics and Technology Assessment Subcommittee of the American Academy of Neurology 1996a).

In a study of 20 patients with persistent postconcussion syndrome after mild head injury, magnetic source imaging (MSI), a combination of MRI and magnetoencephalography, detected brain dysfunction in 65% compared to 5% of normal controls and 10% from those with a complete recovery (Lewine et al. 1999). MSI was more sensitive than either EEG or MRI. Replication of this study in a larger number of subjects will be of interest.

Neuropsychological testing is frequently performed to evaluate cognitive complaints. However, there are numerous problems with test sensitivity, specificity, reliability, and confounding subject characteristics (Prigatano 1996; Report of the Therapeutics and Technology Assessment Subcommittee of the American Academy of Neurology 1996b). The physician should be wary: patients are often misdiagnosed as brain injured (Stuss 1995). The psychologist should be familiar with findings in malingering and exaggerated memory deficits (Binder 1993).

## Study Design Variables

Study designs also vary. Some studies have prospective designs (Rutherford et al. 1977, 1978; Cartlidge 1977; Rimel et al. 1981; Dikmen et al. 1986; Edna 1987; Levin et al. 1987b), while others are retrospective (Denker 1944; Denny-Brown 1945). Retrospective studies may have incomplete baseline data and have varying lengths of follow-up for individual subjects. In studies of both types, the length of follow-up varies from weeks to months to years. Techniques for assessing the presence of symptoms and signs differ. Some studies have used spontaneous volunteering of symptoms, whereas others have had subjects respond to a checklist. Directed interviews and physical exams have been used, although other studies have obtained follow-up only by a questionnaire sent through the mail. More recent studies have used controls matched by sex, education, geographic location, and socioeconomic level. This is particularly important, since so many of the symptoms of postconcussion syndrome are frequent in the general population. The symptoms assessed vary as well. Finally, the number of subjects used is a notable variable.

## Subject Variables

Multiple subject variables influence the usefulness of the prognostic studies. The cause is important because of different mechanisms of head injury and the circumstances which may influence the outcome. For example, compare a motor vehicle accident involving an inertial-loading injury where another person is at fault with a contact phenomena sports injury. Subjects who are hospitalized might have different outcomes than patients seen in outpatient clinics and sent home with milder injuries. The cultural background and geographical location of subjects may be significant.

Sir Charles Symonds observed, "The symptom picture depends, not only upon the kind of injury, but upon the kind of brain" (Symonds 1937). Preexisting psychopathology and premorbid personality are certainly important (Keshaven et al. 1981; Cicerone and Kalmar 1997). The socioeconomic status, educational level, age, and sex of subjects are critical variables. Rimel et al. (1981) reported that significant predictors for return to work by 3 months included older age; higher level of education, employment, and socioeconomic status; and greater income. By 3 months, 100% of executives and business managers had returned to work compared to 68% of skilled laborers and 57% of unskilled laborers. Ruffolo et al. (1999) also found that those who have jobs with greater decision-making latitude are more likely to return to work by 6 to 9 months.

Although the degree of initial impairment of information processing speed is not related to intelligence, high-IQ patients recover faster than low-IQ patients (Gronwall 1976). This may illustrate the greater motivation of high achievers. Older age (> 40 years) has been reported as a risk factor for increased duration and number of postconcussion symptoms (Denker 1944; Hernesniemi 1979; Edna 1987; Rothweiler et al. 1998) and slower recovery of cognitive deficits (Barth et al. 1983; Gronwall 1989). The gender of the patient is an important variable, since late symptoms occur more often in women (Rutherford 1977, 1978; Edna 1987; Bazarian et al. 1999).

A history of prior head injuries or prior use of alcohol and illicit drugs compounds the effects of even mild head injury. Prior head injury is a risk factor for persistence and number of postconcussion symptoms (Gronwall and Wrightson 1975; Carlsson 1987) and is consistent with the neuropathological concept of cumulative diffuse axonal injuries and contusions. A history of alcohol abuse may increase the number of post-traumatic sequelae and may also be related to additional slowing of reaction time (Carlsson et al. 1987). Alcohol intoxication makes the initial assessment of patients with head injury more difficult (Brismar

et al. 1983) and is also a risk factor for neurosurgical sequelae.

Multiple trauma can cause additional functional impairment, depression, anxiety, and stress (Carlsson et al. 1987; Berrol 1989). Multiple trauma with associated orthopedic soft tissue injuries also contributes to the persistence and frequency of postconcussion symptoms (Dikmen et al. 1986).

The incidence of postconcussion syndrome is lower in those with injuries due to sports than by other mechanisms (Bazarian et al. 1999). This may be due to a higher force of impact in other injuries such as motor vehicle accidents or differences in the motivation of individuals.

Litigation that is pending or completed is a significant variable and is discussed in a subsequent section. Attrition of subjects can skew results. Patients without persisting symptoms may not wish to participate in serial evaluations.

## Prognosis of Postconcussion Symptoms

Because of the many variables in prognostic studies, the percentage of patients with symptoms following mild head injury varies often (Table 23-3). The percentage of patients with headaches at 1 month varies from 31.3% (Minderhoud et al. 1980) to 90% (Denker 1944) and at 3 months from 47% (Levin et al. 1987b) to 78% (Rimel et al. 1981). Edna (1987) found that 24% of the patients had persisting headaches at 4 years. The frequency of dizziness also varies considerably, ranging from 19% (Cartlidge 1978) to 53% (Levin et al. 1987b) at 1 week. At 2 years, 18% of patients report continuing dizziness (Denker 1944; Cartlidge 1978) and 18% at 4 years (Edna 1987). Memory problems are reported in 18.8% at 1 month (Minderhoud et al. 1980), 59% at 3 months (Rimel et al. 1981), 15.3% at 6 months (Minderhoud et al. 1980), and 19% at 4 years (Edna 1987). Irritability is reported in 24.7% of patients at 1 month (Minderhoud et al. 1980) and 5.3% at 1 year (Rutherford et al. 1978).

Since the symptoms of postconcussion syndrome are so common in the general population, comparison to controls is very important. Dikmen et al. (1986) studied 20 consecutive patients hospitalized with mild head injury and compared them to carefully matched controls. At 1 month

**Table 23-3.** Percentage of Patients With Persistence Of Symptoms After Mild Head Injury

| | 1 Week | 1 Month | 6 Weeks | 2 Months | 3 Months | 6 Months | 1 Year | 2 Years | 3 Years | 4 Years | 5 Years |
|---|---|---|---|---|---|---|---|---|---|---|---|
| Headache | 71[i] | 90[a] | 24.8[d] | 31.5[b] | 78[g] | 21.6[f] | 35[a] | 22[a] | 20[a] | 24[h] | |
| | 36[e] | 31.3[f] | | | 47[i] | 27[e] | 8.4[d] | 24[e] | | | |
| | | 56[i] | | | | | 18[e] | | | | 12[c] (Headaches and/or dizziness) |
| Dizziness | 53[i] | 12[a] | 14.5[d] | 23[b] | 22[i] | 13.1[f] | 26[a] | 18[a] | 16[a] | 18[h] | |
| | 19[e] | 21.9[f] | | | | 22[e] | 4.6[d] | 18[e] | | | |
| | | 35[i] | | | | | 14[e] | | | | |
| Memory Problems | | 18.8[f] | 8.3[d] | | 59[g] | 15.3[f] | 3.8[d] | | | 19[h] | |
| Irritability | | 24.7[f] | 9[d] | | | 19.6[f] | 5.3[d] | | | | |

[a] Denker (1944).
[b] Denny-Brown (1945).
[c] Steadman and Graham (1969).
[d] Rutherford et al. (1978).
[e] Cartlidge (1977).
[f] Minderhoud et al. (1980).
[g] Rimel et al. (1981).
[h] Edna (1987).
[i] Levin et al. (1987).

following injury, the following symptoms were endorsed by subjects and controls, respectively: headaches, 51% and 38%; memory difficulties, 52% and 6%; dizziness, 41% and 11%; fatigue, 68% and 41%; noise sensitivity, 52% and 10%; light sensitivity, 32% and 28%; difficulty concentrating, 42% and 21%; and irritability, 68% and 42%. These results demonstrate that although these nonspecific symptoms are common in controls, they are still more frequent in patients with mild head injury.

## Neoropsychological Deficits

Following mild head injury, deficits in cognitive functioning have been described including a reduction in information processing speed, attention, reaction time, and memory for new information. For information processing speed, recovery is seen within 3 months in most patients (Gronwall and Wrightson 1974; Levin et al. 1987b; Hugenholtz et al. 1988). Memory for new information also recovers within 1 to 3 months (Dikmen et al. 1986; Levin et al. 1987b), although persisting impairment in visual memory and performance of digit span has been noted (Levin et al. 1987b). Reaction time has been reported to be abnormal between 6 weeks (MacFlynn

1984) and 3 months (Hugenholtz et al. 1988) with recovery occurring within about 6 months (MacFlynn 1984). Attention deficits show persisting impairment at 3 months (Levin et al. 1987b; Gentilini et al. 1989). Dikmen et al. (1986) found recovery of cognitive impairment by 1 year compared to controls, although a minority had ongoing impairment preventing return to normal activities.

Resolution of cognitive impairment on testing does not necessarily imply resolution of subjective symptoms. In the Levin et al. (1987b) study, although testing showed nearly complete neuropsychological recovery at 3 months following injury, headaches were still present in 47% of subjects, dizziness in 22%, and decreased energy in 22%.

Even in patients with complete resolution of cognitive deficits and subjective symptoms, there may be residual brain impairment. Ewing et al. (1980) compared university students who made a full recovery from mild head injury 1 to 3 years previously to matched controls. The two groups were tested at ground level and at a simulated altitude of 12,500 feet. Although both groups performed similarly at ground level, the mild head injury group showed significant impairment in tests of memory and vigilance performed with the mild hypoxia. This study suggests that patients considered completely recovered may demonstrate impairment with environmental stress. Other physical and psychosocial stressors may cause similar impairment. As noted previously, the effects of mild head injury even in persons fully recovered are cumulative, which also suggests permanent brain damage.

Although most patients with mild head injury do not have neuropsychological sequelae after 3 months, a significant subgroup exists with persistent postconcussion difficulties and neuropsychological deficits. Leininger et al. (1990) compared 53 patients with mild head injury who had persisting symptoms after 1 or more months to matched controls. Exclusion criteria included prior history of significant head trauma, substance abuse, or low academic achievement. Thirty-two percent of the patients were dazed without loss of consciousness and 58% were unconscious for 20 minutes or less. Testing was performed from 1 to 22 months following injury. Tests of reasoning, information processing, and verbal learning revealed the most deficits. Controls performed better than the patients on reproduction of a complex geometric design. The loss of consciousness, per se, compared to being dazed, was not predictive for neuropsychological sequelae. Test results were similar in those patients assessed within 3 months of the injury as compared to the others tested after 3 months.

In a pilot study, Waterloo et al. (1997) obtained serum protein S-100 levels (a calcium binding protein synthesized in astroglial cells and used as an index of active cell injury) in seven patients within 12 hours of mild head injury and from seven age- and sex-matched controls. Elevated levels were found to be predictive of neurocognitive abnormalities 12 months following injury. It will be of interest if these findings can be replicated in a larger study.

However, in a larger study with 50 patients, elevated S-100 levels correlated with poorer results on the neuropsychological tests although the association did not reach statistical significance (Ingerbrigsten et al. 1999).

The use of cognitive retraining for cognitive complaints after mild head injury is controversial (Levin 1990; Malec 1996; NIH Consensus Development Panel 1999). In view of the expense, prospective studies demonstrating efficacy are needed before routine application can be recommended.

## The Effect Of Litigation

Litigation as a cause of the postconcussion syndrome has been a topic of debate during the last century. As a matter of routine, defense attorneys still cite Miller's work (1961) and invariably raise questions of secondary gain and malingering. However, studies of the last 30 years demonstrate that secondary gain and malingering certainly exist, but are usually minor elements of the overall picture.

### Are Litigants Different from Nonlitigants?

Patients with litigation are quite similar to those without litigation. Both groups have similar symptoms improving with time (Merskey and Woodford 1972; McKinlay et al. 1983; Leininger et al. 1990), similar types of headaches (Haas 1996), and similar cognitive test results (McKinlay et al. 1983; Leininger et al. 1990). Both groups also respond similarly to appropriate treatment as suggested by a study on post-traumatic migraine (Weiss et al. 1991).

### Compensation Neurosis and Malingering

Miller (1961) reported on 200 consecutive cases seen for medicolegal examination in Newcastle-upon-Tyne, England, with an average interval between the head injury and the first examination of 14 months. Forty-seven of the 200 patients were perceived to have gross and unequivocally psychoneurotic complaints. The patients exhibited characteristic behaviors during the consultation. They frequently arrived late and were accompanied by a family member who took an active part in the interview process. The patients displayed an attitude of "martyred gloom" and were very defensive. An obvious dramatization of symptoms was reported to be present in more than one-half of the patients such as avoiding the ophthalmoscope, performing grip testing inconsistently, or slumping forward while holding their face in their hands. Miller (1961) reports: "The most consistent feature is the subject's unshakable conviction of unfitness for work, a conviction quite unrelated to overt disability, even if his symptomatology is accepted at its face value. At a later stage, the patient will declare his fitness for light work, which is often not available. Another cardinal feature is an absolute refusal to admit any degree of symptomatic improvement."

Miller's study can be criticized for several reasons. He describes a biased sample; the patients were referred specifically for medicolegal consultation. Although his behavioral observations may have some validity, they are by necessity quite subjective and judgmental. Miller dismisses symptoms as being minor but does not give information on the percentage of patients with various complaints such as headaches, dizziness, and memory problems at the time of the examination. In the same paper Miller states, "The consistency of the post-concussional syndrome of headache, postural dizziness, irritability, failure of concentration, and intolerance of noise, argues a structural or at least a pathophysiological basis." Miller's study has stimulated many other investigators to explore further issues of compensation.

Guthkelch (1980) in Pittsburgh, Pennsylvania, reported on 398 consecutive head injury patients he examined in connection with a claim for compensation. All were employed at the time of the injury. Accident neurosis was often defined by bizarre and inconsistent complaints, exaggeration of length of initial unconsciousness, and attention-seeking behaviors. About one-half of the patients returned to work but left work within a few days complaining of headaches and noise intolerance. About one-half of the patients did not return to work until their compensation claim had been settled or they were turned down for disability. Accident neurosis was more common in manual workers sustaining accidents at work than in nonmanual workers. Psychiatric treatment was not found to be helpful. Guthkelch concluded, "Accident neurosis is not particularly common; even in this series, which was exclusively composed of patients with a compensation problem, it was identified in only 6.8% of patients."

The end of litigation does not mean the end of symptoms or return to work for many claimants. Fee and Rutherford (1988) reported that 34% of patients were still symptomatic 1 year after settlement of claims. Many litigating patients, particularly those who are older or employed in more dangerous occupations, do not return to work after settlement (Kelly and Smith 1981). Packard (1992) interviewed 50 patients who had persistent posttraumatic headaches when litigation was settled.

At the time of follow-up, an average of 23 months after settlement, all 50 patients continued to report persistent headache symptoms, with an improvement in the headache pattern reported by only four patients.

Pending litigation may increase the level of stress for some claimants and may result in an increased frequency of symptoms after settlement (Mendelson 1982; Fee and Rutherford 1988). Skepticism of many physicians about persisting symptoms (Evans et al. 1994) may accentuate this level of stress.

However, Miller (1961) and Guthkelch (1980) make several excellent observations about patients who exaggerate or malinger with which clinicians can readily agree. Certainly physicians should consider a patient's motivation when litigation is involved. Clinical evaluation must include consideration of the effect of financial incentives on symptoms and disability (Binder and Rohling 1996). Since most patients who sustain mild closed head injuries have a good outcome, when severe cognitive deficits are still present months later, the strong possibility of malingering or another nonorganic explanation should be considered (Youngjohn et al. 1995; Binder and Rohling 1996). Patients with premorbid neuroticism or psychosocial problems may exaggerate symptoms.

Ruff et al. (1993) have suggested potential indicators of malingering following mild head injury that include the following: premorbid factors (antisocial and borderline personality traits, poor work record, and prior claims for injury); behavioral characteristics (uncooperative, evasive, or suspicious); test performance (missing random items, giving up easily, inconsistent test profile, or frequently stating "I don't know"); postmorbid complaints (describing events surrounding the accident in great detail or reporting an unusually large number of symptoms); and miscellaneous items (engaging in general activities not consistent with reported deficits, having significant financial stressors, resistance, and exhibiting a lack of reasonable follow-through on treatments). In a medicolegal setting, subjective criteria for making a diagnosis of postconcussion syndrome should be clearly delineated from objective findings. However, since some patients with seemingly hysterical signs and symptoms may actually have underlying organic disease (Gould et al.

1986), the diagnosis of accident neurosis, malingering, or conversion neurosis should be made with a great deal of caution.

In 1934, Strauss and Savitsky came to the following conclusion, which is still warranted:

The harshness, injustice, and brutal disregard of complaints shown by the physicians and representatives of insurance companies and their ready (assumptions) of intent to swindle do not foster wholesome patterns of reaction in injured persons. The frequent expression of unjustifiable skepticism on the part of examiners engenders resentment, discouragement, and hopelessness and too often forces these people to resort to more primitive modes of response (hysterical). (Strauss and Savitsky 1934)

## Conclusions

The postconcussion syndrome refers to a large number of symptoms and signs that may occur alone or in combination following usually mild head trauma. Headaches, dizziness, fatigue, irritability, anxiety, insomnia, loss of concentration and memory, and noise sensitivity are the most common complaints. Mild head injury and the postconcussion syndrome are major public health concerns, since mild head injury has an annual incidence of about 15O per 100,000 population and accounts for 75% or more of all head injuries.

Many physicians, lay persons, and interested third parties have serious doubts about the existence of the postconcussion syndrome. An important contributor to these doubts has been the frequent portrayal of head injury in motion pictures and on television as innocuous without sequelae or as humorous (e.g., the Hollywood head injury myth). Educational efforts can include examples of such media misinformation; familiar counterexamples from boxing (such as technical knockouts, knockouts, and punch-drunk syndrome), football, hockey, and soccer; and summarizing the evidence demonstrating organicity.

A growing body of evidence documents the organicity of the postconcussion syndrome. Abnormalities have been reported in neuropathological, neuroimaging, neuropsychological, and neurophysiological studies. Despite differences in definition of mild head injury, use of testing, study design, selection of subjects, and use of controls, prognostic studies clearly substantiate the existence of a postconcussion syndrome and the persistence of symptoms over time as compared to controls. For future studies, the use of a standardized definition of mild head injury such as the one proposed earlier in the chapter is critical to ensure studying similar types of injuries without confounding variables.

The symptoms and signs of the postconcussion syndrome are common and resolve in most patients by 3 to 6 months after the injury. However, a distinct minority of patients may have persisting symptoms and cognitive deficits for additional months or years.

Risk factors for persisting sequelae include age over 40 years; lower educational, intellectual, and socioeconomic level; female gender; alcohol abuse; prior head injury; and multiple trauma. Duration of post-traumatic amnesia, EEG, and auditory brain stem response studies are not predictive of sequelae. Lesions present on MRI scans of the brain do have predictive value for cognitive impairment.

Compensation neurosis or malingering in patients with compensation claims is quite uncommon. Patients with persisting symptoms frequently seek redress because they do have persisting symptoms. Physicians should educate patients, their families, and other interested parties at all stages following injury. As our knowledge increases, it is hoped that treatments will be discovered that favorably improve outcome.

## References

Abdel-Dayem, H. M.; Abu-Dudeh, H.; Kumar, M.; et al. SPECT brain perfusion abnormalities in mild or moderate traumatic brain injury. Clin. Nucl. Med. 23:309–317; 1998.

Annegers, J. F.; Grabow, J. D.; Kurland, L. T.; Laws, E. R. The incidence, causes, and secular trends of head trauma in Olmsted County, Minnesota, 1935–1974. Neurology 30:912–919; 1980.

Annegers, J. F.; Hauser, W. A.; Coan, S. P.; Rocca, W. A. A population-based study of seizures after traumatic brain injuries. N. Engl. J. Med. 338:20–24; 1998.

Ashikaga, R.; Araki, Y.; Ishida, O. MRI of head injury using FLAIR. Neuroradiolology 39:239–242; 1997.

Aubrey, J.; Dobbs, A. R.; Rule, B. G. Laypersons' knowledge about the sequelae of minor head injury and whiplash. J. Neurol. Neurosurg. Psychiatry 52:842–846; 1989.

Barry, E.; Krumhjolz, A.; Bergey, G. K.; et al. Nonepileptic posttraumatic seizures. Epilepsia 39:427–431; 1998.

Barth, J. T.; Macciocchi, S. N.; Giordani, B.; Rimel, R.; Jane, J. A.; Boll, T. J. Neuropsychological sequelae of minor head injury. Neurosurgery 13:529–533; 1983.

Bazarian, J. J.; Wong, T.; Harris, M. Epidemiology and predictors of post-concussive syndrome after minor head injury in an emergency population. Brain Inj. 13:173–189; 1999.

Bernstein, D. M. Recovery from mild head injury. Brain Inj. 13:151–172; 1999.

Berrol, S. Other factors: age, alcohol, and multiple injuries. In: Hoff, J. T.; Anderson, T. E.; Cole, T. M., eds. Mild to moderate head injury. Boston: Blackwell; 1989; p. 135–142.

Biary, N.; Cleeves, L.; Findley, L.; et al. Post-traumatic tremor. Neurology 39:103–106; 1989.

Binder, L. M. Assessment of malingering after mild head trauma with the Portland Digit Recognition Test. J. Clin. Exp. Neuropsychol. 15:170–183; 1993.

Binder, L. M.; Rohling, M. L. Money matters: a meta-analytic review of the effects of financial incentives on recovery after closed-head injury. Am. J. Psychiatry 153:7–10; 1996.

Blumbergs, P. C.; Jones, N. R.; North, J. B. Diffuse axonal injury in head trauma. J. Neurol. Neurosurg. Psychiatry 52:838–841; 1989.

Bohnen, N.; Twijnstra, A.; Wijnen, G.; et al. Tolerance for light and sound of patients with persistent post-concussional symptoms six months after mild head injury. J. Neurol. 238:443–446; 1991.

Brismar, B.; Engstrom, A; Rydberg, U. Head injury and intoxication: a diagnostic and therapeutic dilemma. Acta Chir. Scand. 149:11–14; 1983.

Bruce, D. A. Delayed deterioration of consciousness after trivial head injury in childhood. Br. Med. J. 289:715–716; 1984.

Bryant, R. A.; Harvey, A. G. Relationship between acute stress and posttraumatic stress disorder following mild traumatic brain injury. Am. J. Psychiatry 155:625–629; 1998.

Busch, C. R.; Alpern, H. P. Depression after mild traumatic brain injury: a review of current research. Neuropsychol. Rev. 8:95–108; 1998.

Capruso, D. X.; Levin, H. S. Neurobehavioral outcome of head injury. In: Evans, R. W., ed. Neurology and trauma. Philadelphia: W. B. Saunders Co.; 1996: p. 201–221.

Carlsson, G. S.; Svardsudd, K.; Welin, L. Long-term effects of head injuries sustained during life in three male populations. J. Neurosurg. 67:197–205; 1987.

Cartlidge, N. E. F. Postconcussional syndrome. Scot. Med. J. 23:103; 1977.

Cicerone, K. D.; Kalmar, K. Does premorbid depression influence post-concussive symptoms and neuropsychological functioning? Brain Inj. 11:643–648; 1997.

Couban, S.; Maxner, C. E. Cerebral venous sinus thrombosis presenting as idiopathic intracranial hypertension. Can. Med. Assoc. J. 145:657–659; 1991.

Couch, J. R.; Bearss, C. Chronic daily headache in the post-head injury syndrome (PHIS). Headache 34:296; 1994.

Culotta, V. P.; Sementilli, M. E.; Gerold, K.; Watts, C. C. Clinicopathological heterogeneity in the classification of mild head injury. Neurosurgery 38:245–250; 1996.

de Morsier, C. Les encephalopathies traumatiques. Etude neurologique. Schweiz. Arch. Neurol. Neurochir. Psychiat. 50:161; 1943.

Denker, P. G. The postconcussion syndrome: prognosis and evaluation of the organic factors. N. Y. State J. Med. 44:379–384; 1944.

Denny-Brown, D. Disability arising from closed head injury. JAMA 127:429–436; 1945.

Dikmen, S.; McLean, A.; Temkin, N. Neuropsychological and psychosocial consequences of minor head injury. J. Neurol. Neurosurg. Psychiatry 49:1227–1232; 1986.

Dow, R. S.; Ulett, G.; Raak, J. Electroencephalographic studies immediately following head injury. Am. J. Psychiatry 101:174–183; 1944.

Drake, M. E.; Weate, S. J.; Newell, S. A. Auditory evoked potentials in postconcussive syndrome. Electromyogr. Clin. Neurophysiol. 36:457–462; 1996.

Edna, T. -H.; Cappelen, J. Late postconcussional symptoms in traumatic head injury. An analysis of frequency and risk factors. Acta Neurochir. (Wien) 86:12–17; 1987.

Edna, T. -H. Disability 3–5 years after minor head injury. J. Oslo City Hosp. 37:41–48; 1987.

Erichsen, J. E. On concussion of the spine: nervous shock and other obscure injuries of the nervous system in their clinical and medico-legal aspects. London: Longmans Green; 1882.

Evans, R. W. The postconcussion syndrome and the sequelae of mild head trauma. Neurol. Clin. 10:815–847; 1992.

Evans, R. W. The post-concussion syndrome: 130 years of controversy. Semin. Neurol. 14(1):32–39; 1994a.

Evans, R. W.; Evans, R. I.; Sharp, M. The physician survey on the post-concussion and whiplash syndromes. Headache 34:268–274; 1994b.

Evans, R. W. The postconcussion syndrome and the sequelae of mild head injury. In: Evans, R. W., ed. Neurology and trauma. Philadelphia: W. B. Saunders Co.; 1996a: p. 91–116.

Evans, R. W. Chronic post-traumatic headaches are not a myth. Cephalalgia 16:461; 1996b.

Ewing, R.; McCarthy, D.; Gronwall, D.; Wrightson, P. Persisting effects of minor head injury observable during hypoxic stress. J. Clin. Neuropsychol. 2:147–155; 1980.

Fee, C. R. A.; Rutherford W. H. A study of the effect of legal settlement on postconcussion symptoms. Arch. Emerg. Med. 5:12–17; 1988.

Gama, J. H. P. Traite des plaies de tete et de l'encephalite. Paris; 1835.

Gentilini, M.; Nichelli, P.; Schoenhuber, R. Assessment of attention in mild head injury. In: Levin, H. S.; Eisenberg, H. M.; Benton, A. L., eds. Mild head injury. New York: Oxford University Press; 1989: p. 163–175.

Gordon, W. A.; Brown, M.; Sliwinski, M. The enigma of "hidden" traumatic brain injury. J. Head Trauma Rehabil. 13:39–56; 1998.

Gould, R.; Miller, B. L.; Goldberg, M. A.; Benson, D. F. The validity of hysterical signs and symptoms. J. Nerv. Ment. Dis. 174:593–597; 1986.

Graham, D. I.; McIntosh, T. K. Neuropathology of brain injury. In: Evans, R. W., ed. Neurology and trauma. Philadelphia: W. B. Saunders Co., 1996.; p. 53–90.

Gronwall, D. Concussion: does intelligence help? N. Z. Psychologist 5:72–78; 1976.

Gronwall, D. Cumulative and persisting effects of concussion on attention and cognition. In: Levin, H. S.; Eisenberg, H. M.: Benton, A. L., eds. Mild head injury. New York: Oxford University Press; 1989: p. 153–162.

Gronwall, D.; Wrightson, P. Delayed recovery of intellectual function after minor head injury. Lancet 2:605–609; 1974.

Gronwall, D.; Wrightson, P. Cumulative effects of concussion. Lancet 2:995–997; 1975.

Guthkelch, A. N. Posttraumatic amnesia, postconcussional symptoms, and accident neurosis. Eur. Neurol. 19:91–102; 1980.

Haas, D. C. Chronic post-traumatic headaches classified and compared with natural headaches. Cephalalgia 16:486–493; 1996.

Headache Classification Committee of the International Headache Society. Classification and diagnostic criteria for headache disorders, cranial neuralgias and facial pain. Cephalalgia 88:S1–96; 1988.

Hernesniemi, J. Outcome following head injuries in the aged. Acta Neurochir. 49:67–79; 1979.

Hesselink, J. R.; Dowd, C. F.; Healy, M. E.; et al. MR imaging of brain contusions: a comparative study with CT. AJR Am. J. Roentgenol 150:1133–1142; 1988.

Hugenholtz, H.; Stuss, D. T.; Stethem, L. L.; et al. How long does it take to recover from a mild concussion? Neurosurgery 22:853–858; 1988.

Ingebrigtsen, T.; Waterloo, K.; Jacobsen, EA.; et al. Traumatic brain damage in minor head injury: relation of serum S-100 protein measurements to magnetic resonance imaging and neurobehavioral outcome. Neurosurg 45:468–476; 1999.

Jankovic, J. Post-traumatic movement disorders. Central and peripheral mechanisms. Neurology 44: 2006–2014; 1994.

Jennett, B.; Frankowski, R. F. The epidemiology of head injury. In: Brinkman, R., ed. Handbook of clinical neurology. Vol. 13. New York: Elsevier; 1990: p. 1–16.

Jensen, O. K.; Nielsen, F. F. The influence of sex and pretraumatic headache on the incidence and severity of headache after head injury. Cephalalgia 10: 285–293; 1990.

Jeret, J. S.; Mandell, M.; Anziska, B.; et al Clinical predictors of abnormality disclosed by computed tomography after mild head trauma. Neurosurgery 32:9–16; 1993.

Juni, J. E. Taking brain SPECT seriously: reflections on recent clinical reports in The Journal of Nuclear Medicine. J. Nucl. Med. 35:1891–1895; 1994.

Kant, R.; Smith-Seemiller, L.; Isaac, G.; Duffy, J. Tc-HMPAO SPECT in persistent post-concussion syndrome after mild head injury: comparison with MRI/CT. Brain Inj. 11:115–124; 1997.

Keane, J. R.; Baloh, R. W. Post-traumatic cranial neuropathies. In: Evans, R. W., ed. Neurology and trauma. Philadelphia: W. B. Saunders. Co.; 1996: p. 117–132.

Kelly, J. P.; Rosenberg, J. H. Diagnosis and management of concussion in sports. Neurology 48: 574–580; 1997.

Kelly, R.: Smith, B. N. Posttraumatic syndrome: another myth discredited. J. R. Soc. Med. 74:275–277; 1981.

Keshavan, M. S.; Channabasavanna, S. M.; Narayana Reddy, G. N. Post-traumatic psychiatric disturbances: patterns and predictors of outcome. Br. J. Psychiatry 138:157–160; 1981.

Kraus, J. F.; Black, M. A.; Hessol, N. The incidence of acute brain injury and serious impairment in a defined population. Am. J. Epidemiol. 119:186–201; 1984.

Kraus, J. F.; Nourjah, M. S. The epidemiology of mild, uncomplicated brain injury. J. Trauma. 28: 1637– 1643; 1988.

Lee, S. T.; Lui, T. N. Early seizures after mild closed head injury. J. Neurosurg. 76:435–439; 1992.

Leininger, B. E.; Gramling, S. E.; Farrell, A. D.; Kreutzer, J. S.; Peck, E. A. Neuropsychological deficits in symptomatic minor head injury patients after concussion and mild concussion. J. Neurol. Neurosurg. Psychiatry 53:293–296; 1990.

Lesser, I. M.; Mena, I.; Boone, K. B.; et al Reduction of cerebral blood flow in older depressed patients. Arch. Gen. Psychiatry 51:677–686; 1994.

Levin, H. S. Neurobehavioral outcome of mild to moderate head injury. In: Hoff, J. T.; Anderson, T. E.; Cole, T. M., eds. Mild to moderate head injury. Boston: Blackwell; 1989: p. 153–185.

Levin, H. S. Cognitive rehabilitation: unproved but promising. Arch. Neurol. 47:223–224; 1990.

Levin, H. S.; Amparo, E. G.; Eisenberg, H. M.; Williams, D. H.: High, W. M.: McArdle, C. B.; Weiner, R. L. Magnetic resonance imaging and computerized tomography in relation to the neurobehavioral sequelae of mild and moderate head injuries. J. Neurosurg. 66:706–713; 1987.

Levin, H. S.; Gary, H. E.; High, W. M.; et al. Minor head injury and the postconcussional syndrome: methodological issues in outcome studies. In: Levin, H. S.; Grafman, J.; Eisenberg, H. M., eds. Neurobehavioral recovery from head injury. New York: Oxford University Press; 1987a: p. 262–275.

Levin, H. S.; Mattis, S.; Ruff, R. M.; et al. Neurobehavioral outcome following minor head injury: a three-center study. J. Neurosurg. 66:234–243; 1987b.

Levin, H. S.; Williams, D. H.; Eisenberg, H. M.; High, W. M.; Guinto, F. C. Serial MRI and neurobehavioural findings after mild to moderate closed head injury. J. Neurol. Neurosurg. Psychiatry 55: 255– 262; 1992.

Lewine, J.D.; Davis, J.T.; Sloan, J.H.; et al. Neuromagnetic assessment of pathophysiologic brain activity induced by minor head trauma. AJNR 20:857–866; 1999.

Lorenzoni, E. Electroencephalographic studies before and after head injuries. Electroencephalogr. Clin. Neurophysiol. 28:216; 1970.

MacFlynn, G.; Montgomery, E. A.; Fenton, G. W., et al. Measurement of reaction time following minor head injury. J. Neurol. Neurosurg. Psychiatry 47: 1326–1331; 1984.

Malec, J. F. Cognitive rehabilitation. In: Evans, R. W., ed. Neurology and trauma. Philadelphia: W. B. Saunders. Co.; 1996; p. 231–248.

Martland, H. S. Punch-drunk. JAMA 19:1103–1107; 1928.

Matser, J. T.; Kessels, A. G. H.; Jordan, B. D.; et al. Chronic traumatic brain injury in professional soccer players. Neurology 51:791–796; 1998.

Matthews, W. B. Footballer's migraine. Br. Med. J. 2:326–327; 1972.

McCrory, P. R.; Berkovic, S. F. Second impact syndrome. Neurology 50:677–683; 1998.

McKinlay, W. W.; Brooks, D. N.: Bond, M. R. Postconcussional symptoms, financial compensation, and outcome of severe blunt head injury. J. Neurol. Neurosurg. Psychiatry 46:1084–1091; 1983.

McMordie, W. R. Twenty-year follow-up of the prevailing opinion on the posttraumatic or postconcussional syndrome. Clin. Neuropsychol. 2:198–212; 1988.

Mendelson, G. Not "cured by a verdict": effect of legal settlement on compensation claimants. Med. J. Aust. 2:132–134; 1982.

Merskey, H.; Woodforde, J. M. Psychiatric sequelae of minor head injury. Brain 95:521–528; 1972.

Miller, H. Accident neurosis. Br. Med. J. 1:919–925, 992–998; 1961.

Minderhoud, J. M.; Boelens, M. E. M.; Huizenga, J.; Saan, R. J. Treatment of minor head injuries. Clin. Neurol. Neurosurg. 82:127–140; 1980.

Mitchener, A.; Wyper, D. J.; Patterson, J., et al. SPECT, CT, and MRI in head injury: acute abnormalities followed up at six months. J. Neurol. Neurosurg. Psychiatry 62:633–636, 1997.

Mittl, R. L.; Grossman, R. I.; Hiehle, J. F.; et al Prevalence of MR evidence of diffuse axonal injury in patients with mild head injury and normal head CT findings. Am. J. Neuroradiol. 15:1583–1589; 1994.

NIH Consensus Development Panel on Rehabilitation of Persons with Traumatic Brain Injury. Rehabilitation of persons with traumatic brain injury. JAMA 282: 974–983; 1999

Nuwer, M. Assessment of digital EEG, quantitative EEG, and EEG brain mapping: report of the American Academy of Neurology and the American Clinical Neurophysiology Society. Neurology 49: 277–292; 1997.

Nuwer, M. R.; Hauser, H. M. Erroneous diagnosis using EEG discriminant analysis. Neurology 44: 1998–2000; 1994.

Ochagavia, A. R.; Boque, M. C.; Torre, C.; et al. Dural venous sinus thrombosis due to cranial trauma. Lancet 347:1564; 1996.

Oppenheimer, D. R. Microscopic lesions in the brain following head injury. J. Neurol. Neurosurg. Psychiatry 31:299–306; 1968.

Packard, R. C. Posttraumatic headache: permanence and relationship to legal settlement. Headache 32: 496–500; 1992.

Packard, R. C. Posttraumatic headache. Semin. Neurol. 14:40–45; 1994.

Packard, R. C.; Ham, L. P. Promising techniques in the assessment of mild head injury. Semin. Neurol. 14:74–83; 1994.

Perlis, M. L.; Artiola, L.; Giles, D. E. Sleep complaints in chronic postconcussion syndrome. Percept. Mot. Skills 84:595–599; 1997.

Povlischock, J. T.; Coburn, T. H. Morphopathological change associated with mild head injury. In: Levin, H. S.; Eisenherg, H. M.; Benton, A. L., eds. Mild head injury. New York: Oxford University Press; 1989; p. 37–53.

Practice parameter The management of concussion in sports (summary statement). Report of the Quality Standards Subcommittee. Neurology 48:581–585; 1997.

Report of the Therapeutics and Technology Assessment Subcommittee of the American Academy of Neurology. Assessment of brain SPECT. Neurology 46:278–285; 1996a.

Report of the Therapeutics and Technology Assessment Subcommittee of the American Academy of Neurology. Assessment: neuropsychological testing of adults. Considerations for neurologists. Neurology 47:592–599; 1996b.

Rigler, I. Ueber die Verletzungen auf Eisenbahnen lnsbesondere der Verletzungen des Rueckenmarks. Berlin: Reimer; 1879.

Rimel, R. W.; Giordani, B.; Barth, J. T.; et al. Disability caused by minor head injury. Neurosurgery 9: 221–228; 1981.

Robertson, A. The postconcussional syndrome then and now. Aust. N. Z. J. Psychiatry 22:396–402; 1988.

Ross, R. J.; Col, M.; Thompson, J. S.; et al. Boxers—computer tomography, EEG, and neurological evaluation. JAMA 249:211–213; 1983.

Rothweiler, B.; Temkin, N. R.; Dikmen, S. S. Aging effect on psychosocial outcome in traumatic brain injury. Arch. Phys. Med. Rehabil. 79:881–887; 1998.

Roy, C. W.; Pentland, B.; Miller, J. D. The causes and consequences of minor head injury in the elderly. Injury 17:220–223; 1986.

Ruff, R. M.; Crouch, J. A.; Troster, A. I.; et al. Selected cases of poor outcome following a minor brain trauma: comparing neuropsychological and positron emission tomography assessment. Brain Inj. 8:297–308; 1994.

Ruff, R. M.; Wylie, T.; Tennant, W. Malingering and malingering-like aspects of mild closed head injury. J. Head Trauma Rehabil. 8:60–73; 1993.

Ruffolo, C. F.; Friedland, J. F.; Dawson, D. R.; et al. Mild traumatic brain injury from motor vehicle accidents: factors associated with return to work. Arch. Phys. Med. Rehabil. 80:392–398; 1999.

Russell, M. B.; Olesen, J. Migraine associated with head trauma. Eur. J. Neurol. 3:424–428; 1996.

Rutherford, W. H.; Merrett, J. D.; McDonald, J. R. Sequelae of concussion caused by minor head injuries. Lancet 1:1–4; 1977.

Rutherford, W. H.; Merrett, J. D.; McDonald, J. R. Symptoms at 1 year following concussion from minor head injuries. Injury 10:225–230; 1978.

Schoenhuber, R.; Gentilini, M.; Orlando, A. Prognostic value of auditory brain stem responses for late postconcussion symptoms following minor head injury. J. Neurosurg. 68:742–744; 1988.

Sheth, R. D.; Riggs, J. E.; Bodensteiner, J. B. Acute confusional migraine: variant of transient global amnesia. Pediatr. Neurol. 12:129–131; 1995.

Steadman, J. H.: Graham, J. G. Rehabilitation of the brain-injured. Prog. R. Soc. Med. 63:23–28; 1969.

Stein, S. C.; Ross, S. E. Mild head injury: a plea for routine early CT scanning. J. Trauma 33:11–13; 1992.

Strauss, I.; Savitsky, N. Head injury: neurologic and psychiatric aspects. Arch. Neurol. Psychiatry 31: 893–955; 1934.

Stuss, D. T. A sensible approach to mild traumatic brain injury. Neurology 45:1251–1252; 1995.

Symonds, C. The assessment of symptoms following head injury. Guys Hospital Gazette 51:464; 1937.

Symonds, C. Concussion and its sequelae. Lancet 1: 1–5; 1962.

Thatcher, R. W.; Walker, R. A.; Gerson, I; et al. EEG discriminant analyses of mild head injury. Clin. Neurophysiol. 73:94–106; 1989.

Trimble, M. Post-traumatic neurosis: from railway spine to the whiplash. Chichester: Wiley; 1981.

Tysvaer, A. T.; Storli, O. V.; Bachen, N. I. Soccer injuries to the brain. A neurologic and electroencephalographic study of former players. Acta Neurol. Scand. 80:151–156; 1989.

Van der Naalt, J.; van Zomeren, A. H.; Sluiter, W. J.; Minderhoud, J. M. One year outcome in mild to moderate head injury: the predictive value of acute injury characteristics related to complaints and return to work. J. Neurol. Neurosurg. Psychiatry 66: 207–213; 1999.

Waterloo, K.; Ingebrigtsen, T.; Romner, B. Neuropsychological function in patients with increased serum levels of protein S-100 after minor head injury. Acta Neurochir. (Wien) 139:26–32; 1997.

Weinstock, A.; Rothner, A. D. Trauma-triggered migraine: a cause of transient neurologic deficit following minor head injury in children. Neurology 45 (suppl. 4):A347–348; 1995.

Weiss, H. D.; Stern, B. J.; Goldberg, J. Posttraumatic migraine: chronic migraine precipitated by minor head or neck trauma. Headache 31:451–456; 1991.

Wrightson, P. Management of disability and rehabilitation services after mild head injury. In: Levin, H. S.; Eisenberg, H. M.; Benton. A. L., eds. Mild head injury. New York: Oxford University Press; 1989: p. 245–256.

Wrightson, P.; Gronwall, D. Time off work and symptoms after minor head injury. Injury 12:445–454; 1981.

Yokota, H.; Kurokawa, A; Otsuka, T.; et al. Significance of magnetic resonance imaging in acute head injury. J. Trauma 31:351–357; 1991.

Youngjohn, J. R.; Burrows, L.; Erdal, K. Brain damage or compensation neurosis? The controversial post-concussion syndrome. Clin. Neuropsychol. 9: 112–123; 1995.

# 24

# Spinal Cord Injury

ROBERT J. JACKSON AND DAVID S. BASKIN

Five thousand years ago, an Egyptian physician noted in the Edwin Smith Papyrus the features of spinal cord injury and concluded that this was "an ailment not to be treated" (Breasted 1930). This pessimistic view was held by many through the early 20th century. The eminent neurosurgeon Harvey Cushing found that approximately 80% of WWI casualties who sustained spinal cord injuries died within 2 weeks of injury (Cushing 1927). With the introduction of antibiotics and specialized centers for spinal cord injury near the end of WWII, it became apparent that a spinal cord–injured patient could survive with aggressive treatment. Guttmann promoted the concept that with special care and training, patients with spinal cord injury are able to re-enter society as productive members and care for themselves (Guttmann 1976). More recently, effective bladder management has significantly reduced mortality. Although life expectancy following spinal cord injury has continued to improve, it is far from normal, especially in the more severely injured. With increasing survival, the devastating effects of permanent paralysis became more apparent. Attention has therefore turned from survival to improving quality of life and functional outcome. Despite increased survival and functional outcome, a treatment to aid recovery of the

injured human spinal cord was not clinically demonstrated until 1990, when the results of the National Acute Spinal Cord Injury Study II (NASCIS II) were published (Bracken et al. 1990). Numerous other neuroscientists are working on spinal cord regeneration and transplantation. The prognosis and outcome following spinal cord injury have dramatically improved since Cushing's time. Spinal cord injury, prognosis, and functional outcome are reviewed.

## Epidemiology

The incidence of spinal cord injury (SCI) in the United States is approximately 30 to 40 cases per 1 million persons, or approximately 10,000 new cases per year (Bracken et al. 1981; Kraus et al. 1975). With prevalence rate of 500 to 1000 per million, there are approximately 200,000 to 250,000 individuals with spinal cord injury residing in the United States. Although figures on gender vary, 82.2% of all persons enrolled in the National Spinal Cord Injury Database are male (Stover and Fine 1986). SCI occurs most commonly in teenagers and young adults between the ages of 16 and 30 (Griffin et al. 1985; Kraus et al. 1975; Stover and Fine 1986). In the National SCI Database, more SCIs occur in the 16- to 30-year age group than in all other groups combined. The etiology of SCI varies, but motor vehicle crashes remain the leading cause (50%), followed by falls (20%), interpersonal violence (15% to 20%), and sports and recreation (10% to 15%) (Lobosky 1996). Unfortunately, gunshot wounds are responsible for more traumatic SCIs than automobile crashes in some urban areas (Graham and Weingarden 1989).

## Acute Spinal Cord Injury

An accurate clinical assessment of the neurological injury followed by detailed imaging of the spine and spinal cord are essential for the management of the patient with spinal cord injury. The neurological examination provides the most information for determining the prognosis, although thorough imaging may yield additional information regarding outcome. In order to accurately evaluate baseline SCI and to ensure that serial examinations are capable of assessing improvement or deterioration in a reproducible fashion in an individual and between institutions, a classification system was developed by the American Spinal Injury Association (ASIA) and the International Medical Society of Paraplegia (IMSOP) in 1992 (American Spinal Injury Association 1992) (Fig. 24-1). The ASIA/IMSOP impairment scale contains five grades of impairment, with grade A denoting a complete injury; grades B, C, and D indicating various levels of incomplete injury; and grade E indicating normal motor and sensory function of the spinal cord (Table 24-1). This classification method is based on the Frankel classification (Frankel et al. 1969), and is now considered the international standard.

Initial neurological assessments of the patient with acute spinal cord injury may be confusing due to spinal shock. This condition is thought to be related to temporary axonal and neuronal membrane dysfunction, and is more likely to occur with the more severe and rostral injuries. Spinal shock is characterized by a loss of somatic motor (paralysis, flaccidity, areflexia), sensory (anesthesia) and sympathetic autonomic function (hypotension, bradycardia, skin hyperemia). This temporary and reversible condition may be of variable duration and therefore difficult to separate from pathology producing permanent damage to the cord. To avoid confusion, Tator recommends the

following guidelines: assume that somatic motor and sensory deficits lasting than more than 1 hour after injury are due to pathological changes in the cord rather than spinal shock, and that reflex and autonomic components of spinal shock persist for days to months (Tator 1996).

Individual prognosis from spinal cord injury is based on the magnitude of force delivered to the spinal cord at the time of the traumatic incident, as well as secondary injury such as manipulation at the time of rescue or during transfers, inflammatory responses, and other physiological factors. Physicians can indirectly influence the number of spinal cord injuries through preventative programs such as "Think First" (sponsored by the American Association of Neurological Surgeons and Congress of Neurological Surgeons, 1986). Modifications of football tackling rules based on the input of physicians resulted in a significant decrease of cervical spine injuries in that sport (Torg et al. 1985). Following a traumatic injury to the spinal cord, we can help prevent or reduce secondary injury through careful immobilization, maintaining adequate perfusion and oxygenation, pharmacological methods, and surgery. Surgical decompression as well as internal or external stabilization procedures are indicated in some cases of spinal cord injury to reduce secondary injury. Early surgical intervention may improve neurological outcome (Mirza 1999). Currently, a large multicenter neurosurgical trial is underway to assess the benefits of emergent surgical decompression in acute SCI.

Trauma to the spinal cord initiates a cascade of inflammatory responses to injury, presumably designed to clean up cellular debris and repair injury. These complex mechanisms involve cellular membrane breakdown with the release of arachidonic acid, free radicals, excitatory transmitters, and calcium that in turn cause additional damage. Methylprednisolone (MPS) has been shown to reduce secondary spinal cord injury in the NASCIS II, by suppressing lipid peroxidation and hydrolysis. NASCIS II was a randomized, double-blind, placebo-controlled study that unequivocally demonstrated improved neurological recovery in patients with both complete and incomplete spinal cord injuries treated with MPS in the acute period (Bracken et al. 1990; Bracken et al. 1992). Treatment with MPS more than doubled the probability that patients would convert from quadriplegia or

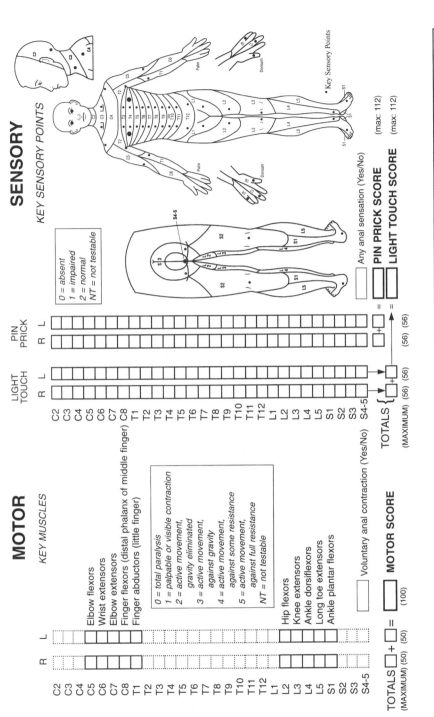

**Figure 24-1.** Standard neurological classification of spinal cord injury.

## MOTOR

*KEY MUSCLES*

| | R | L | |
|---|---|---|---|
| C2 | | | |
| C3 | | | |
| C4 | | | |
| C5 | | | Elbow flexors |
| C6 | | | Wrist extensors |
| C7 | | | Elbow extensors |
| C8 | | | Finger flexors (distal phalanx of middle finger) |
| T1 | | | Finger abductors (little finger) |
| T2 | | | |
| T3 | | | |
| T4 | | | |
| T5 | | | |
| T6 | | | |
| T7 | | | |
| T8 | | | |
| T9 | | | |
| T10 | | | |
| T11 | | | |
| T12 | | | |
| L1 | | | |
| L2 | | | Hip flexors |
| L3 | | | Knee extensors |
| L4 | | | Ankle dorsiflexors |
| L5 | | | Long toe extensors |
| S1 | | | Ankle plantar flexors |
| S2 | | | |
| S3 | | | |
| S4-5 | | | |

```
0 = total paralysis
1 = palpable or visible contraction
2 = active movement,
    gravity eliminated
3 = active movement,
    against gravity
4 = active movement,
    against some resistance
5 = active movement,
    against full resistance
NT = not testable
```

Voluntary anal contraction (Yes/No) [ ]  **MOTOR SCORE** [ ] (100)

TOTALS [ ] + [ ] = [ ]
(MAXIMUM) (50) (50)

## SENSORY

*KEY SENSORY POINTS*

```
0 = absent
1 = impaired
2 = normal
NT = not testable
```

| | LIGHT TOUCH R | LIGHT TOUCH L | PIN PRICK R | PIN PRICK L |
|---|---|---|---|---|
| C2 | | | | |
| C3 | | | | |
| C4 | | | | |
| C5 | | | | |
| C6 | | | | |
| C7 | | | | |
| C8 | | | | |
| T1 | | | | |
| T2 | | | | |
| T3 | | | | |
| T4 | | | | |
| T5 | | | | |
| T6 | | | | |
| T7 | | | | |
| T8 | | | | |
| T9 | | | | |
| T10 | | | | |
| T11 | | | | |
| T12 | | | | |
| L1 | | | | |
| L2 | | | | |
| L3 | | | | |
| L4 | | | | |
| L5 | | | | |
| S1 | | | | |
| S2 | | | | |
| S3 | | | | |
| S4-5 | | | | |

• Key Sensory Points

TOTALS { [ ]+[ ]   [ ]+[ ] }
(MAXIMUM) (56) (56)   (56) (56)

Any anal sensation (Yes/No) [ ]

**PIN PRICK SCORE** [ ] (max: 112)
**LIGHT TOUCH SCORE** [ ] (max: 112)

| **NEUROLOGICAL LEVEL** | R | L | **COMPLETE OR INCOMPLETE?** | |
|---|---|---|---|---|
| The most caudal segment with normal function | | | Incomplete = Any sensory or motor function in S4-S5 | |
| SENSORY | [ ] | [ ] | | |
| MOTOR | [ ] | [ ] | **ASIA IMPAIRMENT SCALE** [ ] | |

| **ZONE OF PARTIAL PRESERVATION** | | R | L |
|---|---|---|---|
| Partially innervated segments | SENSORY | [ ] | [ ] |
| | MOTOR | [ ] | [ ] |

This form may be copied freely but should not be altered without permission from the American Spinal Injury Association.

Version 4p
GHC 1996

**Table 24-1.** ASIA / IMSOP Impairment Scale

| Grade A | Complete | No motor or sensory function is preserved in the sacral segments S4–S5 |
|---|---|---|
| Grade B | Incomplete | Sensory but no motor function is preserved below the neurological level and extends through the sacral segments S4–S5 |
| Grade C | Incomplete | Motor function is preserved below the neurological level, and the majority of key muscles below the neurological level have a muscle grade less than 3 |
| Grade D | Incomplete | Motor function is preserved below the neurological level, and the majority of key muscles below the neurological level have a muscle grade greater than or equal to 3 |
| Grade E | Normal | Motor and sensory function are normal |

paraplegia to quadriparesis or paraparesis, analgesia to hypalgesia, and anesthesia to hypesthesia (Young and Bracken 1992). Other pharmacological interventions that have shown beneficial effects in animal models and/or human studies include: tirilizad, $GM_1$ ganglioside, $N$-methyl-D-apartate (NMDA) receptor antagonists, and 4-aminopyridine (Greene et al. 1996; Zeidman et al. 1996). Readers are encouraged to refer to Amar and Levy (1999) for a comprehensive review of the pathogenesis and pharmacological strategies for mitigating damage in acute spinal cord injury.

Hypotension and hypoxia are thought to cause additional secondary injury in SCI. These factors have been associated with significantly increased morbidity and mortality in head injury, subarachnoid hemorrhage, and stroke (Chestnut et al. 1993; Miller et al. 1978; Strandgaard 1976). Patients managed with volume expansion and hypertensive therapy have improved neurological outcomes as compared to those who do not (Kassell et al. 1982; Miller and Diringer 1995; Montgomery et al. 1981; Origitano et al. 1990; Pritz et al. 1978; Solomon et al. 1988). In an effort to maintain spinal cord blood flow and prevent secondary injury, Vale and colleagues (Vale et al. 1997) have applied this therapy to SCI by maintaining mean arterial blood pressure (MABP) above 85 mm Hg with volume therapy, utilizing vasopressors as needed, along with Swan-Ganz catheterization. In patients with complete cervical SCIs, 60% improved at least one ASIA grade and

30% regained the ability to walk. At the 12 month follow-up, 92% and 88% of incomplete cervical and thoracic spinal cord injuries, respectively, regained the ability to walk. In patients with complete thoracic SCIs, 33% improved at least one ASIA grade, and 10% regained the ability to walk. About half of the walking patients had an ambulatory capacity of less than 200 feet and required a walker, crutches, and/or lower extremity braces. The neurological recovery of patients in this study of aggressive volume resuscitation and blood pressure management is superior to other comparable studies (Ditunno et al. 1995; Stover and Fine 1986; Waters et al. 1992, 1993, 1994b) as we shall see below.

**Prognosis**

It is difficult to predict the neurological outcome for any particular individual following an acute spinal cord injury. We can look at large numbers of patients with acute spinal cord injury, follow them for a certain length of time, and assess outcome for various groups. Basic generalizations can be extrapolated from these data. The prognosis for neurological recovery is much better for incomplete cord injuries as compared to complete cord injuries. The greatest rate of recovery occurs early (hours to weeks) and then generally plateaus in 6 months to 1 year following SCI. Examinations performed at greater lengths of time after injury can more accurately predict recovery, although we strive to find accurate early predictors to guide therapy and expectations.

Prediction of functional abilities after SCI generally follows the degree of motor function (Woolsey 1998). In the National SCI Database, the majority (89%) of patients admitted within 24 hours after sustaining complete motor and sensory SCI (ASIA A), remain ASIA A at time of discharge. Approximately 5%, 3%, and 3% of patients will progress to grades B, C, and D, respectively (Fig. 24-2). For patients admitted ASIA grade A greater than 24 hours following injury, 94% remain so at the time of discharge (Ditunno et al. 1995). Motor scores in patients with complete tetraplegia improved a mean of 6 points from 24 hours to the 3- to 6-month follow-up in the National Database (Ditunno et al. 1995), 4.5 points from admission to 6-months (Curt et al. 1998), 8.6 points from 1 month to 1 year (Waters

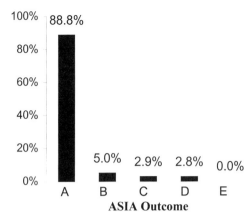

**Figure 24-2.** ASIA outcome for those ASIA A on admission.

et al. 1993), and 24 points from admission to 6-month follow-up in a small group of patients treated with hypervolemic and hypertensive therapy (Vale et al. 1997). Key muscles such as the biceps, wrist extensors, and triceps that have a strength of grades 1 to 2/5 at 72 hours generally improved to grade 4/5 within 4 months of injury (Ditunno et al. 1997). Waters and colleagues (Waters et al. 1993) reported similar findings in 97% of patients when measured at 1 month and 1 year. The next distal key muscle which had grade zero strength recovered to greater than or equal to 3/5 in 27% of patients by 1 year. Only 1% of patients had significant improvement from 0/5 to greater than or equal to 3/5 in a muscle group two levels below by 1 year (Waters et al. 1993). Although 94% of those with complete injuries remain complete, several large series of patients with acute SCI include a small percentage of initially complete cases who recover lower extremity function (Hansebout 1982). Vale and colleagues' (Vale et al. 1997) study of aggressively managed patients with acute SCI found significant improvement, 60% improved at least one Frankel grade, and 30% became ambulatory.

The recovery in complete paraplegia is less than that of complete cervical injuries. In patients with complete paraplegia, Waters and colleagues (Waters et al. 1992) found an ASIA motor index increase of 7.8 points from admission to 1 year, and with time 5% became ambulatory in the community on a limited basis. Approximately 96% remain complete at 1 year (Waters et al. 1991, 1994a).

Although it is more difficult to predict the long-term outcome, the prognosis for incomplete SCI is significantly better than that of complete SCI. In the National SCI Database, approximately 49% of grade B patients remained grade B, 16% progressed to grade C, 28% progressed to grade D, and 5% regressed to grade A (Ditunno et al. 1995) (Fig. 24-3). ASIA motor index scores in patients with incomplete tetraplegia improved by a mean of 13 points from 24 hours to the 3- to 6-month follow-up in the National Database (Ditunno et al. 1995), 28 points in 1 month to 6 months (Curt et al. 1998), 23.5 points in 1 month to 1 year (Waters et al. 1994b), and approximately 45 points from prior to 24 hours to 1 year (Vale et al. 1997). Among those with incomplete injuries, bilateral sacral pinprick sensation is associated with a better prognosis (Curt et al. 1998; Waters et al. 1994b; Foo et al. 1981; Jacobs et al. 1995). This is probably related to the close proximity of the lateral corticospinal tract to the spinothalamic tract, which is presumably intact in those with preserved bilateral pinprick sensation. Approximately 36% to 46% of Frankel grade B patients become ambulatory in the community (Curt et al. 1998; Waters et al. 1994b). However, of those with intact bilateral sacral pinprick sensation, approximately 88% became ambulatory as compared to 11% of those without bilaterally intact pinprick sensation. Less than 50% of those without bilaterally intact pinprick sensation improved one Frankel grade, compared to an improvement of two Frankel grades in most with intact bilateral pinprick sensation. Looking at individual muscles in those

**Figure 24-3.** ASIA outcome for those ASIA B on admission.

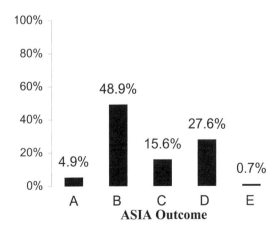

with incomplete cord injuries, nearly all muscles that were 2/5 at 1 month improved to greater than or equal to 3/5, 75% of those muscles with 1/5 strength improved to greater than or equal to 3/5, and 20% of the 0/5 strength muscles improved to greater than or equal to 3/5 (Waters et al. 1994b).

Prognosis is naturally better for the Frankel grade C and D patients. Of the admission grade C patients in the National Database, 41% remained grade C, 53% improved to grade D, and 1.3% improved to grade E (Fig. 24-4). In the admission grade D patients, 90% remained grade D and 6.5% improved to grade E (Fig. 24-5). Approximately 64% to 88% of patients with acute SCI and an initial exam grade of ASIA/Frankel C, and nearly all those initially grade D, have become functional ambulators (Crozier et al. 1991; Jacobs et al. 1995; Vale et al. 1997; Waters et al. 1994b). Hussey and Stauffer (1998) studied and classified ambulatory function in patients with SCI and concluded that quadriceps function was an important determinant in the level of ambulation achieved. Jacobs et al. (1995) found that all SCI patients with greater than 0/5 quadriceps strength on initial examination became ambulatory. Likewise, Crozier et al. (1991) reported that all patients with quadriceps strength greater than or equal to 3/5 at 2 months became ambulatory.

Patients with incomplete paraplegia clearly have a better prognosis than those with complete injuries. Overall, 76% of patients with incomplete paraplegia became ambulatory at 1 year as compared to 5% for those with complete paraplegia. For patients with complete paraplegia, the level of

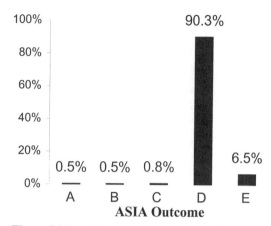

**Figure 24-5.** ASIA outcome for those ASIA D on admission.

injury is significantly associated with potential for future ambulation (Yarkony et al. 1990; Waters et al. 1992). Patients with an initial neurological level of injury (NLI) above T9 did not regain lower extremity motor function, whereas 38% of those with an initial NLI at or below T9 had some return of lower extremity function. Of those with an initial NLI below T12, 22% became ambulatory (Waters et al. 1992).

Additional useful information regarding prognosis can be obtained from magnetic resonance imaging (MRI) in the acute period following spinal cord injury (Selden et al. 1999). Ramon and colleagues (1997) have correlated the MRI cord findings with the neurological examination at presentation and follow-up in 55 patients with spinal cord injuries. MRI cord findings can be divided into five groups. The first group is that of cord transection. The next is that of hemorrhagic contusion—within the first 72 hours, the cord on $T_1$-weighted images (T1WI) is heterogeneous, while on $T_2$-weighted images (T2WI) there is a large central area with low signal intensity surrounded by a thin high-intensity peripheral ring of extracellular methemoglobin. In this group, the cord shows hyperintensity on T1WI and T2WI at 72 hours to 1 week. The third group is that of contusion, with a normal T1WI, and a small central area of cord isointensity and a thick peripheral ring of hyperintensity on T2WI. A fourth group is that of edema, with a normal T1WI and high intensity on T2WI. The final group is that of a normal appearance. Cord transection ($n = 2$) and hemorrhagic contusion ($n = 15$) were associated with a

**Figure 24-4.** ASIA outcome for those ASIA C on admission.

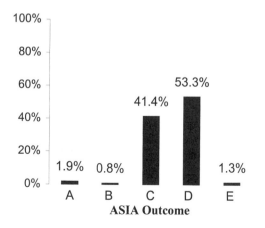

poor prognosis in all cases, and were ASIA grade A at admission and at last follow-up examination, which averaged 17.4 months from admission. Others have found neurological improvement in patients with hemorrhagic cord contusion on MRI (Wasenko et al. 1997). The cord contusion pattern was generally associated with cord injuries ranging from ASIA grades A through C at presentation and at follow-up (Ramon et al. 1997; Silberstein et al. 1992). The cord edema pattern is associated with mostly incomplete injuries and a relatively good prognosis, mostly ASIA grades C and D on follow-up examination (Ramon et al. 1997; Silberstein et al. 1992; Yamashita et al. 1991). As expected, normal cord findings on MRI are associated with the best prognosis. A small number of patients with normal MRI presented with clinical evidence of cord injury ASIA grades C and D and at last follow-up achieved an ASIA grade E (Ramon et al. 1997).

Discussion of prognosis with patients is always difficult, although it is the authors' experience that most patients prefer honesty. Along with an honest assessment, one should provide hope, avoid gloom, and leave the door open for future breakthroughs. The prognosis will likely improve in the future as research in spinal cord regeneration progresses. Since 1928 when Ramon y Cajal (Ramon y Cajal 1928) found that injured spinal neurons may sprout for a millimeter but fail to successfully regrow or regenerate, central nervous system regeneration has challenged many neuroscientists. A variety of tissues and cells have been transplanted into the injured spinal cord with varying degrees of success. Transplantation of fetal spinal cord tissue, or perhaps cultured fetal spinal cord neurons, into animal models has been the most promising to date (Bregman 1987; Zompa et al. 1997). Various studies have demonstrated survival of the transplanted material, extended axon regrowth, and improved motor function and locomotion. Nerve growth inhibitory proteins have been found to prohibit axon growth following spinal cord injury (Caroni and Schwab 1988; Savio and Schwab 1989). Treatment with antibodies (IN-1) to neutralize these inhibitory proteins has been shown to allow increased axon regrowth over longer distances, and to improve function in animal models (Caroni and Schwab 1988; Savio and Schwab 1989; Bregman et al. 1995). Fortunately, it does not appear necessary to have complete axonal regeneration, as it has been shown that a small number of axons (5% to 10%) can support locomotor recovery (Blight 1983; Windle et al. 1958). With acute interventions, such as MPS decreasing secondary injury, and regenerative techniques, we are hopeful that even more effective therapy for spinal cord injury will be available in the future.

## Functional Outcome

Each level of the spinal cord controls specific muscles and transmits sensory information from a particular dermatome. Because the distributions of myotomes and dermatomes are similar between individuals, we can predict the functional ability for various levels of spinal cord injury. Several levels of spinal cord injury can be grouped together for simplicity because the expectations for each group are similar, although we can expect the more caudal levels of each group to perform better than the more rostral levels. Functional outcomes for musculoskeletal, bowel, bladder, and sexual function are described below.

### C1–C4 Tetraplegia

Patients with severe high cervical spinal cord injury have impairment of the intercostal muscles and diaphragm, which leads to respiratory compromise. Spinal cord injuries of C1 through C3 are quickly fatal acutely, unless respiratory assistance is provided in the acute setting following the injury. Permanent assisted ventilation or implanted phrenic nerve pacing is required for all C1 and C2, and many C3 patients. A patient with a C4 level may only require nighttime assisted ventilation. Patients with C1–C4 levels usually require tracheostomies for more comfortable ventilation, and to control tracheobronchial secretions. The tracheostomy can be closed in patients with recovery of paralysis (Sannohe et al. 1996).

Power wheelchairs may allow greater independence for the C1–C4 level patients. These chairs operate by chin, mouth, breath, or voice controls. In a similar fashion, environmental control units allow a patient to access a telephone, radio, television, lights, computer, and so forth from one location. These patients are dependent for transfers, feeding, grooming, dressing, bathing, bowel, and bladder routine and therefore require a full-time trained attendant.

## C5 Tetraplegia

Patients with a C5 level have shoulder and elbow flexion, but no wrist or hand function. The use of the biceps can improve functional ability significantly. With practice and orthotic devices, the patient can eat or drink a prepared meal tray, dress the upper body when provided with clothing, and perform facial grooming activities (Yarkony et al. 1988). An electric wheelchair with a hand control is the primary means of mobility. Bowel and bladder routine, bathing, and transfers require full assistance. A full-time attendant is necessary to assist with most functions, but does not need to be with the patient at all times.

## C6 Tetraplegia

Active wrist dorsiflexion enhances the functional capabilities of patients with C6 tetraplegia. Eating skills and catheterization are possible with a wrist-driven flexor-hinge orthosis, which allows forceful thumb-to-index-finger opposition. Patients with C6 tetraplegia are usually able to feed themselves, write, and perform oral/facial hygiene. However, total dressing and personal hygiene usually require an attendant. Transfers are difficult because of inadequate triceps function, although transfers in and out of bed and on and off a toilet can be achieved with a sliding board. Self-catheterization above the C8 level requires assistance; therefore, many choose an indwelling suprapubic or urethral catheter. Manual wheelchair propulsion is independent on smooth surfaces, and may be enhanced with wheelchair projections. A specially adapted van with modified hand controls and a lift may allow independent driving. Despite more independent function, people with C6 tetraplegia are rarely able to live alone.

## C7–C8 Tetraplegia

Triceps function greatly enhances transfers and mobility. Wheelchair skills and propulsion are enhanced. Due to grip weakness, wheelchairs may still require modifications such as friction tape or projections on the wheel rims. Finger extension and tenodesis splints are helpful for self-care activities. Dressing can be achieved with clothing modifications such as Velcro or snaps as opposed to buttons, which can cause difficulty. The C7 level is generally the most rostral level for which living without an attendant is feasible.

Flexor digitorum profundus function allows individuals with C8 tetraplegia greater hand function, although it remains subnormal without the function of T1. Wheelchair skills, transfers, and self-care are enhanced. Intermittent self-catheterization is possible in the individual with function of the C8 level.

## Thoracic Paraplegia

Individuals who sustain thoracic level spinal cord injuries generally have a significant potential for functional independence. With training, most are independent with self-care skills, intermittent self-catheterization and bowel routine, and transfers. Hand controls and sometimes external trunk support in those with higher lesions are required for driving an automobile. The higher the thoracic level, the greater the loss of abdominal, intercostal, and back musculature, necessary for trunk support and coughing. Patients with higher level injuries in the thoracic spine are at a greater risk for developing respiratory infections, particularly those with lung disease or who are smokers.

Yarkony and colleagues reviewed 184 patients with complete thoracic paraplegia and found no significant differences in self-care scores, modified Barthel Index scores, mobility subscores, and length of rehabilitation stay between high (T1–T6) and low (T7–T12) paraplegic patients. Low paraplegic patients were more likely to ambulate than high paraplegic patients (Yarkony et al. 1990). Bipedal ambulation with knee-ankle-foot orthosis and crutches is possible, particularly at the lower levels, but requires a large expenditure of energy, and is generally not functional. Typically, the wheelchair remains the main mode of ambulation.

## Lumbar Paraplegia

Key muscles in the lumbar region include hip flexion at the L2 level, knee extension at L3, foot dorsiflexion at L4, and extensor hallucis longus (great toe dorsiflexion) at L5. In the sacral region, gastrocnemius and soleus at the S1 level allow foot plantar flexion. Independent functional ambulation indoors with knee-ankle-foot orthosis and a walker or forearm crutches is possible at the L2 level. Community ambulation is possible at the L3–S1 level, with the assistance of ankle-foot orthoses and crutches at the upper levels, and possibly a cane at the lower levels. Below S1–S2, only bowel, bladder, and sexual function are affected. Patients with upper levels of lumbar para-plegia require hand controls for driving an auto-mobile. These patients are typically independent in the remainder of their activities; an attendant is usually not necessary.

## Bowel and Bladder Function

Patients with injury rostral to the sacral cord and cauda equina tend to have hyper-reflexic ure-thral and anal sphincters. Involuntary tone will keep these sphincters in the closed position. In the acute phase following injury, the spinal-cord-injured patient is managed with an indwelling catheter. As the patient improves, intermittent catheterization is recommended and is the pre-ferred method of bladder management. Inter-mittent self-catheterization is possible in the individual with function of the C8 level. Self-catheterization above the C8 level requires assis-tance; therefore, many choose an indwelling sup-rapubic or urethral catheter. However, with an indwelling catheter there are increased risks of in-fection, bladder stones, urethral injury, and blad-der carcinoma (Hollander and Diokno 1993). Some men may wish to avoid catheterization and elect to have a sphincterotomy in order to void without excessive bladder pressure. All patients with spinal cord injury should undergo urological evaluation to assess function and to optimize bladder management.

Elimination may be accomplished by abdomi-nal pressure if the sphincteric pressures are not too great. An anal stretch maneuver (Kiviat et al. 1989), which consists of manually dilating the anal sphincter, which secondarily relaxes the urethral sphincter, may allow bladder emptying. Typically, patients with upper motor neurogenic bowels re-quire digital rectal stimulation or suppositories, and patients with lower motor neuron injuries re-quire manual removal of feces. Adequate fiber and fluid intake is essential in the management of a neurogenic bowel.

## Sexual Function

Many individuals with spinal cord injury have ac-tive sex lives. The production of sex hormones, and feelings of sexual attraction to others are es-sentially undisturbed by spinal cord injury, al-though certain other functions can be affected. Erection, ejaculation, and vaginal lubrication may often be impaired, as well as mobility, necessitat-ing modification of sexual technique.

In general, parasympathetic nerves (S2–S4) control erection, sympathetic nerves (T11–L2) mediate seminal emission, and somatic nerves allow forceful ejaculation. There is some evi-dence that erections are not purely parasympa-thetically mediated, but involve noncholinergic-nonadrenergic mechanisms of both systems, referred to as co-transmission (Yarkony 1990). Reflex erections can occur with an intact sacral segment, and psychogenic erections are cere-brally mediated in association with lower motor nerve lesions. Seminal emission mediated by sympathetic nerves is more likely to occur with lower lesions, which may impair forceful ejacula-tion. In general, erections are more likely to occur and be sustained in the higher lesions, while emis-sion is more likely to occur in the lower lesions. Courtois et al. (1993) found 100% of men with high lesions maintain penile response to reflexo-genic stimulation, and nearly 90% of those with lower lesions respond to psychogenic stimulation, with the latter group having seminal emissions in 100% of cases when their lesion is confined to the conus. Forceful ejaculation rarely appears in men with complete lesions at any level.

Impaired or absent erection and or ejaculation can be treated successfully. Mechanical stimula-tion, intracavernous injections of prostaglandins or papaverine, external vacuum systems, or semi-rigid or inflatable prostheses have been used to restore erection. In a double-blind, placebo-controlled study, sildenafil (Viagra) has been found to improve the quality of erections and satisfaction with sex life in men with erectile dysfunction caused by a spinal cord injury (Derry et al. 1998; Maytom et al. 1999). Penile stimula-tion with an electric or battery-operated vibrator or electroejaculation have been used to achieve ejaculation in spinal cord injured patients. Vibra-tor assisted ejaculation is generally preferable to electroejaculation, as it may be performed in the home, and without risk of rectal mucosa damage. Sonksen et al. (1997) found a 100% ejaculation rate in spinal-cord-injured men using vibratory assistance (79%) as a first option followed by electroejaculation (21%) as a second option. With these and other fertility assistance techniques, the pregnancy rate for spinal-cord-injury couples approaches that of noninjured couples.

As with spinal-cord-injured men, women with spinal cord injuries may develop sensory areas of heightened erotic significance such as the transition zone between normal sensation and no sensation, or if the lesion is incomplete some areas below the main level of paralysis may have heightened erotic feeling (Donovan 1992). Vaginal lubrication may be impaired or inconsistent, often necessitating additional lubrication. Amenorrhea may be present initially but typically resumes within 3 to 12 months following injury. Fertility is generally undisturbed by spinal cord injury. Those with lesions above T6 have an increased risk for developing autonomic dysreflexia, particularly during labor (Yarkony 1992). A woman with spinal cord injury needs close medical attention during pregnancy.

## Employment

Traditionally, return to employment has been considered one of the most important rehabilitation goals. The re-employment figures following spinal cord injury vary widely (13% to 60%) between different studies (Dijkers et al. 1995; Kraus 1992; Stover and Fine 1986; Trieschmann 1988). It is not surprising that the employment rates are so different, due to the sample demographics and injury-related characteristics. A more meaningful employment rate can be ascertained by looking at key sample or individual characteristics.

Educational history has been the most consistent predictor of employment outcome. Individuals with more years of education are more likely to work following spinal cord injury. For those with 16 or more years of education the rate of employment was approximately 52.9% at 1 year following injury (Dijkers et al. 1995), with 69% currently employed in a large study with a mean of 18.6 years following injury (Kraus 1992). This high rate of employment drops precipitously to 3.9% to 3% in those with less than 9 and 12 years of education, respectively, in the two studies above (Dijkers et al. 1995; Kraus 1992).

The age of the patient, time following injury, and the level of injury are additional variables related to potential employment. Age at time of injury is strongly associated with employment. Individuals who are the youngest at time of injury are more likely to work, and more likely to work more hours per week than older individuals. The age figures vary between studies but generally the likelihood of employment and hours worked per week decrease after age 38 at time of injury (Kraus 1992). Employment rates increase steadily to reach

a peak at approximately 10 to 11 years following injury (Dijkers et al. 1995). Intuitively, persons with paraplegia are more likely to be employed than those with tetraplegia. However, several studies indicate only a slight increase (approximately 5%) in employment in individuals with paraplegia as compared to those with tetraplegia (Dijkers et al. 1995; Kraus 1992; Stover and Fine 1986).

## The Future

No discussion of the prognosis of spinal cord injury is complete without some mention of the future, for there is every reason to expect that the outcome of such injuries will continue to improve. The successful completion and publication of NASCIS II represented an exciting milestone. For the first time ever, pharmacological intervention was clearly shown to alter outcome in humans. Further research is ongoing to determine how this therapy can be improved. The consensus of opinion is that the primary mechanism of action of methylprednisolone in the SCI patient is via the inhibition of lipid peroxidation.

Additional promising drugs are currently being studied to explore what early intervention can do in terms of preventing progressive secondary damage. The 21-amino steroids are a new class of synthetically derived nonglucocorticoid steroids that have been found to provide even greater antioxidant activity than methylprednisolone. Tirilazad mesylate (U74006F) has been selected for clinical study in a third clinical trial of human spinal cord injury (NASCIS III), in which the drug is being compared to methylprednisolone.

Gangliosides, acidic glycolipids, are another class of drugs under current study. These compounds are a major component of the cell's outer lipid bilayer of the plasma membrane (Geisler et al. 1992). They are derived from sphingosine, an amino alcohol that contains a long unsaturated hydrocarbon chain. $GM_1$ ganglioside has been used most commonly in clinical application. Exogenous gangliosides are assumed to be incorporated into the lipid bilayer and mimic endogenous gangliosides.

Gangliosides have been found to augment neuronal growth in vitro and induce regeneration and restoration of neuronal functions in vivo. Animal models have shown that these compounds stimulate the growth of nerve cells in damaged tissue

(Geisler et al. 1992). Other possible functions may include enhancing neuronal survival in white matter tracts and limiting the neurotoxic effect of excitatory amino-acid-induced cell death (Skaper and Leon 1992).

An initial clinical study with GM₁ yielded promising results (Geisler et al. 1991). SCI patients were given 100 mg/d of GM₁ sodium salt or placebo intravenously within the first 72 hours after injury, and treatment was continued for 18 to 32 doses. Significant improvement was noted in the GM₁-treated patients in the ASIA motor score and Frankel grades from baseline at a 1-year follow-up examination. Further studies in a multicenter setting are needed to validate this compound's efficacy in acute SCI.

Other drugs under study include calcium channel blocking agents and both competitive and noncompetitive antagonists at the NMDA receptor. Methylprednisolone therapy has so rapidly become the standard of care that all future studies can no longer use a control group with no therapy; rather, the control group now comprises patients treated with the standard methylprednisolone protocol for 24 hours. Work in spinal cord regeneration is also showing promising results, with partial anatomical restoration being the rule rather than the exception.

Based on the above, it appears that the future holds great promise. One of the challenges facing clinicians treating spinal-cord-injured patients will be to keep abreast of such research, in order to continue to deliver state-of-the-art care.

## Conclusions

With approximately 10,000 new cases per year, traumatic spinal cord injury remains a devastating and debilitating condition, which mostly affects young and active individuals. Accurate clinical and radiological assessment is essential in the management of these patients, and are essential in order to accurately determine prognosis. Individual prognosis is based on initial trauma and secondary injury, which can be reduced with immobilization, pharmacological, and medical-surgical intervention. Overall survival and functional outcomes are improving and are significantly better for incomplete versus complete cord injuries, although even patients with initially complete cord injuries can become ambulatory. Once the rate of recovery stabilizes, we can more accurately predict the functional ability for those with complete injury. The functional outcome for an individual with incomplete injury is difficult to prognosticate, although those with some sparing of motor function and those with a relatively rapid recovery enjoy a better prognosis. Intensive neurosurgical management combined with early rehabilitation is necessary to prevent secondary injury to the spinal cord as well as to prevent complications that are known to occur in those with spinal injury.

## References

Amar, A. P.; Levy, M. L. Pathogenesis and pharmacological strategies for mitigating secondary damage in acute cord injury. Neurosurgery 44:1027–1040; 1999.

American Spinal Injury Association, International Medical Society of Paraplegia. International standards for neurological and functional classification of spinal cord injury. Chicago, IL: American Spinal Injury Association; 1992.

Blight, A. R. Cellular morphology of chronic spinal cord injury in the cat: analysis of myelinated axons by line sampling. Neuroscience 10:521–543; 1983.

Bracken, M. B.; Freeman, D. H.; Hallebrand, K. Incidence of acute traumatic hospitalized spinal cord injuries in the United States, 1970–77. Am. J. Epidemiol. 113:615–622; 1981.

Bracken, M. B.; Shepard, M. J.; Collins, W. F.; Holford, T. R.; Young, W.; Baskin, D. S.; Eisenberg, H. M.; Flamm, E.; Leo-Summers, L.; Maroon, J.; Marshall, L. F.; Perot, P. L.; Piepmeier, J.; Sonntag, V. K. H.; Wagner, F. C.; Wilberger, J. E.; Winn, H. R. A randomized, controlled trial of methylprednisolone or naloxone in the treatment of acute spinal-cord injury. Results of the Second National Acute Spinal Cord Injury Study [see comments]. N. Engl. J. Med. 322:1405–1411; 1990.

Bracken, M. B.; Shepard, M. J.; Collins, W. F.; Holford, T. R.; Baskin, D. S.; Eisenberg, H. M.; Flamm, E.; Leo-Summers, L.; Maroon, J.; Marshall, L. F.; Perot, P. L.; Piepmeier, J.; Sonntag, V. K. H.; Wagner, F. C.; Wilberger, J. E.; Winn, H. R.; Young, W. Methylprednisolone or naloxone treatment after acute spinal cord injury: 1-year follow-up data. J. Neurosurg. 76:23–31; 1992.

Breasted, J. H. The Edwin Smith Surgical Papyrus. Chicago: University of Chicago Press; 1930.

Bregman, B. S. Spinal cord transplants permits the growth of serotonergic axons across the site of neonatal spinal cord transection. Dev. Brain Res. 34:265–279; 1987.

Bregman, B. S.; Kunkel-Bagden, E.; Schnell, L.; Dai, H. N.; Gao, D.; Schwab, M. E. Recovery from spinal cord injury mediated by antibodies to neurite growth inhibitors [see comments]. Nature 378:498–501; 1995.

Caroni, P.; Schwab, M. E. Two membrane protein fractions from rat central myelin with inhibitory properties for neurite growth and fibroblast spreading. J. Cell Biol. 106:1281–1288; 1988.

Chesnut, R. M.; Marshall, L. F.; Klauber, M. R. The role of secondary brain injury in determining outcome from severe head injury. J. Trauma 34:216–222; 1993.

Courtois, F. J.; Charvier, K. F.; Leriche, A.; Raymond, D. P. Sexual function in spinal cord injury men. I. Assessing sexual capability. Paraplegia 31:771–784; 1993.

Crozier, K. S.; Cheng, L. L.; Graziani, V.; Zorn, G.; Herbison, G.; Ditunno, J. F., Jr. Spinal cord injury: prognosis for ambulation based on quadriceps recovery. Paraplegia 30:762–767; 1992.

Crozier, K. S.; Graziani, V.; Ditunno, J. F. J.; Herbison, G. J. Spinal cord injury: prognosis for ambulation based on sensory examination in patients who are initially motor complete. Arch. Phys. Med. Rehabil. 72:119–121; 1991.

Curt, A.; Keck, M. E.; Dietz, V. Functional outcome following spinal cord injury: significance of motor-evoked potentials and ASIA scores. Arch. Phys. Med. Rehabil. 79:81–86; 1998.

Cushing, H. Care of head injuries and injuries to the spine and peripheral nerves in forward hospitals. In: Medical Department of the U.S. Army in World War. Vol. 11. Anonymous. Washington, DC: General Printing Office; 1927: p. 755–758.

Derry, F. A.; Dinsmore, W. W.; Fraser, M.; et al. Efficacy and safety of oral sildenafil (Viagra) in men with erectile dysfunction caused by spinal cord injury. Neurology 51:1629–1633; 1998.

Dijkers, M. P.; Abela, M. B.; Gans, B. M.; Gordon, W. A. The aftermath of spinal cord injury. In: Stover, S. L.; DeLisa, J. A.; Whiteneck, G. G., eds. Spinal cord injury: clinical outcomes from model systems. Gaithersburg, MD: Aspen Publishers; 1995: p. 185–212.

Ditunno, J. F.; Cohen, M. E.; Formal, C. S.; Whiteneck, G. G. Functional outcomes. In: Stover, S. L.; DeLisa, J. A.; Whiteneck, G. G.; eds. Spinal cord injury; clinical outcomes from the model systems. Gaithersburg, MD: Aspen Publishers; 1995: p. 170–184.

Ditunno, J. F.; Graziani, V.; Tessler, A. Neurological assessment in spinal cord injury. Adv. Neurol. 72:325–333; 1997.

Donovan, W. H. Spinal cord injury. In: Evans, R. W.; Baskin, D. S.; Yatsu, F. M., eds. New York: Oxford University Press; 1992: p. 109–118.

Foo, D.; Subrahmanyan, T. S.; Rossier, A. S. Post-traumatic acute anterior spinal cord syndrome. Paraplegia 19:201–205; 1981.

Frankel, H. L.; Hancock, D. O.; Hyslop, G.; et al. The value of postural reduction in the initial management of closed injuries of the spine with paraplegia and tetraplegia. I. Paraplegia 7:179–192; 1969.

Geisler, F. H.; Dorsey, F. C.; Coleman, W. P. Recovery of motor function after spinal cord injury: a randomized placebo-controlled trial with GM-1 ganglioside. N. Engl. J. Med. 324:1829–1838, 1991.

Geisler, F. H.; Dorsey, F. C.; Coleman, W. P. GM-1 ganglioside in human spinal cord injury. J. Neurotrauma 9(suppl.):S165–S172; 1992.

Graham, P. M.; Weingarden, S. I. Victims of gun shootings. J. Adolesc. Health Care 10:534–536; 1989.

Greene, K. A.; Marciano, F. F.; Sonntag, V. K. Pharmacological management of spinal cord injury: current status of drugs designed to augment functional recovery of the injured human spinal cord. J. Spinal Disord. 9:355–366; 1996.

Griffin, M. R.; Opitz, J. L.; Kurland, L. T.; Ebersold, M. J.; O'Fallon, W. M. Traumatic spinal cord injury in Olmsted County, Minnesota, 1935–1981. Am. J. Epidemiol. 121:884–895; 1985.

Guttmann, L. Spinal cord injuries: comprehensive management and research. London: Blackwell Scientific; 1976.

Hansebout, R. R. A comprehensive review of methods of improving cord recovery after acute spinal cord injury. In: Tator, C. H., ed. Early management of acute spinal cord injury. New York: Raven Press; 1982: p. 181–196.

Hollander, J. B.; Diokno, A. C. Urinary diversion and reconstruction in the patient with spinal cord injury. Urol. Clin. North Am. 20:465–474; 1993.

Hussey, R. W.; Stauffer, E. S. Spinal cord injury: requirements for ambulation. Arch. Phys. Med. Rehabil. 54:544–547; 1998.

Jacobs, S. R.; Yeaney, N. K.; Herbison, G. J.; Ditunno, J. F., Jr. Future ambulation prognosis as predicted by somatosensory evoked potentials in motor complete and incomplete quadriplegia Arch. Phys. Med. Rehabil. 76:635–641; 1995.

Kassell, N. F.; Peerless, S. J.; Durward, Q. J.; Beck, D. W.; Drake, C. G.; Adams, H. P. Treatment of ischemic deficits from vasospasm with intravascular volume expansion and induced arterial hypertension. Neurosurgery 3:337–343; 1982.

Kiviat, M. D.; Zimmerman, T. A.; Donovan, W. H. Spinchter stretch: a new technique resulting in continence and complete voiding in paraplegics. J. Urol. 141:549–550; 1989.

Kraus, J. F.; Franti, C. E.; Riggins, R. S. Incidence of traumatic spinal cord lesions. J. Chronic Dis. 28:471–492; 1975.

Kraus, J. S. Employment after spinal cord injury. Arch. Phys. Med. Rehabil. 73:163–169; 1992.

Lobosky, J. M. Epidemiology of spinal cord injury. In: Narayan, R. K.; Wilberger, J. E., Jr.; Povlishock, J. T., eds. Neurotrauma. New York: McGraw-Hill; 1996: p. 1049–1058.

Maytom, M. J.; Derry, F. A.; Dinsmore, W. W.; et al. A two-part pilot study of sildenafil (Viagra) in men with erectile dysfunction caused by spinal cord injury. Spinal Cord 37:110–116; 1999.

Miller, J.; Diringer, M. Management of aneurysmal subarachnoid hemorrhage. Neurol. Clin. 13:451–478; 1995.

Miller, J. D.; Sweet, R. C.; Narayan, R. K. Early insults to the injured brain. JAMA 240:439–442; 1978.

Mirza, S. K.; Krengel, W. F., 3rd; Chapman, J. R.; et al. Early versus delayed surgery for acute cervical spinal cord injury. Clin. Orthop. 359:104–114; 1999.

Montgomery, E. B. J.; Grubb, R. L. J.; Raichle, M. E. Cerebral hemodynamics and metabolism in postoperative cerebral vasospasm and treatment with hypertensive therapy. Ann. Neurol. 9:502–506; 1981.

Origitano, T. C.; Wascher, T. M.; Reichman, O. H.; Anderson, D. E. Sustained increased cerebral blood flow with prophylactic hypertensive hypervolemic hemodilution after subarachnoid hemorrhage. Neurosurgery 5:729–740; 1990.

Pritz, M. B.; Gianotta, M. D.; Kindt, G. W.; McGillicuddy, J. E.; Prager, R. L. Treatment of patients with neurological deficits associated with cerebral vasospasm by intravascular volume expansion. Neurosurgery 3:364–368; 1978.

Ramon y Cajal, S. Degeneration and regeneration of the nervous system. London: Oxford University Press; 1928.

Ramon, S.; Dominguez, R.; Ramirez, L.; et al. Clinical and magnetic resonance imaging correlation in acute spinal cord injury. Spinal Cord 35:664–673; 1997.

Sannohe, A.; Harata, S.; Ueyama, K.; et al. The prognosis and the treatment of patients with a C3/4 spinal cord injury. Spinal Cord 34:486–487; 1996.

Savio, T.; Schwab, M. E. Rat CNS white matter, but not gray matter, is nonpermissive for neuronal cell adhesion and fiber outgrowth. J. Neurosci. 9:1126–1133; 1989.

Selden, N. R.; Quint, D. J.; Patel, N.; et al. Emergency magnetic resonance imaging of cervical spinal cord injury: clinical correlation and prognosis. Neurosurgery 44:785–793, 1999.

Silberstein, M.; Tress, B. M.; Hennessy, O. Prediction of neurologic outcome in acute spinal cord injury: the role of CT and MR. Am. J. Neuroradiol. 13:1597–1608; 1992.

Skaper, S. D.; Leon, A. Monosialogangliosides, neuroprotection and neuronal repair processes. J. Neurotrauma 9(suppl.):S507–S516; 1992.

Solomon, R. A.; Fink, M. E.; Lennihan, L. Early aneurysm surgery and prophylactic hypervolemic hypertensive therapy for the treatment of aneurysmal subarachnoid hemorrhage. Neurosurgery 23:699–704; 1988.

Sonksen, J.; Sommer, P.; Bieringsorensen, F.; et al. Pregnancy after assisted ejaculation procedures in men with spinal cord injury. Arch. Phys. Med. Rehabil. 78:1059–1061; 1997.

Stover, S. L.; Fine, P. R. Spinal cord injury: the facts and figures. Birmingham: University of Alabama at Birmingham; 1986.

Strandgaard, S. Autoregulation of cerebral blood flow in hypertensive patients. Circulation 53:720–727; 1976.

Tator, C. H. Classification of spinal cord injury based on neurological presentation. In: Narayan, R. K.; Wilberger, J. E., Jr.; Povlishock, J. T., eds. Neurotrauma. New York: McGraw-Hill; 1996: p. 1059–1073.

Torg, J. S.; Vegso, J. J.; Sennett, B.; Das, M. The national football head and neck registry. JAMA 254:3439–3443; 1985.

Trieschmann, R. B. Spinal cord injuries: psychological, social, and vocational rehabilitation. New York: Demos Publications; 1988.

Vale, F. L.; Burns, J.; Jackson, A. B.; Hadley, M. N. Combined medical and surgical treatment after acute spinal cord injury: results of a prospective pilot study to assess the merits of aggressive medical resuscitation and blood pressure management. J. Neurosurg. 87:239–246; 1997.

Wasenko, J. J.; Hochhauser, L.; Holsapple, J. W.; et al. MR of post traumatic spinal cord lesions—unexpected improvement of hemorrhagic lesions. Clin. Imaging 21:246–251; 1997.

Waters, R. L.; Adkins, R. H.; Yakura, J. Definition of complete spinal cord injury. Paraplegia 29:573–581; 1991.

Waters, R. L.; Adkins, R. H.; Yakura, J. S.; Sie, I. Motor and sensory recovery following complete tetraplegia. Arch. Phys. Med. Rehabil. 74:242–247; 1993.

Waters, R. L.; Adkins, R. H.; Yakura, J. S.; Sie, I. Motor and sensory recovery following incomplete paraplegia. Arch. Phys. Med. Rehabil. 75:67–72; 1994a.

Waters, R. L.; Adkins, R. H.; Yakura, J. S.; Sie, I. Motor and sensory recovery following incomplete tetraplegia.; Arch. Phys. Med. Rehabil. 75:306–311; 1994b.

Waters, R. L.; Yakura, J. S.; Adkins, R. H.; Sie, I. Recovery following complete paraplegia. Arch. Phys. Med. Rehabil. 73:784–789; 1992.

Windle, W. F.; Smart, J. O.; Beers, J. J. Residual function after subtotal spinal cord transection in adult cats. Neurology 8:518–521; 1958.

Woolsey, R. M. Rehabilitation outcome following spinal cord injury. Arch. Neurol. 42:116–119; 1998.

Yamashita, Y.; Takahashi, M.; Matsuno, Y.; et al. Acute spinal cord injury: magnetic resonance imaging correlated with myelopathy. Br. J. Radiol. 64:201–209; 1991.

Yarkony, G. M. Enhancement of sexual function and fertility in spinal cord-injured males. Am. J. Phys. Med. 69:81–86; 1990.

Yarkony, G. M. Spinal cord injured women: sexuality, fertility, and pregnancy. In: Goldstein, P. J.; Stern, B. J., eds. Neurological disorders of pregnancy. Mount Kisco, NY: Futura Publishing; 1992: p. 203–222.

Yarkony, G. M.; Roth, E.; Lovell, L.; Heinemann, A.; Katz, R. T.; Wu, Y. Rehabilitation outcomes in complete C5 quadriplegia. Am. J. Phys. Med. Rehabil. 67:73–76; 1988.

Yarkony, G. M.; Roth, E. J.; Meyer, P. R.; Lovell, L. L.; Heinemann, A. W. Rehabilitation outcomes in patients with complete thoracic spinal cord injury. Am. J. Phys. Med. Rehabil. 69:23–27; 1990.

Young, W.; Bracken, M. B. The Second National Acute Spinal Cord Injury Study. J. Neurotrauma 9(suppl. 1):S397–S405; 1992.

Zeidman, S. M.; Ling, G. S.; Ducker, T. B.; Ellenbogen, R. G. Clinical applications of pharmacologic therapies for spinal cord injury. J. Spinal Disord. 9:367–380; 1996.

Zompa, E. A.; Cain, L. D.; Everhart, A. W.; et al. Transplant therapy—recovery of function after spinal cord injury. J. Neurotrauma 14:479–506; 1997.

# 25

# Peripheral Nerve Injury

NORBERT ROOSEN AND DAVID G. KLINE

Peripheral nerve injuries have important morbidity because of the loss of neurological function and/or the pain syndromes that can accompany them. The examination, treatment, and follow-up of nerve injuries that occurred during both world wars earlier this century, and during other military conflicts of the past, have led to a vast amount of experience and knowledge as regards the incidence, the therapeutic options, and the prognosis of the different types of traumatic lesions involving the peripheral nervous system (PNS). It is on this basis that more research in and further development of the therapy of peripheral nerve injury has been built, be it conservative or be it surgical treatment.

Expanding upon a previous review on prognostic aspects of peripheral nerve injuries (Lowder and Kline 1992), different types of diseases and lesions involving the PNS will be reviewed with emphasis on incidence, etiology, therapeutic options, and prognosis. At the end of this review a compilation of tables summarizing mainly the experience at the Louisiana State University Medical Center (LSUMC) Department of Neurosurgery in New Orleans will assist in judging the prognosis for the more common nerve lesions and their treatment.

## General Classification, Pathological Anatomy, and Physiology of Peripheral Nerve Injury and Regeneration

A detailed knowledge of the anatomy, physiology, and pathology of peripheral nerves is of paramount importance to adequately manage patients with injuries of the PNS and to fully appreciate the factors that influence the prognosis of the multitude of injury types that can affect the PNS. Only an abbreviated overview can be given here, and the interested reader is referred to publications in the recent literature for several excellent treatises on this topic (Gelberman 1991; Kline and Hudson 1995, 1996; Dyck et al. 1993).

### Regeneration after Injury to the Peripheral Nervous System

Nerve injury leads to an attempt at regeneration by the nervous tissue, that may or may not be successful to a variable degree depending on a number of different factors. This regenerative response ultimately requires reconstitution of axonal function to be effective. How elaborate the mechanisms for restitution of normal nervous structure and function need to be will depend on the extent and severity of the initial injury. Injuries to the

PNS, especially those of traumatic etiology, have been categorized by Seddon (1943) and Sunderland (1968), and their relatively similar classifications still form the basis for our present understanding of the prognosis of nerve lesions. Seddon (1943) distinguished three different degrees of severity of nerve injury (i.e., neurapraxia, axonotmesis, and neurotmesis), whereas Sunderland (1968) described five degrees of nerve injury.

### Neurapraxia

Neurapraxia, fully reversible within hours or at the latest within a few weeks, is characterized by a temporary and reversible local conduction block but normal distal conduction. There are no important structural tissue changes, no or at most minimal wallerian degeneration, but some segmental demyelinating changes and biochemical disturbances may be present transiently (Spinner 1978; Gentili and Hudson 1985). Neurapraxia involves preferentially large fibers subserving motor and proprioceptive functions, less so touch and pain sensation, and tends to spare autonomic function (Sunderland 1968). This is not usually a surgical lesion, and the prognosis for full recovery is excellent with conservative management. Neurapraxia corresponds to Sunderland's first-degree injury (Sunderland 1968), and clinical examples of this type of nerve dysfunction are Saturday night palsy, tourniquet palsy, and some entrapment-compression neuropathies.

### Axonotmesis

Axonotmesis, comparable to Sunderland's second-degree and mild third-degree injuries (Sunderland 1968), is characterized by complete loss of axon and myelin sheath continuity with relative preservation of the endoneurial tube's connective tissue, which will guide axonal regrowth distally into the nerve. Marked morphological changes can be found: wallerian degeneration distally, and reduction in axon diameter and myelin sheet thickness proximally (Cragg and Thomas 1961; Gentili and Hudson 1985). This type of lesion results in complete abolishment of all functions in the nerve's territory, and neuronal conduction will disappear distally as an indication of axonal disintegration. The injury, generally caused by moderate stretch or contusion, such as seen in association with skeletal trauma, is in continuity, and because of the preserved endoneurial framework that will guide

sprouting, regenerating axons towards their appropriate innervation sites, the prognosis is rather good. Recovery can be complete but will take a long time depending on the distance the axons need to grow prior to establishing reinnervation: 18 to 36 months is the usual time frame (Seddon 1943; Sunderland 1968). The prime difficulty in decision making for the clinician is the differentiation of this injury from neurotmesis, which will be described below. Indeed, the spontaneous recovery from axonotmesis is definitely superior in all respects to the recovery seen after resection and/or suture of neurotmetic lesions. Distinguishing both is of utmost importance, because neurotmetic lesions require surgical therapy within a relatively short time period after the injury for optimal results (Kline and Hudson 1990). Unfortunately, this differentiation can be very difficult.

### Neurotmesis

Sunderland's fourth-degree (in-continuity) and fifth-degree (transection) injuries (Sunderland 1968) are equivalent to what Seddon called neurotmesis (Seddon 1943). This is the most devastating type of injury, demonstrating loss of continuity not only of the axon and its myelin covering, but to variable degrees of the peri- and epineurial connective tissue as well. Initially, the clinical and electrodiagnostic findings are the same as in axonotmesis. The essential difference between both injury types is the optimal guidance for axonal regrowth that is offered by the axonotmetic nerve's preserved endoneurial tube system as opposed to the absence of any endoneurial guidance in the neurotmetic nerve, which results in chaotic, inefficient, and largely unsuccessful attempts of axonal growth cones to re-establish connections between the proximal and distal parts of the severed nerve and the more distal sensory and motor end organs. (Lundborg 1982, 1987; Thomas and Olson 1984).

### Pathology and Evolution of Nerve Transection Injury

One of the simplest forms of peripheral nerve injury is transection of a nerve. Nonetheless, transection does cause a complex response within the distal and proximal nerve ends, the neuron, and the end-organ such as muscle.

The nerve end distal from the section site undergoes wallerian degeneration (Waller 1850) with Schwann cell proliferation, and phagocytosis of myelin and axonal breakdown products by Schwann cells (Griffin and Hoffman 1993), that may take up to 1 to 3 months for completion. Finally, after collapse of the endoneurial tubes the Schwann cells will rearrange themselves into virtual tubular structures forming a meshwork that will be entered by the axonal sprouts from the proximal end. The axonal growth cones will follow the tubular structures distally towards the end-organ. The growing axon stump with its collateral and terminal sprouts all together comprise a regeneration unit. The process of axonal growth, target searching, and maturation may be facilitated by neurotrophic factors, neurite-promoting factors, and contact guidance. The regenerating axonal sprouts may enter a variable number of tubular structures, some of them reaching appropriate effector cells (e.g., motor axons towards muscle fibers), whereas other sprouting axons will grow towards the wrong end-organs (e.g., motor fibers into sensory branches). This whole degenerative and regenerative process is rather slow, with a regeneration rate between 1 and 4 mm/d, but happens predictably after surgical repair too. Attempts to give more detailed estimates of the axonal growth rate have proven to be difficult (Bateman 1962; Groff and Houtz 1945). Sunderland (1968) and Pollock and Davis (1933) have published some of the most detailed tables on the regeneration and return of function for the different nerves of the PNS.

A degenerative and reparative process identical to wallerian degeneration happens in the proximal nerve stump after transection: traumatic degeneration, which will occur for a variable distance upstream of the lesion site (Griffin and Hoffman 1993). It sometimes reaches the neuronal soma and results in cell death (Horch 1978; Kristensson 1981).

The neuronal body's response to severing its axon is predictable, and both anterior horn motoneurons and dorsal root sensory ganglion neurons behave in an identical fashion. The earliest morphological change (i.e., chromatolysis) can be observed within a few hours following injury: slight increase in neuron body size with a more rounded appearance, Nissl substance breakdown, and nuclear relocation towards the cell's periphery. Protein metabolism is increased, and neurotransmitter metabolism is decreased. Depending on the proximity of the axonal lesion to the neu-

ron, actual cell death may ensue (Horch 1978; Kristensson 1981).

The reactions of the peripheral tissues to nerve section need to be considered too. Muscle fibers will undergo atrophy within several weeks, and intercellular fibrosis develops within 12 to 24 months, thereby severely limiting the amount of recovery achievable by reinnervation. The synaptic plate of the muscle cells, however, will still show synaptic folds for more than 1 year following denervation. The acetylcholine receptors, though, will redistribute along the muscle membrane, paralleling a diffuse increase in membrane excitability (Gorio and Carmignoto 1981). The regenerating axons upon reaching the muscle cell's myoneural junction area will reinnervate the muscle cell, sprout to innervate adjacent cells, and will determine the muscle fiber type irrespective of the predenervational fiber type. Experimental and clinical studies have shown that neurotization of some denervated muscles (i.e., reinnervation) merely by implanting the transected end of a motor nerve, is feasible albeit not as successful as neurolysis, direct repair, or nerve graft interpositioning (McNamara et al. 1987). Cutaneous sensory receptors also undergo postdenervational changes. The non-nervous receptor components can survive denervation for a very long period of time, and from that point of view the prognosis for development of protective cutaneous sensation is relatively good. Much information on cutaneous reinnervation has been obtained by studying transplanted skin flaps and transplanted digits such as in toe-to-thumb transfers (Davis 1934; Kredel and Evans 1933; Adeymo and Wyburn 1957; Mannerfelt 1962; Dellon 1986).

## Etiology and Incidence of Peripheral Nerve Injury

A variety of pathogenetic mechanisms can cause injury to the PNS: acute or chronic trauma, compression, infection, ischemia, neoplasms, immunological disorders and autoimmune diseases, and the like. Some of these lesions will cause polyneuropathy, but many of them will involve only single nerves or sometimes several nerves in close anatomical proximity to each other. We will consider predominantly those types of injury from a point of view of prognosis, that involve surgical decision making and treatment.

## Acute Trauma

Acute trauma to peripheral nerves can be in the form of sharp or blunt transections. Transections made up only about 30% of all peripheral nerve lesions seen in a tertiary referral center (Kline and Hudson 1995), with most remaining injuries being related to a contusive and stretching mechanism. Acute noncontusive injuries that are clean and resulted in nerve segments with neat transection surfaces will benefit tremendously from early (within 72 hours) surgical revision and end-to-end neuropathy. This will allow the surgeon to reapproximate the nerve segments without need to take care of secondary changes related to scar formation. In addition, the nerve segments will not have had the opportunity for retraction into the wounded tissues, thereby obviating the necessity for nerve grafting and thus permitting end-to-end nerve suture in the majority of cases. The prognosis in this kind of injury is generally good. By comparison, a blunt transected nerve is best repaired after a delay of several weeks when the amount of trimming needed to reach healthy nerve will be obvious. Almost 15% of the nerves injured by a potentially transecting mechanism, however, will not be completely disconnected and therefore prone to develop a neuroma-in-continuity (Kline 1977; Kline and Hudson 1995). Management of such neuromas-in-continuity will depend upon the extent of neurological symptoms, and will involve a combination of conservative treatment, serial clinical and electromyographic evaluation, with nerve action potential (NAP) recording, neurolysis, suture, and/or grafting (Kline and Hudson 1995).

Diffuse contusions are seen in gunshot wounds (GSWs), whereas stretch and traction injury can be related to car or motorcycle accidents, be caused by birth injury, or be due to operative positioning trauma. Traction injuries often involve a large segment of nerve thereby making spontaneous recovery difficult, although stretch lesions of the brachial plexus, for example, can recover significantly in about 40% of cases with conservative management (Nagano et al. 1984). This is less so in patients with involvement of two or more roots, however. Stretch injuries to the plexus distal to clavicle and thus in infraclavicular plexus have a somewhat better prognosis, with about 60% spontaneous functional recovery

(Alnot 1984; Leffert 1985). Nevertheless, it is our opinion that brachial plexus lesions need to be treated rather aggressively and require liberal consideration of operative exploration with intraoperative NAP recording, neurolysis, repair, and grafting, or other forms of substitutive or reconstructive procedures (Gilbert et al. 1988; Kline et al. 1986; Kline and Hudson 1995; Millesi 1984b). This is despite the frequent need for long grafts to operatively bridge the gap made by resection of diseased or injured nerve (Kline and Hudson 1995).

Acute compartment syndromes following blunt injury to the forearm or the lower leg may rapidly cause extensive peripheral nerve injury secondary to raised compartmental pressure and neural ischemia. These conditions carry a grave prognosis with regard to extremity function if not treated expeditiously with fasciotomy. Acute neural decompression is paramount when there is compression by acute hematomas, traumatic aneurysms, and compartment syndromes. In cases of lumbosacral plexus compression secondary to a retroperitoneal hematoma the prognosis for spontaneous recovery, however, may be good and surgical exploration is not always recommended (Hudson et al. 1987; Kline and Hudson 1987). Nonetheless, we have had to operate on such clots in several instances because of their size and the severity of the neurological loss as well as their associated pain symptoms.

Contaminated wounds and most nerve injuries with a contusive or a blunt laceration require initial wound debridement, marking and local fixation of the nerve stumps, and delayed surgical repair within a few weeks. This is called secondary neurorrhaphy (Kline and Judice 1983; Kline and Hackett 1975). At that time an adequate assessment of the necessary resection length of nonfunctional nerve will be possible. Nerve grafting will often be necessary and prognosis will depend mainly on the extent of the injury and the resection and therefore the length of graft needed. The location of the injury is of importance too and, interestingly, sharp transections tend to occur more peripherally in the PNS than bluntly lacerated nerves, thereby adding to the gravity of the prognosis of the latter ones. Associated soft tissue and bone trauma may delay surgical repair or may promote scarring in cases of diffuse injury (Frykman and Cally 1988; McQuarrie 1985). Repair

6 months after injury seems in general to lead to inferior results (Frykman and Waylett 1981).

### Gunshot Wounds

The incidence of peripheral nerve injuries associated with GSWs is not negligible. Large series of conservatively managed peripheral nerve injury due to GSWs have accumulated in the past. Especially the experience during the many past military conflicts, including both world wars, has been very productive in providing us with the results of peripheral nerve injury management (Bzik and Bellamy 1984; Campbell 1959; Rothberg et al. 1983; Woodhall and Beebe 1956; Omer 1991). In civilian practice, too, nerve injuries secondary to GSWs are not uncommon: upper extremity nerves are more often involved than lower extremity nerves, and more multiple nerve injuries occur in the arms than in the legs. There is usually major damage to surrounding soft tissues that may include arteries and/or veins, making the treatment of these lesions in the acute setting a challenge for the surgeon. In fact, GSW damage varies somewhat depending on the type of weapon; the bullet caliber, construction, and shape, the velocity of the projectile, the type of tissues injured; and the distance of the gun from the victim (Fackler 1986, 1988; Luce 1978). Higher velocity injuries are usually more frequently seen in military combat and lower velocity injuries in civilian life. Only in about 15% of the cases is the nerve directly hit by the bullet (Kline and Hudson 1995). Most nerves injured by a gunshot are still in continuity even if there is an immediate loss of function. This is the result of the cavitation shock pressure wave that the projectile causes in the traversed tissues. This type of nerve injury is best cared for conservatively initially: about 67% of high-velocity gunshot wounds as opposed to only about 40% of low-velocity gunshot wounds will show significant recovery of function, whereas the remainder will require operative revision (Gentili and Hudson 1985; Kline 1989; Omer 1980, 1982, 1991). In fact, as early as 1917, Tinel had reported greater than 50% spontaneous recovery of peripheral nerve injuries as evidenced by his experience with GSWs during World War I (Tinel 1917). He characterized surgical intervention before 6 months as impatience. Foerster's retrospective analysis of 3907 GSWs to peripheral nerves showed spontaneous recovery in 68% of cases (Foerster 1929). A prospective analysis of GSWs to peripheral nerves during the Vietnam conflict revealed 69% recovery with conservative management (Omer 1982). Serious GSWs to the brachial plexus, however, are more likely to require operative exploration to achieve maximum benefit (Kline 1989).

### Orthopedic Injury

The true incidence of nerve injury related to fractures and dislocations is unknown, but some estimates are available. In children, for example, Hanlon and Estes (1954) reported that 2.5% of extremity fractures are associated with nerve injuries. Dormans et al. (1995) and Brown and Zinar (1995) reported an incidence of about 9.5% to 15% neural injuries, some of them iatrogenic, in 200 and 162 supracondylar humeral fractures, respectively. The incidence seems to be higher following dislocations as compared to fractures, and the vast majority (80% to 90%) of nerve injuries are associated with upper extremity fractures (Omer 1974). The radial nerve suffers most commonly of all, and is involved in about 16% of all upper arm fractures (Pollock et al. 1981).

### Thermal and Electrical Trauma

Patients with burns, due to either thermal injury or chemical or caustic agents, can have direct neural injury. Sometimes a delayed loss secondary to eschar formation, especially in cases of circumferential burns, occurs. Initial debridement needs to be thorough and needs to extend well into nonburned areas. Nerve reconstruction as such is delayed because at the time of escharotomy the extent of nerve injury cannot be judged definitively. Unfortunately, for these patients, long segments of nerve tend to be involved, requiring lengthy grafts and therefore prognosis is not good (Bateman 1962; Rosen 1981; Salisbury and Dingeldein 1982; Salzberg and Salisbury 1991; Salisbury et al. 1998).

Electrical injury secondary to exposure to a high-voltage source can cause major soft tissue damage that may include damage to peripheral nerves (Salisbury et al. 1998). Our knowledge of these injuries is limited because of a paucity of reports. Our own experience with seven cases shows that spontaneous improvement over time is seldom the case. A combination of lengthy nerve resection and graft placement as well as early reconstructive orthopedic and plastic procedures seems to give the best results. Useful reinnervation is difficult to obtain secondary to the severe coagulative injuries to muscle and the development of dense disfiguring scar to all soft tissues. These patients, as well as burn patients, may be candidates for more advanced, experimental surgical procedures such as free neurovascular muscle flaps.

### Radiation Injury

Radiation can potentially cause significant injury to all elements of the PNS (Salisbury et al. 1998). Pathogenetically this may be secondary to direct damage in acute peripheral nerve radiation injury, to autoimmune demyelination in early-delayed injury, to fibrosis in focal late-delayed injury, to hypothyroidism in diffuse late-delayed injury, and to radiation-induced carcinogenesis in neoplastic late-delayed peripheral nerve radiation injury (Posner 1995). For the present discussion, localized radiation injury such as in focal delayed-injury is more important, and is exemplified by radiation plexitis.

### Chronic Trauma

Chronic trauma usually involves some kind of compression or irritation to nerve(s) either continuously and ongoing or with repetitive exacerbations. This might be in the form of callus formation after fracture, of traumatic aneurysm, of soft tissue hematoma or position-related pressure such as habitual leg crossing, or in a form of repetitive irritation such as often discussed with entities like carpal tunnel syndrome. Damage in changes in conduction are most likely due to mechanical deformation (Dahlin 1986). Localized ischemia may play a role in the development of nerve injury in this setting of chronic compression. Overall, however, the blood supply to nerves is excellent, with a rich network of longitudinal collaterals (Lundborg 1975). This actually allows the experienced surgeon to mobilize large segments of nerve without any danger of ischemic damage (Kline et al. 1972). Chronic compression of nerve fibers leads to paranodal changes in myelination, axonal thinning, and even segmental demyelination, whereas wallerian degeneration occurs in more advanced and severe cases (Fullerton and Gilliatt 1967a, 1967b). These conditions have a rather good prognosis provided the causative factor(s) are removed in a timely fashion by surgical decompression (e.g., thoracic

outlet syndrome and carpal tunnel syndrome) or surgical transposition (e.g., ulnar nerve compression at the olecranon notch or cubital tunnel) (Hardy and Wilbourn 1985; Hudson et al. 1987; Kline and Hudson 1985; Rengachary 1985).

Nonetheless, even an entrapment nerve has the potential to disable some patients to the extent that they are not able to earn a living (Rayan 1998).

### Infectious Injury

#### Bacterial Disease With Special Consideration of Hansen's Disease

Infectious injury to peripheral nerve is relatively rare because the connective tissue layers of nerves are rather resistant to invasion by micro-organisms. Most infections are related to wound contamination. If the offending organisms do invade the epineurial and endoneurial tissues, extensive neural necrosis can ensue. This will ultimately require lengthy graft placement in addition to antibiotic therapy.

Some bacteria involve the nerves directly, such as *Mycobacterium leprae* in Hansen's disease, leading to abscess formation or other types of peripheral nerve injury requiring surgical treatment such as abscess incision, resection, neurolysis, or nerve grafting (Enna and Jacobson 1974; Dastur 1978, 1983; Pandya 1983; Salafia and Chauhan 1996). The lepra bacillus can be found in various cellular elements of the peripheral nerve, including Schwann cells, axons, endothelium, and perineurial cells (Boddingius 1974; Dastur et al. 1973; Yoshizumi and Asbury 1974; Minauchi and Igata 1987). The most frequently involved peripheral nerves are, in order of decreasing incidence, the ulnar nerve especially at the elbow level, the median nerve particularly in the distal forearm just proximal to the carpal tunnel, the common peroneal nerve at the fibular head, the tibial nerve at the tarsal tunnel, and less frequently, the radial nerve (Enna 1998). The superficial location of these nerves makes them particularly vulnerable, perhaps because of a combination of a more favorable temperature for Hansen's bacillus in these subcutaneous locations and of these sites' well-known predilection to chronic compressive injury and entrapment syndromes (Shepard 1965; Pandey and Singh 1974). In tuberculoid leprosy of peripheral nerves, an active inflammatory response by the host leads to intense tissue reaction and destruction with the formation of granulomas and nodules with often caseating necrosis (Boddingius 1974; Dastur et al. 1973; Yoshizumi and Asbury 1974).

### Viral Disease Including Human Immunodeficiency Virus Infection

Viral infections often affect the PNS, and a well-known example is herpes zoster, which usually involves a nerve root with its ganglion cells and axons extending into the peripheral nerves. Zoster radiculitis can cause a pain syndrome but may cause paresis too (Merchut and Gruener 1996), which initially may lead to diagnostic confusion. Most cases of zoster have a good prognosis for recovery, although up to 10% to 20% of patients have a persistent and difficult-to-treat pain syndrome sometimes lasting for many years (Johnson 1997).

Human immunodeficiency virus (HIV) can have a multitude of PNS symptoms (Simpson and Berger 1996; Price 1996). From our viewpoint, the progressive polyradiculopathy resulting in a progressively developing cauda equina syndrome, although rare in itself (Fuller et al. 1993), is most important because it can mimic serious surgical disease. Mononeuropathies can mimic surgical disease as well. Such neuropathies can often involve the lateral femoral cutaneous nerve, and the ulnar or median or other nerves typically prone to entrapment, particularly in patients with weight loss (Fuller et al. 1993; Sotaniemi 1984).

### Idiopathic Brachial and Lumbosacral Plexopathy

The pathogenesis of idiopathic brachial plexopathy, also known by synonyms such as Parsonage-Turner syndrome (Parsonage and Turner 1948), neuralgic shoulder amyotrophy, acute brachial radiculitis, acute shoulder girdle neuritis, is unknown, but a relationship to postvaccination, toxic, and hereditary brachial plexopathies has been discussed (Schaumburg et al. 1992; Wilbourn 1993). This condition needs to be differentiated from other affections of the brachial plexus, especially neoplasm, as well as from radicular disease such as secondary to cervical spine spondylosis and disc herniations. Overall the prognosis is rather good, with total recovery occurring in 90% of cases (Schaumburg et al. 1992; Wilbourn 1993). Lower brachial plexus or complete brachial plexus involvement carries a more severe prognosis (Schaumburg et al. 1992; Wilbourn 1993). A similar condition may be found in the lumbosacral plexus. Idiopathic lumbar plexopathy is, however, much more uncommon than idiopathic brachial plexopathy (Schaumburg et al. 1992; Wilbourn 1993). The differential diagnosis includes lumbar disc herniation, and cauda equina and pelvic tumors.

### Iatrogenic Injury

Iatrogenic nerve lesions are particularly distressful because of their potential damaging effect on the patient-physician relationship, which should be one of trust and confidence. These incidents should be openly discussed with the goal of assuring the patient of a renewed therapeutic relationship (Applegate 1986). Iatrogenic injuries include nerve injuries related to positioning, to injection, or to orthopedic procedures such as traction pin application or plaster casting. In general, they should be treated (i.e., sharp vs. blunt, in-continuity vs. not in continuity) using the same timing and other management guidelines as used for noniatrogenic injuries.

### Positioning Injury

Operating room–related peripheral nerve injuries have been noted for many years but were not always interpreted correctly. Indeed, some authors believed they were due to neurotoxic effects of anesthetic medications, although more recently, the importance of correct positioning of patients in the operating room has been appreciated (Büdinger 1894; Britt and Gordon 1964; Britt et al. 1983; Jackson and Keats 1965; Butler et al. 1984; Parks 1973). The mechanism of injury can be ischemic by continuous compression of the smallest vessels within the nerve or may be related to stretch (Cooper et al. 1988; Denny-Brown and Doherty 1945). Direct compression injury of a peripheral nerve is possible whenever a hard surface is in apposition to the nerve such as the ulnar nerve in the olecranon region, the common peroneal nerve at the fibular head, the lateral femoral cutaneous nerve at the inguinal ligament, or positioning and overspreading of retractors such as in sternotomy-related brachial plexopathy. The lithotomy, Trendelenburg, and prone positions are most notorious for positioning-related nerve injury (Cooper 1991).

Fortunately, better education has contributed to an overall decrease in the incidence of these lesions, which is now less than 1% (Cooper 1991). The most commonly injured nerves are the brachial plexus and the peroneal nerve. In general, the recovery of positioning-related lesions is relatively good, but the brachial plexus and the peroneal nerve are among those that have the highest incidence of permanent deficit (5% to 22% and 10% to 27%, respectively) (Cooper 1991). The association with other causes of neuropathy such as diabetes mellitus, malnutrition, alcoholism, or renal insufficiency makes recovery less likely in some of these patients. The treatment of these cases is primarily expectant and conservative, although in cases without recovery, an operation should be considered.

### Iatrogenic Spinal Accessory Neuropathy

Most injuries to the spinal accessory nerve are iatrogenic, especially those relating to lymph node biopsy or other operations in the posterior triangle of the neck. Other etiologies, although less frequent, have been reported (Donner and Kline 1993). About 50% of these patients will require operative exploration (Kline and Hudson 1995). One-third have lesions-in-continuity necessitating end-to-end repair or use of grafts. Most patients with a neurolysis do well if therapy is based on a positive NAP recording, while those with nerve graft procedures recover significantly in about 70% of cases (Kline and Hudson 1995).

### Injection Injury

The incidence of injection injuries to peripheral nerves is not known, but is fortunately low considering the large number of injections given. Greenblatt and Allen (1978) found local complications of intramuscular injections in 0.4% of 12,095 patients who received at least one intramuscular drug injection during their hospitalization. Injection injuries of peripheral nerves are very tragic and their devastating consequences have been documented in detail (Gentili et al. 1980a; Villarejo and Pascual 1993; Fremling and Mackinnon 1996). Most involve the radial or sciatic nerves (Kline and Hudson 1995). Apart from direct trauma to the nerve by a needle, the mechanism of injury appears to involve a direct toxic, necrotizing effect of the injected compound on neural tissue, followed by connective tissue proliferation, scar formation, and usually frustrating attempts to regenerate axons through this dense, fibrotic tissue (Broadbent et al. 1949; Mackinnon et al. 1982; Pizzolato and Mannheimer 1961; Gentili et al. 1980b; Kolb and Gray 1946). External neurolysis has been advocated in the past (Matson 1950), although it has not been agreed upon as a treatment for this condition. A few patients have a lesion resulting from injection around the nerve or even some distance away from the nerve, but this is relatively uncommon, with only about 10% of cases showing a significant delay of up to several days in developing any symptoms at all (Kline and Hudson 1995). Recent progress with internal neurolysis, resection, and grafting has given patients with nerve injection injuries some hope for a better outcome (Frederick et al. 1992; Hudson 1984; Fremling and Mackinnon 1996; Kasten and Louis 1996; Kline and Hudson 1995). Best surgical results seem to be obtained by immediate intervention when the injury was received in an area of the nerve that is predisposed to entrapment, such as the median nerve at the carpal tunnel (Mackinnon and Dellon 1988), although such an immediate surgical approach with open irrigation is often not practical in the acute setting. If the nerve has retained some function, an expectant attitude is justifiable unless pain is a major symptom. Persisting complete deficit requires exploration, which should include NAP recording, external and internal neurolysis, and possibly resection with nerve grafting (Midha et al. 1998). In case there is evidence of partial damage to the nerve, a split repair of only the injured fascicles with resection and grafting as outlined above may be attempted. This may be the case, for example, in some sciatic nerve injection injuries that not uncommonly show differential involvement of the tibial and peroneal components (Kline and Hudson 1995).

## Type of Nerve and Specific Nerve Injured

Of the different kinds of nerves, pure sensory nerves such as the antebrachial cutaneous, the superficial sensory radial, and the sural have the best prognosis for spontaneous regeneration after nontransecting injury (Kline and Hudson 1995). Nerves that are predominantly motor have a somewhat lesser prognosis due to the difficulties in reinnervating the target organs, and secondary to disuse and denervation atrophy of muscle. This is especially so if the target muscles are small and concerned with fine movements like the hand interossei (Kline and Hudson 1995). In the case of mixed nerves, an added difficulty is the potential mixing of motor and sensory fibers depending on the actual fascicular make-up of the nerve. This changes along the course of the nerve; for example, the median nerve is composed of 94% sensory fibers at the wrist level but only 66% sensory fibers at the elbow level (Doyle 1980; Kline and Hurst 1984; Millesi 1979). Usually there is a greater chance of adverse mixture of motor and sensory fibers in proximal than in distal lesions because segregation of the different fibers into fascicles with specific motor or sensory function is more likely as one goes distal in the system.

Some nerves recover better than others regardless of the kind of injury afflicted and whether spontaneous regeneration or surgical repair is considered. At the brachial plexus level (e.g., C5 and C6) plexus roots conjoining to form the upper trunk have the best prognosis (Kline and Hudson 1995). The middle trunk and its C7 root have a less favorable prognosis, whereas the outcome is worst for lesions involving the C8 and T1 roots, or the lower trunk. More distally in the brachial plexus, the lateral cord fares better than the posterior cord, which in turn has better outcome than the medial cord when seriously injured. Finally, lesions of the infraclavicular part of the plexus have a better outlook than supraclavicular injuries. Motor return is overall relatively poor, but functionally useful results can be obtained by appropriate neurolysis and grafting procedures within the plexus as well as between plexus elements and more peripheral neural structures, whereas sensory recovery can be rather good even in lower root and trunk repair (Bateman 1962). Return of intrinsic hand muscle function after complete injury is, however, rare (Alnot 1984; Frykman et al. 1981; Kline 1989).

The prognosis for recovery in upper extremity nerve lesions is probably related to distance of regeneration required and to the specific muscles that need reinnervation. Results are best for the musculocutaneous and radial nerves, whereas the median nerve has an intermediate prognosis for recovery of function, and the ulnar nerve has the worst prognosis (Miller 1987; Millesi 1981; Kline and Hudson 1995).

The tibial nerve and the peroneal nerve, the two major lower extremity nerves forming the sciatic nerve, have a very different prognosis, with the tibial nerve doing much better than the peroneal (Kline and Hudson 1996; Sunderland 1968). Prognosis for return of plantar flexion and sensation on the sole of the foot is quite good, for these functions depend on tibial nerve regeneration. Recovery of dorsiflexion, which depends on the peroneal nerve, is very poor. The third major nerve of the leg is the femoral nerve and its regenerative potential is quite good as well (Kline 1985; Seddon 1972; Kline and Hudson 1995; Kin and Kline 1997), the major difficulty being that this nerve tends to divide rather proximally in the thigh into different branches supplying the quadriceps femoris muscle making some operative repairs at thigh level more difficult (Kline 1985; Seddon 1972).

## Age of the Patient

There is a well-defined and long-known prognostic advantage of young age versus older age in the recovery of peripheral nerve lesions (Matson 1969; Tupper et al 1988; Spinner 1978; Seddon 1972). Various reasons for this phenomenon have been discussed. Regeneration rates in children may be faster, although this is not uncontroversial (Sunderland 1968). Axons may tend to sprout more prolifically in children than in adults. The distances that regenerating axons have to bridge are shorter in smaller children as compared to adults. Although the changes and reparative processes in regenerating peripheral nerves are rather similar in young and adult animals (Almquist et al. 1983), the young nervous system has a greater plasticity than the adult's, particularly in the central nervous system (CNS). Centrally occurring changes may be very important for improved prognosis in children (Kalaska and Pomeranz 1979; McKinley et al. 1987). Indeed, the capacity for cortical reorganization is marked at a very young age and this might very well influence the improved perception of peripheral structures within the areas of damaged and repaired nerves in children (Kaleska et al. 1979; McKinley et al. 1987). There is no consensus on the effect of advanced age: is the geriatric population at a distinct disadvantage for neural regeneration as compared with younger adults (Doyle 1980; Kline and Hurst 1984; Lundborg 1982;

Sunderland 1968)? Numbers are small but tend to support the hypothesis that older adults are less likely to achieve satisfactory results (Steinberg and Koman 1991), but anecdotal evidence of very good recoveries can be found in the literature (Dellon 1981; Mackinnon and Dellon 1988; Marble et al. 1942).

## Obstetrical Palsy

Particularly interesting from the point of view of the age effect on prognosis of peripheral nerve injuries are birth palsies; that is, upper plexus lesions (Erb-Duchenne) and lower plexus lesions (Dejerine-Klumpke). This is a very controversial topic in peripheral nerve surgery, management recommendations varying from a purely conservative approach to a more aggressive opinion favoring early operative revision of these lesions. The pathophysiological cause for the paralysis is a stretch injury of the brachial plexus secondary to dystocia. The forces involved are usually less than in traumatic injury at a later age and this as well as the young age of the patients might help explain why there seems to be a higher incidence of recovery in these birth palsies. Gilbert and Tassin (1987) were the first authors systematically stressing the potential important role of surgical repair for babies with obstetrical palsy. Return of biceps function was emphasized in deciding on a surgical or nonsurgical treatment (Gilbert et al. 1988). The time period given for the biceps musculature to show evidence of reinnervation was 3 months (Meyer 1986). More reports have followed these initial publications on surgery of the brachial plexus in obstetrical palsy (Alanen et al. 1986; Boome and Kaye 1988; Kline and Hudson 1995; Laurent and Lee 1994; Laurent et al. 1990; Metaizeau et al. 1984; Narakas 1981; Terzis et al. 1987a). At LSUMC, a relatively large percentage of cases have had, to date, significant spontaneous improvement, although this was not always evident in the early months after birth (Kline and Hudson 1995). It was often more conspicuous by 9 to 12 months of age. Children were operated between 9 and 36 months of age, with acceptable results. From our series, it is also clear that return of biceps function by 3 months may not be as decisive to prognosticate the need for surgery as originally thought (Gilbert and Tassin 1987; Kline and Hudson 1995). A rather large percentage of children did not have biceps recov-

ery by 3 or 4 months of age, yet had acceptable return of biceps and then other function later on. We feel that the major determinants for prognosis and the need for surgery are the persistence of complete loss of function in one or more of the distributions of C5, C6, and/or C7 and the upper or middle trunks that can be helped by a surgical procedure. In addition, the neonate's and young infant's brachial plexus has a potential for recovery and regeneration that is not to be underestimated despite a longer delay between injury and operation. This is so much different from the situation in older children and adults. For these reasons, we favor a relatively conservative approach in obstetrical brachial plexus palsy, with fairly strict indications for surgical revision which, when done, is usually done after 9 months of age.

## Clinical Evaluation of Peripheral Nerve Injury

A detailed and careful history is of prime importance in the evaluation of peripheral nerve injury and will give valuable information for prognosis. Many of the prognostic variables will be evident from thorough questioning of the patient. To the same extent, a detailed clinical examination is of utmost importance and will give many useful hints as to the eventual prognosis. Often, serial examination of the patient will be absolutely necessary to evaluate the course of recovery and to judge in a more detailed fashion prognosis.

Tinel's sign (Tinel 1915, 1917) is of interest because distal progression along the anatomical course of an injured nerve suggests the presence of young regenerating axons. This, however, does not necessarily guarantee recovery of significant function. The absence of a Tinel's sign distal to an injury site months after the initial trauma is much more significant, indicating poor regrowth even of fine axons.

End-organ examination helps in assessment of the progression of reinnervation. The area of denervated muscle bellies will at first develop diffuse hypersensitivity and pain to palpation as a sign of early recovery. The first sensory modalities to recover are those depending on small-fiber regeneration (e.g., high-threshold hyperpathic response to pinprick). This is a diffuse, unpleasant sensation of discomfort. Restitution of sweating and focal pain sensation signify small-fiber regeneration, whereas large-fiber functions such as proprioception, pallesthesia, and two-point discrimination will recover the last. An improved prognosis for recovery can be assumed if the autonomous zone of an injured nerve shows some signs of sensory reinnervation or if there is recovery of autonomic function such as sweating. These signs, however, do not provide a guarantee for complete recovery and thus repetitive follow-up is necessary. Programs in sensory re-education will assist the patient considerably in achieving maximal recovery and thereby improving prognosis (Carter-Wilson 1991).

Evaluation of motor regeneration may well give the physician the best appreciation of how good spontaneous recovery and/or repair is. A thorough exam of all muscles in the distribution of the nerve(s) involved needs to be performed with careful clinical grading of muscle strength. Early significant improvement will support further conservative management (Groff and Houtz 1945). The pattern of motor loss will help evaluate the lesion site. For example, in brachial plexus injuries, preservation of rhomboid, serratus anterior, supraspinatus, and infraspinatus muscles will indicate a better prognosis than loss of these muscles. Even taking into account favorable factors with regard to the nature of the lesion, its level, the age of the patient, and the nerves involved, complete motor recovery is the exception rather than the rule (Hudson and Tranmer 1985; Kline and Judice 1983; Millesi 1984a; Sedel 1984).

## Ancillary Examinations in Peripheral Nerve Injury

Radiological and imaging studies are indispensable. Indeed, even plain x-rays can be very helpful in drawing the physician's attention to concomitant injuries such as spine or long bone fractures or dislocation(s), callus formation, abnormal bony structures such as a cervical rib or a supracondylar humeral process, and so forth. Angiography should be considered in cases with potential vascular pathology such as arteriovenous fistulae, traumatic aneurysms, and in a few patients with thoracic outlet syndrome. Myelography plays an important role in evaluation of brachial plexus lesions, especially if there is a component of stretch/contusion, because it can demonstrate post-traumatic meningoceles, spinal cord swelling, or atrophy, all of which indicate in-

juries with a poor prognosis for restoration of function (Campbell 1970; Murphey et al. 1947; Robles 1968). These lesions often mean nerve root involvement potentially with nerve root avulsion from the spinal cord, which Sunderland (1974) feels more easily involves the motor than the sensory rootlets. Despite this, nerve root injury in cases of brachial plexus stretch injury can be present without meningocele and, conversely, a meningocele can be present without nerve root injury, especially with early myelography (Heon 1965; Kline and Hudson 1996; Nagano et al. 1984; Simond and Sypert 1983; Sunderland 1968). Computed tomography (CT)–assisted myelography can supplement a traditional myelogram but cannot replace it (Kline and Hudson 1995). The importance of CT-myelography and of additional intraoperative histological studies for nerve root myelinization to assess the presence of nerve root avulsion and to avoid using avulsed nerve root as an axon outflow source has been stressed by Meyer et al. (1995) and Meyer (1998). Carvalho et al. (1997) recommended even intradural exploration as the final definitive method to evaluate nerve root avulsion. New advances in magnetic resonance imaging (MRI) are being made at an ever-increasing speed, and the MRI capabilities for brachial plexus examination are improving continuously (Collins et al. 1998). Examination of the peripheral nerves at the extremity level is another area of future potential for the MRI technique (Iyer et al. 1996; Mukherji et al. 1996). At the present time, however, MRI examinations do not replace myelography in the evaluation of traumatic brachial plexus injuries (Kline and Hudson 1995; Panasci et al. 1995).

Neurophysiological studies are of great assistance in the evaluation of the patient with a peripheral nerve lesion (Kimura 1993). They should be used pre-, intra-, and postoperatively (Kline and Hudson 1995). The findings on electromyography (EMG) help the physician in differentiating various degrees of injuries such as neurapraxia, axonotmesis, and neurotmesis. Fibrillations are few or rare in neurapraxic injuries, whereas they develop frequently along with denervation potentials within 2 to 4 weeks in more severe injuries. Nerve conduction studies using electroneurography (ENG) will help the examiner too: neurapraxia does not cause loss of nerve conduction with stimulation and recording distal to the lesion but axonotmesis and neurotmesis will. EMG and ENG will show characteristic changes depending on the success of regeneration within the injured nerve. Return of insertional activity, decreasing denervation potentials, and increasing nascent potentials speak in favor of regeneration such as seen with axonotemesis. ENG will reveal NAPs at sites along a regenerating nerve and progressively more distant from the original lesion. Absence of an operative NAP across a lesion 2 to 3 months following injury is a poor prognostic sign that suggests a neurotmetic lesion (Kline 1982; Kline and Hackett 1985). EMG changes can precede clinical recovery by a number of weeks, but if there is no progression to clinical movement within the paralyzed muscles, a largely neurotmetic lesion should be suspected. ENG helps in differentiating a pre- from a postganglionic lesion at a nerve root level. Indeed, the presence of large amplitude, rapidly conducting sensory NAPs over nerves such as ulnar and median distal to the brachial plexus without concomitant clinical function and with absent motor conduction strongly suggests a preganglionic lesion. Sensory fibers are spared distal to the sensory nerve root ganglion, but the sensory root or rootlets proximally are damaged close to the spinal cord. This circumstance suggest an extremely poor prognosis. Further refinement in the use of ENG and NAP methodology included the introduction of somatosensory evoked potentials (SSEPs) and motor evoked potentials (MEPs). These techniques can assist in differentiating pre- from postganglionic lesions and in detecting combined pre- and postganglionic lesions (Kondo et al. 1985; Sugioka et al. 1982). It needs to be kept in mind, however, that recording a spinal or cortical SSEP requires only a few hundred intact nerve fibers, and a positive response therefore might have less significance than a negative one (Zhao et al. 1993). Furthermore, the usual stimulation site is distal on the extremity and evaluation of regeneration might be difficult if new fibers associated with a regenerating plexus lesion have not yet reached the stimulated area of the limb. In addition, this technique is very sensitive to reinnervation from surrounding areas. By comparison, intraoperative SSEPs, especially with stimulation of proximal nerve elements such as intraforaminal spinal nerves and roots, can be very useful (Kline and Hudson 1990; Sugioka et al. 1982). A combination of neurophysiological studies and clinical evaluation will often be necessary for optimal diagnosis, especially in areas of great complexity such as the brachial and lumbosacral plexuses.

## Technique of Nerve Repair in Peripheral Nerve Injury

### Techniques of Nerve Anastomosis

Nerve repair can be done with different techniques such as epineurial sutures through the epineurial sheath only, a combination of a few sutures through the fascicular bundles with epineurial sutures, or perineurial sutures involving only single fascicles. Epineurial repair is prognostically the better choice for acute as well as for delayed repair. Fascicular repair should be used for injuries that leave the integrity of some fascicles intact (i.e., split repair). Interfascicular grafts, however, are best for delayed repair of lengthy lesions.

Most peripheral nerve surgeons will use microsutures to perform nerve anastomosis. Innovative approaches to nerve approximation have focused on sutureless techniques such as the use of fibrin glue, the use of tubulation techniques with either synthetic bioabsorbable tubes, nonabsorbable silicone tubes, or vein grafts; the application of lasers; and the adaptation of classical suture techniques to more elaborate techniques such as epineurial splinting (Brunelli et al. 1994; Diao and Peimer 1991; Jabaley 1991; Chiu 1998; Almquist 1998).

### *Suture Tension and the Need for Nerve Grafts*

Suture tension should be as minimal as possible (Millesi 1981; 1986). On the other hand, a single suture line such as in direct end-to-end nerve repair will be more favorable than the use of a graft that necessitates the use of two-suture lines. In order to achieve these goals, mobilization of the nerve ends is often necessary (Kline et al. 1972; Lundborg 1975; Sunderland 1968). An interesting but still experimental approach to increase the length of nerve available for suturing and thereby achieving end-to-end suture without need for a graft is nerve lengthening by gradual balloon expansion, which can be used if nerve grafting per se is expected to have an unfavorable outcome, or if there is not enough autologous nerve graft donor material available (Van Beek and Hoffman 1998). Nerve lengthening is a two-stage procedure and requires careful patient selection.

The technical details of nerve grafting influence the prognosis of this procedure. Several different techniques are being used presently or have been used in the past. They have advantages and disadvantages that may be obvious on purely theoretical grounds but seldom on the basis of hard clinical evidence. Clinical studies are often difficult to analyze because of the many variables involved. Grafting has been firmly advocated by Millesi (1979), even for relatively small gaps. The bulk of the evidence seems to indicate, however, that the difference in outcome between grafting and nongrafting for small gaps is nonexistent or at best not significant (Bratton et al. 1979; Kline and Hudson 1985; McNamara et al. 1987). On the other hand, it is very evident that grafts are the preferred method of repair where end-to-end suture cannot be done with minimal tension and where distraction is a possibility. It is generally agreed that grafts should be less than 5 mm in diameter to ensure optimal vascularization of the graft material. Also, graft length should be about 10% to 15% longer than gap distance. Furthermore, the longer the grafts, the worse the prognosis. If the graft length is more than 10 cm the outlook is generally poor from a prognostic point of view, although some nerves might still do reasonably well, such as the musculocutaneous, radial, and tibial nerves (Frykman and Cally 1988; Kline and Hudson 1996; Kline 1983; Lundborg 1982; McQuarrie 1985; Sunderland 1968). Severity of the nerve injury and length of graft needed for repair are usually interrelated, and this helps explain why longer grafts (i.e., longer defects) have a poorer prognosis, with a reported 6% loss of functional recovery for every centimeter of gap that requires repair (Woodhall and Beebe 1956; Millesi 1998).

*Neurolysis*

Neurolysis (i.e., freeing of scarred nerve from the sometimes encasing fibrotic reaction possibly responsible for pain or, less frequently, a progressive neurological deficit) is usually performed externally. If done carefully, neurolysis should not compromise the nerve's vasculature. Such a neurolysis is usually necessary before NAP recordings and decisions for or against resection can be made (Frykman et al. 1981; Kline et al. 1972; Millesi 1981; Woodhall and Beebe 1956). Omer (1982) reported improvement in 60% of a large

series of missile-injured patients. Today, intraoperative evaluation, especially with the use of NAP's, is essential for the management of these lesions. If an NAP can be recorded across the lesion intraoperatively, thereby demonstrating continuity with the potential for further regrowth, useful recovery will subsequently occur more than 90% of the time. Even if the distal loss has been clinically complete for the first 10 months after the injury, neurolysis alone has been associated with recovery in most cases where an NAP is recordable (Kline 1989).

Internal neurolysis remains controversial. It requires the careful dissection and separation of the intraneural fascicles; therefore, there may be a functional price to be paid for the achievement of its goal (i.e., rapid and more complete decompression). It is usually done for severe, neuritic pain or for nerve lesions that require a split repair because injury involves various portions of the nerve to a different extent. It has been recommended especially for cases of revision (Broudy et al. 1978). The risk of recurrent and even more severe fibrosis than existed prior to the internal neurolysis is very real too. Proximal lesions are much less amenable to this type of intervention, since the fascicles have more interfascicular connecting fibers. Research into internal neurolysis has revealed decreased blood flow and increased intraneural adhesions following the procedure, and clinical studies have not shown convincing evidence of its superiority over external neurolysis (Goth 1987; Graf et al. 1986; Rydevik et al. 1976; Lowry and Follender 1988; Nielsen et al. 1980).

*Operative NAP Studies*

Clinically, symptomatic lesions may present without discontinuity on surgical exploration, although there might be localized swelling, localized intraneural fibrosis, or clinical evidence of intraneural damage: this is a lesion or a neuroma-in-continuity (Kline and Hudson 1995). These incontinuity lesions account for approximately 60% of lesions in civilian series. The introduction of intraoperative recording techniques for the evaluation of NAPs has enhanced the surgeon's capability to judge these lesions. Indeed, physical inspection alone frequently gives a false impression about a lesion's physiological severity, or extent of ongoing recovery (Kline 1977; Kline and

Hackett 1985; Kline and Hudson 1985, 1995). Neurophysiological evaluation of conduction by means of NAP recording allows the surgeon to classify the lesion more accurately and to decide more easily on the correct course of action to be taken (i.e., external neurolysis, split repair, or resection with suture and/or grafts) (Kline 1985; Kline and Hackett 1985; Kline and Hudson 1985, 1995). Regenerating lesions will not be resected unnecessarily and resections will be more complete, therefore improving future prognosis for regeneration of the reanastomosed nerve. Indeed, the most important cause of failure of nerve repair is inadequate resection, and this is much less the case when intraoperative NAP studies are performed.

### Neurotization by Nerve Transfer

Neurotization or nerve transfer has been proposed in cases in which the proximal nerve stump is not available for suture. Examples include brachial plexus lesions with nerve root avulsion or proximal plexus root injury (Narakas 1991). Several approaches have been used. Donor nerves for neurotization have included intercostal nerves, cervical plexus elements, the accessory nerve, the medial pectoral nerve, the phrenic nerve, and the dorsal scapular nerve. Some results have been obtained in 30% to 60% of patients with intercostal donor nerve neurotization, but the amount of useful recovery was limited and involved only one single function such as arm flexion or shoulder abduction but not both (Narakas 1991). Neurotization of the musculocutaneous nerve was much more favorable than neurotization of other nerves such as the radial, median, or ulnar nerve (Narakas 1991). Using the spinal accessory nerve Narakas (1991) obtained relatively good results when neurotizing the suprascapular nerve (80%) but much poorer outcomes when the posterior cord, axillary nerve, or radial nerve was the receiving end for such neurotization procedures (42%). It has been the general experience that it is very difficult to recover multiple functions by these procedures, and if at all feasible a direct repair of the nerve or plexus element involved offers the best outlook to accomplish this (Kline and Hudson 1995). More complex neurotization procedures have been reported by Chuang (1995) using the spinal accessory, phrenic, and/or motor branches of the cervical plexus to neurotize the upper brachial plexus with the goal of obtaining shoulder abduction, using three intercostal nerves to directly neurotize the musculocutaneous nerve to obtain elbow flexion, or using a combination of C5 and C6 plexus roots, and contralateral C7 plexus root, and intercostal and/or spinal accessory nerves to neurotize median and ulnar nerves (Chuang 1995). Excellent results using upper cervical roots and their outflow to cervical plexus as donors for brachial plexus elements have been reported by Yamada et al. (1996). Despite these complicated procedures, results for functional recovery distally in the upper extremity remain poor, and the surgeon will need to plan on additional reconstructive procedures to help his or her patients.

Nerves have been directly implanted into muscles such as biceps and gastrocnemius, but the value of these techniques is still unclear (Heineke 1914; Kline and Hudson 1996; McNamara et al. 1987). Clinically, investigational procedures were initially aimed at innervating muscles paralyzed by poliomyelitis, and results were very inconsistent (Brunelli 1991). Later, muscles paralyzed by peripheral nerve injury were used as the target for this technique if the interval since the denervating injury was not too long. Brunelli and Brunelli (1998) have reported good results for 50 of 56 neurotizations. Included were 15 reinnervation procedures for forearm extensors and 14 reinnervation procedures for extensors of the leg, as well as direct muscle neurotization in trapezius (seven cases), biceps brachii (seven cases), deltoid (six cases), thenar muscles (four cases), tongue (two cases), and extensor pollicis longus muscles (one case). These authors advocate the use of direct muscle neurotization as the only direct solution to a destruction of the neuromuscular junction. It should be cautioned, however, that most workers have not had useful results with direct nerotization into muscle.

### Vascularized Nerve Grafts

Vascularized nerve grafts have been used (Taylor and Ham 1976; Millesi 1991; Breidenbach 1998). The use of a vascularized graft including the ulnar nerve and the superior collateral ulnar artery was reported to have excellent recovery (Terzis et al. 1987b). The ulnar nerve has been used in this way also by other authors, with encouraging results (Bonney et al. 1984, 1987; Alnot and Benfrech 1989). The median nerve and tibial nerve have been repaired with some success using free vascularized nerve grafts (Oberlin et al. 1989). An attempt at neurotization of muscles by this method was also performed by Millesi (1991).

The main advantages of vascularized grafts are related to immediate vascularization and the decreased sensitivity to tension and traction (Millesi 1991). Whether these considerations are relevant to the clinical practice of nerve grafting and how far they translate into better results is open for debate (Millesi 1991). Clinical studies have tended to show an advantage of vascularized nerve grafts over non-vascularized grafts but, due to small numbers of cases, absence of controls, and individual variations between the series, overall conclusions are difficult to make (Taylor and Ham 1976; Taylor 1978; Fachinelli et al. 1981; Bonney et al. 1984; Rose and Kowalski 1985; Rose et al. 1989). Doi et al. (1992) reported results that support the benefits of vascularized nerve grafts over nonvascularized grafts for particular indications. They also expanded the typical indications for vascularized nerve grafting from the presence of a scarred recipient bed, the presence of proximal losses, and the presence of large defects, to include also smaller defects in minimally scarred beds.

### Intraoperative Differentiation of Motor and Sensory Fascicles

To better approximate motor and sensory fascicles in mixed nerves, some authors advocate the use of histochemical and biochemical methods during surgery (Lang et al. 1991; Hurst and Badalamente 1998). The correct identification of the motor or sensory function of proximal and distal fascicles has the advantage of suturing fascicles with the same function. It needs to be kept in mind, however, that distal nerve stump histochemical staining gives reliable results only during the first 7 to 10 days after the acute nerve injury, whereas proximal nerve stump staining is effective for more prolonged periods of time. The overall usefulness of these techniques has not been established: currently such techniques are still a clinical research tool, but conceptually they are very promising (Lang et al. 1991; Hurst and Badalamente 1998). When distal nerves are repaired acutely and especially when this is done in the awake patient, simple stimulation can be used to sort out the receptor and sensory fascicles on the distal as well as proximal stump.

### Timing of Peripheral Nerve Repair

Timing of repair of peripheral nerve lesions has been discussed as a prognostic factor since the very beginnings of peripheral nerve surgery. In general, the debate ranges between primary versus secondary repair. Primary repair (i.e., within 72 hours after injury) can be thought of as repair prior to healing of the associated soft tissue wounds and is indicated for all sharp transections of a peripheral nerve or plexus element. The major difficulty with this type of repair for all injuries is how to decide if there is not actually more widespread and extensive injury to a nerve than is seen on inspection. This is especially the case when there is a component of contusion and/or stretch during the injury, a fact that may or may not be appreciated from the beginning but which influences the prognosis tremendously. Therefore, in cases of doubt or in cases with an obvious contusive or stretch component, repair of even a transected nerve should be delayed for several weeks, allowing an exact delineation of the injured part of the nerve. Resection of the nerve segment and nerve suture with or with-out nerve graft(s) will then involve optimally prepared nerve stumps. Some research reports seem to suggest that the nerve's potential to generate efficient axonal sprouting is highest a few weeks after the initial lesion (McQuarrie 1985). Delayed surgery would therefore capitalize on the neuron's natural peak of regenerative biochemical activity. Negative aspects of delayed surgery for peripheral nerve injuries are the scarring of the operative field and the scar-induced distortion of normal anatomy, the fibrotic changes in the peripheral nerve and its stumps, and the overall increased difficulty of rebuilding a well-functioning myoneural junction (Kline and Hackett 1975; McNamara et al. 1987; Seddon 1972).

In general, primary repair is indicated for sharp, clean transections of nerve elements as well as for injuries to small nerves such as the digital nerves. In most other cases delayed repair will be preferable over primary repair (Ducker 1985; Kline 1982; McGillicuddy 1985).

If care is given to the indications and appropriate patient selection for primary and secondary repair, and if secondary repairs are performed within a reasonable time frame, then the results of both repair strategies are comparable (Braun 1982; Millesi 1980; Seddon 1943; Snyder 1981; Sunderland 1968; Zachary and Holmes 1946).

## Postoperative Care

Postoperative care influences the outcome of all surgery in general and of peripheral nerve surgery in particular. The healing of the wound and the potential development of infection are important factors. Infection can increase scar formation, can damage suture lines, and can prolong time needed for regeneration. Appropriate physical therapy with the goal of improving deficits caused by peripheral nerve lesions is critical. Continuous mobilization should be performed from the very beginning unless this is contraindicated by concurrent lesions such as some fractures. In general, it can be said that nerve lesions do not heal better with immobilization. Mobilization improves muscle tone, joint mobility, and prevents immobilization-induced pain. Sensory re-education is very helpful in improving the efficiency of the patient's recovery. The efficacy of external electrical muscle stimulation to prevent atrophy in denervated muscle is a subject of considerable debate, although there is some evidence that significant beneficial biochemical, electrophysiological, and biomechanical changes are induced by this form of stimulation (Williams 1998). Promising research with implantable and continuously stimulating devices is currently being performed to counteract the postdenervational process in skeletal muscle (Williams 1998).

Sensory loss affecting the limbs puts these at jeopardy for developing skin breakdown and ulcers. It needs to be understood that the main reason for these complications is inadequate care in combination with the absence of the protective feeling of pain by the patient (Brand 1998). These complications can be avoided by appropriate attention to preventive measures.

Psychological or psychiatric support may also be necessary to help distraught or discouraged patients rehabilitate themselves.

## Follow-up and Outcome Reporting

Assessment of recovery and outcome is difficult to standardize, and several scales often based on the British Medical Research Council gradation scales have been devised (Omer and Bell-Krotoski 1998). Nevertheless, a good appreciation of recovery and of functional rehabilitation is of paramount importance to evaluate the different therapeutic modalities that are applied to a particular injury and to evaluate the cost efficiency of these treatments. Standardization should enable physicians and allied health personnel to formulate a prognosis and to better compare the results of different series reported in the literature. Terms such as *useful recovery, moderate recovery, good recovery,* or *superior recovery* should be abandoned. In the literature, more emphasis has been placed generally on motor rehabilitation than on sensory recovery. Sensation, though, has special significance in particular areas of the body such as the thumb and index finger, or the sole of the foot, innervated by the median and tibial nerves, respectively. Furthermore, it is very important to make the patient aware of the fact that full regeneration and thus extent of recovery after peripheral nerve injury and/or repair can take 3 to 6 years to be completed. Even physicians are not always knowledgeable about the very long time periods required for regrowth.

Highet's scheme (Highet and Holmes 1942) has been modified by Zachary and Holmes (1946) to be used in providing prognostic evidence for selected nerve injuries, and this was further refined in the British Medical Research Council Rating Scale (Seddon 1954). At LSUMC, a similar tabulation has been devised (Table 25-1). Tables 25-2 through 25-8, based on Kline and Hudson's 1995 data and Moneim and Omer's 1998 report, should provide some help in forming a prognosis for selected peripheral nerve injuries.

## Pain

A particularly distressful phenomenon for the patient with nerve injury is the frequent association with pain. Usually, this pain finds its origin within the nervous system, but part of many pain syndromes can also be explained by prolonged and often unnecessary immobilization of a limb. An unused extremity can lead to a pain syndrome that can be very difficult to influence positively with therapy. Even considering potential distraction of the repair site and tension at the repair site, immobilization should seldom extend beyond 3 weeks, the time required to develop maximum

**Table 25-1.** Louisiana State University Medical Center (LSUMC) Grading System for Individual Muscles, for Sensation, and for Whole Nerve Function*

| Individual Muscle Grades | | |
|---|---|---|
| Grade | Evaluation | Description |
| 0 | Absent | No contraction |
| 1 | Poor | Trace contraction |
| 2 | Fair | Movement against gravity only |
| 3 | Moderate | Movement against gravity and some (mild) resistance |
| 4 | Good | Movement against moderate resistance |
| 5 | Excellent | Movement against maximal resistance |

| Sensory Grades | | |
|---|---|---|
| Grade | Evaluation | Description |
| 0 | Absent | No response to touch, pin, or pressue |
| 1 | Bad | Testing gives hyperesthesia or paresthesia; deep-pain recovery in autonomous zones |
| 2 | Poor | Sensory response sufficient for grip and slow protection; sensory stimuli mislocalized with over-response |
| 3 | Moderate | Response to touch and pin in autonomous zones; sensation localized and not normal; with some over-response |
| 4 | Good | Response to touch and pin in autonomous zones; response localized but not normal; no over-response |
| 5 | Excellent | Normal response to touch and pin in entire field, including autonomous zones |

| Whole Nerve Grades | | | |
|---|---|---|---|
| Grade | Evaluation | Motor Description | Sensory Description |
| 0 | Absent | No muscle contraction | Absent sensation |
| 1 | Poor | Proximal muscles contract with grade 0 or 1 | Sensory grade 0 or 1 |
| 2 | Fair | Proximal muscles contract with grade 2 Distal muscles do not contract | Sensory grade 0, 1, or 2 |
| 3 | Moderate | Proximal muscles contract with grade 3 Distal muscles contract with grade 2 | Sensory grade 3 |
| 4 | Good | All proximal muscles contract with grade 3 Some distal muscles contract with grade 3 | Sensory grade 3, 4, or 5 |
| 5 | Excellent | All muscles contract with grade 4, or 5 | Sensory grade 4, or 5 |

* Adapted from Kline and Hudson (1995).

tensile strength at the suture site (Liu et al. 1948; Tarlov 1947). In addition, it has been shown in experimental studies that suture sites with time tend to have greater strength than intact nerve (Bora et al. 1980), which is favorable for early mobilization as well (Grewal et al. 1996).

### Regeneration Pain

With a regenerating nerve, the patient may experience a variety of strange and unaccustomed feelings such as paresthesias, dysesthesia, numbness, electric shock-like feelings, and sometimes even sensations with a somewhat burning character. These regenerative sensations tend to be especially bothersome during the first few months after a peripheral nerve injury or repair (Ochoa 1982; Ochs et al. 1989). Although some burning component may be present, this pain is not to be mistaken for neuritic pain or causalgia. Regenerative pain is usually self-limited. Pharmacologically, this type of pain can usually be influenced by drugs like amitriptyline, carbamazepine, phenylhydantoin, or gabapentin (Kline and Hudson 1995). Repetitive use of the involved limb is to be encouraged and will help desensitize it (Haines 1996).

### Denervation Pain

In the acute stage, denervation leads to denervational pain in muscles. Although potentially very intense, this will tend to subside and will diminish to a tolerable level or will disappear completely as the atrophic process completes itself (Noordenbos 1959).

**Table 25-2.** Grading Results* of Surgery on the Median Nerve (LSUMC Series)†

Traumatic Median Nerve Lesions at All Levels ($N = 202$)

| Causes | Number of Cases | | Number of Cases | |
|---|---|---|---|---|
| | With Operation | Result: Grade 3 or Better | Without Operation | Result: Grade 3 or Better |
| Laceration | 54 | 46 (85%) | 14 | 13 (93%) |
| Gunshot wound | 22 | 19 (86%) | 12 | 11 (92%) |
| Fracture | 12 | 11 (92%) | 5 | 4 (80%) |
| Contusion | 16 | 15 (94%) | 12 | 11 (92%) |
| Compression | 14 | 11 (79%) | 8 | 7 (88%) |
| Injection | 10 | 10 (100%) | 7 | 6 (86%) |
| Electrical | 3 | 2 — | 2 | 2 — |
| Volkmann | 2 | 2 — | 1 | 0 — |
| Burn scar | 1 | 1 — | 4 | 2 — |
| Stretch | 3 | 2 — | 0 | 0 — |
| Total | 137 | 119 (87%) | 65 | 56 (86%) |

Carpal Tunnel Level Median Nerve ($N = 376$) with Operation: Carpal Tunnel Release by Palmar Incision

| Complaints and Symptoms | Number | % |
|---|---|---|
| Prominent pain improved | 246 of 282 | 87% |
| Prominent paresthesias improved | 230 of 249 | 92% |
| Significant numbness improved | 82 of 146 | 56% |
| Significant weakness improved | 20 of 48 | 42% |
| Patients satisfied with result | 303 of 340 | 89% |
| Major symptoms persisted | 23 of 376 | 6% |
| Deficit increased | 5 of 376 | 1% |
| Required repeat operation | 3 of 376 | 1% |
| Complications | | |
| Wound hematoma | 1 case | |
| Superficial wound infection | 3 cases | |
| Reflex sympathetic dystrophy | 1 case | |
| Average follow-up, 18.5 Months | | |

* Grading according to the LSUMC grading system for whole nerve (Kline and Hudson 1995)
† Adapted from Kline and Hudson (1995).

## Neuritic Pain

A usually severe type of pain is neuritic pain, which occurs in the typical distribution of the injured nerve. A common feature is local tenderness and a Tinel's sign. It is associated with paresthesias and hyperesthesia in hypesthetic areas as well as with a burning type of pain (Campbell et al. 1988; Devor 1994). Pharmacological treatment includes the same medications already mentioned earlier: tricyclic antidepressants and/or various types of antiepileptic drugs. Neuritic pain may often be helped by surgical procedures on the nerve itself, which may lead not only to an improved pain situation but to some restoration of function as well. Re-exploration with correction of any lesion found is often useful. Sometimes the nerve is not continuous as evidenced by NAP recording, the neuritic pain can then be related to regrowth of fine non-myelinated axons into a neuroma in-continuity, and resection with repair may be very helpful. If all these measures fail, stimulating electrodes, dorsal root entry zone lesions, or more central neurosurgical pain procedures may be considered (Nash-old and Ostahl 1979; Zorub et al. 1974; Ray 1998). Sympathectomy typically does not influence neuritic pain and usually should not be done.

## Causalgia, Reflex Sympathetic Dystrophy, Sympathetically Maintained Pain, and Complex Regional Pain Syndromes

Causalgia (i.e., burning pain), first described by Mitchell et al. (1864), (1872) following observations during the American Civil War, is characterized by a very typical intense and exquisite, burning pain that initially begins in the anatomical territory of an affected nerve, usually a major

**Table 25-3.** Grading Results* of Surgery on the Ulnar Nerve (LSUMC Series)[†]

Traumatic Ulnar Nerve Lesions at All Levels ($N = 119$)

| Operation | Number of Cases | Recovery to Grade 3 or Better[†] |
|---|---|---|
| **Transection ($n = 38$)** | | |
| Primary suture | 16 | 9 (56%) |
| Secondary repair | | |
| Suture | 14 | 10 (71%) |
| Secondary graft | 5 | 2 (40%) |
| Split Repair | 3 | 3 (100%) |
| Total | 38 | 24 (63%) |
| **In-continuity injuries ($n = 81$)** | | |
| Positive NAP ($n = 54$) | | |
| Neurolysis | 54 | 51 (94%) |
| Negative NAP ($n = 27$) | | |
| Suture | 15 | 11 (73%) |
| Grafts | 12 | 5 (42%) |
| Total | 81 | 71 (88%) |

Ulnar Nerve Entrapment ($N = 144$)

| Operation | Number of Grades Improved Postoperatively | Number of Cases |
|---|---|---|
| **No prior surgery** | 1 | 43 (51%) |
| **($N = 84$)** | 2 | 22 (26%) |
| | 3 or 4 | 8 (10%) |
| | No change | 10 (12%) |
| | Worse | 1 (1%) |
| **With prior surgery** | 1 | 32 (53%) |
| **($N = 60$)** | 2 | 10 (17%) |
| | 3 or 4 | 1 (2%) |
| | No change | 17 (28%) |

* Grading according to the LSUMC grading system for whole nerve (Kline and Hudson 1995).

† Adapted from Kline and Hudson (1995).

mixed motor-sensory nerve such as the median, the ulnar, or the tibial nerve, but then gradually spreads out over the borders of this territory to involve progressively larger areas of the limb. This pain is accompanied by intense hyperesthesia and by autonomic disturbances. The affected body part is religiously shielded from all contact. It cannot be touched or manipulated even when the attention of the patient is distracted. The pain syndrome and to a somewhat lesser extent the autonomic dysfunction too, react very favorably to sympathetic block and to sympathectomy. Nowadays, however, the designation of causalgia is being used too loosely and given to too many patients with other types of nerve pain. When applying strict criteria, approximately 2% to 2.5% of patients with severe nerve

injuries may develop causalgia. Reflex sympathetic dystrophy (RSD) was first mentioned in the literature by Evans in 1946. It describes a pain syndrome that develops following soft tissue damage that is often relatively minor and usually with distal small nerve involvement or without nerve injury at all. It is characterized by diffuse burning pain and hyperalgesia not confined to known anatomical areas of innervation, but associated with changes in blood flow and sweating, changes of active and passive movements, and trophic changes of the skin and subcutaneous tissues. It may be responsive to sympathetic block and sympathectomy (Atasoy and Kleinert 1998).

Different clinical types of sympathetically maintained pain (SMP), a term first introduced by Roberts (1986), have been widely recognized, although there is overlap in their definitions and clinical manifestations, and considerable discussion exists among pain specialists as to their exact nature. Causalgia usually is used to denote RSD or SMP involving and thought to be caused by nerve injury. Clinicians tend to make a distinction between major causalgia, involving damage to a major nerve, and minor causalgia, with less severe symptoms and involvement of a more peripheral nerve such as digital nerves. Then there is minor and major traumatic dystrophy, forms of RSD that are thought to result from injury to the soft tissues, joints, or bones, rather than to a specific peripheral nerve.

Because of all the controversy surrounding causalgia, RSD, and SMP, the International Association for the Study of Pain (IASP) in a consensus committee paper proposed a new nomenclature (i.e., complete regional pain syndromes [CRPS] to replace the previously used terms and to better indicate the description of the pain syndromes without invoking pathogenetic mechanisms (Stanton-Hicks et al. 1995). CRPS type I (formerly RSD) follows an initiating noxious event; the pain is spontaneous, out of proportion to the initiating event, and transgresses the known anatomical distribution of a single peripheral nerve. There is evidence of edema, blood flow alterations, and changes in sudomotor activity. There is no other coexisting condition that would explain the patient's symptoms. CRPS type II (formerly causalgia) follows peripheral nerve injury and is identical to CRPS type I in all other respects, especially also by the fact that pain is not

**Table 25-4.** Grading Results* of Surgery on the Radial Nerve (LSUMC Series)†

Traumatic Radial Nerve Lesions at All Levels (N = 155)

| | Number of Cases | | Number of Cases | |
|---|---|---|---|---|
| Causes | With Operation | Result of Grade 3 or Better | Without Operation | Result of Grade 3 or Better |
| Laceration | 26 | 24 (92%) | 2 | 2 — |
| Gunshot wound | 14 | 13 (93%) | 9 | 9 (100%) |
| Fracture | 43 | 38 (88%) | 27 | 25 (93%) |
| Contusion | 15 | 12 (80%) | 8 | 8 (100%) |
| Injection | 7 | 7 (100%) | | |
| Volkmann | | — | 2 | 1 — |
| Total | 107 | 94 (88%) | 48 | 45 (94%) |

Superficial Sensory Radial Nerve Neuroma (N = 23)

| Operation | Number of Cases | Number with Significant Relief of Pain |
|---|---|---|
| Laceration | | |
| Excision | 9 | 6 (67%) |
| Neurolysis | 0 | 0 — |
| Contusion | | |
| Excision | 3 | 3 (100%) |
| Neurolysis | 2 | 0 — |
| Prior suture | | |
| Excision | 2 | 2 (100%) |
| Neurolysis | 0 | 0 — |
| **No operation** | | |
| | 7 | 2 (29%) |

* Grading according to the LSUMC grading system for whole nerve (Kline and Hudson 1995).
† Adapted from Kline and Hudson (1995).

limited to the innervational area of the nerve involved. It is our feeling that as long as we do not know the exact pathogenetic and pathophysiological details of these pain and dystrophy states, this field will suffer from confusion, and agreed upon descriptive terms are to be preferred above a nomenclature that suggests etiology.

Diagnosis of CRPS is very much a clinical one, but can be supported with other modalities, particularly radionuclide three-phase bone scanning (Fournier and Holder 1998; Sintzoff et al. 1997). Therapy for RSD can be very frustrating for patient and physician alike despite trials with vasodilatation therapy, sympathetic blockade, free radical scavenger treatment, physical therapy, and intense psychological and social support (Van Der Laan and Goris 1997). The patient's pain should be addressed first and treated, followed by encouragement to use the affected extremity as much as possible. Indeed, there is no good substitute for the repetitive use of the arm or leg in this condition once the pain is controlled. The help of a physician experienced in the management of difficult pain syndromes can be a great advantage for these patients (Schultz 1998).

### Neuroma Pain

Severance of peripheral nerves regularly leads to neuroma formation, which can be rather painful in up to 30% of cases (Nelson 1977). The neuroma is a mass of tissue primarily composed of sprouting axon cylinders that are arranged in a completely chaotic way and usually interspersed with heavy collagen (Burger et al. 1991). The axis cylinders may be unmyelinated or only slightly enveloped by myelin. Although some neuromas can simulate schwannomas with their cellularity and compactness, the difference is usually easy to make because of the presence of many well-defined but haphazardly oriented axon cylinders within a collagenous stroma in a neuroma and the orientation of the few persisting axons along the long axis of the lesion in schwannomas (Burger et al. 1991). Neuromas can be conveniently classified as

**Table 25-5.** Grading Results* of Surgery on the Tibial and Peroneal Nerve (LSUMC Series)*†

Traumatic Tibial (N = 139) and Peroneal (N = 310) Nerve or Division Lesions at All Levels

Tibial Nerve or Division

| Causes | Number of Cases | | Number of Cases | |
|---|---|---|---|---|
| | With Operation | Result of Grade 3 or Better | Without Operation | Result of Grade 3 or Better |
| Laceration | 27 | 25 (93%) | 4 | 2 — |
| Gunshot wound | 35 | 32 (91%) | 7 | 6 (86%) |
| Fracture | 19 | 18 (95%) | 12 | 10 (83%) |
| Contusion | 7 | 6 (86%) | 14 | 11 (79%) |
| Compression | 4 | 4 (100%) | 1 | 0 (0%) |
| Iatrogenic | 5 | 4 (80%) | 4 | 3 (75%) |
| Total | 97 | 89 (92%) | 42 | 32 (76%) |

Peroneal Nerve or Division

| Causes | Number of Cases | | Number of Cases | |
|---|---|---|---|---|
| | With Operation | Result of Grade 3 or Better | Without Operation | Result of Grade 3 or Better |
| Laceration | 42 | 25 (60%) | 8 | 5 (63%) |
| Gunshot wound | 43 | 30 (70%) | 11 | 8 (73%) |
| Fracture | 35 | 22 (63%) | 18 | 6 (33%) |
| Contusion | 61 | 32 (53%) | 38 | 14 (37%) |
| Compression | 16 | 13 (81%) | 10 | 6 (60%) |
| Iatrogenic | 7 | 5 (71%) | 10 | 5 (50%) |
| Total | 204 | 127 (62%) | 106 | 44 (42%) |

* Grading according to the LSUMC grading system for whole nerve (Kline and Hudson 1995).
† Adapted from Kline and Hudson (1995).

neuromas-in-continuity in incompletely severed nerves, or badly stretched contused nerve and neuromas as such in completely severed nerves (Nath and Mackinnon 1996). Neuromas-in-continuity can involve all or only part of a nerve, the latter sparing some fascicles. This type of neuroma is sometimes called lateral neuroma (Herndon and Hess 1991). After failure of conservative measures such as physical therapy, desensitization, pain medication, transcutaneous electrical nerve stimulation (TENS), or local steroid injection, and after detailed and repetitive discussion of the surgical options and chances for success with the patient, operative procedures can be performed with

**Table 25-6.** Grading Results* of Surgery on the Femoral Nerve (LSUMC Series)†

Traumatic Femoral Nerve Lesions at All Levels (N = 75)

| Causes | Number of Cases | | Number of Cases | |
|---|---|---|---|---|
| | With Operation | Result of Grade 3 or Better | Without Operation | Result of Grade 3 or Better |
| Laceration | 5 | 5 (100%) | 1 | 1 (100%) |
| Gunshot wound | 2 | 1 (50%) | 2 | 1 (50%) |
| Fracture | 12 | 8 (67%) | 6 | 3 (50%) |
| Iatrogenic | 32 | 26 (80%) | 15 | 7 (47%) |
| Total | 51 | 40 (78%) | 24 | 12 (50%) |

* Grading according to the LSUMC grading system for whole nerve (Kline and Hudson 1995).
† Adapted from Kline and Hudson (1995).

**Table 25-7.** Grading Results* of Surgery on the Brachial Plexus (LSUMC Series)[†]

Lacerating Injury to the Brachial Plexus ($N = 47$) with Operation for Elements ($N = 142$) Preoperatively Diagnosed as Complete Loss

| Causes<br>Procedures | Number of Cases | Recovery to<br>Grade 3 or Better |
|---|---|---|
| **One or more elements in continuity** | | |
| Operated brachial plexus cases | 11 | |
| Operated brachial pexus elements | 30 | 24 (80%) |
| **Sharp transection of one or more elements** | | |
| Operated brachial plexus cases | 18 | |
| Operated brachial pexus elements | 60 | 38 (63%) |
| **Blunt transection of one or more elements** | | |
| Operated brachial plexus cases | 18 | |
| Operated brachial pexus elements | 52 | 25 (48%) |
| **Totals for one or more elements in continuity,** | | |
| **with sharp, and with blunt transection** | | |
| Operated brachial plexus cases | 47 | |
| Operated brachial pexus elements | 142 | 87 (61%) |

Gunshot Wounds to the Brachial Plexus ($N = 221$ Injured Elements)

| | NAP Findings | | Neurolysis if<br>NAP Present | Suture | Graft |
|---|---|---|---|---|---|
| | Present | Absent | | | |
| **166 lesions with complete loss** | | | | | |
| **55 lesions with incomplete loss** | | | | | |
| In continuity lesions with complete loss | 29% | (71%) | 91% | 65% | 53% |
| In continuity lesions with incomplete loss | 87% | (13%) | 94% | 83% | 100% |
| Transections | 0% | (0%) | 0% | 50% | 64% |
| Elements thought to be favorable for repair | 30% | (70%) | 96% | 69% | 66% |
| Elements thought to be unfavorable for repair | 27% | (73%) | 79% | 44% | 32% |

Supraclavicular Stretch-Injured Brachial Plexus Postoperative Results ($N = 204$ Patients)

| | Number<br>of Cases | Postoperative<br>Grade 3 or More | |
|---|---|---|---|
| **Complete initial loss** | | | |
| C5/C6 | 35 | 30 | (85%) |
| C5/C6/C7 | 47 | 40 | (85%) |
| C5/C6/C7/C8/T1 | 106 | 37 | (35%) |
| C5/C6/C7/C8 | 2 | 2 | (100%) |
| C6/C7/C8/T1 | 4 | 3 | (75%) |
| C7/C8/T1 | 2 | 1 | (50%) |
| C8/T1 | 4 | 0 | (0%) |
| **Incomplete initial loss** | | | |
| C8/T1 | 2 | 2 | (100%) |
| C7/C8/T1 | 2 | 2 | (100%) |
| **All lesions** | 204 | 117 | (57%) |

Infraclavicular Stretch-Injured Brachial Plexus Postoperative Results ($N = 335$ Patients) (Results displayed as: number of cases/averaged grade of recovery achieved)

| | Initial Partial<br>Function and<br>Neurolysis | Complete<br>Loss and<br>Neurolysis | Complete<br>Loss<br>and Suture | Complete<br>Loss<br>and Grafts | Complete<br>Loss and<br>Split Repair | Repair<br>Impossible |
|---|---|---|---|---|---|---|
| **Cords** | | | | | | |
| Lateral | 3/4.6 | 4/4.2 | 2/4.3 | 6/3.8 | 3/4.0 | 0 |
| Medial | 8/4.1 | 3/3.5 | 2/2.2 | 7/1.2 | 4/3.6 | 2/0 |
| Posterior | 5/4.5 | 4/3.8 | 2/3.6 | 5/3.0 | 3/3.5 | 1/0 |

(continues)

**Table 25-7.** (Continued)

| Initial Partial | Complete Function and Neurolysis | Complete Loss and Neurolysis | Complete Loss and Suture | Complete Loss and Grafts | Loss and Split Repair | Repair Impossible |
|---|---|---|---|---|---|---|
| **Cords to Nerves** | | | | | | |
| Lateral | | | | | | |
| to Musculocutaneous | 7/4.7 | 8/4.0 | 0 | 29/3.8 | 0 | 0 |
| to Median | 14/4.5 | 8/3.5 | 1/4.0 | 14/3.0 | 0 | 2/0 |
| Medial | | | | | | |
| to Median | 6/4.7 | 11/4.1 | 1/4.0 | 9/3.0 | 0 | 2/0 |
| to Ulnar | 14/4.2 | 11/3.1 | 1/0 | 8/1.4 | 1/2.3 | 3/0 |
| Posterior | | | | | | |
| to Radial | 16/4.8 | 5/3.3 | 1/0 | 27/2.7 | 2/3.5 | 1/0 |
| to Axillary | 10/4.7 | 11/4.7 | 1/3.0 | 44/3.5 | 1/4.0 | 2/0 |
| **Totals** | | | | | | |
| Cases/results | 83/4.5 | 65/3.8 | 11/2.8 | 149/3.2 | 14/3.3 | 13/0 |

* Based on a grade 3 or better recovery in the distribution of the brachial plexus element examined: grading according to the LSUMC grading system for whole nerve (Kline and Hudson 1995).

† Adapted from Kline and Hudson (1995).

the goal of treating the pain of the neuroma and/or sometimes restoring neurological function of the nerve (Herndon and Hess 1991; Nath and Mackinnon 1996). Resection of the neuroma may be followed by nerve repair if both proximal and distal nerve ends are still available, by free-tissue transfers including nerve grafting if functionally very important areas are involved, or by local treatment of the nerve stump with the goal of decreasing neuroma recurrence. Unfortunately, no single treatment is ideal and there is a long list of procedures that have been devised to manage this problem, including but not limited to nerve crush-

**Table 25-8.** Combined Results of Acute Nerve Repair of the Median and Ulnar Nerve*

| End-to-End Sutures | | |
|---|---|---|
| **Motor grade†** | | |
| M4 or better | 22 of 32 nerve injuries | 62% |
| Less than M4 | 10 of 32 nerve injuries | 38% |
| **Sensory grade†** | | |
| S3 or better | 27 of 32 nerve injuries | 84% |
| Less than S3 | 5 of 32 nerve injuries | 16% |

| Nerve Grafting Procedures | | |
|---|---|---|
| **Motor grade†** | | |
| M4 or better | 7 of 25 nerve injuries | 28% |
| Less than M4 | 18 of 25 nerve injuries | 72% |
| **Sensory grade†** | | |
| S3 or better | 15 of 25 nerve injuries | 60% |
| Less than S3 | 10 of 25 nerve injuries | 40% |

* After Moneim and Ome (1998).

† British Medical Research Council Rating Scale (Seddon 1954)

ing and ligation (Stevenson 1950; Chavannaz 1940), epineural ligation (Chapple 1918; Martini and Fromm 1989), nerve stump coagulation and sclerosing by physical or chemical means (Herndon and Hess 1991), nerve end capping with a variety of synthetic materials of which silicone is probably the most widely and successfully used (Swanson et al. 1977), neurocampsis (Ashley and Stallings 1988), cross-union of nerve terminal ends and centrocentral anastomosis (Wood and Mudge 1987; Seckel 1984), intramuscular (Moszkowicz 1918; Dellon and Mackinnon 1986b) or intraosseous implantation of the nerve end (Goldstein and Sturim 1985), vascularized island transfer (Tada et al. 1987), and translocation (Laborde et al. 1982). We generally prefer to treat neuromas by sharp, clean sectioning of the nerve 5 to 10 cm proximal to the neuroma, sealing the individual fascicles carefully with bipolar coagulation, and burying the treated end beneath muscle or other soft tissues that are available (Kline and Hudson 1995). Covering the nerve end with adequate soft tissue, especially muscle, seems to be a very important therapeutic strategy.

## Reconstructive Surgery for Peripheral Nerve Injury

Reconstructive surgery on the joints and tendomuscular apparatus is a valid option for rehabilitation of patients with peripheral nerve injuries, and a wide variety of procedures have been devised (Omer 1998a; Gould and Curry 1998). Usually, however, we feel this option should be used later rather than earlier in the course of the disease process. Nerves regenerate slowly and it will take a long time, sometimes up to more than 5 years, to ultimately be able to do a final evaluation after peripheral nerve surgery. Nevertheless, in selected cases, it may be advisable to do relatively early tendon transfers for the purpose of internal splinting (Omer 1998a). This will allow the patient to be splint-free during the time of axon regrowth after peripheral nerve suture, and will often help the patient to adjust to a less than optimal recovery of muscle strength. If the neurorrhaphy is unsuccessful, the tendon transfer will become the permanent substitute (Burkhalter 1993).

In general, tendon transfers (Almquist 1991) are a favored reconstructive approach, but should be performed after correction of deformities due to contracture. As a rule, muscles are used that have the same or similar actions as the ones that are being replaced and that achieve a straight pull vector in the intended direction of action. The tendons are commonly inserted onto other tendons in the upper extremity, whereas they are inserted onto bone in the lower extremity. During the preoperative evaluation, the intended functional active motion should be easily obtainable by passive motion of the involved joints and the muscle-tendon(s) to be transferred must contract with enough strength to make sure that an operative procedure will be worthwhile.

Upper extremity reconstruction after irreparable lesions of the brachial plexus or after failed nerve repair will focus first on distal functions such as hand and wrist tendon balance, elbow flexion, and then on proximal functions such as shoulder motility (Richards 1991). Reasons for this distal-to-proximal concept in operative reconstruction of the upper extremity include the pivotal role of the hand in upper extremity functioning and the fact that more proximal procedures to obtain flexion, sometimes fixed flexion, in the elbow or to obtain shoulder arthrodesis will make hand and wrist surgery technically more difficult. Those muscles that have not been previously paralyzed are the better donor candidates for tendon transfer. Unfortunately, many patients with plexus palsies do not have enough or suitable muscle sparing for tendon transfers. If shoulder movement is paralyzed

secondary to a brachial plexus injury, a shoulder arthrodesis may be of considerable advantage to the patient by helping to position the arm, by increasing the possibility for active shoulder movement, and by encouraging more effective distal arm movements. The best position for shoulder arthrodesis has been found to be 30 degrees of flexion, 30 degrees of abduction, and 30 degrees of endorotation. Shoulder arthrodesis should be considered in patients with a flail shoulder who either have good hand function or have an orthosis, or who are considering amputation and prosthesis fitting (Richards 1991). The procedure is very helpful, although the ultimate result will depend to a large part on the associated hand and distal arm function. Patients with shoulder pain or with more distal neurogenic pain will not experience a change in their pain and should be made aware of this prior to any surgical procedure.

Patients with a complete brachial plexus palsy that is not regaining any function at all despite all previously mentioned treatment measures will need to decide for themselves between amputation and prosthetic fitting, use of an orthosis, or continuing a permanently one-armed life.

Microneurovascular free muscle transfer is an attractive alternative if a motor nerve with adequate axonal outflow can be secured to attach to the free muscle graft (Manktelow 1998; Van Beek and Siddiqui 1998). This is a more elaborate reconstructive treatment option that can be used in selected cases to obtain functional reconstruction (Manktelow 1991). This type of procedure has been used primarily in the upper extremity for reconstruction of various functions such as finger flexion or extension, upper arm flexion (biceps replacement), or shoulder mobility (deltoid replacement). Although the operation is complex and considerable time is needed for full clinical recovery secondary to the inherently required nerve regeneration, the majority of patients feel that the procedure is successful (Manktelow 1991, 1998).

Recently, increasing attention is directed to the application of reconstructive surgery to regenerate useful sensation by the transfer of sensate flaps to the hands and the weight-bearing areas of the body such as the sole of the foot (Boyd 1998). The territorial supply of tissues by not only arteries and veins but nerves as well is a very important concept in this context (Taylor et al. 1994). The reconstructive surgeon's knowledge of the existing "neurotomes" is crucial for the correct planning and performance of such sensate flaps.

## Rehabilitation After Peripheral Nerve Injury

The goal of rehabilitation after peripheral nerve injury is to obtain maximal functional recovery for the patient. This involves sympathetic, motor, and sensory function (Mackin and Byron 1991).

The immediate and persistent loss of sudomotor activity in the innervated region with its absent sweating and decreased sebaceous secretion makes the skin dry and therefore impedes function. Appropriate physical measures need to be taken to correct these deficiencies and help mobility and function of the afflicted parts (Brand and Hollister 1993).

Motor deficits will lead to muscle atrophy and finally fibrosis. They often cause joint instability, but then inevitably secondary to nonuse, joint stiffening and a reduced range of motion. This may provoke more pain upon efforts to mobilize, which then will lead to even less use of the joint by the patient to prevent pain from occurring: a vicious circle ensues. The joints need to be mobilized as early as possible to prevent stiffening, and if mobilization is contraindicated because of accompanying injuries or because of nerve-lengthening procedures, the joints should be immobilized for the shortest period of time needed, preferentially in a physiological position (Kline and Hudson 1995). Splinting may help in restoration of function but depends on the preservation of passive joint mobility and adequate positioning of paretic or paralyzed muscles. Functional splints such as the Colditz tenodesis splint (Colditz 1987) will substitute for movements normally performed by the paralyzed muscles. While splints restore externally the balance, position, and sometimes also the dynamics of an injured limb, functional training of the muscles needs to start at an early point in time. Biofeedback systems can be very useful in this regard (Basmajian 1989).

Sensibility evaluation performed during follow-up examinations can suggest recovery by using threshold tests, two-point discrimination tests, and sensory localization tests. Pick-up tests will help evaluate tactile gnosis and the practical use of the neurologically impaired hand. The LSUMC sensory evaluation relies on comparison of responses to touch and pinprick between affected and normal areas. Ability to utilize touch and pinprick are also felt to be important parameters. Sensory re-education forms part of the rehabilitation process and depends to a large extent on cortical plasticity, which is present to a remarkable extent even in the adult (Mackinnon and Dellon 1988). Sensory re-education happens in three phases. In stage one emphasis is placed on protection and desensitization. The patient is taught how to compensate for the loss of protective sensibility, and is helped to cope with the unpleasant and often painful sensations of regenerating nerve. The second stage of sensory re-education will try to re-educate specific perceptions such as moving touch, constant touch, pressure, and localization. Although some misinterpretations by the patient can be attributed to regeneration of nerve fibers into inappropriate directions, here too the plasticity of the brain can compensate and correct to a remarkable extent (Horch and Burgess 1979; Paul et al. 1972; Wall et al. 1986). The third phase in sensory re-education follows after moving and constant touch are well perceived. The goal of this stage is to regain a functional, tactile gnosis. Exercises are specific, very intense, and given during short periods of time because of the extraordinary concentration required. They are performed in a sequence with, without, and again with visual control to help in giving feedback to the patient with the goal of retraining use of the limb.

Patients who have participated in a formal program of retraining constantly achieve better results and obtain these results faster than those who did not have the opportunity for such a rehabilitation program (Carter-Wilson 1991; Imai et al. 1989).

## Conclusions

Peripheral nerve injuries are among the most devastating that can occur. The loss of neurological function and the pain that often accompanies these lesions can alter the patient's vocational, social, and private life completely. It is the task of the physician taking care of these patients to offer them as much help, support, and guidance as possible. Fortunately, medical science has made enormous progress in the understanding and management of these conditions and we are now able to improve the outlook for many but not all patients with lesions and injuries of the peripheral nervous system considerably. The current state of the art is not optimal yet, and many patients would be grateful for further advances in understanding nerve injury and regeneration, and its practical application. This review has outlined some of the basic concepts of the etiology, pathogenesis, and treatment of peripheral nerve lesions with a focus on the factors that influence prognosis.

# References

Adeymo, O.; Wyburn, G. M. Innervation of skin grafts. Transplant. Bull. 4:152–153; 1957.

Alanen, M.; Halonen, J. P., Katevuo, K.; Vilkki, P. Early surgical exploration and epineurial repair in birth brachial palsy. Z. Kinderchir. 41:335–337; 1986.

Almquist, E. Adjuncts to suture repair of peripheral nerves: laser, glue, and other techniques. In: Omer, G. E., Jr., Spinner, M.; Van Beek, A. L., eds. Management of peripheral nerve problems. 2nd ed. Philadelphia: W. B. Saunders Co.; 1998: p. 311–318.

Almquist, E. E. Principles of tendon transfers. In: Gelberman, R. H., ed. Operative nerve repair and reconstruction. Philadelphia: J. B. Lippincott; 1991: p. 689–696.

Almquist, E. E., O. A.; Fry, L. Nerve conduction velocity, microscopic, and electron microscopy studies compairing repaired adult and baby monkey median nerves. J. Hand Surg. [Am.] 8-A:406–410; 1983.

Alnot, J. Y. Infraclavicular lesions. Clin. Plast. Surg. 11:127–131; 1984.

Alnot, J. Y.; Benfrech, E. Les autogreffes nerveuses. Problèmes techniques actuels. Ann. Chir. Main 8:291–295; 1989

Applegate, W. B.; Physician management of patients with adverse outcomes. Arch. Intern. Med. 146:2249–2252; 1986.

Ashley, L.; Stallings, J. O. End-to-side nerve flap for treatment of painful neuroma: a 15-year follow-up. J. Am. Osteopath. Assoc. 88:621–624; 1988.

Atasoy, E.; Kleinert, H. E. Surgical sympathectomy and sympathetic blocks for the upper and lower extremities, and local and plexus levels. In: Omer, G. E., Jr.; Spinner, M.; Van Beek, A. L. eds. Management of peripheral nerve problems. 2nd ed. Philadelphia: W. B. Saunders Co.; 1998: p. 157–171.

Basmajian, J. V., ed. Biofeedback. Principles and practice for clinicians, 3rd ed. Baltimore: Williams & Wilkins; 1989.

Bateman, J. E. Results and assessment of disability; iatrogenic nerve injuries. In: Bateman, J. E., ed. Trauma to nerves in limbs. Philadelphia: W. B. Saunders Co.; 1962: p. 285–305.

Bernhardt, M. Neuropathologische Beobachtungen. Dsch. Arch. Klin. Med. 22:362; 1878.

Boddingius, J. The occurrence of Mycobacterium leprae within axons of peripheral nerves. Acta Neuropathol. (Berl.) 27:257–270; 1974.

Bonney, G.; Birch, R.; Jamieson, A. M.; Eames, R. A. Experience with vascularized nerve grafts. Clin. Plast. Surg. 11:137–142; 1984.

Bonney, G.; Birch, R.; Jamieson, A. M.; Eames, R. A. Experience with vascularized nerve grafts. In: Terzis, J. K., ed. Microreconstruction of nerve injuries. Philadelphia: W. B. Saunders Co.; 1987: p. 403–414.

Boome, R. S.; Kaye, J. C. Obstetric traction injuries of the brachial plexus. Natural history, indications for surgical repair and results. J. Bone Joint Surg. [Br.] 70-B:571–576; 1988.

Bora, F. W., Jr.; Richardson, S.; Black, J. The biomechanical responses to tension in a peripheral nerve. J. Hand Surg. [Am.] 5-A:21–25; 1980.

Boyd, J. B. Sensation-bearing flaps. In: Omer, G. E., Jr.; Spinner, M.; Van Beek, A. L., eds. Management of peripheral nerve problems. 2nd ed. Philadelphia: W. B. Saunders Co.; 1998: p. 745–761.

Brand, P. W.; Hollister, A. Clinical mechanics of the hand. 2nd ed. St. Louis: Mosby Year Book; 1993.

Brand, P. W. Management of sensory loss in the extremities. In: Omer, G. E., Jr.; Spinner, M.; Van Beek, A. L., eds. Management of peripheral nerve problems. 2nd ed. Philadelphia: W. B. Saunders Co.; 1998: p. 762–766.

Bratton, B. R.; Kline, D. G.; Coleman, W.; Hudson, A. R. Experimental interfascicular nerve grafting. J. Neurosurg. 51:323–332; 1979.

Braun, R. M. Epineurial nerve suture. Clin. Orthop. 163:50–56; 1982.

Britt, B. A.; Gordon, R. A. Peripheral nerve injuries associated with anaesthesia. Can. Anaesth. Soc. J. 11: 514–536; 1964.

Britt, B. A.; Joy, N.; Mackay, M. B. Positioning trauma. In: Orkin, F. K.; Cooperman, L. H., eds. Complications in anesthesiology. Philadelphia: J. B. Lippincott; 1983: p. 646–670.

Broadbent, T. R.; Odom, G. L.; Woodhall, B. Peripheral nerve injuries from administration of penicillin. Report of four clinical cases. JAMA 140:1008–1010; 1949.

Brown, I. C.; Zinar, D. M. Traumatic and iatrogenic neurological complications after supracondylar humerus fractures in children. J. Pediatr. Orthop. 15:440–443; 1995.

Brunelli, G. A. Direct muscular neurotization. In: Gelberman, R. H., ed. Operative nerve repair and reconstruction. Philadelphia: J. B. Lippincott; 1991: p. 783–791.

Brunelli, G. A.; Brunelli, G. R. Direct muscle neurotization. In: Omer, G. E., Jr.; Spinner, M.; Van Beek, A. L., eds. Management of peripheral nerve problems, 2nd ed. Philadelphia: W. B. Saunders Co.; 1998: p. 393–397.

Brunelli, G. A.; Vigasio, A.; Brunelli, G. R. Different conduits in peripheral nerve surgery. Microsurgery 15:176–178; 1994.

Büdinger, K. Ueber Lähmungen nach Chloroformnarkosen. Arch. Klin. Chir. 47:121–145; 1894.

Burger, P. C.; Scheithauer, B. W.; Vogel, F. S. Surgical pathology of the nervous system and its coverings. 3rd ed. New York: Churchill Livingstone; 1991.

Burkhalter, W. E. Median nerve palsy. In: Green, D. P., ed. Operative hand surgery. 3rd ed. New York: Churchill Livingstone; 1993: p. 1419–1448.

Butler, V. M.; Dean, L. S.; Little, J. R. Positioning the neurosurgical patient in the operating room: 'a team effort'. J. Neurosurg. Nurs. 16:89–95; 1984.

Bzik, K. D.; Bellamy, R. F. A note on combat casualty statistics. Mil. Med. 149:229–230; 1984.

Campbell, E. H., Jr. The Mediterranean (formerly North African) theater of operations. In: Coates, J. B., Jr.; Spurling, R. G.; Woodhall, B.; McFetridge, E. M., eds. Surgery in World War II. Neurosurgery. Vol. II. Washington, DC: Office of the Surgeon General, Department of the Army; 1959: p. 231–238.

Campbell, J. B. Peripheral nerve repair. Clin. Neurosurg. 17:77–98; 1970.

Campbell, J. N.; Raja, S. N.; Meyer, R. A.; Mackinnon, S. E. Myelinated afferents signal the hyperalgesia associated with nerve injury. Pain 32:89–94; 1988.

Carter-Wilson, M. Sensory re-education. In: Gelberman, R. H., ed. Operative nerve repair and reconstruction. Philadelphia: J. B. Lippincott; 1991: p. 827–844.

Carvalho, G. A.; Nikkhah, G.; Matthies, C.; Penkert, G.; Samii, M. Diagnosis of root avulsions in traumatic brachial plexus injuries: value of computerized tomography myelography and magnetic resonance imaging. J. Neurosurg. 86:69–76; 1997.

Chapple, W. A. Prevention of nerve bulbs in stumps. Br. Med. J. 1:399; 1918.

Chavannaz, G. A propos de la technique de l'amputation de cuisse. La ligature du nerf grand sciatique. Bull. Acad. Nat. Med. 123:123; 1940.

Chiu, D. T. W. Autogenous and synthetic conduits for nerve repair. In: Omer, G. E., Jr.; Spinner, M.; Van Beek, A. L., eds. Management of peripheral nerve problems. 2nd ed. Philadelphia: W. B. Saunders Co.; 1998: p. 305–310.

Chuang, D. C.-C. Neurotization procedures for brachial plexus injuries. Hand Clin. 11:633–645; 1995.

Colditz, J. C. Splinting for radial nerve palsy. J. Hand Ther. 1:18–22; 1987.

Collins, J. D.; Shaver, M. L.; Disher, A. C.; Miller, T. Q. Bilateral magnetic resonance imaging of the brachial plexus and peripheral nerve imaging: technique and three-dimensional color. In: Omer, G. E., Jr.; Spinner, M.; Van Beek, A. L., eds. Management of peripheral nerve problems. 2nd ed. Philadelphia: W. B. Saunders Co.; 1998: p. 82–93.

Cooper, D. E. Nerve injury associated with patient positioning in the operating room. In: Gelberman, R. H., ed. Operative nerve repair and reconstruction. Philadelphia: J. B. Lippincott; 1991: p. 1231–1242.

Cooper, D. E.; Jenkins, R. S.; Bready, L.; Rockwood, C. A., Jr. The prevention of injuries to the brachial plexus secondary to malposition of the patient during surgery. Clin. Orthop. 228:33–41; 1988.

Cragg, B. G.; Thomas, P. K. Changes in conduction velocity and fiber size proximal to peripheral nerve lesions. J. Physiol. 157:315–327; 1961.

Dahlin, L. B.; McLean, W. G. Effects of graded experimental compression on slow and fast axonal trans-

port in rabbit vagus nerve. J. Neurol. Sci. 72:19–30; 1986.

Dastur, D. K. Leprosy (an infectious and immunological disorder of the nervous system). In: Vinken, P. J.; Bruyn, G. W.; Klawans, H. L., eds. Infections of the nervous system, part I. Handbook of clinical neurology. Vol. 33. Amsterdam: North-Holland Publishing Company; 1978: p. 421–468.

Dastur, D. K. Pathology and pathogenesis of predilective sites of nerve damage in leprous neuritis. Nerves in the arm and the face. Neurosurg. Rev. 6:139–152; 1983.

Dastur, D. K.; Ramamohan, Y.; Shah, J. S. Ultrastructure of lepromatous nerves. Neural pathogenesis in leprosy. Int. J. Lep. Other Mycobact. Dis. 41:47–80; 1973.

Davis, L. The return of sensation to transplanted skin. Surg. Gynecol. Obstet. 59:533–543; 1934.

Dellon, A. L. Evaluation of sensibility and re-education of sensation in the hand. Baltimore: Williams & Wilkins; 1981.

Dellon, A. L. Sensory recovery in replanted digits and transplanted toes: a review. J. Reconstruct Microsurg. 2:123–129; 1986.

Dellon, A. L.; Mackinnon, S. E. Treatment of the painful neuroma by neuroma resection and muscle implantation. Plastic Reconstr. Surg. 77:427–438; 1986.

Denny-Brown, D.; Doherty, M. M. Effects of transient stretching of peripheral nerves. Arch. Neurol. Psychiatry 54:116–129; 1945.

Devor, M. The pathophysiology of damaged peripheral nerves. In: Wall, P. D.; Melzack, R., eds. Textbook of pain. 3rd ed. Edinburgh: Churchill Livingstone; 1994: p. 79–100.

Diao, E.; Peimer, C. A. Sutureless methods of nerve repair. In: Gelberman, R. H., ed. Operative nerve repair and reconstruction. Philadelphia: J. B. Lippincott; 1991: p. 305–314.

Doi, K.; Tamaru, K.; Sakai, K.; Kuwata, N.; Kurafuji, Y.; Kawai, S. A comparison of vascularized and conventional sural nerve grafts. J. Hand Surg. [Am.] 17-A:670–676; 1992.

Donner, T. R.; Kline, D. G. Extracranial spinal accessory nerve injury. Neurosurgery 32:907–910; 1993.

Dormans, J. P.; Squillante, R.; Sharf, H. Acute neurovascular complications with supracondylar humerus fractures in children. J. Hand Surg. [Am.] 20-A:1–4; 1995.

Doyle, J. R. Factors affecting clinical results in nerve sutures. In: Jewett, D. L.; McCarroll, H. R., Jr., eds. Nerve repair and regeneration. Its clinical and experimental basis. St. Louis: C. V. Mosby; 1980: p. 263–266.

Ducker, T. B. Pathophysiology of peripheral nerve trauma. In: Wilkins, R. H.; Rengachary, S. S., eds. Neurosurgery. New York: McGraw-Hill; 1985: p. 1812–1816.

Dyck, P. J.; Thomas, P. K.; Griffin, J. W.; Low, P. A.; Poduslo, J. F., eds. Peripheral neuropathy. 3rd ed. Philadelphia: W. B. Saunders Co.; 1993.

Enna, C. D. The management of leprous neuritis. In: Omer, G. E., Jr.; Spinner, M.; Van Beek, A. L., eds. Management of peripheral nerve problems. 2nd ed. Philadelphia: W. B. Saunders Co.; 1998: p. 615–621.

Enna, C. D.; Jacobson, R. R. A clinical assessment of neurolysis for leprous involvement of the ulnar nerve. Int. J. Lepr. Other Mycobact. Dis. 42:162–164; 1974.

Evans, J. A. Reflex sympathetic dystrophy. Surg. Clin. North Am. 26:780–790; 1946.

Fachinelli, A.; Masquelet, A.; Restrepo, J.; Gilbert, A. The vascularized sural nerve. Int. J. Microsurg. 3:57; 1981.

Fackler, M. L. Ballistic injury. Ann. Emerg. Med. 15:1451–1455; 1986.

Fackler, M. L. Wound ballistics. A review of common misconceptions. JAMA 259:2730–2736; 1988.

Foerster, O. In: Bumke, O.; Foerster, O., eds. Handbuch der neurologie. Berlin: Julius Springer Verlag; 1929.

Fournier, R. S.; Holder, L. E. Reflex sympathetic dystrophy: diagnostic controversies. Semin. Nucl. Med. 27:116–123; 1998.

Frederick, H. A.; Carter, P. R.; Littler, J. W. Injection injuries to the median and ulnar nerves at the wrist. J. Hand Surg. [Am.] 17-A:645–457; 1992.

Fremling, M. A.; Mackinnon, S. E. Injection injury to the median nerve. Ann. Plast. Surg. 37:561–567; 1996.

Frykman, G. K.; Adams, J.; Bowen, W. W. Neurolysis. Orthop. Clin. North Am. 12:325–342; 1981.

Frykman, G. K.; Cally, D. Interfascicular nerve grafting. Orthop. Clin. North Am. 19:71–80; 1988.

Frykman, G. K.; Waylett, J. Rehabilitation of peripheral nerve injuries. Orthop. Clin. North Am. 12:361–379; 1981.

Fuller, G. N.; Jacobs, J. M.; Guiloff, R. J. Nature and incidence of peripheral nerve syndromes in HIV infection. J. Neurol. Neurosurg. Psychiatry 56:372–381; 1993.

Gelberman, R. H., ed. Operative nerve repair and reconstruction. Philadelphia: J. B. Lippincott; 1991.

Gentili, F.; Hudson, A. R. Peripheral nerve injuries: types, causes, grading. In: Wilkins, R. H.; Rengachary, S. S., eds. Neurosurgery. New York: McGraw-Hill; 1985: p. 1802–1812.

Gentili, F.; Hudson, A. R.; Hunter, D. Clinical and experimental aspects of injection injuries of peripheral nerves. Can. J. Neurol. Sci. 7:143–151; 1980a.

Gentili, F.; Hudson, A. R.; Hunter, D.; Kline, D. G. Nerve injection injury with local anesthetic agents: a light and electron microscopic, fluorescent microscopic, and horseradish peroxidase study. Neurosurgery 6:263–272; 1980b.

Gilbert, A.; Razaboni, R.; Amar-Khodja, S. Indications and results of brachial plexus surgery in obstetrical palsy. Orthop. Clin. North Am. 19:91–105; 1988.

Gilbert, A.; Tassin, J. L. Obstetrical palsy: a clinical, pathologic, and surgical review. In: Terzis, J., ed. Microreconstruction of nerve injuries. Philadelphia: W. B. Saunders Co.; 1987: p. 529–553.

Goldstein, S. A.; Sturim, H. S. Intraosseous nerve transposition for treatment of painful neuromas. J. Hand Surg. [Am.] 10-A:270–274; 1985.

Gorio, A.; Carmignoto, G. Reformation, maturation and stabilization of neuromuscular junctions in peripheral nerve regeneration. In: Gorio, A.; Millesi, H.; Mingrino, S., eds. Postraumatic peripheral nerve regeneration. New York: Raven Press; 1981: p. 481–492.

Goth, D. Tierexperimentelle Untersuchungen zur Neurolyse peripherer Nerven. Handchir. Mikrochir. Plast. Chir. 19:212–216; 1987.

Graf, P.; Hawe, W.; Biemer, E. Gefäßversorgung des N. ulnaris nach Neurolyse im Ellenbogenbereich. Handchir. Mikrochir. Plast. Chir. 18:204–206; 1986

Grewal, R.; Xu, J.; Sotereanos, D. G.; Woo, S. L. Biomechanical properties of peripheral nerves. Hand Clin. 12:195–204; 1996.

Griffin, J. W.; Hoffman, P. N. Degeneration and regeneration in the peripheral nervous system. In: Dyck, P. J.; Thomas, P. K.; Griffin, J. W.; Low, P. A.; Poduslo, J. F., eds. Peripheral neuropathy. 3rd ed. Philadelphia: W. B. Saunders Co.; 1993: p. 361–376.

Groff, R. A.; Houtz, S. J. Recovery and regeneration. In: Groff, R. A.; Houtz, S. J., eds. Manual of diagnosis and management of peripheral nerve injuries. Philadelphia: J. B. Lippincott; 1945: p. 33–35.

Haines, B. L. Rehabilitation of the painful upper extremity. Hand Clin. 12:801–816; 1996.

Hanlon, C. R.; Estes, W. L. Fractures in childhood—a statistical analysis. Am. J. Surg. 87:312–323; 1954.

Heineke, P. Die direkte Einpflanzung des Nerven in den Muskel. Zentralbl. Chir. 41:465; 1914.

Heon, M. Myelogram: a questionable aid in diagnosis and prognosis in avulsion of brachial plexus components by traction injuries. Conn. Med. 29:260–262; 1965.

Herndon, J. H.; Hess, A. V. Neuromas. In: Gelberman, R. H., ed. Operative nerve repair and reconstruction. Philadelphia: J. B. Lippincott; 1991: p. 1525–1540.

Highet, W. B.; Holmes, W. Traction injuries to the lateral popliteal nerve and traction injuries to peripheral nerves after suture. Br. J. Surg. 30:212–233; 1942.

Horch, K. Central responses of cutaneous sensory neurons to peripheral nerve nerve crush in the cat. Brain Res. 151:581–586; 1978.

Horch, K. W.; Burgess, P. R. Functional specificity and somatotopic organization during peripheral nerve regeneration. In: Jewett, D. L.; McCarroll, H. R., Jr., eds. Nerve repair and regeneration. Its clinical and experimental basis. St. Louis: C. V. Mosby; 1979: p. 105–109.

Hudson, A. R. Nerve injection injuries. Clin. Plast. Surg. 11:27–30; 1984.

Hudson, A. R.; Tranmer, B. Brachial plexus injuries. In: Wilkins, R. H.; Rengachary, S. S., eds. Neurosurgery. New York: McGraw-Hill; 1985: p. 1817–1832.

Hurst, L. C.; Badalamente, M. A. Histochemical aids to control specificity in peripheral nerve repair. In: Omer, G. E., Jr.; Spinner, M.; Van Beek, A. L., eds.

Management of peripheral nerve problems, 2nd ed. Philadelphia: W. B. Saunders Co.; 1998: p. 243–247.

Imai, H.; Tajima, T.; Natsuma, Y. Interpretation of cutaneous pressure threshold (Semmes-Weinstein monofilament measurement) following median nerve repair and sensory re-education in the adult. Microsurgery 10:142–144; 1989.

Iyer, R. B.; Fenstermacher, M. J.; Libshitz, H. I. MR imaging of the treated brachial plexus. AJR Am. J. Roentgenol. 167:225–229; 1996.

Jabaley, M. E. Modified techniques of nerve repair: epineurial splint. In: Gelberman, R. H., ed. Operative nerve repair and reconstruction. Philadelphia: J. B. Lippincott; 1991; p. 315–326.

Jackson, L.; Keats, A. S. Mechanism of brachial plexus palsy following anesthesia. Anesthesiology 26:190–194; 1965.

Johnson, R. W. Herpes zoster and postherpetic neuralgia. Optimal treatment. Drugs Aging 10:80–94; 1997.

Kalaska, J.; Pomeranz, B. Chronic paw denervation causes an age-dependent appearance of novel responses from forearm in "paw cortex" of kittens and adult cats. J. Neurophysiol. 42:618–633; 1979.

Kasten, S. J.; Louis, D. S. Carpal tunnel syndrome: a case of median nerve injection injury and a safe and effective method for injecting the carpal tunnel. J. Fam. Pract. 43:79–82; 1996.

Kimura, J. Nerve conduction studies and electromyography. In: Dyck, P. J.; Thomas, P. K.; Griffin, J. W.; Low, P. A.; Poduslo, J. F., eds. Peripheral neuropathy. 3rd ed. Philadelphia: W. B. Saunders Co.; 1993: p. 598–644.

Kline, D. G. Physiological and clinical factors contributing to the timing of nerve repair. Clin. Neurosurg. 24:425–455; 1977.

Kline, D. G. Timing for exploration of nerve lesions and evaluation of the neuroma-in-continuity. Clin. Orthop. 163:42–49; 1982.

Kline, D. G. Diagnostic determinants for management of peripheral nerve lesions. In: Rand, R. W., ed. Microneurosurgery. 3rd ed. St. Louis: C. V. Mosby; 1985: p. 707–726.

Kline, D. G. Civilian gunshot wounds to the brachial plexus. J. Neurosurg. 70:166–174; 1989.

Kline, D. G.; Hackett, E. R. Reappraisal of timing for exploration of civilian peripheral nerve injuries. Surgery 78:54–65; 1975.

Kline, D. G.; Hackett, E. R. Management of the neuroma in continuity. In: Wilkins, R. H.; Rengachary, S. S., eds. Neurosurgery. New York: McGraw-Hill; 1985: p. 1864–1871.

Kline, D. G.; Hackett, E. R.; Davis, G. D.; Myers, M. B. Effect of mobilization on the blood supply and regeneration of injured nerves. J. Surg. Res. 12:254–266; 1972.

Kline, D. G.; Hackett, E. R.; Happel, L. H. Surgery for lesions of the brachial plexus. Arch. Neurol. 43:170–181; 1986.

Kline, D. G.; Hudson, A. R. Complications of nerve injury and nerve repair. In: Greenfield, L. J., ed. Com-

plications in surgery and trauma. Philadelphia: J. B. Lippincott; 1990: p. 746–759.

Kline, D. G.; Hudson, A. R. Selected recent advances in peripheral nerve injury research. Surg. Neurol. 24:371–376; 1985.

Kline, D. G.; Hudson, A. R. Nerve injuries. In: Horwitz, N. H.; Rizzoli, H. V., eds. Postoperative complications of extracranial neurological surgery. Baltimore: Williams & Wilkins; 1987: p. 243–259

Kline, D. G.; Hudson, A. R. Acute injuries of peripheral nerves. In: Youmans, J., ed. Neurological surgery. A comprehensive reference guide to the diagnosis and management of neurosurgical problems. 4th ed. Philadelphia: W. B. Saunders Co.; 1996: p. 2103–2181.

Kline, D. G.; Hudson, A. R. Nerve injuries. Operative results for major nerve injuries, entrapments, and tumors. Philadelphia: W. B. Saunders Co.; 1995.

Kline, D. G.; Hurst, J. Prediction of recovery from peripheral nerve injury. Neurol. Neurosurg. Updated Series 5:2–8; 1984.

Kline, D. G.; Judice, D. J. Operative management of selected brachial plexus lesions. J. Neurosurg. 58: 631–649; 1983.

Kolb, L. C.; Gray, S. J. Peripheral neuritis as a complication of penicillin therapy. JAMA 132:323–326; 1946.

Kondo, M.; Matsuda, H.; Miyawaki, Y.; Yoshimura, M., Shimazu, A. A new method of electrodiagnosis during operations on the brachial plexus and peripheral nerve injuries. The value of motor nerve action potentials evoked by trans-skull motor area stimulation. Int. Orthop. 9:115–121; 1985.

Kredel, F. E.; Evans, J. P. Recovery of sensation in denervated pedicles and free skin grafts. J. Neurol. Neurosurg. Psychiatry 19:1203–1221; 1933.

Kristensson, K. Retrograde signalling of nerve cell body response to trauma. In: Gorio, A.; Millesi, H.; Mingrino, S., eds. Postraumatic peripheral nerve regeneration. New York: Raven Press; 1981: p. 27–34.

Laborde, K. J.; Kalisman, M.; Tsai, T. M. Results of surgical treatment of painful neuromas of the hand. J. Hand Surg. [Am.] 7-A:190–193; 1982.

Lang, D. H.; Lister, G. D.; Jevans, A. W. Histochemical and biochemical aids to nerve repair. In: Gelberman, R. H., ed. Operative nerve repair and reconstruction. Philadelphia: J. B. Lippincott; 1991: p. 259–271.

Laurent, J. P.; Lee, R. T. Birth-related upper brachial plexus injuries in infants: operative and nonoperative approaches. J. Child Neurol. 9:111–117; 1994.

Laurent, J. P.; Schenaq, S.; Lee, R. Upper brachial plexus birth injuries. A neurosurgical approach. Concepts Pediatr. Neurosurg. 10:156–162; 1990.

Leffert, R. D. Brachial plexus injuries. New York: Churchill Livingstone; 1985.

Liu, C. T.; Benda, C. E.; Lewey, F. H. Tensile strength of human nerves. Arch. Neurol. Psychiatry 59:322–336; 1948.

Lowder, C. E.; Kline, D. G. Peripheral nerve injury. In: Evans, R. W.; Baskin, D. S.; Yatsu, F. M.; eds. Prognosis of neurological disorders. New York: Oxford University Press; 1992: p. 389–404.

Luce, E. A.; Griffen, W. O. Shotgun injuries of the upper extremity. J. Trauma 18:487–492; 1978.

Lundborg, G. Structure and function of the intraneural microvessels as related to trauma, edema formation, and nerve function. J. Bone Joint Surg. 57-A:938–948; 1975.

Lundborg, G. Regeneration of peripheral nerves—a biological and surgical problem. Scand. J. Plast. Reconstr. Surg. Suppl. 19:38–44; 1982.

Lundborg, G. Nerve regeneration and repair. A review. Acta Orthop. Scand. 58:145–169; 1987.

Lundborg, G. Nerve injury and repair. Edinburgh: Churchill Livingstone; 1988.

Mackinnon, S. E.; Dellon, A. L. Surgery of the peripheral nerve. New York: Thieme Medical Publishers; 1988.

Mackinnon, S. E.; Hudson, A. R.; Gentilli, F.; Kline, D. G.; Hunter, D. Peripheral nerve injection injury with steroid agents. Plast. Reconstr. Surg. 69:482–490; 1982.

Manktelow, R. T. Free muscle transfer for functional reconstruction. In: Gelberman, R. H., ed. Operative nerve repair and reconstruction. Philadelphia: J. B. Lippincott; 1991: p. 775–781.

Manktelow, R. T Microneurovascular free muscle transfer. Background and clinical application. In: Omer, G. E., Jr.; Spinner, M.; Van Beek, A. L., eds. Management of peripheral nerve problems. 2nd ed. Philadelphia: W. B. Saunders Co.; 1998: p. 731–734.

Mannerfelt, L. Evaluation of functional sensation of skin grafts in the hand area. Br. J. Plast. Surg. 15:136–154; 1962.

Marble, H. C.; Hamlin, E., Jr.; Watkins, A. L. Regeneration in the ulnar, median, and radial nerves. Am. J. Surg. 55:274–294; 1942.

Martini, A.; Fromm, B. A new operation for the prevention and treatment of amputation neuromas. J. Bone Joint Surg. Br. 71-B:379–382; 1989.

Matson, D. D. Early neurolysis in the treatment of injury of the peripheral nerves due to faulty injection of antibiotics. N. Engl. J. Med. 242:973–975; 1950.

Matson, D. D. Neurosurgery of infancy and childhood. 2nd ed. Springfield, IL: Charles C Thomas; 1969.

McGillicuddy, J. E. Techniques of nerve repair. In: Wilkins, R. H.; Rengachary, S. S., eds. Neurosurgery. New York: McGraw-Hill; 1985: p. 1871–1881.

McKinley, P. A.; Jenkins, W. M.; Smith, J. L.; Merzenich, M. M. Age-dependent capacity for somatosensory cortex reorganization in chronic spinal cats. Brain Res. 428:136–139; 1987.

McNamara, M. J.; Garrett, W. E., Jr.; Seaber, A. V.; Goldner, J. L. Neurorrhaphy, nerve grafting, and neurotization: a functional comparison of nerve grafting techniques. J. Hand Surg. [Am.] 12:354–360; 1987.

McQuarrie, I. G. Clinical signs of peripheral nerve regeneration. In: Wilkins, R. H.; Rengachary, S. S., eds. Neurosurgery. New York: McGraw-Hill; 1985: p. 1881–1884.

Merchut, M. P.; Gruener, G. Segmental zoster paresis of limbs. Electromyogr. Clin. Neurophysiol. 36:369–375; 1996.

Metaizeau, J. P.; Prevot, J.; Lascombes, P. Les paralysies obstétricales. Evolution spontanée et résultats du traitement précoce par microchirurgie. Ann. Pediatr. (Paris) 31:93–102; 1984.

Meyer, R. Treatment of obstetrical palsy. In: Omer, G. E., Jr.; Spinner, M.; Van Beek, A. L., eds. Management of peripheral nerve problems. 2nd ed. Philadelphia: W. B. Saunders Co.; 1998: p. 454–458.

Meyer, R.; Claussen; G. C., Oh; S. J. Modified trichrome staining technique of the nerve to determine proximal nerve viability. Microsurgery 16:129–132; 1995.

Meyer, R. D. Treatment of adult and obstetrical brachial plexus injuries. Orthopedics 9:899–903; 1986.

Midha, R.; Guha, A.; Gentili, F.; Kline, D. G.; Hudson, A. R. Peripheral nerve injection injury. In: Omer, G. E., Jr.; Spinner, M.; Van Beek, A. L., eds. Management of peripheral nerve problems. 2nd ed. Philadelphia: W. B. Saunders Co.; 1998: p. 406–413.

Miller, R. G. AAEE Minimonograph #28: injury to peripheral motor nerves. Muscle Nerve 10:698–710; 1987.

Millesi, H. Microsurgery of peripheral nerves. World J. Surg. 3:67–79; 1979.

Millesi, H. Interfascicular nerve repair and secondary repair with nerve grafts. In: Jewett, D. L.; McCarrol, H. R., Jr., eds. Nerve repair and regeneration. Its clinical and experimental basis. St. Louis: C. V. Mosby; 1980: p. 299–319.

Millesi, H. Reappraisal of nerve repair. Surg. Clin. North Am. 61:321–340; 1981.

Millesi, H. Nerve grafting. Clin. Plast. Surg. 11:105–113; 1984a.

Millesi, H. Brachial plexus injuries. Management and results. Clin. Plast. Surg. 11:115–120; 1984b.

Millesi, H. The nerve gap. Theory and clinical practice. Hand Clin. 2:651–663; 1986.

Millesi, H. Indications and techniques of nerve grafting. In: Gelberman, R. H., ed. Operative nerve repair and reconstruction. Philadelphia: J. B. Lippincott; 1991: p. 525–543.

Millesi. H. Nerve grafts: indications, techniques, and prognosis. In: Omer, G. E., Jr.; Spinner, M.; Van Beek, A. L., eds. Management of peripheral nerve problems. 2nd ed. Philadelphia: W. B. Saunders Co.; 1998: p. 280–289.

Minauchi, Y.; Igata, A. Leprous neuritis. In: Vinken, P. J.; Bruyn, G. W.; Matthews, W. B., eds: Neuropathies. Handbook of clinical neurology. Vol. 51, Revised Series 7. Amsterdam: Elsevier Science Publishers; 1987.

Mitchell, S. W. Injuries of Nerves and Their Consequences. Philadelphia: J. B. Lippincott; 1872; reprinted 1965, New York: Dover Publications.

Mitchell, S. W.; Morehouse, G. R.; Keen, W. W., Jr. Gunshot wounds and other injuries to nerves. Philadelphia: J. B. Lippincott; 1864.

Moneim, M. S. A.; Omer, G. E., Jr. Clinical outcome following acute nerve repair. In: Omer, G. E., Jr.; Spinner, M., Van Beek, A. L., eds. Management of peripheral nerve problems. 2nd ed. Philadelphia: W. B. Saunders Co.; 1998: p. 414–420.

Moszkowicz, L. P. Zur Behandlung der schmerzhaften Neurome. Zentralb. Chir. 45:547; 1918.

Mukherji, S. K.; Castillo, M.; Wagle, A. G. The brachial plexus. Semin. Ultrasound CT MR 17:519–538; 1996.

Murphey, F.; Hartung, W.; Kirklin, J. Myelographic demonstration of avulsion injury of the brachial plexus. Am. J. Epidemiol. 58:102–105; 1947.

Nagano, A.; Tsuyama, N.; Hara, T.; Sugioka, H. Brachial plexus injuries. Prognosis of postganglionic lesions. Arch. Orthop. Trauma Surg. 102:172–178; 1984.

Narakas, A. Brachial plexus surgery. Orthop. Clin. North Am. 12:303–323; 1981.

Narakas, A. O. Neurotization in the treatment of brachial plexus injuries. In: Gelberman, R. H., ed. Operative nerve repair and reconstruction. Philadelphia: J. B. Lippincott; 1991: p. 1329–1358.

Nashold, B. S., Jr.; Ostdahl, R. H. Dorsal root entry zone lesions for pain relief. J. Neurosurg. 51:59–69; 1979.

Nath, R. K.; Mackinnon, S. E. Management of neuromas in the hand. Hand Clin. 12:745–756; 1996.

Nelson, A. W. The painful neuroma: the regenerating axon versus the epineural sheath. J. Surg. Res. 23: 215–221; 1977.

Noordenbos, W. Pain. Amsterdam: Elsevier; 1959.

Oberlin, C.; Alnot, J. Y.; Comtet, J. J. Les greffes nerveuses tronculaires vascularisées. Techniques et résultats de vingt-sept cas. Ann. Chir. Main 8:316–323; 1989.

Ochoa, J. Pain in local nerve lesions. In: Culp, W. J.; Ochoa, J., eds. Abnormal nerves and muscles as impulse generators. New York: Oxford University Press; 1982: p. 568–587.

Ochs, G.; Schenk, M.; Struppler, A. Painful dysaesthesias following peripheral nerve injury: a clinical and electrophysiological study. Brain Res. 496:228–240; 1989.

Omer, G. E., Jr. Injuries to nerves of the upper extremity. J. Bone Joint Surg. [Am.] 56-A:1615–1624; 1974.

Omer, G. E., Jr. Past experience with epineurial repair: primary, secondary, and grafts. In: Jewett, D. L.; McCarroll, H. R., Jr., eds. Nerve repair and regeneration. Its clinical and experimental basis. St. Louis: C. V. Mosby; 1980: p. 267–276.

Omer, G. E., Jr. Results of untreated peripheral nerve injuries. Clin. Orthop. 163:15–19; 1982.

Omer, G. E., Jr. Nerve injuries associated with gunshot wounds of the extremities. In: Gelberman, R. H., ed. Operative nerve repair and reconstruction. Philadelphia: J. B. Lippincott; 1991: p. 655–670.

Omer, G. E., Jr. Reconstruction of the forearm and hand after peripheral nerve injuries. In: Omer, G. E., Jr.; Spinner, M., Van Beek, A. L., eds. Management of peripheral nerve problems. 2nd ed. Philadelphia: W. B. Saunders Co.; 1998a: p. 675–705.

Omer, G. E., Jr.; Bell-Krotoski, J. The evaluation of clinical results following peripheral nerve suture. In: Omer, G. E., Jr.; Spinner, M., Van Beek, A. L., eds. Management of peripheral nerve problems. 2nd ed. Philadelphia: W. B. Saunders Co.; 1998: p. 340–349.

Omer, G. E., Jr.; Spinner, M.; Van Beek, A. L., eds. Management of peripheral nerve problems. 2nd ed. Philadelphia: W. B. Saunders Co. 1998.

Panasci, D. J.; Holliday, R. A.; Shpizner, B. Advanced imaging techniques of the brachial plexus. Hand Clin. 11:545–553; 1995.

Pandey, S.; Singh, A. K. Treatment of neural involvement in lepra. Lepr. India 46:83; 1974.

Pandya, S. S. Surgery on the peripheral nerves in leprosy. Neurosurg. Rev. 6:153–154; 1983.

Parks, B. J. Postoperative peripheral neuropathies. Surgery 74:348–357; 1973.

Parsonage, J. M.; Turner, J. W. A. Neuralgic amyotrophy. The shoulder-girdle syndrome. Lancet i:973–978; 1948.

Paul, R. L.; Goodman, H.; Merzenich, M. Alterations in mechanoreceptor input to Brodmann's area 1 and 3 of the postcentral hand area of *Macaca mulatta* after nerve section and regeneration. Brain Res. 39:1–19; 1972.

Pizzolato, P.; Mannheimer, W. Histopathologic effects of local anesthetic drugs and related substances. Springfield, IL: Charles C Thomas; 1961.

Pollock, L. J.; Davis, L. Peripheral nerve injuries. New York: Paul B. Hoeber; 1933.

Pollock, F. H.; Drake, D.; Bovill, E. G.; Day, L.; Trafton, P. G. Treatment of radial neuropathy associated with fractures of the humerus. J. Bone Joint Surg. [Am.] 63-A:239–243; 1981.

Posner, J. B. Neurologic complications of cancer, contemporary neurology series. Vol. 45. Philadelphia: F. A. Davis Company; 1995.

Price, R. W. Neurological complications of HIV infection. Lancet 348:445–452; 1996.

Ray, C. D. Spinal cord and peripheral nerve stimulation for management of peripheral pain. In: Omer, G. E., Jr.; Spinner, M.; Van Beek, A. L., eds. Management of peripheral nerve problems. 2nd ed. Philadelphia: W. B. Saunders Co.; 1998: p. 135–145.

Rayan, G. M.; Asal, N. R.; Bohr, P. C. Epidemiology and economic impact of compression neuropathy. In: Omer, G. E., Jr.; Spinner, M., Van Beek, A. L., eds. Management of peripheral nerve problems. 2nd ed. Philadelphia: W. B. Saunders Co.; 1998: p. 488–493.

Richards, R. R. Operative treatment for irreparable lesions of the brachial plexus. In: Gelberman, R. H., ed. Operative nerve repair and reconstruction. Philadelphia: J. B. Lippincott; 1991: p. 1303–1327.

Roberts, W. J. A hypothesis on the physiological basis for causalgia and related pains. Pain 24:297–311; 1986.

Robles, J. Brachial plexus avulsion. A review of diagnostic procedures and report of six cases. J. Neurosurg. 28:434–438; 1968.

Rose, E. H.; Kowalski, T. A. Restoration of sensibility to anesthetic scarred digits with free vascularized nerve grafts from the dorsum of the foot. J. Hand Surg. [Am.] 10-A:514–521; 1985.

Rose, E. H.; Kowalski, T. A., Norris, M. S. The reversed venous arterialized nerve graft in digital nerve reconstruction across scarred beds. Plast. Reconstr. Surg. 83:593–604; 1989.

Rosen, J. M. Concepts of peripheral nerve repair. Ann. Plast. Surg. 7:165–171; 1981.

Rothberg, J. M.; Tahmoush, A. J.; Oldakowski, R. The epidemiology of causalgia among soldiers wounded in Vietnam. Mil. Med. 148:347–350; 1983.

Rydevik, B.; Lundborg, G.; Nordborg, C. Intraneural tissue reactions induced by internal neurolysis. An experimental study on the blood-nerve barrier, connective tissues and nerve fibres or rabbit tibial nerve. Scand. J. Plast. Reconstr. Surg. 10:3–8; 1976.

Salafia, A.; Chauhan, G. Nerve abscess in children and adults leprosy patients: analysis of 145 cases and review of the literature. Acta Leprol. 10:45–50; 1996.

Salisbury, R. E.; Bevin, A. G.; Lombardo, A. A. Burninduced peripheral nerve injury. In: Omer, G. E., Jr., Spinner, M.; Van Beek, A. L., eds. Management of peripheral nerve problems. 2nd ed. Philadelphia: W. B. Saunders Co.; 1998: p. 623–629.

Salisbury, R. E.; Dingeldein, G. P. Peripheral nerve complications following burn injury. Clin. Orthop. 163:92–97; 1982.

Salzberg, C. A.; Salisbury, R. E. Thermal injury of peripheral nerve. In: Gelberman, R. H., ed. Operative nerve repair and reconstruction. Philadelphia: J. B. Lippincott; 1991: p. 671–678.

Schaumburg, H. H.; Berger, A. R.; Thomas, P. K. Disorders of Peripheral Nerves. 2nd ed. Contemporary Neurology Series, Vol. 36. Philadelphia: F. A. Davis Company; 1992.

Schultz, D. Indications for utilization of a pain clinic. In: Omer, G. E., Jr.; Spinner, M., Van Beek, A. L., eds. Management of peripheral nerve problems. 2nd ed. Philadelphia: W. B. Saunders Co.; 1998: p. 120–133.

Seckel, B. R. Discussion: treatment and prevention of amputation neuromas in hand surgery, by Gorkisch, K.; Boese-Landgraf, J.; Vaubel, E. Plast. Reconst. Surg. 73:297–299; 1984.

Seddon, H. J. Three types of nerve injury. Brain 66:237–288; 1943.

Seddon, H. J., ed. Peripheral nerve injuries, Medical Research Council Special Report Series No. 282. London: Her Majesty's Stationary Office; 1954.

Seddon, H. Results of repair of nerves. In: Seddon, H., ed. Surgical disorders of the peripheral nerves. Baltimore: Williams & Wilkins; 1972.

Sedel, L. The management of supraclavicular lesions. Clin. Plast. Surg. 11:121–126; 1984.

Shepard, C. C. Temperature optimum of *Mycobacterium leprae* in mice. J. Bacteriol. 90:1271–1275; 1965.

Simond, J.; Sypert, G. Closed traction avulsion injuries of the brachial plexus. Contemp. Neurosurg. 50:1–6; 1983.

Simpson, D. M.; Berger, J. R. Neurologic manifestations of HIV infection. Med. Clin. North Am. 80:1363–1394; 1996.

Sintzoff, S.; Sintzoff, S., Jr.; Stallenberg, B.; Matos, C. Imaging in reflex sympathetic dystrophy. Hand Clin. 13:431–442; 1997.

Snyder, C. C. Epineurial repair. Orthop. Clin. North Am. 12:267–276; 1981.

Spinner, M. Factors affecting return of function following nerve injury. In: Spinner, M., ed. Injuries to the major branches of peripheral nerves of the forearm. 2nd ed. Philadelphia, W. B. Saunders Co.; 1978: p. 42–51.

Stanton-Hicks, M.; Janig, W.; Hassenbusch, S.; Haddox, J. D.; Boas, R.; Wilson, P. Reflex sympathetic dystrophy: changing concepts and taxonomy. Pain 63:127–133; 1995.

Steinberg, D. R.; Koman, L. A. Factors affecting the results of peripheral nerve repair. In: Gelberman, R. H., ed. Operative nerve repair and reconstruction. Philadelphia: J. B. Lippincott; 1991: p. 349–364.

Stevenson, G. H. Amputations, with special reference to phantom limb sensation. Edinb. Med. J. 57:44–56; 1950.

Sugioka, H.; Tsuyama, N.; Hara, T.; Nagano, A.; Tachibana, S.; Ochiai, N. Investigation of brachial plexus injuries by intraoperative cortical somatosensory evoked potentials. Arch. Orthop. Trauma Surg. 99:143–151; 1982.

Sunderland, S. Nerves and nerve injuries. Baltimore: Williams & Wilkins; 1968.

Sunderland, S. Mechanisms of cervical root avulsion in injuries of the neck and shoulder. J. Neurosurg. 41:705–714; 1974.

Swanson, A. B.; Boeve, N. R.; Lumsden, R. M. The prevention and treatment of amputation neuromata by silicone capping. J. Hand Surg. [Am.] 2-A:70–78; 1977.

Tada, K.; Nakashima, H.; Yoshida, T.; Kitano, K. A new treatment of painful amputation neuroma: a preliminary report. J. Hand Surg. [Br.] 12-B:273–276; 1987.

Tarlov, I. M. How long should an extremity be immobilized after nerve suture? Ann. Surg. 126:366–376; 1947.

Taylor, G. I. Nerve grafting with simultaneous microvascular reconstruction. Clin. Orthop. 133:56–70; 1978.

Taylor, G. I.; Ham, F. J. The free vascularized nerve graft. A further experimental and clinical application of microvascular techniques. Plast. Reconstr. Surg. 57:413–426; 1976.

Taylor, G. I.; Gianoutsos, M. P.; Morris, S. F. The neurovascular territories of the skin and muscles: anatomic study and clinical implications. Plast. Reconstr. Surg. 94:1–36; 1994.

Terzis, J. K.; Liberson, W. T.; Levine, R. Our experience in obstetrical brachial plexus palsy. In: Terzis, J. K., ed. Microreconstruction of nerve injuries. Philadelphia: W. B. Saunders Co.; 1987a; p. 513–528.

Terzis, J. K.; Liberson, W. T.; Maragh, H. A. Motorcycle brachial plexopathy. In: Terzis, J. K., ed. Microreconstruction of nerve injuries. Philadelphia: W. B. Saunders Co.; 1987b; p. 361–384.

Thomas, P. K.; Olsson, Y. Microscopic anatomy and function of the connective tissue components of peripheral nerve In: Dyck, P. K.; Thomas, P. K.; Lambert, E. H.; Bunge, R., eds. Peripheral neuropathy. 2nd ed. Philadelphia: W. B. Saunders Co.; 1984: p. 97–120.

Tinel, J. Le signe du "fourmillement" dans les lésions des nerfs périphériques. Presse Med. 23:388–389; 1915.

Tinel, J. Nerve wounds. Symptomatology of peripheral nerve lesions caused by war wounds. London: Baillière, Tindall and Cox; 1917.

Tupper, J. W.; Crick, J. C.; Matteck, L. R. Fascicular nerve repairs. A comparative study of epineurial and fascicular (perineurial) techniques. Orthop. Clin. North Am. 19:57–69; 1988.

Van Beek, A. L.; Hoffman, J. A. Nerve lengthening using balloon expansion. In: Omer, G. E., Jr.; Spinner, M.; Van Beek, A. L., eds. Management of peripheral nerve problems. 2nd ed. Philadelphia: W. B. Saunders Co.; 1998: p. 290–293.

Van Beek, A. L.; Siddiqui, A. Microneurovascular free muscle transfer. Microvascular fine muscle transfer technique. In: Omer, G. E., Jr.; Spinner, M.; Van Beek, A. L., eds. Management of peripheral nerve problems. 2nd ed. Philadelphia: W. B. Saunders Co.; 1998: p. 734–743.

Van Der Laan, L.; Goris, R. J. A. Reflex sympathetic dystrophy. An exaggerated regional inflammatory response? Hand Clin. 13:373–385; 1997.

Villarejo, F. J.; Pascual, A. M. Injection injury of the sciatic nerve (370 cases). Childs Nerv. Syst. 9:229–232; 1993.

Wall, J. T.; Kaas, J. H.; Sur, M.; Nelson, R. J.; Fellman, D. J.; Merzenich, M. M. Functional reorganization in somatosensory cortical areas 3b and 1 of adult monkeys after median nerve repair: possible relationship to sensory recovery in humans. J. Neurosci. 6:218–233; 1986.

Waller, A. V. Experiments on the section of the glossopharyngeal and hypoglossal nerves of the frog, and observations of the alterations produced thereby in the structure of their primitive fibres. Phil. Trans. R. Soc. Lond. 140:423–429; 1850.

Wilbourn, A. J. Brachial plexus disorders. In: Dyck, P. J.; Thomas, P. K.; Griffin, J. W., Low, P. A.; Poduslo, J. F., eds. Peripheral neuropathy. 3rd ed. Philadelphia: W. B. Saunders Co.; 1993: p. 911–950.

Williams, H. B. Electrical stimulation of denervated muscles. In: Omer, G. E., Jr.; Spinner, M.; Van Beek, A. L., eds. Management of peripheral nerve problems. 2nd ed. Philadelphia: W. B. Saunders Co.; 1998: p. 669–674.

Wood, V. E.; Mudge, M. K. Treatment of neuromas about a major amputation stump. J. Hand Surg. [Am.] 12-A:302–206; 1987.

Woodhall, B.; Beebe, G. W., eds. Peripheral nerve regeneration. A follow-up study of 3,656 World War II injuries. VA Medical Monograph. Washington, DC: U.S. Government Printing Office; 1956.

Yamada, S.; Lonser, R. R.; Iacono, R. P.; Morenski, J. D.; Bailey, L. Bypass coaptation procedures for cervical nerve root avulsion. Neurosurgery 38:1145–1152; 1996.

Yoshizumi, M. O.; Asbury, A. K. Intra-axonal bacilli in lepromatous leprosy. A light and electron microscopic study. Acta Neuropathol. (Berl.) 27:1–10; 1974.

Zachary, R. B.; Holmes, W. Primary suture of nerves. Surg. Gynecol. Obstet. 82:632–651; 1946.

Zhao, S.; Kim, D. H.; Kline D. G.; Beuerman, R. W.; Thompson, H. W. Somatosensory evoked potentials induced by stimulating a variable number of nerve fibers in rat. Muscle Nerve 16:1220–1227; 1993.

Zorub, D. S.; Nashold, B. S., Jr.; Cook, W. A., Jr. Avulsion of the brachial plexus: I. A review with implications on the therapy of intractable pain. Surg. Neurol. 2:347–353; 1974.

# PART VIII

# NEOPLASTIC DISORDERS

# 26

# Neoplasms

MORRIS D. GROVES AND VICTOR A. LEVIN

Historically, patients diagnosed with brain tumors anticipate a poor prognosis with severe disability and short survival. The actual prognosis for these patients is specific for the age and performance status of each patient, and the histology and location of the tumor. Depending on these factors, the extent of resection, radiation dose, and chemotherapeutic responsiveness of each tumor may also play a role in prognosis. Modern imaging and surgical advances have resulted in improved prognosis for most patients with brain tumors. Also, advances in chemotherapy for brain tumors has improved survival in a number of central nervous system (CNS) malignancies, including primary CNS lymphoma, medulloblastoma, oligodendroglioma, anaplastic astrocytoma, and intracranial germ-cell tumors. Patients with glioblastoma have yet to see significant benefit from newer chemotherapies.

Patients diagnosed with brain tumors can look forward to continuing improvement in diagnostic imaging, preoperative and intraoperative localization and mapping techniques, and microsurgical techniques, resulting in less treatment-related morbidity. Chemotherapeutic options are broadening for these patients, and in the future these options will include less toxic biological response modifiers, growth factor inhibitors, and anti-invasion and antiangiogenic agents. Additionally,

small molecules that block signal transduction pathways activated in tumor cells will be targets of therapies in the future. Gene therapy is in its infancy, but will likely have a role in the treatment of some patients with brain tumors. As the biology of these tumors is better understood, tailored treatments aimed specifically at the mutated genes and altered gene products of an individual patient's tumor, in the setting of the patient's genomic substrate, should become a reality.

## Cerebral Gliomas

Gliomas represent the largest group of primary CNS neoplasms. Histologically, they vary in malignancy from the juvenile pilocytic astrocytomas of childhood to the most aggressive, glioblastoma multiforme (GBM). While most gliomas are astrocytomas, oligodendrogliomas, ependymomas, and various combinations of two or more cell types occur in this broad grouping. Among the gliomas, each subtype and level of malignancy is associated with age-specific prevalence patterns.

## Treatment

Treatment is multimodality incorporating surgery, radiation therapy, chemotherapy, and biological response modifiers in selected cases. Surgery is

**429**

necessary for histological diagnosis and grading of malignancy as well as to debulk tumor. Radiation therapy is of significant value for high-grade gliomas and for many low-grade gliomas.

The use of chemotherapy is more controversial. This is primarily because adjuvant chemotherapy following radiation therapy is given for periods of 1 year or longer and is associated with continual morbidity during treatment. In addition, except for a limited number of earlier trials by the Brain Tumor Study Group (BTSG) and the Radiation Treatment Oncology Group (RTOG), adjuvant chemotherapy is usually not currently randomized against radiation therapy alone.

Controlled clinical trials have demonstrated the efficacy of a number of drugs when combined with irradiation as adjuvant therapy. Efficacy has been shown for carmustine (BCNU), lomustine (CCNU), 1-(2-chloroethyl)-3-(2,6-dioxo-3-piperidyl)-1-nitrosourea (PCNU); procarbazine, streptozotocin, and the combination of lomustine, procarbazine, and vincristine. Lesser activity has been shown for other agents such as aziridinylbenzoquinone (AZQ) and spiromustine. The consensus has been that adjuvant chemotherapy following surgery and radiotherapy for glioblastoma and anaplastic astrocytomas modestly increases both time to tumor progression and survival (Fazekas, 1977; Kramer, 1983; Leibel et al, 1975; Levin et al. 1997; Walker et al. 1978, 1979). A meta-analysis of adult malignant glioma patients treated with adjuvant chemotherapy after radiation therapy reported by Fine et al. (1993) showed the magnitude of the absolute survival advantage in the chemotherapy-treated patients to be only 10.1% and 8.6% at 12 and 24 months after resection, respectively. The relative survival advantage was more impressive at 23.4% and 52.4% at 12 and 24 months, respectively, due to the poor overall survival of patients with malignant gliomas.

## Prognosis

Survival is generally well correlated to histological diagnosis, although more advanced patient age at the time of tumor onset can be an extremely powerful deterrent to long-term survival, regardless of age (McKeever et al. 1997; Davis et al. 1998). The occasional younger patient with glioblastoma multiforme will survive for extended periods of over 10 years (Pollak et al. 1997). Between age and histology, however, there is overlap in that younger patients usually have lower grade gliomas.

Despite attempts to use immunocytochemical markers that may be more predictive of prognosis (BrdU, MIB-1/Ki-67, PCNA), these markers have not been consistently shown to be more predictive than standard histopathological diagnostic criteria (McKeever et al. 1997), although MIB-1 and other proliferation markers may be of use where clinical or histopathological criteria are incomplete or ambiguous. Recently, mdm2 protein (a nuclear protein that can form complexes with the $p53$ tumor suppressor gene product and inhibit its function) overexpression was identified as a strong negative prognostic factor in patients with grade III and IV gliomas (Rainov et al. 1997). In that study, significantly more glioblastoma patients than anaplastic astrocytoma patients demonstrated mdm2-positive staining tumors (46% vs. 13%). Within the glioblastoma group (70 patients) median survival was approximately 10 months in mdm2-positive patients versus approximately 18 months in mdm2-negative patients ($p = .02$). Additional genetic markers that assist in prognosis are being identified. New therapies may ultimately be based upon these findings. The recently identified MMAC/PTEN tumor suppressor gene, when expressed in higher levels in the tumors of glioma patients, results in significantly better prognosis (Sano et al. 1999).

Gliomas occur more frequently in males than females, but survival is not affected by sex. Similarly, while gliomas are less common among blacks than other races, survival appears to be unrelated to race (Simpson et al. 1996). Aside from occupational patterns, survival is unaffected by the geographical location of patients.

Typically, patients with a long history of symptoms, particularly seizures, live longer after histological diagnosis than those with shorter histories (Smith et al. 1991). This is probably due to the higher incidence of low-grade tumors in these patients.

In patients with anaplastic astrocytomas less than 50 years of age, abnormal mental status is associated with a poorer prognosis when compared to patients with normal mental status, 18.4 months median survival versus 58.6 months, respectively (Curran et al. 1993).

Performance status is predictive of prognosis (Curran et al. 1993). In GBM patients less than 50 years of age, Karnofsky performance score (KPS) of 90 to 100 was associated with a median survival time (MST) of 17.6 months, whereas a KPS of less than 90 was associated with an MST of 10.7 months. In the same study, in patients with GBM and greater than 50 years of age, KPS above 70 versus below 70 had MSTs of 10.3 versus 5.3 months, respectively.

Location of tumor has not been found to be of prognostic value in an analysis of a large group of malignant glioma patients (Curran et al. 1993), although analysis of the GBM patients from this same database did reveal frontal lobe tumor location to be predictive of significantly improved survival. Median survivals for GBM patients with frontal versus temporal versus parietal tumor locations were 11.4 versus 9.1 versus 9.6 months, respectively ($p = .01$) (Simpson et al. 1993). Furthermore, with regard to tumor location, a recent report (Stelzer et al. 1997) identified corpus callosum involvement seen on preoperative imaging as predictive of a shorter survival in a subgroup of young (<50 years), good perfomance status (Karnofsky performance >70), high-grade astrocytoma patients. In that analysis, corpus callosum involvement was associated with a decrease in median survival from 105 to 57 weeks, and in 2-year suvival from 56% to 35%. These survival numbers held true for patients with enhancing and nonenhancing tumor in the corpus callosum.

Tumor volume closely reflects tumor cell burden and postsurgical tumor volume correlates inversely with survival for gliomas (Andreou et al. 1983; Levin et al. 1980). For patients receiving postsurgery radiation and chemotherapy, there is an approximate twofold difference in survival for patients whose residual tumor volumes are in the lower 10% versus those with residual volumes in the upper 90% (Levin et al. 1980). Most large cooperative group trials of radiation-chemotherapy regimens show a correlation between the extent of surgical resection and subsequent survivals in patients with the more malignant astrocytomas (Levin et al. 1990; Simpson et al. 1993; Walker et al. 1978, 1979). Simpson and associates (1993) reporting on the results of treatment of 645 patients with glioblastoma multiforme found that patients undergoing total resection, partial resection, or biopsy had median survivals of 11.3, 10.4, or 6.6 months, respectively.

Prognosis in low-grade gliomas is influenced by many of the same factors as higher grade tumors. Younger age is a prognostic factor that predicts longer survival; adult patients with low-grade gliomas have median survival times ranging from 7 to 9 years (Philippon et al. 1993; Smith et al. 1991; Piepmeier, 1987; Bahary et al. 1996). Reported negative prognostic factors in low-grade glioma patients include poor performance status (Soffietti et al. 1989; Philippon et al. 1993), mental dysfunction, and focal neurological deficits. In a recently published study (Lote et al. 1997) of a group of 379 low-grade glioma (including astrocytomas, oligodendrogliomas and mixed gliomas) patients, the median survival of all patients was 100 months, with age being inversely related to survival. The age group 0 to 19 years ($n = 41$) had a median survival of 226 months; age group 20 to 49 years ($n = 263$), 106 months, age group 50 to 59 years ($n = 49$), 76 months; and for older patients ($n = 26$), median survival was 39 months. In this heterogeneous group of low-grade glioma patients, projected survival at 10 and 15 years was 42% and 29%, respectively.

Gross total surgical resection was among the dominant factors favoring longer survival in a large series of patients with low-grade astrocytomas treated at the Mayo Clinic (Laws et al. 1984). This has been reconfirmed in more recent studies (Soffietti et al. 1989; Philippon et al. 1993; Bahary et al. 1996), although there is not a clear concensus that a greater extent of resection improves overall survival (Berger and Rostomily 1997).

The benefit of postoperative radiation therapy for low-grade astrocytomas is shown by 5-year survival rates of 13% to 19% for incomplete surgical resection versus 41% to 46% with the addition of postoperative radiotherapy (Fazekas 1977; Leibel et al. 1975) Laws and colleagues (1984) report a 5-year survival rate of 49% for patients who received at least 40 Gy versus 34% ($p = .05$) for those with lesser doses or no irradiation. With standard therapy, survival of low-grade glioma patients is 50% to 60% at 5 years. Ten-year survival rates of 6% to 48% have been reported, depending on extent of resection and whether radiotherapy was used following resection (Bloom 1982; Laws et al. 1984; Leibel et al. 1975;

McCormack et al. 1992). In a study published by Levin and associates (1995), low grade contrast-enhancing astrocytomas were treated with BrdU during radiation and followed by PCV (lomustine, procarbazine, vincristine) chemotheraphy; they found a 79% 6-year survival.

For the more anaplastic gliomas, radiation therapy is clearly beneficial. The most telling randomized clinical trial in which patients with malignant gliomas were randomized to receive or not to receive postoperative radiotherapy was carried out by the U.S. BTSG (Walker et al. 1978). Of 222 patients, 90% had glioblastoma multiforme and 9% anaplastic astrocytoma. The median survival was 14 weeks without radiotherapy versus 36 weeks with ($p = .001$). The 12-month survival rates were 24% percent with radiotherapy and 3% without. Combining data from several BTSG clinical trials demonstrated that 60 Gy in 6 to 7 weeks yielded a better survival than did 50 Gy in 5 to 6 weeks (Walker et al. 1979). No additional improvement in survival was noted when the total dose was escalated from 60 Gy to 70 Gy.

For anaplastic gliomas, an RTOG/Eastern Cooperative Oncology Group (ECOG) prospective randomized trial of 626 patients found a median survival time of 28 versus 8 months for anaplastic astrocytoma versus glioblastoma multiforme, and 15% survival at 18 months for glioblastoma multiforme. Comparable differences have also been reported for anaplastic astrocytoma (or malignant astrocytoma) and glioblastoma multiforme using data from older retrospective studies (Kramer, 1983; Marsa et al. 1975; Sheline 1975).

Chemotherapy programs are not reviewed here, but it is apparent that some regimens are more effective than others. For example, postirradiation BCNU has been compared to the PCV combination (Levin et al. 1990). The last analysis showed, for glioblastoma multiforme patients, that 50% of patients survived 50 weeks with PCV versus 59 weeks for BCNU; 25% survived 94 and 71 weeks, respectively (Phillips et al. 1991). This was more significant ($p = .009$), however, for anaplastic tumors. Fifty percent of PCV patients survived 157 weeks versus 82 weeks for BCNU patients; 25% of patients were alive at greater than 320 weeks with PCV while only 214 weeks with BCNU (Levin et al. 1995).

## Brain Stem Gliomas

Gliomas of the brain stem are usually classified as either diffuse, focal, cervicomedullary with or without exophytic components extending into the fourth ventricle, peripontine cisterns, or both locations. Focal lesions carry a better prognosis (Edwards et al. 1989). In addition, patients with exophytic components in the fourth ventricle do better than those with infiltrative central lesions (Stroink et al. 1987; Khatib et al. 1994). There is evidence that dorsally exophytic tumors are more likely to have the histopathology of a juvenile pilocytic astrocytoma (Khatib et al. 1994). As with cerebral gliomas, juvenile pilocytic astrocytomas and lower grade anaplastic tumors do better than higher grade anaplastic tumors (Albright et al. 1986; Edwards et al. 1994). Gangliogliomas and ependymomas can present in the brain stem (Epstein and Farmer 1993)

### Treatment

Surgery for brain stem tumors is of limited value. By virtue of location, these tumors rarely are totally excised. An exception is surgery for exophytic tumors that appears to be benefical (Epstein and Wisoff 1988; Albright et al. 1986). Diffuse pontine tumors can frequently be biopsied, but the risk of creating transient or permanent neurological deterioration is significant. Ventriculoperitoneal shunting for obstructive hydrocephalus can provide symptomatic improvement in patients in whom tumor blocks the fourth ventricle.

Radiation remains the standard therapy for all brain stem tumors more malignant than juvenile pilocytic astrocytoma. The use of chemotherapy to treat patients failing radiation therapy is palliative.

### Prognosis

Usually the natural history of brain stem gliomas is steady progression to death, with median survivals of 4 to 15 months (Fulton et al. 1981; Lassman and Arjona 1967; Panitch and Berg 1970; Stroink et al. 1987). Actuarial 5-year survival rate is 30% (Petronio and Edwards 1989). Generally, patients with longer clinical histories prior to diagnosis, and those with focal lesions, especially cervicomedullary and midbrain, have better long-term survival. The early appearance of cranial nerve palsies predicts poorer survival, with 1-, 2-, and 6-year actuarial predicted survival rates of

43%, 20%, and 9.5%, respectively, in patients with this finding, compared to 84%, 71%, and 61% in patients without cranial nerve palsies (Albright et al. 1986). Those patients with cranial nerve palsies were also more likely to have histologically malignant tumors. In the same study, if a tumor was reported as malignant, chance of survival to 2.1 years was 14.1%, but if biopsy showed a low-grade (benign) tumor, chance of survival to 2.1 years was 65.8%.

In a small study of 12 children with midbrain tectal tumors (Squires et al. 1994), gadolinium enhancement and extension of the tumor beyond the tectal plate conferred a less favorable prognosis. The overall median progression-free survival of this small group was 24 months (range, 8 to 264), while the median survival was 50 months (range, 15 to 264) with all patients alive at the time of the publication.

Extent of tumor on computed tomography (CT) scan and the presence of a hypodense area in the brain stem prior to contrast enhancement are associated with length of survival. Survival to 2.1 years was 40.4% versus 14% in groups of children with tumor localized to the midbrain or pontomedullary region versus the whole brain stem. In that same group, if brain stem hypodensity was present versus not, 2.1-year survival was 18.3% versus 60.1% (Albright et al. 1986). However, contrast enhancement or it's lack on magnetic resonance imaging (MRI) scans has not been shown to correlate to prognosis (Moghrabi et al. 1995).

In a small study with five patients with histologically proven brain stem juvenile pilocytic astrocytomas treated with radiation to 54 Gy, four of the five are free of tumor 4 ½ to 8 years following irradiation. The fifth patient had 50% reduction in tumor size and follow-up is less than 1 year. The poor results obtained with conventional radiation dose schedules, with (median survival, 44 weeks) or without (median survival, 35 weeks) chemotherapy (Fulton et al. 1981; Jenkin 1983; Levin et al. 1984), led to hyperfractionation radiation treatments that deliver higher total doses. Studies utilizing 1 Gy were given twice daily to a total dose of 72 to 78 Gy (Edwards et al. 1989; Packer et al. 1994; Prados et al. 1995a). Results from this hyperfractionation program initially found a 50% increase in survival among children when compared to other regimens (median survival, 47 to 64 compared to

35 weeks). It was also shown that those 18 years or older did better than children with hyperfractionated radiotherapy, with median survivals of 70 to 92 weeks in the adults (Edwards et al. 1989; Prados et al. 1995a). Further evidence that brain stem gliomas in adults may be less aggressive than the same tumor in children comes from a retrospective study of 19 adults demonstrating a median survival of 54 months (range, 3 to 98 months) and a 5-year survival of 45% (Landolfi et al. 1998).

Adjuvant chemotherapy has not been shown to be advantageous, although chemotherapy for recurrent or progressive brain stem gliomas has demonstrated some palliative benefit in the range of 15% to 20% of patients (Fulton et al. 1981; Rodriguez et al. 1988; Chamberlain 1993; Allen and Siffert 1996).

## Cerebellar Astrocytomas

In general, these tumors carry a better prognosis than cerebral or brain stem gliomas. They occur at a younger age and are more likely to be low grade (Allen et al. 1986). These tumors are sometimes associated with neurofibromatosis.

### Treatment

The treatment of choice is gross total surgical resection regardless of histology; if this is not possible, extensive subtotal resection is advocated. For tumors more malignant than juvenile pilocytic astrocytoma, radiation therapy is advocated, since it substantially improves the survival for patients with incompletely resected highly anaplastic gliomas (Allen et al. 1986; Chamberlain et al. 1990).

Chemotherapy has been used infrequently, and its efficacy is difficult to evaluate. For highly anaplastic gliomas that recur or progress following radiation therapy, chemotherapy can provide palliation.

### Prognosis

Cure is achievable, but not guaranteed, for patients with fully resected low-grade cerebellar astrocytomas. Factors associated with improved survival include gross total resection, lack of brain stem invasion, and nonmalignant histology (Campbell and Pollack 1996; Sgouros et al. 1995; Pencalet et al. 1999). Five-year survivals of children with cerebellar astrocytomas of 91% have been reported (Duffner et al. 1986). When seen in adulthood, low-grade tumors have a similar prognosis to those seen in children (Hassounah et al. 1996). Chemotherapy at recurrence can provide palliation with relapse-free survivals in 50% of patients at 18 months; and 25% of patients who received chemotheraphy survived for more than 32 months (Chamberlain et al. 1990).

## Oligodendrogliomas

Oligodendrogliomas represent between 4% and 15% of all primary intracranial gliomas and are usually considered to be equally distributed between the genders, although there may be an increased incidence in males (Couldwell and Hinton 1995). They occur most commonly in young and middle-aged adults, with a median age at diagnosis of 40 to 50 years (Peterson and Cairncross 1996). Most oligodendrogliomas occur in the cerebral hemispheres, with a possible predisposition for the frontal lobes (Kros et al. 1996). Approximately 10% disseminate through the cerebrospinal fluid (CSF) pathways and carry a worse prognosis (Levin et al. 1997). Even though oligodendrogliomas can be grossly resected, they frequently recur in the previous operative site and require reoperation.

### Treatment

As in astrocytic tumors, extensive resection improves survival. In the report of the Mayo Clinic experience (Shaw et al. 1992), patients with gross total resections achieved median survivals of 12.6 years, and 5- and 10-year survival rates of 74% and 59%. While patients who had subtotal resections had a median survival time of 4.9 years, and 5- and 10-year survival rates of 46% and 23%. No prospective controlled studies of radiation or chemotherapy for oligodendrogliomas have been published. Five- and 10-year survival rates of up to 100% and 56% can be achieved for patients who receive radiotherapy versus up to 54% and 36% for those who do not (Chin et al. 1980; Wallner et al. 1988; Gannett et al. 1994). Improved 5-year (up to 62% to 78%) and 10-year (up to 31% to 56%) survival has been achieved with radiation doses above 45 to 50 Gy versus doses below this level or no radiotherapy (39% to 54% and 18% to 20%) (Wallner et al. 1988; Shaw et al. 1991). The bulk of published reports supports a role for postoperative radiotherapy in the treatment of oligodendrogliomas, particularly in the setting of a subtotal resection. Controversy still exists in that not all reports have demonstrated a benefit of the therapy (Kros et al. 1994), and there are long-term hazards to brain irradiation. The survival curves for patients with irradiated mixed tumors (i.e., oligodendroglioma-astrocytoma) is virtually identical to that for the irradiated pure tumors (Wallner et al. 1988).

Chemotherapy for recurrent or progressive disease appears to be of benefit (Cairncross and MacDonald 1988; Levin et al. 1997; Rajan et al. 1994; Peterson et al. 1996). These tumors appear to respond to several chemotherapeutic agents, including CCNU, AZQ, melphalan, platinum-based agents, and thiotepa (Peterson and Cairncross 1996; Rajan et al. 1994). A nitrosourea-based chemotherapy program such as PCV can produce a median relapse-free survival of approximately 1.4 years (Levin et al. 1997). A recently published study of 24 oligodendroglioma patients treated at recurrence with either a nitrosourea plus platinum or a nitrosourea with or without other agents demonstrated a 45% 1-year suvival rate, with 10 of 24 (42%) patients achieving a partial or complete response (Rajan et al. 1994). PCV chemotherapy has also been shown to be of benefit in patients with high-grade oligoastrocytomas and anaplastic oligodendrogliomas. Kim and colleagues (1996a) demonstrated a 91% response rate in 32 treated patients. Median times to progression for patients with grade 3 oligoastrocytomas, grade 4 oligoastrocytomas, and anaplastic oligodendrogliomas were 13.8 months, 12.4 months, and 63.4 months, respectively. From the start of therapy, median survival for these patients was 49.8 months, 16 months, and 76 or more months, respectively.

### Prognosis

Changes in diagnostic and treatment procedures since the mid-1970s have resulted in improved survival for oligodendroglioma patients (Davis et al. 1998). Like astrocytomas, oligodendrogliomas vary in malignancy, and survival is closely coupled to histology (Chin et al. 1980; Ludwig et al. 1986). Frontal lobe tumor location is associated with improved 5-year survival, 40% versus 10% in nonfrontal tumor patients (Kros et al. 1996), and probably reflects that the former patients had tumors that were more readily resectable. Patients with oligodendrogliomas designated grades A and B have longer survival than those considered grades C and D (Ludwig et al. 1986; Kros et al. 1996); some believe that a three-tiered histological grading system is sufficient (Bullard et al. 1987; Chin et al. 1980).

As with astrocytomas, progression to glioblastoma multiforme can occur in oligodendroglioma patients, and this progression carries a worse prognosis. A recent study reported a 35% 5-year survival with an MIB-1 LI of less than 0.1 compared to a 14% 5-year survival with an MIB-1 LI of greater than 0.2 (Kros et al. 1996). Prognostication and prediction of chemosensitivity in patients with anaplastic oligodendrogliomas has recently been enhanced. In 39 patients with anaplastic oligodendrogliomas, Caincross and colleagues found that allelic loss (or loss of heterozygosity) of chromosome 1p is a statistically significant predictor of chemosensitivity, and that combined loss involving chromosomes 1p and 19q is statistically significantly associated with both chemosensitivity and longer recurrence-free survival after chemotherapy. Furthermore, losses involving both chromosomes 1p and 19q were strongly associated with longer overall survival. Additionally, in the same study, CDKN2A gene deletions and tumor ring enhancement on neuroimaging were associated with a significantly worse prognosis (Cairncross et al. 1998).

## Ependymoma

Ependymomas occur intracranially above the tentorium cerebelli, infratentorially, and along the spinal axis. The ratio of spinal axis-intracranial ependymomas is approximately 1:2 (Helseth and Mrk 1989). In a recent series of 62 patients, 35% were supratentorial, 33% were infratentorial, and 30% were intramedullary spinal cord tumors. These groups had mean ages of 17, 7, and 41 years, respectively, at the time of first symptoms (Rawlings et al. 1988). Extension into the subarachnoid space occurs in up to 50% and carries a worse prognosis. Anaplastic ependymomas are more likely to disseminate through the CSF pathways. Differentiated or grade 2 (WHO classification) ependymomas occur twice as frequently as anaplastic ependymomas (grade 3) (Ernestus et al. 1989).

## Treatment

Surgery is the major treatment modality for both cranial and spinal axis tumors. Following complete surgical resection of differentiated ependymomas, radiation is usually not given. Following recurrence and for incompletely resected tumors, radiation therapy is advocated (Hulshof et al. 1993). For the treatment of anaplastic ependymomas following surgery, radiation therapy is required; the place of postirradiation chemotherapy awaits validation.

The use of chemotherapy is experimental. Palliation with BCNU (Levin et al. 1997) and dibromodulcitol (Levin et al. 1984) has been observed. In infants with malignant ependymomas, the "eight-drugs-in-1-day" regimen has shown some activity, resulting in a 3-year progression-free survival of 26% (Geyer et al. 1994). Chemotherapeutic activity in an adjuvant setting with radiation therapy has been noted in children (Kun et al. 1988).

## Prognosis

Prognosis is dependent on patient age, tumor location, and histology and the therapy administered. In a report of 34 intraspinal ependymoma patients, the 10-year actuarial survival rate was 91%, with no difference between those patients undergoing complete resections as compared to those with subtotal resections followed by postoperative irradiation (mean dose, 49 Gy) (Hulshof et al. 1993). In the same report, there was recurrence in seven patients with a 5-year actuarial recurrence rate of 25%. Five- and 10-year actuarial survivals of 83% and 75% for patients with spinal cord ependymomas have also been reported, patients with well-differentiated tumors faring better than those with intermediate or poorly differentiated tumors (5-year cause-specific survivals of 97% and 71%, respectively) (Waldron et al. 1993).

In a recent multivariate analysis of 92 children with supra-and infratentorial ependymomas, only radical resection was a significant factor for predicting long-term overall survival (OS) and progression-free survival (PFS) (Perilongo et al. 1997). There, children with complete resections achieved a 10-year OS and PFS of 69.8% and 57.2%, respectively, versus 32.5% and 11.1% for children undergoing subtotal resections. The administration of radiation, on multivariate analysis, reached only marginal statistical significance for PFS and not for OS. On univariate analysis age less than 5 years was significant in predicting poorer survival, and more malignant histology reached only marginal significance in predicting poorer PFS. With regard to radiotherapy, these data are at variance with the report from the Institut Gustave Roussy group (Rousseau et al. 1994) that reported on 80 children with intracranial ependymomas and a 5-year survival rate of 63% with and 23% without radiotherapy. The 5-year event-free survival rates were 45% and 0% with and without radiotherapy, respectively.

Age of the patient and duration of symptoms before diagnosis has also been shown predictive of prognosis. In a study of 40 children with intracranial ependymomas (Pollack et al. 1995), patients less than 3 years of age fared poorer, with 5-year PFS and OS of 12% and 22%, respectively, compared to older children with 5-year PFS of 60% and OS of 75%. Patients with duration of symptoms before diagnosis of less than 1 month (5-year PFS and OS of 33% and 33%, respectively), had a worse outcome than those with a more protracted course (5-year PFS and OS of 53% and 64%, respectively).

The 5- and 10-year survival rates for those who received more than 45 Gy is 61% to 75% and 58%, respectively (Shaw et al. 1987; Wallner et al. 1986). For anaplastic ependymomas, 5-year survival rates range from 10% to 50%. The 5-year survival rate for patients with spinal axis ependymoma was 89% in contrast to 24% for patients with intracranial ependymoma (Helseth and Mrk 1989).

The risk of CNS dissemination along CSF pathways from intracranial ependymomas depends on the site of origin and grade of malignancy, with a 50% incidence in cases with high-grade lesions situated in the posterior fossa (Bloom et al. 1990). Survivals at 5, 10, and 15 years in 51 children were 51%, 40%, and 31%, respectively. Mean time from tumor diagnosis to dissemination in 16 patients was 6.8 years of a total group of 140 ependymoma patients, and dissemination occurred in younger patients with subtotal resections, and those with myxopapillary or high-grade tumors (Rezai et al. 1996).

Although some argue that histology does not influence survival (Ross and Rubinstein 1989), most believe that marked survival differences exist (Nazar et al. 1990). The 5-year survival rate without recurrence was 57.4% in grade 2 ependymomas as compared to 24.1% in grade 3 ependymomas (DiMarco et al. 1988). MIB-1 proliferation index greater than 20%, or a high Ki-67 labeling index (Ki-67 LI), both of which are measures of growth fraction, are associated with poorer outcomes in children with ependymomas (Bennetto et al. 1998; Ritter et al. 1998).

## Primary CNS Lymphoma

Most primary CNS lymphomas are currently considered to be B-cell lymphomas of the histiocytic (large cell or large cell immunoblastic) type (Hochberg and Miller 1988). These tumors occur in immunocompromised hosts, especially renal transplant patients, acquired immunodeficiency syndrome (AIDS) victims, and patients with inherited disorders of the immune system (Rosenblum et al. 1988). Three percent of AIDS patients will develop this tumor either prior to AIDS diagnosis or during their subsequent course. Approximately 8% of primary CNS lymphomas occur in patients with prior known malignancies (Reni et al. 1997). Typically, these tumors can involve multiple areas of the neuraxis, the eye, and multiple intracranial sites without obvious evidence of systemic lymphoma (Hochberg and Miller 1988).

### Treatment

Since a tissue diagnosis is essential and surgery is not curative, patients may receive only a CT-guided stereotactic biopsy. The treatment of primary CNS lymphoma is evolving and chemotherapy with or without radiotherapy is becoming the standard of care (Chamberlain et al. 1998). Radiotherapy alone leads to a prompt response, but results in median survival times averaging only 17 months (Nelson et al. 1992) and 5-year disease-free survival rates of only 3% (Leibel and Sheline 1987). Combined chemotherapy (single-agent methotrexate or multiagent regimens including methotrexate systemically and intrathecally) and radiotherapy have improved median survivals up to 30 to 45 months (Cher et al. 1996; DeAngelis et al. 1992; DeAngelis 1995; Glass et al. 1994). Hydroxyurea with irradiation followed by PCV has been used to achieve similar survivals (Chamberlain and Levin 1992). Chemotherapy at diagnosis and reservation of radiotherapy for relapse has been advocated in the elderly to avoid or postpone the toxicity associated with CNS irradiation (Freilich et al. 1996). For widespread disease associated with leptomeningeal spread, craniospinal axis irradiation is indicated.

## Prognosis

Radiation therapy is of proven value, although the duration of improvement may last only 12 to 24 months (Hochberg and Miller 1988). The 1- and 5-year survival rates are 66% and 7%. Prognostic factors shown to be associated with longer survival in immunocompetent patients include age less than 60, KPS greater than 70, symptom duration greater than 4 weeks, radiation dose greater than 55 Gy, and a negative CSF cytology (Kim et al. 1996b). The impact of age was demonstrated in one study of 22 human immunodeficiency virus (HIV)-negative patients (Schaller and Kelly 1996), which reported a median survival of 5.4 years in patients less than 45 years of age compared to a median survival of 9 months for those patients greater than 45 years old ($p = .03$).

AIDS-related CNS lymphomas appear to respond to irradiation in a fashion similar to other CNS lymphomas; however, AIDS patients are more likely to die of other causes.

Karnofsky performance status greater than 70, age less than 35, and irradiation dose greater than 39 Gy were associated with a better prognosis in AIDS patients with CNS lymphoma, median survivals in these groups being 181, 162, and 162 days, respectively (Corn et al. 1997).

Positive CSF cytology or simultaneous intracranial and spinal lesions both carry a poorer prognosis. Recurrent disease complicated by lymphomatous meningitis can be treated with radiotherapy, systemic chemotherapy, and/or intrathecal chemotherapy. In a recent report (Chamberlain et al. 1998), 4 of 14 such patients (28.6%) are disease free and have durable responses (median, 36 months; range, 22 to 56 months) after being treated with either irradiation, systemic chemotherapy, or intrathecal chemotherapy (methotrexate, cytosine arabinoside, or thiotepa). Ten patients (71.4%) had died with a median survival of 5.5 months (range, 3 to 12 months). In this study leukoencephalopathy was present in the disease-free survivors.

## Primative Neuroectodermal Tumors

Primarily a disease of early childhood, primitive neuroectodermal tumors (PNETs) represent a controversial nosology of primitive tumors. Some authors divide them into the following classification schema: medulloepithelioma, neuroblastoma, spongioblastoma, ependymoblastoma, pineoblastoma, and medulloblastoma. With the exception of the medulloblastoma, primitive neuroectodermal tumors are rare. For the purposes of discussion, we will restrict PNETs to only those tumors located in the cerebral hemisphere, and are composed of predominantly undifferentiated neuroectodermal tumor with or without glial or neuronal differentiation.

## Treatment

The initial therapy for primitive neuroectodermal tumors is surgical bulk reduction whenever feasible. It is well documented in the literature that PNETs do metastasize and these patients should be staged and treated like medulloblastoma and given craniospinal axis irradiation. Most specialists treat these patients as "poor-risk" medulloblastomas. Pre- or postirradiation chemotherapy is frequently given (Gaffney et al. 1985) and may prolong survival. A number of different chemotherapeutic regimens have been utilized; vincristine plus cyclophosphamide alternating with carboplatin plus etoposide has shown activity (Gaze et al. 1994). CCNU plus vincristine and prednisone after radiotherapy or the eight-drugs-in-1-day regimen in the midst of radiotherapy have also been utilized (Cohen et al. 1995). Daily oral etoposide is active in recurrent PNETs (Needle et al. 1997).

## Prognosis

The prognosis of these patients is usually poor, but has been improving due to more aggressive resections and chemotherapeutic advances. There are some reports of long-term survival, usually coincident with radical resection (Duffner et al. 1981; Gaffney et al. 1985; Halperin et al. 1993). There is evidence of a trend towards longer survival in those patients with a more complete surgical resection (Albright et al. 1995; Dirks et al. 1996). In the Albright study of 1995, 27 patients with supratentorial PNETs were all treated with surgery, irradiation, and chemotherapy, with

5-year overall and progression-free survivals of 34% and 31%, respectively. Progression-free survival was worse in children aged 1.5 to 3 years of age and those with evidence of tumor dissemination at the time of diagnosis. Pineal site of tumor involvement is associated with better 3-year overall and progression-free survivals (73% and 61%, respectively) than tumor location in other areas of the supratentorium (Cohen et al. 1995). Additionally, patients with posterior fossa PNETs tend to have a better prognosis than those with supratentorial PNETs (Albright et al. 1995).

In a small group of 18 patients referred for radiotherapy, 3- and 5-year survival rates were 29% and 25%, respectively (Gaffney et al. 1985). In that series, patients with tumors containing a larger percentage of undifferentiated tumor tissue had a poorer survival. Dirks et al. reported a series of 36 children with supratentorial PNETs treated with biopsy or surgery, 26 receiving adjuvant radiation and 13 receiving chemotherapy. Median survival was 23 months, and 2-, 3-, and 5-year survivals were 50%, 34%, and 18%, respectively. Berger and colleagues (1983) reviewed the results of treatment for 11 patients with cerebral neuroblastoma and found that of six patients with cystic tumors, none had recurrence, while four of the five solid tumor patients had recurrences.

## Medulloblastoma

Initially localized to the cerebellum, these tumors can spread down the spinal axis and outside the neuraxis; 7% to 10% of all patients present with extraneural metastases (Leo et al. 1997). Some studies indicate that up to 30% of cases will have positive cytology or myelographic evidence of spinal metastasis at diagnosis (Allen et al. 1986; Bloom 1982b). Medulloblastoma occurs in children and adults with a ratio of approximately 2:1 in some series. A short duration of symptoms is often associated with more advanced disease at the time of diagnosis (Halperin and Friedman 1996).

### Treatment

Surgery should be aggressive and seek to remove as much tumor as possible. Greater extent of tumor resection correlates with better survival in patients older than 3 years of age without tumor dissemination (Albright et al. 1996). Conventional radiation therapy is given to the craniospinal axis with

a "boost" to the posterior fossa (Bloom 1982b; Bloom et al. 1982). There is good evidence that decreasing the dose of neuraxis radiation from 36 Gy in 20 fractions to 23.4 Gy in 13 fractions increases the risk of early relapse in good prognosis, newly diagnosed patients (Deutsch et al. 1996).

Chemotherapy following radiation therapy as well as prior to radiation continues to be evaluated in an effort to improve survival (Levin et al. 1988; Loeffler et al. 1988; Packer et al. 1988). Medulloblastomas are responsive to a wide variety of antineoplastic agents including vincristine, nitrosoureas, procarbazine, dibromodulcitol, cyclophosphamide, methotrexate, cisplatinum, etoposide, and various drug combinations (Allen et al. 1986; Friedman and Schold 1985; Levin et al. 1983; van Eys et al. 1988; Chamberlain and Kormanik 1997). Many patients treated with craniospinal irradiation have reduced bone marrow reserves, which can reduce the dose frequency and intensity of chemotherapy.

For recurrent disease, surgery clearly benefits some patients (Balter-Seri et al. 1997). Similarly, chemotherapy with single agents and combinations is efficacious. While controversy surrounds the use of autologous stem-cell or bone marrow rescue, some benefit in patients with recurrent disease has been shown (Dunkel et al. 1998; Mahoney et al. 1996).

### Prognosis

Due to advances in surgical technique, radiotherapy, and chemotherapy, prognosis in medulloblastoma patients has been improving if one compares 1970s data to that from the 1990s (Davis et al. 1998). Prognosis is defined, to an extent, by staging criteria. Poor-risk is defined as (1) less than a 75% resection; (2) metastasis to spinal cord, cerebrum, leptomeninges, or seeding of the cerebellum; (3) positive CSF cytology 2 weeks after surgery; (4) invasion of the brain stem; and (5) age under 4 years (Bloom et al. 1982; Allen et al. 1986; Levin et al. 1988). Markers of increased cellular proliferation are also associated with a poorer prognosis (Gilbertson et al. 1997).

Poor-risk associated with those younger than 4 years of age is due to the fact that radiation therapists do not treat with full doses of craniospinal irradiation at this age. To prevent radiation-induced toxicity, chemotherapy alone is being used in some young children. A recent series of 19 patients

(18 treated with only chemotherapy) under 3 years of age reported a survival of 8 of 19 (42.1%) at a mean follow-up of 86 months (Di Rocco et al. 1997). Ater and associates (1997) reported a median survival of 10.6 years in 8 of 12 medulloblastoma patients under 3 years of age treated with MOPP chemotherapy (mechlorethamine, vincristine, procarbazine, and prednisone) without irradiation, with a reduction in treatment-related neurodevelopmental sequelae. A recent randomized study of 203 children with untreated, high-stage medulloblastoma demonstrated that vincristine, lomustine (CCNU), and prednisone (VCP) plus external radiation therapy (XRT) is a superior adjuvant combination when compared with 8-in-1 chemotherapy plus XRT. Five-year PFS rates for VCP versus 8-in-1 of 63% versus 45% ($p = .006$), respectively, were achieved (Zeltzer et al. 1999).

The 5-year survival of poor-risk patients with craniospinal irradiation with or without chemotherapy has been reported at 25% to 40% (Allen et al. 1986; Bloom et al. 1982; Evans et al. 1990; Park 1983). The impact of the extent of resection in patients with brain stem involvement by tumor is explored in a recent report of 40 patients with brain stem invasion undergoing either gross-total, near-total or subtotal resections with a postirradiation PFS of 61% at a median of 4 years' follow-up (Gajjar et al. 1996). In this group there was no significant difference in outcome between the surgical subsets. The 1999 Zeltzer study demonstrated that for patients with M0 tumors, residual tumor bulk (not extent of resection) is a predictor for PFS. Patients with M0 tumors, 3 years of age or greater with no more than 1.5 cm$^2$ residual tumor, had a 78% ± 6% 5-year PFS rate.

Good-risk patients, on the other hand, have 5-year survivals of 66% to 70% (Allen et al. 1986; Bloom et al. 1982; Evans et al. 1990; Levin et al. 1988). Results of the multi-institutional randomized trials conducted by the Children's Cancer Study Group (CCSG) demonstrated 5-year event-free survival rates of 59% with and 50% without the chemotherapy.

Survival for adult medulloblastoma patients is comparable to the pediatric population (Le et al. 1997). In this study of 34 adult medulloblastoma patients, 5-year posterior fossa control and overall survival rates were 61% and 58%, respectively. 5-year survival for females versus males was 92% versus 40%, and 5-year survival for patients with localized versus disseminated disease was 67% versus 25%. Adult 10-year survival rates up to 41% are reported (Frost et al. 1995). Prados and associates (1995b) treated 47 adult medulloblastoma patients with biopsy or resection followed by radiotherapy; 32 of 47 patients received chemotherapy. Median survival of the poor-risk patients was 282 weeks (5.3 years). Five-year overall survival and disease-free survival in the good-risk versus poor-risk patients was 81% and 58% versus 54% and 38%, respectively. Median survival from the time of recurrence was 77 weeks.

Survival of patients presenting with extraneural metastases, usually skeletal or lymph node, is poor: 5 months in children and 10 months in adults (Rochkind et al. 1991). There are rare reports of long-term (up to 120 months) remissions obtained with chemotherapy in patients with extraneural medulloblastoma metastases (Leo et al. 1997).

The prognosis for patients with recurrent disease is generally poor (Le et al. 1997), although a possible role for high-dose chemotherapy with carboplatin, thiotepa, and etoposide with autologous stem-cell rescue (ASCR) was recently reported (Dunkel et al. 1998). In that study of 23 recurrent medulloblastoma patients treated with ASCR, three died from treatment-related toxicities, seven (30%) are event-free survivors at a median of 54 months after ASCR (range, 24 to 78 months), and Kaplan-Meier estimates of event-free and overall survivals are 34% and 46%, respectively, at 36 months after ASCR.

Long-term childhood survivors can develop neuropsychological dysfunction, decreased cognition, impaired growth of the spine, and pituitary-hypothalamic dysfunction. Growth hormone deficiency is the most frequent endocrine dysfunction following irradiation.

Neurocognitive deficits in long-term adult survivors have also been reported (Kramer et al. 1997).

## Metastatic Cancer

Widespread dissemination is the life-limiting factor for most patients afflicted with cancer. Control of hematogenous spread or local extension into other vital organs determines prognosis. Cancer of lung, breast, and skin (melanoma) account for the bulk of brain metastases (Sawaya and Bindal 1995). While brain metastases are frequently just one more manifestation of end-stage cancer, their presence often significantly affects quality and length of survival.

For each type of primary cancer, a pattern of central nervous system involvement can be defined. In gynecology, cancers of ovarian and cervical origin rarely metastasize to the brain (<1%) and, when detected, durable remissions still can be achieved. Brain metastases in stage IV melanoma is seen in up 72% of patients. In breast cancer, 26% of patients will develop metastatic disease within 10 years of diagnosis. Brain metastasis is documented in 16% of patients with metastatic cancer, but this represents only 4.2% of the entire population of patients with a breast primary. While the synchronous discovery of the lung primary and brain metastasis is not uncommon, breast and colorectal cancers rarely present with CNS signs and symptoms as the initial manifestation of disease.

### Treatment

The treatment plan is dictated by the need to provide immediate palliation of neurological signs and symptoms, the desire to achieve durable remissions, and the status of the patient's systemic disease and overall performance status. Surgery is indicated for diagnosis when in doubt. Resection of a symptomatic tumor provides immediate palliation and may enhance the durability of subsequent therapy; coordination of surgery with other treatment modalities is of key importance (Lang and Sawaya 1998).

Whole-brain radiotherapy (WBRT) has been the standard treatment of brain metastases and, when combined with steroids, may provide adequate symptomatic control. Stereotactic radiosurgery (SRS) has recently been shown feasible and beneficial for patients with surgically inaccessible metastatic lesions less than 3.5 cm in diameter (Young 1998) and even in patients with more than one lesion (Breneman et al. 1997). With the advent of improved surgical techniques and stereotactic radiation, the continued utility of whole-brain radiotherapy and its accompanying morbidity is being reassessed (Vermeulen 1998). Patients who are bedridden at the time of brain metastases are not likely to benefit from any form of therapy.

While controversial (Wagner 1997), limited-stage small cell lung cancer patients who completely respond to induction therapy and are treated with prophylactic cranial irradiation (PCI) have been shown to have reduced rates of brain metastasis and increase brain metastasis-free survival, but a nonsignificant increase in overall survival compared to those not received PCI (Gregor et al. 1997; Arriagada et al. 1995).

### Prognosis

In a review of 729 patients with metastatic lesions to the brain from various primary sources, Nussbaum and associates found a median duration from presentation of brain metastases until death of 4 months, ranging from 3 months in patients with small cell lung cancer (SCLC) to 13 months for patients with prostate carcinoma. Median survival for patients with single lesions was 5 months, compared to 3 months in patients with multiple lesions. Median survival for patients with single metastases treated with surgery was 11 months, compared to 3 months for those not treated with surgery, and surgery did not significantly influence survival in patients with multiple lesions. A recent retrospective report of 1292 patients with brain metastases from a variety of primary cancers found an overall median survival of 3.4 months, with 6-month, 1-year, and 2-year survival percentages of 36%, 12%, and 4%, respectively. Survival was significantly different between treatment modalities, with median survival of 1.3 months in patients treated with steroids only, 3.6 months in patients treated with radiotherapy, and 8.9 months in patients treated with neurosurgery followed by radiotherapy ($p < .0001$). Performance status, response to steroid treatment, systemic tumor activity, and serum lactate dehydrogenase were independent prognostic factors with the strongest impact on survival, while site of primary tumor, patient age, and number of brain metastases were also identified as prognostic factors, although with lesser importance. (Lagerwaard et al. 1999).

### *Lung Adenocarcinoma*

Patient selection will markedly enhance the length of survival in patients who undergo specific treatments. For example, Patchell and associates (1986) report a 19-month median survival in lung cancer patients operated on for a single brain metastasis. All of these patients had no active systemic disease, but they represented only 9% of the patients seen with metastatic lung cancer. Thus their impact on the expected survival of the entire group was only modest. At M. D. Anderson Cancer Center, the median survival for patients who underwent craniotomy for removal of one or more metastases was slightly less than 12 months. However, durable remissions lasting more than 3 years were observed in up to 20% of patients (Moser and Johnson 1989).

In a randomized trial, surgical resection, followed by radiation resulted in longer survival, fewer recurrences, and better quality of life than similar patients treated with radiotherapy alone (Patchell et al. 1990), although this has not been confirmed in all randomized studies (Mintz et al. 1996). Infrequently, non–small cell lung cancer patients can achieve very-long-term remissions (>10 years) after resection of the primary tumor and the brain metastasis (Shahidi and Kvale 1996).

### Breast Adenocarcinoma

In a study of 28 patients with a single brain metastasis as first site of distant metastasis from a breast primary, overall median survival was 16 months. Median survival in the primarily surgical and radiotherapy-treated patients was 23 months compared to 9 to 10 months in the non–surgically treated group Boogerd et al. 1997). In 20 non–surgically treated patients with multiple brain metastases as first site of recurrence from a breast primary, median survival was 4 months. In a study of 61 patients undergoing surgery for brain metastases from breast cancer, median survival was 16 months and 5-year survival rate was 17% (Pieper et al. 1997). Rarely, patients can survive up to 10 years after brain metastases from breast cancer when treated aggressively with surgery, radiation, and hormonal therapy (Nieder et al. 1996).

### Melanoma

In a large review of 702 patients with brain metastases from melanoma, overall median survival of these patients from the time of diagnosis of the brain metastasis was 113.2 days (Sampson et al. 1998). Median survival of the patients given palliative chemotherapy alone was 39 days, for patients receiving whole-brain radiotherapy, median survival was 120 days, for those patients undergoing surgical resection alone, median survival was 194.6 days, and for those patients undergoing surgical resection followed by radiotherapy, median survival was 268 days. The difference in survival between the surgical group receiving radiotheraphy versus the group not receiving radiotherapy was not significant. A primary lesion located in the head or neck region was associated with a shorter survival time, while a single brain metastasis, the absence of visceral metastases, and initial presentation of melanoma with brain metastasis was associated with a better prognosis.

### Colorectal Adenocarcinoma

In a series of 100 patients with brain metastases from colorectal carcinoma, median survival was 1 month if treatment was steroids alone, 3 months for those who received radiotherapy, and 9 months for those undergoing surgery (Hammoud et al. 1996). The extent of noncerebral systemic disease was not correlated with survival in that study. A recent retrospective report of 73 colon cancer patients who underwent surgical resection for brain metastases found 1-year and 2-year survival rates of 31.5% and 6.8%, respectively. In the same study, infratentorial tumor location was associated with a poorer survival compared with supratentorial tumor location. (5.1 months vs. 9.1 months; $p < .002$)(Wronski and Arbit 1999).

### Thyroid Adenocarcinoma

When brain metastases from thyroid cancer are identified, median survival is 4.7 months, 12.4 months with a differentiated tumor. Resection of one or more lesions is associated with a median survival of 16.7 months, compared to 3.4 months in patients not undergoing resection, independent of the presence of multiple brain lesions (Chiu et al. 1997).

Thus, in patients with a good performance status and potentially treatable systemic disease, surgery, radiation, and in some situations, chemotherapy can result in both immediate palliation and durable symptom-free remissions. The source of the primary tumor is of importance in determining both therapy and prognosis.

## Germ Cell Tumors

### Germinomas

Germinomas are the most common intracranial germ cell tumor and are histologically indistinguishable from testicular seminoma. They represented 0.2% of all primary intracranial tumors documented in the United States during the years 1980 and 1985 (Mahaley et al. 1989). This low number contrasts to a much higher reported incidence in Japan (Matsutani et al. 1997) and certain regions of Germany where 4.5% to 10% of tumors are called germinomas. Men (73.1%) were more likely to develop a germinoma and the mean age at diagnosis was 19.8 years (Dehner 1983). Most germinomas arise in the midline axis from the suprasellar cistern to the pineal region. Local leptomeningeal dissemination and spinal metastases are seen.

## Treatment

The role of surgery, beyond biopsy for tissue diagnosis, remains controversial (Moser and Backlund 1984). Though the concept of surgical cytoreduction is attractive, resection exposes the patient to the operative risks and the possibility of regional tumor dissemination. Germinomas are exquisitely sensitive to both ionizing radiation and chemotherapy. The presence of a relatively homogeneous, well-circumscribed, extra-axial, enhancing pineal region mass in a young male is so characteristic of a germinoma that diagnostic radiotherapy can be justified. In such a situation, the patient receives 20 Gy over 2 weeks. A reduction in the tumor diameter of more than 50% is consistent with the diagnosis of this highly radiosensitive tumor and a complete course of radiation (craniospinal up to 22 Gy and tumor region to 50 Gy) is administered. Patients should have a ventricular drain placed if acutely ill from obstructive hydrocephalus and the CSF analyzed for human chorionic gonadotropin (HCG) and α-fetoprotein (AFP). If a definite reduction is not seen, then surgical resection should be considered as the next step. In the modern era of microsurgical technique, a limited needle biopsy can be reserved for those situations where open exploration is not feasible. Accurate staging of the disease requires CSF cytology and MRI spinal imaging.

In order to diminish radiation-induced neurotoxicity, induction chemotherapy with cisplatin or carboplatin, and etoposide, plus ifosfamide, followed by reduced volume irradiation is being evaluated with promising early results (Sawamura et al. 1998; Baranzelli et al. 1997).

## Prognosis

The prognosis for intacranial germinomas is good and has been improving. Since the beginning of the CT era, 5- and 10-year survivals have risen to better than 90% (Haddock et al. 1997; Huh et al. 1996) after treatment with radiotherapy. A 20-year survival rate of 80.6% in 63 patients has been reported, with no added benefit when chemotherapy was given after radiation (Matsutani et al. 1997). Previously, survival following radiation alone or combined with initial surgery ranged from 60% to 79% (Amendola et al. 1984; Jenkin et al. 1978; Packer et al. 1984; Sano and Matsutani, 1981; Sung et al. 1978). Outcome is adversely affected by tumor dissemination within the neuraxis.

Modern reports of 5-year actuarial disease-free and overall survivals of 97% after treatment with lower dose radiation (<25.5 Gy whole brain, < 50 Gy to primary site, 22 Gy to the spine) with or without chemotherapy exist (Hardenbergh et al. 1997).

In a small series of eight patients initially treated with carboplatin, etoposide, and bleomycin who later recurred, high-dose cyclophosphamide followed by craniospinal irradiation with a boost to the site of recurrence resulted in no failures at a median follow-up of 32 months (range, 16 to 47 months) (Merchant et al. 1998). A recently published study by the French Society of Pediatric Oncology (Baranzelli et al. 1997) of 29 patients treated with pre-irradiation chemotherapy consisting of carboplatin, etoposide, and ifosfamide followed by 40 Gy to the original tumor volume had only one recurrence at 3 years which is again in a second complete remission. Twenty-eight of 29 patients are in a first complete remission at a median follow-up of 32 months (range, 7 to 68 months) and the 4-year survival rate is 100%.

## Teratoma

Of primary intracranial tumors, 0.5% are teratomas, but in children the incidence is higher (Zulch 1986). The majority of tumors are found along the midline. Teratomas are heterogeneous on imaging studies, reflecting the cysts, cartilage, hair, teeth, and other products of the germ cell layers present. Sarcomatous or malignant germ cell tissue is present in the teratoid malignant tumors (Rubinstein 1971).

## Treatment

Complete surgical removal should be attempted if possible. The benign (mature) teratoma may have an very indolent clinical course. If symptomatic mass effect is present, radiation therapy will not reduce the tumor burden (Stein 1979). If malignant germ cell tumor (choriocarcinoma, embryonal carcinoma, or endodermal sinus) is present within a teratoma, it should be treated aggressively with both radiation and chemotherapy. The chemotherapeutic agents ifosfamide, vincristine, etoposide, cisplatin, carboplatin, bleomycin, and dactinomycin have been used in patients with immature teratomas (Garre et al. 1996; Kobayashi et al. 1989), but these tumors are sometimes refractory to chemotherapy (Yoshida et al. 1993).

### Prognosis

In contrast to pure germinomas, the 5-year survival for the teratoma patient is only 35% (Jennings et al. 1985), although, in a more recent report, 10-year survivals of 30 patients with either mature teratoma or malignant teratoma were 92.7% and 80.6%, respectively (Matsutani et al. 1997). Though complete surgical removal and long-term survival are well known, the persistence of tumor mass effect in some patients and the presence of malignant tissue in others probably accounts for the mortality encountered.

### Embryonal Carcinoma, Choriocarcinoma, and Yolk Sac Tumor

These tumors are rare and represent the malignant correlate of the embryonal pluripotent stem cells and extraembryonic derivatives. They are found most often in the pineal region and specific serological and immunohistochemical markers (HCG or AFP) can be demonstrated (Edwards et al. 1988; Matsutani et al. 1997).

### Treatment

These tumors require aggressive multimodality therapy. Complete surgical excision should be attempted. In most situations, the patient should receive local radiation and systemic chemotherapy using those agents most active against the same corresponding systemic cancer, although systemic chemotherapy has not been shown to add benefit to radiotherapy in all studies (Matsutani et al. 1997). Children under the age of 4 should be considered for chemotherapy alone and radiation reserved for relapse.

### Prognosis

A poor prognosis exists for these patients, this is particularly true for those with choriocarcinoma. Extensive resection is associated with better long-term survival than partial resection or biopsy. 1-, 3-, and 5-year survival rates are 45.5%, 27.3%, and 27.3%, respectively (Matsutani et al. 1997).

## PINEAL CELL TUMORS

### Pineocytoma

Pineocytomas are rare tumors that represent less than 1% of intracranial tumors. They are seen in all age groups and equally distributed in men and women. Neoplasms arising from the pineal parenchyma represent 20% to 30% of pineal region tumors (Donat et al. 1978). Neoplastic pineal parenchymal cells are capable of differentiation into tumors with astrocytic and ganglionic components (Rubinstein 1977).

### Treatment

The tumors tend to be well encapsulated, and complete macroscopic resection can frequently be achieved. Durable remissions have been reported following surgery alone (Lapras 1984). Radiation therapy has been used to treat pineocytomas (Disclafani et al. 1989). Occasionally, widespread CNS metastases occur, and treatment may then include craniospinal irradiation and chemotherapy (D'Andrea et al. 1987).

### Prognosis

In patients with documented pineocytoma, long-term survival is usually only expected in patients whose tumors are completely resected. The presence of astrocytic or neuronal differentiation may also be associated with a better prognosis. In a recent report of nine patients with pineocytoma, none of whom had a gross total resection, 5-year survival was 86% (Schild et al. 1996). Disclafani and colleagues (1989) report six cases treated with 45 to 54 Gy radiation. Survival ranged up to 29 years with a median of 9 years. Mena and associates (1995) report 21 patients with pineocytomas; two died before surgery, two died immediately postoperatively, and the remaining 15 of 17 patients not lost to follow-up had 100% survival at a median follow-up of 38 months (range, 6 to 118 months) after surgery.

### Pineoblastoma

Of pineal parenchymal neoplasms, this tumor is the least differentiated and is considered a primitive neuroectodermal tumor. It occurs most frequently in the first 2 decades of life and there is no sexual predilection.

### Treatment

As with other primitive neuroectodermal tumors, a gross total removal may enhance the durability of remissions. Surgery alone is never definitive. Craniospinal radiation is indicated for children older than 3 years of age and additional chemotherapy should be considered. In younger children, chemotherapy should be utilized prior to radiation. High-dose cyclophosphamide has shown activity against these tumors (Ashley et al. 1996), although a combination of cyclophosphamide, vincristine, cisplatinum, and etoposide, used in an attempt to delay radiation in 11 infants with pineoblastoma, was not found to be effective in treating the primary tumor site or in treating or preventing leptomeningeal spread (Duffner et al. 1995). The eight-drugs-in-1-day regimen without radiotherapy has also been felt to be ineffective in young children with pineoblastomas (Jakacki et al. 1995).

### Prognosis

Few long-term survivors have been documented. For children more than 18 months of age treated with craniospinal radiation and chemotherapy, the estimated 3-year progression-free survival is 61%, which is superior to that of children with other supratentorial PNETs (Jakacki et al. 1995).

Extent of disease at diagnosis appears to be an important prognostic factor in adult pineoblastoma patients (Chang et al. 1995). In this report by Chang and colleagues of 11 patients, one refused further therapy after surgery and died 6 months later, and five patients with positively staged disease had a median overall survival after surgery of 30 months. This group progressed at a median of 10 months after surgery and died 1 to 20 months after recurrence. Of the five negatively staged patients, all were alive at a median of 26 months follow-up.

High-dose chemotherapy with autologous stem cell transplantation (ASCT) has been utilized in pineoblastoma patients with some success. Of seven patients treated, two for recurrence suffered progressive disease soon after ASCT. Four of five patients who underwent ASCT before the development of recurrence remain disease-free 28+ to 49+ months after ASCT (Graham et al. 1997).

## Pituitary Adenoma

### Nonsecreting Pituitary Tumors

Nonsecreting adenomas comprise 25% to 30% of pituitary tumors. Patients most commonly present with macroadenomas producing symptoms related to mass effect on the optic chiasm, hypothalamus, and adjacent pituitary tissue.

### Treatment

The primary therapy for these tumors is surgical resection. Trans-sphenoidal decompression is the treatment of choice. Postoperative conventional radiotherapy is appropriate when residual disease is present and shows evidence of progression on follow-up MRI scans (Pistenma et al. 1975; McCutcheon 1996; Zierhut et al. 1995). Gamma-knife treatment of these tumors has also been reported (Motti et al. 1996).

### Prognosis

Improvement in neurological functions compromised by the tumor mass will occur in the majority of patients following surgical decompression. Radiation therapy may influence the development of hypopituitarism if not already present. Progressive tumor growth has been documented in 18% of patients irradiated for postoperative residual tumor and 12% of patients treated with only surgery. In a recently published retrospective study of 120 patients who had undergone radiotherapy for nonfunctional pituitary adenomas, actuarial tumor control rates at 10, 20, and 30 years were $87.5 \pm 3.6\%$, $77.6 \pm 6.3\%$, and $64.7 \pm 12.9\%$, respectively. Tumor progression after radiotherapy occurred significantly more than ($p = .039$) in patients with the so-called oncocytoma than in patients with nononcocytic null cell adenoma (Breen et al. 1998). With the exception of the few patients with very aggressive and destructive tumors of the skull base, durable, disease-free survival is the rule (Ebersold et al. 1986).

### Secreting Pituitary Tumors

These tumors secrete prolactin, thyrotropin, gonadotropin, growth hormone, and adrenocorticotropic hormone (ACTH). Hormone secretion from the pituitary gland depends on the intimate association between the hypothalamus and pituitary (Challa et al. 1985). The pathogenesis of pituitary tumors remains unknown. There is evidence for and against the hypothesis that secretory tumors arise as the result of hypothalamic dysregulation (Kovacs and Horvath 1987). For each of the hormones, 80% to 90% appear to arise de novo within the pituitary. The prolactinomas are most common, while the thyrotropin-secreting tumors are rare (Kleinberg et al. 1997). Gonadotropin cell adenomas occur frequently and are generally seen in middle-aged men.

### Treatment

For prolactinomas, medical therapy with a dopamine agonist is generally safer and more effective than surgery or pituitary irradiation (Parl et al. 1986). Even very large tumors can shrink dramatically in response to bromocriptine (Pelkonin et al. 1981). In a report of 409 patients undergoing transsphenoidal resection for prolactin-secreting pituitary adenomas, recurrence of hyperprolactinemia occurred in 47% of all patients, but only 16% of those with a single surgical procedure, histology of prolactinoma, and postoperative prolactin levels of 5 ng/ml or less (Feigenbaum et al. 1996).

The other secreting tumors are best treated by trans-sphenoidal excision and postoperative irradiation if invasive residual tumor is present (Jennings et al. 1977; Tyrrell et al. 1978). Dopamine agonist and somatostatin analogues may have a role in growth hormone–secreting tumors (Lamberts et al. 1985). Heavy particle irradiation and stereotactic radiosurgery have been used in the treatment of ACTH-producing tumors (Kjellberg and Kliman 1980). Metyrapone and aminoglutethimide have also been used in the medical therapy of Cushing's disease (Kreiger 1979). Octreotide therapy has a high success rate when surgery fails in thyrotropin-secreting pituitary adenomas (Beck-Peccoz et al. 1996).

When a patient has evidence of a pituitary tumor, a serum thyroxine ($T_4$) and thyroid-stimulating hormone (TSH) level must be obtained (Hamilton et al. 1970). In primary hypothyroidism, secondary pituitary enlargement will spontaneously resolve when thyroid replacement is administered.

### Prognosis

Long-term survival is the rule for patients with functioning pituitary tumors. Severe systemic sequelae from acromegaly, Cushing's disease, hyperthyroidism, and treatment-induced panhypopituitarism can be seen. These conditions can have a profound effect on the quality of life, but with good medical management, a satisfactory level of function can be maintained.

## Tumors of Meningeal and Related Tissues

### Meningioma

These tumors include a number of histopathological categories, including meningotheliomatous, fibrous, transitional, psammomatous, angiomatous, hemangioblastic, papillary, anaplastic, and malignant. In the American College of Surgeons' brain tumor survey, meningiomas and anaplastic meningiomas represented 21.9% and 1.2% of tumors reported, respectively (Mahaley et al. 1989). The mean age of all meningioma patients was 59, and 68% were women. In some series, malignant meningiomas can comprise up to 10% of the total meningioma cases (Jaaskelainen et al. 1986). Anaplastic and malignant meningiomas occur more commonly in men than in women. The tumor occurs in children and adolescents in approximately 2 % of cases. Meningiomas are found most commonly along the falx cerebri, sphenoid ridges, parasellar region, and cerebral convexities. Tumors less frequently arise in the optic nerve sheath, foramen magnum, cerebellopontine angles, pineal region, and ventricular system. Meningiomas in bone and paranasal sinuses are rarely seen (Batsakis, 1979). Meningiomas generally are firm and well demarcated. When they invade the pia mater, edema is seen in the adjacent brain. To some degree, meningiomas can be graded. Meningotheliomatous, fibrous, transitional, psammomatous, angiomatous, hemangioblastic meningiomas are considered grade I or benign (Kepes 1982). Papillary meningiomas are more prone to malignancy, though any histological subtype may transform into a malignant phenotype (Ludwin et al. 1975).

### Treatment

Surgical removal is the treatment of choice for symptomatic tumors. It provides a diagnosis, immediate palliation, and the potential for cure. Recurrences are seen in 3% to 5% at 5 years and up to 32% at 15 years postoperatively after a gross total removal of a benign meningioma is performed (Jaaskelainen et al. 1986; Mirimanoff et al. 1985). This may represent residual microscopic disease or possible multicentric tumor origin.

After the subtotal resection of histologically benign meningiomas, rates of progression are as high as 37%, 55%, and 91% at 5, 10, and 15 years, respectively (Mirimanoff et al. 1985). The en plaque meningiomas of the skull base rarely are resected completely. Angiomatous, anaplastic, and malignant meningiomas have higher recurrence rates. When anaplastic tumors recur, transformation into a malignant meningioma may occur, 26% of the time in a recent report (Palma et al. 1997).

Radiation therapy should be used for incomplete tumor resections where the likelihood of symptomatic recurrence is expected (Carella et al. 1982; Barbaro et al. 1987; Taylor et al. 1988). In anaplastic, malignant, and angiomatous meningiomas, radiation is usually considered part of the primary therapy. This is suggested by a number of studies, but has not been evaluated in a prospective randomized trial (Salazar 1988; Rodriguez et al. 1989; Goldsmith et al. 1994). Higher radiation doses of greater than 53 Gy are probably indicated for the more aggressive meningioma phenotypes (Goldsmith et al. 1994; Forbes and Goldberg 1984). Not all reports support the use of radiotherapy in atypical and malignant meningioma patients (Jaaskelainen et al. 1986; Younis et al. 1995). Cytotoxic chemotherapy with agents active against soft tissue sarcomas is often utilized for recurrent tumors following surgery and radiation therapy, although outcomes are usually poor. The use of less aggressive therapies such as hydroxyurea or interferon-$\alpha$ has recently been reported with some associated success (Schrell et al. 1997; Kaba et al. 1997).

*Prognosis*

The 5-year survival for meningiomas and anaplastic meningiomas is 91% and 61% respectively (Mahaley et al. 1989). In the incompletely resected benign meningiomas, radiation therapy suppresses regrowth in approximately 50% of patients, with a reported 28% to 54% reduction in the rate of recurrence (Barbaro et al. 1987; Taylor et al. 1988). There is no prognostic difference between the benign subtypes (Skullerud and Loken 1974).

In a recently published study of 71 atypical and malignant meningioma patients, 5- and 10-year survival in atypical meningioma patients was 95% and 79%, respectively, while 64.3% and 34.5%, respectively, in malignant meningioma patients (Palma et al. 1997). In this study, a Simpson grade I resection (gross total resection of tumor, dural attachments, and abnormal bone) and convexity location were associated with a better clinical course.

## Meningeal Sarcomas

These tumors include fibrosarcoma, polymorphic cell sarcoma, meningeal sarcomatosis, rhabdomyosarcoma, mesenchymal chondrosarcoma, and malignant fibrous histiocytoma.

Frank sarcomatous neoplasms of meningeal origin comprise approximately 1.2% of intracranial tumors (Zulch 1986). In addition to the fibrosarcomas, the polymorphic cell sarcomas, and the primary meningeal sarcomatosis, other sarcomas are associated with the blood vessels within the brain parenchyma (Kernohan and Uhlheim 1962; Lukes et al. 1983). Meningeal sarcomas, particularly fibrosarcomas, may arise as the result of previous radiation therapy (Gonzales-Vitale et al. 1976).

*Treatment*

In all cases, complete surgical removal is the treatment of choice. Radiation therapy to the involved region may reduce the rate of recurrence. Chemotherapy may play a role in the management of these tumors. Sarcomas can respond to the standard frontline drugs most active against the systemic version of the tumor.

*Prognosis*

Most of these tumors are so rare that no valid information is available regarding patient outcomes. Long-term survivors have been reported for most of the sarcomas mentioned (Simpson et al. 1986), and this likely reflects the fact that some of these tumors are well circumscribed and amenable to curative resection.

In one report, eight of nine patients with fibrosarcomas of the brain or meninges died, with a median survival of 7.5 months (range, 1 day to 96 months) (Gaspar et al. 1993). Meningeal sarcomatosis has been reported to have an extremely poor prognosis of only days to a few weeks after diagnosis (Budka et al. 1975). Primary intracranial rhabdomyosarcoma is reported to have a median survival of 8 to 10 months (Tomei et al. 1989). Based on the experience with other organ system sarcomas, multimodality therapy, including aggressive surgery, radiation, and chemotherapy, will result in improved survival.

## Tumors of Nerve Sheath Cells

### Neurilemoma and Neurofibroma

The acoustic nerve is the most common site for development of a neurilemoma. Rarely, the trigeminal and glossopharyngeal nerves are involved as a solitary finding. Other cranial nerves and bilateral acoustic nerve involvement are generally associated with neurofibromatosis type 2 (NF2). Tumors can arise in the dorsal spinal nerve roots and grow large in the paraspinal soft tissue. Recent studies have demonstrated allelic losses on chromosome 22q, which encodes a protein known as merlin or schwannomin, which functions as a tumor suppressor (Lutchman and Rouleau 1996). The Commission on Cancer reported that in 1980 and 1985, less than 4% of primary intracranial tumors were neurilemomas, and the mean age at diagnosis was 50 years (Mahaley et al. 1989). The tumor occurs more frequently in females (57%) and has been seen in young children.

Neurofibromatosis type 1 (NF1), also known as von Recklinghausen's disease, is a common (1 per 3500 population), autosomal dominantly inherited disease that is associated with mutations and deletions in the *NF1* gene on chromosome 17q, which encodes the protein *Neurofibromin* which functions as a tumor suppressor. NF1 is manifested by dermal abnormalities, optic gliomas, and peripheral nerve tumors, or neurofibromas. Neurofibromas can grow intracranially or intraspinally, and are generally multiple in number. Sarcomatous transformation of neurofibromas may occur.

### *Treatment*

Surgical resection is the treatment of choice in most situations. Since the tumors are histologically benign and may behave in a clinically indolent manner, no treatment may be indicated for the asymptomatic, elderly, or frail patient. Small, intracranial tumors in NF2, generally less than 2 cm, have been treated using single-dose, highly focused ionizing radiation (stereotactic radiosurgery). Peripheral tumors are resected when disability occurs due to neural compression, intractable pain ensues, or sarcomatous transformation appears likely. When sarcomatous transformation occurs, treatment with radiation is usually administered, and chemotherapeutic agents such as cyclophosphamide, vincristine, Adriamycin, and DTIC have shown some activity against these tumors (Yap et al. 1980).

### *Prognosis*

The expected outcome for most patients with NF2 is quite favorable. The 5-year survival for patients with acoustic neurilemoma operated in 1980 was 96.3%. Hearing loss is the most common early neurological finding, but the frequency of this and other operative morbidity is diminishing due to modern microsurgical techniques and intraoperative monitoring. Complete resection is obtainable in 99% of cases and is nearly always followed without recurrence. Incomplete resections can result in tumor regrowth (Gormley et al. 1997). The few deaths seen are usually the result of large recurrent tumors where the surgical complication and mortality rates are much higher. Modern diagnostic imaging allows for the detection of smaller lesions resulting in minimal surgical morbidity and better preservation of cranial nerve functions.

When sarcomatous transformation occurs in a peripheral neurofibroma in NF1, the prognosis is poor, and patients often succumb to metastatic disease. Reports are few, but survival for more than 24 months is unusual.

## Malformative Tumors

### Craniopharyngioma

Craniopharyngiomas are most frequently associated with childhood and adolescence, though they may remain asymptomatic until late adulthood. These tumors are thought to arise from the vestigial remnants of Rathke's pouch (other names for this tumor have included tumors of Rathke's cleft or the hypophyseal duct). They arise exclusively in the sellar region and may be contained solely within the sella or more frequently in the suprasellar space. The tumors may expand as predominately solid or cystic lesions. The cyst may be multiloculated and be responsible for the majority of the mass effect when present. Though they may expand into the sphenoid sinus, they usually grow into the suprasellar region displacing the optic apparatus and effacing the ventricular system.

Craniopharyngiomas generally grow slowly, although cyst enlargement can be quite dramatic over a few months. The solid cellular component consists of stratified squamous epithelium arranged in various bands, cords, or papillary structures surrounding the vascularized connective tissue stroma (Russell and Rubinstein 1977). Histologically apparent malignant transformation is not associated with this type of tumor, though aggressive biological activity is seen.

### Treatment

The optimal management of these tumors remains controversial. Complete tumor removal of small intrasellar and suprasellar tumors with minimal morbidity and a durable remission can be expected. Larger tumors that distort the floor of the third ventricle or expand into its lumen can elicit a reactive gliosis and become enmeshed in the ventricular wall. In this situation, removal frequently is associated with significant hypothalamic dysfunction. Cyst drainage and removal of all solid tumor without stripping all of the cyst wall from adjacent brain tissue and vessels will provide immediate decompression and restoration of neurological function and greatly reduce the surgical morbidity. The addition of ionizing radiation in older children and adults may maximize the opportunity for a durable symptom-free remission (Amacher 1980). Stereotactic radiosurgery is being used for recurrent or residual tumors in some centers (Kobayasi et al. 1994). Some authors recommend observation after a complete resection and radiotherapy at the time of recurrence (Wara et al. 1994).

### Prognosis

The biological behavior of these tumors generally is indolent. They may be found as an incidental mass and followed for years with no symptoms or radiographic progression. As surgical morbidity declines, improved postoperative endocrine support, in cases of panhypopituitarism, can permit a near-normal life. Despite their benign histology,

death or significant disability from progressive tumor and the cumulative toxicity of treatment are frequent. Radical tumor resections are associated with recurrences in 17.6% to 23% of cases (Villani et al. 1997; Shapiro et al. 1979). Local control rates after complete resection, subtotal resection, or incomplete resection and postoperative irradiation are 70%, 26%, and 75%, respectively (Wen et al. 1989). Villani et al. reported a recurrence rate of 42.8% in patients treated with limited surgery plus radiotherapy. The 10-year survival rates are better for patients treated with surgery and radiation (70% to 77%) than with surgery alone (50%) (Sung et al. 1981; Wara et al. 1994). A 20-year survival rate of 66% has been reported in patients treated with limited surgery followed by radiotherapy (Rajan et al. 1993), and radiation doses in excess of 54 Gy are associated with decreased rates of recurrence, 16% versus 44% (Regine et al. 1993).

Neurobehavioral abnormalities are common in children with craniopharyngioma, 17 of 20 patients manifesting abnormal neurobehavioral testing in one report (Anderson et al. 1997). Small stature, obesity, headache, visual impairment, and emotional and sexual disturbances are common despite pharmacological treatment (Villani et al. 1997).

### References

Albright, A. L.; Guthkeltch, A. N.; Packer, R. J.; Price, R. A.; Rourke, L. B. Prognostic factors in pediatric brain-stem gliomas. J. Neurosurg. 65:751–755; 1986.

Albright, A. L.; Wisoff, J. H.; Zeltzer, P.; Boyett, J.; Rorke, L. B.; Stanley, P. Effects of medulloblastoma resections on outcome in children: a report from the Children's Cancer Group. Neurosurgery 38:265–271; 1996.

Albright, A. L.; Wisoff, J. H.; Zeltzer, P.; Boyett, J.; Rorke, L. B.; Stanley, P.; Geyer, J. R.; Milstein, J. M. Prognostic factors in children with supratentorial (nonpineal) primitive neuroectodermal tumors. A neurosurgical perspective from the Children's Cancer Group. Pediatr. Neurosurg. 22:1–7; 1995.

Allen, J. C.; Bloom, J.; Ertel, I.; Evans, A.; Hammond, D.; Jones, H.; Levin, V.; Jenkin, D.; Sposto, R.; Wara, W. Brain tumors in children: current cooperative and institutional chemotherapy trials in newly diagnosed and recurrent disease. Semin. Oncol. 13:110–122; 1986.

Allen, J. C.; Siffert, J. Contemporary chemotherapy issues for children with brainstem gliomas. Pediatr. Neurosurg. 24:98–102; 1996.

Amacher, A. L. Craniopharyngioma: the controversy regarding radiotherapy. Childs Brain 6:57–64; 1980.

Anderson, C. A.; Wilkening, G. N.; Filley, C. M.; Reardon, M. S.; Kleinschmidt-DeMasters, B. K. Neurobehavioral outcome in pediatric craniopharyngioma. Pediatr. Neurosurg. 26:255–260; 1997.

Arriagada, R.; Le Chevalier, T.; Borie, F.; Riviere, A.; Chomy, P.; Monnet, I.; Tardivon, A.; Viader, F.; Tarayre, M.; Benhamou, S. Prophylactic cranial irradiation for patients with small-cell lung cancer in complete remission. J. Natl. Cancer Inst. 87:183–190; 1995.

Ashley, D. M.; Longee, D.; Tien, R.; Fuchs, H.; Graham, M. L.; Kurtzberg, J.; Casey, J.; Olson, J.; Meier, L.; Ferrell, L.; Kerby, T.; Duncan-Brown, M.; Stewart, E.; Colvin, O. M.; Pipas, J. M.; McCowage, G.; McLendon, R.; Bigner, D. D.; Friedman, H. S. Treatment of patients with pineoblastoma with high dose cyclophosphamide. Med. Pediatr. Oncol. 26: 387–392; 1996.

Ater, J. L.; van Eys, J.; Woo, S. Y.; Moore, B., III; Copeland, D. R.; Bruner, J. MOPP chemotherapy without irradiation as primary post-surgical therapy for brain tumors in infants and young children. J. Neurooncol. 32:243–252; 1997.

Bahary, J. P.; Villemure, J. G.; Choi, S.; Leblanc, R.; Olivier, A.; Bertrand, G.; Souhami, L.; Tampieri, D.; Hazel, J. Low-grade pure and mixed cerebral astrocytomas treated in the CT scan era. J. Neurooncol. 27:173–177; 1996.

Balter-Seri, J.; Mor, C.; Shuper, A.; Zaizov, R.; Cohen, I. J. Cure of recurrent medulloblastoma: the contribution of surgical resection at relapse. Cancer 79: 1241–1247; 1997.

Baranzelli, M. C.; Patte, C.; Bouffet, E.; Couanet, D.; Habrand, J. L.; Portas, M.; Lejars, O.; Lutz, P.; Le Gall, E.; Kalifa, C. Nonmetastatic intracranial germinoma: the experience of the French Society of Pediatric Oncology. Cancer 80:1792–1797; 1997.

Barbaro, N. M.; Gutin, P. H.; Wilson, C. B.; Sheline, G. E.; Boldrey, E. B.; Wara, W. M. Radiation therapy in the treatment of partially resected meningiomas. Neurosurgery 20:525–528; 1987.

Beck-Peccoz, P.; Persani, L.; Mantovani, S.; Cortelazzi, D.; Asteria, C. Thyrotropin-secreting pituitary adenomas. Metabolism 45(8 suppl. 1): 75–79; 1996.

Bennetto, L.; Foreman, N.; Harding, B.; Hayward, R.; Ironside, J.; Love, S.; Ellison, D. Ki-67 immuno-labelling index is a prognostic indicator in childhood posterior fossa ependymomas. Neuropathol. Appl. Neurobiol. 24:434–440; 1998.

Berger, M. S.; Edwards, M. D.; Wara, W. M.; Levin, V. A. Primary cerebral neuroblastoma: long-term follow-up review and therapeutic guidelines. J. Neurosurg. 59:418–423; 1983.

Berger, M. S.; Rostomily, R. C. Low grade gliomas: functional mapping resection strategies, extent of resection, and outcome. J. Neurooncol. 34:85–101; 1997.

Bloom, H. J.; Glees, J.; Bell, J. The treatment and long-term prognosis of children with intracranial tumors: a study of 610 cases, 1950–1981. Int. J. Radiat. Oncol. Biol. Phys. 18:723–745; 1990.

Bloom, H. J. G. Intracranial tumors: response and resistance to therapeutic endeavors 1970–1980. Int. J. Radiat. Oncol. Biol. Phys. 8:1083–1113; 1982a.

Bloom, H. J. G. Medulloblastoma in children: increasing survival rates and further prospects. Int. J. Radiat. Oncol. Biol. Phys. 8: 2023–2027; 1982b.

Bloom, H. J. G.; Thornton, H.; Schweisguth, O. SIOP medulloblastoma and high grade ependymoma therapeutic clinical trials: preliminary results (1975–1981). In: Raybaud, C.; Clement, R.; Lebreuli, G.; Bernard, J. L., eds. Pediatric oncology. Amsterdam: Excerpta Medica; 1982: p. 309.

Boogerd, W., Hart, A. A.; Tjahja, I. S. Treatment and outcome of brain metastasis as first site of distant metastasis from breast cancer. J. Neurooncol. 35: 161–167; 1997.

Breen, P.; Flickinger, J. C.; Kondziolka, D.; Martinez, A. J. Radiotherapy for nonfunctional pituitary adenoma: analysis of long-term tumor control. J. Neurosurg. 89:933–938; 1998.

Breneman, J. C.; Warnick, R. E.; Albright, R. E., Jr.; Kukiatinant, N.; Shaw, J.; Armin, D.; Tew, J., Jr. Stereotactic radiosurgery for the treatment of brain metastases. Results of a single institution series. Cancer 79:551–557; 1997.

Budka, H.; Pilz, P.; Guseo, A. Primary leptomeningeal sarcomatosis. Clinicopathological report of six cases. J. Neurol. 211:77–93; 1975.

Bullard, D. E.; Rawlings, C. E., III; Phillips, B.; Cox, E. B.; Schold, S. C., Jr.; Burger, P.; Halperin, E. C. Oligodendroglioma. An analysis of the value of radiation therapy. Cancer 60:2179–2188; 1987.

Cairncross, J. G.; Macdonald, D. R. Successful chemotherapy for recurrent malignant oligodendroglioma. Ann. Neurol. 23:360–364; 1988.

Cairncross, J. G.; Ueki, K.; Zlatescu, M. C.; Lisle, D. K.; Finkelstein, D. M.; Hammond, R. R.; Silver, J. S.; Stark, P. C.; Macdonald, D. R.; Ino, Y.; Ramsay, D. A.; Louis, D. N. Specific genetic predictors of chemotherapeutic response and survival in patients with anaplastic oligodendrogliomas. J. Natl. Cancer Inst. 90:1473–1479; 1998.

Campbell, J. W.; Pollack, I. F. Cerebellar astrocytomas in children. J. Neurooncol. 28:223–231; 1996.

Challa, V. R.; Marschall, R. B.; Hopkins, M. B., III; Kelly, D. L., Jr.; Civantos, F. Pathobiologic study of pituitary tumors: report of 62 cases with a review of the recent literature. Hum. Pathol. 16:873–884; 1985.

Chamberlain, M. C. Recurrent brainstem gliomas treated with oral VP-16. J. Neurooncol. 15:133–139, 1993.

Chamberlain, M. C.; Kormanik, P. A. Chronic oral VP-16 for recurrent medulloblastoma. Pediatr. Neurol. 17:230–234; 1997.

Chamberlain, M. C.; Kormanik, P.; Glantz, M. Primary central nervous system lymphoma complicated by lymphomatous meningitis. Oncol. Rep. 5:521–525; 1998.

Chamberlain, M. C.; Levin, V. A. Primary central nervous system lymphoma: a role for adjuvant chemo-therapy. J. Neurooncol. 14:271–275; 1992.

Chamberlain, M. C.; Silver, P.; Levin, V. A. Poorly differentiated gliomas of the cerebellum. A study of 18 patients. Cancer 65:337–340; 1990.

Chang, S. M.; Lillis-Hearne, P. K.; Larson, D. A.; Wara, W. M.; Bollen, A. W.; Prados, M. D. Pineoblastoma in adults. Neurosurgery 37:383–390; 1995.

Cher, L.; Glass, J.; Harsh, G. R.; Hochberg, F. H. Therapy of primary CNS lymphoma with methotrexate-based chemotherapy and deferred radiotherapy: preliminary results. Neurology 46:1757–1759; 1996.

Chin, H. W.; Hazel, J. J.; Kim, T. H.; Webster, J. H. Oligodendrogliomas. I. A clinical study of cerebral oligodendrogliomas. Cancer 45:1458–1466; 1980.

Chiu, A. C; Delpassand, E. S.; Sherman, S. I. Prognosis and treatment of brain metastases in thyroid carcinoma. J. Clin. Endocrinol. Metab. 82:3637–3642; 1997.

Cohen, B. H.; Zeltzer, P. M.; Boyett, J. M.; Geyer, J. R.; Allen, J. C.; Finlay, J. L.; McGuire-Cullen, P.; Milstein, J. M.; Rorke, L. B.; Stanley, P.; et al. Prognostic factors and treatment results for supratentorial primitive neuroectodermal tumors in children using radiation and chemotherapy: a Childrens Cancer Group randomized trial. J. Clin. Oncol. 13: 1687–1696; 1995.

Corn, B. W.; Donahue, B. R.; Rosenstock, J. G.; Hyslop, T.; Brandon, A. H.; Hegde, H. H.; Cooper, J. S.; Sherr, D. L.; Fisher, S. A.; Berson, A.; Han, H.; Abdel-Wahab, M.; Koprowski, C. D.; Ruffer, J. E.; Curran, W. J., Jr. Performance status and age as independent predictors of survival among AIDS patients with primary CNS lymphoma: a multivariate analysis of a multi-institutional experience. Cancer J. Sci. Am. 3:52–56; 1997.

Couldwell, W. T.; Hinton, D. R. Oligodendroglioma. In: Kaye, A. H.; Laws, E. R., Jr., eds. Brain tumors. New York: Churchill Livingstone; 1995: p. 479–491.

Curran, W. J. Jr.; Scott, C. B.; Horton, J.; Nelson, J. S.; Weinstein, A. S.; Fischbach, A. J.; Chang, C. H.; Rotman, M.; Asbell, S. O.; Krisch, R. E.; Nelson, D. F. Recursive partitioning analysis of prognostic factors in three radiation therapy oncology group malignant glioma trials. J. Natl. Cancer Inst. 85: 704–710; 1993.

D'Andrea, A. D.; Packer, R. J.; Rorke, L. B.; Bilaniuk, L. T.; Sutton, L. N.; Bruce, D. A.; Schut, L. Pineocytomas of childhood. A reappraisal of natural history and response to therapy. Cancer 59:1353–1357; 1987.

Davis, F. G.; Freels, S.; Grutsch, J.; Barlas, S.; Brem, S. Survival rates in patients with primary malignant brain tumors stratified by patient age and tumor histological type: an analysis based on Surveillance, Epidemiology, and End Results (SEER) data, 1973–1991. J. Neurosurg. 88:1–10; 1998.

DeAngelis, L. M. Current management of primary central nervous system lymphoma. Oncology (Huntingt.) 9:63–71; 1995.

DeAngelis, L. M.; Yahalom, J.; Thaler, H. T.; Kher, U. Combined modality therapy for primary CNS lymphoma. J. Clin. Oncol. 10:635–643; 1992.

Dehner, P. L. Gonadal and extragonadal germ cell neoplasia of childhood. Hum. Pathol. 14:493–511; 1983.

Deutsch, M.; Thomas, P. R.; Krischer, J.; Boyett, J. M.; Albright, L.; Aronin, P.; Langston, J.; Allen, J. C.; Packer, R. J.; Linggood, R.; Mulhern, R.; Stanley, P.; Stehbens, J. A.; Duffner, P.; Kun, L.; Rorke, L.; Cherlow, J.; Freidman, H.; Finlay, J. L.; Vietti, T. Results of a prospective randomized trial comparing standard dose neuraxis irradiation (3,600 cGy/20) with reduced neuraxis irradiation (2,340cGy/13) in patients with low-stage medulloblastoma. A Combined Children's Cancer Group–Pediatric Oncology Group Study. Pediatr. Neurosurg. 24:167–176; 1996.

DiMarco, A.; Campostrini, F.; Pradella, R.; Reggio, M.; Palazzi, M.; Grandinetti, A.; Garusi, G. F. Postoperative irradiation of brain ependymomas. Analysis of 33 cases. Acta Oncol. 27:261–267; 1988.

Dirks, P. B.; Harris, L.; Hoffman, H. J.; Humphreys, R. P.; Drake, J. M.; Rutka, J. T. Supratentorial neuroectodermal tumors in children. J. Neurooncol. 29:75–84; 1996.

Di Rocco, C.; Iannelli, A.; Papacci, F.; Tamburrini, G. Prognosis of medulloblastoma in infants. Childs Nerv. Syst. 13:388–396; 1997.

Disclafani, A.; Hudgins, R. J.; Edwards, M. S.; Wara, W.; Wilson, C. B.; Levin, V. A. Pineocytomas. Cancer 63:302–304; 1989.

Duffner, P. K.; Cohen, M. E.; Heffner, R. R.; Freeman, A. I. Primitive neuroectodermal tumors of childhood. An approach to therapy. J. Neurosurg. 55:376–381; 1981.

Duffner, P. K.; Cohen, M. E.; Myers, M. H.; Heise, H. W. Survival of children with brain tumors: SEER Program, 1973–1980. Neurology 36:597–601; 1986.

Duffner, P. K.; Cohen, M. E.; Sanford, R. A.; Horowitz, M. E.; Krischer, J. P.; Burger, P. C.; Friedman, H. S.; Kun, L. E. Lack of efficacy of postoperative chemotherapy and delayed radiation in very young children with pineoblastoma. Pediatric Oncology Group. Med. Pediatr. Oncol. 25:38–44; 1995.

Dunkel, I. J.; Boyett, J. M.; Yates, A.; Rosenblum, M.; Garvin, J. H. Jr.; Bostrom, B. C.; Goldman, S.; Sender, L. S.; Gardner, S. L.; Li, H.; Allen, J. C.; Finlay, J. L. High-dose carboplatin, thiotepa, and etoposide with autologous stem-cell rescue for patients with recurrent medulloblastoma. Children's Cancer Group. J. Clin. Oncol. 16:222–228; 1998.

Ebersold, M. J.; Quast, L. M.; Laws, E. R.; Scheithauert, B.; Randall, R. V. Long-term results in transsphenoidal removal of nonfunctioning pituitary adenomas. J. Neurosurg. 64:713–719; 1986.

Edwards, M. S.; Hudgins, R. J.; Wilson, C. B.; Levin, V. A.; Wara, W. M. Pineal region tumors in children. J. Neurosurg. 68:689–697; 1988.

Edwards, M. S. B.; Wara, W. M.; Ciricillo, S. F.; Barkovich, A. J. Focal brain-stem astrocytomas causing symptoms of involvement of the facial nerve nucleus: long-term survival in six pediatric cases. J. Neurosurg. 80:20–25; 1994.

Edwards, M. S.; Wara, W. M.; Urtasun, R. C.; Prados, M.; Levin, V. A.; Fulton, D.; Wilson, C. B.; Hannigan, J.; Silver, P. Hyperfractionated radiation therapy for brain-stem glioma: a phase I-II trial. J. Neurosurg. 70:691–700; 1989.

Epstein, F. J.; Farmer, J-P. Brain-stem glioma growth patterns. J. Neurosurg. 78:408–412; 1993.

Epstein, F.; Wisoff, J. H. Intrinsic brain-stem tumors in childhood: surgical indications. J. Neurooncol. 6: 309–317; 1988.

Ernestus, R. I.; Wilcke, O.; Schroder, R. Intracranial ependymomas: prognostic aspects. Neurosurg. Rev. 12:157–163; 1989.

Evans, A. E.; Jenkin, R. D. T.; Sposto, R.; Ortega, J. A.; Wilson, C. B.; Wara, W.; Ertel, I. J.; Kramer, S.; Chang, C. H.; Leikin, S. L.; Hammond, G. D. The treatment of medulloblastoma. J. Neurosurg. 72: 572–582; 1990.

Fazekas, J. T. Treatment of grade I and II brain astrocytomas. The role of radiotherapy. Int. J. Radiat. Oncol. Biol. Phys. 2:661–666; 1977.

Feigenbaum, S. L.; Downey, D. E.; Wilson, C. B.; Jaffe, R. B. Transsphenoidal pituitary resection for preoperative diagnosis of prolactin-secreting pituitary adenoma in women: long term follow-up. J. Clin. Endocrinol. Metab. 81:1711–1719; 1996.

Fine, H. A.; Dear, K. B. G.; Loeffler, J. S.; Black, P. McL.; Canellos, G. P. Meta-analysis of radiation therapy with and without adjuvant chemotherapy for malignant gliomas in adults. Cancer 71:2585–2597; 1993.

Forbes, A. R.; Goldberg, I. D. Radiation therapy in treatment of meningiomas: the Joint Center for Radiation Therapy experience 1970 to 1982. J. Clin. Oncol. 10:1139–1143; 1984.

Freilich, R. J.; Delattre, J. Y.; Monjour, A.; DeAngelis, L. M. Chemotherapy without radiation therapy as initial treatment for primary CNS lymphoma in older patients. Neurology 46:435–439; 1996.

Friedman, H. S.; Schold, S. C., Jr. Rational approaches to the chemotherapy of medulloblastoma. Neurol. Clin. 3:843–853; 1985.

Frost, P. J.; Laperierre, N. J.; Wong, C. S.; Milosevic, M. F.; Simpson, W. J.; Pintilie, M. Medulloblastoma in adults. Int. J. Radiat. Oncol. Biol. Phys. 32: 951–957; 1995.

Fulton, D. S.; Levin, V. A.; Wara, W. M.; Edwards, M. S. Chemotherapy of pediatric brain stem tumors. J. Neurosurg. 54: 721–725; 1981.

Gaffney, C. C.; Sloane, J. P.; Bradley, N. J.; Bloom, H. J. Primitive neuroectodermal tumours of the cerebrum. Pathology and treatment. J. Neurooncol. 3: 23–33; 1985.

Gajjar, A.; Sanford, R. A.; Bhargava, R.; Heideman, R.; Walter, A.; Li, Y.; Langston, J. W.; Jenkins, J. J.; Muhlbauer, M.; Boyett, J.; Kun, L. E. Medulloblastoma with brain stem involvement: the impact of gross total resection on outcome. Pediatr. Neurosurg. 25:182–187; 1996.

Gannett, D. E.; Wisbeck, W. M.; Silbergeld, D. L.; Berger, M. S. The role of postoperative irradiation in the treatment of oligodendroglioma. Int. J. Radiat. Oncol. Biol. Phys. 30:567–573; 1994.

Garre, M. L.; El-Hossainy, M. O.; Fondelli, P.; Gobel, U.; Brisigotti, M.; Donati, P. T.; Nantron, M.; Ravegnani, M.; Garaventa, A.; De Bernardi, B. Is chemotherapy effective therapy for intracranial immature teratoma? A case report. Cancer 77:977–982; 1996.

Gaspar, L. E.; Mackenzie, I. R.; Gilbert, J. J.; Kaufmann, J. C.; Fisher, B. F.; Macdonald, D. R.; Cairncross, J. G. Primary cerebral fibrosarcomas. Clinicopathologic study and review of the literature. Cancer 72:3277–3281; 1993.

Gaze, M. N.; Smith, D. B.; Rampling, R. P.; Simpson, E.; Barrett, A. Combination chemotherapy for primitive neuroectodermal and other malignant brain tumours. Clin. Oncol. (R. Coll. Radiol.) 6:110–115; 1994.

Geyer, J. R.; Zeltzer, P. M.; Boyett, J. M.; Rorke, L. B.; Stanley, P.; Albright, A. L.; Wisoff, J. H.; Milstein, J. M.; Allen, J. C.; Finlay, J. L.; Ayers, G. D.; Shurin, S. B.; Stevens, K. R.; Bleyer, W. A. Survival of infants with primitive neuroectodermal tumors or malignant ependymomas of the CNS treated with eight drugs in 1 day: a report from the childrens cancer group. J. Clin. Oncol. 12: 1607–1615; 1994.

Gilbertson, R. J.; Jaros, E.; Perry, R. H.; Kelly, P. J.; Lunec, J.; Pearson, A. D. Mitotic percentage index: a new prognostic factor for childhood medulloblastoma. Eur. J. Cancer 33:609–615; 1997.

Glass, J.; Gruber, M. L.; Cher, L.; Hochberg, F. H. Preirradiation methotrexate chemotherapy of primary central nervous system lymphoma: long-term outcome. J. Neurosurg. 81:188–195; 1994.

Goldsmith, B. J.; Wara, W. M.; Wilson, C. B.; Larson, D. A. Postoperative irradiation for subtotally resected meningiomas. A retrospective analysis of 140 patients treated from 1967 to 1990. J. Neurosurg. 80:195–201; 1994.

Gonzales-Vitale, J. C.; Slavin, R. E.; McQueen, J. D. Radiation induced intracranial malignant fibrous histiocytoma. Cancer 37:2960–2963; 1976.

Gormley, W. B.; Sekhar, L. N.; Wright, D. C.; Kamerer, D.; Schessel, D. Acoustic neuromas: results of current surgical management. Neurosurgery 41:50–58; 1997.

Graham, M. L.; Herndon, J. E, II; Casey, J. R.; Chaffee, S.; Ciocci, G. H.; Krischer, J. P.; Kurtzberg, J.; Laughlin, M. J.; Longee, D. C.; Olson, J. F.; Paleologus, N.; Pennington, C. N.; Friedman, H. S. High-dose chemotherapy with autologous stem-cell rescue in patients with recurrent and high-risk pediatric brain tumors. J. Clin. Oncol. 15:1814–1823; 1997.

Gregor, A.; Cull, A.; Stephens, R. J.; Kirkpatrick, J. A.; Yarnold, J. R.; Girling, D. J.; Macbeth, F. R.; Stout, R.; Machin, D. Prophylactic cranial irradiation is indicated following complete response to induction therapy in small cell lung cancer: results of a multi-centre randomised trial. United Kingdom Coordinating Committee for Cancer Research (UKCCCR) and the European Organization for Research and Treatment of Cancer. Eur. J. Cancer 33:1752–1758; 1997.

Haddock, M. G.; Schild, S. C.; Scheithauer, B. W.; Schomberg, P. J. Radiation therapy for histologically confirmed primary central nervous system germinoma. Int. J. Radiat. Oncol. Biol. Phys. 38:915–923; 1997.

Halperin, E. C.; Friedman, H. S. Is there a correlation between duration of presenting symptoms and stage of medulloblastoma at the time of diagnosis? Cancer 78:874–880; 1996.

Halperin, E. C.; Friedman, H. S.; Schold, S. C. Jr.; Fuchs, H. E.; Oakes, W. J.; Hochenberger, B.; Burger, P. C. Surgery, hyperfractionated craniospinal irradiation, and adjuvant chemotherapy in the management of supratentorial embryonal neuroepithelial neoplasms in children. Surg. Neurol. 40:278–283; 1993.

Hamilton, C. R., Jr.; Adams, L. C.; Maloof, F. Hyperthyroidism due to the thyrotropin-producing pituitary chromophobe adenoma. N. Engl. J. Med. 280: 1077–1080; 1970.

Hammoud, M. A.; McCutcheon, I. E.; Elsouki, R.; Schoppa, D.; Patt, Y. Z. Colorectal carcinoma and brain metastasis: distribution, treatment, and survival. Ann. Surg. Oncol. 3:453–463; 1996.

Hardenbergh, P. H.; Golden, J.; Billet, A.; Scott, R. M.; Shrieve, D. C.; Silver, B.; Loeffler, J. S.; Tarbell, N. J. Intracranial germinoma: the case for lower dose radiation therapy. Int. J. Radiat. Oncol. Biol. Phys. 39:419–426; 1997.

Hassounah, M.; Siqueira, E. B.; Haider, A.; Gray, A. Cerebellar astrocytoma: report of 13 cases aged over 20 years and review of the literature. Br. J. Neurosurg. 10:365–371; 1996.

Helseth, A.; Mrk, S. J. Primary intraspinal neoplasms in Norway, 1955 to 1986. A population-based survey of 467 patients. J. Neurosurg. 71:842–845; 1989.

Hochberg, F. H.; Miller, D. C. Primary central nervous system lymphoma. J. Neurosurg. 68:835–853; 1988.

Huh, S. J.; Shin, K. H.; Kim, I. H.; Ahn, Y. C.; Ha, S. W.; Park, C. I. Radiotherapy of intracranial germinomas. Radiother. Oncol. 38:19–23; 1996.

Hulshof, M. C. C. M.; Menten, J.; Dito, J. J.; Dreissen, J. J. R.; van den Bergh, R.; Gonzalez Gonzalez, D. Treatment results in primary intraspinal gliomas. Radiother. Oncol. 29:294–300; 1993.

Jaaskelainen, J.; Haltia, M.; Servo, A. Atypical and anaplastic meningiomas: radiology, surgery, radiotherapy, and outcome. Surg. Neurol. 25:233–242; 1986.

Jakacki, R. I.; Zeltzer, P. M.; Boyett, J. M.; Albright, A. L.; Allen, J. C.; Geyer, J. R.; Rorke, L. B.; Stanley, P.; Stevens, K. R.; Wisoff, J.; et al. Survival and prognostic factors following radiation and/or chemotherapy for primitive neuroectodermal tumors of the pineal region in infants and children: a report of the Children's Cancer Group. J. Clin. Oncol. 13: 1377–1383; 1995.

Jenkin, D. Posterior fossa tumors in childhood: radiation treatment. Clin. Neurosurg. 30:203; 1983.

Jennings, A. S.; Liddle, G. W.; Orth, D. N. Results of treating childhood Cushing's disease with pituitary irradiation. N. Engl. J. Med. 297:957–962; 1977.

Jennings, M. T.; Gelman, R.; Hochberg, F. Intracranial germ-cell tumors: natural history and pathogenesis. J. Neurosurg. 63:155–167; 1985.

Kaba, S. E.; DeMonte, F.; Bruner, J. M.; Kyritsis, A. P.; Jaeckle, K. A.; Levin, V. A.; Yung, W. K. The treatment of recurrent unresectable and malignant meningiomas with interferon alpha 2-B. Neurosurgery 40:271–275; 1997.

Kepes, J. J. Meningiomas: biology, pathology, and differential diagnosis. New York: Masson; 1982.

Kernohan, J. W.; Uhlheim, A. Sarcomas of the brain. Springfield, IL: Charles C Thomas; 1962.

Khatib, Z. A.; Heideman, R. L.; Kovnar, E. H.; Langston, J. A.; Sanford, R. A.; Douglas, E. C.; Ochs, J.; Jenkins, J. J.; Faircloth, D. L.; Greenwald, C.; et al. Predominance of pilocytic histology in dorsally exophytic brain stem tumors. Pediatr. Neurosurg. 20: 2– 10; 1994.

Kim, L.; Hochberg, F. H.; Thornton, A. F.; Harsh, G. R.; Patel, H.; Finkelstein, D.; Louis, D. N. Procarbazine, lomustine, and vincristine (PCV) chemotherapy for grade III and grade IV oligoastrocytomas. J. Neurosurg. 85:602–607; 1996a.

Kim, D. G.; Nam, D. H.; Jung, H. W.; Choi, K. S.; Han, D. H. Primary central nervous system lymphoma: variety of clinical manifestations and survival. Acta Neurochir. (Wien) 138:280–289; 1996b.

Kjellberg, R. N.; Kliman, B. Radiosurgery therapy for pituitary adenoma. In: Post, K. D.; Jackson, I. M. D.; Reichlin, S., eds. The pituitary adenoma. New York: Plenum; 1980: p. 459–478.

Kleinberg, D. L.; Noel, G. L.; Frantz, A. G. Galactorrhea: a study of 235 cases, including 48 with pituitary tumors. N. Engl. J. Med. 296:588–600; 1977.

Kobayashi, T.; Tanaka, T.; Kida, Y. Stereotactic gamma radiosurgery for craniopharyngiomas. Pediatr. Neurosurg. 21 (suppl. 1): 69–74; 1994.

Kobayashi, T.; Yoshida, J.; Ishiyama, J.; Noda, S.; Kito, A.; Kita, Y. Combination chemotherapy with cisplatin and etoposide for malignant intracranial germ-cell tumors. An experimental and clinical study. J. Neurosurg. 70:676–681; 1989.

Kovacs, K.; Horvath, E. Pathology of pituitary tumors. In: Endocrinology and metabolism clinics of north america, 16: 3. Philadelphia: W.B. Saunders Co.; 1987: p. 529–551.

Kramer, J. H.; Crowe, A. B.; Larson, D. A.; Sneed, P. K.; Gutin, P. H.; McDermott, M. W.; Prados, M. D. Neuropsychological sequelae of medulloblastoma in adults. Int. J. Radiat. Oncol. Biol. Phys. 38:21–26; 1997.

Kreiger, D. T. Pharmacological therapy of Cushing's disease and Nelson's syndrome. In: Linfoot, J. A., ed. Recent advances in the diagnosis and treatment of pituitary tumors. New York: Raven Press; 1979: p. 337–340.

Kros, J. M.; Hop, W. C. J.; Godschalk, J. J. C. J.; Krishnadath, K. K. Prognostic value of the proliferation-related antigen Ki-67 in oligodendrogliomas. Cancer 78:1107–1113; 1996.

Kros, J. M.; Pieterman, H.; van Eden, C. G.; Avezaat, C. J. J. Oligodendroglioma: the Rotterdam-Dijkzigt experience. Neurosurgery 34:959–966; 1994.

Kun, L. E.; Kovnar, E. H.; Sanford, R. A. Ependymomas in children. Pediatr. Neurosci. 14:57–63; 1988.

Lagerwaard, F. J.; Levendag, P. C.; Nowak, P. J.; Eijkenboom, W. M.; Hanssens, P. E.; Schmitz, P. I. Identification of prognostic factors in patients with brain metastases: a review of 1292 patients. Int. J. Radiat. Oncol. Biol. Phys. 43:795–803; 1999.

Lamberts, S. W.; Uitterlinden, J. P.; Verschoor, L.; van Dongen, K. J.; del Pozo, E. Long-term treatment of acromegaly with the somatostatin analogue SMS 201-995. N. Engl. J. Med. 313:1576–1580; 1985.

Landolfi, J. C.; Thaler, H. T.; DeAngelis, L. M. Adult brainstem gliomas. Neurology 51:1136–1139; 1998.

Lang, F. F.; Sawaya, R. Surgical treatment of metastatic brain tumors. Semin. Surg. Oncol. 14:53–63; 1998.

Lapras, C. Surgical therapy of pineal region tumors. In: Neuwelt, E., ed. Diagnosis and treatment of pineal region tumors. Baltimore: Williams & Wilkins; 1984: p. 289—299.

Lassman, L. P.; Arjona, V. E. Pontine gliomas of childhood. Lancet 1: 913–915; 1967.

Laws, E. R.; Taylor, W. F.; Bergstrahl, E. J.; Okazaki, H.; Clifton, M. B. The neurosurgical management of low-grade astrocytoma. J. Neurosurg. 61: 665–673; 1984.

Le, Q. T.; Weil, M. D.; Wara, W. M.; Lamborn, K. R.; Prados, M. D.; Edwards, M. S.; Gutin, P. H. Adult medulloblastoma: an analysis of survival and prognostic factors. Cancer J. Sci. Am. 3: 238–245; 1997.

Leibel, S. A.; Sheline, G. E. Radiation therapy for neoplasms of the brain. J. Neurosurg. 66:1–22; 1987.

Leibel, S. A.; Sheline, G. E.; Wara, W. M.; Boldrey, E. B.; Nielsen, S. L. The role of radiation therapy in the treatment of astrocytomas. Cancer 35: 1551–1557; 1975.

Leo, E.; Schlegel, P. G.; Lindemann, A. Chemotherapeutic induction of long-term remission in metastatic medulloblastoma. J. Neurooncol. 32:149–154; 1997.

Levin, V. A.; Edwards, M. S. B.; Gutin, P. H.; Vestnys, P.; Fulton, D.; Seager, M.; Wilson, C. B. Phase II evaluation of dibromodulcitol in the treatment of recurrent medulloblastoma, ependymoma, and malignant astrocytoma. J. Neurosurg. 61:1063–1068; 1984.

Levin, V. A.; Edwards, M. S.; Wara, W. M.; Allen, J.; Ortega, J.; Vetsnys, P. S. 5-fluorouracil and CCNU followed by hydroxyurea, misonidazole and irradiation for brain stem gliomas: a pilot study of the Brain Tumor Research Center and the Childrens Cancer Group. Neurosurgery 14:679–681; 1984.

Levin, V. A., Hoffman, W., Heilbron, D. C., Norman, D., Wilson, C. B. Prognostic significance of the pre-treatment CT scan on time to progression for patients with malignant gliomas. J. Neurosurg. 52:642–647; 1980.

Levin, V. A.; Prados, M. R.; Wara, W. M.; Davis, R. L.; Gutin, P. H.; Philips, T. L.; Lamborn, K.; Wilson, C. B. Radiation therapy with bromodeoxyuridine followed by CCNU, procarbazine, and vincristine (PCV) chemotherapy for the treatment of anaplastic gliomas. Int. J. Radiat. Oncol. Biol. Phys. 32(1): 75–83; 1995.

Levin, V. A.; Rodriguez, L. A.; Edwards, M. S.; Wara, W.; Liu, H. C.; Fulton, D.; Davis, R. L.; Wilson, C. B.; Silver, P. Treatment of medulloblastoma with procarbazine, hydroxyurea, and reduced radiation doses to whole brain and spine. J. Neurosurg. 68: 383–387; 1988.

Levin, V. A.; Leibel, S. A.; Gutin, P. H. Neoplasms of the central nervous system. In: DeVita, V. T., Jr.; Hellman, S., Rosenberg, S. A., eds. Cancer: principles and practice of oncology. 5th ed. Philadelphia: Lippincott-Raven; 1997: p. 2022–2082.

Levin, V. A.; Silver, P.; Hannigan, J.; Wara, W. M.; Gutin, P. H.; Davis, R. L.; Wilson, C. B. NCOG 6G61 final report: superiority of post-radiotherapy adjuvant chemotherapy with CCNU, procarbazine, and vincristine (PCV) over BCNU for anaplastic gliomas. Int. J. Radiat. Oncol. Phys. Biol. 18: 321– 324; 1990.

Levin, V. A.; Vestnys, P. S.; Edwards, M. S.; Wara, W. M.; Fulton, D.; Barger, G.; Seager, M.; Wilson, C. B. Improvement in survival produced by sequential therapies in the treatment of recurrent medulloblastoma. Cancer 51:1364–1370; 1983.

Loeffler, J. S.; Kretschmar, C. S.; Sallan, S. E.; LaVally, B. L.; Winston, K. R.; Fischer, E. G.; Tarbell, N. J. Pre-radiation chemotherapy for infants and poor prognosis children with medulloblastoma. Int. J. Radiat. Oncol. Biol. Phys. 15:177–181; 1988.

Lote, K.; Egeland, T.; Hager, B.; Stenwig, B.; Skullerud, K.; Berg-Johnsen, J.; Storm-Mathisen, I.; Hirschberg, H. Survival, prognostic factors, and therapeutic efficacy in low-grade glioma: a retrospective study in 379 patients. J. Clin. Oncol. 15: 3129–3140; 1997.

Ludwig, C. L.; Smith, M. T.; Godfrey, A. D.; Armbrustmacher, V. W. A clinicopathologic study of 323 patients with oligodendrogliomas. Ann. Neurol. 19: 15–21; 1986.

Ludwin, S. K.; Rubinstein, L. J.; Russell, D. S. Papillary meningioma: a malignant variant of meningioma. Cancer 36:1363–1373; 1975.

Lukes, A.; Wollmann, R.; Stefannson, K. Meningeal sarcomatosis and multiple astrocytomas. Arch. Neurol. 40:179–182; 1983.

Lutchman, M.; Rouleau, G. A. Neurofibromatosis type 2: a new mechanism of tumor suppression. Trends Neurosci. 19:373–377; 1996.

McCormack, B. M.; Miller, D. C.; Budzilovich, G. N. Treatment and survival of low-grade astrocytoma in adults—1977–1988. Neurosurgery 31:636–642; 1992.

McCutcheon, I. E. Pituitary tumors. In: Levin, V. A., ed. Cancer in the nervous system. New York: Churchill Livingstone; 1996: p. 231.

McKeever, P. E.; Ross, D. A.; Strawderman, M. S.; Brunberg, J. A.; Greenberg, H. S.; Junck, L. A comparison of the predictive power for survival in gliomas provided by MIB-1, bromodeoxyuridine and proliferating cell nuclear antigen with histopathologic and clinical parameters. J. Neuropathol. Exp. Neurol. 56:798–805; 1997.

Mahaley, M. S.; Mettlin, C.; Natarajan, N.; Laws, E. R.; Peace, B. National survey of patterns of care of brain tumor patients. J. Neursurg. 71:826–836; 1989.

Mahoney, D. H., Jr.; Strother, D.; Camitta, B.; Bowen, T.; Ghim, T.; Pick, T.; Wall, D.; Yu, L.; Shuster, J. J.; Friedman, H. High-dose melphalan and cyclophosphamide with autologous bone marrow rescue for recurrent/progressive malignant brain tumors in children: a pilot pediatric oncology group study. J. Clin. Oncol. 14:382–388; 1996.

Matsutani, M.; Sano, K.; Takakura, K.; Fujimaki, T.; Nakamura, O.; Funata, N.; Seto, T. Primary intracranial germ cell tumors: a clinical analysis of 153 histologically verified cases. J. Neurosurg. 86:446–455; 1997.

Mena, H.; Rushing, E. J.; Ribas, J. L.; Delahunt, B.; McCarthy, W. F. Tumors of pineal parenchymal cells: a correlation of histological features, including nucleolar organizer regions, with survival in 35 cases. Hum. Pathol. 26:20–30; 1995.

Merchant, T. E.; Davis, B. J.; Sheldon, J. M.; Leibel, S. A. Radiation therapy for relapsed germinoma after primary chemotherapy. J. Clin. Oncol. 16:204–209; 1998.

Mintz, A. H.; Kestle, J.; Rathbone, M. P.; Gaspar, L.; Hugenholtz, H.; Fisher, B.; Duncan, G.; Skingley, P.; Foster, G.; Levine, M. A randomized trial to assess the efficacy of surgery in addition to radiotherapy in patients with a single cerebral metastasis. Cancer 78:1470–1476; 1996.

Mirimanoff, R. O.; Dosoretz, D. E.; Linggood, R. M. Meningioma: analysis of recurrence and progression following neurosurgical resection. J. Neurosurg. 62:18–24; 1985.

Moghrabi, A.; Kerby, T.; Tien, R. D.; Friedman, H. S. Prognostic value of contrast-enhanced magnetic resonance imaging in brainstem gliomas. Pediatr. Neurosurg. 23:293–298; 1995.

Moser, R. P.; Backlund, E. O. Stereotactic techniques in the diagnosis and treatment of pineal region tumors. In: Neuwelt, E., ed. Diagnosis and treatment of pineal region tumors. Baltimore: Williams & Wilkins; 1984: p. 236–253.

Moser, R. P.; Johnson, M. L. Surgical management of brain metastases: how aggressive should we be? Oncology 3:123–134; 1989.

Motti, E. D.; Losa, M.; Pieralli, S.; Zecchinelli, A.; Longobardi, B.; Giugni, E.; Ventrella, L. Stereotactic radiosurgery of pituitary adenomas. Metabolism 45 (8 suppl. 1):111–114; 1996.

Nazar, G. B.; Hoffman, H. J.; Becker, L. E.; Jenkin, D.; Humphreys, R. P.; Hendrick, E. B. Infratentorial ependymomas in childhood: prognostic factors and treatment. J. Neurosurg. 72:408–417; 1990.

Needle, M. N.; Molloy, P. T.; Geyer, J. R.; Herman-Liu, A.; Belasco, J. B.; Goldwein, J. W.; Sutton, L.; Phillips, P. C. Phase II study of daily oral etoposide in children with recurrent brain tumors and other solid tumors. Med. Pediatr. Oncol. 29:28–32; 1997.

Nelson, D. F.; Martz, K. L.; Bonner, H.; Nelson, J. S.; Newall, J.; Kerman, H. D.; Thomson, J. W.; Murray, K. J. Non-Hodgkin's lymphoma of the brain: can high dose, large volume radiation therapy improve survival? Report on a prospective trial by the Radiation Therapy Oncology Group (RTOG): RTOG 8315. Int. J. Radiat. Oncol. Biol. Phys. 23:9–17; 1992.

Nieder, C.; Walter, K.; Nestle, U.; Schnabel, K. Ten years disease-free survival after solitary brain metastasis from breast cancer. J. Cancer. Res. Clin. Oncol. 122:570–572; 1996.

Nussbaum, E. S.; Djalilian, H. R.; Cho, K. H.; Hall, W. A. Brain metastases. Histology, multiplicity, surgery, and survival. Cancer 78:1781–1788; 1996.

Packer, R. J.; Boyett, J. M.; Zimmerman, R. A.; Albright, A. L.; Kaplan, A. M.; Rorke, L. B.; Selch, M. T.; Cherlow, J. M.; Finlay, J. L.; Wara, W. M. Outcome of children with brain stem gliomas after treatment with 7800 cGy of hyperfractionated radiotherapy. A Childrens Cancer Group Phase I/II Trial. Cancer 74:1827–1834, 1994.

Packer, R. J.; Sutton, L. N.; Rorke, L. B.; Rosenstock, J. G.; Zimmerman, R. A.; Littman, P.; Bilaniuk, L. T.; Bruce, D. A.; Schut, L. Intracranial embryonal cell carcinoma. Cancer 54:520–524; 1984.

Packer, R. J.; Siegel, K. R.; Sutton, L. N.; Evans, A. E.; DAngio, G.; Rorke, L. B.; Bunin, G. R.; Schut, L. Efficacy of adjuvant chemotherapy for patients with poor-risk medulloblastoma: a preliminary report. Ann. Neurol. 24:503–508; 1988.

Palma, L.; Celli, P.; Franco, C.; Cervoni, L.; Cantore, G. Long-term prognosis for atypical and malignant meningiomas: a study of 71 surgical cases. J. Neurosurg. 86:793–800; 1997.

Panitch, H. S.; Berg, B. O. Brain stem tumors of childhood and adolescence. Am. J. Dis. Child. 119:465–472; 1970.

Park, T. S.; Hoffman, H. J.; Hendrick, E. B.; Humphreys, R. P. Medulloblastoma: clinical presentation and management. Experience at the Hospital For Sick Children, Toronto, 1950–1980. J. Neurosurg. 58:543–552; 1983.

Parl, F. F.; Cruz, V. E.; Cobb, C. A.; Bradley, C. A.; Aleshire, S. L. Late recurrence of surgically removed prolactinomas. Cancer 57:2422–2426; 1986.

Patchell, R. A.; Cirrincione, C.; Thaler, H. T.; Galicich, J. H.; Kim, J. H.; Posner, J. B. Single brain metastases: surgery plus radiation or radiation alone. Neurology 36:447–453; 1986.

Patchell, R. A.; Tibbs, P. A.; Walsh, J. W.; Dempsey, R. J.; Maruyama, Y.; Kryscio, R. J.; Markesbery,

W. R.; MacDonald, J. S.; Young, B. A randomized trial of surgery in the treatment of single metastases to the brain. N. Engl. J. Med. 322:494–500; 1990.

Pelkonen, R.; Grahne, B.; Hirvonen, E.; Karonen, S.; Salmi, J.; Tikkanen, M.; Valtonen, S. Pituitary function in prolactinoma: effect of surgery and postoperative bromocriptine therapy. Clin. Endocrinol. 14:335–348; 1981.

Pencalet, P.; Maixner, W.; Sainte-Rose, C.; Lellouch-Tubiana, A.; Cinalli, G.; Zerah, M.; Pierre-Kahn, A.; Hoppe-Hirsch, E.; Bourgeois, M.; Renier, D. Benign cerebellar astrocytomas in children. J. Neurosurg. 90:265–273; 1999.

Perilongo, G.; Massamino, M.; Sotti, G.; Belfontali, T.; Masiero, L.; Rigobello, L.; Garre, L.; Carli, M.; Lombardi, F.; Solero, C.; Sainati, L.; Canale, V.; del Prever, A. B.; Giangaspero, F.; Andreussi, L.; Mazza, C.; Madon, E. Analyses of prognostic factors in a retrospective review of 92 children with ependymoma: Italian Pediatric Neuro-oncoloy Group. Med. Pediatr. Oncol. 29:79–85; 1997.

Peterson, K.; Cairncross, J. G. Oligodendroglioma. Cancer Invest. 14:243–251; 1996.

Peterson, K.; Paleologos, N.; Forsyth, P.; Macdonald, D. R.; Cairncross, J. G. Salvage chemotherapy for oligodendroglioma. J. Neurosurg. 85:597–601; 1996.

Petronio, J. A.; Edwards, M. S. B. Management of brainstem tumors in children. Contemp. Neurosurg. 11:1–6; 1989.

Philippon, J. H.; Clemenceau, S. H.; Fauchon, F. H.; Foncin, J. F. Supratentorial low-grade astrocytomas in adults. Neurosurgery 32:554–559; 1993.

Phillips, T. L.; Levin, V. A.; Ahn, D. K.; Gutin, P. H.; Davis, R. L.; Wilson, C. B.; Prados, M. D.; Wara, W. M.; Flam, M. S. Evaluation of bromodeoxyuridine in glioblastoma multiforme: a Northern California Cancer Center phase II study. Int. J. Radiat. Oncol. Biol. Phys. 21:709–714; 1991.

Pieper, D. R.; Hess, K. R.; Sawaya, R. E. Role of surgery in the treatment of brain metastases in patients with breast cancer. Ann. Surg. Oncol. 4: 481–490; 1997.

Pollack, I. F.; Gerszten, P. C.; Martinez, A. J.; Lo, K.; Shultz, B.; Albright, A. L.; Janosky, J.; Deutsch, M. Intracranial ependymomas of childhood: long-term outcome and prognostic factors. Neurosurgery 37: 655–667; 1995.

Pollak, L.; Gur, R.; Walach, N.; Reif, R.; Tamir, L.; Schiffer, J. Clinical determinants of long-term survival in patients with glioblastoma multiforme. Tumori 83:613–617; 1997.

Prados, M. D.; Wara, W. M.; Edwards, M. S.; Larson, D. A.; Lamborn, K.; Levin, V. A. The treatment of brain stem and thalamic gliomas with 78 Gy of hyperfractionated radiation therapy. Int. J. Radiat. Oncol. Biol. Phys. 32:85–91; 1995a.

Prados, M. D.; Warnick, R. E.; Wara, W. M.; Larson, D. A.; Lamborn, K.; Wilson, C. B. Medulloblastoma in adults. Int. J. Radiat. Oncol. Biol. Phys. 32: 1145–1152; 1995b.

Rainov, N. G.; Dobberstein, K-U.; Bahn, H.; Holzhauzen, H-J.; Lautenschlager, C.; Heidecke, V.; Burkert, W. Prognostic factors in malignant glioma: influence of the overexpression of oncogene and tumor-suppressor gene products on survival. J. Neurooncol. 35:13–28; 1997.

Rajan, B.; Ashley, S.; Gorman, C.; Jose, C. C.; Horwich, A.; Bloom H. J.; Marsh, H.; Brada, M. Craniopharyngioma—a long-term results following limited surgery and radiotherapy. Radiother. Oncol. 26: 1–10; 1993.

Rajan, B.; Ross, G.; Lim, C. C.; Ashley, S.; Goode, D.; Traish, D.; Brada, M. Survival in patients with recurrent glioma as a measure of treatment efficacy: prognostic factors following nitrosourea chemotherapy. Eur. J. Cancer 30A:1809–1815; 1994.

Rawlings, C. E., III; Giangaspero, F.; Burger, P. C.; Bullard, D. E. Ependymomas: a clinicopathologic study. Surg. Neurol. 29:271–281; 1988.

Regine, W. F.; Mohiuddin, M.; Kramer, S. Long-term results of pediatric and adult craniopharyngiomas treated with combined surgery and radiation. Radiother. Oncol. 27:13–21; 1993.

Reni, M.; Ferreri, A. J.; Zoldan, M. C.; Villa, E. Primary brain lymphomas in patients with a prior or concomitant malignancy. J. Neurooncol. 32: 135–142; 1997.

Rezai, A. R.; Woo, H. H.; Lee, M.; Cohen, H.; Zagzag, D.; Epstein, F. J. Disseminated ependymomas of the central nervous system. J. Neurosurg. 85:618–624; 1996.

Ritter, A. M.; Hess, K. R.; McLendon, R. E.; Langford, L. A. Ependymomas: MIB-1 proliferation index and survival. J. Neurooncol. 40:51–57; 1998.

Rochkind, S.; Blatt, I.; Sadeh, M.; Goldhammer, Y. Extracranial metastases of medulloblastoma in adults: literature review. J. Neurol. Neurosurg. Psychiatry 54:80–86; 1991.

Rodriguez, L. A; Prados, M.; David, R.; Gutin, P.; Wilson, C. B. Malignant meningiomas: an analysis of 35 cases (abstract #36). J. Neurosurg. 70:318A; 1989.

Rodriguez, L.; Prados, M.; Fulton, D.; Edwards, M. S. B.; Silver, P.; Levin, V. A. Treatment of recurrent brain stem glioma and other CNS tumors with 5-fluorouracil, CCNU, hydroxyurea, and 6-mercaptopurine. Neurosurgery 22:691–693; 1988.

Rosenblum, M. L.; Levy, R. M.; Bredesen, D. E.; So, Y. T.; Wara, W.; Ziegler, J. L. Primary central nervous system lymphomas in patients with AIDS. Ann. Neurol. 23(suppl.):13–16; 1988.

Ross, G. W.; Rubinstein, L. J. Lack of histopathological correlation of malignant ependymomas with postoperative survival. Neurosurgery 70:31–36; 1989.

Rousseau, P.; Habrand, J. L.; Sarrazin, D.; Kalifa, C.; Terrier-Lacombe, M. J.; Rekacewicz, C.; Rey, A. Treatment of intracranial ependymomas of children: review of a 15-year experience. Int. J. Radiat. Oncol. Biol. Phys. 28:381–384; 1994.

Rubinstein, L. Tumors of the central nervous system. Atlas of tumor pathology. 2nd Series, Fascicle 6. Washington, DC: AFIP; 1970.

Rubinstein, L. J. Sarcomas of the nervous system. In: Minckler, J., ed. Pathology of the nervous system. Vol. 2. New York: McGraw-Hill; 1977: p. 2144–2164.

Russell, D. S.; Rubinstein, L. J. Pathology of tumors of the nervous system, 4th ed. Baltimore: Williams & Wilkins; 1977.

Salazar, O. M. Ensuring local control in meningiomas. Int. J. Radiat. Oncol. Biol. Phys. 15:501–504; 1988.

Sampson, J. H.; Carter, J. H.; Friedman, A. H.; Seigler, H. F. Demographics, prognosis, and therapy in 702 patients with brain metastases from malignant melanoma. J. Neurosurg. 88:11–20; 1998.

Sano, T.; Lin, H,; Chen, X.; Langford, L. A.; Koul, D.; Bondy, M. L.; Hess, K. R.; Myers, J. N.; Hong, Y. K.; Yung, W. K.; Steck, P. A. Differential expression of MMAC/PTEN in glioblastoma multiforme: relationship to localization and prognosis. Cancer Res. 59:1820–1824; 1999.

Sawamura, Y.; Shirato, H.; Ikeda, J.; Tada, M.; Ishii, N.; Kato, T.; Abe, H.; Fujieta, K. Induction chemotherapy followed by reduced-volume radiation therapy for newly diagnosed central nervous system germinoma. J. Neurosurg. 88:66–72; 1998.

Sawaya, R.; Bindal, R. K. Metastatic brain tumors. In: Kaye, A. H.; Laws, E. R., Jr., eds. Brain tumors. Edinburgh: Churchill Livingstone; 1995: p. 924.

Schaller, C.; Kelly, P. J. Primary central nervous system non-Hodgkin's lymphoma (PCNSL): does age and histology at presentation affect outcome? Zentralbl. Neurochir. 57:156–162; 1996.

Schild, S. E.; Scheithauer, B. W.; Haddock, M. G.; Wong, W. W.; Lyons, M. K.; Marks, L. B.; Norman, M. G.; Burger, P. C. Histologically confirmed pineal tumors and other germ cell tumors of the brain. Cancer 78:2564–2571; 1996.

Schrell, U. M.; Rittig, M. G.; Anders, M.; Koch, U. H.; Marschalek, R.; Kiesewetter, F.; Fahlbusch, R. J. Hydroxyurea for treatment of unresectable and recurrent meningiomas. II. Decrease in the size of meningiomas in patients treated with hydroxyurea. Neurosurgery 86:840–844; 1997.

Sgouros, S.; Fineron, P. W.; Hockley, A. D. Cerebellar astrocytoma of childhood: long-term follow-up. Childs Nerv. Syst. 11:89–96; 1995.

Shahidi, H.; Kvale, P. A. Long-term survival following surgical treatment of solitary brain metastasis in non-small cell lung cancer. Chest 109:271–276; 1996.

Shapiro, K.; Till, K.; Grant, D. N. Craniopharyngiomas in childhood: a rational approach to treatment. J. Neurosurg. 50:617–623; 1979.

Shaw, E. G.; Evans, R. G.; Scheithauer, B. W.; Ilstrup, D. M.; Earle, J. D. Postoperative radiotherapy of intracranial ependymoma in pediatric and adult patients. Int. J. Radiat. Oncol. Biol. Phys. 13: 1457–1462; 1987.

Shaw, E. G.; Scheitauer, B. W.; O'Fallon, J. R. Management of supratentorial low-grade gliomas. Semin. Radiat. Oncol. 1:23; 1991.

Shaw, E. G.; Scheitauer, B. W.; O'Fallon, J. R.; Tazelaar, H. D.; Davis, D. H. Oligodendrogliomas: the Mayo Clinic experience. J. Neurosurg. 76:428–434; 1992.

Sheline, G. E. Radiation therapy of primary tumors. Semin. Oncol. 2:29; 1975.

Simpson, J. R.; Horton, J.; Scott, C.; Curran, W. J.; Rubin, P.; Fischbach, J.; Isaacson, S.; Rotman, M.; Asbel, S. O.; Nelson, J. S.; Weinstein, A. S.; Nelson, D. F. Influence of location and extent of surgical resection on survival of patients with glioblastoma multiforme: results of three consecutive radiation therapy oncology group (RTOG) clinical trials. Int. J. Radiat. Oncol. Biol. Phys. 26:239–244; 1993.

Simpson, J. R.; Scott, C. B.; Rotman, M.; Curran, W. J.; Constine, L. S., III; Fischbach, J.; Asbel, S. O. Race and prognosis of brain tumor patients entering multicenter clinical trials. Am. J. Clin. Oncol. 19: 114–120; 1996.

Simpson, R. H.; Phillips, J. I.; Miller, P.; Hagen, D.; Anderson, J. E. M. Intracerebral malignant fibrous histiocytoma. Clin. Neuropathol. 5:185–189; 1986.

Skullerud, K.; Loken, A. C. The prognosis in meningioma. Acta Neuropathol. (Berl.) 29:337–344; 1974.

Smith, D. F.; Hutton, J. L.; Sandemann, D.; Foy, P. M.; Shaw, M. D. M.; Williams, I. R.; Chadwick, D. W. The prognosis of primary intracranial tumours presenting with epilepsy: the outcome of medical and surgical management. J. Neurol. Neurosurg. Psychiatry 54:915–920; 1991.

Soffietti, R.; Chio, A.; Giordana, M. T.; Vasario, E.; Schiffer, D. Prognostic factors in well-differentiated cerebral astrocytomas in the adult. Neurosurgery 24: 686–692; 1989.

Squires, L. A.; Allen, J. C.; Abbott, R.; Epstein, F. J. Focal tectal tumors: management and prognosis. Neurology 44:953–956; 1994.

Stein, B. M. Supracerebellar-infratentorial approach to pineal tumors. Surg. Neurol. 11:331–337; 1979.

Stelzer, K. J.; Sauve, K. I.; Spence, A. M.; Griffin, T. W.; Berger, M. S. Corpus callosum involvement as a prognostic factor for patients with high-grade astrocytoma. Int. J. Radiat. Oncol. Biol. Phys. 38: 27–30; 1997.

Stroink, A. R.; Hoffman, H. J.; Hendrick, E. B.; Humphreys, R. P.; Davidson, G. Transependymal benign dorsally exophytic brain stem gliomas of childhood: diagnosis and treatment recommendations. Neurosurgery 20:439–444; 1987.

Sung, D. I.; Chang, C. H.; Harisiades, L.; Carmel, P. W. Treatment results of craniopharyngiomas. Cancer 47:847–852; 1981.

Taylor, B. W., Jr.; Marcus, R. B., Jr.; Friedman, W. A.; Ballinger, W. E., Jr.; Million, R. R. The meningioma controversy: prospective radiotherapy. Int. J. Radiat. Oncol. Biol. Phys. 15:299–304; 1988.

Tomei, G.; Grimaldi, N.; Cappricci, E.; Sganzerla, E. P.; Gaini, S. M.; Villani, R.; Masini, B. Primary intracranial rhabdomyosarcoma: report of two cases. Childs Nerv. Syst. 5:246–249; 1989.

Tyrrell, J. B.; Brooks, R. M.; Fitzgerald, P. A.; Cofoid, P. B.; Forshaw, P. H.; Wilson, C. B. Selective transsphenoidal resection of pituitary adenomas. N. Engl. J. Med. 298:753–758; 1978.

van Eys, J.; Baram, T. Z.; Cangir, A.; Bruner, J. M.; Martinez-Prieto, J. Salvage chemotherapy for recurrent primary brain tumors in children. J. Pediatr. 113: 601–606; 1988.

Vermeulen, S. S. Whole brain radiotherapy in the treatment of metastatic brain tumors. Semin. Surg. Oncol. 14:64–69; 1998.

Villani, R. M.; Tomei, G.; Bello, L.; Sganzerla, E.; Ambrosi, B.; Re, T.; Giovanelli Barilari, M. Long-term results of treatment for craniopharyngioma in children. Childs Nerv. Syst. 13:397–405; 1997.

Wagner, H., Jr. Prophylactic cranial irradiation for patients with small cell lung cancer. An enduring controversy. Chest Surg. Clin. North Am. 7:151–166; 1997.

Waldron, J. N.; Laperriere, N. J.; Jaakkimainen, L.; Simpson, W. J.; Payne, D.; Milosevic, M.; Wong, C. S. Spinal cord ependymomas: a retrospective analysis of 59 cases. Int. J. Radiat. Oncol. Biol. Phys. 27:223–229; 1993.

Walker, M. D.; Alexander, E., Jr.; Hunt, W. E.; MacCarty, C. S.; Mahaley, M. S., Jr.; Mealey, J., Jr.; Norrell, H. A.; Owens, G.; Bansohoff, I.; Wilson, C. B.; Gehan, E. A.; Strike, T. A. Evaluation of BCNU and/or radiotherapy in the treatment of anaplastic gliomas. A cooperative clinical trial. J. Neurosurg. 49:333–343; 1978.

Walker, M. D.; Strike, T. A.; Sheline, G. E. An analysis of dose-effect relationship in the radiotherapy of malignant gliomas. Int. J. Radiat. Oncol. Biol. Phys. 5:1725–1731; 1979.

Wallner, K. E.; Gonzales, M.; Sheline, G. E. Treatment of oligodendrogliomas with or without postoperative irradiation. J. Neurosurg. 68:684–688; 1988.

Wallner, K. E.; Wara, W. M.; Sheline, G. E.; Davis, R. L. Intracranial ependymomas: results of treatment with partial or whole brain irradiation without spinal irradiation. Int. J. Radiat. Oncol. Biol. Phys. 12: 1937–1941; 1986.

Wara, W. M.; Sneed, P. K.; Larson, D. A. The role of radiation therapy in the treatment of craniopharyngioma. Pediatr. Neurosurg. 21(suppl. 1): 98–100; 1994.

Wen, B. C.; Hussey, D. H.; Staples, J.; et al. A comparison of the roles of surgery and radiation therapy in the management of craniopharyngiomas. Int. J. Radiat. Oncol. Biol. Phys. 16:17–24; 1989.

Wronski, M.; Arbit, E. Resection of brain metastases from colorectal carcinoma in 73 patients. Cancer 85:1677–1685; 1999.

Yap, B. S.; Baker, L. H.; Sinkovics, J. G.; Rivkin, S. E.; Bottomley, R.; Thigpen, T.; Burgess, M. A.; Benjamin, R. S.; Bodey, G. P. Cyclophosphamide, vincristine, adriamycin, and DTIC (CYVADIC) combination chemotherapy for the treatment of advanced sarcomas. Cancer Treat. Rep. 64:93–98; 1980.

Yoshida, J.; Sugita, K.; Kobayashi, T.; Takakura, K.; Shitara, N.; Matsutani, M.; Tanaka, R.; Nagai, H.; Yamada, H.; Yamashita, J.; et al. Prognosis of intracranial germ cell tumors: effectiveness of chemotherapy with cisplatin and etoposide (CDDP and VP-16). Acta Neurochir. (Wien) 120:111–117; 1993.

Young, R. F. Radiosurgery for the treatment of brain metastases. Semin. Surg. Oncol. 14:70–78; 1998.

Younis, G. A.; Sawaya, R.; DeMonte, F.; Hess, K. R.; Albrecht, S.; Bruner, J. M. Aggressive meningeal tumors: review of a series. J. Neurosurg. 82:17–27; 1995.

Zeltzer, P. M.; Boyett, J. M.; Finlay, J. L.; Albright, A. L.; Rorke, L. B.; Milstein, J. M.; Allen, J. C.; Stevens, K. R.; Stanley, P.; Li, H.; Wisoff, J. H.; Geyer, J. R.; McGuire-Cullen, P.; Stehbens, J. A.; Shurin, S. B.; Packer, R. J. Metastasis stage, adjuvant treatment, and residual tumor are prognostic factors for medulloblastoma in children: conclusions from the Children's Cancer Group 921 randomized phase III study. J. Clin. Oncol. 17:832–845; 1999.

Zierhut, D.; Flentje, M.; Adolph, J.; Erdmann, J.; Raue, F.; Wannenmacher, M. External radiotherapy of pituitary adenomas. Int. J. Radiat. Oncol. Biol. Phys. 33:307–314; 1995.

Zulch, K. J. Brain tumors. Their biology and physiology. 3rd ed. New York: Springer; 1986.

# 27

# Paraneoplastic Diseases of the Nervous System

JOSEP O. DALMAU AND S. CLIFFORD SCHOLD, JR.

Paraneoplastic diseases of the nervous system are definable, nonmetastatic neurological syndromes that occur in association with systemic malignancy (Henson and Urich 1982; Posner 1995). These conditions are rare, and they should be considered only after the more common causes of neurological dysfunction in patients with cancer have been excluded (Table 27-1) (Dalmau 1997). These "remote effects" of cancer on the nervous system can be organized according to the anatomical site of predominant involvement (Table 27-2). Although some paraneoplastic disorders are incompletely described or are recognized in only a few case reports, enough is known in other cases to permit a discussion of the prognosis of both the paraneoplastic syndrome (PNS) and the coexisting cancer.

Paraneoplastic syndromes of the nervous system influence a patient's prognosis in several ways. First, the remote effect itself may lead to death or severe disability because of neurological dysfunction. Second, recognition of the PNS may precede identification of the underlying malignancy, permitting earlier diagnosis and therefore perhaps more successful treatment of the tumor. Sometimes, the activity of the PNS parallels that of the tumor, providing a clinical "marker" of the neoplastic disease and allowing early recognition

of disease reactivation and again leading to earlier therapy. Finally, the presence of a PNS may be associated with an altered course of the underlying malignancy. This last consideration reflects the presence of complex immune responses, usually characterized by the presence of antineuronal antibodies, in an increasing number of paraneoplastic disorders (Posner 1995) (Table 27-3). In some syndromes, such as neuromyotonia and the Lambert-Eaton myasthenic syndrome (LEMS), the neurological symptoms result from a direct interaction of specific antibodies with target antigens (Lang and Vincent 1996). In other syndromes, the pathogenic role of antineuronal antibodies remains unproven, but they are used as reliable markers of specific neurological syndromes and distinct types of cancer (Dalmau 1997).

## Brain

Paraneoplastic encephalomyelitis is an inflammatory disorder that is characterized pathologically by perivascular lymphocytic infiltrates, astrocytosis, and neuronal loss (Henson et al. 1965). The predominant site of involvement and the most severely affected structures dictate the specific nomenclature and the signs and symptoms of this syndrome. Thus, in limbic encephalitis, the cin-

458

**Table 27-1.** Causes of Neurological Dysfunction
in Patients With Cancer

Metastatic nervous system disease
Metabolic derangements
Nutritional deficiencies
Opportunistic infections
Coagulopathy and cerebrovascular disorders
Complications of therapy
Paraneoplastic syndromes

gulate cortex, hippocampus, and amygdaloid nuclei are involved, and seizures, marked impairment in recent memory, mood changes, and confusion progressing to dementia constitute the clinical syndrome (Alamowitch et al. 1997; Brennan and Craddock 1983; Carr 1982; Corsellis et al. 1968; Dalmau et al. 1992; Halperin et al. 1981; Henson et al. 1965; Henson and Urich 1982; Kaplan and Stabashi 1974; Markham and Abeloff 1982) Involvement of the medullary and (to a lesser extent) pontine and mesencephalic nuclei produces a brain stem encephalitis with corresponding cranial nerve dysfunction. The basis for

**Table 27-2.** Paraneoplastic Nervous System Disorders

Brain
    Paraneoplastic encephalomyelitis* (limbic encephalitis, brain stem encephalitis, myelitis)
    Paraneoplastic cerebellar degeneration
    Paraneoplastic opsoclonus-myoclonus
    Visual paraneoplastic syndromes (cancer-associated retinopathy; optic neuritis)
Spinal cord
    Paraneoplastic necrotizing myelopathy
    Motor neuron syndromes (subacute motor neuronopathy, lower motor neuron, ALS)
Peripheral nerves
    Paraneoplastic sensory neuronopathy
    Sensorimotor neuropathies associated with plasma cell dyscrasias (POEMS, myeloma, Waldenström's macroglobulinemia)
    Acute polyradiculoneuropathy
    Brachial neuritis
    Vasculitis of nerve and mucle
    Subacute or chronic sensorimotor peripheral neuropathy
    Autonomic neuropathy
    Neuromyotonia
Neuromuscular junction
    Lambert-Eaton myasthenic syndrome
    Myasthenia gravis and thymoma
Muscle
    Polymyositis/dermatomyositis
    Acute necrotizing myopathy
    Carcinoid myopathy
    Cachectic myopathy
    Carcinomatous neuromyopathy

* Can include cerebral and cerebellar symptoms, autonomic dysfunction, and sensory neuronopathy.

this anatomical variability of what is considered a single disease entity is unknown.

The cerebrospinal fluid (CSF) in patients with paraneoplastic encephalomyelitis generally shows lymphocytosis, with an elevated protein concentration, intrathecal synthesis of immunoglobulin G (IgG), and oligoclonal bands. In patients with small cell lung cancer (SCLC) and paraneoplastic encephalomyelitis, serum and CSF studies usually demonstrate the presence of anti-Hu antibodies; these antibodies are less often found in association with neuroblastoma, and rarely with other tumors, even though the clinical syndromes are identical (Dalmau et al. 1992). In patients with limbic encephalitis, magnetic resonance imaging (MRI) studies often reveal abnormalities (usually with $T_2$-weighted images) in the medial aspect of the temporal lobes, with variable patchy areas of contrast enhancement (Dirr et al. 1990; Glantz et al. 1994). The electroencephalogram (EEG) may show bitemporal (or generalized) slowing with epileptiform activity in limbic encephalitis.

Age at onset and sex reflect the epidemiology of the underlying tumor—usually SCLC, less commonly non–small cell lung cancer, breast, testicular, ovarian, gastric, or uterine cancer or Hodgkin's disease. In two-thirds of the cases, presentation of the neurological disease precedes recognition of the tumor (Alamowitch et al. 1997; Brennan and Craddock 1983; Carr 1982; Corsellis et al. 1968; Dalmau et al. 1992; Halperin et al. 1981; Henson et al. 1965; Kaplan and Stabashi 1974; Markham and Abeloff 1982). The onset of symptoms (except seizures) is subacute, and a course of 2 to 24 months (average, 10.5 months) before diagnosis is typical. Rarely, effective treatment of the underlying malignancy results in neurological stability or improvement (Burton et al. 1988).

Paraneoplastic cerebellar degeneration (PCD) can be another form of presentation of paraneoplastic encephalomyelitis. In nearly 60% of patients, PCD also presents before recognition of an associated cancer (Anderson et al. 1988a; 1988d; Brain and Wilkinson 1965; Greenberg 1984; Greenlee and Brashear 1983; Greenlee and Lipton 1986; Mason et al. 1997; Peterson et al. 1992). Intervals of 1 month to 8 years between the onset of the neurological illness and the diagnosis of cancer have been reported, with a mean interval of about 6 months. SCLC, breast and ovarian cancers, and Hodgkin's disease are most commonly

**Table 27-3.** Antineuronal Antibodies Associated With Paraneoplastic Neurological Disorders

| Antibody | Antigen | Symptoms | Tumor* |
|---|---|---|---|
| Anti-Yo | 34 and 62 kDa (cytoplasm of Purkinje cells) | Cerebellar degeneration | Ovary, breast, Fallopian tube |
| Anti-Ri | 55 and 80 kDa (nuclei of neurons) | Opsoclonus, ataxia | Breast, SCLC |
| Anti-Hu | 35–40 kDa (nuclei of neurons) | Sensory neuronopathy, encephalomyelitis | SCLC Neuroblastoma |
| Anti-retinal | 23 (recoverin) 65, 145 205 kDa | Cancer-associated retinopathy | SCLC |
| Anti-VGCC | P/Q-type voltage-gated calcium channels MysB, synaptotagmin | LEMS | SCLC |
| Anti-Tr | Purkinje cells | Cerebellar degeneration | Hodgkin's |
| Anti-amphiphysin | 128 kDa (neuronal synapse) | Stiff-man | Breast, SCLC |
| Anti-CV2 | 66-kDa glial protein | Encephalomyelitis, cerebellar degeneration | SCLC, others |
| Anti-VGKC | α-Subunit of several VGKC | Neuromyotonia (Isaac's syndrome) | Thymoma, others |

* Most frequently associated tumor.

associated. Dramatic, selective loss of cerebellar Purkinje cells and frequently perivascular mononuclear infiltrates in the deep cerebellar white matter are identified at autopsy. Clinically, diffuse cerebellar dysfunction, with prominent dysarthria, gait ataxia, and eye movement abnormalities (nystagmus, ocular dysmetria, occasionally opsoclonus) develop over days to weeks. A mild lymphocytic pleocytosis, elevated protein concentration, oligoclonal bands, and an increased IgG index are the usual findings (Peterson et al. 1992). In contrast to other forms of paraneoplastic encephalomyelitis, patients with PCD often have anti-Yo (rather than anti-Hu) antibodies in their serum or CSF.

Cerebellar atrophy on computed tomography (CT) or MRI appears late in the course of the disease (Greenberg 1984; Mason et al. 1997). There have been a few reports of spontaneous arrest (rarely reversal) of this condition as well as rare instances of apparent response to vitamin supplementation, plasmapheresis, and other forms of immunosuppression (Anderson et al. 1988b; Auth

and Chodoff 1957; Batson et al. 1992; Cocconi et al. 1985; Counsell et al. 1994;Eekhof 1985; Kearsley et al. 1985; Paone and Jeyasingham 1980). As in other forms of paraneoplastic encephalomyelitis, there are reports in a few patients of remission of PCD following successful antineoplastic therapy, and recurrent cerebellar symptoms heralded the return of the tumor (Anderson et al. 1988d). Most often, the syndrome progresses to significant neurological disability, independent of age, sex, tumor type, CSF findings, or course of the underlying cancer.

Several other antineuronal antibodies have been demonstrated in the serum and CSF of patients with PCD (Table 27-4). In addition, the different antibodies are specifically associated with certain histological types of tumors, and their detection has prognostic significance (Mason et al. 1997; Voltz et al. 1997). For example, the detection of anti-Hu antibodies in a patient with presenting symptoms of cerebellar dysfunction indicates that the underlying disease is a diffuse paraneoplastic encephalomyelitis and that symptoms will likely

**Table 27-4.** Subtypes of Paraneoplastic Cerebellar Dysfunction

| Antibody | Sex | Tumor* | Onset[†] | Clinical findings |
|---|---|---|---|---|
| Anti-Yo | F | Ovary, breast | Before | Subacute pancerebellar symptoms |
| Anti-Hu | F > M | SCLC | Before | Sensory neuronopathy, encephalomyelitis[‡] |
| Anti-Ri | F | Breast | Before/after | Opsoclonus, truncal ataxia, myoclonus |
| Anti-Tr | M > F | Hodgkin's | After | May remit, less severe than other subtypes |
| PCD-LEMS Anti-VGCC | M = F | SCLC | Before | Pancerebellar symptoms with proximal weakness; decreased reflexes (LEMS may be overlooked) |

* Tumor most commonly associated.

† Onset of symptoms *before* or *after* the tumor diagnosis.

‡ A cerebellar syndrome can be the form of presentation of anti-Hu–associated encephalomyelitis and sensory neuronopathy.

progress to involve other areas of the nervous system. These patients frequently die as a result of the neurological dysfunction. In contrast, the presence of other antibodies (e.g., anti-Yo or anti-Tr) does not usually imply progression to other parts of the nervous system. Some patients with anti-Tr antibodies improve with treatment or spontaneously (Graus et al. 1997b).

The most common form of paraneoplastic encephalomyelitis in children is the opsoclonus-myoclonus syndrome seen in association with neuroblastoma. Between 2% and 3% of children with neuroblastoma are afflicted with this clinically striking syndrome (Altman and Baehner 1976; Pranzatelli et al. 1996; Rosen et al. 1984). Gait and limb ataxia, opsoclonus, and myoclonus constitute the clinical triad of this disorder. There are no consistent pathological abnormalities in the few autopsied cases, and elevated urinary or serum catecholamines do not influence the presentation or course of this disorder. Affected children are almost always 2 years old or younger at the onset of the neurological disorder, and the symptoms nearly always precede recognition of the associated tumor by 1 week to 4 years (Altman and Baehner 1976; Bray et al. 1969; Moe and Nellhaus 1970; Pranzatelli 1996; Rosen et al. 1984); Spontaneous remissions and relapses occur, and treatment with adrenocorticotropic hormone (ACTH) mitigates the neurological disorder in at least two-thirds of patients.

Successful treatment of the tumor is associated with resolution of the opsoclonus-myoclonus syndrome in up to 75% of cases. Nevertheless, residual ataxia and mental retardation are common (Russo et al. 1997). The tumor, when accompanied by opsoclonus-mycoclonus, generally is more benign, histologically (ganglioneuroma) and clinically (Evans stages I, II, or IV-S) and, even for tumors of the same stage, is associated with a notably better prognosis (Altman and Baehner 1976). The presence of a single copy of n-*myc* in neuroblastoma of most patients with opsoclonus, compared with the presence of multiple copies of this oncogene in the tumor of patients without opsoclonus, may explain the better tumor prognosis in the paraneoplastic patients (Cohn et al. 1988; Hiyama et al. 1994). Although, several antibodies have been detected in the serum of these patients (Antunes et al. 1997; Connolly et al. 1997), a reliable specific marker has not yet been identified.

A related syndrome, consisting of opsoclonus, myoclonus (predominantly truncal), ataxia, and encephalopathy, has been described as a complication of small cell carcinoma of the lung (more than half of the cases), non–small cell lung cancer and tumors of the bladder, thyroid, and bone (Anderson et al. 1988b). Onset is acute to subacute (2 weeks to 2 months) and precedes the diagnosis of cancer by 2 to 12 weeks (average, 3.5 weeks) in approximately 50% of patients. The CSF formula is similar to that in paraneoplastic encephalomyelitis, but autopsy findings and antibody studies generally have been unrevealing. Complete or partial remissions or a remitting and relapsing course occur in nearly two-thirds of patients, and some responses may have been related to treatment with clonazepam, thiamine, or effective cancer chemotherapy. Steroids have not been beneficial.

Patients with ataxia and opsoclonus associated with breast and gynecological cancers frequently develop antibodies (anti-Ri), which can be used as marker of the paraneoplastic disorder (Luque et al. 1991). Some of these patients improve with immunosuppression (Dropcho et al. 1993).

## Spinal Cord

Patients with anti-Hu–associated paraneoplastic encephalomyelitis may present with symptoms of spinal cord or lower motor neuron dysfunction (Forsyth et al. 1997; Verma et al. 1996). However, soon after initial presentation, these patients usually develop other symptoms that suggest more widespread neurological disease. There is no reason to believe that this syndrome differs pathophysiologically from the more common forms of encephalitis that are associated with the anti-Hu antibody.

Numerous case reports describe a paraneoplastic motor neuropathy affecting the lower motor neurons and occurring in patients with Hodgkin's and non-Hodgkin's lymphomas (Rowland and Schneck 1963; Schold et al. 1979; Walton et al. 1968). The clinical course is marked by generalized or asymmetrical muscle weakness, atrophy, fasciculations, and reduced tendon reflexes. The lower extremities often are more severely affected than the upper extremities. Bulbar involvement can occur; sensory symptoms if present are mild. Pathologically, anterior horn cell loss with variable (usually mild or absent) inflammation is seen.

Some loss of cells in Clarke's column also may occur. The onset of neurological symptoms followed the diagnosis of hematological malignancy by 2 to 7 months in 10 of 13 reported cases. Neurological improvement, sometimes a complete resolution of symptoms, occurred from 3 months to 3 years in eight of these cases, independent of the course of the cancer. Treatment with steroids has been ineffective. On the other hand, treatment of the underlying malignancy with vincristine may produce a temporary exacerbation of symptoms.

Patients with lymphoproliferative disorders may develop a combination of upper and lower motor neuron signs (Younger et al. 1991) indicating neurological dysfunction that is not restricted to anterior horn cells. In a prospective study, in which all patients with motor neuron disease had bone marrow biopsy, there was a higher than expected incidence of lymphoproliferative disorders (Rowland et al. 1992). However, treatment of the lymphoproliferative disease does not usually result in neurological improvement, and the relationship between the neurological and lymphoproliferative syndromes remains elusive.

Otherwise typical motor neuron disease has also been reported associated with tumors other than SCLC. No paraneoplastic markers have been identified in these patients. Although in most cases the association of neurological disease and cancer is probably coincidental, there are a few reports of patients whose motor neuron deficits improved or resolved after cancer treatment (Evans et al. 1990; Rosenfeld and Posner 1995).

A rare, fulminant spinal cord disorder has been reported in the setting of lymphoma; leukemia; and carcinomas of the lung, breast, prostate, kidney, stomach, thyroid, and ovary. This condition, which is called subacute necrotizing myelopathy, is characterized pathologically by indiscriminant spinal cord necrosis, most prominently in the mid-thoracic region (Gieron et al. 1987; Handforth et al. 1983; Ojeda 1984). Vasculopathy and inflammatory changes are absent. In one-third of cases, the onset of pain, ascending lower extremity weakness, paresthesias, and sphincter dysfunction precede the diagnosis of cancer. Red blood cells, white blood cells, and an elevated protein concentration usually are seen in the CSF. Myelography and CT of the spine are reliably normal. One case report (with autopsy confirmation of the diagnosis) describes increased $T_2$ signal on MRI without swelling or mass effect, corresponding to pathologically involved areas of the cervical spinal cord (Gieron et al. 1987). In another patient with non-SCLC and spinal cord biopsy suggestive of necrotizing myelopathy, the MRI demonstrated increased $T_2$ signal and patchy contrast enhancement in the mid and upper thoracic spinal cord (Glantz et al. 1994). The course is relentlessly progressive, and death, usually directly related to the neurological syndrome, occurs in an average of 5 weeks. The pathophysiology is unknown, and no known treatment alters the natural history. Acute necrotizing myelopathy may result in some instances from viral infections, particularly of the herpes group (Iwamasa 1989).

## Peripheral Nerves and Nerve Roots

Subacute sensory neuropathy (SSN), a pure sensory neuropathy that is analogous to the paraneoplastic inflammatory disorders of more rostral central nervous system (CNS) structures (limbic system, brain stem), is another well-described remote effect of cancer (Chalk et al. 1992; Wilkinson and Zeromski 1965; Dalmau et al. 1992; Denny-Brown 1948; Horwich et al. 1977). Pathologically, this condition is a dorsal root ganglionitis, resulting in the loss of neurons in the posterior root ganglia and wallerian degeneration of the posterior columns of the spinal cord and sensory fibers in peripheral nerves. In 70% of patients there is clinical or pathological evidence of a similar inflammatory process concurrently involving motor neurons, brain stem, cerebellum, or limbic structures. Pain, paresthesias, and a sensory ataxia dominate the clinical picture. The face and trunk can be affected, and sphincter dysfunction is rare. CSF protein concentration is elevated in most patients. SCLC is the most commonly associated tumor, although other lung cancers and cancers of the breast, ovary, esophagus, stomach, colon, and bladder are also represented. When the associated tumor is SCLC, anti-Hu antibodies are almost always present in the patient's serum (Anderson et al. 1988c; Budde-Steffen et al. 1988; Dalmau et al. 1992; Graus et al. 1985, 1986, 1987). Consequently, this disorder can be considered to be in the spectrum of paraneoplastic inflammatory conditions that are associated with anti-Hu antibodies.

In general, the signs and symptoms of SSN usually precede the diagnosis of cancer (approximately two-thirds of the cases) by 1 to 46 months. The course is subacute, with peak disability attained over several weeks to months. Spontaneous arrest of the disease process after months to 1 year leaves most patients moderately to severely impaired. The course of SSN, except in two case reports, (Sagar and Read 1982), is unrelated to the activity of the associated cancer and is unaltered by steroids, vitamins, immunomodulation (plasma exchange, intravenous immunoglobulin), or antineoplastic therapy (Graus et al. 1992; Posner 1995; Uchuya et al. 1996). Survival depends on the virulence of the underlying malignancy.

The prognosis of all forms of paraneoplastic conditions associated with the anti-Hu antibody is a subject of considerable interest and importance (Voltz et al. 1997). In general, the tumors of these patients are less aggressive than those not associated with anti-Hu antibodies. However, the neurological deficits may be severe and when there is a diffuse, widespread encephalomyelitis they are a common cause of death (Dalmau et al. 1992). Patients with a better prognosis are those whose symptoms remain confined to a sensory neuropathy and do not progress to encephalomyelitis. In some patients the sensory deficits are stable and indolent (Graus et al. 1994). Exceptional cases of spontaneous improvement (Byrne et al. 1997) and response to steroids (Oh et al. 1997) have been reported.

A prominent sensorimotor polyneuropathy, distinguished by concurrent dysfunction in multiple organ systems, and associated with plasma cell dyscrasia (usually osteosclerotic plasmacytomas) also has been reported (Bardwick et al. 1980; Kelly et al. 1983; Miralles et al. 1992; Resnick et al. 1981). In these patients, polyneuropathy, organomegaly, multiple endocrinopathies, M-proteins, skin changes (hyperpigmentation, anasarca), and papilledema (POEMS) may be seen. Features of this PNS precede (by 2 to 24 months on average) the diagnosis of a plasmacytoma in three-fourths of patients. The neurological component of the syndrome is the sole or prominent presenting symptom in most patients. A distal, symmetrical, sensorimotor polyneuropathy with gradual spread proximally is seen. Except for papilledema (present in about 40% of cases), cranial nerves are spared. The CSF protein concentration character-

istically is elevated, and nerve conduction velocities are markedly slowed. When the underlying disorder is an osteosclerotic myeloma, the neuropathy (and the other manifestations of POEMS syndrome) frequently improves or resolves following successful treatment of the tumor with local irradiation or surgery. Cross-reactivity between the tumor-derived abnormal protein and a component of peripheral myelin represents the likely pathogenic mechanism of this PNS (Mendell et al. 1985).

An ill-defined subacute or chronic sensorimotor polyneuropathy can occur in association with any malignancy, but it is most commonly seen with lung cancer (Croft et al. 1967). Patients develop symmetrical, distal paresthesias, sometimes associated with pain. There is loss of deep tendon reflexes and with time atrophy of the distal musculature. In most patients, symptoms are slowly progressive, and the motor weakness develops late. Less often, some patients may have remitting and relapsing symptoms. Electrodiagnostic and pathological studies demonstrate axonal degeneration, segmental demyelination, and less commonly, a combination of both. The underlying pathophysiology is not clear, and the neuropathy may be multifactorial. Generally, the neuropathy is not reversible unless a specific cause can be identified and corrected, but mortality is usually due to the underlying cancer and not to the neurological syndrome.

## The Neuromuscular Junction

The Lambert-Eaton myasthenic syndrome (LEMS) is an autoantibody-mediated neuromuscular disorder that occurs as a remote effect of cancer in two-thirds of affected patients and without a known associated cancer in the remainder (Engel 1984; Lambert et al. 1956; O' Neill et al. 1988). When cancer is present, SCLC of the lung is most common, and the tumor becomes clinically evident within 2 years of onset of the PNS in nearly all cases (O'Neill et al. 1988). Cancers of the breast, prostate, kidney, stomach, and rectum also have been reported, but they may reflect chance associations. In both groups, an increased incidence of other autoantibodies, systemic autoimmune disorders, and the HLA-B8 haplotype are seen (Newsom-Davis 1985; O'Neill et al. 1988). The onset of symptoms usually precedes the diagnosis of tumor by weeks or months. Proximal muscle weakness, myalgias, paresthesias, loss of tendon reflexes, dry mouth, blurred vision, sphincter dysfunction, and impotence are typical clinical manifestations (Brown and Johns 1974; Heath et al. 1988; Lambert et al. 1956; O'Neill et al. 1988; Rubenstein et al. 1979). Facilitation of strength often is difficult to demonstrate clinically, but the electrophysiological correlate, an incremental response to high-frequency repetitive stimulation, is a cornerstone of diagnosis. Autoantibodies directed against voltage-gated calcium channels (VGCC) play a pathophysiological role (Kim and Neher 1988; Lang et al. 1981). A highly sensitive and specific assay detecting antibodies against P/Q-type VGCC is available as a diagnostic marker (Motomura et al. 1995). In patients with cancer, treatment should be directed against the tumor, and successful treatment usually results in neurological improvement (Chalk et al. 1990; Clamon et al. 1984; Jenkyn et al. 1980). Removal of the antibodies with plasma exchange is also highly effective (Arnason et al. 1986; Dau and Denys 1982; Newsom-Davis and Murray 1984). The use of intravenous immunoglobulin may improve symptoms as well (Bain et al. 1996). Corticosteroids or a combination of corticosteroids and immunosuppressive agents often provide relief (Dau and Denys 1982; Vroom and Engel 1969). For long-term treatments, the use of 3,4-diaminopyridine should be considered (Lundh et al. 1984; McEvoy et al. 1989).

## Muscle

Controversy persists regarding the status of polymyositis and dermatomyositis as paraneoplastic conditions. Most authors agree that polymyositis alone is associated with malignancy only by chance, while cancer underlies dermatomyositis in 7% to 40% of cases (Callen 1984; Dalakas 1991; Henson and Urich 1982; Lakhanpal et al. 1986). This association is further strengthened by excluding patients younger than 50. About 15% of patients with dermatomyositis develop cancer which, in contrast to polymyositis, is usually diagnosed shortly before the onset of the neurological disease. These patients are more often female (Sigurgeirsson et al. 1992) and the most commonly associated tumors are cancer of the breast, lung, ovary, and stomach, with a few patients

reported with Hodgkin's lymphoma (Posner 1995).

Clinically, cutaneous manifestations include a heliotrope rash and periungual erythema or telangiectasia. Symmetrical, predominantly proximal muscle weakness and atrophy are the neurological hallmarks. Muscle tenderness is less common. In some series, there has been a greater incidence of dysphagia (Pearson 1963) and respiratory insufficiency (Talbott 1980) in patients with cancer-associated dermatomyositis. Laboratory abnormalities include elevated serum muscle enzymes (in approximately 95% of cases) and erythrocyte sedimentation rate (50% of cases). Electromyography demonstrates brief, low-amplitude polyphasic waves, increased insertional activity, and fibrillation potentials. None of these findings influences prognosis.

Spontaneous arrests and remissions occur occasionally, and improvement following successful surgery or chemotherapy directed at the underlying malignancy is common. Treatment with corticosteroids produces clinical improvement in most patients (Pearson 1966; Rowland et al. 1977). The addition of other immunosuppressive agents may enhance the response (Bunch et al. 1980; Dalakas 1991; Jacobs 1977; Metzger et al. 1974). At least three-fourths of patients achieve a significant clinical and laboratory response with these measures. Refractory patients have been treated successfully with intravenous immunoglobulin (Dalakas et al. 1993). Dysphagia and profound weakness at the time of presentation are poor prognostic signs (Benbassat et al. 1985; Bohan et al. 1977; Carpenter et al. 1977).

A rare type of paraneoplastic myopathy is specifically associated with carcinoid tumors (Berry et al. 1974; Lederman et al. 1985; Swash et al. 1975). Patients present with proximal muscle weakness and may complain of muscle cramps and tenderness in the shoulder muscles. The disorder develops long after the diagnosis of cancer has been established, and it may respond to treatment with serotonin antagonists (Moertel et al. 1991).

In patients with cancer, a much more common myopathy is that associated with cachexia. Growth factors such as epidermal growth factor and cytokines including tumor necrosis factor and interleukin-6 play a role in the pathogenesis of paraneoplastic cachexia (Black et al. 1991; Strassmann et al. 1993; Yoneda et al. 1991). This myopathy is clinically and pathologically identical to the myopathy associated with other chronic debilitating diseases. Despite significant muscle wasting, strength is often preserved until late in the course of the neoplastic disease. Myoedema (mounding phenomenon) is often present. There is no evidence of inflammation or nerve degeneration.

## Conclusions

Many paraneoplastic neurological syndromes, mediated indirectly by a variety of extraneural malignancies, have been identified. The prognosis of the paraneoplastic syndrome and its associated neoplasm may be related in one of several ways. The neurological disorder may follow a relentlessly progressive course, oblivious to the course of the underlying tumor. In this group are most cases of subacute cerebellar degeneration, subacute necrotizing myelopathy, encephalomyelitides (limbic, brain stem, spinal cord), and sensory neuronopathy (dorsal root ganglionitis). In other cases, succesful antineoplastic therapy results in improvement of the neurological syndrome. The neuropathy of POEMS is the best example. Sometimes spontaneous resolution occurs or specific therapy is available for the remote effect. This occurs in opsoclonus-myoclonus, LEMS, subacute motor neuronopathy, dermatomyositis, neuromyotonia, and carcinoid myopathy. The discovery that some antineuronal antibodies are reliable markers of specific paraneoplastic syndromes and characteristic neoplasms has provided the opportunity for earlier diagnosis and more effective cancer treatment (Dalmau 1997). Finally, the presence of some paraneoplastic disorders and associated antibodies is associated with a more benign course of the underlying malignancy. Opsoclonus-myoclonus and some antibody-related paraneoplastic disorders (e.g., anti-Hu, anti-Yo) fall into this category.

The cases marked by inexorable progression underscore the incomplete knowledge of the pathogenesis of the remote effect. When direct therapeutic intervention is possible or when treatment of the underlying cancer improves the paraneoplastic syndrome, a known or suspected immune-mediated process of the peripheral nervous system is usually at work. Cases in which the presence of a paraneoplastic neurological disorder is associated with improved tumor prognosis remain perplexing. Shared antigens between the tumor and the host's nervous system tissue may create a situation in which a vigorous immune response effectively controls the cancer but produces a disabling remote effect on the nervous system (Bell and Seetharam 1977, 1979; Bell et al. 1976; Furneaux et al. 1990; Graus et al. 1997a; Peterson et al. 1992; Voltz et al. 1997). A better understanding of this relationship may offer greater control over the outcomes of both the tumor and the paraneoplastic syndrome.

## References

Alamowitch, S.; Graus, F.; Uchuya, M.; Reñé, R.; Bescansa, E.; Delattre, J.-Y. Limbic encephalitis and small cell lung cancer: clinical and immunological features. Brain 120:923–928; 1997.

Altman, A. J.; Baehner, R. L. Favorable prognosis for survival in children with coincident opso-myoclonus and neuroblastoma. Cancer 37: 846–852; 1976.

Anderson, N. E.; Budde-Steffen, C.; Rosenblum M. K.; Graus, F.; Ford, D.; Synek, B. J. L.; Posner, J. B. Opsoclonus, ataxia, and encephalopathy in adults with cancer: a distinct paraneoplastic syndrome. Medicine 67:100–109; 1988b.

Anderson, N. E.; Budde-Steffen, C.; Wiley, R. G.; Thurman, L.; Rosenblum, M. K.; Nadeau, S. E.; Posner, J. B. A variant of the anti-Pukinje cell antibody in a patient with paraneoplastic cerebellar degeneration. Neurology 38:1018–1026; 1988a.

Anderson, N. E.; Rosenblum, M. K.; Graus, F.; Wiley, R. G.; Posner, J. B. Autoantibodies in paraneoplastic syndromes associated with small cell lung cancer. Neurology 38: 1391–1398; 1988c.

Anderson, N. E.; Rosenblum, M. K.; Posner, J. B. Paraneoplastic cerebellar degeneration: clinical-immunological correlations. Ann. Neurol. 24: 559–567; 1988d.

Antunes, N. L.; Khakoo. Y.; Stram, D. O.; Seeger, R. C.; Matthay, K. K.; Dalmau, J. Antineuronal antibodies in patients with neuroblastoma (NBT) and paraneoplastic opsoclonus myoclonus (POM). Ann. Neurol. 42:534–535; 1997.

Arnason, B. G.; Areen, J.; et al. Consensus Conference. The utility of therapeutic plasmapheresis for neurological disorders. JAMA 256:1333–1337; 1986.

Auth, T. L.; Chodoff, P. Transient cerebellar syndrome from extracerebral carcinoma. Neurology 7: 370–372; 1957.

Bain, P. G.; Motomura, M.; Newsom-Davis, J.; Misbah, S. A.; Chapel, H. M.; Lee, M. L.; et al. Effects of intravenous immunoglobulin on muscle weakness and calcium-channel autoantibodies in the Lambert-Eaton myasthenic syndrome. Neurology 47:678–683; 1996.

Bardwick, P. A.; Zvailfler, N. J.; Gill, G. N.; Newman, D.; Greenway, G. D.; Resnick, D. L. Plasma cell dyscrasia with polyneuropathy, organomegaly, endocrinopathy, M protein, and skin changes: the POEMS syndrome. Report on two cases and a review of the literature. Medicine 59:311–322; 1980.

Batson, O. A.; Fantle, D. M.; Stewart, J. A. Paraneoplastic encephalomyelitis. Dramatic response to chemotherapy alone. Cancer 69:1291–1293; 1992.

Bell, C. E.; Seetharam, S. Identification of the Schwann cell as a peripheral nervous system cell possessing a differentiation antigen expressed by a human lung tumor. J. Immunol. 118:826–831; 1977.

Bell, C. E.; Seetharam, S. Expression of endodermally derived and neural crest-derived differentiation antigens by human lung and colon tumors. Cancer 44:13–18; 1979.

Bell, C. E.; Seetharam, S.; McDaniel, R. C. Endodermally-derived and neural crest-derived differentiation antigens expressed by a human lung tumor. J. Immunol. 116:1236–1243; 1976.

Benbassat, J.; Gefel, D.; Larholt, K.; Sukenik, S.; Morgenstern, V.; Zlotnick, A. Prognostic factors in polymyositis/dermatomyositis: a computer-assisted analysis of ninety-two cases. Arthritis Rheum. 28:249–255; 1985.

Berry, E. M.; Maunder, C.; Wilson, M. Carcinoid myopathy and treatment with cyproheptadine (periactin). Gut 15:34–38; 1974.

Black, K.; Garrett, I. R.; Mundy, G. R. Chinese hamster ovarian cells transfected with the murine interleukin-6 gene cause hypercalcemia as well as cachexia, leukocytosis and thrombocytosis in tumor-bearing nude mice. Endocrinology 128:2657–2659; 1991.

Bohan, A.; Peter, J. B.; Bowman, R. L.; Pearson, C. M. A computer-assisted analysis of 153 patients with polymyositis and dermatomyositis. Medicine 56:255–286; 1977.

Brain, R.; Wilkinson, M. Subacute cerebellar degeneration associated with neoplasms. Brain 88:465–478; 1965.

Bray, P. F.; Ziter, F. A.; Lahey, M. E.; Myers, G. G. The coincidence of neuroblastoma and acute cerebellar encephalopathy. J. Pediatr. 75:983–990; 1969.

Brennan, L. V.; Craddock, P. R. Limbic encephalitis as a non-metastatic complication of oat cell lung cancer. Am. J. Med. 75:518–520; 1983.

Brown, J. C.; Johns, R. J. Diagnostic difficulties encountered in the myasthenia syndrome sometimes associated with carcinoma. J. Neurol. Neurosurg. Psychiatry 37:1214–1224; 1974.

Budde-Steffen, C.; Anderson, N. E.; Rosenblum, M. K.; Posner, J. B. Expression of an antigen in small cell lung carcinoma lines detected by antibodies from patients with paraneoplastic dorsal root ganglionitis. Cancer Res. 48:430–434; 1988.

Bunch, T. W.; Worthington, J. W.; Combs, J. J.; Ilstrup, M. S.; Engel, A. G. Azathioprine with prednisone for polymyositis. Ann. Intern. Med. 92:365–369; 1980.

Burton, G. V.; Bullard, D. E.; Walther, P. J.; Burger, P. C. Paraneoplastic limbic encephalopathy with testicular carcinoma: a reversible neurologic syndrome. Cancer 62:2248–2251; 1988.

Byrne, T.; Mason, W. P.; Dalmau, J.; Posner, J. B. Spontaneous neurological improvement in anti-Hu associated encephalomyelitis J. Neurol. Neurosurg. Psychiatry 62:276–278; 1997.

Callen, J. P. Myositis and malignancy. Clin. Rheum. Dis. 10:117–131; 1984.

Carpenter, J. R.; Bunch, T. W.; Engel, A. G.; O'Brien, P. Survival in polymyositis: corticosteroids and risk factors. J. Rheumatol. 4:207–214; 1977.

Carr, I. The Ophelia syndrome: memory loss in Hodgkin's disease. Lancet 1:844–845; 1982.

Chalk, C. H.; Murray, N. M.; Newsom-Davis, J.; O'Neill, J. H.; Spiro, S. G. Response of the Lambert-Eaton myasthenic syndrome to treatment of associated small-cell lung carcinoma. Neurology 40:1552–1556; 1990.

Chalk, C. H.; Windebank, A. J.; Kimmel, D. W.; McManis, P. G. The distinctive clinical features of paraneoplastic sensory neuronopathy. Can. J. Neurol. Sci. 19:346–351; 1992.

Clamon, G. H.; Evans, W. K.; Shepherd, F. A.; Humphrey, J. G. Myasthenic syndrome and small cell cancer of the lung: variable response to antineoplastic therapy. Arch. Intern. Med. 144:99–100; 1984.

Cocconi, G.; Ceci, G.; Juvarra, G. Successful treatment of subacute cerebellar degeneration in ovarian carcinoma with plasmapheresis. A case report. Cancer 56:2318–2320; 1985.

Cohn, S. L.; Salwen, H.; Herst, C. V.; et al. Single copies of the N-myc oncogene in neuroblastomas from children presenting with the syndrome of opsoclonus-myoclonus. Cancer 62:723–726; 1988.

Connolly, A. M.; Pestronk, A.; Metha, S. Serum autoantibodies in childhood opsoclonus-myoclonus syndrome: an analysis of antigenic targets in neural tissues. J. Pediatr. 130:878–884; 1997.

Corsellis, J. A. N.; Goldberg, G. J.; Norton, A. R. "Limbic encephalitis" and its association with carcinoma. Brain 91:481–497; 1968.

Counsell, C. E.; McLeod, M.; Grant, R. Reversal of subacute paraneoplastic cerebellar syndrome with intravenous immunoglobulin. Neurology 44:1184–1185; 1994.

Croft, P. B.; Urich, H.; Wilkinson, M. Peripheral neuropathy of sensorimotor type associated with malignant disease. Brain 90:31–66; 1967.

Dalakas, M. C. Polymyositis, dermatomyositis, and inclusion-body myositis. N. Engl. J. Med. 325:1487–1498; 1991.

Dalakas, M. C.; Illa, I.; Dambrosia, J. M.; Soueidan, S. A.; Stein, D. P.; Otero, C.; Dinsmore, S. T.; McCrosky, S. A controlled trial of high-dose intravenous immune globulin infusions as treatment for dermatomyositis. N. Engl. J. Med. 329:1993–2000; 1993.

Dalmau, J. Paraneoplastic syndromes of the nervous system: general pathogenic mechanisms and diagnostic approaches. In: Vinken, P. J.; Bruyn, G. W., eds. Handbook of clinical neurology. Vol. 25, Neuro-oncology, Vecht, C. J., ed. Amsterdam: Elsevier; 1997: p. 319–328.

Dalmau, J.; Graus, F.; Rosenblum, M. K.; Posner, J. B. Anti-Hu-associated paraneoplastic encephalomyelitis/ sensory neuronopathy. A clinical study of 71 patients. Medicine 71:59–72; 1992.

Dau, P. C.; Denys, E. H. Plasmapharesis and immuno-suppressive drug therapy in the Eaton-Lambert syndrome. Ann. Neurol. 11:570–575; 1982.

Denny-Brown, D. Primary sensory neuropathy with muscular changes associated with carcinoma. J. Neurol. Neurosurg. Psychiatry 11:73–87; 1948.

Dirr, L. Y.; Elster, A. D.; Donofrio, P. D.; Smith, M. Evolution of brain MRI abnormalities in limbic encephalitis. Neurology 40:1304–1306; 1990.

Dropcho, E. J.; Kline, L. B.; Riser, J. Antineuronal (anti-Ri) autoantibodies in a patient with steroid-responsive opsoclonus myoclonus. Neurology 43:207–211; 1993.

Eekhof, J. L. A. Remission of a paraneoplastic cerebellar syndrome. Clin. Neurol. Neurosurg. 87:133–134; 1985.

Engel, A. G. Myasthenia gravis and myasthenic syndromes. Ann. Neurol. 16:519–534; 1984.

Evans, B. K.; Fagan, C.; Arnold, T.; et al. Paraneoplastic motor neuron disease and renal cell carcinoma: improvement after nephrectomy. Neurology 40:960–962; 1990.

Forsyth, P. A.; Dalmau, J.; Graus, F.; Posner, J. B. Paraneoplastic motor neuron disease (MND). Ann. Neurol. 34:277; 1997.

Furneaux, H. M.; Rosenblum, M. K.; Dalmau, J.; et al. Selective expression of Purkinje-cell antigens in tumor tissue from patients with paraneoplastic cerebellar degeneration. N. Engl. J. Med. 322:1844–1851; 1990.

Gieron, M. A.; Margraf, L. R.; Korthals, J. K.; Gonzalvo, A. A.; Murtagh, R. F.; Hvizdala, E. V. Progressive necrotizing myelopathy associated with leukemia: clinical, pathologic, and MRI correlation. J. Child Neurol. 2:44–49; 1987.

Glantz, M. J.; Biran, H.; Myers, M. E.; Gockerman, J. P.; Friedberg, M. H. The radiographic diagnosis and treatment of paraneoplastic central nervous system disease. Cancer 73:168–175; 1994.

Graus, F.; Bonaventura, I.; Uchuya, M.; Valls-Solé, J.; Reñe, R.; Leger, J. M.; et al. Indolent anti-Hu-associated paraneoplastic sensory neuropathy. Neurology 44:2258–2261; 1994.

Graus, F.; Cordon-Cardo, C.; Posner, J. B. Neuronal antinuclear antibody in sensory neuronopathy from lung cancer. Neurology 35:538–543; 1985.

Graus, F.; Dalmau, J.; Reñe, R.; Torá, M.; Malats, N.; Verschuuren, J. J.; Cardenal, F.; Viñolas, N.; Garcia del Muro, J.; Vadell, C.; Mason, W. P.; Rosell, R.; Posner, J. B.; Real, F. X. Anti-Hu antibodies in patients with small cell lung cancer: association with complete response to therapy and improved survival. J. Clin. Oncol. 15:2866–2872; 1997a.

Graus, F.; Dalmau, J.; Valldeoriola, F.; Ferrer, I.; Reñé, R.; Marin, C.; Vecht, Ch. J.; Arbizu, T.; Targa, C.; Moll, J. W. B. Immunological characterization of a neuronal antibody (anti-Tr) associated with paraneoplastic cerebellar degeneration and Hodgkin's disease. J. Neuroimmunol. 74:55–61; 1997b.

Graus, F.; Elkon, K. B.; Cordon-Cardo, C.; Posner, J. B. Sensory neuronopathy and small cell lung cancer: antineuronal antibody that also reacts with the tumor. Am. J. Med. 80:45–52; 1986.

Graus, F.; Elkon, K. B.; Lloberes, P.; Ribalta, T.; Torres, A.; Ussetti, P.; Valls, J.; Obach, J.; Agusti-Vidal, A. Neuronal antinuclear antibodies (anti-Hu) in paraneoplastic encephalomyelitis simulating acute polyneuritis. Acta Neurol. Scand. 75:249–252; 1987.

Graus, F.; Vega, F.; Delattre, J. Y.; et al. Effect of plasmapheresis and antineoplastic treatment in CNS paraneoplastic syndromes with antineuronal autoantibodies. Neurology 42:536–540; 1992.

Greenberg, H. S. Paraneoplastic cerebellar degeneration. J. Neurooncol. 2:377–382; 1984.

Greenlee, J. E.; Brashear, H. R. Antibodies to cerebellar Purkinje cells in patients with paraneoplastic cerebellar degeneration and ovarian carcinoma. Ann. Neurol. 14:609–613; 1983.

Greenlee, J. E.; Lipton, H. L. Anticerebellar antibodies in serum and cerebrospinal fluid of a patient with oat cell carcinoma of the lung and paraneoplastic cerebellar degeneration. Ann. Neurol. 19:82–85; 1986.

Halperin, J. J.; Richardson, E. P.; Ellis, J.; Ross, J. S.; Wray, S. H. Paraneoplastic encephalomyelitis and neuropathy: report of a case. Arch. Neurol. 38:773–775; 1981.

Handforth, A.; Nag, S.; Dharp, D.; Robertson, D. M. Paraneoplastic subacute necrotic myelopathy. Can. J. Neurol. Sci. 10:204–207; 1983.

Heath, J. P.; Ewing, J. P.; Cull, R. E. Abnormalities of autonomic function in the Lambert Eaton myasthenic syndrome. J. Neurol. Neurosurg. Psychiatry 51:436; 1988.

Henson, R. A.; Hoffman, H. L.; Urich, H. Encephalomyelitis with carcinoma. Brain 88:449–464; 1965.

Henson, R. A.; Urich, H. Cancer and the nervous system: the neurological manifestations of systemic malignant disease. Oxford: Blackwell Scientific Publications; 1982; p. 422–426.

Hiyama, E.; Yokoyama, T.; Ichikawa, T.; et al. Poor outcome in patients with advanced stage neuroblastoma and coincident opsomyoclonus syndrome. Cancer 74:1821–1826; 1994.

Horwich, M. S.; Cho, L.; Porro, R. S.; Posner, J. B. Subacute sensory neuropathy: a remote effect of carcinoma. Ann. Neurol. 2:7–19; 1977.

Iwamasa, T.; Utsumi, Y.; Sakuda, H.; et al. Two cases of necrotizing myelopathy associated with malignancy caused by herpes simplex virus type 2. Acta Neuropathol. 78:252–257; 1989.

Jacobs, J. C. Methotrexate and azathioprine for treatment of childhood dermatomyositis. Pediatrics 59:212–218; 1977.

Jenkyn, L. R.; Brooks, P. L.; Forcier, R. J.; Maurer, L. H.; Ochoa, J. Remission of Lambert-Eaton syndrome and small cell anaplastic carcinoma of the lung induced by chemotherapy and radiation therapy. Cancer 46:1123–1127; 1980.

Kaplan, A. M.; Stabashi, H. H. Encephalitis associated with carcinoma: central hypoventilation syndrome +

cytoplasmic inclusion bodies. J. Neurol. Neurosurg. Psychiatry 37:1166–1176; 1974.

Kearsley, J. H.; Johnson, P.; Halmagyi, M. Paraneoplastic cerebellar disease. Remission with excision of the primary tumor. Arch. Neurol. 42: 1208– 1210; 1985.

Kelly, J. J.; Kyle, R. A.; Miles, J. M.; Dyck, P. J. Osteosclerotic myeloma and peripheral neuropathy. Neurology 33:202–210; 1983.

Kim, Y. I.; Neher, E. IgG from patients with Lambert-Eaton syndrome blocks voltage-dependent calcium channels. Science 239:450–458; 1988.

Lakhanpal, S.; Bunch, T. W.; Ilstrup, D. M.; Melton, L. J., III. Polymyositis-dermatomyositis and malignant lesions: does an association exist? Mayo Clin. Proc. 61:645–653; 1986.

Lambert, E. H.; Eaton, L. M.; Rooke, E. D. Defect of neuromuscular transmission associated with malignant neoplasms. Am. J. Physiol. 187:612–613; 1956.

Lang, B.; Newsom-Davis, J.; Wray, D.; Vincent, A. Autoimmune etiology for myasthenic (Eaton-Lambert) syndrome. Lancet 2:224–226; 1981.

Lang, B.; Vincent, A. Autoimmunity to ion-channels and other proteins in paraneoplastic disorders. Curr. Opin. Immunol. 8:865–871; 1996.

Lederman, R. J.; Bukowski, R. M.; Nickerson, P. Carcinoid myopathy. Neurology 35:165; 1985.

Lundh, H.; Nilsson, O.; Rosen, I. Treatment of Lambert-Eaton sundrome: 3,4-diaminopyridine and pyridostigmine. Neurology 34:1324–1330; 1984.

Luque, F. A.; Furneaux, H. M.; Ferziger, R.; et al. Anti-Ri: an antibody associated with paraneoplastic opsoclonus and breast cancer. Ann. Neurol. 29:241–251; 1991.

Markham, M.; Abeloff, M. D. Small cell lung cancer and limbic encephalitis. Ann. Intern. Med. 96:785; 1982.

Mason, W. P.; Graus, F.; Lang, B.; Honnorat, J.; Delattre, J.-Y.; Valldeoriola, F.; Antoine J. C.; Rosenblum, M. K.; Rosenfeld, M. R.; Newsom-Davis, J.; Posner, J. B.; Dalmau, J. Small-cell lung cancer, paraneoplastic cerebellar degeneration and the Lambert-Eaton myasthenic syndrome. Brain 120: 1279–1300; 1997.

McEvoy, K. M.; Windebank, A. J.; Daube, J. R.; Low, P. A. 3,4-diaminopyridine in the treatment of Lambert-Eaton myasthenic syndrome. N. Engl. J. Med. 321:1567–1571; 1989.

Mendell, J. R.; Sahenk, Z.; Whiaker, J. N.; Trapp, B. D.; Yates, A. J.; Griggs, R. C.; Quarles, R. H. Polyneuropathy and IgM monoclonal gammopathy: studies on the pathogenic role of anti-myelin-associated glycoprotein antibody. Ann. Neurol. 17:243– 254; 1985.

Metzger, A. L.; Bohan, A.; Goldberg, L. S.; Bluestone, R. Polymyositis and dermatomyositis: combined methotrexate and corticosteroid therapy. Ann. Intern. Med. 81:182–189; 1974.

Miralles, G. D.; O'Fallon, J. R.; Talley, N. J. Plasma-cell dyscrasia with polyneuropathy. N. Engl. J. Med. 327:1919–1923; 1992.

Moe, P. G.; Nellhaus, G. Infantile polymyoclonia-opsoclonus syndrome and neural crest tumors. Neurology 20:756–764; 1970.

Moertel, C. G.; Kvols, L. K.; Rubin, J. A study of cyproheptadine in the treatment of metastatic carcinoid tumor and the malignant carcinoid syndrome. Cancer 67:33–36; 1991.

Motomura, M.; Johnston, I.; Lang, B.; Vincent, A.; Newsom-Davis, J. An improved diagnostic assay for Lambert-Eaton myasthenic syndrome. J. Neurol. Neurosurg. Psychiatry 58:85–87; 1995.

Newsom-Davis, J. Lambert-Eaton myasthenic syndrome. Springer Semin. Immunopathol. 8:129–140; 1985.

Newsom-Davis, J.; Murray, N. M. P. Plasma exchange and immunosuppression drug therapy in the Lambert-Eaton myasthenic syndrome. Neurology. 34: 480–485; 1984.

Oh, S. J.; Dropcho, E. J.; Claussen, G. C. Anti-Hu associated paraneoplastic sensory neuropathy responding to early aggressive immunotherapy: report of two cases and review of the literature. Muscle Nerve 20:1576–1582; 1997.

Ojeda, V. J. Necrotizing myelopathy associated with malignancy: a clinicopathologic study of two cases and literature review. Cancer 53:1115–1123; 1984.

O'Neil, J. H.; Murray, N. M. F.; Newsom-Davis, J. The Lambert-Eaton myasthenic syndrome: a review of 50 cases. Brain 111:577–596; 1988.

Paone, J. F.; Jeyasingham, K. Remission of cerebellar dysfunction after pneumonectomy for bronchogenic carcinoma. N. Engl. J. Med. 302:156–157; 1980.

Pearson, C. M. Patterns of polymyositis and their response to treatment. Ann. Intern. Med. 59:827–838; 1963.

Pearson, C. M. Polymyositis. Annu. Rev. Med. 17: 63–82; 1966.

Peterson, K.; Rosenblum, M. K.; Kotanides, H.; Posner, J. B. Paraneoplastic cerebellar degeneration. I. A clinical analysis of 55 anti-Yo antibody-positive patients. Neurology 42:1931–1937; 1992.

Posner, J. B., ed. Paraneoplastic syndromes. Neurologic complications of cancer. Philadelphia: FA Davis; 1995: p. 353–385.

Pranzatelli, M. R. The immunopharmacology of the opsoclonus-myoclonus syndrome. Clin. Neuropharmacol. 19:1–47; 1996.

Resnick, D.; Greenway, G. D.; Bardwick, P. A.; Zvaifler, N. J.; Gill, G. N.; Newman, D. R. Plasma cell dyscrasia with polyneuropathy, organomegaly, M-protein, and skin changes: the POEMS syndrome. Distinctive radiographic abnormalities. Radiology 140:17–22; 1981.

Rosen, E. M.; Cassady, J. R.; Frantz, C. N.; Kretschmar, C.; Levey, R.; Sallan, S. E. Neuroblastoma: the Joint Center for Radiation Therapy/Dana-Farber Center Institute/Children's Hospital experience. J. Clin. Oncol. 2:719–732; 1984.

Rosenfeld, M. R.; Posner, J. B. Paraneoplastic motor neuron disease. Adv. Neurol. Amyotrophic Lateral Sclerosis Other Motor Neuron Dis. 56:445–459; 1995.

Rowland, L. P.; Clark, C.; Olarte, M. Therapy for dermatomyositis and polymyositis. Adv. Neurol. 17: 63–97; 1977.

Rowland, L. P.; Sherman, W. H.; Latov, N.; Lange, D. J.; McDonald, T. D.; Younger, D. S.; Murphy, P. L.; Hays, A. P.; Knowles, D. Amyotrophic lateral sclerosis and lymphoma: bone marrow examination and other diagnostic tests. Neurology 42: 1101–1102; 1992.

Rowland, L. P.; Schneck, S. A. Neuromuscular disorders associated with malignant neoplastic disorders. J. Chron. Dis. 16:777–795; 1963.

Rubenstein, A. E.; Horowitz, S. H.; Bender, A. N. Cholinergic dysautonomia and Eaton-Lambert syndrome. Neurology 29:720–723; 1979.

Russo, C.; Cohn, S. L.; Petruzzi, M. J.; Alarcon, P. A. Long-term neurologic outcome in children with opsoclonus-myoclonus associated with neuroblastoma: a report from the Pediatric Oncology Group. Med. Pediatr. Oncol. 29:284–288; 1997.

Sagar, H. J.; Read, D. J. Subacute sensory neuropathy with remission: an association with lymphoma. J. Neurol. Neurosurg. Psychiatry 45: 83–85; 1982.

Schold, S. C., Jr.; Cho, L.; Somasundarum, M.; Posner, J. B. Subacute motor neuronopathy: a remote effect of lymphoma. Ann. Neurol. 5: 271–287; 1979.

Sigurgeirsson, B.; Lindelof, B.; Edhag, O.; Allander, E. Risk of cancer in patients with dermatomyositis or polymyositis. A population-based study. N. Engl. J. Med. 326:363–367; 1992.

Strassmann, G.; Jacob, C. O.; Fong, M.; Bertolini, D. R. Mechanisms of paraneoplastic syndromes of colon-26: involvement of interleukin 6 in hypercalcemia. Cytokine 5:463–468; 1993.

Swash, M.; Fox, K. P.; Davidson, A. R. Carcinoid myopathy: serotonin-induced muscle weakness in man? Arch. Neurol. 32:572–574; 1975.

Talbott, J. H. Acute dermatomyositis-polymyositis and malignancy. Semin. Arthritis Rheum. 6:305–360; 1980.

Uchuya, M.; Graus, F.; Vega, F.; Reñé, R.; Delattre, J. Y. Intravenous immunoglobulin treatment in paraneoplastic neurological syndromes with antineuronal autoantibodies. J. Neurol. Neurosurg. Psychiatry 60:388–392; 1996.

Verma, A.; Berger, J. R.; Snodgrass, S.; Petito, C. Motor neuron disease: a paraneoplastic process associated with anti-Hu antibody and small cell lung carcinoma. Ann. Neurol. 40:112–116; 1996.

Voltz, R. D.; Graus, F.; Posner, J. B.; Dalmau, J. Paraneoplastic encephalomyelitis: an update of the effects of the anti-Hu immune response on the nervous system and tumor (editorial). J. Neurol. Neurosurg. Psychiatry 63:133–136; 1997.

Vroom, F. O.; Engel, W. K. Non-neoplastic steroid-responsive Lambert-Eaton myasthenic syndrome. Neurology 19:281; 1969.

Walton, J. N.; Tomlinson, B. E.; Pearce, G. W. Subacute "poliomyelitis" and Hodgkin's disease. J. Neurol. Sci. 6:435–445; 1968.

Wilkinson, P. C.; Zeromski, J. Immunofluorescent detection of antibodies against neurons in sensory carcinomatous neuropathy. Brain 88:529–538; 1965.

Yoneda, Y.; Alsina, M. M.; Watatani, K.; Bellot, F.; Schlessinger, J.; Mundy, G. R. Dependence of a human squamous carcinoma and associated paraneoplastic syndromes on the epidermal growth factor receptor pathway in nude mice. Cancer Res. 51: 2438–2443; 1991.

Younger, D. S.; Rowland, L. P.; Latov, N.; et al. Lymphoma, motor neuron diseases, and amyotrophic amyotrophic lateral sclerosis. Ann. Neurol. 29:1, 78–86; 1991.

# PART IX

# NEUROMUSCULAR DISORDERS

# 28

# Neuromuscular Junction and Muscle Disease

HANS E. NEVILLE AND STEVEN P. RINGEL

In the last decade the prognosis of various neuro-muscular disorders has received increasing attention by investigators designing therapeutic trials. It is now well accepted that the natural history of a disease must be defined clearly if investigators are to demonstrate any positive effect of therapeutic intervention (Brooke et al. 1983; Munsat et al. 1988; Ringel et al. 1993). For example, in Duchenne's dystrophy, a relatively homogenous disorder with a linear progression of weakness, the Clinical Investigations in Duchenne Dystrophy (CIDD) group has shown there is a significant variation in the rate at which weakness develops. The situation is much more complicated for myotonic dystrophy, facioscapulohumeral dystrophy, and amyotrophic lateral sclerosis (see Chapter 30). In general, the degree of weakness and rate of progression is highly variable among individuals with the same disease and even among such individuals in the same family. Such extensive variability is highlighted below, so that the reader will develop an understanding of the spectrum of each neuromuscular illness.

The emphasis of this chapter is on the more common, chronic disorders that affect the neuromuscular junction and voluntary skeletal muscles, including myasthenia gravis, the inflammatory myopathies, various muscular dystrophies, con-genital myopathies, mitochondrial myopathies, and several other muscle disorders resulting from metabolic abnormalities. We have chosen not to cover some of the very rare myopathies because the small numbers of reported cases precludes any accurate description of natural history and prognosis.

## Myasthenia Gravis

Myasthenia gravis (MG) is characterized by fluctuating weakness in cranial, respiratory, and limb muscles. The disease results from an immunological abnormality in which immunoglobulin G (IgG) antibodies and complement interact with acetylcholine receptor protein to cause progressive destruction of the neuromuscular junction (Engel 1994a). The antibodies are produced from activated B cells located in the thymus, which is usually hyperplastic. The diagnosis of myasthenia gravis is confirmed in several ways: (1) the finding of serum *acetylcholine receptor antibodies* (the presence of these antibodies is variable; they are present in 50% of purely ocular MG; 84% of generalized MG; and in 24% of patients in remission (Tindall 1981); (2) a *decrement* in the compound muscle action potential following repetitive electrical stimulation; (3) a *positive edrophonium chloride* or *Tensilon* test whereby there is improvement of objectively demonstrated muscle weakness when edrophonium chloride is injected intravenously (ptosis or a paretic eye muscle are the best endpoints); (4) the finding of *increased jitter with single-fiber electromyography* (EMG). The disease has a coexisting thymoma in 10% of cases, thyroid disease in 13%, and other autoimmune diseases in at least 3% (Genkins et al. 1987; Christensen et al. 1995).

Myasthenia is associated with HLA types A1, B7, and DRw3 in patients younger than 40 years and types A3, B7, and DRw3 in those older than 40 years (Compston et al. 1980). This association suggests that HLA class II molecules associated with myasthenia gravis are more likely to bind peptides that will activate T cells and lead to MG antibody production (Abbas et al. 1991).

Myasthenia gravis may occur at any age. It is more prevalent in women (57%), particularly if the onset is before the age of 40 (Grob et al. 1987). After 40 years of age, the disease characteristics shift to a male predominance, increased severity, and different HLA correlates (Compston et al. 1980). The disease frequently starts with purely ocular symptoms. In untreated cases, based on reports in the 1920s and 1930s before specific drug therapy was available, patients typically developed increasing complaints of limb, speech, swallowing, and breathing weakness with death in over 50% due to respiratory failure and pneumonia. In the past 3 decades new therapies have been introduced and used, usually with limited objective clinical measurements and often without adequate controls. The best summary of disease course and response to treatment from 1940 to the mid-1980s is to be found in the paper by Grob and collaborators (1987). Since then many smaller series have reported on patients undergoing thymectomy and immunosuppressive therapy, all of which have led to improved patient outcomes.

## Ocular and Generalized Myasthenia Gravis

### Ocular Myasthenia Gravis

This is a relatively benign form of the disease at onset and is seen more commonly in males. Complaints of ptosis or double vision occur as the initial symptom in slightly over 50% of MG patients and, if not treated, weakness becomes generalized within 2 years (Grob et al. 1987; Donaldson et al.

1990). If weakness remains localized to the eyes for more than 2 years, only 10% to 20% progress to more generalized myasthenia (Grob et al. 1987).

In patients with ocular complaints alone and no clinically demonstrable limb or diaphragm weakness, the edrophonium chloride test will be positive in 95%. In this same group an EMG decremental response to repetitive stimulation in limb muscles (even in the presence of normal strength) and elevated acetylcholine receptor antibody titers are seen in only 50% (Evoli et al. 1988; Tindall 1981). In several series it has been shown that ocular MG will respond initially to anticholinesterase agents but probably less than half the patients so treated become entirely asymptomatic (Evoli et al. 1988). Increasingly, treating physicians are advocating that ocular MG be treated with corticosteroids and, sometimes, thymectomy (Evoli et al. 1988; Schumm et al. 1985). Recently, Sommer et al. (1997) reported that early use of immunosuppressive therapy for purely ocular MG results in limitation of symptoms and signs to the eyes in 69% of their patients followed over a 5-year period. This is a remarkable result considering that previous authors had been able to limit symptoms to the eyes with immunosuppression in only 14% to 31% (Grob et al. 1987; Oosterhuis 1989). In any event, immunosuppression must be maintained for extended periods of time if ocular or generalized symptoms are to be controlled.

### Generalized Myasthenia Gravis

Throughout the 1920s and 1930s when MG was clearly defined as a clinical entity, supportive therapy was inadequate, since modern pulmonary assistance was only being developed. Consequently, 40% to 70% of patients died, with survivers experiencing varying degrees of limb and bulbar weakness. With more sophisticated observations and treatments in the 1930s through 1950s, it became apparent that limb and bulbar muscle weakness reached maximal severity in over 50% of patients during the first year and in 85% of patients within 3 years (Grob et al. 1987). During this time when treatment was limited to anticholinesterase agents, positive pressure ventilation, and tracheostomy, death occurred in nearly 30% within 3 years, improvement was seen in about 30%, remission occurred in 10%, and 30% remained unchanged.

The high mortality and low remission rate was altered in the period 1960 to 1985, with several series reporting a beneficial effect of immunosuppressive therapy, thymectomy, and improved critical care therapy. The longest series reported for this time showed a drop in mortality rate to 7%, an improvement in nearly 50%, no change in about 30%, with remissions staying the same at about 10% (Grob et al. 1987). Jaretzki et al. (1988) followed 72 myasthenic patients after maximal thymectomy and found a 45% drug-free remission rate. They estimated an 81% remission rate at 89 months by life-table analysis. One view has been that 65% to 85% of treated patients will improve or go into complete remission with modern therapy (Rowland 1980). A more recent retrospective study demonstrated complete remission in only 35% of patients followed over 5 years (Mantegazza et al. 1990).

## Treatment

Treatment of myasthenia gravis requires the use of anticholinesterase agents, prednisone or other immunosuppressives, thymectomy, plasmapheresis, and immune globulin.

*Anticholinesterase* medications improve the strength of some myasthenics, but are inadequate for patients with more severe disease. Such agents are most useful in patients with purely ocular complaints, very mild generalized weakness, in patients unable to tolerate immunosuppression or who cannot undergo thymectomy.

*Immunosuppressive* agents have been used now for 3 decades with prednisone most commonly employed to reduce the severity of symptoms or induce remission in patients with generalized myasthenia gravis. Johns (1987) using prednisone at doses of 60 to 80 mg/d reported improvement or complete remission in 80% of treated patients. After variable periods of time the majority of patients were successfully maintained on low-dose alternate-day prednisone, and 15% who were off all medication were totally asymptomatic. In John's (1987) series, thymectomy had no effect on clinical response or medication requirements. In contrast, another series showed a better response and less medication needed in patients undergoing thymectomy (Donaldson et al. 1990). Sommer et al. (1997) proposed that early immunosuppression with prednisone and azathioprine is helpful in reducing the develop-

ment of generalized MG in patients presenting with ocular complaints. Up to 50% of myasthenic patients on long-term steroids, however, incur significant side effects, the commonest being weight gain in 40%, cataracts in 19%, and infections in 18% (Donaldson et al. 1990). Clinical improvement may be attained in patients given a variety of immunosuppressive medications, including azathioprine, cyclophosphamide, and cyclosporin A (Niaken et al. 1986; Tindall et al. 1987). Usually these agents are added later in the course of MG treatment in order to minimize prednisone side effects.

*Thymectomy* has become standard therapy in many centers. Although several series and anecdotal reports support its effectiveness, the benefit from thymectomy has not been demonstrated in a well-controlled prospective study (Rowland 1980; McQuillin and Leone 1977). Whereas Grob et al. (1987) could see little benefit of thymectomy in patients during the era 1958 through 1985, Olanow and coworkers (1987) promoted the approach of plasmapheresis followed by thymectomy without the use of corticosteroids. After 3 years, 80% of patients had an excellent response, with 55% being off all medicines and 38% of patients never receiving any medical therapy. Others have argued that thymectomy offers no additional benefit to other therapies (McQuillen and Leone 1977). Somnier (1994) disagreed with this view in a small prospective series which showed that thymectomy for a hyperplastic thymus gland led to clinical improvement and a drop in acetylcholine receptor antibody levels. In that same series, patients with thymoma were observed to develop worsening MG for up to 1 year and then a return of symptoms to preoperative levels (Somnier 1994). In two longer retrospective studies, thymectomy was done in 72% of 1152 (Mantegazza et al. 1990) and 65% of 165 (Donaldson et al. 1990) patients followed on average of 5 and 8 years. Remission was seen in 35% and 26%, respectively, leading the authors to conclude that thymectomy improved the course of the disease when combined with immunosuppression.

*Plasmapheresis and immune globulin* are used in life-threatening situations where symptoms cannot be controlled quickly with conventional immunosuppression. Beneficial effects are short-term, lasting 3 to 6 weeks in most patients (Seybold 1987; Cosi et al. 1991).

## Congenital Myasthenia Gravis

This is a rare, heterogeneous group of disorders mimicking the more common acquired, immunological based disease described above (Engel 1994b). Congenital MG may be due to one of several genetic mutations that cause structural or functional abnormalities of the acetylcholine receptor protein channel or an absence of acetylcholinesterase. Most patients develop myasthenic symptoms at an early age, but one subtype is not symptomatic until the teenage years. Electrophysiological tests confirm a neuromuscular junction defect. Antiacetylcholine receptor antibodies are not found in these conditions and the edrophonium chloride test is usually negative. Patients have little disease progression and remission does not occur. Congenital myasthenia may respond to anticholinesterase agents but corticosteroids are of no use (Engel 1994b).

## Neonatal Myasthenia Gravis

Transient neonatal myasthenia occurs in approximately 12% of infants born to mothers who have myasthenia gravis, regardless of the mother's disease severity. These infants typically develop poor feeding, weakness, and respiratory difficulty during the first day of life. Passively transferred maternal acetylcholine receptor antibodies (and possibly independently produced antibodies) detectable in the infant's sera account for transient weakness in the child. Symptoms last an average of 18 days but may persist up to 47 days until passively transferred maternal antibodies are metabolized (Lefvert and Osterman 1983). Vigorous short-term supportive therapy is indicated in these infants, since the syndrome is transient.

## Dermatomyositis and Polymyositis

Dermatomyositis (DM) and polymyositis (PM) are inflammatory muscle diseases of unknown etiology. Immune hyper-reactivity is evident, which in DM is considered to be a humorally mediated vasculitis and in PM which is due, most likely, to cell-mediated responses directed at muscle fibers.

These inflammatory diseases may begin at any age. In children DM has a peak age of onset between years 5 and 14 and is 10 to 20 times more common than PM. In adults, PM or DM are more common from 45 to 64 years (Bohan et al.

1977; Mastaglia and Ojeda 1985). Most estimates of disease incidence vary from 2 to 5 per 1 million population, with PM being more common than DM (Medsger et al. 1970; Rose and Walton 1966). Women outnumber men in most series (Bohan et al. 1977; DeVere and Bradley 1975). The most prominent clinical feature is symmetrical proximal muscle weakness, accompanied by myalgias and dysphagia. Facial, extraocular, and distal skeletal muscles rarely are involved.

More than 90% of patients with DM have a rash at the time of presentation (Bohan et al. 1977). The characteristic DM rash appears as a lilac discoloration of the eyelids, and can be accompanied by facial and neck erythema, as well as erythematous, atrophic, scaly changes over extensor surfaces of joints. The rash precedes muscle weakness in at least half of patients. Changes in the rash do not correlate with disease activity (Barwick and Walton 1963; Bohan et al. 1977; Bohan 1988; Eaton 1954; Logan et al. 1966).

The symptoms of myositis progress insidiously in most patients for weeks to months, although spontaneous remissions have been described (Rosenberg 1988). Rarely, the disease may present acutely over the course of 1 to 3 weeks with rapidly progressive weakness, severe myalgias, dysphagia, and, occasionally myoglobinuria, or respiratory insufficiency.

Serum creatine kinase (CK) is elevated in 66% to 95% of active or untreated cases of myositis (Bohan et al. 1977; DeVere and Bradley 1975). Abnormal antibodies include antinuclear antibodies (ANA) (16% to 40% of PM; 24% to 60% of DM cases), anti-Jo-1 (20% of PM; less frequent in DM), and signal recognition protein (SRP) seen only in PM and occurring in only 5% of cases (Amato and Barohn 1997). Electromyography demonstrates short-duration, small-amplitude polyphasic motor unit potentials in 90% of cases, fibrillation potentials and positive sharp waves in 74%, and complex repetitive discharges in 38% (Bohan et al. 1977). Abnormalities occasionally are isolated to paraspinous muscles. The spontaneous activity often decreases after effective treatment (Kimura 1983).

During the course of PM and DM, organs other than skeletal muscle may be involved. A review of ten series demonstrated an average of 21% of patients with another definable connective tissue disorder (Rosenberg and Ringel 1988). The most common overlapping diseases were systemic lupus erythematosus, progressive systematic sclerosis, Sjögren's syndrome, rheumatoid arthritis, and mixed connective tissue disease (Isenberg 1984).

Many types of malignancy have been associated with the inflammatory myopathies, with a frequency ranging from 3% to 60% (Callen 1994). Most reported series are simply too small to give reliable percentages. The most recent large series found malignancy in 15% of DM and 9% of PM patients (Sigurgeirsson et al. 1992). Whether these frequencies exceed those expected for the normal population remain uncertain, since valid age-matched controls were not included (Engel et al. 1994). Malignancy may occur prior to or at any time in the course of myositis (Cailen 1982).

Symptomatic cardiac involvement is uncommon (Bohan et al. 1977) but, with sophisticated cardiac assessment, subtle abnormalities are found in more than 70% of patients (Denbow et al. 1979; Gottdiener et al. 1978). Creatine kinase (CK)-MB fractions should be interpreted with caution because they may be elevated in the absence of cardiac pathology (Adornato and Engel 1977; Larca et al. 1981).

Detailed pulmonary accesssment can demonstrate interstitial lung disease with restrictive characteristics in more than 30% of patients, but symptomatic disease with radiographic changes occurs in less than 10% (Dickey and Myers 1984). An anti-Jo-1 antibody, present in 20% of cases, is associated with interstitial lung disease and is useful for predicting that complication (Yoshida et al. 1983). Interstitial lung disease is associated with a reduced response to therapy and predicts a poor long-term prognosis (Bohan 1988, Joffe et al. 1993). Diagnostic confusion of interstitial lung disease may occur with aspiration pneumonia, opportunistic infections, and methotrexate-induced pneumonitis (Rosenberg and Ringel 1988).

Dysphagia from pharyngeal or esophageal dysfunction increases the risk of aspiration and pneumonia (Bohan 1988; Kagen et al. 1985). Respiratory insufficiency secondary to fulminant muscle weakness occurs occasionally and improves if the underlying myositis responds to immunosuppression (Dickey and Myers 1984).

Children with DM develop unique complications, including subcutaneous calcifications and gastrointestinal hemorrhages. Calcinosis occurs in 20% to 50% of children, is refractory to treatment,

and may lead to skin ulcerations and secondary infections (Bohan 1988; Sarnat 1988). The necrotizing vasculitis results in symptoms of systematic illness, bowel hemorrhage and infarction, and vasculitic skin and nail bed changes (Banker and Victor 1966). Early contractures of extremities and growth retardation are common in childhood cases.

If untreated, both DM and PM have a very poor prognosis with a progressive downhill course. A mortality rate of 50% was recorded in a group of patients before the availability of prednisone or other immunosuppressive medications (O'Leary and Waisman 1940). At present most clinicians agree that corticosteroids are the treatment of choice in DM and PM. Most series demonstrate significant clinical improvement with the chronic administration of corticosteroids, although virtually all reports are retrospective, and have no adequate control group. Corticosteroids lead to improvement of strength in nearly 100% of DM cases and over 80% with PM (Joffe et al. 1993). Some patients are refractory to treatment or have only a partial return of function (Henriksson and Sanstedt 1982, Oddis 1994; Rose and Walton 1966; Vignos et al. 1964). This incomplete response, resulting from steroid resistance, an insufficient time of treatment, or permanent muscle injury, is not predictable prospectively (Rosenberg and Ringel 1988).

In addition to corticosteroids, a variety of other drugs are used in the treatment of DM and PM (Oddis 1994; Amato and Barohn 1997). These include the following.

*Azathioprine* (Bunch 1981) is a steroid-sparing agent that is introduced after symptoms are controlled with corticosteroids. The goal is to replace the immunosuppression of steroids and gradually reduce steroid dosage to minimize side effects of these agents. Unwanted azathioprine side effects are rare but include leukopenia, fever, rash, induction of malignancy, liver toxicity, and gastrointestinal intolerance.

*Methotrexate* (Fischer et al. 1979) can be used like azathioprine for the purpose of lowering prednisone requirements. The agent has similar hazards as azathioprine and may, in addition, cause interstitial lung disease.

*Cyclophosphamide* (Currie and Walton 1971) is used less often in PM or DM (Oddis 1994) and carries the same risks as the two agents described above as well as hemorrhagic cystitis.

*Chlorambucil* (Ansell 1984) is used infrequently in PM and DM and has considerable risks of bone marrow suppression and induction of malignancies.

*Cyclosporine* (Bendtzen et al. 1984) has been used when all other agents are either ineffective or not usable for any reason. Intense monitoring is necessary primarily because of its nephrotoxicity.

*Total-body irradiation* (Kelly et al. 1984) has been reported to help in a small number of DM and PM refractory to all other treatments.

*Plasma Exchange, and leukapheresis* (Miller et al. 1992) is without effect in DM and PM.

*Immune globulin* (Dalakas et al. 1993), although expensive, may be beneficial in DM refractory to all other treatments.

In terms of prognosis, an associated malignancy is the feature most closely correlated with poor outcome. The increased mortality is related to tumor spread rather than any failure of myositis to respond to corticosteroids (Bohan et al. 1977; Engel and Askansas 1976). Other factors predicting a worse prognosis include an acute fulminant course, dysphagia, cardiac involvement, acute pulmonary infiltration, and black race (Rosenberg and Ringel 1988). The presence of SRP antibodies in PM is particularly ominous, since such patients usually have a very abrupt onset, are resistant to immunosuppression, and show only a 25% survival at 5 years (Joffe et al. 1993). Factors predicting a better outcome include early intervention for better strength maintenance (Fafalak et al. 1994; Lilley et al. 1994) and age under 50 (Lilley et al. 1994).

## Inclusion Body Myositis

Inclusion body myositis (IBM) is an idiopathic, slowly progressive inflammatory myopathy with selective early weakness of wrist/finger flexors, foot dorsi flexors, and lower leg extensors (Lotz et al. 1989; Amato et al. 1996). Muscle biopsy light microscopic findings include characteristic basophilic rimmed vacuoles, subsarcolemmic eosinophilic cytoplasmic deposits in fibers, and patches of macrophages and CD8+ lymphocytes. Using ultrastructural methods, characteristic tubular filaments can be found in the nucleus (12 to 15 nM) and/or cytoplasm (15 to 19 nM). Amyloid and ubiquitin reactivity is present in the areas of rimmed vacuoles (Carpenter 1996). In some IBM biopsies typical "ragged red" fibers due to collections of abnormal mitochondria are seen. The mitochondria contain DNA mutations, and can be detected in 73% of IBM patients, a figure nearly double that found in normal patients and disease controls (Santorelli et al. 1996). Whether this is an aging effect, is related to inflammation, or is unique to IBM awaits further clarification.

Following its initial description by Chou (1967), IBM has become recognized as a major cause of acquired inflammatory disease in adults, occurring almost as frequently as DM or PM. The disease is seen in both sexes and is most common in men over the age of 50. It typically progresses so insidiously that an average of 6.5 years transpires from first weakness until diagnosis (Chou 1988; Ringel et al. 1987; Sawchek and Kula 1988). Patients with proximal limb weakness can be suspected of having DM or PM, but the finding of less severe but definite distal hand weakness and asymmetrical patterns greatly raise the possibility of IBM in the patient prior to biopsy (Amato et al. 1996). Dysphagia occurs in 40% of patients and facial weakness in about one-third. Electromyography reveals mixed neurogenic and myopathic features and the CK is commonly elevated but only minimally (Amato and Barohn 1997). Diagnosis is confirmed by muscle biopsy.

Immunosuppressive therapy with prednisone or other agents has little or no effect on the disease progression (Amato et al. 1996; Barohn 1997). recent trial of intravenous immune globulin (IVIG) for IBM patients failed to show any statistically significant outcome differences between the drug and placebo groups (Dalakas et al. 1997). Treatment of these patients must be directed at symptomatic measures including bracing and other assistive devices, wheelchairs, and scooters. In contrast to DM and PM there is no increased risk of interstitial lung disease or malignancy. Patients should be advised that although IBM produces progressive limb weakness and is resistant to drug therapy, a normal life span can be expected.

## MUSCULAR DYSTROPHIES

### Background

This heterogenous group of muscle diseases has undergone extensive reclassification in light of recent advancements in molecular biology. Until the advent of modern molecular genetic techniques, classification was only possible based on patterns of muscle weakness and rates of disease progression. Many of the disorders, though differing clinically, had similar pathological change on muscle biopsy so that clinicians had no means of identifying features helpful in predicting progression rates. In the mid-1980s a variety of dystrophin gene mutations were found to be associated with total absence of or abnormalities in dystrophin, a key muscle membrane-associated protein. Depending on the nature of the gene defect on the X chromosome, the patient could manifest either Duchenne's muscular dystrophy (DMD) or the closely related Becker's dystrophy (BMD) (Hoffman et al. 1988). Further research has shown that other muscle membrane-associated proteins such as the sarcoglycans, dystroglycans, and laminins, when absent or defective, may well underlie previously well-described clinical patterns in patients with limb girdle dystrophy (Ozawa et al. 1998), facioscapulohumeral dystrophy (van Deutekom et al. 1996b), or congenital dystrophy (Pegoraro et al. 1996). The following section will correlate clinical disease patterns with the known gene mutations in this rapidly changing field.

## Dystrophies Due to Dystrophin or Dystrophin-Associated Membrane Protein Defects

### X-Linked Duchenne's and Becker's Muscular Dystrophy

DMD and BMD type muscular dystrophy are similar disorders based on the inheritance of a defective gene located at the Xp21 locus of the X chromosome (Griggs et al. 1995). The Duchenne's form occurs with an incidence of about 30 per 100,000 live births and the Becker's form at about 3 per 100,000 births. The DMD form of the disorder occurs in young boys who develop weakness of shoulder and pelvic girdle muscles, usually before the age of 5. Calf hypertrophy, progressively clumsy gait, and need for wheelchair ambulation by the age of 8 to 10 is common, as is scoliosis and slowed intellectual development. In the majority, death due to pulmonary or cardiac failure occurs by the age of 20. The Becker's form of the disease is less severe but shares many of the findings seen in DMD. Becker's children develop symptoms after the age of 5, progress more slowly, can walk

as late as the age of 15 to 20 (and in some instances even into their 30s), and survive well into their 40s and 50s before succumbing to respiratory and cardiac complications. Both DMD and BMD are expressed in males but rare "manifesting carrier" females with symptom severity ranging from that seen in severe DMD of males to very minimal weakness have been reported (Pegoraro et al. 1995).

The gene at Xp21, which consists of 2000 kilobases, normally programs for a very large protein, dystrophin, whose molecular weight is 427 kDa. The dystrophin molecule in normal individuals is located just beneath the muscle cell membrane where it provides a bridging structure between intracellular actin filaments and several cell membrane proteins, the dystroglycans and sarcoglycans (Ozawa et al. 1998). In DMD patients the absence of dystrophin from the cell membrane is associated with progressive muscle cell breakdown and clinical weakness. In BMD, dystrophin is present, but its abnormal molecular structure contributes to premature muscle breakdown. Specific molecular defects in dystrophin do not always predict clinical symptomatology (Hoffman et al. 1988).

The symptoms of DMD may not be apparent clinically until age 4 or 5 and are characterized by falling, waddling gait, persistent toe walking, and the need for support to rise from the floor (Brooke 1986). Individual muscles continue to decline in strength at a uniform rate of 0.40 strength units per year on a 0 to 10 strength scale (Brooke et al. 1983) (Fig. 28-1). Functional decline is less linear (Allsop and Ziter 1981). Some affected children appear to improve their ambulation between ages 3 and 6, even while losing objective muscle strength. After age 8, ambulation typically deteriorates rapidly. In one assessment of natural history, all children walked until age 8, and 60% of children at age 12 were using a wheelchair (Brooke et al. 1983) (Fig. 28-2). Clinical experience with this prevalent disease and natural history studies have provided reliable information concerning course and prognosis (Scott et al. 1982). The most complete data are from a comprehensive analysis by the CIDD group (Brooke et al. 1983; Brooke 1986).

BMD may be considered a slower and less malignant form of DMD where the same clinical features appear but at a slower rate. With new molecular diagnostic techniques, the diagnosis of

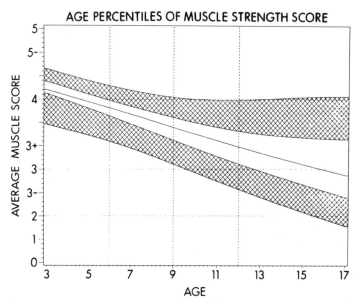

**Figure 28-1.** Graphic representation of the change in muscle strength with the age of a child. The data come from a multicenter study of 150 patients with Duchenne's muscular dystrophy: (From Brooke 1983.) The "average muscle score" is the mean Medical Research Council (MRC) grade of 34 separate muscles. The center line represents the 50% percentile, the upper hatched area the 75 to 95 percentiles, and the lower area the 5 to 25 percentiles.

BMD can be defined early on, which should allow for better treatment, counseling, and accurate natural history studies. Some cases previously described as BMD may, in fact, represent other types of muscle disease. The variable course reported previously, including the fact that some patients with dystrophies ambulate well into middle-age or beyond, needs confirmation, now that BMD cases can be identified with certainty (Ringel et al. 1977).

**Figure 28-2.** Graphic representation of the ages at which functional milestones are lost by patients with Duchenne's muscular dystrophy. (From Brooke 1989.)

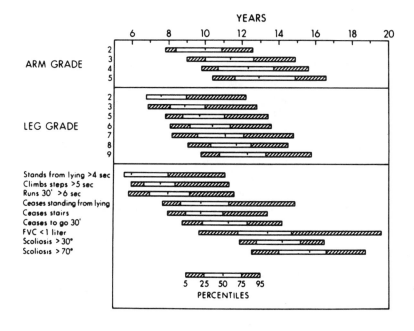

The diagnosis of DMD or BMD relies on characteristic clinical features and confirmatory laboratory studies. The serum creatinine kinase levels are elevated 20 to 100 times normal but gradually diminish with age (Brooke et al. 1983). Muscle biopsy, previously the definitive diagnostic test for DMD, should show fiber size variation, opaque fibers, increased fat and connective tissue, necrotic fibers with some infiltrating mononuclear cells, split fibers, and increased internal nuclei. With the discovery of absent or abnormal dystrophin, molecular analytic techniques are now used to confirm the diagnosis. Frozen sections of muscle biopsy material when layered with solutions of antidystrophin antibodies (immunostaining) will display an absence of dystrophin reactivity (DMD) or a spotty pattern of reactivity (BMD). Since only a few laboratories are equipped to carry out this immunostaining dystrophin analysis reliably, an alternative is Western blot analysis, for confirming the diagnosis. This technique uses a sample of muscle tissue to detect altered dystrophin size or reduced or absent dystrophin (Hoffman et al. 1988). DNA analysis of patient blood by polymerase chain reaction (PCR) or Southern blot is also useful, although it can detect deletions or duplications in only about 65 % of patients with Duchenne's or Becker's dystrophy. For carrier testing in females (Pegoraro et al. 1995), blood DNA can be screened for a dystrophin abnormality. Prenatal detection of a DNA mutation is possible during pregnancy using samples of amniotic fluid which contain fetal cells.

Drug treatment of Duchennes dystrophy has been disappointing. Prednisone has been shown to cause an initial strength improvement in Duchenne's patients, but the rate of decline thereafter over 6 months' follow-up is nearly the same as controls (Griggs et al. 1991). Side effects of weight gain, retardation of growth, and behavioral changes, even with alternate-day dosing, limit its use in clinical practice (Griggs et al. 1991; Mendell et al. 1991; Fenichel et al. 1991). Recent trials of the prednisolone derivative deflazacort (Angelini et al. 1994) and the anabolic steroid oxandrolone (Fenichel et al. 1997) have reported slight slowing of Duchenne's dystrophy progression, but both studies were on small numbers of patients. Attempts at gene replacement therapy using transplanted myoblasts have shown no clinical effect following extremely labor-intensive studies in a small number of patients (Mendell et al. 1995). Studies using viral vectors to carry dystrophin DNA replacement into muscle cells are now ongoing.

Children with DMD or BMD exhibit the same general patterns of muscle weakness, with the Becker's form progressing at a much slower rate. With increasing leg muscle weakness there is a propensity for tripping and falling, particularly in the setting of active children at play in school or at home. There is a disproportionate and increasing weakness of hip extensors and foot dorsi flexors, accompanied by antagonist muscles pulling disproportionately in the opposite direction. Over several years this leads to a compensatory lumbar lordosis and tendency to toe walking. Contractures reduce the range of limb motion so that the posture becomes increasingly permanent. Gradually, the combination of increasing weakness and contractures leads to such gait instability that the DMD child may begin to use a wheelchair for safety reasons from age 6 or 7 onward. The development of contractures can be slowed with a sensible stretching program and some increase of strength can be obtained with active exercise (Brooke at al. 1989). Such a program is only successful when parents and child agree that continued independent standing and walking are desirable goals. In some families where motivation for walking is great, the use of long leg braces can extend the time that the child walks safely. For these children, Achilles tendon releases may be needed to restore markedly plantar flexed feet to a stabilized neutral position which is then held fixed by lower leg braces. Extensions of the brace envelope the thigh so that knee joint fixation is accomplished, allowing the child to walk in a "stiff legged" manner (Siegal 1986). One series reports that with a comprehensive program of stretching, standing, tenotomies, and orthoses, patients were able to walk until a mean age of 13.6 years (Vignos et al. 1996). Such an outcome requires enthusiasm and the full cooperation of family and child in the setting of a multidisciplinary rehabilitation unit. Eventually, the progressive weakness, increasing difficulty walking, and increasing falls will convince the family and child that the majority of waking hours are safer if spent in a wheelchair.

The majority of DMD children exhibit slow intellectual development and many will require special education classes (Brooke 1986). This further complicates the family situation, where the physical difficulties experienced by the child already consume great blocks of time by parents and other family members. School authorities need to be made aware of the special needs of the Duchenne's child so that a reasonable, adequately paced educational plan can be developed.

Once wheelchair confined, problems other than skeletal muscle weakness become most apparent in DMD patients (Brooke 1986). Progressive kyphoscoliosis develops in up to 80% of children who are no longer ambulatory and may further compromise a weakening diaphragm (Brooke 1986; Smith et al. 1987). Orthotic devices and specialized wheelchair supports can delay the progression of scoliosis. Spinal bracing with polypropylene body jackets is probably not of any use (Brooke et al. 1989). Certainly these jackets tend to decrease vital capacity in many patients and should therefore not be used during respiratory infections or in patients with a very low vital capacity (Noble-Jamieson et al. 1986). Surgical correction of scoliosis using the technique of L-rod segmental stabilization has become popular (Luque 1982). There are conflicting data as to whether this procedure slows the decline of vital capacity (Kurz et al. 1983; Smith et al. 1987; Brook et al. 1996). In spite of any of these therapies, respiratory decline continues, and death typically occurs in the DMD patient by the late second or early third decade from pulmonary infection or respiratory insufficiency (Inkley et al. 1976). A refractory cardiomyopathy occasionally is the primary cause of death.

Proper nutrition to maintain a moderate weight is important, since obesity or low weight from malnutrition can cause impaired respiratory function (Smith et al. 1987). Prompt treatment of acute respiratory infections with antibiotics, physiotherapy, postural drainage, and assistive ventilation is imperative. An annual influenza vaccination also is recommended. Long-term assisted ventilation with tracheostomy may not be needed until the vital capacity drops to as low as 10% (Fukunaga et al. 1993). This is used, at first, only at night but eventually becomes a full-time requirement for the remainder of the child's life, which can be extended into the third decade (Rideau et al. 1983; Rideau 1986). Assisted ventilation is increasingly being used, but much remains to be learned in selecting the appropriate patients to receive this in-

tervention There are substantial disagreements regarding the ethical and financial questions of long-term assistive ventilation of patients with advanced DMD (Smith et al. 1987). A recent study has shown that noninvasive intermittent positive-pressure ventilation (Bi-Pap) substantially reduced hospitalization time and prolonged survival in DMD patients compared to those undergoing tracheostomy/ventilator support (Bach et al. 1997). The authors favor Bi-Pap, since it is less invasive, less labor intensive, and far cheaper as a method of pulmonary support.

### Limb Girdle Muscular Dystrophy

Limb girdle dystrophy (LGMD) is the designation given to a distinctive subgroup within the muscular dystrophies as delineated by Walton and Natrass (1954). It is now apparent that several different diseases were included under LGMD as originally defined solely by clinical features. The disease occurs in both sexes, becomes clinically obvious in childhood or young adults, and is transmitted as an autosomal dominant or recessive trait. With newer genetic techniques, subtypes of LGMD have been identified so that the collection of various clinical observations is now becoming organized into more clinically useful groupings based on DNA mutations and abnormal proteins.

The most benign form of LGMD seen in adults usually presents in the early teens or twenties with proximal leg weakness, and, within a few years proximal arm weakness. Scapular winging is generally an early finding, progression is slow, and the need for assisted ambulation may not be obvious for 20 or 30 years after symptom onset. Facial weakness does not occur.

Muscle biopsy changes in any of the adult-onset LGMDs are nonspecific and include fiber size variation, increased central muscle, scattered hypertrophied fibers, and some increase in connective tissue. A characteristic lobulated appearance on biopsies of LGD patients in several Dutch kindreds have been termed by some as "Bethlem myopathy" after the author first describing the condition, but the term is not universally accepted.

Cases in adults are usually based on autosomal recessive inheritance. One type designated LGMD 2B has been linked to a gene mutation on chromosome 2. Cases of the adult form are autosomal recessive. In two large kindreds (one from the island of Reunion and the other in Amish of northern Illinois) transmission of this autosomal recessive disease (designated LGMD 2A) results from a gene mutation on chromosome 15, leading to an abnormality of the nonstructural muscle protein, calpain.

Another form termed LGMD1A slowly manifests progressive muscle weakness and is transmitted as an autosomal dominant abnormality due to a gene mutation on chromosome 5 (Speer et al. 1992). Several other LGMD types designated as "Erb type" and "Leyden-Mobius type" based on clinical features alone may not be forms of LGMD at all and, consequently, the terms are not in general use (Shields 1994).

A less frequent but very serious form of LGMD termed severe childhood autosomal recessive muscular dystrophy or (SCARMD) occurs early in childhood. It is known to result from defects in one or more of the transmembrane proteins termed sarcoglycans (Ozawa et al. 1998). In normal skeletal muscle, these sarcoglycans are closely linked to another membrane protein group, the dystroglycans and together they form a bridge between the extracellular basal lamina protein laminin and subsarcolemmal dystrophin. The commonest pattern in these SCARMD patients is to find normal dystrophin immunostaining accompanied by a reduction or absence of immunostaining for α-sarcoglycan (Duggan et al. 1997). Further analysis will show an underlying primary gene mutation of DNA coding for α-(LGMD 2D, chromosome 17), β-(LGMD 2E, chromosome 4) or γ-(LGMD 2G, chromosome 13) sarcoglycan (Onggan et al. 1997; Eymard et al. 1997). Generally speaking, any of these mutations is associated with low levels of all sacroglycans (Straab and Campbell 1997). A fourth sarcoglycan mutation, δ sarcoglycan, is recognized as due to a mutation on chromosome 5 (LGMD 2F). One hopes that the "nomenclature wars" over LGMD have ended so that clinicians can become comfortable with this bewildering maze of chromosome mutations, disease types, and protein defects.

Before modern molecular genetic tests were available, males with SCARMD were thought to have DMD. The presence of normal dystrophin in muscle and occurrence in both sexes greatly changed that early impression. Onset varies from early to late childhood. Children manifest proximal arm and leg weakness, calf hypertrophy, a waddling gait, and early loss of walking in a pattern like DMD or BMD. Use of a wheelchair because of weakness varies from age 7 to 8 to late teens. Intellect is usually normal in these children. Most of the kindreds reported demonstrate consanguinity. The serum creatine kinase is elevated usually in excess of 10,000 and muscle biopsy changes are very similar to those seen in DMD (Ben Hamida et al. 1983).

In any of the LGMDs, cardiac involvement with arrhythmias and congestive failure may be seen, but these manifestations are typically much milder than in Duchenne's muscular dystrophy (Hoshio et al. 1987; Hunter 1980; Welsh et al. 1963). Diaphragmatic and intercostal muscle weakness produce alveolar hypoventilation in a few severely affected patients (Kilburn et al. 1959; Newsom-Davis 1980). Severe low back pain may develop as a consequence of lumbar and abdominal muscle weakness (Brooke 1986). Rehabilitation treatment for any of the LGMD syndromes employs the same methods as for Duchenne's muscular dystrophy.

Great variability exists with age of onset, and progression of LGMD. Generally, the clinical features are predictable only within the specific kindreds reported and studied to date (Duggan et al. 1997). Before a diagnosis of limb girdle dystrophy can be made, other muscle disease must be excluded utilizing electrical studies, muscle biopsy and, when indicated, screening for dystrophin and specific sarcoglycan defects (Shields 1994).

### Congenital Muscular Dystrophy

This rare neuromuscular disorder contains two types: the classical occidental form affecting muscle only and the Fukuyama form in which CNS abnormalities are prominent.

In classical congenital muscular dystrophy (CMD), at birth, abnormalities noted include hypotonia, hip dislocation, respiratory problems, and are severe weakness. These children show developmental delay but are intellectually normal. Creatine kinase levels are usually elevated substantially, brain MRI may show a few scattered white matter lesions, and the muscle biopsy shows moderate to severe dystrophic changes and, in some rare cases, inflammation (Pegoraro et al. 1996). Immunostaining for membrane proteins reveals normal dystrophin levels, but in about half the CMD cases merosin cannot be detected

(Kobyashi et al. 1996; Pegoraro et al. 1996). Merosin ($\alpha_2$-laminin) is the heavy chain part of the extracellular matrix protein laminin, which is linked to intracellular dystrophin by the transmembrane dystroglycan/sarcoglycan complex. Merosin absence in CMD is an unfavorable prognostic sign, since these children rarely gain the ability to walk. Patients in whom merosin is present are generally less severely affected, develop the ability to stand and walk (although a wheelchair may be needed later in life), and are intellectually normal. Merosin absence has been linked to a gene mutation on chromosome 6.

In the *Fukuyama* form of CMD, seen primarily in Japan, patients are more seriously affected at birth and, in addition, have mental retardation, seizures and rarely survive beyond the age of 10 years. A chromosome 9 defect is thought to underlie abnormalities of laminin in these cases.

There is no specific drug treatment for any form of CMD. An active rehabilitation program is vital for minimizing contractures, and assistive devices such as wheelchairs and braces should be utilized as needed.

## Other Dystrophies

### Myotonic Dystrophy

Myotonic dystrophy is an autosomal dominant disease resulting from an unstable CTG trinucleotide (triplet) repeat in a noncoding region (intron) on the long arm of chromosome 19. Normal individuals have 5 to 25 of these triplet repeats. The disease is variably expressed depending on the number of repeats present—mildly affected patients may have only 50 to 80 repeats, but above that number clinical manifestations of the disease are increasingly severe. The most seriously affected patients can have up to 4000 triplet repeats (Fu et al. 1992). The intron repeats are thought to interfere somehow with coding for 71- and 80-kDa protein kinases (myotonin) which, to date, has been localized to the terminal cisternae of the sarcoplasmic reticulum in skeletal muscle, cardiac intercalated discs, and at the neuromuscular junction (Maeda et al. 1995). The normal function of this protein is poorly understood. The disease is manifested by progressive muscle weakness and myotonia as well as abnormalities of other organ systems. A prevalence rate of 5 per 100,000 makes myotonic dystrophy the most common dystrophy in the general population (Harper and Rudel 1994).

The age of clinical onset and the severity of symptoms vary greatly. Occasionally, adult carriers of the gene are unaware of their disease, although careful clinical evaluation usually demonstrates signs of myotonic dystrophy by late adolescence (Bundey 1974).

The first signs of myotonic dystrophy may be behavioral and cognitive as the patient shows poor school performance, and bizarre, if not genuinely antisocial behavior and indifference to tasks at hand, work, family responsibilites, and so forth. Patients frequently seek medical help when the disease is well established, complaining of grip and foot dorsiflexion weakness accompanied by weakness and atrophy of facial, temporalis, masseter, and sternocleidomastoid muscles. There may be a characteristic expressionless facial appearance with ptosis, hollowing at the temples and jaw (hatchet-face), a thin, swan-like neck, and frontal balding. Early in the disease weakness is confined to distal muscles but, with time, proximal weakness occurs. Although grip myotonia is easily demonstrated in a typical patient, only rarely is it troublesome to the patient. Muscle weakness is the major patient complaint and is progressive in all patients as recently reported (Griggs et al. 1989).

A peculiarly severe form of the disease is seen during infancy and is almost exclusively of children born to myotonic dystrophy mothers (Harper and Rudel 1994). These infants are hypotonic with weak facial muscles and feeding difficulties. Respiratory insufficiency may occur and often results in pulmonary infection or death. As these children develop, they are more likely to have severe respiration problems (25% dying within 18 months of birth), bowel dysfunction, mental retardation, and premature death, with only 50% surviving into their thirties (Reardon et al. 1993). The reason for such "anticipation" of symptoms in subsequent generations is now understood. The expanded portion of the gene containing triplet repeats is unstable during meiosis and liable to further amplification, particularly in the female gamete. Thus, a large amplification is more likely to occur when the abnormal gene is passed from the mother. The result, almost invariably, is a child with very advanced symptoms of myotonic dystrophy at birth.

Involvement of organ systems other than skeletal muscle occurs in most myotonic dystrophy patients and can cause severely disabling problems as follows:

1. Electrocardiographic (ECG) changes occur in up to 90% of patients (Church 1967). Progressive conduction defects and cardiac arrhythmias are noted in over half of patients tested and may be responsible for occasional sudden deaths (Florek et al. 1990; Hawley et al. 1991). Yearly ECGs are advised when following these patients, looking for first-degree heart block or other changes within the conduction system. Patients may or may not complain of dizzy spells or fainting, but in the presence of such symptoms, cardiac pacemaker placement should be considered.

2. Breathing difficulties may occur in the myotonic patient manifested either by excessive daytime sleepiness, much less commonly nocturnal sleep disturbance (van der Meche et al. 1994). The resulting alveolar hypoventilation is due to respiratory muscle weakness and/or impaired central ventilatory response (Carroll et al. 1977; Martin 1984). For some patients with demonstrable hypercapnia, night-time assisted ventilation should be considered as well as low-dose methylphenidate (van der Meche et al. 1994). Although often asymptomatic, these respiratory abnormalities combined with cardiac defects lead to an increased risk with general anesthetics and hypersensitivity to other respiratory depressants (Ravin et al. 1975).

3. Cataracts eventually develop in almost all patients (Brooke 1986) and are treated with removal if clinically indicated.

4. The mental status of myotonic dystrophy patients often is bizarre and many seem argumentative, lack insight, are demanding, and have difficulty getting along with others. Although mental retardation occurs in a minority of patients (Harper and Rudel 1994), changes on psychometric and behavioral testing are much more frequent (Bird et al. 1983). These findings may account for the high incidence of unemployment and low motivation described in many patients (Woodward et al. 1982).

5. Gastrointestinal tract problems are seen in a high proportion of patients, and in one study were rated by patients as their most disabling complication (Ronnblom et al. 1996). Symptoms include abdominal pain, swallowing difficulties, esophageal motility problems, diarrhea, and anal sphincter incontinence. Metoclopromide may be helpful for symptomatic relief (Horowitz et al. 1987).

Other abnormalities noted during the course of the disease include cholelithiasis, hyperinsulinemia, testicular atrophy, polyhydramnios, and spontaneous abortions in women (Brooke 1986; Marshall 1959; Stuart et al. 1977; Swick et al. 1981).

Specific drug treatments for the systemic disorder have not been developed, since so little is known of underlying disease mechanisms. A trial of testosterone, based on its anabolic effect on muscle and the observation of low testosterone in myotonics, did not result in any measurable improvement of strength (Griggs et al. 1989). At present, treatment is limited to providing ankle/foot orthoses for the foot drop in patients and monitoring of the other systems noted above in order to provide timely intervention. Since myotonia is virtually never a complaint in these patients, there is rarely a need for symptomatic relief. When treatment is requested for myotonia, phenytoin should be given and quinine or procainamide avoided because they tend to prolong the cardiac conduction P-R interval.

## Facioscapulohumeral Dystrophy

The clinical features of facioscapulohumeral dystrophy (FSHD) was defined in the classic paper on muscular dystrophies by Walton and Nattrass (1954). FSHD is a genetically determined disease transmitted as an autosomal dominant trait with full penetrance but variable degrees of expression (Padberg et al. 1991). Prevalence is 1 case per 100,000 population.

Key features of FSHD are covered in the review by Padberg et al. (1991). Symptoms begin in childhood or teens/twenties with weakness initially in facial muscles but with sparing of masseter, temporalis, and extraocular muscles. Progressive facial weakness and laxity lead to the characteristic appearance of an expressionless, smooth, drooping face and protruding lips or *bouche de tapir*. Patients will be unable to puff their cheeks out adequately, will have weakness of forced eyelid closure, and often admit to a lifelong history of difficulty blowing up balloons or drinking from straws. Attempts to smile show poor horizontal movement of the angles of the mouth with dimpling. Weakness and wasting of shoulder girdle muscles, usually in an asymmetrical fashion, occurs early in the disease, to produce prominent scapular winging, and marked inability to abduct the arm at the shoulder. Due to serratus weakness the scapulae become displaced laterally and slightly downward, resulting in prominent anterior axillary folds and the clavicles, rather than angling slightly upward, assume a position parallel to the floor. Initially, most patients are aware of the scapular winging but are bothered by difficulty in raising their arms over their head. To compensate, patients may resort to a "flinging" movements to elevate the arms. If the scapula is held forcefully against the chest wall by the examiner, the deltoid muscle strength will be found to be nearly normal, allowing the patient to carry out full arm abduction and elevation of their arm over their head. Later in the course, selective and asymmetrical involvement of biceps, triceps, and peroneal groups can be seen. Weakness of the anterior tibialis muscles will lead to a slapping, footdrop gait. Abdominal muscle weakness may lead to any inability to do a conventional sit-up, and with such weakness a positive Beaver's sign may be seen. A minority of patients, usually around 20%, and only after many years, develop such extensive weakness that rising from a chair is no longer possible and walking so precarious and difficult that a wheelchair or power-driven scooter is needed.

The time of symptom onset varies greatly in FSHD. Symptoms are commonly noted in late adolescence or early adulthood in most patients (Walton and Nattrass 1954; Padberg et al. 1991). Several studies, however, document that at least 30% of affected family members may be unaware of their disease, even during adulthood (Zundel and Tyler 1965). Uncommonly, symptoms may begin during infancy, and these children typically have more severe weakness and occasionally other associated abnormalities, such as nerve deafness, retinal telangiectasia/detachment (Coat's disease), and lumbar lordosis. The disease is very slowly progressive and may remain confined to the upper extremities in up to 50% of affected people (Munsat 1986). Lifespan is not reduced (Padberg et al. 1991). A few cases that begin with

isolated facial weakness and rapidly progress to profound generalized weakness over a period of months have been noted, but they are poorly documented (Brooke 1986).

Diagnosis of the disorder is based on the characteristic clinical feature, the exclusion of other disorders producing proximal weakness, and a positive family history, although nearly one-third of patients may be unaware of similarly affected relatives. The serum CK is usually only moderately elevated. Muscle biopsy shows mild, nonspecific changes such as increased central nuclei, fiber size variation, split fibers, and minimal amounts of increased connective tissue. In a small number of biopsies inflammatory infiltrates are present. Since biopsy is usually obtained from less severely affected "conventional sites" (quadriceps, biceps, or deltoid), the lack of more striking abnormalities is not surprising. Diagnostic biopsy of the more clinically involved supraspinatus muscle has been suggested by some, but the procedure is technically more difficult and not commonly done (Bodensteiner and Schochet 1986).

Treatment of FSHD is entirely symptomatic. Most patients eventually need polypropylene ankle-foot orthoses for the footdrop difficulty. Since progression is slow and the disease not fatal in itself, patients in their forties to sixties may eventually need wheelchairs or scooters. For progressive hand weakness, an occupational therapist will be vital in introducing adaptive equipment for eating, dressing, toileting, and other aids to daily living. For individuals demonstrating inflammatory muscle biopsies, particularly severe juvenile cases, there is no response to prolonged corticosteroid therapy (Munsat et al. 1972; Munsat and Bradley 1977; Wulff et al. 1982). A recent trial of prednisone for 12 weeks in eight FSHD patients failed to improve strength (Tawil et al. 1997), but trials with albuterol, a β-adrenergic agent, are promising and ongoing. Surgical fixation of the scapula to the thoracic wall may allow greater functional use of the arms in selected cases (Letournel et al. 1990).

FSHD is transmitted as an autosomal dominant trait resulting from a gene abnormality on chromosome 4. The actual gene locus and gene product have not yet been defined. Disease expression seems to be related to variably sized deletions within a repetitive element near the telomeric portion of the long arm of chromosome 4. These deletions, by a process termed "position effect variegation," are postulated to repress gene transcription to produce the human disease (van Deutekom et al. 1996a). There are numerous uncertainties about the actual gene for FSHD, but genetic testing to look for distal telomeric deletions can be carried out on patients and families having the disorder (Tawil et al. 1998). For the estimated 10% of new sporadic mutations occurring, genetic verification may also be possible. The latest reports suggests that specific deletions are found in 86% to 95% of cases with disease (van Deutekom et al. 1996b).

### *Scapuloperoneal Syndrome*

This category of rare muscle disorders has become even smaller as gene analysis and other diagnostic techniques place patients into more precise groups such as FSHD and LGMD. Unlike FSHD, scapuloperoneal syndrome (SPS) patients develop weakness initially in the shoulder girdle muscles by the teenage years with slow progression to involve foot dorsiflexors and eventually pelvic girdle weakness. Minimal facial weakness may occur but it is seen late in the disease (Feigenbaum and Munsat 1970; Kaeser 1965), unlike FSHD, where it is an early and striking feature. Many other diseases mimic this pattern of muscle weakness, including spinal muscular atrophies, some unusual polyneuropathies, and other myopathies (Harding and Thomas 1980; Kaeser 1965). SPS can be sporadic or may be transmitted in an autosomal dominant or recessive manner (Munsat 1986; Thomas et al. 1975). To date, no candidate gene or chromosome locus has been identified. Nerve deafness also may be associated with this syndrome (Ansher et al. 1989). Laboratory studies are abnormal but not diagnostic, there being a mild elevation of CK and either neurogenic or myopathic changes seen on muscle biopsy.

Emery-Dreifuss muscular dystrophy (EDMD) has many of the clinical features of SPS starting with biceps, triceps, and anterior tibial weakness in childhood with scapular winging later. Unique features of EDMD, however, include (1) the development of early joint contractures, especially at the elbows and toes to give affected children a very characteristic phenotypic appearance; (2) cardiac conduction defects; and (3) an X-linked inheritance pattern. (Emery and Dreifuss 1966; Rowland et al. 1979). Because of the cardiac conduction block and arrhythmias, sudden death may occur if the cardiac disturbance is not recognized and treated promptly with pacemaker placement (Grim and Janka 1994). The muscle weakness pattern is slowly progressive. Treatment is limited to symptomatic measures.

### *Oculopharyngeal Dystrophy*

This rare autosomal dominant disorder, first described in a French-Canadian kindred, is found in virtually every ethnic group in the world. It is characterized clinically by progressive ptosis, limitation of extraocular movements with eventual complete paralysis of eye muscles, and progressive swallowing difficulties. Commonly, symptoms do not begin until about age 50. Arm and leg weakness is rarely a feature except in some Japanese kindreds. Patients may deny any family involvement at first, suggesting other diagnoses such as myasthenia gravis but, eventually, involvement of others in the family is discovered. Muscle biopsy reveals characteristic rimmed vacuoles in small, angular fibers. The CK levels are two to three times normal, and electromyographic (EMG) studies may show mild myopathic changes in limb muscles. The disorder is passed as an autosomal dominant trait due to a mutation of the gene responsible for coding of a cardiac myosin heavy chain on chromosome 14.

Oculopharyngeal dystrophy (OPD) symptoms progress gradually over many years, and patients tend to develop similar degrees of incapacity as seen in those affected in previous generations. Since there is no specific drug treatment for the disorder, patients can receive only symptomatic therapy, which includes corrective surgery for the ptosis and, in rare instances, cricopharyngeal myotomy to assist with the swallowing difficulty. A small number of patients will require a feeding gastrostomy tube.

## Other Muscle Diseases

### Congenital Myopathies

These disorders are relatively rare and present in early infancy or childhood with muscle weakness and hypotonia and are characterized by a variety of unique changes on muscle biopsy. Virtually all were discovered and described in the past 40 years using histochemical and electron microscopic techniques. A few of the conditions have known genetic mutations, and in several there are prominent accumulations of desmin and vimentin (Goebel 1996).

Clinically, all can present at birth with hypotonia, difficulty feeding and breathing, and with a stormy neonatal course and early death (Bodensteiner 1988). Differentiation from spinal muscular atrophy or a glycogen storage disease is not possible without a muscle biopsy. More commonly, children exhibit delayed motor milestones which bring them to a pediatrician and eventually to specialists for diagnosis. On examination the child shows slowness in running, difficulty getting up from the floor, and mild limb weakness. Laboratory studies may show a normal or slightly elevated CK. Electrical studies are only rarely abnormal. For a specific diagnosis, muscle biopsy is recommended to detect the unique features of a congenital myopathy and to exclude an inflammatory disorder or neurogenic disease such as spinal muscular atrophy. Once diagnosed, the course of the vast majority, with a few exceptions to be noted below, is relatively benign. The child continues to show muscle strength development below the level of peers, may do poorly in games requiring physical skills, but is generally intellectually normal or even above average and can grow into adulthood within the limitations of the muscle weakness.

Three of the congenital myopathies manifest special features that differentiate them from the generic description given above (Bodensteiner 1988; Goebel 1996):

### Nemaline Myopathy

These children may have striking dysmorphic features, including an elongated, thin head, and a high arched palate. Skeletal abnormalities are common and include kyphoscoliosis, pectus excavatum, high arched foot, and other foot deformities. If the disease is not associated with early death in infancy, the course is relatively benign, although a minority of patients develop increasing respiratory insufficiency requiring Bi-Pap ventilation or even tracheostomy/ventilator. The disease is thought to be due to a gene mutation on chromosome 1 (Laing et al. 1992) and is transmitted as an autosomal dominant disorder with low penetrance or, rarely, as an autosomal recessive trait. There is no specific treatment for this disorder, but skeletal abnormalities may be helped by appropriate surgical therapies.

### Central Core Disease

Skeletal abnormalities are similar to those of nemaline myopathy but also include congenital hip dislocation and an increased incidence of malignant hyperthermia (MH). Since the gene mutation for this autosomal dominant disease is on chromosome 19 (Mulley et al. 1993), the higher risk for MH may be due to the fact that the ryanodine receptor maps to the same region (Frank et al. 1980). These children generally follow a clinical course described in the initial part of this section, with survival commonly into adulthood. Rarely, adult patients may require canes, crutches, or wheelchairs.

### Centronuclear (Myotubular) Myopathy

The neonatal form of the this disease, marked by severe weakness and extraocular movement paralysis, is rapidly fatal and is due to a gene defect on the X chromosome (Starr et al. 1990). Two other forms whose gene locus is unknown exhibit less severe patterns of weakness: the late infantile/early childhood form is transmitted as an autosomal recessive trait, exhibits diffuse muscle weakness with delayed milestones and, in addition, extraocular muscle weakness; the late childhood/adult type has no extraocular involvement, may appear as a limb girdle syndrome, and is transmitted as an autosomal dominant trait.

## Other Congenital Myopathies

The remainder of the congenital myopathies are extremely rare and are defined by muscle biopsy changes in a child presenting with mild weakness covered in the initial description above. An excellent summary of these various conditions is to be found in the text by Griggs, Mendell and Miller (1995) and review by Goebel (1996).

### Metabolic Muscle Disorders

These disorders, based on a number of biochemical abnormalities, are clinically characterized by exercise intolerance, muscle pain and, in some cases, muscle breakdown resulting in release of myoglobin into the blood and urine. In normal skeletal muscle, the energy needed in the contractile process is provided by hydrolysis of adenosine triphosphate (ATP), which is constantly replenished by complex reactions within the cell cytoplasm and mitochondria. To produce and maintain adequate quantities of ATP, skeletal muscle utilizes certain "fuels" depending on the intensity and duration of muscle action. During brief, high-intensity muscle contraction, glycogen is degraded into glucose, which is anaerobically metabolized to lactate to produce ATP. Other anaerobic sources, phosphocreatine, and processes of the purine nucleotide cycle contribute ATP to a lesser extent. During more prolonged exercise there is a shift to aerobic glycogen metabolism to produce ATP from pyruvate entering the citric acid cycle and long-chain fatty acids undergoing β oxidation within mitochondria. If any of the ATP-producing pathways are defective, excess substrates may accumulate to produce morphological abnormalities within skeletal muscle. These can vary widely and include striking accumulations of lipid, autophagic vacuoles, or glycogen. In other instances, large numbers of bizarrely shaped mitochondria may be seen. The specific enzyme defect underlying any one of the diseases in this heterogeneous group may be assayed using specific biochemical tests. Despite current detailed knowledge of such enzyme defects and the gene locus for many of the conditions, treatment remains symptomatic. Several of the more common disorders will be described.

## Myophosphorylase Deficiency

The most common glycogen storage disease of muscle is myophosphorylase deficiency (McArdle's disease), most frequent in males and transmitted as an autosomal recessive disorder (DiMauro and Tsujino 1994) due to several gene mutations on chromosome 11 (Vorgerd et al. 1998). Rarely, it can occur as an autosomal dominant trait (Chu and Munsat 1976). Because of muscle myophosphorylase deficiency, glycogen cannot be degraded to glucose for anaerobic metabolism to produce the ATP necessary in short, intense exercise. Patients while exercising may develop muscle pain, stiffness, and early fatigue. In extreme cases, patients may develop painful and sustained muscle contraction (termed "contractures," which by EMG are electrically silent) and myoglobinuria. A "second wind" phenomenon or lessening of pain and fatigue occurring with continued exercise may be seen due to a shift to aerobic metabolism as adequate fuel is provided in the form of fatty acids entering the mitochondria. Onset of symptoms has been reported during infancy and as late as age 60 (DiMauro and Tsujino 1994; Kost and Verity 1980). In one large series, 85% of patients developed symptoms younger than 15 years (DiMauro and Tsujino 1994).

With exercise, only 50% of patients ever develop myoglobinuria, and 60% of these have less than three episodes. Renal failure has been reported to occur in nearly 50% of affected patients, but the figure is probably much lower as the full spectrum of the condition has become better known (Penn et al. 1994). Most patients learn to prevent severe contractures and myoglobinuria by limiting exercise when they first notice muscle fatigue. More frequent exacerbations have been documented secondary to vascular insufficiency and other unknown factors (Kost and Verity 1980; Wheeler and Brooke 1983).

A minority of patients develop fixed proximal muscle weakness, typically after many years of symptoms (Schmid and Hammer 1961). Cardiac muscle involvement is rare due to preserved activity of the cardiac isoenzyme of phosphorylase (Miranda et al. 1979).

The diagnosis of a glycogen storage disorder can be confirmed by performing a forearm ischemic exercise. A failure to show lactic acid buildup in venous blood following exercise is highly indicative of the disorder. Final confirmation can be obtained by muscle biopsy, which will show a specific absence of phosphorylase either by standard histochemical methods or by a specific enzyme assay that is available commercially. Other rarer enzyme defects can only be diagnosed by commercially available enzyme assays.

Several therapies have been used to improve exercise tolerance, including oral fructose, intravenous glucose, isoproterenol, fasting, and exercise training (DiMauro and Tsujino 1994). The effects generally have been mild and not beneficial in all patients. If exercise is avoided, further symptoms can be prevented and progressive weakness will not occur.

## Primary Muscle Carnitine Deficiency

Although several myopathies showing lipid excess in muscle are known, these disorders occur so infrequently that a description of the pathogenesis of each is not practical. One example, primary muscle carnitine deficiency, is a clinical syndrome defined by progressive muscle weakness, lipid storage in muscle, and decreased free carnitine levels demonstrable only in skeletal muscle (Carroll 1988; Engel and Angelini 1973). Another example is primary systemic carnitine deficiency, an exceedingly rare condition that presents with heart failure due to a cardiomyopathy. It is thought that high-affinity carnitine receptors are missing from cells (DiDonato 1994). Without these receptors, carnitine is reduced or absent from cells and most likely from mitochondrial membranes as well. This would be a critical defect, since carnitine acts as a carrier protein to transport long-chain fatty acids across the mitochondrial membrane to enter the process of $\beta$ oxidation. The process also requires two active enzymes, carnitine palmitoyl transferase I and II (CPT I and CPT II) (DiDonato 1994).

Carnitine deficiency probably occurs more commonly as a secondary phenomenon seen with organic acidurias, respiratory chain defects, Fanconi's syndrome, dialysis, and valproate therapy (DiDonato 1994). An autosomal recessive inheritance has been suggested (DiMarco et al. 1985).

Whether primary or secondary, the onset of symptoms in carnitine deficiency typically begins in childhood but can be seen as early as age 18 months and up to as late as 38 years. Exercise intolerance is an early symptom in patients (Willner 1979). A slowly progressive proximal muscle weakness develops in most patients (DiMarco et al. 1985). The weakness may fluctuate and sometimes will progress rapidly (Bradley et al. 1978; Carroll 1988). Several patients have been described with cardiomyopathy, which may lead to early death (Hart et al. 1978). Some patients have been reported to improve with oral carnitine, corticosteroids, riboflavin, or propranolol, while others are unresponsive to treatment (Angelini et al. 1976; Carroll et al. 1980; 1981; Engel and Siekert 1972; Isaacs et al. 1986).

## Carnitine Palmitoyl Transferase Deficiency

This disorder is due to an absence of either CPT I or II from the mitochondrial membrane. As a result, fatty acids cannot cross into the mitochondrial matrix to be used in $\beta$ oxidation. Patients can utilize the normally functioning glucose metabolism system for short-term exercise but, with sustained activity, symptoms appear as the required changeover to fatty acid metabolism fails to occur. Symptoms of muscle pain, stiffness, and tightness result during prolonged exercise. The most alarming result of continued exercise is muscle breakdown, which can lead to myoglobinuria, renal failure, and death if not treated appropriately. Other precipitating factors besides exercise include a low-carbohydrate/high-fat diet, fasting, exposure to cold, and infection (Galdi and Clark 1989). The disorder is transmitted as an autosomal recessive trait due to a gene defect on chromosome 1. Diagnosis is by enzyme assay of skeletal muscle for CPT I or II. Skeletal muscle biopsy shows the muscle to be entirely normal with no evidence of lipid storage, unlike the findings in carnitine deficiency. Symptoms of the disorder, which is the commonest cause of recurrent myoglobinuria, can be prevented by avoidance of precipitating factors, particularly exercise. A low-fat, high-carbohydrate diet is also recommended. There is no residual weakness after episodes of myoglobinuria and the development of fixed weakness does not occur.

## Mitochondrial Myopathies

These disorders share the common feature of a genetic defect in mitochondrial DNA (mDNA) that leads to mitochondrial-specific metabolic abnormalities. Clinical features that show a wide variation include slowly progressive proximal muscle weakness beginning in older adults, the appearance of ptosis and extraocular weakness in younger individuals and, in a few, a rapidly fatal metabolic disorder of infants and children. The diagnosis of these disorders depends on the clinician having a high index of suspicion in patients with typical features and recognizing the need to obtain confirmatory tests that can verify a specific condition. Muscle biopsy will show abnormal fibers containing accumulations of mitochondria (ragged red fibers) and fibers that fail to stain with the cytochrome oxidase reaction.

Genetic transmission of mDNA is nonmendelian in that the disease is always passed from the maternal line. Normal muscle cell mitochondria contain double-stranded DNA, mtDNA, consisting of 16,569 base pairs which code for transfer RNAs, ribosomal RNAs, and subunits of the respiratory chain enzymes. Deletions or point mutations of mDNA produce defects in mitochondrial protein, failure of metabolic function in the electron transport chain, and clinical disease. Normally, during meiosis, each daughter cell produced retains one-half of the total mitochondrial content of the original ovum. Some of the mitochondria may contain mutated DNA. If the segregation of mitochondria results in the bulk of mitochondria with mutated DNA going to one of the daughter cells, a disproportionate number of all subsequent mitochondria produced by future cells will carry the mutation. This, in turn, will be expressed as a mitochondrial-based disorder of the electron transport chain. To further complicate matters, some fragments of mitochondrial protein may be coded for by *nuclear* DNA, the template being carried via messenger RNA into the mitochondria where final protein assembly with mtDNA-coded protein subunits is carried out. In these very rare instances a defective mitochondrial protein is produced that is based not on maternal inheritance at all but, rather, on an autosomal dominant pattern within a kindred (Shoubridge 1996).

Distinctive clinical syndromes can result from deletions of mDNA sequence as seen in the Kearns-Sayres (KSS) syndrome and familial progressive external ophthalmoplegia (familial PEO). Point mutations of mtDNA underlie the relatively rare MELAS, MERFF, and MNGIE syndromes.

Clinically, KSS is characterized by ptosis, retinal pigmentary degeneration, and progressive ophthalmoplegia beginning in late childhood or teenage years. Cardiac conduction block is often an early feature along with mild proximal weakness, limb and gait ataxia, hearing loss, short stature, and subnormal mental functioning. The triad of ophthalmoplegia, pigmentary retinal degeneration, and heart block are key diagnostic features. Some patients exhibit only these three features, while others show varying combinations and severity. The disorder progresses slowly, but the cardiac arrhythmia is life threatening and may require pacemaker placement as a life-saving measure.

The familial PEO syndrome due to maternal inheritance, generally a more benign condition than KSS, is marked by varying degrees of limb weakness and ophthalmoparesis. Depressed ventilatory drive may occur, requiring pulmonary intervention with Bi-Pap or other assistive methods. Several forms of PEO exhibiting autosomal dominant inheritance may have more severe symptoms including tremor, ataxia, peripheral neuropathy, and hearing loss (Zeviani et al. 1990).

MELAS, MERFF, and MNGIE are very rare maternally inherited syndromes, all of which show abnormal accumulations of muscle mitochondria and varying clinical presentation with associated lactic acid accumulation. For details see Griggs et al. (1995).

Finally, a small group of patients over 69 years of age with mild proximal muscle weakness have shown excessive mitochondria and cytochrome oxidase–negative fibers in the presence of multiple mtDNA deletions (Johnston et al. 1995). The authors propose that these mtDNA mutations are an exaggeration of what normally occurs during the aging process. As with other abnormalities of muscle mitochondria, treatment is symptomatic.

## References

Abbas, A. K.; Litchman, A. H.; Pober, J. S. Cellular and molecular immunology. Philadelphia: W. B. Saunders Co.; 1991.

Adornato, B. T.; Engel, W. K. MB-creatine phosphokinase isoenzyme elevation not diagnostic of myocardial infarction. Arch. Intern. Med. 137: 1089–1090; 1977.

Allsop, K. G.; Ziter, F. A. Loss of strength and functional decline in Duchenne's dystrophy. Arch. Neurol. 38:406–411; 1981.

Amato, A. A.; and Barohn, R. J. Idiopathic inflammatory myopathies, Neurol. Clin. 15: 615–648; 1997.

Amato, A. A.; Gronseth, G. S.; Jackson, C. E.; Wolfe, G. I.; Katz, J. S.; Bryan, W. W.; Barohn, R. J. Inclusion body myositis; clinical & pathological boundaries. Ann. Neurol. 40:581–586; 1996.

Angelini, C.; Pegoraro, E.; Turella E.; Intino, M. T; Pini, A.; Costa, C; Deflazacort in Duchenne dystrophy: study of long-term effect. Muscle Nerve 17:386–391; 1994.

Angelini, C.; Lucke, S.; Cantarutti, F. Carnitine deficiency of skeletal muscle: report of a treated case. Neurology 26:633–637; 1976.

Ansell, B. M. Management of polymyositis and dermatomyositis. Clin. Rheum. Dis. 10:205–213; 1984.

Ansher, M.; Smith, L. D.; Ringel, S. P. Autosomal dominant scapuloperoneal syndrome with sensorineural hearing loss. Otolaryngol. Head Neck Surg. 100:242–244; 1989.

Bach, J. R., Ishikawa, Y.; Kim, H. Prevention of pulmonary morbidity for patients with Duchenne muscular dystrophy. Chest 112:1024–1028; 1997.

Barohn, R. J. The theraputic dilema of inclusion body myositis. Neurology 48:567–568; 1997.

Banker, B. Q.; Victor, M. Dermatomyositis (systemic angiopathy) of childhood. Medicine 45:261–288; 1966.

Barwick, D. D.; Walton, J. N. Polymyositis. Am. J. Med. 35:646–660; 1963.

Bendtzen, K.; Tuede, N.; Andersen, V.; Bendixen, G. Cyclosporin for polymyositis. Lancet 1:792–793; 1984.

Ben Hamida, M.; Fardeau, M.; Attia N. Severe childhood muscular dystrophy affecting both sexes and frequent in Tunecin. Muscle Nerve 6:469; 1983.

Bird, T. D.; Follett, C.; Griep, E. Cognitive and personality function in myotonic muscular dystrophy. 1. Cognitive function 2. Personality profiles. J. Neurol. Neurosurg. Psychiatry 46:971–980, 1983.

Bodensteiner, J. B.; Schochet, S. S. FSH dystrophy: the choice of a biopsy site. Muscle Nerve 9:544–547; 1986.

Bodensteiner, J. B. Congenital myopathies. Neurol. Clin. 3:499–518; 1988.

Bohan, A. Clinical presentation and diagnosis of polymyositis and dermatomyositis. In: Dalakas, M., ed. Polymyositis and dermatomyositis. Boston: Butterworth; 1988: p. 19–36.

Bohan, A.; Peter, J. B.; Bowman, R. L.; Pearson, C. M. A computer assisted analysis of 153 patients with PM & DM. Medicine 56:255–286; 1977.

Bradley, W. G.; Tomlinson, B. E.; Hardy, M. Further studies of mitochondrial and lipid storage myopathies. J. Neurol. Sci. 35:201–210; 1978.

Brook, P. D., Kennedy, J. D., Stern, L. M., Sutherland, A. D., Foster, B. K., Spinal fusion in Duchenne's muscular dystrophy. J. Pediatr. Orthop. 16:324–331; 1996.

Brooke, M. H.; Fenichel, G. M.; Griggs, R.; Mendell, J. R.; Moxley, R.; Miller, J.; Philip, A. B.; Province, M. A. Clinical investigation in Duchenne dystrophy: 2. determination of the "power" of therapeutic trials based on natural history. Muscle Nerve 6:91–103; 1983.

Brooke, M. H. A clinician's view of neuromuscular disease. 2nd ed. Baltimore: Williams & Wilkins; 1986.

Brooke, M. H.; Fenichel, G. M.; Griggs, R. C.; Mendell, J. R.; Moxley, R.; Florence, J.; King, W. M.; Pandya, S.; Robinson, J.; Schierbecker, P. T.; Signore, R. N.; Miller, J. P.; Gilder, B. F.; Kaiser, K. K.; Mandel, S.; ArEken, C. Duchenne muscular dystrophy: patterns of clinical progression and effects of supportive therapy. Neurology 39:475–481; 1989.

Bunch, T. W. Prednisone and azathioprine for polymyositis: long-term follow-up. Arthritis Rheum. 24:45–48; 1981.

Bundey, S. Detection of heterozygates for myotonic dystrophy. Clin. Genet. 5: 107–109; 1974.

Callen, J. P.; Relationships of cancer to inflammatory muscle disease. Rheum. Dis. Clin. North Am. 20:943–953; 1994.

Cailen, J. P. The value of malignancy evaluation in patients with dermatomyositis, J. Acad. Dermatol. 6:253–259; 1982.

Carpenter, S.; Inclusion body myositis: J. Neuropathol. Exp. Neurol 55:1105–1114; 1996.

Carroll, J. E.; Zwillich, C. W.; Weil, J. V. Ventilatory response in myotonic dystrophy. Neurology 27:1125–1128; 1977.

Carroll, J. E.; Brooke, M. H.; De Vivo, D. C.; Shumata, J. B.; Kratz, R.; Ringel, S. P.; Hagberg, J. M. Carnitine "deficiency": lack of response to carnitine therapy. Neurology 30:618–626; 1980.

Carroll, J. E.; Shumate, J. B.; Brooke, M. H.; Hagberg, J. M. Riboflavin-responsive lipid myopathy and carnitine deficiency. Neurology 31:1557–1559; 1981.

Carroll, J. E. Myopathies caused by disorders of lipid metabolism. Neurol. Clin. 6(3):563–574; 1988.

Chou, S. M. Myositis-like structures in a case of human chronic polymyositis. Science 158:1453–1455; 1967.

Chou, S. M. Viral myositis. In: Mastaglia, F., ed. Inflammatory diseases of muscle. Oxford: Blackwell Scientific; 1988: p. 125–153.

Chu, L. A.; Munsat, T. L. Dominant inheritance of McArdle syndrome. Arch. Neurol. 33:636–641; 1976.

Church, S. C. The heart in myotonia atrophica. Arch. Intern. Med. 119:176–181; 1967.

Christensen, P. B.; Jensen, T. S.; Tsiropoulos, I.; et al. Associated autoimmune diseases in myasthenia gravis. Acta Neurol. Scand. 91(3):192–195; 1995.

Compston, D. A. S.; Vincent, A.; Newsom Davis, J.; Batchelor, J. R. Clinical, pathological, HLA antigen and immunological evidence for disease heterogeneity in myasthenia gravis. Brain 103:579–601; 1980.

Cosi, V.; Lombardi, M.; Piccolo, G.; et al. Treatment of myasthenia gravis with high-dose intravenous immunoglobulin. Acta Neurol. Scand. 84:81; 1991.

Currie, S.; Walton, J. N. Immunosuppressive therapy in polymyositis. J. Neurol. Neurosurg. Psychiatry 34:447–452; 1971.

Dalakas, M. C.; Illa, I; Dambrosia, J. M.; et al. A controlled trial of high dose IVIG infusions as treatment for dermatomyositis. N. Engl. J. Med. 329:1993–2000; 1993.

Dalakas, M. C.; Sonier, B.; Dambrosia, J. M.; et al; Treatment of IBM with IVIG. A double blind, placebo controlled study. Neurology 48:712–716; 1997.

Denbow, C. E.; Lie, J. T.; Tancredi, R. G.; Bunch, T. W. Cardiac involvement in polymyositis: a clinicopathologic study of 20 autopsied patients. Arthritis Rheum. 22:1088–1092; 1979.

DeVere, R.; Bradley, W. G. Polymyositis: its presentation, morbidity and mortality Brain 98:637–666; 1975.

Dickey, B. F.; Myers, A. R. Pulmonary disease in polymyositis/dermatomyositis. Semin. Arthritis Rheum. 14:60–76; 1984.

DiDonato, S. Disorder of lipid metabolism affecting skeletal muscle: carnitine deficiency syndromes. In: Engel, A. G.; Franzini-Armstrong, C. L., eds. Myology. New York: McGraw-Hill; 1994: p. 1587–1609.

DiMarco, A. P.; DiMarco, M. S.; Jacobs, L.; Shields, R.; Altase, M. D. The effects of inspiratory resistive maining of respiratory muscle for patients with muscular dystrophy. Muscle Nerve 8:284–290; 1985.

DiMauro, S.; Tsujino, S. Nonlysosomal glycogenoses. In: Engel, A. G.; Frazini-Armstrong, C., eds. Myology. New York: McGraw-Hill; 1994: p. 1554–1576.

Donaldson, D. H.; Ansher, M.; Horan, S.; Rutherford, R. B.; Ringel, S. P. The relationship of age to outcome in myasthenia gravis. Neurology 40:786–790; 1990.

Duggan, D. J., Gorospe, J. R., Fanin, M., Hoffman, E. P.; and Angelini, C. Mutation of the sarcoglycan gene in patients with myopathy, N. Engl. J. Med. 336:618–624; 1997.

Eaton, L. M. The perspective of neurology in regard to polymyositis: a study of 41 cases. Neurology 4:245–263; 1954.

Emery, A. E. H.; Dreifuss, F. E. Unusual type of benign x-linked muscular dystrophy. J. Neurol. Neurosurg. Psychiatry 29:338–342; 1966.

Engel, A. G. Myasthenic syndromes. In: Engel, A. G.; Franzini-Armstrong, C. A., eds. Myology. New York: McGraw-Hill; 1994a: p. 1769–1797.

Engel, A. G. Congential myasthenic syndromes. In: Engel, A. G.; Franzini-Armstrong, C., eds. Myology. New York, McGraw-Hill; 1994b: p. 1806–1835.

Engel, A. G.; Hohelfeld, R.; Banker, B. Q. PM and DM associated with malignancy. In: Engel, A. G.; Franzini-Armstrong, C., eds. Myology. New York: McGraw-Hill; 1994: p. 1339–1340.

Engel, A. G.; Siekert, R. G. Lipid storage myopathy responsive to prednisone. Arch. Neurol. 27:174–181; 1972.

Engel, A. G.; Angelini, C. Carnitine deficiency of human skeletal muscle with associated lipid storage myopathy. Science 179:899–902; 1973.

Engel, W. K.; Askansas V. Remote effects of focal cancer on the neuromuscular system. In: Thompson, R. A.; Green, J. R., eds. Advances in neurology. New York: Raven Press; 1976: p. 119–148.

Eymard, B., Romero, N. B., Leturcq, F.; et al. Primary sarcoglycanopathy (alpha sarcoglycanopathy). Neurology 48:1227–1234; 1997.

Evoli, A.; Tonali, P.; Bestorcian, E.; Manoco, M. L. Ocular myasthenia: diagnosis and therapeutic problems. Acta. Neurol. 77:31–35; 1988.

Fafalak, R. G.; Peterson, M. G.; Kagen, L. T. Strength in IM and DM; but outcomes in patients treated early. J. Rheum. 21:643–648; 1994.

Feigenbaum, J. A.; Munsat, T. L. A neuromuscular syndrome of scapuloperoneal distribution. Bull. Los Angeles Neurol. Soc. 35:47–57; 1970.

Fenichel, G. M.; Mendell, J. R.; Moxley, R. T.; et al. A comparison of daily and alternate day prednisone therapy in the treatment of Duchenne muscular dystrophy. Arch. Neurol. 48:575–579; 1991.

Fenichel, G.; Pestronk, A.; Florence, J.; Robinson, V.; Hemelt, V. A beneficial effect of oxandralone in the treatment of Duchenne muscular dystrophy. Neurology 48:1225–1226; 1997.

Fischer, T. J.; Rachelefsky, G. S.; Klein, R. B.; Paulus, H. E.; Steihm, E. R. Childhood dermatomyositis and polymyositis: treatment with methotrexate and prednisone. Am. J. Dis. Child. 133:386–389; 1979.

Florek, R. C.; Triffon, D. W.; Mann, D. E.; Ringel, S. P.; Reiter, M. J. Prevalence and progression of electrocardiographic abnormalities in patients with myotonic dystrophy. West. J. Med. 153:24–27; 1990.

Frank, J. P.; Harat, Y.; Butler, L. J.; Nelson, T. E.; Scott, C. I. Central core disease and malignant hyperthermia syndrome. Ann. Neurol. 7:11–17; 1980.

Fu, Y.; Pizzuta, A; Fenwick, R. G.; et al. An unstable triplet repeat in a gene related to myotonic dystrophy. Science 255:1256–1258; 1992.

Fukunaga, H.; Okubo, R.; Moritoyo, T.; et al. Long term follow-up of patients with Duchenne muscular dystrophy receiving ventilatory support. Muscle Nerve 16:554–558; 1993.

Galdi, A. P.; Clark, J. B. An unusual case of carnitine palmitoyl transferase deficiency. Arch. Neurol. 46: 819; 1989.

Genkins, G.; Kornfeld, A.; Papatestas, A. L.; Bender, A. N.; Mattas, R. J. Clinical experience in more than 2000 patients with myasthenia gravis. Ann. N. Y. Acad. Sci. 505:500–513; 1987.

Goebel, H. H.; Congential myopathies. Semin. Pediatr. Neurol. 3:152–161; 1996.

Gottdiener, J. S.; Sherberg, H. S.; Hawley, R. L.; Engel, W. K. Cardiac manifestations in polymyositis. Am. J. Cardiol. 41:1141–1149; 1978.

Griggs, R. C.; Pandya, S.; Florence, J. M.; Brooke, M. H.; Kingston, W.; Miller, J. P.; Chutkow, J.; Herr, B. E.; Moxley, R. T., III. Randomized controlled trial of testosterone in myotonic dystrophy. Neurology 39:219–222; 1989.

Griggs, R. C.; Moxley, R. T.; Mendell, J. R.; et al. Prednisone in Duchenne dystrophy. A randomized, controlled trial defining the time course and dose response. Arch Neurol. 48:383; 1991.

Griggs, R. C.; Mendell, J. R.; Miller, R. G. Evaluation and treatment of myopathies. Philadelphia: F. A. Davis; 1995.

Grim, T.; Janka, M. Emory Dreifuss muscular dystrophy. In: Engel, A. E.; Franzini-Armstrong, C., eds. Myology. New York: McGraw-Hill; 1994: p. 1188–1191.

Grob, D.; Arsuie, E. L.; Brunner, N. G.; Namba, T. The course of myasthenia and therapies affecting outcome. Ann. N. Y. Acad. Sci. 505:472–499; 1987.

Harding, A. E.; Thomas, P. K. Distal and scapular peroneal distribution of muscle involvement occurring within a family with type I hereditary motor and sensory neuropathy. J. Neurol. 224(1):17–23; 1980.

Harper, P. S.; Rudel, R. Myotonic dystrophy. In: Engel, A. G.; Franzini-Armstrong, C., eds. Myology. New York: McGraw-Hill; 1994: p. 1207.

Hart, Z. H.; Chang, C. H.; DiMauro, S.; Farooki, Q.; Ayyar, R. Muscle carnitine deficiency and fatal cardiomyopathy. Neurology 28:147–151; 1978.

Hawley, R. J.; Milner, M. R.; Gottdiener, J. S.; Cohen, A. Myotonic heart disease. Neurology 41:259–262; 1991.

Henriksson, K. G.; Sandstedt, P. Polymyositis—treatment and prognosis: a study of 107 patients. Acta. Neurol. Scand. 65:280–300; 1982.

Hoffman, E. P.; Fischbeck, K. H.; Brown, R. H., et al. Characterization of dystrophin in muscle-biopsy specimens from patients with Duchenne's or Becker's muscular dystrophy. N. Engl J. Med 318: 1363–1368; 1988.

Horowitz, M; Maddox, A; Maddern, G. J.; Wishart, J.; Collins, P. J.; Shearman, D. J. Gastric and esophageal emptying in dystrophia myotonica: effect of metoclopramide. Gastroenterology 92:570; 1987.

Hoshio, A.; Kotake, H.; Saitoh, M.; Ogino, K.; Fujimoto, Y. Cardiac involvement in a patient with limb girdle muscular dystrophy. Heart Lung 16(4):439–441; 1987.

Hunter, S. The heart in muscular dystrophy. Br. Med. Bull. 36:133–134; 1980.

Inkley, S.; Oldenberg, F.; Vignos, P. J., Jr. Pulmonary function in Duchenne muscular dystrophy related to stage of disease. Am. J. Med. 6:297–306; 1976.

Isaacs, H., Heffron, J. J. A.; Badenhorst, M.; Pickering, A. Weakness associated with the pathological presence of lipid in skeletal muscle: a detailed study of a patient with carnitine deficiency. J. Neurol. Neurosurg. Psychiatry 39:1114–1123; 1976.

Isenberg, D. Myositis in other connective tissue disorders. Clin. Rheum. Dis. 10:151–175; 1984.

Jaretzki, A., III; Penn, A.; Younger, D.; Wolff, M.; Olarte, M. R.; Lovelace, R. E.; Rowland, L. P. Maximal thymectomy for myasthenia gravis. J. Thorac. Cardiovasc. Surg. 95:747–757; 1988.

Joffe, M. M.; Love, L. A.; Leff, R. L. Drug therapy of idiopathic inflammatory myopathies: predictors of response to prednisone, azathiaprine, and methotrexate and a comparison of their efficacy. Am. J. Med. 94:379–387; 1993.

Johns, T. R. Long-term corticosteroid treatment of myasthenia gravis. Ann. N. Y. Acad. Sci. 505:568–583; 1987.

Johnston, W.; Karpati, G.; Carpenter, S.; Arnold, D.; Shoubridge, A. Late onset mitochondrial myopathy. Ann. Neurol. 37:16–23, 1995.

Kaeser, H. E. Scapuloperoneal muscular atrophy. Brain 88:407–418; 1965.

Kagen, L. J.; Hochman, R. B.; Strong, E. W. Cricopharyngeal obstruction in inflammatory myopathy (polymyositis/dermatomyositis): report of three cases and review of the literature. Arthritis Rheum. 28: 630–636; 1985.

Kelly, J. J.; Madoc-Jones, H.; Adelman, L. R.; Munsat, T. L. Treatment of refractory polymyositis with total body irradiation. Neurology 34(suppl. 1):80; 1984.

Kilburn, K. H.; Eagan, J. T.; Sieker, H. O.; Heyman, A. Cardiopulmonary insufficiency in myotonic and progressive muscular dystrophy. N. Engl. J. Med. 261:1089–1096; 1959.

Kimura, J. Electrodiagnosis of nerve and muscle. Philadelphia: F. A. Davis; 1983.

Kobayashi, O.; Hayashi, Y.; Arahata, K.; Ozawa, E.; Nonaka, I.; Congential muscular dystrophy. Neurology 46:815–818; 1996.

Kost, G. J.; Verity, M. A. A new variant of late-onset myophosphorylase deficiency. Muscle Nerve 3:195–201; 1980.

Kurz, L. T.; Mubeersade, S. J.; Schultz, P.; Park, S. M.; Lead, J. Correlation of scoliosis and pulmonary function in DMD. J. Pediatr. Orthop. 3:347–153; 1983.

Laing, N. G.; Majda, B. T.; Akkari, P. A.; et al. Assignment of a gene (NEMI) for autosomal dominant nemaline myopathy to chromosome the number 1. Am. J. Hum. Genet. 50:320; 1992.

Larca, L. J.; Coppola, J. T.; Honig, S. Creatine kinase MS isoenzyme in dermatomyositis: a noncardiac source. Ann. Intern. Med. 94:341–343; 1981.

Lefvert, A. K.; Osterman, P. O. Newborn infants to myasthenic mothers: a clinical study and an investigation of acetylcholine receptor antibodies in 17 children. Neurology 33:133–138; 1983.

Letournel, E.; Fardeau, M.; Lytle, J. O.; et al. Scapulothoracic arthrodesis for patients who have FSH dystrophy. J. Bone Joint Surg. 72:78–84; 1990.

Lilley, H.; Dennett, X.; Byrne, E. Biopsy proven PM in Victoria 1982–87; analysis of prognostic factors. J. R. Soc. Med. 87:323–326, 1994.

Logan, R. G.; Bandera, J. M.; Mikkelsen, W. M. Polymyositis: a clinical study. Ann. Intern. Med. 65:996–1007; 1966.

Lotz, B. P.; Engel, A. G.; Niskino, H.; et al. Inclusion body myositis: observation in 40 patients. Brain 112:727–747; 1989.

Luque, E. R. Segmental spinal instrumentation for correction of scoliosis. Clin. Orthop. 163:192–198; 1982.

Maeda, M.; Taft, C. S.; Buch, E. H.; et al. Identification of tissue specific expression and sub-cellular localization of the 80 and 71kDa forms of myotonic dystrophy kinase protein. J. Biol. Chem. 270:20246–20249; 1995.

Mantegazza, R.; Beghi, E.; Pareyson, D.; et al. A multicentre follow-up study of 1152 patients with myasthenia gravis in Italy. J. Neurol. 237: 339–344; 1990.

Marshall, J. Observations on endocrine function in dystrophia myotonica. Brain 82:221–231; 1959.

Martin, R. J. Cardiorespiratory disorders during sleep. New York: Futura; 1984.

Mastaglia, F. L.; Ojeda, V. J. Inflammatory myopathies. Ann. Neurol. 17:215–217; 317–323; 1985.

McQuillen, M. P.; Leone, M. G. A treatment carol: thymectomy revisited. Neurology 27:1103–1106; 1977.

Medsger, T. A.; Dawson, W. N.; Masi, A. T. The epidemiology of polymyositis. Am. J. Med. 48:715–723; 1970.

Mendell, J. R.; Moxley, R. T.; Griggs, R. C.; et al. Randomized, double blind six-month trial of prednisone in Duchenne's muscular dystrophy. N. Engl J. Med. 320:1592–1597; 1991.

Mendell, J.; Kissel, J. T.; Amato, A. A.; et al. Myoblast transfer in the treatment of Duchenne's muscular dystrophy. N. Engl J. Med. 333:832–838; 1995.

Miller, F. W.; Leitman, S. F.; Cronin, M. E.; et al. Controlled trial of plasma exchange and leukopheresis in PM & DM. N. Engl. J. Med. 326:1380–1384; 1992.

Miranda, A. F.; Nette, E. G.; Hartlage, P. L.; DiMauro, S. Phosphorylase isoenzymes in normal and myophosphorylase-deficient human heart. Neurology 29:1538–1540; 1979.

Mulley, J. C.; Koxman, H. M.; Phillips, H. A. et al. Refined genetic localization for central core disease. Am. J. Hum. Genet. 52:398; 1993.

Munsat, T. L.; Piper, D.; Cancilla, P.; Mednick, J. Inflammatory myopathy with facioscapulohumeral dystrophy. Neurology 22:335–347; 1972.

Munsat, T. L.; Bradley, W. G. Serum creatine phosphokinase levels and prednisone treated muscle weakness. Neurology 27:96–97; 1977.

Munsat, T. L. Facioscapulohumeral dystrophy and the scapuloperoneal syndrome. In: Engel, A.; Banker, B. Q., eds. Myology. New York: McGraw-Hill; 1986; p. 1251–1265.

Munsat, T. L.; Andres, P. L.; Finison, L.; Conlon, T.; Thibodeau, L. The natural history of motorneuron loss in amyotrophic lateral sclerosis. Neurology 38:409–413; 1988.

Newsom-Davis, J. The respiratory system in muscular dystrophy. Br. Med. Bull. 36:135–137; 1980.

Niaken, E.; Hasati, Y.; Rolak, L. Immunosuppressive drug therapy in myasthenia gravis. Arch. Neurol. 43:155–156; 1986.

Noble-Jamieson, C. M.; Heckmett, J. Z.; Dubowitz, V.; Silverman, M. Effects of posture and spinal bracing on respiratory function in neuromuscular disease. Arch. Dis. Child. 61:178–181; 1986.

Oddis, C. V. Therapy of inflammatory myopathy. Rheum. Dis. Clin. North Am. 20:899–918; 1994.

O'Leary, P. A.; Waisman, M. Dermatomyositis: a study of 40 cases. Arch. Dermatol. Syph. 41:1001–1019; 1940.

Olanow, C. W.; Wechsler, A. S.; Sirotkin-Roses, M.; Stajich, J.; Roses, A. D. Thymectomy as primary therapy in myasthenia gravis. Ann. N. Y. Acad. Sci. 505:595–605; 1987.

Oosterhuis, H. J. G. H. The natural course of myasthenia gravis. J. Neurol. Neurosurg. Psychiatry 52:1121–1127; 1989.

Ozawa, E.; Noguchi, S.; Mizuno, Y.; Hagiwara, Y.; Yoshida, M. From dystrophinopathy to sarcoglycanopathy. Muscle Nerve 21:421–438; 1998.

Padberg, G.; Lunt, P. W.; Fardeau, M. Diagnostic criteria for FSH. Neuromuscul. Disord. 1:231–234; 1991.

Pegoraro, E.; Schimke, R. N.; Garcia, C.; Stern, H.; Cadaldini, M.; Angelini, C.; Barbosa, E.; Carroll, J.; Marks, W. A.; Neville, H. E.; Marks, H.; Appleton, S.; Toriello, H.; Wessell, H. B.; Donnely, J.; Bernes, S. M.; Taber, J. W.; Weiss, L.; Hoffman, E. P. Genetic and biochemical normalization in female carriers of Duchenne muscular dystrophy: evidence for failure of dystrophin production-competent myonuclei. Neurology 45:677–690; 1995.

Pegoraro, E.; Mancias, P.; Swerdlow, S. H.; et al. Congential muscular dystrophy with primary laminin alpha 2 (merosin) deficiency presenting as inflammatory myopathy. Ann. Neurol. 40:782–791, 1996.

Penn, A. Myoglobinuria. In: Engel, A. G.; Franzini-Armstrong, C., eds. Myology. New York: McGraw-Hill; 1994: p. 1679–1696.

Reardon, W.; Newcombe, R.; Fenton, I.; Sibert, J.; Harper, P. S. The natural history of congenital myotonic dystrophy; mortality and long term clinical aspects. Arch. Dis. Child. 68:177–181; 1993.

Ravin, M.; Newmark, Z.; Saviello, G. Myotonia dystrophica: an anesthetic hazard: two case reports. Anesth. Analg. 54:216–218; 1975.

Rideau, Y.; Gatin, G.; Bach, J.; Gines, G. Prolongation of life in Duchenne's muscular dystrophy. Acta. Neurol. (Napol.) 5:118–124; 1983.

Rideau, Y. The Duchenne muscular dystrophy child: case of wheelchair dependent patient: death prevention (abstract). Muscle Nerve 9(suppl.):86; 1986.

Ringel, S. P.; Carroll, J.; Schold, C. The spectrum of mild x-linked recessive muscular dystrophy. Arch. Neurol. 34:408–416; 1977.

Ringel, S. P.; Kenny, C. E.; Neville, H. E.; Giorno, R.; Carly, M. R. Spectrum of inclusion body myositis. Arch. Neurol. 44:1154–1157; 1987.

Ringel, S. P.; Murphy, J. R.; Alderson, M. K; Bryan, W.; England, J. D.; Miller, R. G.; Petajan, J. H.; Smith, S. A.; Roelofs, R. I.; Ziter, F.; Lee, M. Y.; Brinkmann, J. R.; Almada, A.; Gappmaier, E.; Graves, J.; Herbelin, L.; Mendoza, M.; Mylar, D.; Smith, P.; Yu, P. The natural history of amyotrophic lateral sclerosis. Neurology 43:1316–22; 1993.

Ronnblom, A.; Forsberg, H.; Danielson, A. GI symptoms in myotonic dystrophy. Scand J. Gastroenterol. 31:654–657; 1996.

Rose, A. L.; Walton, J. N. Polymyositis: a survey of 89 cases with particular reference to treatment and prognosis. Brain 89:747–768; 1966.

Rosenberg, N. L.; Ringel, S. P. Adult polymyositis and dermatomyositis. In: Mastaglia, F., ed. Inflammatory diseases of muscle. Oxford: Blackwell Scientific Publications; 1988: p. 87–106.

Rowland, L. P.; Fetell, M.; Olarte, M.; Hayes, A.; Singh, N.; Wanat, F. E. Emery-Dreifuss muscular dystrophy. Ann. Neurol. 5:111–117; 1979.

Rowland, L. P. Controversies about the treatment of myasthenia gravis. J. Neurol. Neurosurg. Psychiatry 43(7):644–659; 1980.

Santorelli, M. D.; Scicco, M. D.; Tanji M. D.; et al. Multiple mitochondrial DNA deletions in sporadic IBM: a study of 56 patients. Ann. Neurol. 39:789–795; 1996.

Sarnat, H. B. Juvenile dematomyositis. In: Mastaglia, F., ed. Inflammatory disease of muscle. Oxford: Blackwell Scientific Publications; 1988: p. 71–86.

Sawcheck, I. A.; Kula, R. W. Inclusion body myositis. In: Dalakas, M., ed. Polymyositis and dermatomyositis. Boston: Butterworth; 1988: p. 121–132.

Schmid, R.; Hammer, L. Hereditary absence of muscle phosphorylase (McArdle's syndrome). N. Engl. J. Med. 264:223–225; 1961.

Schumm, F.; Wietholter, H.; Fatch-Moghadam, A.; Dichgans, J. Thymectomy in myasthenia with pure ocular symptom. J. Neurol. Neurosurg. Psychiatry 48:332–337; 1985.

Scott, W.; Hyde, S. A.; Goddard, C. M.; Dubowitz, V. Quantitation of muscle function in children: a prospective study in Duchenne muscular dystrophy. Muscle Nerve 5:291–301; 1982.

Seybold, M. Plasmapheresis in myasthenia gravis. Ann. N. Y. Acad. Sci. 505:584–587; 1987.

Shields, R. W. Limb girdle syndromes. In: Engel, A. G.; Franzini-Armstrong, C., eds. Myology. New York: McGraw Hill; 1994: p. 1258–1274.

Shoubridge, E. A. Autosomal dominant chronic progressive external ophthalmoplegia; a tale of two genomes. Ann. Neurol. 40:693–694; 1996.

Siegal, L. M. Orthopedic management of muscle disease. In: Maloney, F. P.; Burks, J. S.; Ringel, S. P., eds. Interdisciplinary rehabilitation of multiple sclerosis and neuromuscular disorders. Philadelphia: J. B. Lippincott; 1986: p. 277–295.

Sigurgeirsson, B.; Liudelof, B.; Edhag, O.; et al. Risk of cancer in patients with dermatomyositis or polymyositis. N. Engl. J. Med. 326:363–367, 1992.

Smith, E. M.; Calvesley, P. M.; Edwards, R. H.; Evans, G. A.; Campbell, E. J. Practical problems in the respiratory care of patients with muscular dystrophy. N. Engl. J. Med. 316:1197–1204; 1987.

Sommer, N.; Sigg, B.; Melms, A.; et al. Ocular myasthenia gravis: response to long term immunosuppressive therapy. J. Neurol. Neurosurg. Psychiatry 62:156–162; 1997.

Somnier, F. E. Exacerbation of myasthenia gravis after removal of thymomas Acta Neurol. Scand. 90(1): 56–66; 1994.

Speer, M. C.; Yamaoka, L. H.; Gilchist, J. H.; et al. Confirmation of genetic heterogenity in limb girdle dystrophy: linkage of an autosomal dominant form to chromosome, 5g. Am. J. Hum. Genet. 50:1211; 1992.

Starr, J.; Lamont, M.; Iselins, L.; et al. A linkage study of large pedigree with X-linked centronuclear myopathy. J. Med. Genet. 27:281; 1990.

Straub, V.; Campbell, K. Muscular dystrophies and the dystrophin-glycoprotein complex. Curr. Opin. Neurol. 10:168–175; 1997.

Stuart, C. A.; Armstrong, R.; Provow, S.; Plishker, G. A. Insulin resistance in patients with myotonic dystrophy. Neurology 33:679–685; 1977.

Swick, H. M.; Werlin, S. L.; Dodds, W. J.; Hogan, W. J. Pharyngo-esophageal motor function in patients with myotonic dystrophy. Ann. Neurol. 10:454–457; 1981.

Tawil, R.; McDermott, M. P.; Pandya, S.; King, W.; Kissel, J.; Mendell, J. R.; Griggs, R. C. A pilot trial of prednisone in facioscapulohumeral muscular dystrophy. Neurology 48:46–49; 1997.

Tawil, R.; Figlewics, D. A.; Griggs, R. C.; et al. Facioscapulohumeral dystrophy: a distinct regional myopathy with a novel molecular pathogenesis. Ann. Neurol. 43:279–282; 1998.

Thomas, P. K.; Calne, D. B.; Elliot, C. F. X-linked scapuloperoneal syndrome. J. Neurol. Neurosurg. Psychiatry 35:208–215; 1975.

Tindall, R. S. A. Humoral immunity in myasthenia gravis: biochemical characterization of acquired antireceptor antibodies and clinical correlation. Ann. Neurol. 10:437–447; 1981.

Tindall, R. S. A.; Rollins, J.; Phillips, T.; Greenlee, R. G.; Wells, L.; Belendiak, G. Preliminary results of a double-blind, randomized, placebo-controlled trial of cyclosporine in myasthenia gravis. N. Engl. J. Med. 361:719–724; 1987.

van Deutekom, J. C.; Lemmers, R. J.; Grewal, P. K.; et al. Identification of the first gene (FRG1) from the FSHD region on human chromosome 4q35. Hum. Mol. Genet. 5(5):581–590; 1996a.

van Deutekom, J. C.; Bakker, E., et al. Evidence for subtelomeric exchange of 3.3 kb tandemly repeated units between chromosomes 4q35 and 10q26: implications for genetic counselling and etiology of FSHD1. Hum. Mol. Genet. 5:1997–2003; 1996b.

van der Meche, F. G. A.; Bogaard, J. M.; Van der Sluys J. C. M.; et al. Daytime sleep in myotonic dystrophy is not caused by sleep apnea. J. Neurol. Neurosurg. Psychiatry 57: 626–628; 1994.

Vignos, P. J.; Bowling, G. F.; Watkins, M. P. Polymyositis: effect of corticosteroids on final results. Arch. Intern. Med. 114:263–267; 1964.

Vignos, P. J.; Wagner, M. B.; Karlinchak, B. Evaluation of program for long term treatment of Duchenne muscular dystrophy. J. Bone Joint Surg. 78:1844–1852; 1996.

Vorgerd, M.; Kubisch, C.; Burwinkel, B.; Reichmann, H.; Mortier, W.; Tettenborn, B.; Pongratz, D.; Lindemuth, R.; Tegenthoff, M.; Malin J.-P.; Kilimann, M. W. Mutation analysis of myophosphorylase deficiency (McArdle's disease). Ann. Neurol. 43:326–331; 1998.

Walton, J. N.; Nattrass, F. J. On the classification, natural history and treatment of the myopathies. Brain 77:169–231; 1954.

Welsh, J. D.; Lynn, T. N.; Haase, G. R. Cardiac findings in 73 patients with muscular dystrophy. Arch. Intern. Med. 112:199; 1963.

Wheeler, S. D.; Brooke, M. H. Vascular insufficiency in McArdle's disease. Neurology 33(2):249–250; 1983.

Willner, J. H.; DiMauro, S.; Hays, A.; Roohi, F.; Lovelace, R. Muscle carnitine deficiency: genetic heterogeneity. J. Neurol. Sci. 41:235–246; 1979.

Woodward, W. B.; Keaton, R. K.; Simon, D. B.; Ringel, S. P. Neuropsychological defects in myotonic dystrophy. J. Clin. Neuropsych. 4:335–342; 1982.

Wulff, J. D.; Lin, J. T.; Kepes, J. J. Inflammatory facioscapulohumeral muscular dystrophy and Coats syndrome. Ann. Neurol. 12:398–401; 1982.

Yoshida, S.; Akizuki, M.; Mimori, T.; Yamagata, H.; Inada, S.; Homma, M. The precipitating antibody to an acidic nuclear protein antibody, the Jo-1, in connective tissue disease: a marker for a subset of polymyositis with interstitial pulmonary fibrosis. Arthritis Rheum. 26:604–611; 1983.

Zeviani, M.; Bresolin, N.; Gellera, C.; et al. Nucleus-driven multiple large-scale deletions of the human mitochondrial genome: a new autosomal dominant disease. Am. J. Hum. Genet. 47:904; 1990.

Zundel, W. S.; Tyler, F. H. The muscular dystrophies. Parts I and II. N. Engl. J. Med. 273:537, 596; 1965.

# 29

# Peripheral Nervous System

PRAFUL KELKAR AND GARETH J. PARRY

There are a number of factors that influence prognosis in diseases of peripheral nerves, the most important of which is whether the neuropathy is characterized primarily by segmental demyelination or axonal degeneration. Other factors that play a role in determining the prognosis in neuropathy include etiology, severity, rapidity of evolution, and location and distribution of the nerve injury.

## Etiologic Factors

### Axonal Degeneration Versus Demyelination

In the aquired demyelinating neuropathies there is the potential for rapid and complete recovery of function by remyelination, which is an efficient and rapid process. These neuropathies are characterized, for the most part, by macrophage-mediated attack on myelin, which is multifocal in its distribution. The Schwann cell itself is not a target and retains its capacity to proliferate. Following an episode of demyelination, Schwann cells from the demyelinated segment of nerve rapidly proliferate and lay down new myelin in the demyelinated segment. In experimental animals with acute monophasic demyelination, this process begins within a few days and is complete within a

matter of weeks (Saida et al. 1980). In humans with Guillain-Barre syndrome (GBS), the quintessential acute demyelinating neuropathy, the time course is not much more protracted: in mild cases with pure demyelination, complete recovery occurs within weeks (Berger et al. 1988). In GBS, prognosis is almost entirely related to the degree of associated axonal degeneration. In the chronic inflammatory demyelinating polyradiculoneuropathies (CIDP), this process of remyelination may somehow be frustrated and recovery is less rapid and less assured. Even so, potential for recovery with treatment in CIDP is largely a function of the degree of associated axonal degeneration. In the inherited demyelinating neuropathies, demyelination is a much more indolent process. It may arise as the result of pathological processes directed at the Schwann cell, rather than at myelin, or may be secondary to axonal disease. Remyelination in this instance is ineffective, although Schwann cell proliferation is still active, and very thinly myelinated axons are surrounded by redundant Schwann cell processes (onion bulbs). Nonetheless, even in this situation, the functional prognosis may be primarily dependent on the degree of associated axonal degeneration. Even in early childhood, severe demyelination with onion bulb formation is seen without any clinically detectable abnormality of function. Progressive loss of function later in life is closely paralleled by progressive axonal degeneration, rather than any change in the state of myelination (Dyck et al. 1989).

By contrast, recovery in neuropathies in which the primary pathological process is axonal degeneration is less assured. If the cause of the neuropathy can be removed, axons do have the ability to sprout and elongate, provided the perikaryon is intact. Therefore, in distal axonopathies, in which there is dying back of axons from their receptor or effector organ, some recovery of function by way of axonal regeneration can be expected. However, wallerian degeneration from proximal sites invariably carries a poor prognosis.

## Severity

It may appear self-evident that more severe neuropathies have a worse prognosis, but this is not inevitably the case. In GBS, complete flaccid quadriplegia with respiratory and bulbar paralysis may recover quickly and completely if there is little associated axonal degeneration. However, in general, prognosis is directly related to severity. In the aforementioned example of GBS, significant associated axonal degeneration would usually occur and recovery would likely be slow and incomplete. With axonal degeneration, prognosis is highly dependent on severity. Recovery of function may take place by two mechanisms, namely, axonal regeneration and collateral sprouting. If there is only partial loss of axons, recovery may take place by collateral sprouting from the preterminal nodes of Ranvier of surviving axons. In this situation, elongation of these preterminal sprouts occurs over very short distances before synaptic contact is made. The process of recovery is therefore quick and effective, taking place over weeks to months, and the chance for aberrant innervation is negligible. In muscle, complete restoration of normal function is possible, even when as much as 70% of the motor axons are lost (Daube 1985). When there is severe axonal degeneration that exceeds the capacity of the motor neuron to reinnervate by collateral sprouting, recovery by way of axonal regeneration is possible but functional recovery is usually limited. Not only do axons regenerate poorly but the more axons that are damaged, the

more likely that misdirected regeneration could occur. Therefore, the primary determinant of recovery in axonal degeneration is the severity of the damage.

## Location

There is limited potential for recovery when axonal degeneration occurs at the proximal segments of peripheral nerves for several reasons. First, axonal injury in close proximity to the perikaryon may result in cell death. Second, axons regenerate slowly, elongating at less than 1 mm/d, and they regenerate poorly over long distances. Third, there is an increased probability of misdirected regeneration that may impair the quality of functional recovery even when significant numbers of axons successfully regenerate. Finally, with an attack on the dorsal root, there is degeneration of the central processes of the sensory neurons and regeneration into the central nervous system (CNS) does not occur.

## Acute Versus Chronic Neuropathies

With acutely evolving neuropathies, the patient is likely to seek medical advice early, before pathological changes have become advanced or irreversible. Therefore, if the cause can be treated or removed, potential for recovery is greater. By contrast, with chronic neuropathies, the insidious onset and progression enables maximal compensation to occur during the evolution and the patient may not present clinically until the severity of the neuropathy has already exceeded the individual's ability to compensate. In such situations, the best that can be expected is prevention of further progression.

## Etiology

Recovery from peripheral neuropathies is highly dependent on being able to remove the cause, which is often impossible, since 25% to 40% of neuropathies are idiopathic. Even when the etiology is apparent, there may be no effective treatment. In general, idiopathic and untreatable neuropathies are inexorably progressive but usually at a slow pace. If the cause can be removed or treated, progression will usually halt and some recovery then occurs, the rapidity and efficacy of which is determined by the factors discussed above.

## Role of Electrodiagnosis in Determining Prognosis

As stated above, the primary determinant of prognosis in neuropathies is the relative proportion of demyelination and axonal degeneration. The only reliable means by which this can be determined is the electrodiagnostic evaluation. In addition, the electrophysiological studies provide invaluable information regarding localization, severity, and acuteness that may not be available by other means. The presence of conduction block, differential dispersion of responses, and severe conduction slowing all point toward a primary demyelinating process and indicate the potential for excellent recovery. Low-amplitude responses without dispersion or conduction block and relatively preserved conduction velocity are the characteristic nerve conduction changes seen with axonal degeneration. Furthermore, on needle electromyography (EMG), the presence of fibrillation potentials indicates recent or ongoing denervation. Large-amplitude, long-duration, polyphasic motor unit potentials indicate the presence of partial denervation with reinnervation by collateral sprouting or regeneration, indicating the chronicity of the neuropathy. Highly polyphasic, extremely long-duration motor unit potentials, usually of low amplitude (nascent units), may be seen in muscles in which the degree of denervation has exceeded the ability of the nerve to reinnervate by collateral sprouting. These nascent units reflect reinnervation by regeneration and are usually seen only following severe wallerian degeneration lesions (trauma, infarction). The electrodiagnostic changes can also be evaluated in a semiquantitative manner to provide some objectivity in the assessment of severity and are invaluable in the longitudinal assessment of improvement or deterioration in patients with neuropathy. Finally, the presence of covert changes in both nerve conduction studies and EMG allows for refinement of the clinical localization. In most neuropathies, the clinical manifestations are distally accentuated, particularly in the legs. However, the clinical picture may be very similar in distal axonopathy, sciatic neuropathy, or even multiple lumbosacral radiculopathies, all of which may cause distally accentuated weakness and sensory loss. In such cases, there may be denervation in muscles innervated by the posterior primary ramus of the ventral root (erector spinae) or of proximal muscles of a myotome or peripheral nerve distribution even when strength is normal.

Prognosis is very different over the wide range of different disorders that involve the peripheral nerves. The clinical presentation of neuropathy ranges from acute fulminant paralysis with respiratory impairment to slow onset with evolution over half a century. The manifestations may be mainly motor, mainly sensory, or combined motor and sensory and/or autonomic. Generally, symptoms are most prominent distally, but there are exceptions. Neuropathy may even be asymptomatic, demonstrated only by neurophysiological testing. Depression of ankle jerks might be the only finding to alert the clinician of a likely neuropathy. In this chapter the acutely evolving neuropathies have been separated from those that are more likely to present with a subacute or chronic evolution, and discuss prognosis in selected examples of each.

The terms *polyneuropathy, polyneuritis, peripheral neuropathy,* and *neuropathy* are synonymous. Multiple mononeuropathy or mononeuritis multiplex occurs when multiple focal lesions randomly affect different nerves or roots. These lesions, whether ischemic or demyelinating, are generally asymmetrical.

## Acutely Evolving Polyneuropathies

### Guillain-Barré Syndrome

GBS is an acute inflammatory demyelinating polyradiculoneuropathy that is characterized clinically by acutely evolving paralysis, usually heralded by paresthesiae, and often accompanied by autonomic instability. Weakness involves proximal and distal muscles but is usually distally accentuated. Severity may range from minimal limitation of function to complete flaccid paralysis, including respiratory and bulbar muscles. Although sensory symptoms are often prominent, objective sensory loss is minimal, although areflexia or hyporeflexia is almost invariable. About 70% of patients report an antecedent viral illness, usually gastroenteritis or an upper respiratory infection. The most commonly identified viruses are cytomegalovirus and Epstein-Barr virus, although the offending organsim is usually not identified. Other antecedent events include other infections, surgery, vaccination, and a variety of systemic diseases. Neurological symptoms typically appear within 7 to 10 days of the preceding event and evolve rapidly, reaching a nadir within 2 to 3 weeks. The cardinal feature that has long been used to define the syndrome is albuminocytological dissociation in the cerebrospinal fluid (CSF). However, this is not invariable. CSF pleocytosis is not uncommon and is the rule with human immunodeficiency virus (HIV)-associated disease and normal protein may be seen, particularly early. The diagnosis can almost always be confirmed with nerve conduction studies, which may show blocking of F waves, conduction slowing, or multifocal conduction blocks. The pronounced pathological changes are lymphocytic infiltration associated with segmental foci of demyelination in ventral roots, limb girdle plexuses, and proximal nerve trunks; changes also occur in dorsal roots, autonomic ganglia, and distal peripheral nerves.

GBS usually is a monophasic illness with a very low mortality, and complete or partial recovery almost always occurs with time. In a retrospective study of 40 patients collected over 42 years, Kennedy et al. (1978) found complete recovery, as judged by return to all former activities, in 31 and partial recovery in 7 of the 38 patients who survived the acute illness. Andersson and Siden (1982) also found a high rate of recovery, with 54 of 56 survivors making a complete functional recovery, 30% within 3 months, 73% within 6 months, and the remainder by 18 months. Several other studies (Ravn 1967; Wiederholt et al. 1964; Marshall 1963; Loffel et al. 1977; The Italian GBS study group 1996; Vedeler et al. 1997) have reported complete functional recovery in about 75% of cases. In contrast, McLeod et al. (1976), based on an epidemiological study, found that less than 50% of 18 patients recovered completely, although only four had significant disability. When these patients were examined prospectively many had only mild abnormalities of neurological examination such as absent ankle reflexes and impaired two-point discrimination, abnormalities that are unlikely to have functional significance.

Although most patients make an excellent recovery, about 15% are left with a significant disability. The most important determinant of rate and efficacy of recovery is the degree of axonal degeneration that accompanies the demyelination. Remyelination is an efficient and rapid process that is usually completed within 4 to 6 months of the nadir of the illness. Thus, even severe neurological disability resulting solely from demyelination may recover completely within approximately 6 months of the onset of clinical disease. Conversely, axonal regeneration is a slow and inefficient process, with elongation of regenerating sprouts occurring at a rate of less than 1 mm/d. Therefore, recovery occurs over many months and may not be maximal for up to 2 years. Furthermore, even if regeneration occurs, the axon may fail to make synaptic contact with an appropriate receptor or effector organ, so functional recovery fails. Additionally, synaptic contact may be made with inappropriate end organs (aberrant regeneration) resulting in abnormal function.

Several studies have sought to identify factors that might enable a prediction of outcome at the time of the acute illness. It has been suggested that CSF pleocytosis (Kaeser 1964), severe sensory loss or a prolonged progressive phase (Osler and Sidell 1960; Loffel et al. 1977), and papilledema (Morely and Reynolds 1966) all carry an ominous prognosis. However, others (Forster et al. 1941; Duvoison 1960; Pleasure et al. 1968; Miller et al. 1988) have disputed these claims. Winer et al. (1985) and Miller et al. (1998) found that the most powerful and reliable clinical predictor of poor outcome was the need for ventilator assistance during the acute illness and Ravn et al. (1967) and Loffel et al. (1977) noted that severe maximum motor impairment, not surprisingly, carried a poorer prognosis.

Children with GBS have been felt to have a significantly higher incidence of permanent and significant neurological sequelae (Ravn 1967; Peterman et al. 1959) and yet, paradoxically, the mortality in children is lower (Peterman et al. 1959; Berglund 1954). More recent reports suggest that GBS may be milder in children than in adults (Hart et al. 1994; Korinthenberg and Monting 1996).

The most reliable overall predictor of outcome in GBS is the result of nerve conduction studies and EMG. Miller et al. (1988), Cornblath et al. (1988), McKhann et al. (1988), and Ropper et al. (1990) all found that a low-amplitude compound muscle action potential (CMAP), even when recorded during the early stages of the disease, carried an ominous prognosis. In the former study, 60 patients who were bedfast, 22 of which were ventilator dependent, were analyzed retrospectively to see which factors correlated significantly with inadequate recovery. The only electrophysiological parameter that correlated significantly was the low CMAP amplitude. They found no significant correlation between poor outcome and density of fibrillation potentials found with needle EMG. The studies of Cornblath and McKhann report the results of the North American multicenter trial of plasmapheresis for GBS, in which no needle EMG data was gathered. Again the only significant correlation with poor outcome was low-amplitude CMAP. However, even in those patients in whom the CMAP amplitude was 0% to 20% of normal, outcome was still improved with plasmapheresis (The Guillain-Barré Study Group 1985).

Pleasure et al. (1968) were the first to suggest that the presence of fibrillation potentials in weak muscles at the nadir of weakness predicted a poor outcome. Their observations were confirmed in more extensive studies by Eisen and Humphries (1974) and McLeod et al. (1976). However, Miller et al. found no such correlation. Ropper et al. found widespread fibrillation in 10 of 113 patients, most of whom were studied in the first 3 weeks of illness. Only the two patients in whom the CMAP amplitude was severely reduced failed to make complete recovery. Since recovery is primarily dependent on the degree of axonal degeneration, it is hardly surprising that patients with electrodiagnostic evidence of severe axonal degeneration should have a worse outcome. Fibrillation of muscle indicates loss of the trophic influence of axons on muscle fibers and indicates axonal degeneration. A low-amplitude CMAP may be due to acute axonal degeneration conduction block in distal intramuscular nerve twigs and can give the same result, although the CMAP is usually dispersed and the distal motor latency prolonged as well. Nonetheless, if the amplitude is reduced to less than 10% of normal, regardless of whether it is initially due to severe conduction block or axonal degeneration, the end result is invariably severe axonal degeneration and carries a poor prognosis.

GBS associated with either *Campylobacter jejuni* or cytomegalovirus (Schmitz and van Doorn, 1996) infections in general carries poorer prognosis, and delayed recovery is most likely related to the greater degree of axonal loss associated with these infections (Yuki et al. 1990; Visser et al. 1996).

Although, as strictly defined, GBS is a monophasic illness, a few patients do relapse. Some of these go on to develop a relapsing chronic demyelinating neuropathy. Overall, about 5% of patients have a single relapse and yet never develop a chronic disorder. Osterman et al. (1988) and Ropper et al. (1988) suggested that relapses were more likely in patients treated with plasmapheresis. However, neither the North American nor French multicenter studies of several hundred cases found a significant difference in the relapse rates between treated and untreated patients (French Cooperative Group on Plasma Exchange in Guillain-Barre Syndrome 1987). Similarly, relapses may be more common in patients treated with intravenous gammaglobulins, although relapses respond with equal effectiveness to treatment (Kleyweg and van der Meche 1991).

## Acute Sensory Neuronopathy

An acutely evolving syndrome of patchy sensory loss, predominantly affecting functions subserved by large myelinated axons, may also occur as an infectious or postinfectious syndrome (Sterman et al. 1980; Windebank et al. 1990). Although there are often complaints of weakness, objective strength testing is normal. Symptoms typically appear within days of the viral illness and are of acute onset and progression, reaching a nadir within a week. A subacute disorder, identical except for its rate of progression, may occur as a paraneoplastic syndrome (Horwich et al. 1977) and with Sjögren's syndrome (Malinow et al. 1986), and a chronic sensory neuronopathy occurs with pyridoxine intoxication (Parry and Bredesen 1985).

In acute sensory neuronopathy, prognosis is poor although some patients do make a complete recovery. In one series (Windebank) 8 of 42 patients made a complete recovery and an additional 22 made sufficient recovery to return to work. The remainder were severely disabled. The subacute form has an even worse outlook with few, if any, patients improving, in part because the cause is difficult or impossible to treat. In the chronic form, associated with pyridoxine intoxication, there is steady improvement after stopping the pyridoxine. The degree of recovery depends primarily on the severity of the neuropathy. Patients with severe sensory ataxia, particularly if it involves the arms, seldom return completely to normal. The persistent abnormalities may be due to degeneration of the central projections of the sensory neurons in the rostral portion of the posterior columns, where regeneration cannot take place.

## Acute Inflammatory Autonomic Neuropathy (Pandysautonomia)

Acute inflammatory autonomic neuropathy is a rare condition whose etiology is not understood, but it may be the autonomic counterpart of GBS. Postural hypotension, cramping, abdominal pain, and varying amounts of diarrhea are the principal symptoms. It may run a relapsing course.

Prognosis for full recovery in acute dysautonomia is guarded. Young et al. (1975) emphasized the good prognosis in their cases who all made excellent recovery. However, Hart and Kanter (1990), in their review of the literature, noted that only 40% of reported cases recovered completely, although another 48% made partial recovery. Time course for recovery is protracted, taking several months to 2 years.

## Brachial Neuritis

Brachial neuritis is an idiopathic, acute, painful paralysis of the arm. It most commonly involves the muscles of the shoulder girdle but involvement of more distal (e.g., anterior interosseus) and more proximal (e.g., spinal accessory) nerves may be seen. It is occasionally bilateral but is always markedly asymmetrical. Recurrent and familial forms are seen. An analogous neuropathy involving the lumbosacral plexus may occasionally occur.

The prognosis for recovery is generally good. The pain, which may be severe, almost invariably resolves over a period of weeks. However, treatment with narcotic analgesics is usually needed. Although corticosteroids do not influence the rate or efficacy of recovery from the paralysis, it has been suggested that they may shorten the painful phase (Sumner 1990). Recovery from the paralysis is less predictable but is usually good. In one study (Tsiaris et al. 1972), 80% of patients fully recovered and another 18% were still improving at the time of follow-up. Similarly, Devathasan and Tong (1980) found complete recovery of motor function in 18 of 19 patients followed for 2 years; 12 within 6 months and an additional five by a year. In general, the most reliable predictor of outcome is the severity of the paralysis. With mild to moderate weakness and survival of 10% to 30% of motor units on EMG, full functional recovery can occur over 3 to 6 months. With complete or near-complete denervation, prognosis is much more guarded. However, some cases with severe weakness and atrophy still make a remarkable recovery, perhaps reflecting the site of pathology. It has been suggested that the lesion in brachial neuritis is located very distally (England and Sumner 1987), perhaps in the intramuscular nerve terminals (Kraft 1969), so that recovery by regeneration over these short distances is possible.

## Porphyria

The dominantly inherited hepatic porphyrias (acute intermittent porphyria, variegate porphyria [V.P], and coproporphyria) may also present with an acute neuropathy mimicking GBS (Ridley 1984). Manifestations usually begin at puberty. Abdominal, loin, or back pain followed by restlessness, crying, and hysterical or neurotic behavior occur. Barbiturates worsen the situation. In VP and hereditary coproporphyria (HCP), cutaneous photosensitivity (unrelated to the attacks) may occur. Motor involvement can be acute and symmetrical and may involve respiratory muscles and cranial nerves. Sensory symptoms can be distal or proximal with a "bathing trunk" or "long johns" distribution. Muscle pain and aching may be prominent. Tendon reflexes are unpredictable but are usually diminished or absent. There may be prominent autonomic instability and also signs of CNS involvement with encephalopathy and seizures. The CSF is acellular with a modest elevation of protein. The predominant pathology is distal axonopathy with preferential involvement of short motor axons, but there may be some secondary paranodal demyelination.

Although porphyric neuropathy is primarily an axonal degeneration neuropathy, prognosis for recovery of function is good. There is a significant mortality during the acute phase, probably exacerbated by delayed diagnosis in many instances. This early mortality is mainly related to autonomic failure. Those patients who survive the acute attack steadily improve and even those with severe paralysis usually recover functionally over many months, although some weakness may be permanent (Sorensen and With 1971).

## Polyarteritis Nodosa

The neuropathy associated with polyarteritis nodosa (PAN) is the quintessential acute, multifocal axonal neuropathy and results from nerve infarction secondary to necrotizing vasculitis. Similar ischemic neuropathies occur with the other vasculitides (e.g., rheumatoid arthritis, systemic lupus erythematosis, Sjögren's syndrome) but are usually less severe and tend to be more chronic in their evolution. Although PAN is rare, neuropathy occurs in approximately two-thirds of cases and may be the presenting feature (Lovelace 1964). Additional clinical features include abdominal pain, purpura, ulcers, asthma, arthralgia, hypertension, renal sediment abnormalities, and anemia. Extensive arterial involvement precedes neuropathy. The mononeuropathies are abrupt in onset, with pain and numbness in the distribution of the affected nerve, quickly followed by weakness. Confluence of multiple nerve lesions can result in a symmetrical sensorimotor polyneuropathy (Parry 1985). Hepatitis B surface antigen has been found in 10% to 50% of patients. Complement levels are usually normal but may be depressed (mixed cryoglobulinemia). Proteinuria or red cell casts suggest renal involvement. Muscle and whole sural nerve biopsies can be useful, and visceral angiography should be considered if biopsy does not show necrotizing vasculitis. An acutely evolving axonal mononeuropathy multiplex is a clear indication for high-dose corticosteroids, which probably should be combined with cyclophosphamide.

Prognosis for recovery from systemic necrotizing vasculitis itself is guarded. Early recognition and aggressive treatment of the underlying disease will limit the extent of neurological damage. Recovery from the associated mononeuropathies is determined primarily by the severity of the axonal degeneration. With partial nerve infarcts, some recovery of function occurs by two mechanisms. First, with mild nerve infarcts, there may be ischemic conduction block that resolves rapidly over days to weeks (Parry and Linn 1988). This usually accounts for only a very small proportion of the clincial deficit, but some rapid resolution may be seen. The second mechanism involves reinnervation by terminal collateral sprouting of surviving motor axons. Up to a third of motor axons may be lost and yet full strength restored by this mechanism (Daube 1985). Therefore, full recovery of function may occur with mild lesions. Because these distal branches need only elongate a very short distance before establishing synaptic contact, recovery of some function may occur within weeks to months. Reinnervation by regeneration is unlikely in ischemic nerve lesions, perhaps because of ischemic damage to Schwann cells and the perineurium. As a result, recovery is poor in more severe lesions. Although recovery of neurological function is poor, the pain associated with these acute nerve infarcts almost invariably resolves spontaneously, although it may take several months and sometimes as long as 2 years.

## Toxic Neuropathies

Toxic neuropathies may be an acute, but delayed, result of massive exposure to a neurotoxin but are more commonly subacute or chronic, secondary to more protracted exposure. Causes of acute delayed neuropathy include organophosphates, arsenic, and thallium. Subacute and chronic toxic neuropathies may occur with many toxins, including many medications. An important phenomenon that occurs with some toxic neuropathies is "coasting" (Schaumburg and Spencer 1984). That is, after exposure to the neurotoxin is stopped there is continuing worsening of the neurological signs and symptoms for days to weeks before recovery begins. This obviously has important implications for prognosis. Most toxic neuropathies are distal axonopathies (Cavanaugh 1985; Schaumburg and Spencer 1984), usually with both central and peripheral axonal degeneration. With some acute, massive exposures there may be multifocal demyelination as well, presumably from a direct toxic effect on Schwann cells, but severe axonal degeneration always predominates (Donofrio 1987). Clinical features of toxic neuropathy seldom are sufficiently specific or characteristic to identify the toxic etiology or the specific toxin. Sensory, motor, and autonomic features occur in varying proportions, but sensory usually predominates, often with severe pain. There may be evidence of involvement of other organs, including the CNS, which may provide a clue to the etiology.

Prognosis following identification of an intoxication is related to a number of factors. Involvement of other organs, particularly liver and kidney, may be fatal or severely disabling. CNS involvement may also limit the extent and rapidity of recovery. With regard to the neuropathic features, since these are mainly distal axonopathies, the principal determinant of recovery is the extent of the axonal degeneration. When there has been minimal "dying-back," regeneration with re-establishment of appropriate contact with receptor or effector organs occurs within weeks. As mentioned above, some continued deterioration of neurological function may occur even after the toxin is removed, so it is important to recognize a toxic neuropathy as soon as possible so that irreversible changes are minimized. With more severe neuropathies, some improvement will occur with time, but sensory abnormalities may persist indefinitely because of the central degeneration in the rostral portion of the posterior columns.

## Bell's Palsy

Bell's palsy is an acute idiopathic facial paralysis that evolves over hours to days. It is commonly preceded by pain in or behind the ear. There is often an accompanying subjective numbness of the face but no objective sensory loss. Occasionally, with very proximal facial nerve involvement, there is hyperacusis, xerostomia, and xerophthalmia. It is important to distinguish Bell's palsy from facial paralysis associated with geniculate herpes zoster, since the latter has a much worse prognosis.

Prognosis for recovery from Bell's palsy is excellent (Katusic et al. 1986). Without treatment, 75% recover completely within 2 to 4 weeks or occasionally longer. An additional 15% make an excellent functional recovery with only subtle facial asymmetry apparent on examination. The remainder are left with varying degrees of facial weakness. Even in these patients, slow improvement may continue over many months. However, there is a significant risk of developing aberrant regeneration resulting in facial synkinesis and occasionally lacrimation induced by eating (crocodile tears). Controlled trials indicate that treatment with high-dose prednisone accelerates recovery and reduces the incidence of aberrant regeneration (Wolf et al. 1978). Prognosis is related closely to the severity of the axonal degeneration. Electrodiagnostic testing 3 to 5 days after the onset of the paralysis can provide useful prognostic information. If there is partial or complete preservation of the evoked motor response, voluntary motor unit potentials, and a paucity of fibrillations with needle EMG, prognosis is better. Furthermore, the rate of recovery is proportional to the amplitude of the evoked motor response (Albers and Bromberg 1990). Prognosis for recovery is considerably worse when the compound action potential is reduced to less than 50% as compared to the asymptomatic side (Danielides et al. 1996).

## Subacutely Evolving Neuropathies

### Alcoholic Neuropathy

There is a close association between alcoholism and peripheral nerve disease. Symptoms may be subacute or slowly progressive (Walsh and McLeod 1970; Tabaraud et al. 1990). Alcohol neuropathy may be caused by lack of thiamine and other vitamins, but alcohol itself might be neurotoxic. The neuropathy can be asymptomatic with mild leg thinness, muscle tenderness, ankle reflex depression, and subtle loss of distal sensation. Mild calf ache, discomfort of the soles, distal paresthesia, pain, and weakness are common. The legs are invariably affected before the arms. Motor and sensory symptoms usually occur together, although the sensory features usually predominate. One-quarter of patients have distressing pain, paresthesia, and burning feet. The entire leg may become sensitive to the touch. The condition is usually accompanied by excessive perspiration. Distal weakness and atrophy are usually present, but proximal weakness and even bulbar involvement may also occur and may be ascribed erroneously to alcoholic myopathy. Postural hypotension and bladder symptoms are common. Muscle tenderness is characteristic. Lower limb ataxia from alcohol-induced anterior cerebellar vermis atrophy may also be present. CSF is usually normal but the protein may be elevated. Other signs of alcoholism and nutritional deprivation are common, particularly Korsakoff's psychosis.

Alcoholic neuropathy is primarily a distal axonopathy, although the commonly associated malnutrition may produce significant associated demyelination. Two factors are important in determining prognosis, the most important of which is the ability of the patient to stop drinking. If alcohol intake can be stopped, the neuropathy will improve and the amount of improvement that occurs is then related to the severity of the neuropathy. Some numbness of the feet is usually permanent with the more severe, cases but the pain usually subsides over several months.

## Chronically Evolving Neuropathies

### Chronic Inflammatory Demyelinating Polyneuropathy

CIDP may run a relapsing or inexorably progressive course. It shares many clinical and pathological features with GBS. Onset can be at any age. The neuropathy usually evolves over months or years, and relapses or steps with progression can occur. Sensory complaints are as common as weakness. Generally, weakness is out of proportion to atrophy, providing a clinical clue to the underlying pathology. Cranial nerves may be involved. Signs of CNS involvement, such as extensor plantar responses and papilledema, may occasionally be seen. CSF protein is usually elevated and there may be an associated paraproteinemia.

Electrodiagnostic studies show the characteristic features of demyelination, and the amount of associated axonal degeneration is extremely variable. Particularly in the relapsing form, axonal degeneration may be minimal, while in some cases of indolently evolving CIDP there is so much axonal degeneration that it may be difficult to recognize the primary underlying pathology. In such cases, nerve biopsy can be diagnostically helpful.

CIDP is a potentially treatable neuropathy. Most cases will respond to some form of immune manipulation. Both high-dose corticosteroids and plasmapheresis have been shown in controlled studies to benefit CIDP more than no treatment (Dyck et al. 1978, 1982, 1986). Several randomized studies have established intravenous gammaglobulin as an effective treatment of CIDP (Faed 1989; van Doorn et al. 1990, Dyck et al. 1994; Hahn et al. 1996).

Prognosis in CIDP is primarily dependent on the ability to control the immune-mediated demyelination. If the immune attack on myelin can be halted, dramatic recovery by way of remyelination can occur. Improvement is sometimes seen within hours and continues over subsequent days to weeks. If there is significant associated axonal degeneration, recovery is more protracted and is often incomplete. The not infrequent involvement of nerve roots makes full recovery impossible if there is significant axonal degeneration at this level. There is a small mortality from complications of the neuropathy. In the series of Dyck et al. (1975), 11% of patients died from complications, but a lower mortality is usually found (Austin 1958). A few cases eventually go into complete remission, either as a result of treatment or spontaneously. Only 4% of Dyck's series recovered. However, treatment was either not given or was less than optimal. About 60% of the patients will be able to return to or continue to work. The remainder will be disabled, some confined to bed or wheelchair.

There is no similar long-term follow-up of patients with CIDP who have received optimal treatment, but our experience suggests that this rather gloomy prognosis can be improved. In one study with long-term follow-up of 30 patients treated with intravenous immunoglobulin (IVIG) with mean follow-up of 6.5 years van der Meche and von Doorn (1995) reported a 60% remission rate, while 40% required intermittent IVIG. In our combined experience of more than 75 patients over the last 15 years there have been no deaths and most patients continue in their former activities.

The chronic demyelinating neuropathy associated with monoclonal gammopathies may have a worse prognosis, although up to 66% of patients were reported to improve with treatment (Gorson et al. 1997). However, chronic demyelinating neuropathy associated with a solitary plasmacytoma can be cured with complete removal of the tumor.

## Diabetic Neuropathies

The diabetic neuropathies have considerable clinical heterogeneity, and the prognosis differs for different syndromes. Broadly, these neuropathies can be divided into two categories (Dyck et al. 1987). Focal or multifocal neuropathies have an acute or subacute onset, are overtly asymmetrical, have a predilection for proximal nerves, are most likely the result of nerve ischemia, and have a reasonably good prognosis for complete or partial recovery. These include cranial, truncal, and proximal asymmetrical motor neuropathies and mononeuropathies. Distal neuropathies have a slow onset and insidious progression, are largely symmetrical, are distally accentuated and, in those for which the pathogenesis is obscure, are inexorably progressive. This more common syndrome is what is generally referred to as diabetic neuropathy.

Focal and multifocal neuropathies (Asbury 1987) are characterized clinically by the acute or subacute onset of pain followed by loss of function in the distribution of the affected nerve(s). The maximal clinical deficit is usually reached within hours, or at the most days, although a more subacute course may occur. Cranial neuropathy most commonly affects the third nerve but classically spares pupillary function. Truncal neuropathy appears to have a predilection for the thoracic and upper lumbar spinal nerves, although cervical and lumbar involvement, if it does occur, is more likely to be attributed to spondylosis or disc disease. Proximal motor neuropathy mainly affects the femoral and obturator nerves. The main symptom is pain, which may be severe. Motor abnormalities are equally common but may be missed with truncal neuropathies because focal abdominal paralysis produces negligible clinical symptoms and signs (Parry and Floberg 1989).

Prognosis in each of these focal or multifocal neuropathies is similar. Once the nadir is reached, the condition persists for several weeks and then slowly improves. With oculomotor neuropathy, complete recovery is the rule in 3 to 5 months, and aberrant regeneration is rare. The other focal neuropathies tend to recover more slowly and incompletely. Pain, which may be severe and require narcotic analgesics, always improves but may take several months and sometimes as long as 2 years to subside. Recovery from the motor deficit is also quite good and occurs over about the same time period. Over half the patients regain normal or near normal function over 6 to 12 month period, but the remainder have significant residual disabilities (Garland 1955; Fry et al. 1962; Casey and Harrison 1972; Chad and Bradley 1987). Experience and common sense indicate that the degree of motor recovery is predicated primarily by the severity of the denervation. There is very little information available on the effect of glycemic control on prognosis for recovery, but most recommend attempts to lower blood glucose, since improvement in some cases correlates with good control of hyperglycemia (Casey and Harrison 1972; Chokroverty et al. 1977).

Distal neuropathies constitute a much more common type of neuropathy and are the almost inevitable consequence of long-standing diabetes. After 25 years of diabetes, 50% of patients develop symptomatic neuropathy and the remainder have asymptomatic neuropathy of varying severity (Pirart 1978). Surveys of prevalence indicate that one-third to one-half of patients with diabetes have symptomatic neuropathy and about 15% have significant disability attributable to the neuropathy (Dyck et al. 1987). On rare occasions, death may be attributable to neuropathy, presumably due to autonomic instability.

Prognosis for this type of neuropathy is less optimistic. Inexorable progression is the rule, with the development of sensory, motor, and autonomic disorders in varying combinations. Apart from duration of diabetes, the only factor related to the development and progression of neuropathy is glycemic control (Dahl-Jorgensen 1987). Age, sex, family history, and obesity have no beneficial or adverse effect (Pirart). Severe hyperglycemia in recently diagnosed diabetics (usually type I) may be associated with symptoms of neuropathy and abnormal nerve conduction. When this short-term hyperglycemia is controlled, symptoms resolve and nerve conduction returns to normal. These neuropathic symptoms are probably related to functional metabolic abnormalities of the nerve and are completely reversible. Occasionally, irreversible neuropathy is present at the time of diagnosis of diabetes in older patients with mild type II diabetes, and symptoms of neuropathy may lead to the diagnosis of diabetes. In such cases, mild diabetes has almost certainly been unrecognized for many years. Once established in chronic diabetics, objective evidence of neuropathy cannot be reversed, although symptoms can be improved. Rigid glycemic control, be it with diet, oral hypoglycemic drugs, insulin, or pancreatic transplantation (Kennedy et al. 1990), can only halt or reduce the rate of progression. None of the other treatments suggested for diabetic neuropathy have been shown, in any way, to influence progression (Harati 1987).

## Genetically Determined Neuropathies

There is a diverse group of inherited neuropathies that affect myelin, axons, or both. Peripheral nerves are also often involved in multisystem degenerations. All inherited neuropathies are inexorably progressive and no treatment is available. However, variation in the rate of progression is enormous, not only between genetically distinct types of neuropathy but also within a particular neuropathy type and even within individual kindreds. For example, completely asymptomatic individuals with hereditary motor sensory neuropathy type I may be discovered in late life, only when their children or grandchildren present with severe disease in childhood. Furthermore, siblings with similar age of onset of symptoms may progress at very different rates. Thus it is difficult to anticipate the prognosis of neuropathy in a given individual at the time of diagnosis. Patients with hereditary neuropathy with liability for pressure palsy (HNPP) carry a much better prognosis and many patients are asymptomatic.

## Focal Entrapment Neuropathies

The prognosis in focal entrapment neuropathies is determined by the site of the nerve involvement, type of neuropathological injury (demyelinating vs. axonal), severity, and chronicity of the process. Not all focal entrapment neuropathies carry similar prognosis; for instance, median neuropathy at the wrist or carpal tunnel syndrome (CTS) carries a much better prognosis than ulnar neuropathy at the elbow or cubital tunnel syndrome. These differences may be partly related to the unique predisposition of each nerve toward developing varying degrees of axonal loss associated with compression. We will discuss the prognostic factors in three of the common forms of entrapment neuropathies.

### Carpal Tunnel Syndrome

This is the most common form of entrapment neuropathy which, in general, carries an excellent prognosis. Mild cases or patients with reversible causes such as pregnancy often do well with conservative management with wrist splints. Most patients with moderate to severe symptoms or with progressive symptoms will eventually require surgery.

Surgeries for carpal tunnel are highly successful and most series report between 85% and 96% recovery of symptoms with surgery (Cseuz et al. 1966; Glowacki et al. 1996; Atroshi et al. 1997). Short histories and painful nocturnal paresthesias are good prognostic features (Nau et al. 1988).

Many patients often experience relief of painful sensory symptoms almost immediately post operatively, which has been thought to be related to rapid improvement in the median nerve conduction within minutes and which can be seen with intraoperative electrophysiological studies (Hongel and Mattsson 1971). Such rapid improvement in the electrophysiological studies has been questioned (Yates et al. 1981), and it is suggested that reduction in the spontaneous activity generated by the compressed nerve may be responsible for immediate relief of symptoms.

Once again, the extent of associated axonal injury is the main determinant of the ultimate outcome. Thenar atrophy and duration of symptoms for greater than 7 months suggest worse outcome (Muhlau 1984). Electrodiagnostic evidence of axonal injury suggests a relatively poor prognosis. Marked alterations in the motor unit potentials and their recruitment pattern and signs of chronic muscle denervation suggest worse prognosis for improvement in neurological deficits, although pain relief may be good.

The severity of axonal degeneration is best assessed by electrodiagnostic studies. The extent of axonal injury does affect the outcome (Mahlau and Konath 1984), although the exact role of electrodiagnostic studies in predicting functional recovery or re-employment is debated (Glowacki et al. 1996; Gunnarsson et al. 1997).

Median time until return to work is reported to be 17 days (Atroshi et al. 1997). Economic and psychological variables seem to impact the relief of symptoms and ability to return to work (Kantz et al. 1997) and these include worker's compensation, worse mental health status, work absence preoperatively, involvement of an attorney, and preoperative absence from work.

The prognosis after nonsurgical intervention is not as good. With corticosteroid injections 28% reported improvement in one series (Gelberman et al. 1980). Relapses are common (Goodman and Foster 1962) and many would require surgery at a later date. However, carefully selected patients with mild carpal tunnel syndrome were shown to have 93% symptomatic improvement after injection with steriod (Giannini et al. 1991).

The prognosis in patients with diabetes with carpal tunnel syndrome is good if there are clear focal changes of demyelination in the median nerve across the carpal tunnel. In a retrospective study al-Qattan (1994) found good to excellent results in 15 of 20 patients with diabetes and CTS treated with surgery. The five patients who failed to respond had no clear focal abnormalities in nerve conduction studies.

## Ulnar Neuropathy at the Elbow

The exact site of pathology in idiopathic ulnar neuropathy at the elbow is debated, and it appears that some patients have compression in the cubital tunnel (cubital tunnel syndrome), whereas in others it is damaged in the epicondylar groove. Although these two types of neuropathies are clinically identical, electrophysiological abnormalities (Miller 1979; Brown and Yates 1982) and intraoperative findings can be helpful in making the distinction. It is not known if the different sites of nerve involvement have any bearing on the prognosis.

In mild idiopathic cases the outcome with conservative management, such as wearing an elbow pad, can lead to complete recovery (Eisen and Danon 1974; De Jesus and Steiner 1976). Surgical intervention is indicated for more severe neuropathy or when there is worsening.

Although there is no consensus about the type of surgery outcome with surgical interventions in general is good with improvement in up to 75% of patients. Ulnar nerve transposition is widely regarded as the treatment of choice with excellent results, with improvement in about 75% of patients being reported in most series (Levy and Apfelberg 1972; Glowacki and Weiss 1997; Nouhan and Kleinert 1997). Equally good results have been reported with simple decompression (Chan et al. 1980; Steiner et al. 1996; Bimmler and Meyer 1996) or with medial epicondylectomy (Geutjens et al. 1996).

Complications from surgery include treatment failure, persistent paresthesias and pain, and scar formation leading to further nerve compression (Jackson and Hotchkiss 1996). Submuscular transposition of the ulnar nerve seems indicated for patients with previous failed transpositions (Siegel 1996).

## Peroneal Neuropathy at the Fibular Head

With traumatic peroneal neuropathies, immediate surgical intervention is indicated if the nerve is completely transected, while delayed surgery is indicated for incomplete lesions if spontaneous improvement does not occur within months. Surgery is also recommended for patients with progressive peroneal neuropathy of unknown cause or with lack of improvement with conservative management following an identifiable episode of compressive injury.

Where a definite compressive episode can be identified, most patients improve spontaneously by avoiding further pressure on the nerve. If there is no improvement, surgery is recommended. Mont et al. (1996) reviewed 31 patients who had failed to improve with conservative management and found epineural fibrosis and bands of fibrous tissue constricting the nerve at the fibular head. They found much better prognosis in patients treated with surgical intervention. At a mean of 36 months (range, 12 to 72 months) postoperatively, 30 (97%) of the 31 patients reported subjective and functional improvement and were able to discontinue the use of the ankle-foot orthosis. In contrast, only three of nine patients who had been managed nonoperatively reported subjective and functional improvement ($p < .01$). Similarly, patients with chronic progressive peroneal neuropathies should be explored surgically even if no compressive pathology is identified.

## References

Albers, J. W.; Bromberg, M. B. Bell's palsy. In: Johnson, R. T., ed. Current therapy in neurologic disease—3. Philadelphia: B. C. Decker; 1990: p. 376–380.

al-Qattan, M. M.; Manktelow, R. T.; Bowen, C. V. Outcome of carpal tunnel release in diabetic patients. J. Hand Surg. [Br.] 19(5):626–629; 1994.

Andersson, T.; Siden, A. A clinical study of the Guillain-Barre syndrome. Acta Neurol. Scand. 66: 316–327; 1982.

Asbury, A. K. Focal and multifocal neuropathies of diabetes. In: Dyck, P. J.; Thomas, P. K.; Asbury, A. K.; Winegrad, A. I.; Porte, D., eds. Philadelphia: W. B. Saunders Co.; 1987; p. 45–55.

Atroshi, I.; Johnson, R.; Ornstein, E. Endoscopic carpal tunnel release: prospective assessment of 255 consecutive cases. J. Hand Surg. [Br.] 22(1):42–47; 1997.

Austin, J. H. Recurrent polyneuropathies and their corticosteroid treatment; with five-year observations of a placebo-controlled case treated with corticotrophin, cortisone and prednisone. Brain 81: 157–194; 1958.

Berger, A. R.; Logigian, E. L.; Shahani, B. T. Reversible proximal conduction block underlies rapid recovery in Guillain-Barre syndrome. Muscle Nerve 11:1039–1042; 1988.

Berglund, A. Polyradikulonevriter. Nord. Med. 52: 1091–1095; 1954.

Bimmler, D.; Meyer, V. E. Surgical treatment of the ulnar nerve entrapment neuropathy: submuscular anterior transposition or simple decompression of the ulnar nerve? Long-term results in 79 cases. Ann. Chir. Main Memb. Super. 15(3):148–57; 1996.

Brown, W. F.; Yates, S. K. Percutaneous localization of conduction abnormalities in human entrapment neuropathies. Can. J. Neurol. Sci. 9:391–400; 1982.

Casey, E. B.; Harrison, M. J. G. Diabetic amyotrophy: a follow-up study. Br. Med. J. 1:656–659; 1972.

Cavanagh, J. B. Mechanisms of damage by chemical agents. In: Swash, M.; Kennard, C. eds. Scientific basis of neurology. Edinburgh: Churchill Livingstone; 1985; p. 631–645.

Chad, D. A.; Bradley, W. G. Lumbosacral plexopathy. Semin. Neurol. 7:97–109; 1987.

Chan, R. C.; Paine, K. W. E.; Warughese, G. Ulnar neuropathy at the elbow: comparison of simple decompression and anterior transposition. Neurosurgery 7:545–550; 1980.

Chokroverty, S.; et al: The syndrome of diabetic amyotrophy. Arch. Neurol. 27: 403–407; 1977.

Cornblath, D. R.; Mellits, E. D.; Griffin, J. W.; McKhann, G. M.; Albers, J. W.; Miller, R. G.; Feasby, T. E.; Quaskey, S. A.; and the Guillain-Barre Study Group. Motor conduction studies in Guillain-Barre syndrome: description and prognostic value. Ann. Neurol. 23:354–359; 1988.

Cseuz, K. A.; Thomas, J. E.; Lamber, E. H.; et al. Long-term results of operation for carpal tunnel syndrome. Mayo Clin. Proc. 41:232–241; 1966.

Dahl-Jorgernsen, K. Near-normoglycemia and late diabetic complications. The Oslo study. Acta Endocrinol. 115(suppl. 284):1–38; 1987.

Danielides, V.; Skevas, A.; Van Cauwenberge, P. A comparison of electroneuronography with facial nerve latency testing for prognostic accuracy in patients with Bell's palsy. Eur. Arch. Otorhinolaryngol. 253(1–2):35–38; 1996.

Daube, J. R. Electrophysiologic studies in the diagnosis and prognosis of motor neuron diseases. Neurol. Clin. 3:473–481; 1985.

De Jesus, P. V.; Steiner, J. C. Spontaneous recovery of ulnar neuropathy at the elbow. Electromyogr. Clin. Neurophysiol. 16:608–613; 1976.

Devathasan, G.; Tong, H. I.; Neuralgic amyotrophy: criteria for diagnosis and a clinical with electromyographic study of 21 cases. Aust. N. Z. J. Med. 10: 188–191; 1980.

Donofrio, P. D.; Wilbourn, A. J.; Albers, J. W.; Rogers, L.; Salanga, V.; Greenberg, H. S. Acute arsenic intoxication presenting as Guillain-Barre-like syndrome. Muscle Nerve 10:114–120; 1987.

Duvoisin, R. C. Polyneuritis: clinical review of 23 cases of Landry-Guillain-Barre syndrome. U.S. Armed Forces Med. J. 11:1294–1306; 1960.

Dyck, P. J.; Daube, J. R.; O'Brien, P.; Pineda, A.; Low, P. A.; Windebank, A. J.; Swanson, C. Plasma exchange in chronic inflammatory demyelinating poly-

radiculoneuropathy. N. Engl. J. Med. 314:461–465; 1986.

Dyck, P. J.; Karnes, J.; O'Brien, P. C. Diagnosis, staging, and classification of diabetic neuropathy and associations with other complications. In: Dyck, P. J.; Thomas, P. K.; Asbury, A. K.; Winegrad, A. I.; Porte, D., eds. Diabetic neuropathy. Philadelphia: W. B. Saunders Co.; 1987: p. 36–44.

Dyck, P. J.; Karnes, J. L.; Lambert, E. H. Longitudinal study of neuropathic defects and nerve conduction abnormalities in hereditary motor and sensory neuropathy type I. Neurology 39:1302–1308; 1989.

Dyck, P. J.; Lais, A. C.; Ohta, M.; Bastron, J. A.; Okazaki, H.; Groover, R. V. Chronic inflammatory polyradiculoneuropathy. Mayo Clin. Proc. 50: 621–637; 1975.

Dyck, P. J.; O'Brien, P. C.; Oviatt, K. F.; Bastron, J. A.; Daube, J. R.; Dinapoli, R. P.; Groover, R. V.; Stevens, J. C. Suggestive preliminary evidence from controlled 3-month clinical trials that prednisone improves chronic inflammatory polyradiculoneuropathy. Trans. Am. Neurol. Assoc. 103:26–28; 1978.

Dyck, P. J.; O'Brien, P. C.; Oviatt, K. F.; Dinapoli, R. P.; Daube, J. R.; Bartleson, J. D.; Mokri, B.; Swift, T.; Low, P. A.; Windebank, A. J. Prednisone improves chronic inflammatory demyelinating polyradiculoneuropathy more than no treatment. Ann. Neurol. 11:136–141; 1982.

Dyck, P. J.; Litchy, W. J.; Kratz, K. M.; Suarez, G. A.; Low, P. A.; Pineda, A. A.; Windebank, A. J.; Karnes, J. L.; O'Brien, P. C. A plasma exchange versus immune globulin infusion trial in chronic inflammatory demyelinating polyradiculoneuropathy. Ann. Neurol. 6(6):838–845; 1994.

Eisen, A.; Danon, J. The mild cubital tunnel syndrome: its natural history and indications for surgical intervention. Neurology 24;608–613; 1974.

Eisen, A.; Humphreys, P. The Guillain-Barre syndrome. A clinical and electrodiagnostic study of 25 cases. Arch. Neurol. 30:438–443; 1974.

England, J. D.; Sumner, A. J. Neuralgic amyotrophy: an increasingly diverse entity. Muscle Nerve 10: 60–68; 1987.

Faed, J. M.; Day, B.; Pollock, M.; Taylor, P. K.; Nukada, H.; Hammond-Tooke, G. D. High-dose intravenous human immunoglobulin in chronic inflammatory demyelinating polyneuropathy. Neurology 39:422–425; 1989.

Forster, F. M.; Browm, M.; Merritt, H. H. Polyneuritis with facial diplegia: a clinical study N. Engl. J. Med. 225:51–56; 1941.

French Cooperative Group on Plasma Exchange in Guillain-Barre Syndrome. Efficiency of plasma exchange in Guillain-Barre syndrome: role of replacement fluids. Ann. Neurol. 22:753–761; 1987.

Fry, I. K.; et al. Diabetic neuropathy: a survey and follow-up of 66 cases. Guys Hosp. Rep. 111:113; 1962.

Garland, H. Diabetic amyotrophy. Br. Med. J. 2:1287; 1955.

Gelberman, R. H.; Arnoson, D.; Weissman, M. H. Carpal tunnel syndrome: results of a prospective trial of steroid injection and splinting. J. Bone Joint Surg. [Am.] 62:1181–1184; 1980.

Geutjens, G. G.; Langstaff, R. J.; Smith, N. J.; Jefferson, D.; Howell, C. J.; Barton, N. J. Medial epicondylectomy or ulnar-nerve transposition for ulnar neuropathy at the elbow? J. Bone Joint Surg. [Br.] 78(5):777–779; 1996.

Giannini, F.; Passero, S.; et al. Electrophysiologic evaluation of local steroid injection in carpal tunnel syndrome. Arch. Phys. Med. Rehabil. 72:738–742; 1991.

Glowacki, K. A.; Breen, C. J.; Sachar, K.; Weiss, A. P. Electrodiagnostic testing and carpal tunnel release outcome. J. Hand Surg. [Am.] 22(1):117–121; 1996.

Glowacki, K. A.; Weiss, A. P. Anterior intramuscular transposition of the ulnar nerve for cubital tunnel syndrome. J. Shoulder Elbow Surg. 6(2):89–96; 1997.

Goodman, H. V.; Foster, J. B. Effect of local corticosteroid injection on median nerve conduction in carpal tunnel syndrome. Ann. Phys. Med. 6:287–294; 1962.

Gorson, K. C.; Allam, G.; Ropper, A. H. Chronic inflammatory demyelinating polyneuropathy: clinical features and response to treatment in 67 consecutive patients with and without a monoclonal gammopathy. Neurology 48(2):321–328; 1997.

Gunnarsson, L. G.; Amilon, A.; et al. The diagnosis of carpal tunnel syndrome. Sensitivity and specificity of some clinical electrophysiological tests. J. Hand Surg. [Br.] 22(1):34–37; 1997.

Hahn, A. F.; Bolton, C. F.; Zochodne, D.; Feasby, T. E. Intravenous immunoglobulin treatment in chronic inflammatory demyelinating polyneuropathy. A double-blind, placebo-controlled.; cross-over study. Brain 119(Pt. 4):1067–1077; 1996.

Harati, Y. Diabetic peripheral neuropathies. Ann. Intern. Med. 107:546–559; 1987.

Hart, D. E.; Rojas, L. A.; Rosario, J. A.; Recalde, H.; Roman, G. C. Childhood Guillain-Barre syndrome in Paraguay 1990 to 1991. Ann. Neurol. 36(6):859–863; 1994.

Hart, R. G.; Kanter, M. C. Acute autonomic neuropathy. Two cases and a clinical review. Arch. Intern. Med. 150:2373–2376; 1990.

Hongel, A.; Mattsson, H. S. Neurographic studies before, after, and during operation for median nerve compression in the carpal tunnel. Scand. J. Plast. Reconstr. Surg. 5:103–109; 1971.

Horwich, M. S.; Cho, L.; Porro, R. S.; Posner, J. B. Subacute sensory neuropathy: a remote effect of carcinoma. Ann. Neurol. 2:7–19; 1977.

Jackson, L. C.; Hotchkiss, R. N. Cubital tunnel surgery. Complications and treatment of failures. Hand Clin. 12(2):449–456; 1996.

Kaeser, H. E. Klinische und elektromyographische verlaufsuntersuchungen beim Guillain-Barre-syndrom. Schweiz. Arch. Neurol. Neurochir. Psychiat. 94:278–286; 1964.

Kantz, J. N.; Keller, R. B.; et al. Predictors of return to work following carpal tunnel release. Am. J. Ind. Med. 31(1):85–91; 1997.

Katusic, S. K.; Beard, C. M.; Wiederholt, W. C.; Bergstralh, E. J.; Kurland, L. T. Incidence, clinical features, and prognosis in Bell's palsy, Rochester, Minnesota 1968–1982. Ann. Neurol. 20:622–627; 1986.

Kennedy, R. H.; Danielson, M. A.; Mulder, D. W.; Kurland, L. T. Guillain-Barre syndrome: a 42 year epidemiologic and clinical study. Mayo Clin. Proc. 53:93–99; 1978.

Kennedy, W. R.; Navarro, X.; Goetz, F. C.; Sutherland, D. E. R.; Najarian, J. S. Effects of pancreatic transplantation on diabetic neuropathy. N. Engl. J. Med. 322:1031–1037; 1990.

Kleyweg, R. P.; van der Meche, F. G. A. Treatment related fluctuations in Guillain-Barre syndrome after high-dose immunoglobulins or plasma-exchange. J. Neurol. Neurosurg. Psychiatry 54:957–960; 1991.

Korinthenberg, R.; Monting, J. S. Natural history and treatment effects in Guillain-Barre syndrome: a multicentre study. Arch. Dis. Child. 74(4):281–287; 1996.

Kraft, G. H. Multiple distal neuritis of the shoulder girdle: an electromyographic clarification of "paralytic brachial neuritis." Electroencephalogr. Clin. Neurophysiol. 27:722; 1969.

Levy, D. M.; Apfelberg, D. B. Results of anterior transposition for ulnar neuropathy at the elbow. Am. J. Surg. 123:304–308; 1972.

Loffel, N. B.; Rossi, L. N.; Mumenthaler, M.; Lutschg, J.; Ludin, H.-P. The Landry-Guillain-Barre syndrome. Complications; prognosis and natural history in 123 cases. J. Neurol. Sci. 33:71–79; 1977.

Lovelace, R. E. Mononeuritis multiplex in polyarteritis nodosa. Neurology 14:434–442; 1964.

Malinow, K.; Yannakakis, G. D.; Glusman, S. M.; Edlow, D. W.; Griffin, J.; Pestronk, A.; Powell, D. L.; Ramsey-Goldman, R.; Eidelman, B. H.; Medsger, T. A.; Alexander, E. L. Subacute sensory neuronopathy secondary to dorsal root ganglionitis in primary Sjoegren's syndrome. Ann. Neurol. 20:535–537; 1986.

Marshall, J. The Landry-Guillain-Barre syndrome. Brain 86:55–66; 1963.

McKhann, G. M.; Griffin, J. W.; Cornblath, D. R.; Mellits, E. D.; Fisher, R. S.; Quasket, S. A.; and the Guillain-Barre Study Group. Plasmapheresis and Guillain-Barre syndrome: analysis of prognostic factors and the effects of plasmapheresis. Ann. Neurol. 23:347–353; 1988.

McLeod, J. G.; Walsh, J. C.; Prineas, J. W.; Pollard, J. D. Acute idiopathic polyneuritis. A clinical and electrophysiological follow-up study. J. Neurol. Sci. 27:145–162; 1976.

Miller, R. G. The cubital tunnel syndrome: diagnosis and precise localization. Ann. Neurol. 6:56–59; 1979.

Miller, R. G.; Peterson, G. W.; Daube, J. R.; Albers, J. W. Prognostic value of electrodiagnosis in Guillain-Barre syndrome. Muscle Nerve 11:769–774; 1988.

Mont, M. A.; Dellon, A. L.; Chen, F.; Hungerford, M. W.; Krackow, K. A.; Hungerford, D. S.; Morley,

J. B.; Reynolds, E. H. Papilloedema and the Landry-Guillain-Barre syndrome. Brain 89:205–222; 1966.

Muhlau, G.; Kunath, H. Carpal tunnel syndrome—course and pognosis. J. Neurol. 231:83–86; 1984.

Nau, H. E.; Lange, B.; Lange, S. Prediction of outcome of decompression for carpal tunnel syndrome. J. Hand Surg. 13(4):391–394; 1988.

Nouhan, R.; Kleinert, J. M. Ulnar nerve decompression by transposing the nerve and Z-lengthening the flexor-pronator mass: clinical outcome. J. Hand Surg. [Am.] 22(1):127–131; 1997.

Osler, L. D.; Sidell, A. D. The Guillain-Barre syndrome. The need for exact diagnostic criteria. N. Engl. J. Med. 262:964–969; 1960.

Osterman, P. O.; Fagius, J.; Safwenberg, J.; Wikstrom, B. Early relapse of acute inflammatory polyradiculoneuropathy after successful treatment with plasma exchange. Acta Neurol. Scand. 77:273–277; 1988.

Parry, G. J.; Bredesen, D. E. Sensory neuropathy with low-dose pyridoxine. Neurology 35:1466–1468;1985.

Parry, G. J.; Floberg, J. Diabetic truncal neuropathy presenting as abdominal hernia. Neurology 39:1488–1490; 1989.

Parry, G. J.; Linn, D. J. Conduction block without demyelination following acute nerve infarction. J. Neurol. Sci. 84:265–273; 1988.

Parry, G. J. G. Mononeuropathy multiplex (AAEE case report #11). Muscle Nerve 8:493–498; 1985.

Peterman, A. F.; Daly, D. D.; Dion, R. F.; Keith, H. M. Infectious neuronitis (Guillain-Barre syndrome) in children. Neurology 9:533–539;1959.

Pirart, J. Diabetes mellitus and its degenerative complications: a prospective study of 4400 patients observed between 1947 and 1973 Diabetes Care 1:168–188, 252–263; 1978.

Pleasure, D. E.; Lovelace, R. E.; Duvoisin, R. C. The prognosis of acute polyradiculoneuritis. Neurology 18:1143–1148; 1968.

Ravn, H. The Landry-Guillain-Barre syndrome. A survey and a clinical report of 127 cases. Acta Neurol. Scand. 43(suppl. 30):1–64; 1967.

Ridley, A. Porphyric neuropathy. In: Dyck, P. J.; Thomas P. K.; Lambert, E. H.; Bunge R., eds. Peripheral neuropathy. Philadelphia: W. B. Saunders Co.; 1984: p. 1704–1716.

Ropper, A. H.; Albers, J. W.; Addison, R. Limited relapse in Guillain-Barre syndrome after plasma exchange. Arch. Neurol. 45:314–315;1988.

Ropper, A. H., Wijdicks, E. F. M.; Shahani, B. T. Electrodiagnostic abnormalities in 113 consecutive patients with Guillain-Barre syndrome. Arch. Neurol. 47:881–887; 1990.

Saida, K.; Sumner, A. J., Saida, T., Brown, M. J., Silberberg, D. H. Antiserum-mediated demyelination: relationship between remyelination and functional reecovery. Ann. Neurol. 8:12–24; 1980.

Schaumburg, H. H.; Spencer, P. S. Human toxic neuropathy due to industrial agents. In: Dyck, P. J.; Thomas, P. K.; Lambert, E. H.; Bunge, R., eds. Peripheral neuropathy. Philadelphia: W. B. Saunders Co., 1984: p. 2115–2152.

Schmitz, P. I.; van Doorn, P. A. Cytomegalovirus infection and Guillain-Barre syndrome: the clinical, electrophysiologic, and prognostic features. Dutch Guillain-Barre Study Group. Neurology 47(3):668–673;1996.

Siegel, D. B. Submuscular transposition of the ulnar nerve. Hand Clin. 12(2):445–448;1996.

Sorensen, A. W. S.; With T. K. Persistent paresis after porphyric attacks (special issue). S. Afr. Med. J. 45:101–103;1971.

Steiner, H. H.; von Haken, M. S.; Steiner-Milz, H. G. Entrapment neuropathy at the cubital tunnel: simple decompression is the method of choice. Acta Neurochir. 138(3):308–313;1996.

Sterman, A. B.; Schaumburg, H. H.; Asbury, A. K. The acute sensory neuronopathy syndrome: a distinct clinical entity. Ann. Neurol. 7:354–358;1980.

Sumner, A. J. Brachial neuritis. In: Johnson R. T., ed. Current therapy in neurologic disease—3. Philadelphia: B. C. Decker; 1990: p. 374–375.

Tabaraud, F.; Vallat, J. M.; Hugon, J.; Ramiandrisoa, H.; Dumas M.; Signoret, J. L. Acute or subacute alcoholic neuropathy mimicking Guillain-Barre syndrome. J. Neurol. Sci. 97:195–205;1990.

The Guillain-Barre Study Group. Plasmapheresis and acute Guillain-Barre syndrome. Neurology 35:1096–1104; 1985.

The Italian Guillain-Barre Study Group. The prognosis and main prognostic indicators of Guillain-Barre syndrome. A multicentre prospective study of 297 patients. Brain 119 (Pt. 6):2053–2061; 1996.

Mont, M. A.; Dellon A. L.; Chen, F.; Hungerford, M. W.; Krackow K. A.; Hungerford D. S. The operative treatment of peroneal nerve palsy. J. Bone Joint Surg [Am.] 78(6):863–869; 1996.

Tsiaris, P.; Dyck, P. J.; Mulder, D. W. Natural history of brachial plexus neuropathy. Arch. Neurol. 27:109–117; 1972.

van der Meche, F. G.; van Doorn, P. A. Guillain-Barre syndrome and chronic inflammatory demyelinating polyneuropathy: immune mechanisms and update on current therapies (review). Ann. Neurol. 37 (suppl. 1):S14–S31;1995.

Van Doorn, P. A.; Brand, A.; et al. High-dose intravenous immunoglobulin treatment in chronic inflammatory demyelinating polyneuropathy. A double-blind placebo-controlled crossover study. Neurology 40:209–212; 1990.

Vedeler, C. A.; Wik, E.; Nyland, H. The long-term prognosis of Guillain-Barre syndrome. Evaluation of prognostic factors including plasma exchange. Acta Neurol. Scand. 95(5):298–302; 1997.

Visser, L. H.; van der Meche, F. G.; Meulstee, J.; Rothbarth, P. P.; Jacobs, B. C.; Schmitz, P. I.; van Doorn, P. A. Cytomegalovirus infection and Guillain-Barre syndrome: the clinical, electrophysiologic, and prognostic features. Dutch Guillain-Barre Study Group. Neurology 47:668–673; 1996.

Walsh, J. C.; McLeod, J. G. Alcoholic neuropathy: an electrophysiological and histological study. J. Neurol. Sci. 10:457–469; 1970.

Wiederholt, W. C.; Mulder, D. W.; Lambert, E. H. The Landry-Guillain-Barre-Strohl syndrome or poly-radiculoneuropathy: historical review, report on 97 patients, and present concepts. Mayo Clin. Proc. 39:427–451;1964.

Windebank, A. J.; Blexrud, M. D.; Dyck, P. J.; Daube, J. R.; Karnes, J. L. The syndrome of acute sensory neuropathy: clinical features and electrophysio-logical and pathological changes. Neurology 40: 584–591; 1990.

Winer, J. B.; Greenwood, R. J.; Hughes, R. A. C.; Perkin, G. D.; Healy, M. J. R. Prognosis in Guillain-Barre syndrome Lancet 1:1202–1203; 1985.

Wolf, S. M.; Wagner, J. H.; Davidson, S.; Forsythe, A. Treatment of Bell's palsy with prednisone: a prospec-tive, randomized study. Neurology 28:158–161; 1978.

Yates, S. K.; Hurst, L. N.; Brown, W. F. Physiological observations in the median nerve during carpal tun-nel surgery. Ann Neurol 10:227–229; 1981.

Young, R. R.; Asbury, A. K.; Corbett, J. L.; Adams, R. D. Pure pandysautonomia with recovery. Brain 98:613–636; 1975.

Yuki, N.; Yoshino, H.; Sato, S.; Miyatake, T. Acute ax-onal polyneuropathy associated with anti-GM1 anti-bodies following Campylobactor enteritis. Neurol-ogy 40:1900–1902;1990.

# 30

## Amyotrophic Lateral Sclerosis

STANLEY H. APPEL, R. GLENN SMITH, EUGENE C. LAI,
DENNIS R. MOSIER, AND LANNY J. HAVERKAMP

The term *motoneuron disease* often is used interchangeably with amyotrophic lateral sclerosis
(ALS). (However, motoneuron disease may present as a lower motoneuron syndrome, an upper
motoneuron syndrome, or a combination of the
two. Only the latter is referred to as ALS. The loss
of lower motoneuron function manifests in signs
and symptoms that are clinically categorized as
progressive muscular atrophy (PMA) or spinal
muscular atrophy (SMA). The presence of upper
motoneuron deficits alone is termed primary lateral sclerosis (PLS). When a patient presents with
symptoms and signs of bulbar difficulty manifested by impairment of speech and swallowing,
then he or she is considered to have progressive
bulbar palsy (PBP); and this presentation can
occur either as lower motoneuron or upper motoneuron involvement or a combination of both.

Of these disorders, ALS is the most common,
PBP is the next most common, PMA or SMA is
less common, and PLS is the least common. In one
series (Caroscio et al. 1987), approximately 80%
of the patients with motoneuron disease had ALS,
10% had PBP, 7% had PMA, and 2% had PLS.
These percentages are not an accurate reflection of
the prevalence of the different motoneuron diseases because of referral bias, namely, the potential understatement of cases of SMA because pa-

tients are being referred to an ALS clinic. With the
1200 patients seen at our MDA/ALS clinic at Baylor College of Medicine, approximately 70% had
sporadic disease with evidence of upper and lower
motoneuron involvement; 10% had familial ALS;
9% had lower motoneuron involvement only or
PMA; 3% had upper motoneuron involvement
only or PLS, 5% had possible postpolio; and 4%
had significant other medical problems masking or
simulating motoneuron injury (Haverkamp et al.
1995). Almost all cases with PBP had clinical and
pathological evidence of involvement of upper
and lower motoneurons and thus were considered
to have ALS. In the data provided by Caroscio and
colleagues (1987), the prognosis of patients diagnosed as ALS was not statistically different from
the prognosis of patients with PBP; however, patients with PMA and PLS had a much more benign
course.

### Prognosis of SMA

Because this chapter deals primarily with prognosis in ALS, cases of PMA, SMA, and PLA are
excluded. Nevertheless, it is important to note that
many cases of SMA are inherited and are relatively predictable. This statement applies to the
type I SMA, which appears in infants and has

513

been called acute Werdnig-Hoffmann disease. The manifestations may appear in utero when kicking movements of the fetus may be markedly decreased or absent. Other abnormalities noticed at birth or within the first few days are decreased muscle tone, decreased respiratory function, and a relatively weak cry. Approximately 25% of all cases of SMA represent this acute infantile form. Typically, patients die within the first few years.

When the disease manifests between the acute infantile ages and adolescence, it is referred to as intermediate or type II SMA. In these cases, the prognosis is more variable, and the course is difficult to predict. Even patients with relatively compromised respiratory function may survive until adulthood. Later onset, juvenile SMA is called type III or Kugelberg-Welander disease. This disorder typically presents between ages 5 and 15, although it may begin earlier or later. Weakness usually progresses slowly with some patients able to ambulate 30 years after the onset of the illness; others require a wheelchair in less than 10 years.

## Diagnosis of ALS

It is critical that other conditions associated with slowly progressive proximal weakness, such as limb girdle dystrophy, be ruled out by appropriate electrical, morphological, and genetic analyses. A more difficult task is to assess prognosis in patients who present later in life with predominantly lower motoneuron involvement. The overlap of patients with motor neuropathy and with lower motoneuron syndromes confounds the issue. An additional source of confusion is patients who present early with lower motoneuron signs and later develop evidence of upper motoneuron and bulbar compromise characteristic of ALS. Their prognosis is more difficult to estimate and will depend on the rate of upper motoneuron and bulbar dysfunction. Nevertheless, most patients with motor neuropathy and lower motoneuron compromise who subsequently develop bulbar symptoms follow a less devastating course than patients with more classical ALS.

## Prognosis of ALS

ALS is a relentless, incapacitating neuromuscular disease with an unknown cause and with no known therapy to reverse its course. The incidence of disease is 1 to 2 per 100,000, and the prevalence 4 to 6 per 100,000 (Bobowick and Brody 1973; Kahana et al. 1976; Annegers et al. 1991). The disease is approximately 1.7 times as common in men as in women and has a mean age of onset of 56 years in most series (Appel at al. 1986; Haverkamp et al. 1995). A Kaplan-Meier plot for the disease course is presented in Figure 30-1 reflecting 50% survival at 36 months after first symptom.

Although many specific etiologies, including viral, toxic, endocrine, and genetic, have been associated with upper and lower motoneuron dysfunction, the majority of ALS cases are sporadic and of unknown etiology. The disease usually begins with focal weakness and progresses with worsening disability of limbs or bulbar musculature. One-quarter of the patients exhibited primary bulbar symptoms, though presentation was again strongly correlated with age. (Haverkamp et al. 1995). Below age 30 years, only about 15% of patients exhibit primary bulbar symptoms, while over the age of 70 years, this presentation increased to 43%. This trend of increasing primary bulbar symptoms was seen in both sexes, although it was more pronounced in women, with more than half the female patients past the age of 70 years exhibiting primary bulbar symptoms and signs. Of the primary bulbar patients, the first symptom was speech difficulties for the vast majority (95%) with the remainder first experiencing choking. In addition to the 25% of the population with primary bulbar symptoms, 67.6% first described motor symptoms, 3.9% reported sensory symptoms, and 3.5% both motor and sensory symptoms. Approximately equal numbers of nonbulbar patients exhibited first symptoms in their arms (47.7%) or legs (46.5%), with 5.8% in both arms and legs, overwhelmingly in the distal portions (73%). There was a slight tendency to report first symptoms on the right side (40.9% vs. 35.1% on the left, vs. 22.1% on both sides vs. 1.9% with generalized symptoms). The pattern of progression of neurological deterioration followed a characteristic course. When the difficulty started in the right lower extremity, the next area of involvement was usually the left lower extremity. When the onset was one upper extremity, the next area of involvement in most patients was the contralateral upper extremity. For patients whose onset was bulbar, the next area of involvement was usually an upper extremity. Furthermore,

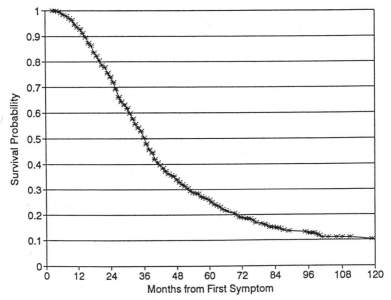

**Figure 30-1.** Kaplan-Meier curve describing survival in ALS. The number of patients known alive at time of entry (date of first symptom) and at yearly intervals thereafter were: 831, 738, 504, 302, 170, 103, 69, 42, 31, 17, 13.

even in patients diagnosed with PBP with no symptomatic involvement of upper or lower extremities, most patients showed electrical or morphological evidence of limb involvement.

## ALS RATING SCALE

To assess the rate of progression of neurological deterioration, the authors devised a rating scale that provides a quantitative estimate of the clinical status of the patient and of disease progression (Appel et al. 1987). The general clinical experience had been to anticipate variability in the musculature involved and in the progression of the disease. For example, a patient may experience rapid deterioration in speech and swallowing and have minimal change in extremity strength, rendering strength tests meaningless in evaluating disease progression. In contrast, pulmonary function alone may be less accurate in patients for whom extremity strength is compromised and bulbar function is spared. The rating scale includes assessment of swallowing and speech function, respiratory function, muscle strength in upper and lower extremities, and function of upper and lower extremities. The total ALS score consists of five group scores: bulbar, respiratory, muscle strength, lower-extremity function, and upper-extremity

function. The bulbar group is composed of the swallowing and speech subgroups, each of which is ranked according to fives degrees of severity; for example, normal swallowing is considered the ability to eat a general diet. Very severe dysfunction means the patient requires a feeding tube or gastrostomy. In the speech subgroup, "normal" indicates clear speech, while maximal dysfunction is characterized by aphonia. With respiration, scoring is graded into five steps based on changes of forced vital capacity expressed as a percent of predicted response. Muscle strength is assessed using the Medical Research Council system of grading, and tests of grip strength and lateral pinch strength. Lower-extremity function is assessed with timed functions and observed functions. Upper-extremity function is evaluated in four tests of timed functions (e.g., assembly of peg units, turning over blocks) and observed functions (e.g., ability to abduct the arms and independence in dressing and feeding).

With this method of monitoring patients for several years, it was apparent that the total ALS score changed in linear fashion with time. Linear regression analysis of the change in ALS scores of 74 patients with time yielded a median correlation coefficient of 0.956, supporting the linearity of progression. Using a quantitative testing battery,

Andress and coworkers (1986) and Munsat and associates (1987) followed 51 patients with ALS for a minimum of 12 months and found that their rates of deterioration were linear, with no plateaus or improvement. Using the total ALS score, progression differed markedly in different patients. When the slope of the regression line was calculated (i.e., the point change per 28 days), there was greater than a 20-fold difference in the rate of progression from the slowest to the most rapid course (Fig. 30-2). During 1 year, 19% of the patients progressed at a slow rate, changing less than 13 points; 77% of patients progressed at an intermediate rate of 13 to 48 points; and 34% of patients progressed at a rapid rate, changing more than 40 points. The study by Jablecki and colleagues (1989) also documented differing rates of progression in different patients with ALS. In their study, they noted a 60-fold difference between the fastest and slowest rates of progression of 194 patients followed for 8 years. In the patients in the author's study, the difference was not due to lower motoneuron disease in the slow category and lower and upper motoneuron disease with severe bulbar involvement in the fast category. This is because all patients in the analysis

had both lower and upper motoneuron involvement with minimal bulbar compromise at entry into the study. Bonduelle (1975) reports that ALS patients presenting with bulbar symptoms and signs deteriorated more quickly than patients presenting initially with limb weakness. Subsequent studies have confirmed the finding but have noted that bulbar presentation is more common in older patients (Kristensen and Melgaard 1977; Rosen 1978). In fact, if survival in patients presenting with bulbar signs was corrected for age of onset, there was no longer a statistical difference in prognosis of these two groups of patients (Daube 1985; Mulder 1984). The studies by Jablecki and associates (1989) suggest that older patients have a shorter survival, regardless of whether the initial presentation is of bulbar or spinal onset. However, in 318 ALS patients in Israel, patients with onset of disease with bulbar signs had a shorter life expectancy (2.2 years) even when corrected for age and sex (Gubbay et al. 1985). Longer survival in Guamanian ALS patients did depend on an early age at onset and male sex (Reed et al. 1975), but neither bulbar nor extremity onset showed a meaningful pattern of association with the duration of illness. In most studies, regardless

**Figure 30-2.** Histogram showing distribution of slopes of the total ALS score. Data were derived from 321 ALS patients having three or more examinations, with the slope derived by a least squares analysis, with units of points per month.

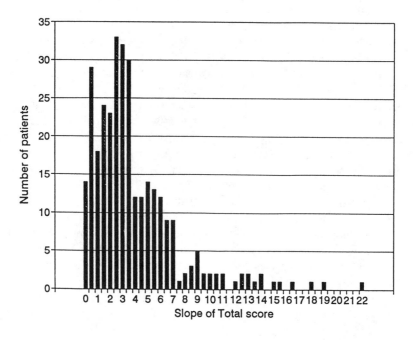

of whether bulbar or extremity signs occur first, the rapid progression of bulbar signs is associated with a poor prognosis. The rapid onset of bulbar signs in patients presenting initially with extremity weakness resulted in death within 1.5 to 2 years in 67% of all spinal cases in the series by Boman and Meurman (1967).

In a detailed analysis, our scoring system permitted a relatively good correlation between the survival as predicted by the slope of the total score, and the actual months survived (Fig. 30-3). When the differences between the predicted and actual survival are viewed as a function of slope, it was apparent that the slow course patients with low slopes most often die sooner than the slopes would predict. Individual subscores of our scoring system were not well correlated with overall disease progress.

Four attributes were apparent as significant covariates of survival: age, rate of change of the total score (the slope described by three or more examinations), rate of change of the respiratory subscore, and the time from first symptom until the first examination (Havnerkamp et al. 1995). The higher the score or the slope of total score or respiratory subscore, or the greater the age, the shorter the survival. Contrarily, duration of first symptom to first examination was negatively related to hazard. Thus, the longer the delay until first examination, the longer the survival. Clearly, the more rapidly the patient deteriorates at an early stage in the disease, the shorter the delay before the patient seeks medical attention and, therefore, the shorter the delay before first examination.

The inclusion of the respiratory subscore as a significant covariate of survival was unexpected. Since it usually contributes about 20% of the total score, it was thought that its predictive value would be subsumed by the more global total score. Furthermore, the slope of the respiratory subscore exhibits poor linearity primarily due to its discontinuous nature. Nevertheless, it is clear that the respiratory subscore is a significant covariate of survival.

The rate of change in total score over time was stable and linear in the majority of patients. More

**Figure 30-3.** Scatter graph showing the relationship between actual months survival from first symptom and months survival predicted by slope of the total ALS score. Prediction is based on assuming death or placement on a respirator at an average of 140 points in the total score. (Although maximum theoretical disability would be reflected in a score of 164, death usually occurs before that score is reached. The score of 140 used here in predicting survival is based on clinical experience; use of a different score would not alter the nature of the relationship between predicted and actual survival.) The straight line shows the region of perfect concordance between actual survival and that predicted by slope. Data are derived from typical ALS patients who received three or more examinations and for whom date of death (or placement on respirator) is certified ($n = 20$).

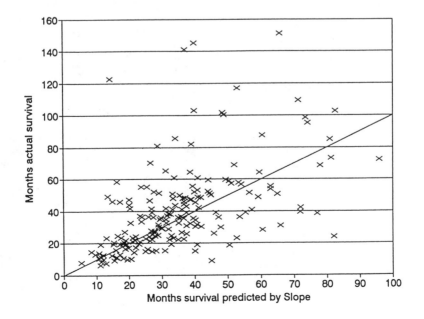

importantly, this rate of change was a significant covariate of survival and provided validation of our ALS rating system as a measure of disease progress. As a method of internal validation of our model, the mean survival probabilities for all patients were derived for a number of time points from 1 to 10 years after the date of first symptom. Plotting these values against the actual Kaplan-Meier survival curves showed the model to fit the data reasonably well. When the patients were stratified into prognostic groups of high risk, medium risk, and low risk, the modeled data for the central 82% of patients gave excellent correspondence between predicted and actual survival probabilities. For high-risk patients, the model tended to overestimate survival, while for low-risk patients the model consistently underestimated survival.

## Management

In almost all cases, the events leading to death were associated with deteriorating respiratory function, which caused increased susceptibility to infection. Difficulty in swallowing can also lead to aspiration and can impair respiration. Early gastrostomy might avoid many of the complications of swallowing. Among the many different noninvasive nasal ventilators developed, the bi-level intermittent positive air pressure (BiPAP) ventilator has proven most effective in ALS. A small prospective study of BiPAP in ALS suggested a median survival of 15 months compared to 2 months in patients not able to use BiPAP (Aboussouan et al. 1997). A more recent study (Kleopas et al. 1999) using Kaplan-Meier analysis demonstrated a greater than fivefold increase in survival rate at 12 months and ninefold increase in survival rate at 18 months in the BiPAP group compared to the control group. Thus BiPAP is emerging as an important measure that could significantly prolong survival and slow the decline of FVC in ALS.

Tracheostomy and ventilatory assistance may be important life supports, but issues of quality of life and financial means should be evaluated carefully. Decisions must be made by the patient and family, based on the unique circumstances of each situation. In the absence of ventilatory support, patients succumb to impaired breathing.

To date, only Riluzole has been approved for ALS by the U. S. Food and Drug Administration

based upon its ability to slightly prolong survival (approximately 10%). Myotrophin awaits approval based on its ability to slow progressing of ALS by 26% (Lai et al. 1998). The authors anticipate that these and other drugs will continue to alter the natural history of ALS and significantly improve the progress in this devastating disorder.

**Acknowledgment.** This study was made possible by the Muscular Dystrophy Association support of the Vicki Appel MDA ALS Clinic. We are grateful to our ALS team and to the many ALS patients and their families who gave of themselves to further our understanding of this devastating condition.

## References

Aboussouan, L. S.; Khan, S. U.; Meeker, D. P.; Stelmach, K.; Mitsumoto, H. Effect of noninvasive positive-pressure ventilation on survival in amyotrophic lateral sclerosis. Ann. Intern. Med. 127: 450–453; 1997.

Andres, P. L.; Hedlund, W.; Finison, L.; Conlon, T.; Felmus, M.; Munsat, T. L. Quantitative motor assessment in amyotrophic lateral sclerosis. Neurology 36:937–941; 1986.

Annegers, J. F.; Appel, S. H.; Lee, J. R.; Perkins, P. Incidence and prevalence of amyotrophic lateral sclerosis in Harris County, Texas, 1985–1988. Arch. Neurol. 49:589–593; 1991.

Appel, S. H.; Stockton-Appel, V.; Stewart, S. S.; Kerman, R. H. Amyotrophic lateral sclerosis-associated clinical disorders and immunological evaluations. Arch. Neurol. 43:234–238; 1986.

Appel, V.; Stewart, S. S.; Smith, G.; Appel, S. H. A rating scale for amyotrophic lateral sclerosis: description and preliminary experience. Ann. Neurol. 22: 328–333; 1987.

Bobowick, A. R.; Brody, J. A. Epidemiology of motor neuron disease. N. Engl. J. Med. 288;1047–1055; 1973.

Boman, K.; Meurman, T. Prognosis of amyotrophic lateral sclerosis. Acta. Neurol. Scand. 43:478–498; 1967.

Bonduelle, M. Amyotrophic lateral sclerosis. In: Vinken, R. J.; Bruyn, G. W., eds. Handbook of clinical neurology. Vol. 22. New York: American Elsevier Company; 1975: p. 281–338.

Caroscio, J. T.; Mulvihill, M. N.; Sterling, R.; Abrams, B. Amyotrophic lateral sclerosis—its natural history. Neurol. Clin. 5:1–8; 1987.

Daube, J. R. Electrophysiologic studies in the diagnosis and prognosis of motor neuron diseases. In: Aminoff, ed. Symposium of electrodiagnosis. Vol. 3. Philadelphia: W. B. Saunders Co.; 1985: p. 477–493.

Gubbay, S. S.; Kahana, E.; Zilber, N.; Cooper, G.; Pintov, S.; Leibowitz, Y. Amyotrophic lateral sclerosis.

A study of its presentation and prognosis. J. Neurol. 232:259–300; 1985.

Haverkamp, L. J.; Appel V.; Appel, S. H. Natural history of amyotrophic lateral sclerosis in a database population. Validation of a scoring system and a model for survival prediction. Brain 118:707–719; 1995.

Jablecki, C. K.; Berry, C.; Leach, J. Survival prediction in amyotrophic lateral sclerosis. Muscle Nerve 12: 833–841; 1989.

Jokelainen, M. The epidemiology of amyotrophic lateral sclerosis in Finland: a study based on the death certificates of 421 patients. J. Neurol. Sci. 20: 55–63; 1976.

Kahana, E.; Alter, M.; Feldman, S. Amyotrophic lateral sclerosis: a population study. Neurology 212: 205–213; 1976.

Kleopa, K. A.; Sherman, M.; Neal, B.; Romano, G. J.; Heiman-Patterson, T. BiPAP improves survival and rate of pulmonary function decline in patients with ALS. J. Neurol. Sci. 164:82–89, 1999.

Kristensen, O.; Melgaard, B. Motor neuron disease. Acta. Neurol. Scand. 56:299–308; 1977.

Lai, E. C.; Felice, K. J.; Festoff, B. W., et al. Effect of recombinant human insulin-like growth factor-I on progression of ALS. Neurology 49:1621–1630; 1997.

Mulder, D. W. Motor neuron disease. In: Dyck, P. J.; Thomas, P. K.; Lambert, S. H.; Bunge, R., eds. Peripheral neuropathy. Philadelphia: W. B. Saunders Co.; 1984: p. 1525–1536.

Munsat, T.; Andres, P. L.; Bumside, S.; et al. The natural history of amyotrophic lateral sclerosis. Ann. Neurol. 18:157; 1987.

Reed, D. M.; Brody, J. A.; Holden, E. M. Predicting the duration of Guam amyotrophic lateral sclerosis. Neurology 25:277–288; 1975.

Rosen, A. D. Amyotrophic lateral sclerosis. Arch. Neurol. 35:638–642; 1978.

PART X

# METABOLIC AND TOXIC DISORDERS

# 31

# Disorders of Consciousness

MELISSA C. PULVER AND FRED PLUM

The term *consciousness* was first defined psychologically by William James in 1890 as awareness of the self and the environment. Consciousness requires a state of both wakefulness and awareness. Coma is the opposite, an eyes-closed unarousable state accompanied by absence of mental capacities. Between the extreme states of consciousness and coma stand a variety of altered state of consciousness: lethargy, delirium, stupor, dementia and ultimately the vegetative state. Disturbances of consciousness can be transient, persistent or permanent. Predicting the chance for recovery depends on a number of variables, which include not only the degree and the duration of the neurological injury but the severity of the underlying illness and the presence or absence of medical complications. Physicians caring for patients with brain damage must know whether and when they can accurately anticipate if the patient will recover or remain permanently overwhelmingly disabled. Prediction of individual outcome is a difficult task with important medical, ethical, and socioeconomic implications. Three general disorders of consciousness are discussed in this chapter: (1) nontraumatic coma, (2) the vegetative state, and (3) transient disturbances of consciousness (syncope and transient global amnesia.)

## Nontraumatic Coma

For centuries coma has been viewed as a near-death state with a corresponding poor prognosis. Because of the perceived hopelessness of the condition, little effort was made to distinguish its causes and to differentiate patients likely to recover from those with a poor prognosis. In recent decades, however, advances in approach to treatment and recording of results have made more prognostic information available to the clinician. These studies indicate that within a few hours or days from the onset of coma many patients show neurological signs that differentiate to a high degree of probability the future extremes of little or no cognitive improvement and the capacity for good recovery. Several studies have shown that the duration and depth of coma strongly predict outcome (Levy et al. 1985; Edgren et al. 1994; Bedell et al. 1983). However, clinical signs or brain images of neurological damage can be as important in predicting outcome of coma as the duration of the state as well as the specific illness or injury that damages the brain (Plum and Posner 1982; Kampfl et al. 1998a).

Coma describes a state of deep, sustained pathological unconsciousness that results from acute dysfunction of the brain stem ascending reticular activating arousal system, its immediately rostral thalamic connections, and their ultimate targets in both cerebral hemispheres. The eyes remain closed and the patient cannot be aroused by either exogenous or endogenous stimulation. To be clearly distinguished from syncope, concussion, or other states of brief transient unconsciousness, coma has been arbitrarily described as persisting for at least 1 hour following a physical or pharmacological insult to the brain. Coma can result from acute injuries, neurodegenerative disorders, metabolic disorders, epilepsy, developmental malformations, soporifics, and a variety of anesthesias, as well as toxic agents.

As accuracy has improved in diagnostic methods, physicians have learned that excessive emphasis on single prognostic variables can be misleading. Some authorities suggest that predictions made only a few days after the brain injury can run the risk of falsely pessimistic recommendations as high as 5% to 10% (Golby et al. 1995; Shewmon and De Giorgio 1989; Bates 1991). It is important to fully consider the patient's underlying condition and any medications, sedatives, or paralytic agents that might have been prescribed prior to the initial neurological exam (Angelopoulos et al. 1995). A combination of clinical factors and electrophysiological, neuroradiological, and biochemical variables have been shown to be more reliable in predicting outcome than any one variable alone (Bassetti et al. 1996; Buunk et al. 1997; Edgren et al. 1987; Madl et al. 1996).

Once unarousability has been established and the airway and the ventilation ensured, neuroophthalmological and brain stem signs become a paramount factor in evaluating the nature of the insult and its potential severity (Fisher 1969). Absence of pupillary responses to light, oculocephalic responses to "doll's head" movements, oculovestibular responses to caloric stimulation, and corneal responses to stimulation all predict an unfavorable course in nonpharmacological coma. For example, the absence of two or more of the preceding signs at the end of the first day of spontaneous nontraumatic coma (mostly cardiac arrest or other forms of oxygen deprivation) identified patients with poor prognosis (Levy et al. 1981). But we must be cautious, as barbiturates and other depressants can reversibly halt spontaneous eye movements and caloric responses, when intentionally self-administered or when administered to the patient prior to the development of unresponsiveness. The nature of spontaneous and noxiously evoked motor response has repeatedly been reported to be an accurate and important part of the clinical exam. Abnormal flexor, abnormal extensor, and predominately flaccid responses lasting 4 days or more following injury denote a poor prognosis. However, paralytic agents are often given to intubated patients that block the ability to evaluate motor reflexes at the time of the examination, irrespective of duration.

The need for a consistent, reliable and sensitive scale led to the development of the Glasgow coma scale (GCS) in 1974 in patients with acute head injuries (Table 31-1). Mullie and associates (1988) used the GCS as a numerical indicator of clinical exam for awaking after out-of-the-hospital cardiac arrest. They reported that the persistence of a GCS score less than 5 for more than 2 to 3 days and of a GCS score less than 8 for more than 1 week all heralded a poor outcome. Sacco and colleagues (1990) reported that the use of the GCS and consideration of etiology yielded the most accurate prediction of 2-week outcome in their study of ten patients with nontraumatic coma.

Many recent efforts have been made to identify electrophysiological tests that would identify brain functional capacity and increase reliability in predicting outcomes (Bassetti et al. 1996; Berek et al.

**Table 31-1.** Glasgow Coma Scale

| Motor Response | | Verbal Response | | Eye Opening Response | |
|---|---|---|---|---|---|
| Obeys commands | 6 | Oriented | 5 | Spontaneous | 4 |
| Localizes | 5 | Disoriented | 4 | To speech | 3 |
| Withdraws | 4 | Inappropriate | 3 | To pain | 2 |
| Flexion | 3 | Incomprehensible | 2 | None | 1 |
| Extension | 2 | None | 1 | | |
| None | 1 | | | | |

Adapted from Jennett; et al. (1979).

1995; Ganes and Lundar 1998; Synek 1990; Rothstein et al. 1991). These methods potentially could overcome the diagnostic limitations in intubated patients and those receiving sedative or paralytic medications. Scolio-Laviazzari and Bassetti (1987) reported that the electroencephalogram (EEG) has a reasonable predictive value in comatose patients, but was not sufficiently reliable to be used alone. Nondrugged patients with the worst prognosis have EEGs that express low-voltage delta, nonreactive alpha, periodic phenomena, or isoelectricity. EEGs suggesting an intermediate prognosis tend to record theta-delta activity without detectable alpha; by contrast, those with theta-delta and reactive alpha have a better prognosis for recovery. Bassetti and Karbowski refined a grading system for EEG and evoked potentials in comatose patients (Table 31-2).

Evoked potentials have been useful as an electrophysiological aid predicting coma outcome especially when used in combination with clinical assessment and etiology, (Kane et al. 1946). Bassetti and colleagues (1996) reported the use of median nerve somatosensory evoked potentials (SEPs) in 56 comatose patients following cardiac arrest. Normal SEPs were recorded in 20 patients, ten of whom had a good recovery. Delayed or low-amplitude SEPs were found in 12 patients, only one of which had a favorable outcome. Cortical SEPs were absent in 23 patients, all of whom had poor outcome. This study reported that the combination of SEP with the GCS was able to predict the risk for bad outcome after cardiopulmonary arrest to 97% at 48 hours (95% confidence level).

Considerable interest has evaluated the effect of clinical and/or electrographic seizure activity as a predictor of outcome from coma. Krumholz and coworkers (1988) reported that only status epilepticus or status myoclonus was associated with a poor outcome in patients with coma from cardiopulmonary arrest. Seizures or myoclonus alone did not predict a worse outcome in comatose patients (Levy et al. 1981). Nevertheless, Wijdicks and associates (1994) reported that generalized myoclonus status in postanoxic coma patients, while suggestive of pronounced neuronal necrosis, generally predicts poor outcome but should not be the sole predictor. They found that patients with myoclonus status were more likely to have burst suppression on EEG, cerebral edema and/or infarcts on neuroimaging, and acute ischemic neuronal changes in all cortical laminae, which all predict uniformly poor outcome.

Multiple attempts have been made to identify biochemical tests that would accurately predict outcome in comatose patients, but none has proved individually accurate. Bassetti et al. (1996) confirmed reports that over 80% of patients with raised serum neuron-specific enolase and decreased ionized calcium have a bad outcome. Longstreth and colleagues (1983) found that comatose patients who had increased serum glucose levels after cardiac arrest did worse than those with lower values. Creatinine kinase and CSF lactate in cerebrospinal fluid (CSF) have been investigated by Longstreth and Edgren, respectively. The prognostic accuracy of these potential markers remains to be confirmed, but presently appears too loose in exactitude.

Several studies report patient age as a predictive variable of outcome. Recorded evidence indicates that the influence is greatest in traumatic coma, in which a young age associates with improved

**Table 31-2.** Grading of EEG and Median Somatosensory Evoked Potentials (SEPs)

| | |
|---|---|
| EEG | |
| Grade I | Dominant normally distributed alpha activity, reactive |
| Grade II | Dominant theta–delta activity, reactive |
| Grade III | Delta–theta activity without alpha activity, reactive or nonreactive |
| Grade IV* | "Alpha–theta coma", nonreactive |
| Grade IV | Burst suppression activity; low-voltage delta activity, nonreactive; periodic general phenomena with isoelectric intervals |
| Grade V | Very-low-voltage EEG; isoelectric EEG |
| SEP | |
| Grade I | Normal N20/P25 response bilaterally |
| Grade II | Abnormal N20/P25 response unilaterally or bilaterally |
| Grade III | Absent N20/P25 bilaterally |

Adapted from Bassetti et al. (1996).

chances of recovery. Jennett and coworkers (1979) found that 78% of patients older than 60 years in traumatic coma either died or became vegetative, as opposed to only 29% of those younger than 20 years. For patients with nontraumatic coma, older age often means less recovery, but in many, this reflects the presence of previous underlying systemic conditions (Levy et al. 1981; Rothweiler et al. 1998).

In 1995, the Study to Understand Prognoses and Preferences for Outcomes and Risks of Treatments (SUPPORT) attempted to develop and validate a simple prognostic scoring system to identify patients in nontraumatic coma at high risk for poor outcomes using data available early in the hospital course: 596 patients were studied at five medical centers. The primary cause of coma was cardiac arrest in 31% and cerebral infarction or intracerebral hemorrhage in 36%. The main outcome measures were death and severe disability at 2 months. Hamel and SUPPORT investigators identified five clinical variables available 3 days after disease onset that associated independently with 2-month mortality. These included abnormal brain stem response, absent verbal response, absent withdrawal response to pain, creatinine level in serum greater than or equal to 132.6 μM/L and age of 70 or greater (Table 31-3).

Patients suffering traumatic coma do much better than those with anoxic unconsciousness: 39% of 1000 patients in traumatic coma for at least 6 hours recovered independent function at 6 months (Jennett et al. 1979), whereas 16% of 500 patients with nontraumatic coma had comparable results at 1 year (Levy et al. 1981). The most common nontraumatic injuries to the central nervous system (CNS) result from drug overdose, cerebrovascular disease, cardiopulmonary arrest, and endogenous metabolic disturbances. Nearly all patients with coma from exogenous poisoning recover fully if treated with prompt supportive care. Levy and colleagues (1981) reported outcomes at 1 year in patients with nontraumatic coma not caused by medically administered pharmacological agents. Coma-inducing cerebrovascular disease (cerebral infarction, parenchymal hemorrhage, or subarachnoid hemorrhage) carried the bleakest prognosis, with only 9% reaching independent function. Twelve percent of cardiac arrest patients regained independent function, as did 33% of patients with nonfulminating hepatic coma (Table 31-4). However, overall outcomes were not favorable; of the 500 patients in the study, 379 (76%) died within the first month and 88% died by the end of the year. In 1990, Sacco evaluated the 2-week outcomes in nontraumatic coma. Seventy-nine percent of those with hypoxic or ischemic coma were dead/comatose, 68% with metabolic or septic coma were dead/comatose, and 66% of those with focal cerebral lesions causing coma were dead/comatose. Patients with general cerebral lesions had a 55% dead/comatose outcome, whereas 27% of drug-induced coma were dead/comatose (Table 31-5). The comparison of these two studies shows that the time of evaluation of outcome is important in considering etiology and prognosis.

Most fatal suicide attempts occur outside the hospital. If pharmacologically overdosed patients reach treatment alive, the overall mortality is reported at no more than 1%. The death rate increases to 5% with increasing depth and severity of coma. Adverse prognostic factors in depressant drug coma include an advanced age of the patient, the presence of complicating medical illnesses, and a long period of coma suffering minimal residual brain damage. Rare exceptions to this rule occur in overdose patients who suffer cardiac arrest.

**Table 31-3.** SUPPORT Variables Correlated with 2-Month Mortality

| Risk Factor Present on Day 3 | 2-Month Mortality, No.(%) | |
|---|---|---|
| | If Factor Present | If Factor Absent |
| Abnormal brain stem response | 88/99 (89) | 83/136 (61) |
| Absent verbal response | 151/175 (86) | 23/57 (40) |
| Absent withdrawal to pain | 122/136 (90) | 52/96 (54) |
| Creatinine ≥ 132.6 μmol/L (1.5 mg/dl) | 82/94 (87) | 99/153 (65) |
| Age ≥70 years | 93/111 (84) | 88/136 (65) |

Adapted from Hamel et al. (1995).

**Table 31-4.** Best Functional State Related to Cause of Coma

| Cause of Coma | Best 1-Year Recovery, % | | | | |
| --- | --- | --- | --- | --- | --- |
| | No Recovery | Vegetative State | Severe Disability | Moderate Disability | Good Recovery |
| All patients ($n = 500$) | 61 | 12 | 11 | 4 | 12 |
| Subarachnoid hemorrhage ($n = 38$) | 74 | 5 | 8 | 10 | 3 |
| Other cerebrovascular disease ($n = 141$) | 74 | 5 | 13 | 3 | 5 |
| Hypoxia-ischemia ($n = 210$) | 58 | 20 | 10 | 2 | 10 |
| Hepatic encephalopathy ($n = 51$) | 49 | 2 | 14 | 8 | 27 |
| Miscellaneous ($n = 58$) | 45 | 9 | 12 | 3 | 31 |

Adapted from Levy et al. (1981).

Bedell and associates (1983) reported that up to 44% of patients who suffer cardiac arrest in the hospital can be successfully resuscitated. Most remained comatose initially and only 10% to 20% made a good recovery. Physicians have correlated outcome following cardiac arrest with the following indicators: duration of anoxia, duration of postanoxic coma, changes in the EEG pattern, and the pattern of motor responses to stimulation, as well as the presence or absence of brain stem reflexes (Hung and Chens 1995). Measurements of cerebral blood flow and oxygenation, cerebral spinal fluid tests, and blood electrolyte changes have not contributed reliable predictions of outcome (Longstreth et al. 1981; Roine et al. 1989; Urban et al. 1988).

Hepatic coma patients studied in the medical coma study had the best chance for recovery of about 33%. The best explanation for the difference in outcome between the cerebrovascular patients, the cardiac arrest patients, and those with hepatic coma is that although hemorrhage or ischemia directly damages brain structures, biochemical mechanisms producing coma in patients with chronic liver disease often fail to injure brain structures. Hepatic coma develops in two forms, either as an inexorable stage in progressive hepatic failure or as a reversible process in patients with portal systemic shunts in whom increased loads of nitrogenous substances suddenly become dumped into the circulation. Prognosis in hepatic coma depends on the etiology of the insult, the acuteness and the severity of the liver failure, and the presence of dysfunction of other organs. In patients with chronic hepatocellular disease, episodes of hepatic encephalopathy usually resolve if the hepatocellular function is well maintained and the precipitating factors can be identified and corrected. However, if no precipitating factor is identified, the mortality rises. About 50% of patients with cirrhosis die within the first year after an incidence of hepatic encephalopathy and 80% die within 5 years as a consequence of their liver disease, not of neurological causes. Bluml et al. (1998) used MR (magnetic resonance) spectroscopy on patients with liver disease, and their results revealed disturbances of cerebral osmoregulation and energy metabolism in the patients with chronic hepatic encephalopathy. In patients with acute fulminant liver failure due to severe hepatitis or

**Table 31-5.** Two-Week Outcome of Nontraumatic Coma and Coma Etiology

| Coma Etiology | 2-Week Outcome, % | | | |
| --- | --- | --- | --- | --- |
| | No. (%) | Awake | Dead | Coma |
| Hypoxic or ischemic | 61 (36.1) | 21.3 | 54.1 | 24.6 |
| Metabolic or septic | 37 (21.8) | 32.4 | 48.7 | 18.9 |
| Focal cerebral | 38 (22.5) | 34.2 | 47.4 | 18.4 |
| General cerebral | 22 (13.0) | 45.4 | 36.4 | 18.2 |
| Drug induced | 11 (6.5) | 72.7 | 0 | 27.3 |
| All | 169 (100) | 33.1 | 44.4 | 21.5 |

Adapted from Sacco et al. (1990).

toxic drugs the mortality is high, especially when coma ensues (Jones and Weissenborn 1997). An acute or chronic increase in intracranial pressure (ICP) in fulminant hepatic failure may augment brain ischemia due to compression of the cerebral vasculature (Cordoba and Blei 1996; Wendon et al. 1994) and/or brain stem herniation (Gazzard et al. 1975; Hanid et al. 1978). Supportive care remains the mainstay of treatment, with liver transplant reserved for select patients (Bernstein and Tripodi 1998).

## Chronic Vegetative State

In 1972, Plum and Jennett described the condition of severe brain damage in patients with coma who had progressed to a state of wakefulness but remained without detectable awareness for at least 4 weeks. They called the condition a persistent vegetative state. Twenty years later the Multi-Society Task Force on Persistent Vegetative State (PVS) was established to review and summarize the outcomes to the condition. The final report in 1994 (Multi-Society Taskforce on PVS 1994a, 1994b) defined the vegetative state as a clinical condition of complete unawareness of the self and the environment, accompanied by sleep-wake cycles with either partial or complete preservation of hypothalamic and brain stem functions. The condition can be transient and evolve during the recovery from coma to consciousness, but its chronic state describes a failure to recover from severe brain damage. In addition to following severe anoxia-asphyxia or traumatic injury, the vegetative state may also emerge as a late progression of neurodegenerative diseases. Infants born with developmental malformations such as anencephaly can also be considered to remain permanently in a vegetative state.

Prognosis for recovery from a persistent vegetative state seldom justifies optimism. Most patients who regain consciousness remain at least somewhat disabled and cannot participate fully in the normal activities of daily living. Age and mechanisms of trauma have predictive value in vegetative patients similar to comatose patients. Those who eventually progress from a trauma-induced injury to a persistent vegetative state may have a chance for nearly complete recovery if they are under 40 years of age (Braakman et al. 1988) and if the cause of the brain injury was trau-

matic versus nontraumatic. Kampfl et al. (1998b) suggest that a cerebral MRI at 6 to 8 weeks after a traumatic brain injury resulting in a vegetative state may help predict poor outcome. They found that corpus callosum lesions and dorsolateral brain stem lesions are highly significant in predicting nonrecovery. However, recovery of consciousness in patients after 12 months from a traumatic injury is unlikely and good recovery from a nontraumatic injury in patients after 3 months is uncommon. Early complicating features of a patient's vegetative course that predict a poorer outcome include: ventilatory dysfunction, lack of early motor reactivity, late-onset epilepsy, or the development of epilepsy (Sazbon et al. 1993).

The most complete review of patient data comes from the Multi-Society Task Force on PVS. Data were reviewed on 434 patients who were in PVS 1 month after traumatic head injury and 169 patients in PVS 1 month after nontraumatic injury (Table 31-6). In the traumatic injury group after 3 months, 33% had recovered consciousness and 67% had died or remained vegetative. The outcome from the patents with nontraumatic injury was much worse at 3 months, with only 11% having recovered consciousness and 89% having died or remaining vegetative. At 12 months, 52% of the 434 traumatic group had regained consciousness, 15% were persistently vegetative, and 33% had died. Conversely, only 15% of the 169 nontraumatic patients had recovered consciousness after 1 year, 32% were still in a persistent vegetative state, and 53% had died. Children's outcomes from PVS are also included in Table 31-6. As can be seen, fewer children die within 12 months, but the percentage of PVS at that time is much higher than in the adult population.

Recovery of consciousness after persistent vegetative states does not correlate automatically with good functional recovery. The Glasgow Outcome Scale was developed to measure recovery. It classifies outcome into five categories: good recovery (ability to resume normal work and social activities with only minor cognitive or physical limitations), moderate disability (can resume most all activities of daily living with some independence), severe disability (unable to participate in social work or activities of daily living and require comprehensive care), persistent vegetative state, and death (Jennett and Bond 1975). Among the 52% of the 434 patients suffering PVS

**Table 31-6.** Incidence of Recovery of Consciousness and Function in Adults in Persistent Vegetative State (PVS) after Traumatic or Nontraumatic Brain Injury

| Outcome and Functional Recovery | 3 Months, % | 6 Months, % | 12 Months, % |
|---|---|---|---|
| **Adults** | | | |
| Traumatic injury ($n = 434$) | | | |
|   Death | 15 | 24 | 33 |
|   PVS | 52 | 30 | 15 |
|   Recovery of consciousness | 33 | 46 | 52 |
|     Severe disability | | | 28 |
|     Moderate disability | | | 17 |
|     Good recovery | | | 7 |
| Nontraumatic injury ($n = 169$) | | | |
|   Death | 24 | 40 | 53 |
|   PVS | 65 | 45 | 32 |
|   Recovery of consciousness | 11 | 15 | 15 |
|     Severe disability | | | 11 |
|     Moderate disability | | | 3 |
|     Good recovery | | | 1 |
| **Children** | | | |
| Traumatic injury ($n = 106$) | | | |
|   Death | 4 | 9 | 9 |
|   PVS | 72 | 40 | 29 |
|   Recovery of consciousness | 24 | 51 | 62 |
|     Severe disability | | | 35 |
|     Moderate disability | | | 16 |
|     Good recovery | | | 11 |
| Nontraumatic injury ($n = 45$) | | | |
|   Death | 20 | 22 | 22 |
|   PVS | 69 | 67 | 65 |
|   Recovery of consciousness | 11 | 11 | 13 |
|     Severe disability | | | 7 |
|     Moderate disability | | | 0 |
|     Good recovery | | | 6 |

Adapted from The Multi-Society Task Force on PVS (1994).

after traumatic brain injury, the outcomes on the Glasgow Outcome Scale for adults after 1 year amounted to 7% with good recovery, 17% with moderate disability, and 28% with severe disability. The 7% with good outcome all showed recovery of consciousness within the first 6 months after injury and most within the first 3 months. In fact, only one patient in the nontraumatic group had a Glasgow Outcome rating of good recovery, two had moderate disability, and three were severely disabled. No patients in the traumatic group showed any recovery after 12 months and no patients in the nontraumatic group developed a good recovery after 3 months. The Multi-Society Task Force on PVS stated that the vegetative state would be considered permanent after 12 months from traumatic injury and after 3 months from nontraumatic injury.

Kampfl et al. (1998) recently have reported the relationship of certain magnetic resonance imaging (MRI) 1.5T findings on patients still vegetative 6 to 8 weeks following head trauma. All patients were followed to either 12 full months following their injuries or died before that time. The mean age of the patients was $25.8 \pm 7.3$ years. At year's end, 42 remained in a PVS and 38 had become conscious, 24 at 3 months, 12 more at 6 months, and two between 6 and 12 months. Six recoverers were described as good outcomes. The number of MRI-detected lesions at 8 weeks were equal between patients with PVS versus non-PVS outcomes. Three factors, however, linked to poor outcome. In the 42 persons still vegetative at 12 months, 41 had damage to the corpus callosum (usually posterior), 31 had damage to the mesencephalic tegmentum, and 24 had prominent damage to the corona radiata. Among awakeners, only nine had callosal damage, ten had injury to the mesencephalic tegmentum, and ten had lesions detected in the corona radiata.

Several anecdotal reports of isolated cases of late recovery from a persistent vegetative state have been reported in the medical literature and in the press. One report described the return of consciousness in a patient who had been persistently vegetative for 30 months. She remained severely disabled, however, (Arts et al. 1985). Six of 93 patients registered in the Traumatic Coma Data Bank recovered consciousness from a vegetative state 1 to 3 years following their trauma. None of the six had full recovery and further follow-up material appears to have been lost (Levin et al. 1991). The total number of patients with late recovery is very small and the functional status of those patients with late recovery has been poor. Therefore, while not out of the realm of possibility, the recovery after 1 year in the persistent vegetative state is highly unlikely. Andrews (1996) reported rehabilitative rescue of seven patients vegetative for longer than 1 year, but no details of the patients' functions or appropriate tests are provided.

Patients who lapse into a vegetative state from neurodegenerative disorders usually are permanently vegetative. Occasionally, underlying infections or medical problems that temporarily worsen neurological function can create temporary vegetative states in patients severely neurologically impaired by degenerative disorders. Children born with anencephaly never attain consciousness because they lack a developed cerebrum. Other severe developmental malformations at birth may yield a vegetative infant. If there is no sign of recovery at 3 months of age, the prognosis for any attainment of consciousness is very poor (Ashwal et al. 1992).

Early estimates categorized the average life expectancy of patients who are in a permanent vegetative state at approximately 2 to 5 years. Overall, the data available from the information reviewed by the task force indicate that the mortality rate for adults in persistent vegetative state after acute brain injury is 82% at 3 years and 95% at 5 years. The data are based on 251 patients in four large series (Minderhoud et al. 1985; Higashi et al. 1981; Sazbon et al. 1993, 1991). In a study of 110 patients the mortality rate increased from 65% to 73% between 3 and 5 years, and 90% of the patients had died within 10 years. The average life expectancy of the 71 patents who died was 38.4 months (Higashi et al. 1981). Among patients with degenerative diseases who enter the vegetative state, survival ranges from 3.5 to 7 years (Walshe and Leonard 1985).

## Syncope

The term *syncope* describes a sudden and temporary loss of consciousness not caused by trauma or seizures. Recovery from syncopal episodes generally occurs swiftly without further cognitive complication. Rather, the problem is gauging the likelihood of subsequent serious medical problems that may increase the patient's risk for sudden death. Important prognostic factors are the etiology of the syncopal attack in combination with the patient's age, family history, and sex.

Syncope results when cerebral arterial perfusion falls below the level required to supply sufficient oxygen to the brain. (The critical blood flow required to maintain effective cerebral activity in humans is about 20 ml/100 gm/min.) Kapoor et al. (1996) evaluated the etiologies of 470 patients with syncope and identified 14.7% with cardiac disease, 49.8% with noncardiac causes, and 35.5% with an unknown etiology. Cardiovascular causes generally consist of electrical arrhythmias endogenously interrupting the heart's endogenous pacemaker or mechanical obstruction of circulation at a cardiac valve or of major vascular structure. Noncardiovascular causes include or are associated with orthostatic hypotension, vasovagal reaction, micturition syncope, carotid sinus hypersensitivity, migraines, psychiatric crises, drugs, cerebral hemorrhages, subarachnoid hemorrhages, and increased intracranial pressure (Farrehi et al. 1995; Kapoor and Hanusa 1996).

Martin and colleagues (1997) identified historical, physical exam, and ECG factors at the initial presentation to the emergency room for a syncopal episode as most helpful in risk assessment for arrhythmias or mortality within 1 year of the attack. If warranted, more thorough workup includes biochemical tests, Holter monitoring, continuous blood pressure monitoring, electrophysiology studies, and head-up tilt-table testing. Sheldon et al. (1997) reported that patients with syncope and either positive or negative tilt-table tests share many pretest and post-test clinical characteristics: number of syncopal spells, durations of symptoms, frequency of spells, age at onset, and peak heart rate during tilt-test. These risk factors better predict outcome than the tilt-table test alone.

Syncope itself is not a risk factor for increased overall and cardiac mortality or cardiovascular events. Kapoor and Hanusa (1996), discovered that the 1-year mortality of patients presenting with syncope is similar to patients without syncope. However, the 1 year follow-up found that patients with previous syncope had a tenfold increased risk of further syncope. No significant differences in cardiovascular outcomes such as myocardial infarction, cerebrovascular events, or cardiac arrest were reported comparing patients with and without syncope. Independent factors that best predict risk for mortality, regardless of a patients' history of syncope, include congestive heart failure and the numerical class of heart disease.

Age, familial tendency, and gender aid in prediction of outcome and recurrence in patients with syncope. In one study (Houdent et al. 1988), the 1 year mortality of patients older than 65 with syncope was nearly 20%. It is generally accepted that new syncope starting after age 55 should be fully evaluated to identify etiology. Mathias et al. (1998) reported a familial tendency in confirmed vasovagal syncope (by tilt-table test), especially when the onset is below the age of 20. Camfield and Camfield (1990) reported a family history of fainting in 27 (90%) of 30 children. Freed and associates (1997) identified gender-based differences in the clinical presentation of syncope for hospital admission in 109 consecutive patients admitted to the Massachusetts General Hospital for syncope. They found that men are more likely to have cardiac syncope and worse cardiac event-free survival when compared with women.

## Transient Global Amnesia

Transient global amnesia (TGA) causes loss of memory but not a loss of consciousness. Patients experience an abrupt, acute onset of anterograde amnesia, usually with repetitive questioning of those around them. During the attack the patient is alert and communicative, with no other apparent cognitive impairment besides the amnesia. Attacks generally resolve within 12 to 24 hours. The patient is usually middle aged with no other risk factors for epilepsy or cerebrovascular or cardiovascular disease. The prognosis of recovery is assured and the chance of recurrence is small. Hodges and Warlow (1990) reported a yearly recurrence of TGA in 3% of patients. The only lasting impairment was a permanent memory gap of the event and several hours preceding it. The interesting aspect about TGA is that until recently the etiology of the disorder has been an enigma.

In the past, the etiology of TGA was attributed to one of the three following categories: thromboembolism, epilepsy, or migraine. The worry of TGA as a precursor to stroke has been cleared by a significantly large group of case controlled studies which proved that TGA has no immediate association with stroke, nor does it carry the same risk of having a transient ischemic attack (Hodges 1991; Melo et al. 1992). No evidence exists to prove that the etiology is thromboembolic. A study of 114 patients detected a small subgroup of patients (ten) who experienced attacks similar to TGA but were clearly epileptiform (Hodges and Warlow 1990). These patients' attacks began upon waking and produced both anterograde and retrograde amnesia, accompanied by repetitive questioning. However, the attacks lasted less than 1 hour and occurred repeatedly. While such patients were awake their EEGs were normal. However, their sleep EEGs all revealed temporal lobe epileptiform activity. These patients also frequently had impairment of retrograde memory.

The studies by Hodges et al. report a higher incidence of migraine headaches in patients who have suffered from transient global amnesia. In the same series of 114 patients, 25% reported classic or common migraine (Hodges and Warlow 1990), a number significantly larger than in matched controls. In the Oxford series, one-third of patients with TGA gave a history suggestive of common or classic migraine (Hodges 1991). In 1997, Inzitari and colleagues reported a systematic evaluation of precipitants and life events in 51 prospectively studied TGA patients: almost 50% were triggered by a precipitant. The link between migraine and TGA, and the relationship to such life stresses, strengthen the "unifying spreading depression hypothesis" for the pathophysiology of TGA, proposed by Oleson and Jorgenson (1986). Several studies suggest that TGA is caused by a disturbance of the function of the limbic structures in the temporal lobe and thalamus but do not resolve the issue of whether the hypoperfusion detected in these areas is primary or secondary to diminished metabolism (Strupp et al. 1998; Kazui et al. 1995; Evans et al. 1993).

## References

Andrews, K.; Murphy, L; Mundag, R; Littlewood, C. Misdiagnosis of the vegetative state: retrospective study in a rehabilitation unit. BMJ 313:13–19; 1996.

Angelopoulos, M.; Gupta, S. R.; Azat Kia, B. Primary intraventricular hemmorhage in adults: clinical features, risk factors, and outcome. Surg. Neurol. 44: 433–436; 1995.

Arts, W. F. M.; Van Dongen, H. R.; Van Hofvanduin, J.; Lammens, E. Unexpected improvement after prolonged posttraumatic vegetative state. J. Neurol. Neurosurg. Psychiatry 48:1300–1303; 1985.

Ashwal, S.; Bale, J. F., Jr.; Coulter, D. L. The persistent vegetative state in children: report of a childhood neurology society ethics commitee. Ann. Neurol 32:570–576; 1992.

Bassetti, C.; Bomio, F.; Mathis, J.; Hess, C. W. Early prognosis in coma after cardiac arrest: a prospective clinical, electrophysiological, and biochemical study of sixty patients. J. Neurol. Neurosurg. Psychiatry 61:610–615; 1996.

Bates, D. Defining prognosis in medical coma. J. Neurol. Neurosurg. Psychiatry 54:569–571; 1991.

Bedell, S. E.; Delbanco, T. L.; Cook, E. F.; Epstein, F. E. Survival after cardiopulmonary resuscitation in the hospital. N. Engl. J. Med. 309:569–576; 1983.

Berek, K.; Lechleitner, P.; Luef, G.; Felber, S.; Salturari, L.; Schinnerl, A.; Traweger, C.; Dienstl, F.; Aichner, F. Early determination of neurologic outcome after prehospital cardiopulmonary resuscitation. Stroke 26:543–549; 1995.

Bernstein, D.; Tripodi, J. Fulminant hepatic failure. Crit. Care Clin. 14:181; 1998.

Bluml, S.; Zuckerman, E.; Tan, J.; Ross, B. D. Proton-decoupled 31-P magnetic resonance spectroscopy reveals osmotic and metabolic disturbances in human hepatic encephalopathy. J. Neurochem. 71: 1564; 1998.

Braakman, R.; Jennett, W. B.; Minderhoud, J. M. Prognosis of the posttraumatic vegetative state. Acta Neurochir. (Wein) 95:49–52; 1988.

Buunk, G.; Van Der Hoveen, J. G.; Meinders, A. E. Cerebrovascular reactivity in comatose patients resuscitated from a cardiac arrest. Stroke 28: 1569– 1573; 1997.

Camfield, P. R.; Camfield, C. S. Syncope in childhood: a case control study of the familial tendency to faint. Can. J. Neurol. Sci. 17:306; 1990.

Cordoba, J.; Blei, E. T. Brain edema and hepatic encephalopathy. Semin. Liver Dis. 16:271–280; 1996.

Edgren, E.; Hedstrand, U.; Kelsey, S.; Sutton-Tyrelle, K.; Safar, P.; and BRCT1 Study Group. Assessment of neurologic prognosis in comatose survivors of cardiac arrest. Lancet 343:1055–1059; 1994.

Edgren, E.; Hedstrand, U.; Nordin, N. Prediction of outcome after cardiac arrest. Crit. Care Med. 15: 820–825; 1987.

Evans, J.; Wilson, B.; Wraight, E. P.; Hodges, J. R. Neuropsychological and SPECT scan findings during and after transient global amnesia: evidence for the differential impairment of remote episodic memory. J. Neurol. Neurosurg. Psychiatry 56:1227–1230; 1993.

Farrehi, P. M.; Santinga, J. T.; Eagle, K. A. Syncope: diagnosis of cardiac and non-cardiac causes. Geriatrics 50:24; 1995.

Fisher, C. M. The neurological examination of the comatose patient. Acta Neurol. Scand. 45:4–56; 1969.

Freed, L. A.; Eagle, K. A.; Mahjoub, Z. A.; Gold, M. R.; Smith, H. A.; Terrell, L. B.; O'Gara, P. T.; Paul, S. D. Gender differences in presentation, management, and cardiac event free survival in patients with syncope. Am. J. Cardiol. 80:1183–1187; 1997.

Ganes, T.; Lundar, T. EEG and evoked potentials in comatose patients with severe brain damage. Electroencephalogr. Clin. Neurophysiol. 69:6–13; 1988.

Gazzard, B. G.; Portman, B.; Murray-Lyon, I. M.; Williams, R. Causes of death in fulminant hepatic failure and relationship to histological assessment of parenchymal damage. Q. J. Med. 44:615–626; 1975.

Golby, A.; McGuire, D.; Bayne, L. Unexpected recovery from anoxic-ischemic coma. Neurology 45:1629; 1995.

Hamel, M. B.; Goldman, L.; Teno, J.; Lynn, J.; Davis, R. B.; Harrell, F. E.; Conners, A. F., Jr.; Califf, R.; Kussin, P.; Bellammy, P.; et al. Identification of comatose patients at high risk for death or severe disability: SUPPORT Investigators. JAMA 273: 1842–1848; 1995.

Hanid, M. A.; Silk, D. B. A.; Williams, R. Prognostic value of the oculovestibular reflex in fulminant hepatic failure. Br. Med. J. I:1029; 1978.

Higashi, K.; Hantanto, M.; Abaiko, S.; Ihara, K.; Katayama, S.; Wakuta, Y.; Okamura, T.; Yamashita, T. Five year follow-up study of patients with persistent vegetative state. J. Neurol. Neurosurg. Psychiatry 44: 552–554; 1981.

Hodges, J. R. Transient global amnesia. London: W. B. Saunders Co., 1991.

Hodges, J. R.; Warlow, C. P. The etiology of transient global amnesia: a case control study of 114 cases with prospective follow-up. Brain 113:639–637; 1990.

Houdent, C.; Morcamp, D.; Sereni, D.; Conroi, C.; Colvez, A.; Delegove, H.; Vincheneux, P.; Pibarot, M. L. One year prognosis of syncope and brief loss of consciousness in patients over sixty-five: a multicenter study of 188 cases. Presse Med. 17:626–629; 1988.

Hung, T. P.; Chen, S. T. Prognosis of deeply comatose patients on ventilators. J. Neurol. Neurosurg. Psychiatry 58:75–80; 1995.

Jennett, B.; Bond, M. Assessment of outcome after severe brain damage. Lancet 1: 480; 1975.

Jennett, B.; Teasdale, G.; Braakman, R.; Minderhound, J.; Heiden, J.; Kurze, T. Prognosis of patients with severe head injury. Neurosurgery 4:283–289; 1979.

Jones, E. A.; Weissenborn, K. Neurology and the liver. J. Neurol. Neurosurg. Psychiatry 63:279–293; 1997.

Kampfl, A.; Franz, G.; Aichner, F.; Pfausler, B.; Haring, H.; Felber, S.; Luz, G.; Schocke, M.; Schmutzard, E. The persistent vegetative state after closed head injury: clinical and magnetic resonance imaging findings in 42 patients. J. Neurosurg. 88:809–816; 1998.

Kampfl, A.; Schutzhard, E.; Franz, G.; Pfaubler, B.; Haring, H. P.; Ulmer, H.; Felber, S.; Golaszewski, S.; Aichner, F. Prediction of recovery from post-traumatic vegetative state with cerebral magnetic-resonance imaging. Lancet 35:1763; 1998b.

Kane, N. M.; Curry, S. H.: Rolands, C. A.; Manara, A. R.; Lewis, T.; Moss, T.; Cummins, B. H.; Butler, S. R. Event related potentials-neurophysiological tools for predicting emergence and early outcome from traumatic coma. Intensive Care Med. 22: 39–46; 1946.

Kapoor, W. N.; Hánusa, B. H. Is syncope a risk factor for poor outcomes? comparison of patients with and without syncope. Am. J. Med. 100:646–655; 1996.

Kazui, H.; Tanabe, H.; Ikeda, M. Memory and cerebral flow in cases of transient global amnesia during and after the attack. Behav. Neurol. 8:93–101; 1995.

Krumolz, A.; Stern, B. J.; Weiss, H. D. Outcome from coma after cardiopulmonary resuscitation: relation to seizures and myoclonus. Neurology 38:401–405; 1988.

Levin, H. S.; Saydjari, C.; Eisenberg, H. M.; et al. Vegetative state after closed head injury: a traumatic coma data bank report. Arch. Neurol. 48:580–585: 1981.

Levy, D. E.; Bates, D.; Caronna, J. J.; Cartlidge, N. E. F.; Knill-Jones, R. P.; Lapinsky, R. H.; Singer, B. H.; Shaw, D. A.; Plum, F. Prognosis in nontraumatic coma. Ann. Intern. Med. 94:293–301; 1981.

Levy, D. E., Carronna, J. J., Singer, B. H.; Lapinski, R. H.; Frydman, H.; Plum, F. Predicting the outcome from hypoxic ischemic coma. JAMA 254:1420–1426; 1985.

Longstreth, W. T., Jr.; Diehr, P.; Inui, T. S. Prediction of awakening after out of hospital cardiac arrest. N. Engl. J. Med. 308:1378–1382; 1983.

Madl, C.; Kramer, L.; Yeganehfar, W.; Eisenhuber, E.; Kranza, A.; Ratheiser, K.; Zauner, C.; Schneider, B.; Grimm, G. Detection of nontraumatic comatose patients with no benefit of intensive care treatment by recording of sensory evoked potentials. Arch. Neurol. 53:512–516; 1996.

Martin, T. P.; Hanusa, B. H.; Kapor, W. N. Risk stratification of patients with syncope. Ann. Emerg. Med. 29:459–466; 1997.

Mathias, C.; Deguchi, K.; Bleasdale-Barr, K.; Kimber, J. Frequency of family history in vasovagal syncope. Lancet 352:33–34; 1998.

Melo, T. P.; Ferro, J. M.; Ferro, H. Transient global amnesia: a case control study. Brain 11:261–270; 1992.

Minderhoud, J. M.; Braakman, R. The vegetative existance. Ned. Tijdschr. Geneeskd. 129:2385; 1985.

Mullie, A.; Buylaert, W.; Michem, N. Predictive value of Glasgow coma scale for awakening after our of hospital cardiac arrest. Lancet 1:137–140; 1988.

Multi-Society Taskforce on PVS. Medical aspects of the persistive vegetative state: part 1. N. Engl. J. Med. 330:1499–1508; 1994a.

Multi-Society Taskforce on PVS. Medical aspects of the persistive vegetative state: part 2. N. Engl. J. Med. 330:1572–1579; 1994b.

Olesen, J.; Jorgensen, M. B. Leao's spreading depression in the hippocampus explains transient global amnesia. Acta Neurol. Scand. 73:219–220; 1986.

Plum, F.; Posner, J. B. Diagnosis of stupor and coma. Philadelphia: F. A. Davis; 1982.

Roine, R. O.; Somer, H.; Kaste, N.; Viinikka, L.; Karonen, S. Neurological outcome after out of hospital cardiac arrest: prediction by cerebrospinal fluid enzyme analysis. Arch. Neurol. 46:753–756;1989.

Rothweiler, B.; Temkin, N. R.; Dikmen, S. S. Aging effect on psychosocial outcome in traumatic brain injury. Arch. Phys. Med. Rehabil. 79:881; 1998.

Rothstein, T. L.; Thomas, E. M.; Sumi, S. M. Predicting outcome in the hypoxic-ischemic coma: a prospective clinical and electrophysiological study. Electroencephalogr. Clin. Neurophysiol. 79:101–107; 1991.

Sacco, R. L.; Vangool, R.; Mohr, J. P.; Hauser, W. A. Nontraumatic coma: Glasgow coma scale and coma etiology as predictors of two week outcome. Arch. Neurol. 47:1181–1184; 1990.

Sazbon, L.; Fuchs, C.; Costeff, H. Pronosis for recovery from prolonged posttraumatic unawareness: logistic analysis. J. Neurol. Neurosurg. Psychiatry 52:149; 1991.

Sazbon, L.; Zagreba, F.; Ronen, J.; Solzi, P.; Costeff, H. Course and outcome of patients in vegetative state of nontraumatic etiology. J. Neurol. Neurosurg. Psychiatry 56: 407–409;1993.

Scolio-Lavizzari, G.; Basetti, C. Prognostic value of EEG in post-anoxic coma after cardiac arrest. Eur. Neurol. 26:161–170; 1987.

Sheldon, R.; Rose, S.; Koshman, M. L. Comparison of patients with syncope of unknown cause having negative or positive tilt-table tests. Am. J. Cardiol. 80: 581–585; 1997.

Shewmon, D. A.; DeGiorgio, C. M. Early prognosis in anoxic coma. Neurol. Clin. 7:823; 1989.

Strupp, M.; Bruning, R.; Wu, R. H.; Deinmling, M.; Reiser, M.; Brandt, T. Diffusion weighted MRI in transient global amnesia colon: elevated signal intensity in the left mesial temporal lobe in seven of ten patients. Ann. Neurol. 43:164–170; 1998.

Synek, V. M. Value of revised EEG coma scale for prognosis after cerebral anoxia and diffuse head injury. Clin. Electroencephalogr. 21:25–30; 1990.

Urban, P.; Scheidegger, G.; Buchman, B.; Barthe, D. Cardiac arrest and blood ionized calcium levels. Ann. Intern. Med. 109:110–113; 1988.

Walshe, T. M.; Leonard, C. Persistent vegetative state: extension of the syndrome to include chronic disorders. Arch. Neurol. 42:1045–1047; 1985.

Wendon, J. A.; Harrison, P. M.; Keayes, R.; Williams, R. Cerebral blood flow and metabolism in fulminant hepatic failure. Hepatology 19:1407–1413; 1994.

Wijdicks, E. F. M.; Parisi, J. E.; Sharbrough, F. M. Prognostic value of myoclonus status in comatose survivors of cardiac arrest. Ann. Neurol. 35:239–243; 1994.

# 32

## Exposure to Industrial Toxins

CHRISTOPHER G. GOETZ

In an industrial and predominantly urban society, the consequences of factory-produced toxins and fumes have been increasingly recognized. Whereas environmentalists must be concerned with the toxic effects on plant and ecological balance, neurologists must focus on the specific effects of industrial chemicals and gases on the human nervous system. In spite of increasing concern, however, the neurological sequelae of acute and chronic exposure to industrial products are incompletely studied. This chapter concentrates on the neurological prognosis of victims exposed to various industrial chemicals by inhalation, skin exposure, and ingestion. Most cases of toxic exposure are inadvertent, but some specific agents are prominent substances of volitional abuse. The topics cover the major organic solvents, gases, and pesticides.

### Methyl Alcohol

Methanol is used as a solvent, a combustible, a component of antifreeze, and an adulterant of alcoholic beverages. Although the compound is only mildly toxic, its oxidation products, formaldehyde and formic acid, induce a severe metabolic acidosis and account for most of the signs of methanol intoxication. To a large extent, the prognosis of the intoxicated patient depends on the degree and duration of acidosis, although both formaldehyde and formate probably have neurotoxic effects independent of acidosis (Fink 1943; Roe 1969). The amount of methanol needed to cause serious effects varies with the individual and may largely depend on concomitant ethanol ingestion. Methanol and ethanol share the same degrading enzyme, alcohol dehydrogenase, so ethanol intoxication tends to diminish the rapid production of toxic formaldehyde and formic acid from methanol.

Because the oxidation and excretion of methanol is slow, toxic signs may not develop for 12 to 48 hours, especially in a patient with cointoxication with ethanol. Acute toxicity may last for several days, and persistent neurological sequelae are well described (Kaplan and Levreault 1944). The visual apparatus, central nervous, gastrointestinal, and respiratory systems are affected by methanol (Mittal et al. 1991).

Early toxic symptoms are nausea, vomiting, generalized weakness, severe abdominal pain, vertigo, and headache. Symptoms similar to ethanol intoxication are restlessness, incoordination, delirium, and hallucinations. Visual disturbance and ocular abnormalities are frequent; visual loss may start within the first hours after ingestion or may be delayed for several days. Amblyopia, scotomas, or total blindness occur, and the pupils become dilated and fail to react to light. Ocular pain is common. Ophthalmoscopic examination may reveal injection of the discs, with blurring of the margins and pericapillary and macular edema (Krolman and Pidde 1968). Photoreceptors, Müller cells, and the retrolaminar portion of the optic nerve appear to be particular targets of methanol (McKellar et al. 1997). Increasing severity of the poisoning may lead to stupor, coma, tonic muscle contractions, hyperactive reflexes, opisthotonos, and generalized convulsions. In severely acidotic patients, death occurs from respiratory failure (Krolman and Pidde 1968). In the acute setting, the severity of neurological symptoms does not clearly correlate with the serum level of methanol, and a better surrogate indicator of severe intoxication is arterial pH (Teo et al. 1996).

Survival prognosis depends mainly on the degree of acidosis and the effectiveness of treatment. Only in unusual cases does the narcotic effect of the methanol or toxicity directly relate to formaldehyde or formic acid mortality (Ritchie 1975). In the largest clinical group of 323 patients reported with methanol exposure to bootleg whiskey, 6.2% died. When acidosis accompanied the methanol intoxication, the mortality rate was higher; when plasma $CO_2$, values were less than 20 mEq. 19% died, and when $CO_2$ values were less than 10 mEq. 50% died (Bennett et al. 1953). Coma and seizures do not always indicate a hopeless prognosis (Schneck 1979). Typical shallow slow respiration, tonic limb contractions, and opisthotonic posturing are considered a likely fatal triad (Roe 1955). In regard to vision, formate appears to be the primary toxic agent (Martin-Amat et al. 1978), and levels of serum formate correlate well with acute signs of neurotoxicity (Osterloh et al. 1986). For prognosis, the absence of pupillary light reflexes is generally associated with a low likelihood of survival (Benton and Calhoun 1952). Patients with severe retinal edema but retained pupillary responses usually are left with some degree of permanent visual loss. Most patients, however, have partial or complete recovery of visual acuity, and the recovery may occur within the first hours after correction of acidosis. If vision has not returned to normal within 6 days, however, full recovery is deemed unlikely (Roe 1953).

In survivors of methanol intoxication, long-term visual impairment and extrapyramidal signs may be prominent. Bradykinesia, low voice volume, masked facies, and tremor occur. Dementia and additional motor signs with increased or decreased reflexes may accompany this clinical picture. In two patients with parkinsonism, bilateral symmetrical infarctions of the frontal and central white matter and putamen were found. In the more severely affected patient, levodopa therapy was attempted but without success. One brain was examined at autopsy and cystic degeneration of the putamen and subcortical white matter accompanied widespread neuronal damage to the brain stem and spinal cord. The prominent putaminal necrosis seen in these patients may have related to decreased venous outflow through the Rosenthal's veins or to a possible accumulation of formic acid and formaldehyde in the putamen (McLean et al. 1980). An alternative presentation is dystonia and severe hypokinesis with putaminal necrosis but without other parkinsonian signs (LeWitt and Martin 1988). In the latter example, dopaminergic drugs were moderately helpful in ameliorating symptoms.

In an attempt to improve prognosis, clinicians use a three-part approach to treatment, involving ethanol infusions, bicarbonate treatment, and hemodialysis. Ethanol administration saturates the alcohol dehydrogenase enzyme and retards the conversion of methanol into its toxic by-products (Lawrence and Haggerty 1971). Massive and rapid alkalinization with bicarbonate may be necessary to correct acidosis, and it must be carried out for several days to avoid relapse (Rumack 1976). Dialysis is advocated when the methanol blood concentration is more than 50 mg/dl, and more recent work suggests that serum formate concentrations may be a better criterion for hemodialysis (Osterloh et al. 1986). The rapidity of therapeutic intervention is important, at least for the protection of vision. The longer the initial visual loss is present prior to the onset of therapy, the less likely full vision will be regained (Krolman and Pidde 1968). Ethanol-enriched bicarbonate-based hemodialysis, along with ethanol intravenous infusion, has been used with success and full neurological recovery (Chow et al. 1997b). Because the half-life of methanol is long (median, 43.1 hours in one series) in the setting of ethanol infusion, hemodialysis should accompany ethanol infusion therapy (Palatnick et al. 1995).

Because methanol presumably remains in the body for a long time, transient correction of acidosis may lead to clinical relapse. In the review by Bennett and coworkers (1953) of more than 300 patients, many were treated in the emergency room with only transiently assured correction of acidosis. On discharge from the emergency room, patients were instructed to consume bicarbonate as outpatients. Six cases returned in relapse: three had mild and easily correctable symptoms; two arrived in a moribund state 12 and 24 hours after discharge; and one had mild symptoms but collapsed suddenly and died. For these reasons, persistent observation for several days is indicated. Bennett and colleagues (1953) also observed that acidotic patients must be treated aggressively regardless of how clinically well they appear. Six acidotic patients who were rational and conversing on admission suddenly became comatose and died within minutes. Therefore, intensive observation of all acidotic patients would presumably improve prognosis (Bennett et al. 1953).

## Ethylene Glycol

Ethylene glycol is commonly used as an antifreeze for automobiles, as a solvent, and as a constituent in the manufacturing of explosives. The toxic dose approximates 100 ml. Ingestion of larger doses has been associated with death, usually from renal or cardiopulmonary damage (Hunt 1932). Ingestion of this solvent results in 40 to 60 deaths per year (Vale et al. 1976). A recent surge of intentional ethylene glycol poisonings occurred in Sweden, with a mortality rate of 17% (Karlson-Stiber and Persson 1993). In Haiti, an epidemic outbreak of diethylene glycol–contaminated glycerine occurred in children (Morbidity and Mortality Weekly Report 1996).

Symptoms of toxicity may appear early or may be delayed for several hours. Initially, the patient becomes restless and agitated. This is followed by somnolence, stupor, coma, and convulsions (Peterson et al. 1981). Death results from respiratory or cardiac failure. Abducens or soft-palate paralysis, aphasia, nystagmus, and fecal or urinary incontinence have been observed (Berger and Ayyar 1981). Hypocalcemia can occur and may be responsible for episodes of tetany.

Following oral ingestion, a portion of ethylene glycol is oxidized to oxalic acid and is excreted in the urine. Calcium oxalate crystals deposited in the kidney are responsible for the prominent renal symptoms (Huhn and Rosenberg 1995). They may also be deposited in the brain or meninges and result in some degree of cellular reaction. It has been suggested that CNS signs may relate directly to the observed deposits of calcium oxalate crystals rather than to the ethylene glycol or its metabolites. In cases of intoxication where a history of ethylene glycol exposure cannot be obtained, the detection of calcium oxalate crystals in the urine can be an important diagnostic finding (Rainey 1992; Huhn and Rosenberg 1995).

Delayed neurological signs may develop as late as 10 days after intoxication and include multiple cranial nerve palsies and sensorimotor polyneuropathies (Lewis et al. 1997; Broadley et al. 1997). Treatment consists chiefly of symptomatic measures, respiratory support, correction of severe metabolic acidosis, and control of hypocalcemia. As with methyl alcohol toxicity, ethylene glycol intoxication can be treated with ethyl alcohol infusions reaching 5 to 10 g/hr. Hemodialysis has been associated with improvement in gait disorders and focal neurological signs, specifically visual and speech (Berger and Ayyar 1981). Outcome depends primarily on the degree of acidosis and not the serum ethylene glycol level (Huhn and Rosenberg 1995). Phosphorus-enriched dialysate prevents the fall in plasma inorganic phosphorus levels (Chow et al. 1997a). In dogs, treatment with 4-methylpyrazole within 8 hours after severe intoxication with ethylene glycol led to excellent recovery, and this treatment may be initiated in human trials (Connally et al. 1996).

## Isopropyl Alcohol

Isopropyl alcohol is a solvent used in the manufacturing of perfumes, cosmetics, and various lacquers and varnishes. It also is commonly used as rubbing alcohol and in tepid sponges to reduce elevated body temperatures (Vivier et al. 1994). The toxicity and narcosis effect of isopropyl alcohol is approximately twice that of ethanol. Dizziness and headache, followed by ataxia, depression, and narcosis usually occur in acute isopropyl alcohol intoxication. At higher levels, patients may present in coma. When hypotension occurs, a poor prognosis is suggested (Adelson 1962). Because isopropyl alcohol has a longer duration of action than ethanol and its major metabolite, acetone, also is a central nervous system (CNS) depressant, hemodialysis is considered a life-saving procedure in severely intoxicated patients (Rosansky 1982). Approximately 27 g of isopropyl alcohol can be removed per hour with hemodialysis, which is 50 times the rate of removal achieved by urinary excretion.

## Benzene

The hydrocarbon benzene is one of the most important of the industrial poisons, ranking second only to tetrachloroethane in the production of serious intoxications. Benzene is widely used in industry, although its use has been curtailed because of toxic reactions. It is used in the processing of rubber, motor fuel, dyes, leather, and paints. Workers in chemical laboratories and in coal tar distilleries are subject to exposure to this toxin.

Acute benzene intoxication can follow oral ingestion in suicide attempts, but commonly it occurs in workers who have been cleaning or repairing leaks in benzene tanks or who have been exposed to toxic concentrations of this substance in the air (Dinberg 1945).

Excessive ventilation of benzene vapor produces euphoria and an alcohol-like inebriation, associated with giddiness, tinnitus, headache, drowsiness, and vomiting. The gait becomes ataxic and muscular twitching appears with severe intoxication. Finally, convulsive seizures and unconsciousness occur. In very severe intoxications, there may be almost immediate loss of consciousness and respiratory depression.

In patients who survive acute effects, recovery usually is complete, although headache, chest pain, shortness of breath, anorexia, nausea, and vomiting may be present for days or weeks. No specific risk factors have been identified to affect prognosis in these acute intoxications.

Chronic benzene intoxication has been observed during benzene treatment for leukemia. CNS symptoms occur as a result of anemia and from direct toxic effects of the compound. Pyramidal tract involvement, hyperesthesia, ataxia, paresthesias, paraplegia, retrobulbar neuritis, peripheral neuropathy, and seizures have been observed (Klein 1950). Recovery in nonfatal cases takes several months.

The best studied of the neurological complications related to chronic benzene intoxication is peripheral neuropathy. However, because toluene often is mixed with benzene, the specificity of benzene neuropathy is not fully established. Six exposed Turkish shoemaker-leather workers were studied neurologically and electrophysiologically and showed slowed conduction velocities and clinical signs of atrophy (Baslo and Aksoy 1982). The severity of residual neurological dysfunction and the duration of nonexposure, that is, the period from last benzene exposure to the neurological evaluation, were inversely correlated. In fact, the two patients with the longest freedom from exposure (as high as 96 months) had minimal or no neurological abnormalities. The degree of pancytopenia associated with benzene exposure did not correlate with neurological prognosis (Kahn and Muzyka 1973).

## Toluene (Methylbenzene)

Toluene is one of the most widely used solvents and is used as a paint and lacquer thinner, a cleaning and dying agent, and a constituent of fuels. It is commonly used in histology laboratories and has been estimated to be the most widely abused solvent (King 1983). Neurological signs occur after exposure to as little as 100 ppm, and with concentrations of 800 ppm, signs may persist for several days. After acute exposure, there is an early exhilaration, followed by fatigue, mild confusion, ataxia, and dizziness; intentional exposure by sniffing glue with the head in a plastic bag may result in blood levels of 6.5 mg/dl. Psychotic behavior, unconsciousness, and death have been reported following such exposure (Winek et al. 1968). In most cases, however, single acute intoxication episodes are associated with no neurological residua.

After chronic toluene abuse, the prognosis is more serious. Tremulousness, unsteadiness, emotional lability, and insomnia are prominent features, and jaw jerk, snout, and other primitive reflexes have been reported in chronically exposed patients months after cessation of exposure (Browning 1937). Cerebellar ataxia with and without optic nerve dysfunction also had been reported with cognitive impairment (Barnes 1967; King 1983). In a 20-patient study of solvent (mainly toluene) abusers, after 4 weeks of solvent abstinence, cognitive impairment persisted in 60%, pyramidal signs in 50%, cerebellar signs in 45%, and brain stem or cranial nerve impairment in 25% (Hormes et al. 1986; Rosenberg et al, 1988). Brain stem auditory evoked responses (BAERs) and magnetic resonance imaging (MRI) scans also showed persistent abnormalities in chronic abusers (Rosenberg et al. 1988). The extent of long-term dementia correlates with the extent of white matter changes detected on MR scans (Filley et al. 1990). Irreversible optic neuropathy can occur, although even severe visual compromise (4/200) can reverse to 20/30 after weeks of complete abstinence from chronic toluene exposure (Keane 1978).

Additionally, a patient may present with a polyneuropathy, symmetrical weakness, and atrophy after chronic toluene exposure. The long-term outcome of these patients, however, has not been well described.

### n-Hexane and Methyl Butyl Ketone

n-Hexane is a component of numerous glues and, like toluene, is a source of major inhalation abuse. The substance is associated with a euphoric effect in patients with acute exposure and a pronounced peripheral neuropathy after chronic intoxication. Although many glues contain a combination of n-hexane and toluene, the independent role of n-hexane has been indicated in cases in which the neuropathy did not develop until the glue sniffer changed to a glue containing n-hexane (Towfighi et al. 1976). The neurotoxic product is probably not hexane, but 2.5 hexanedione (2,5-HD), which also is a metabolite of methyl butyl ketone (MBK) (Spencer et al. 1980). Workers exposed to n-hexane first report headache, nausea, and anorexia. Two to 6 months after initial exposure, victims may demonstrate a neuropathy, including symmetrical, predominantly distal, motor deficits and frequent sensory symptoms that may progress for up to 3 months after exposure ceases. Although clinically detectable neurological abnormalities and sensory symptoms have been reported to persist for 2 to 3 years after exposure ceases, partial or complete recovery is the rule (Bravaccio et al. 1981; Spencer and Schaumburg 1985b). Most neuropathy cases occur after chronic exposure, although acute, high-dose exposure has been reported (Oge et al. 1994). In a series of work-related exposures, the amplitude of the sensory nerve action potentials (SNAP) recorded from the sural and median nerves correlated significantly with the exposure time to n-hexane (Pastore et al. 1994)

More recent concerns regarding n-hexane and petroleum derivatives have focused on parkinsonism. Cases of well-described intoxication have been associated with rigidity, bradykinesia, tremor, and postural reflex compromise (Pezzoli 1989; Tetrud et al. 1990) Furthermore, animal experiments demonstrate that n-hexane exposure lowers brain dopamine and homovanillic acid, the central metabolite of dopamine (Pezzoli et al. 1991). Since n-hexane is a common environmental contaminant and hydrocarbons can be by-products of endogenous metabolic pathways, these compounds are a focus of pathogenic research efforts in movement disorders. Although chemically dissimilar from carbon disulfide, n-hexane is metabolized to the γ-diketone 2,5-hexanedione, which induces similar histological neurofilament-filled swelling in distal axons of the central and peripheral nervous system, very similar to carbon disulfide (Graham et al. 1995). This observation suggests that these two neurotoxins may share some pathogenic features and serve as a unifying model for the study of chemicals that adversely affect both peripheral and central nervous system axons.

MBK is a component of paint thinners, cleaning agents, and solvents for printing. Numerous outbreaks of polyneuropathy have been reported (Teitelbaum 1977). The sensory polyneuropathy is insidious and painless, usually beginning several months after continued chronic exposure. Autonomical and cranial nerve dysfunction also occurs.

As with n-hexane neuropathy, there is no recognized form of treatment for MBK neurotoxicity. The administration of prednisolone and large doses of vitamin B have been tried without effect (Yamamura 1969). Removing the patient from the exposure source generally is associated with a good prognosis, although for the first few weeks or months, the disease may intensify. Only rarely have patients exposed to either hexacarbon shown signs of long-term CNS damage (Spencer and Schaumburg 1985b).

### Gasoline

The composition of gasoline is extremely varied. Originally, it was composed largely of butanes, hexanes, and pentanes, but various other hydrocarbons have been added. Because of its antiknock qualities, tetraethyl lead is present in most gasoline, and triorthocresyl phosphate occasionally is found as well. With the inhalation of toxic quantities of gasoline, inebriation, blurred vision, incoordination, confusion, excitement, and occasionally delirium with visual hallucinations may occur. Voluntary gasoline abusers report that 15 to 20 breaths of gasoline vapors cause a 5- to 6-hour euphoric intoxication (Hartman 1988). These symptoms are followed by depression, headache, lethargy, trembling, staggering, and nausea. In severe cases, symptoms progress to dyspnea, cyanosis, and convulsions. Death has occurred in cases of extreme exposure, but generally recovery is followed by an alcoholic-like "hangover." In a 50-patient study of chronic gasoline sniffers, 92% had abnormal neurological examinations at the time of gasoline sniffing, but all except one case resolved after 8 weeks. Lead chelation was instituted in 39 of these patients. Twenty-seven of the 46 patients had an abnormal electroencephalogram (EEG) with very low voltage and an excess of diffuse slow activity; 10 of the 15 EEGs performed 8 to 12 weeks later were normal. Common neurological signs that resolved were brisk deep tendon reflexes, intention tremor, and ataxia. However, cases of persistent seizure disorders, ataxia, and dementia have been reported (Browning 1937: Valpey et al. 1978). In a patient with susceptibility to malignant hyperthermia, accidental gasoline inhalation led to massive rhabdomyolysis, most likely due to benzine-induced contractions. (Anetseder et al. 1994).

The precise toxic components in gasoline remains undetermined, but some toxicity may relate to solvents and others to tetraethyl lead. Chelation has been used successfully and has been reported to improve long-term clinical outcome, although this has not been tested in controlled trials (Valpey et al. 1978). A chronic encephalopathy can be progressive in patients who persist in gasoline sniffing (Valpey et al. 1978).

## Turpentine and Other Solvent Mixtures

Turpentine is widely used in the paint and varnish industry and has been used medically as an expectorant. Intoxication can occur after inhalation of fumes in industry or after ingestion (accidentally or in attempted suicide). With acute intoxication, patients develop headache and dizziness, followed by confusion, excitement, and delirium. Patients may become ataxic and exhibit visual disturbances. These resolve without sequelae in most cases. In more severely intoxicated cases, renal failure and gastrointestinal irritation occur, along with encephalopathy that may progress to coma and generalized convulsions. In cases in which pneumonia and poor oxygenation may develop, a long-standing posthypoxic encephalopathy also may develop.

Two major toxic syndromes occur in association with chronic mixed solvent exposure: encephalopathy and neuropathy. Cerebellar and myopathic changes have been described but are less common (Pedersen et al. 1980). Chronic encephalopathic symptoms include fatigue, concentration difficulties, impaired memory, and sleep disruption (Eskelinen et al. 1986). Specific neuropsychological impairment of verbal memory and slowed emotional reactivity have been reported. One recent study emphasized long-standing decrements in manual dexterity and executive/ motor functioning (Bolla et al. 1995). In 80 patients exposed to mixed solvents and followed for a mean of 5.8 years after initial chronic exposure, objective clinical signs of CNS dysfunction and evidence of progression (Juntunen 1982) persisted in most cases. In many cases, no neurological abnormality was detected at initial diagnosis, but at follow-up, cerebellar or pyramidal involvement was documented. Of the 10 patients who demonstrated signs of peripheral neuropathy at diagnosis, the long-term prognosis will split in approximately equal numbers between improvement ($n = 4$), no change ($n = 4$), and deterioration ($n = 3$). In a second study specifically aimed at follow-up prognosis, 26 patients chronically exposed to solvents who had shown signs of encephalopathy were removed from the solvents for 2 years and reexamined neurologically, neuropsychologically, and by computed tomography (CT) scans. In general, the encephalopathy persisted in spite of removal of the solvent exposure. In three patients, neurological function deteriorated Bruhn et al. 1981).

Other population studies have compared painters or floor layers with workers not exposed to mixed solvents, such as carpenters and construction workers. These studies show more depression, slower reaction times, and more impaired visual constructive tasks in the solvent-exposed groups (Ekberg et al. 1986; Lindstrom and Marbelin 1982). Patients who voluntarily abuse solvents by soaking a cloth and inhaling the fumes also have been studied for chronic encephalopathy lasting beyond the period of toxic exposure;

results of persistent disability were similar (Berry et al. 1977).

In another follow-up study in which investigators re-examined 26 of their original 50 painters chronically exposed to solvent mixtures for an average of 28 years, subjective complaints of headaches and dizziness declined for most patients, but no one improved in neuropsychological, neurological, or neuroradiological status after 2 years without solvent exposure. Specifically, if cortical atrophy or other objective signs of neurological dysfunction developed, recovery was slow or absent. Exposed workers without objective signs of structural abnormalities or neurological dysfunction appeared to be much more likely to recover (Hartman 1988).

Several studies suggest that chronic exposure, usually longer than 3 years, of mixed solvents (specific constituent not always determined) is associated with an encephalopathy that progresses during exposure and tends to plateau but may progress after removal from the source of intoxication (Spencer and Schaumburg 1985a).

A second neurological syndrome seen in solvent mixtures is referred to as Huffer's neuropathy (Procktop et al. 1974). This disorder was originally described in patients who had inhaled lacquer thinner over several years but became acutely ill when the solvent mixture was changed to another composition. A severe and predominantly motor neuropathy developed and continued to progress for up to 2 months after cessation of exposure. The weakness involved proximal and distal muscles and the muscles of respiration and facial expression. Some patients required respiratory support. Areflexia was the rule, although sensory loss was mild. Most patients showed improvement in motor function after exposure ceased, but many showed persistent deficits. Electromyographical studies demonstrated severely slowed conduction velocities and signs of acute denervation.

## Tetrachloroethane

This solvent is the most dangerous of the chlorinated hydrocarbons and its use often is restricted because of toxicity. It has been marketed commercially under names such as Alanol, cellon, Novania, and Westron. Tetrachloroethane exerts a prolonged narcotic effect, resulting in uncon-

sciousness, loss of corneal reflexes, cyanosis, and death, often within 12 hours. More commonly, however, tetrachloroethane poisoning results from chronic exposure to excess concentrations of the vapor in the air. In such cases, headache, giddiness, anorexia, nausea, and other nonspecific complaints predominate (Browning 1937). Good prognostic studies have not been conducted with this agent. The treatment of toxicity is aimed chiefly at protection of the liver from parenchymal damage (Fairhall 1949).

## Trichloroethylene and Perchloroethylene

Trichloroethylene (TCE) is an important organic solvent used occasionally in medicine as an anesthetic but more widely used in the dry cleaning industry. Deliberate inhalation of TCE induces a rapid state of euphoria, and many workers have become addicted to the fumes (Grandjean et al. 1955). Sudden death associated with bronchial constriction, pulmonary edema, and myocardial irritability have been reported infrequently (Seage and Bruns 1971). Neurologically, cranial and peripheral neuropathies are the most striking feature of TCE toxicity. There is a propensity for trigeminal involvement, both sensory and motor, with facial nerve involvement also a characteristic (Feldman 1979). Neuro-ophthalmological complications, including retrobulbar neuropathy, optic atrophy, and ocular motor disturbance may occur, as well as cerebellar and extrapyramidal dysfunction in the form of tremor and ataxia (Szlatenyi and Wang 1996).

In the first 24 hours after exposure, the entire face usually becomes anesthetic, but by 4 to 8 weeks, the peripheral face generally has returned to normal. Twenty to 30 weeks after exposure, the anesthetic area further retracts to involve only the eyes, nose, and mouth. By 80 weeks, only spotty hypalgesia is noted (Feldman 1979). For diagnosis, blood trichloroethylene levels are more relevant than urinary trichloroacetic acid (Kostrzewski et al. 1993).

In addition to the well-documented cranial neuropathies of TCE exposure, less specific neurasthenic symptoms, including fatigue, insomnia, anxiety, and emotional giddiness, have been reported that may last for several weeks (Spencer and Schaumburg 1985a). A review of deaths attributed to trichloroethylene between 1975 and

1992 showed that all occurred in young men who were usually working in confined work spaces without adequate ventilation (Ford et al. 1995).

Perchloroethylene (PCE) has been widely substituted for TCE in the dry cleaning industry and produces similar clinical problems. Acute intoxication signs, usually dizziness, headache, nausea, and vomiting, clear after removal of the patient from the PCE fumes. After months or years of exposure, an encephalopathy has been described consisting of irritability, labile affect, memory loss, and mild confusion. Even 1 year after cessation of chronic exposure, long-lasting changes in personality and memory loss have been reported (Gold 1969).

## Carbon Tetrachloride

Carbon tetrachloride is widely used for manufacturing refrigerants and insecticides (Hardin 1954). Following oral ingestion, the intoxicated patient develops nausea and vomiting, often associated with abdominal pain and diarrhea. The acute symptoms usually are more severe following inhalation. In the 77-patient study review by Hardin (1954), neurological symptoms, such as headache, dizziness, and convulsions, were the sixth, 10th, and 12th most frequent symptoms after nausea, vomiting, abdominal pain, edema, and jaundice. Staggering gait, confusion, and unconsciousness also may occur during intoxication but were less common (Kazantzis and Bomford 1960). Stewart and Witts (1944) examined 78 industrial workers in an English factory who were exposed intermittently to carbontetrachloride vapors. More than 50% of the workers were discharged from work because of symptoms attributable to gaseous exposure, including insomnia, irritability, nausea and vomiting, abdominal pains, and diarrhea. Objective evidence of hepatic or renal failure was rarely found, and no long-term follow-up information after exposure cessation was reported. Late sequelae of acute exposure can include optic atrophy with amblyopia (listed 14th on Hardin's list), generalized convulsions, and delirium terminating in death. In such cases, the patient usually is the victim of severe hepatic and renal failure (Morgan et al. 1949). After chronic carbon tetrachloride exposure, persisting states of mental confusion, polyneuropathy, and parkinsonism have

been described, although specific population studies have not been performed (Melamed and Levy 1977).

Factors that may alter the toxicity of carbon tetrachloride have been studied. First, ingestion of alcohol concomitant to or preceding exposure to the toxin increases the victim's susceptibility to poisoning (Morgan et al. 1949). Among a group of workers equally exposed to carbon tetrachloride, two workers with a well-established history of alcohol abuse developed severe intoxication that required hemodialysis, whereas the rest of the workers remained asymptomatic (Manno et al. 1996). In spite of their prolonged hepatonephrotoxic syndrome, eventual recovery occurred in both individuals. Furthermore, obesity, diabetes, and prior liver or renal disease also appear to lower the threshold to the toxic effects of carbon tetrachloride (Council of Industrial Health 1946). Evidence from animal studies suggests that phenobarbital may negatively affect prognosis because the drug increases microsomal enzyme activity leading to greater quantities of toxic metabolites. Oxidizing substances, such as vitamin E and selenium, protect against carbon tetrachloride intoxication in animals, although these two therapies have not been studied extensively in humans. Hemodialysis has been recommended in cases of exposure (Fogel 1983).

Any exposure concentration of more than 100 ppm can be associated with severe liver or kidney damage. When hepatic necrosis exists, longstanding cirrhotic changes develop in surviving patients. Hepatoma also has developed in some cases and occasionally has been ascribed to the carbon tetrachloride exposure (Louria and Bogden 1980).

## Carbon Monoxide

Carbon monoxide, an odorless and nonirritating gas, is the most abundant air pollutant in the lower atmosphere. Acute poisoning accounts for more than 3000 accidental or suicidal deaths each year in the United States. The effects of chronic exposure to carbon monoxide, due to inhalation of polluted air, are of increasing concern to scientists and clinicians. The threshold limit of carbon monoxide is 50 ppm, causing a carboxyhemoglobin saturation level of 8% to 10% after an 8-hour exposure. Levels of carboxyhemoglobin that exceed 50% saturation are considered life-threatening, and levels of 70% to 75% usually are fatal. Such saturation levels may occur by exposure to very high acute concentrations or by exposure to relatively lower concentrations for a chronic period. The threshold limit assumes that the carbon monoxide comes from a single source and does not take into account endogenous factors or smoking, which also can increase the victim's baseline saturation.

Mild neurological effects include headache, dizziness, and visual disturbances; more severe toxic reactions include convulsive disorder, pyramidal and extrapyramidal signs, cerebral blindness, and deafness. Such symptoms may be transient to persistent, appearing immediately, days, or weeks after intoxication. Myositis and calcification in the muscles with mild necrosis also may occur; these are related to the direct effects of the toxin on myoglobin and the crushing effect of the patient's own body on muscles.

Behavioral and psychiatric alterations, including irritability and violent behavior, personality disturbances, inappropriate euphoria, confusion, and impaired judgment may occur. In a follow-up study, 3 years after carbon monoxide poisoning, 13% of patients showed gross neuropsychiatric damage, 33% showed a deterioration of personality, and 43% demonstrated impaired memory.

More recent concern over the chronic effects of carbon monoxide focus on patients with continued industrial or urban exposure to the gas. Cigarette smokers also fit into this potential category, although environmental tobacco smoke likely contributes only minor and toxicologically insignificant increments in ambient carbon monoxide concentrations (Mennear 1993). Six patients with leaking exhaust systems in their automobiles were chronically self-exposed to carbon monoxide (McClain and Becker 1975). Over weeks they developed an insidious syndrome of somnolence and mental decline with gait difficulty, incoordination, and slurred speech. When the exhaust system was corrected, their carboxyhemoglobin levels declined and their symptoms resolved. A more focal neurological syndrome reported after acute and chronic exposure to carbon monoxide is parkinsonism (Westerman et al. 1965). Some patients show diffuse neurological involvement associated with parkinsonian features, while others demonstrate purer parkinsonism. This clinical syndrome usually is associated with globus palli-

dal lucency on the CT scan and pallidal atrophy histologically. Patients may respond to levodopa or to anticholinergic drugs, but the response is unpredictable.

If toxic levels of carboxyhemoglobin are determined, the diagnosis of carbon monoxide poisoning is safely made. However, the level of carbon monoxide does not indicate the severity of the poisoning because a patient removed from the intoxicated environment and allowed to breathe fresh air will show a rapid decline in the carboxyhemoglobin levels.

The prognosis for patients with significant carbon monoxide poisoning is difficult to determine immediately after the patient is discovered. Patients with carboxyhemoglobin levels as low as 29% have died after a carbon monoxide poisoning, while others with much higher levels have survived.

Personality change and memory impairment are a particular concern: in a 3-year follow-up study of 63 patients who survived acute carbon monoxide intoxication, eight (12.7%) showed gradual behavioral improvement, 21 (33.3%) showed deterioration, and 27 (43%) reported memory impairment. Personality deterioration and memory impairment correlated, and the degree of depressed consciousness at hospital admission correlated significantly with the development of neuropsychiatric sequelae (Smith and Brandon 1973). Nonneurological morbidity and mortality concerns have primarily focused on the cardiovascular system. Foundry workers exposed to chronic carbon monoxide have shown excess rates of medication treatment for hypertension and deaths due to ischemic heart disease compared to workers without exposure (Koskela 1994).

Treatment is well established and improves survival. Upon discovery of the patient with carbon monoxide poisoning, the physician should immediately remove the patient from the contaminated environment. Fresh air and inactivity are recommended to maintain the tissue demands for oxygen at an absolute minimum. Resuscitation in the contaminated environment may be dangerous to the rescuer and to the patient. If the patient cannot breathe, artificial respiration is indicated. One hundred percent oxygen should be started as soon as possible through an oral or nasal mask. The half-life of carboxyhemoglobin is 40 minutes after the administration of 100% oxygen.

Hyperbaric oxygen reduces the half-life of carboxyhemoglobin to less than 25 minutes. The following are recommendations for hyperbaric oxygen: 46 minutes of 100% oxygen at 3 atm absolute pressure, followed by 2 atm absolute pressure for 2 hours or until the proper carboxyhemoglobin level is achieved (Cohen 1975; Sauerhoff and Michaelson 1973). Hyperbaric oxygen is considered the treatment of choice for carbon monoxide poisoning, and if possible, it should be administered to every patient who presents with signs and symptoms of severe intoxication. In premature infants, the toxicity of oxygen must be considered and weighed against the likelihood of the diagnosis in questionable cases.

To decrease the tissue demand for oxygen, hypothermia also has been advocated, although no controlled studies have determined its effects on prognosis. Patients covered in ice are maintained for 8 to 12 hours at a temperature of 30° to 32°C. Shivering, which increases the metabolic rate, should be prevented and often can be controlled by administering 25 mg of chlorpromazine. If seizures develop. they may be treated with steroids, such as dexamethasone. 16 to 20 mg/d.

## Nitrous Oxide

Volitional inhalation of nitrous oxide has gained increasing popularity, especially among dentists and other health-care workers (Layzer et al. 1978). The gas also is available in various compressed dispenser cartridges and may account for "whipped cream dispenser" polyneuropathy (Sahenk et al. 1978). Nitrous oxide neuropathy may be a predominantly distal polyneuropathy or may follow a radicular pattern. Also, cases of mixed or primarily sensory neuropathy have been described. Cessation of exposure has been associated with gradual clinical improvement, although as late as 6 months after removal from nitrous oxide, mild neuropathic symptoms may persist (Layzer et el. 1978; Sahenk et al. 1978).

In addition to neuropathy, myelopathic signs of upper motor neuron disease also may exist, provoking a picture resembling subacute combined degeneration due to vitamin $B_{12}$ deficiency. In fact, nitrous oxide has been shown to inactivate certain $B_{12}$-dependent enzymes (Chanarin 1982). The gait difficulty, sensory ataxia, paresthesias,

and impotency regress at least partially after removal from exposure (O'Donoghue 1985).

Supplementation with methionine can arrest progression of clinical disease, and patients gained significant recovery (Stacy et al. 1992). It is not clear whether nitrous oxide can provoke this syndrome in patients with normal $B_{12}$ or whether a subclinical vitamin deficiency state must coexist (Nestor and Stark 1996). Exposure to the gas has also been associated with slowing of performance on neuropsychological testing.

## Methyl Chloride

Methyl chloride is primarily a foaming agent for plastics. Acute exposures are associated with a toxic confusional state, involving slurred speech, ataxia, and occasionally convulsions (Kegel et al. 1929). Headache, dizziness, and personality changes also may occur. These changes, however, usually revert to normal, although they may take several weeks or months to clear (MacDonald 1964). During the first months after acute exposure, symptoms have recurred after apparent recovery and without further exposure (Scharnweber et al. 1974).

The most complete follow-up of patients exposed to acute intoxication of methyl chloride is a report by Gudmundsson (1977), who re-evaluated patients 13 years after a refrigeration leak. Of the 15 original patients, four died, one within 24 hours of the episode, and two others committed suicide 11 and 18 months later. The fourth patient was assessed as 75% disabled because of severe neurological and psychiatric disturbances and died 10 years after the accident at age 34. Of the 11 survivors in 1976, ten were examined: six had abnormal neurological examinations, including peripheral neuropathy ($n = 2$), tremor ($n = 3$), paralysis of visual accommodation ($n = 2$), and single cases of muscle atrophy, primitive reflexes, and habit spasms. The degree of disability was less than the evaluation 20 months after the accident, suggesting that with time, very slow improvement occurred. Only one patient showed complete regression of symptoms between the 20-month follow-up and the 7-year follow-up (Gudmundsson 1977).

After chronic methyl chloride exposure, patients may develop an insidious form of dementia and ataxia. Peripheral neuropathy, more common with many other industrial toxins, is less conspicuous with methyl chloride (Scharnweber et al. 1974). Removal of the patients is associated with significant improvement, although some patients' long-term personality changes persisted, and 3 months after cessation of chronic exposure, some patients still showed tremor and nervousness (Scharnweber et al. 1974).

## Carbon Disulfide

Carbon disulfide is used to manufacture viscose, rayon, cellophane, and adhesives. Acute fulminant intoxications can result in toxic psychosis, agitated delirium, and permanent sequelae of mental impairment (Gordy and Trumper 1940). The more important syndrome follows chronic exposure and involves the development of progressive mental impairment with cranial and peripheral neuropathies. Mental changes include irritability, personality changes, and emotional lability. A characteristic cranial nerve dysfunction involving the selective loss of corneal reflexes without facial sensory complaints also has been reported. The peripheral neuropathy is relatively mild, with mixed sensory and motor involvement and predominantly distal distribution. An unusual parkinsonian presentation has been reported after carbon disulfide intoxication and was marked by characteristic resting tremor, rigidity, and bradykinesia. It was associated with peripheral neuropathy and marked mental impairment (Allen 1979). In addition, a subtle parkinsonian finger tremor may develop in workers chronically exposed to carbon disulfide (Chapman et al. 1991). In terms of prognosis, persistent absentmindedness and difficulties in perceptive abilities have been documented even after long-term removal from exposure (Cassitto et al. 1993), and in one proportional mortality analysis of workers exposed to carbon disulfide, an increased risk of strokes was reported (Liss and Finkelstein 1996).

## Ethylene Oxide

Ethylene oxide is a gas used as a precursor to various other industrial chemicals, including ethylene glycol. Generally considered innocuous, this gas recently has been implicated in human toxic peripheral neuropathies, cerebellar dysfunction, and encephalopathy. Signs of acute toxicity in-

volving the nervous system are agitation and confusion, headaches, and drowsiness. With excessive doses, convulsions and death may occur (O'Donoughue 1985). After chronic exposure, a variety of syndromes can develop (Gross et al. 1979). Of four men exposed for 2 months to ethylene oxide at levels of more than 700 ppm, one developed repeated motor seizures, and the other three had a sensory motor peripheral neuropathy. Clinically, the latter patients showed generalized fatigue, weakness of the distal muscles, ataxia, and reduction or loss of the deep tendon reflexes. One man had additional cranial neuropathy, difficulty with memory, and slurred speech. All showed marked improvement within 2 weeks of cessation of exposure (Gross et al. 1979).

The best evaluated series of ethylene oxide intoxication was a cluster of hospital employees who developed toxic symptoms after 5 months of exposure to high levels of ethylene oxide and its by-product, ethylene chlorohydrin. Neuropathy and cognitive impairment were the hallmarks of the syndrome and sural nerve biopsy on a severely affected patient showed axonal injury (Brashear et al. 1996). No long-term follow-up on this group was reported. Experimental studies suggest that there are toxic effects on both CNS and peripheral nerves. In the sensory system, axonal degeneration of myelinated fibers includes not only distal nerves but extends into the gracilis fasciculus. Electron microscopic changes include axonal swelling, accumulation of membrane-bound vesicles, and disruption of microtubules (Garnaas et al. 1991).

## Organophosphates

These chemicals are powerful inhibitors of acetylcholinesterase and pseudocholinesterase (Arlien-Søberg 1985). In humans, the former enzyme is found in nervous tissue, specifically in the brain, spinal cord, and myoneural junctions at preganglionic and postganglionic parasympathetic synapses and preganglionic and some postganglionic sympathetic nerve endings. Excess acetylcholine causes overstimulation and then depolarization blockade of cholinergic transmission (Goetz 1985).

Most reports of major organophosphate poisoning have been due to parathion or methylparathion. Clinically, intoxication may range from latent, asymptomatic poisoning to a life-threatening illness. Toxicity usually is monitored with serum cholinesterase activity. Decreases of 10% to 50% may not be clinically detectable. When levels are moderately depressed (20% of normal), sweating, cramps, tingling of the extremities, and mild bulbar weakness with fasciculation may occur. At 10% of normal, consciousness becomes depressed, and myosis with no pupillary response to light occurs. The patient may become cyanotic from respiratory weakness and pooled secretions may obstruct the airway. Although symptoms generally abate after removal of the causative agent, the resolution may slow; headaches and weakness may persist for 1 month. Eye discomfort has been reported 5 months after exposure (Midtling et al. 1985).

Pralidoxime usually is used intravenously to reverse the acute cholinergic alterations. The major action of this drug is to reactivate organophosphate-inhibited acetylcholinesterase activity. The compound removes the phosphate group bound to the esteratic site (Lotti 1982). Because pralidoxime has a quaternary structure, it does not penetrate the blood-brain barrier well and therefore does not reach high CNS concentrations. However, it has controlled seizures, possibly through its peripheral effect on respiratory and skeletal muscles (Namba et al. 1971). Pancuronium improves the neuromuscular transmission defect most likely by blockade of cholinergic receptors, especially those located on the terminal axon responsible for antidromic backfiring (Besser et al. 1990).

After acute organophosphate intoxication with mortality, death almost always occurs within the first 24 hours in untreated cases and within 10 days in treated cases (Namba et al. 1971). If anoxia does not develop, complete recovery should be expected within 10 days, although EEG abnormalities can be detected weeks after exposure (Wislicki 1960). The use of serum cholinesterase levels as a prognostic sign has been controversial. In a series of 52 subjects with acute organophosphate intoxications, serum cholinesterase levels above 10% of normal values were associated with good recovery (Cunha et al. 1995). However, another smaller study failed to show this association (Nouira et al. 1994). Another prognostic indicator test is the initial electrocardiogram, and among 223 patients with severe intoxication, those with QTc prolongation had a significantly higher mortality and higher incidence of respiratory failure

(Chuang et al. 1996). In a series of 190 subjects admitted to the hospital for organophosphate intoxication from suicide attempts, occupational exposure, and accidental poisoning, the mortality rate was 6.3%, and the chances for recovery were highest when patients were hospitalized at the earliest indications of intoxication (Agawal 1993). Occasionally, mild persistent residua are reported: for example, 25 of 600 acutely exposed victims complained of persistent neurobehavioral symptoms, including confusion, concentration difficulties, muscle aches, and mild diffuse weakness lasting for weeks. Among 128 workers with acute exposure to organophosphates, sustained visual attention and mood assessement were significantly worse at chronic follow-up compared to a referent group (Steenland et al. 1994). Rarely, extrapyramidal signs develop 4 to 40 days after acute exposure and may take the form of dystonia, choreoathetosis, or parkinsonism with rest tremor or cogwheel rigidity (Senanayake and Sanmuganathan 1995). After chronic exposure, residua may be seen more predictably; in a 16-patient study of chronic (months) exposure to organophosphates, eight patients had impaired memory, seven had depression, and five had "schizophrenic reactions" lasting up to 1 year after cessation of exposure (Gershon and Shaw 1961). Extensive follow-up data are not available: however, in Australia, no increase in mental hospital admissions was noted in a region where organophosphates were widely used compared to areas where they were rarely used (Stoller et al. 1965).

Neuropathy is another prominent toxic sign of organophosphate exposure and has been reported as a progressive disorder after both acute and chronic poisoning. In such cases, the acute cholinergic toxicity is followed after several days by a delayed, progressive weakness, including foot drop, absent ankle jerk, and muscle weakness. Bilateral vocal cord paralysis can also occur and be life threatening (Thompson and Stocks 1997). Persisting neuropathy can develop as late as 3 months after exposure ceases (Petry 1952). Pyramidal signs can accompany this syndrome (Senanayake 1982). Examples of responsible compounds include tri-aryl phosphate, nipafox, trichlorfon, and methamidophos. There is no correlation between the potency of acute cholinergic effects and the likelihood of chronic neuropathy (Cherniak 1985). However, for alkyl or mixed alkyl-aryl esters with the structure of R1R2P(O or S)X, factors that increase the relative risk for delayed neurotoxicity compared with acute toxicity include phosphonate or phosphoramidates, rather than phosphates and long chain length (four or five carbon atoms) or hydrophobicity of R1 and R2.

The pathophysiology of the neuropathy does not appear to relate to effects on the cholinergic system. Instead, it relates to a two-step phosphorylation and "aging" of the protein called neuropathy target esterase (NTE) (Lotti 1986).

## Dichlorodiphenyltrichloroethane and Organochloride Insecticides

The chlorinated hydrocarbon insecticides, of which dichlorodiphenyltrichloroethane (DDT) is the prototype, share numerous toxicological properties, although certain individual variations exist. They are all highly soluble in fats and oils and most are extremely enduring in the environment, making chronic toxicity a most serious ecological and clinical problem. Pregnant women pass organochlorines to the fetus, and for humans, food provides 80% of organochlorine exposure. As a group, these compounds are primarily toxic to the nervous system, the major manifestations being tremor and convulsions. Neurobehavioral effects in children born to mothers with high exposure is a second syndrome of concern (Hall 1992). Finally, intentional suicide by organochlorines and other pesticides is an important clinical entity, and in recent mortality figures from England and Wales, pesticides accounted for 44 of approximately 4000 poisoning deaths (Thompson et al. 1995). In general, these compounds are toxic to the nervous system and induce tremor and convulsions. DDT is associated with acute and chronic neurotoxicity. Acutely, patients notice a metallic taste in the mouth, and within 1 hour, they experience dryness of the mouth and extreme thirst. The patient may experience drowsiness or insomnia, eye burning, and a gritty feeling of the eyelids. Muscle spasms, tremor, and stiffness of the jaw may develop later. After chronic low-dose exposure, weakness of the arms may occur, or weakness may be relatively isolated to distal muscles and cause bilateral wrist drop (Garrett 1947). Mononeuropathy, optic neuropathy, and polyneuropathy have been described with chronic intoxication (Committee on Pesticides 1951). When these symptoms result from exposure of the skin to DDT, they may be limited to the limb that was in direct contact with the toxin (Mackerras and West 1946). With chronic high-dose exposure, generalized convulsions, coma, and death may ensue (Globus 1948).

After acute exposure to DDT, motor signs generally abate; however, even months later, objective disability can persist in the form of weakness and poor coordination (Taylor and Calabrese 1979). In cases of retrobulbar neuritis, recovery has been reported after a few months (Campbell 1952).

Chlordecone (Kepone) has not been reported to induce seizures regularly but causes a dramatic irregular postural tremor that is maximal when the limbs are extended but not specifically enhanced by actions. In more severe cases, the tremor is evident at rest. Additionally, opsoclonia is associated with chlordecone exposure and occasionally pseudotumor cerebri (Sanborr et el. 1979; Taylor et al. 1978). In the chlordecone outbreak in Virginia, more than half of the active employees of the affected plant were moderately ill. A few patients required hospitalization for months, but severe toxic signs generally abated when patients were removed from the toxic environment. However, 4 years later, several workers continued to show incapacitating tremor (Taylor et al. 1978).

## Paraquat

Prognosis related to acute paraquat poisoning has been specifically addressed by Bismuth and colleagues (1982) in a 28-patient study. Eleven patients survived, representing a mortality rate of approximately 60%. To determine which factors likely related to survival, they analyzed sex, route of exposure, exposure doses, and pre-existing medical conditions in the survivors and in those who died. They determined that paraquat inhalation is benign because the aerosolized particles do not attain significant alveolar penetration and because patients survived without sequelae when exposed by this route. Percutaneous penetration was more dangerous, but only occasionally were severe intoxications caused by this route. Oral ingestion was the most dangerous, with a mortality rate of 70%. The minimal lethal dose is 35 mg/kg, so one mouthful of a 20% solution may kill a victim. A 50% mortality occurred with one mouthful and 92% mortality with two mouthfuls. In the group with the lower exposure dose, death occurred from pulmonary fibrosis 5 to 31 days after intoxication, whereas the group ingesting the higher dose died within 48 hours from circulatory collapse. In 13 cases, gastric content prior to intoxication could be determined. Only one of five patients poisoned immediately after eating a meal died, whereas seven of eight who were intoxicated at a time unrelated to eating died. Gastric endoscopy was useful in predicting survival because 9 of 14 patients with ulcerations died, and no patient without ulcerations died. Finally, and possibly most important, the plasma level of paraquat was helpful in determining outcome; at 4, 6, 10, 16, and 24 hours after ingestion, patients with levels at or below 2.0, 0.6, 0.3, 0.2, and 0.1 mg/L, respectively, were likely to survive. Renal failure and pulmonary function results had no prognostic value.

Therapeutic interventions that influence prognosis include rapid removal of paraquat from the gastrointestinal tract, although the efficacy of this therapy has not been fully established. Forced renal diuresis does not enhance removal of the herbicide from the blood (Paillard, private communication), and because the pulmonary accumulation of paraquat is so rapid, hemodialysis and hemoperfusion have not regularly improved outcome (Suzuki et al. 1993). Long-term neurological prognosis in the seven survivors of this study was not specified. Because paraquat toxicity relates largely to oxidative-stress mechanisms, antioxidants have been used in experimental models and human treatment, although no detailed studies on relative prognosis have been conducted with these agents (Lheureux et al. 1995). One study showed a significantly reduced degree of respiratory failure and mortality in patients treated with pulse therapy of cyclophosphamide and dexamethasone (Lin et al. 1996). Models based on paraquat toxicological indices and discriminant function scores have been developed to predict prognosis, but have not been tested across multiple populations (Ikebuchi et al. 1993).

## Agent Orange—Dioxin

*Tetrachlorodibenzo-para-dioxin* (TCDD), has been the source of intense controversy in industrial medicine. A large-scale dioxin intoxication occurred in Seveso. Italy, in 1976, although prior episodes had been reported. Dioxin exposure has been associated with skin lesions, including chloracne,

multiple irregularities in blood chemistries, and neurological and psychiatric alterations (Togoni and Bonaccorsi 1982).

Dioxin is a solid substance, insoluble in water, and only slightly soluble in fats and chlorinated solvents. It is a contaminant of such herbicides as Agent Orange. It is highly heat stable and exerts its biological effects at extremely low concentrations. Its half-life in soil is estimated to be approximately 1 year, and microbial degradation rarely occurs. Although there are significant differences in species susceptibility to the toxin, the toxic effect occurs slowly and progresses several days or weeks after a dose. Since the Seveso accident, long-term follow-up has been conducted on intoxicated patients from this group, from a group of 80 patients from Czechoslovakia (Pazderova-Vejlupkova 1981), and from several studies of Vietnam U.S. veterans (Goetz et al. 1994; Committee to Review the Health Effects of Vietnam Veterans of Exposure to Herbicides 1996).

In the Seveso subjects, the earliest symptoms following intoxication were the gradual development of chloracne, a global feeling of sickness, fatigue, and weakness. Usually this occured days or weeks after the initial exposure, but in some patients, these consistent findings did not occur until several months after work with dioxin was completed. In the Czechoslovakian series, 23% of patients exposed to chronic dioxin showed initial evidence by clinical examination or electromyographic study of polyneuropathy. In most cases, the neuropathy progressed and then stabilized after 4 years. In addition, four patients showed signs of facial weakness as evidence of a peripheral seventh cranial nerve lesion. Encephalopathy occurred initially in 7% of the patients and progressed in chronic follow-up to include 9% of those studied. Early psychiatric signs included neurotic symptoms, neurasthenia, and depression occurring in 83% of patients. The latter syndrome tended to decrease in severity and was only present in 58% in long-term follow-up. Other studies have questioned any direct behavioral consequence of dioxin exposure (Hartman 1988).

Importantly, these neuropathic symptoms did not occur initially. Polyneuropathy in some patients occurred only in the third or fourth year after exposure had ceased. The origin of this abnormality and its relation to dioxin exposure are unclear because many of the patients had abnormal glucose tolerance tests and other metabolic abnormalities, including hypercholesterolemia, hyperlipemia, and high pre-beta fractions. Based largely on these findings, and studies of neuropathy in Seveso (Pocchiari et al. 1979) and occupational exposure settings (Sweeney et al. 1984), when an update report on the effects of dioxin on veterans from Vietnam was prepared, subacute/transient peripheral neuropathy was placed in the "Limited/ suggested Evidence of an Association" category (Committee to Review the Health Effects in Vietnam Veterans of Exposure to Herbicides 1997). In contrast, the psychiatric problems were seen early and may have been related to exogenous influences, including fear of death, disfigurement from the cutaneous manifestations, and concerns about job permanency. In a series of patients who were examined by the author (unpublished) and who were exposed to dioxin and other chemicals in an American work setting, 20 to 46 (43%) had an intention tremor, most of the postural type, and more than half had evidence of peripheral neuropathy. Further studies have documented action dystonia that began months or years after chronic exposure started and stabilized thereafter (Klawans 1987). In order to assess long-term outcomes of exposure to dioxin, the Institute of Medicine has regular updates of follow-up on Vietnam veterans.

## References

Adolson, L. Fatal intoxication with isopropyl alcohol (rubbing alcohol). Am. J. Clin. Pathol. 38:144–151; 1962.

Agawal, S. B. A clinical, biochemical, neurobehavioral and sociopsychological study of 190 patients admitted to hospital as a result of acute organophosphorus poisoning. Environ. Res. 62:63–70; 1993.

Allen, N. Solvents and other industrial organic compounds. In: Vinken, P. J.; Bruyn. G., eds. Handbook of clinical neurology. Amsterdam: North Holland; 1979: p. 361–375.

Anetseder, M.; Hartung, E.; Klepper, S.; Reichmann, H. Gasoline vapors induce severe rhabdomyolysis. Neurology 44:2393–2395; 1994.

Arlien-Søberg, P. Chronic effects of organic solvents on the central nervous system and diagnostic criteria. In: Chronic effects of organic solvents on the central nervous system and diagnostic criteria. Copenhagen: World Health Organization: 1985: p. 218–226.

Barnes, R. Poisoning by the insecticide chlordane. Med. J. Aust. 1:972–974; 1967.

Baslo, A.; Aksoy, M. Neurologic abnormalities in chronic benzene poisoning. Environ. Res. 27: 457–465; 1982.

Bennett, I. L.; Cary, F. H.; Mitchell, G. L. Acute methyl alcohol poisoning: a review based on experiences in an outbreak of 323 cases. Medicine 32: 431–463: 1953.

Benton, C. D., Jr.; Calhoun, F. P., Jr. The ocular effects of methyl alcohol poisoning: report of a catastrophe involving three hundred and twenty persons. Trans. Am. Acad. Ophthalmol. Otolaryngol. 56:875–885; 1952.

Berger, J. R.; Ayyar, O. R. Neurological complication of ethylene glycol intoxication. Arch. Neurol. 38: 724–726; 1981.

Berry, G. J.; Heaton, R. K.; Kirby, M. W. Neuropsychological deficits of chronic inhalant abusers. In: Rumack, B. H.; Temple, A. R., eds. Management of the poisoned patient. Princeton: Science Press; 1977: p. 9–31.

Besser, R.; Vogt, T.; Gutmann, L. Pancuronium improves the neuromuscular transmission defect of human organophosphate intoxication. Neurology 40:1275–1277; 1990.

Bismuth, C.; Garnier, R.; Dally, S.; Fournier, P. E. Prognosis and treatment of paraquat poisoning: a review of 28 cases. J. Toxicol. Clin. Toxicol. 19(5): 461–474; 1982.

Bolla, K. I.; Schwartz, B. S.; Stewart, W.; et al. A comparison of neurobehavioral function in workers exposed to a mixture of organic and inorganic lead and in workers exposed to solvents. Am. J. Ind. Med. 27:231–246; 1995.

Brashear, A.; Unverzagt, F. W.; Farber, M. O.; Bonnin, J. M. Ethylene oxide neurotoxicity: a cluster of twelve nurses with peripheral and central nervous system toxicity. Neurology 46:992–998; 1996.

Bravaccio, F.; Ammendola, A.; Barruffo, L.; Carlomagno, S. H-reflex behavior in glue (n-hexane) neuropathy. Clin. Toxicol. 18: 1369–1375; 1981.

Broadley, S. A.; Ferguson, I. T.; Walton, B.; Tomson, C. R. Severe sensorimotor polyneuropathy after ingestion of ethylene glycol. J. Neurol. Neurosurg. Psychiatry 63:261–262; 1997.

Browning, E. Toxicity of industrial organic solvents. London: His Majesty's Stationery Office; 1937.

Bruhn, P.; Arlien-Soborg, A.; Gyldensted, C.; Christensen, E. L. Prognosis in chronic toxic encephalopathy: a two-year follow-up study in 26 house painters with occupational encephalopathy. Acta. Neurol. Scand. 64:259–272; 1981.

Campbell, A. M. G. Neurological complications associated with insecticides and fungicides. Br. Med. J. 2:415–417; 1952.

Cassitto, M. G.; Camerino, D.; Imbriani, M.; Contardi, T. Carbon disulfide and the central nervous system. Environ. Res. 63:252–263; 1993.

Chanarin, I. The effects of nitrous oxide on cobalamins, folates, and other related events. Crit. Rev. Toxicol. 10:179–213; 1982.

Chapman, I. J.; Sauter, S. L., Henning, R. A., Levine, R. L. Finger tremor after carbon disulfide-based pesticide exposures. Arch. Neurol. 48:866–870; 1991.

Cherniak, M. G. Organophosphorus esters and polyneuropathy. Ann. Intern. Med. 104:264–266; 1985.

Chow, M. T.; Chen, J.; Patel, J. S.; Ali, S. Use of a phosphorus-enriched dialysate to hemodialyse patients with ethylene glycol intoxication. Int. J. Artif. Org. 20:101–104; 1997a.

Chow, M. T.; di Silvestro, V. A.; Yng, C. Y.; Nawab, Z. M. Treatment of acute methanol intoxication wth hemodialysis using an ethanol-enriched bicarbonate-based dialysate. Am. J. Kidney Dis. 30:568–570; 1997b.

Chuang, F. R.; Jang, S. W.; Lin, J. L., Chern, M. S. Qtc prolongation indicates a poor prognosis in patients with organophosphate poisoning. Am. J. Emerg. Med. 14:451– 453; 1996.

Cohen, M. M. Neural Toxins. In: Cohen, M. D., ed. Biochemistry of neural disease. Hagerstown, MD: Harper & Row; 1975: p. 220–244.

Committee on Pesticides. Pharmacology and toxicologic aspects of DDT (chlorophenothane, USP). JAMA 145:728–729; 1951.

Committee to Review the Health Effects in Vietnam Veterans of Exposure to Herbicides. Veterans and Agent Orange. Washington, DC: Institute of Medicine; 1997.

Connally, H. E.; Thrall, M. A.; Forney S. D.; Grauer, G. F. Safety and efficacy of 4-methylpyrazole for treatment of suspected or confirmed ethylene glycol intoxication in dogs: 107 cases. J. Am. Vet. Med. Assoc. 209:1880–1883; 1996.

Council of Industrial Health. The recognition and treatment of carbon tetrachloride poisoning. JAMA 132:786–792; 1946.

Cunha, J.; Povoa, P.; Mourao, L.; Santos, A. L. Intoxicacao grave por compostos organofosforados. Acta Med. Port. 8:465–468; 1995.

Dinberg, M. C. Benzene poisoning. Can. Med. Assoc. J. 52:176–179; 1945.

Ekberg, K.; Barregard, L.; Hagberg, S.; Sallsten, S. Chronic and acute effects of solvents on central nervous system functions in floorlayers. Br. J. Ind. Med. 43:101–106; 1986.

Eskelinen, L.; Luisto, M.; Tenkanen, K.; Mattel, O. Neuropsychological methods in the differentiation of organic solvent intoxication from certain neurological conditions. J. Clin. Exp. Neuropsychol. 8: 239–256; 1986.

Fairhall, L. T. Industrial toxicology. Baltimore: Williams & Wilkins: 1949.

Feldman, R. G. Trichloroethylene. In: Vinken, P. J.; Bruyn, G. W., eds. Handbook of clinical neurology. Amsterdam: North Holland; 1979: p. 457–477.

Filley, C. M.; Heston, R. K.; Rosenberg, N. L. White matter dementia in chronic toluene abuse. Neurology 40:532–534; 1990.

Fink, W. H. The ocular pathology of methylalcohol poisoning. Am. J. Ophthalmol. 26:694–698; 1943.

Fogel, R. P. Carbon tetrachloride poisoning treated with hemodialysis and total parenteral nutrition. Can. Med. Assoc. J. 114:560–561; 1983.

Ford, E. S.; Rhodes, S.; McDiarmid, M.; Schwartz, S. L.; Brown, J. Deaths from acute exposure to trichloroethylene. J. Occup. Environ. Med. 37:749–754; 1995.

Garnass, K. R.; Windebank, A. J.; Blexrud, M. D.; Kurtz, S. B. Ultrastructural changes produced in dorsal root ganglia in vitro by exposure to ethylene oxide from hemodialyzers. J. Neuropathol. Exp. Neurol. 50:256–262; 1991.

Garrett, R. M. Toxicity of DDT for man. J. Med. Assoc. State Ala. 17:75–78; 1947.

Gershon, S.; Shaw, F. H. Psychiatric sequelae of chronic exposure to organophosphorus insecticides. Lancet 1:1371–1376; 1961.

Globus, J. H. Histopathologic observations on central nervous system in so-treated monkeys, dogs, cats, and rats. J. Neuropathol. Exp. Neurol. 7:418–422; 1948.

Goetz, C. G. Neurotoxins in clinical practice. New York: SP Medical and Scientific Books; 1985.

Goetz, C. G.; Bolla, K. I.; Rogers, S. M. Neurologic health outcomes and agent orange: Institute of Medicine report. Neurology 44:801–809; 1994.

Gold, J. H. Chronic perchloroethylene poisoning. Can. Psychiatr. Assoc. J. 14:627–630; 1969.

Gordy, S. T.; Trumper, M. Carbon disulfide poisoning. Ind. Med. 9:182–184; 1940.

Graham, D. G.; Amarnath, V.; Valentine, W. M.; Pyle, S. J. Pathogenetic studies of hexane and carbon disulfide neurotoxicity. Crit. Rev. Toxicol. 25:91–112; 1995.

Grandjean, E.; Haas, H. K.; Knoepel, V.; Munchinger, H.; Rosenmund, H.; Turrian, P. A. Investigations into the effects of exposure to trichloroethylene in mechanical engineering. Br. J. Intern. Med. 12:131–138; 1955.

Gross, J. A.; Haas, M. L.; Swift, T. R. Ethylene oxide neurotoxicity: report of four cases and review of the literature. Neurology 29:978–984; 1979.

Gudmundsson, G. Methyl chloride poisoning 13 years later. Arch. Environ. Health 32:236–240; 1977.

Hall, R. H. A new threat to public health: organochlorines and food. Nutr. Health 8:33–43; 1992.

Hardin, B. L., Jr. Carbon tetrachloride poisoning: a review. Ind. Med. 23:93–96; 1954.

Hartman, D. E. Neuropsychological toxicology: identification and assessment of human neurotoxic syndromes. New York: Pergamon Press; 1988.

Hormes, J. T.; Filley, C. M.; Rosenberg, N. L. Neurologic sequelae of chronic solvent vapor abuse. Neurology 36:698–702; 1986.

Huhn, K. M.; Rosenberg, F. M. Critical clue to ethylene glycol poisoning. Can. Med. Assoc. J. 152:193–195; 1995.

Hunt, R. Toxicity of ethylene and prophylene glycol. Ind. Eng. Chem. 24:361–363; 1932.

Ikebuchi, J.; Proudfoot, A. T.; Matsubara, K.; Hampson, E. C. Toxicological index of paraquat: a new strategy for assessment of severity of paraquat poisoning in 128 patients. Forensic Sci. Int. 59:85–87; 1993.

Juntunen, J. Neurological examination and assessment of the syndromes caused by exposure to neurotoxic agents. In: Gilioli, R.; Cassitto, M. G.; Foa, V., eds. Neurobehavioral methods in occupational health. New York: Pergamon Press; 1982: p. 3–10.

Kahn, H.; Muzyka, V. Chronic effect of benzene on porphyrin metabolism. Work Environ. Health 10: 140–143; 1973.

Kaplan, A.; Levreault, G. V. Methyl alcohol poisoning: report of 42 cases. U.S. Navy Med. Bull. 44:1107–1109; 1944.

Karlson-Stiber, C.; Persson, H. Ethylene glycol poisoning: experiences from an epidemic in Sweden. J. Toxicol. Clin. Toxicol. 31:499–500; 1993.

Kazantzis, G.; Bomford, R. R. Dyspepsia due to inhalation of carbon tetrachloride vapor. Lancet 1: 360–364; 1960.

Keane, J. R. Toluene optic neuropathy. Ann. Neurol. 4:390–394; 1978.

Kegel, A. H.; McNally, W. E.; Pope, A. S. Methyl chloride poisoning from domestic refrigerators. JAMA 93:353–358; 1929.

King, M. Long-term neuropsychological effects of solvent abuse. In: Cherry, N.; Waldron, H. A., eds. The neuropsychological effects of solvent exposure. Havant, Hampshire: Colt Foundation; 1983: p. 75–84.

Klawans, H. L. Dystonia and tremor following exposure to 2,3,7,8-Tetrachlorodibenzo-p-dioxin. Mov. Disord. 2:255–261; 1987.

Klein, H. Zur pathologischen Histologie nach akuter Benzinvergiftung. Dtsch. Z. Ges. Gerichtl. Med. 40:76–79; 1950.

Koskela, R. S. Cardiovascular diseases among foundry workers exposed to carbon monoxide. Scand. J. Work Environ. Health 20:286–293; 1994.

Kostrzewski, P.; Jakubowski, M.; Kolacinski, Z. Kinetics of trichloroethylene elimination from venous blood after acute inhalation poisoning. J. Toxicol. Clin. Toxicol. 31:353–363; 1993.

Krolman, G. M.; Pidde, W. J. Acute methyl alcohol poisoning. Can. J. Ophthalmol. 3:270–278; 1968.

Lawrence, R. A.; Haggerty, R. J. Household agents and their potential toxicity. Mod. Treat. 8:511–514; 1971.

Layzer, R. B.; Fishman, R. A.; Schaefer, J. A. Neuropathy following abuse of nitrous oxide. Neurology 28:504–508; 1978.

Lewis, L. D.; Smith, B. W.; Mamourain, A. C. Delayed sequelae after acute overdoses or poisoning: cranial neuropathy related to ethylene glycol ingestion. Clin. Pharmacol. Ther. 61:692–699; 1997.

LeWitt, P. A.; Martin, S. D. Dystonia and hypokinesia with putaminal necrosis after methanol intoxication. Clin. Neuropharmacol. 2: 161–167; 1988.

Lheuruex, P.; Leduc, D.; Vanbinst, R.; Askenasi, R. Survival of a case of massive paraquat ingestion. Chest 107:285–289; 1995.

Lin, J. L.; Wei, M. C.; Liu, Y. C. Pulse therapy with cyclophosphamide and methylprednisolone in patients with moderate to severe paraquat poisoning. Thorax 51:659–660; 1996.

Lindstrom, K.; Marbelin, T. Personality and long-term exposure to organic solvents. Neurobehav. Toxicol. 2:89–100; 1982.

Liss, G. M.; Finkelstein, M. M. Mortality among workers exposed to carbon disulfide. Arch. Environ. Health 51:193–200; 1996.

Lotti, M. Pralidoxine in parathion poisoning. J. Toxicol. Clin. Toxicol. 19:121–124; 1982.

Lotti, M. Biological monitoring for organophosphate-induced delayed polyneuropathy. Toxicol. Lett. 33:167–172; 1986.

Louria, D. B.; Bogden, J. D. The dangers from limited exposure to carbon tetrachloride. Crit. Rev. Toxicol. 72:177–188; 1980.

MacDonald, J. D. C. Methyl chloride intoxication: report of 8 cases. J. Occup. Med. 6: 81–89; 1964.

Mackerras, I. M.; West, R. F. K. DDT poisoning in man. Med. J. Aust. 1:400–414; 1946.

Manno, M.; Rezzadore, M.; Grossi, M.; Sbrana, C. Potentiation of occupational carbon tetrachloride toxicity by ethanol abuse. J. Exp. Toxicol. 15:294–300; 1996.

Martin-Amat, G.; McMartin, K. E.; Hayreh, M. S.; Tephly, R. R. Methanol poisoning: ocular toxicity produced by formate. Toxicol. Appl. Pharmacol. 45:201–205; 1978.

McClain, R. M.; Becker, B. A. Teratogenicity, fetal toxicity and placental transfer of lead nitrate in rats. Toxicol. Appl. Pharmacol. 31: 72–78; 1975.

McKellar, M. J.; Hidajat, R. R.; Elder, M. J. Acute ocular methanol toxicity—clinical and electrophysiological features. Aust. N. Z. J. Ophthalmol. 25:225–230; 1997.

McLean, D. R.; Jacobs, H.; Mielke, B. W. Methanol poisoning. Ann. Neurol. 8:161–167; 1980.

Melamed, E.; Levy, S. Parkinsonism associated with chronic inhalation of carbon tetrachloride. Lancet 1:1015–1117; 1977.

Mennear, J. H. Carbon monoxide and cardiovascular disease: an analysis of the weight of the evidence. Regul. Toxicol. Pharmacol. 17:77–84; 1993.

Midtling, J. E.; Barnett, P. G.; Coye, M. J. Clinical management of field worker organophosphate poisoning. West. J. Med. 142:514–518; 1985.

Mittal, B. V.; Desai, A. P.; Khade, K. R. Methyl alcohol poisoning: an autopsy study of 28 cases. J. Postgrad. Med. 37:9–13; 1991.

Morbidity and Mortality Weekly Report. Fatalities associated with ingestion of diethylene glycol-contaminated glycerin used to manufacture acetaminophen syrup: Haiti. MMWR Morbid. Mortal. Wkly. Rep. 5:649–650; 1996.

Morgan, E. C.; Wyatt, J. P.; Sutherland, R. B. An episode of carbon tetrachloride poisoning with renal complications. Can. Med. Assoc. J. 60:145–148; 1949.

Namba, T.; Nolte, C.; Jackrel, J.; Grob, D. Poisoning due to organophosphate insecticides. Am. J. Med. 50:475–492; 1971.

Nestor, P. J.; Stark, R. J. Vitamin B12 myeloneuropathy precipitated by nitrous oxide anaesthesia. Med. J. Aust. 165:174; 1996.

Nouira, S.; Aboug, F.; Elastrous, S. Prognostic value of serum cholinesterase in organophosphate poisoning. Chest 106:1811–1814; 1994.

O'Donoghue, J. L. Neurotoxicity of industrial and commercial chemicals (2 volumes). Boca Raton, FL: CRC Press; 1985.

Oge, A. M.; Yazici, J.; Boyaciyan, A. Peripheral and central conduction in n-hexane polyneuropathy. Muscle Nerve 17:1416–1430; 1994.

Osterloh, J. D.; Pond, S. M.; Grady, S.; Becker, C. E. Serum formate concentrations in methanol intoxication as a criterion for hemodialysis. Ann. Intern. Med. 104:200–203; 1986.

Palatnick, W.; Redman, L. W.; Sitar, D. S. Methanol half-life during ethanol administration: implications for management of ethanol poisoning. Ann. Emerg. Med. 26:202–207; 1995.

Pastore, C.; Marhuenda, D.; Marti, J.; Cardona, A. Early diagnosis of n-hexane-caused neuropathy. Muscle Nerve 17:981–986; 1994.

Pazderova-Vejlupkova. J. Development and prognosis of chronic intoxication by tetrachlorodibenzo-p-dioxin in men. Arch. Environ. Health 36:5–11; 1981.

Pederson, W.; Nygaard, E.; Nielson, O. Solvent-induced occupational myopathy. Occup. Med. 22: 603–607; 1980.

Peterson, C. D.; Collins, A. J.; Himes, J. M.; Bullock, M. L.; et al. Ethylene glycol poisoning. N. Engl. J. Med. 304:21–23; 1981.

Petry, H. Polyneuritis durch E 605. Zbl Arbeitsmed 1:86. Cited in Arch. Indust. Hyg. 6:461–470; 1952.

Pezzoli, G. Parkinsonism due to n-hexane exposure. Lancet 2:874; 1989.

Pezzoli, G.; Masotto, C.; Perbellini, L.; Mariani, C. B. Are endogenous hydrocarbons associated with Parkinson's disease? Ann. Neurol. 41:121; 1991.

Pocchiari, F.; Silano, V.; Zampieri, A. Human health effects from accidental release of TCDD at Seveso, Italy. Ann. N. Y. Acad. Sci. 320:311–320; 1979.

Procktop, L. D.; Alt. M.; Tison, J. Huffer's neuropathy. JAMA 229:1083–1084; 1974.

Rainey, P. M. Clinical problem solving: the landlady confirms the diagnosis. N. Engl. J. Med. 327:895–896; 1992.

Ritchie, J. M. The aliphatic alcohols. In: Gilman, A. G.; Goodman, L. S., eds. The pharmacological basis of therapeutics. New York: MacMillan Publishing Co.; 1975: p. 372–386.

Roe, O. Past, present and future fight against methanol blindness and death. Trans. Ophthalmol. Soc. U.K. 89:235; 1969.

Roe, O. The metabolism and toxicity of methanol. Pharmacol. Rev. 7:399–412; 1955.

Roe, O. Clinical investigations of methyl alcohol poisoning with special reference to the pathogenesis and treatment of amblyopia. Acta Med. Scand. 113:558–608; 1953.

Rosansky, S. J. Isopropyl alcohol poisoning treated with hemodialysis: kinetics of isoprophyl alcohol and acetone removal. J. Toxicol. Clin. Toxicol. 19(3):265–270; 1982.

Rosenberg, N. L.; Spitz, M. C.; Filley, C. M.; Schaumburg, H. H. Central nervous system effects of chronic toluene inhalation: Clinical. brainstem evokes response, and MRI studies. Neurology 38(suppl.): 113–120; 1988.

Rumack, B. H. Methanol. In: Rumack, B. H., ed. Poisindex. Denver: Micromedex; 1976.

Sahenk, Z.; Mendell, J. R.; Co4uri, D.; Nachman, J. Generalized polyneuropathy: Inhalation of $N_2O$. Neurology 28:485–492; 1978.

Sanberr, G. E.; Selhorst, J. B.; Calabrese, V. P.; Taylor, J. R. Pseudotumor cerebri and insecticide intoxication. Neurology 29:1222–1228; 1979.

Sauerhoff, M. W.; Michaelson, I. A. Hyperactivity and brain catecholamines in lead-exposed developing rats. Science 182:1022–1024; 1973.

Senanayake, N. Acute polyneuropathy after poisoning by a new organophosphate insecticide. N. Engl. J. Med. 306:155–170; 1982.

Senanayake, N.; Sanmuganathan, P. S. Extrapyramidal manifestation complicating organophosphorus insecticide poisoning. Hum. Exp. Toxicol. 14:600–604; 1995.

Scharnweber, H. C.; Spears, G. N.; Cowles, S. R. Chronic methyl chloride intoxication in six industrial workers. J. Occup. Med. 16: 112–118; 1974.

Schneck, S. A. Methyl alcohol. In: Vinken, P. J.: Bruyn, G. W., eds. Handbook of clinical neurology: intoxications of the nervous system. Amsterdam: North-Holland Publishing Company; 1979: p. 351–360.

Seage, A. J.; Bruns, M. W. Pulmonary edema following exposure to trichloroethylene. Med. J. Aust. 2: 484–487; 1971.

Smith, J. S.; Brandon, S. Morbidity from acute carbon monoxide poisoning at three-year follow-up. Br. Med. J. 1:318–321; 1973.

Spencer, P. S.; Couri, D.; Schaumburg, H. H. N-hexane and methyl n-butyl ketone. In: Spencer, P. S.; Schaumburg, H. H., eds. Experimental and clinical neurotoxicology. Baltimore: Williams & Wilkins; 1980: p. 456–475.

Spencer, P. S.; Schaumburg, H. H. Organic solvent neurotoxicity. Facts and research needs. Scand. J. Work Environ. Health 53 (suppl. 1):53–60; 1985a.

Spencer, P. S.; Schaumburg, H. H., eds. Experimental and clinical neurotoxicology. Baltimore: Williams & Wilkins; 1985b.

Stacy, C. B.; Di Rocco, A.; Gould, R. J. Methionine in the treatment of nitrous-oxide induced neuropathy and myeloneuropathy. J. Neurol. 239:401–403; 1992.

Steenland, K.; Jenkins, B.; Ames, R. G.; O'Malley, M. Chronic neurological sequelae to organophosphate pesticide poisoning. AM. J. Public Health 84:731–736; 1994.

Stewart, A.; Witts, L. J. Chronic carbon tetrachloride intoxication. Br. J. Indust. Med. 1:11–40; 1944.

Stoller, A.; Krupinski, J.; Christophers, A. J.; Blanks, G. K. Organophosphorus insecticides and major mental illness. An epidemiological investigation. Lancet 1:1387–1389; 1965.

Sweeney, M. H.; Fingerhut, M. A.; Arezzo, C. Peripheral neuropathy after occupational exposure to TCDD. JAMA 251:2372–2380; 1984.

Suzuki, K.; Takasu, N.; Okabe, T.; Ishimatsu, S. Effect of aggressive haemoperfusion on the clinical course of patients with paraquat poisoning. Hum. Exp. Toxicol. 12:323–327; 1993.

Szlatenyi, C. S.; Wang, R. Y. Encephalopathy and cranial nerve palsies caused by intentional trichloroethylene inhalation. Am. J. Emerg. Med. 14:464–466; 1996.

Taylor, J. R.; Calabrese, V. P. Organochlorine and other insecticides. In: Vinken, P. J.: Bruyn, G. W., eds. Handbook of clinical neurology: intoxications of the nervous system. Amsterdam: North-Holland; 1979; p. 391–455.

Taylor, J. R.; Selhorst, J. B.; Houff, S. A.; Martinez, A. J. Chlordecone intoxication in man. Neurology 28:626–629; 1978.

Teitelbaum, D. T.; Morgan, J.; Gray, G. Nonconcordance between clinical impression and laboratory findings in clinical toxicology. Clin. Toxicol. 10: 417–422; 1977.

Teo, S. K.; Lo, K. L.; Tey, B. H. Mass methanol poisoning: a clinico-biochemical analysis of ten cases. Singapore Med. J. 37:485–487; 1996.

Tetrud, J. W.; Langston, J. W.; Irwin, I. Acute and persistant parkinsonism associated with ingestion of petroleum product mixture. Ana. Neurol. 28:296; 1990.

Thompson, J. P.; Casey, P. B.; Vale, J. A. Deaths from pesticide poisoning in England and Wales 1990–1991. Hum. Exp. Toxicol. 13:437–445; 1995.

Thompson, J. W.; Stocks, R. M. Brief bilateral vocal cord paralysis after insecticide poisoning: a new variant of toxicity syndromes. Arch. Otelaryngol. Head Neck Surg. 123:93–96; 1997.

Togoni, C.; Bonaccorsi, A. Epidemiological problems with TCDD (a critical review). Drug Metab. Rev. 13:447–469; 1982.

Towfighi, J.; Gonatas, N. K.; Pleasure, D.; Cooper, H. S.; McCree, L. Glue sniffer's neuropathy. Neurology 26:238–242; 1976.

Vale, J. A.; Widdop, B.; Bluett, N. H. Ehtylene glycol poisoning. Postgrad. Med. J. 52:598–603; 1976.

Valpey, R.; Sumi, S. M.; Compass, M. K.; Goble, G. J. Acute and chronic progressive encephalopathy due to gasoline sniffing. Neurology 281:507–511; 1978.

Vivier, P. M.; Lewander, W. J.; Martin, H. F.; Linakis, J. G. Isopropyl alcohol intoxication in a neonate through chronic dermal exposure. Pediatr. Emerg. Care 10:91–93; 1994.

Westerman, M. P.; Pfitzer, E.; Ellis, L. D.; Jensen, W. N. Concentration of lead in bones in plumbism. N. Engl. J. Med. 273:1246–1248; 1965.

Winek, C. L.; Wecht, C. H.; Collom, W. D. Toluene fatality from glue sniffing. Pa. Med. 71:81–84; 1968.

Wislicki, L. Differences in the effect of oximes on striated muscle and respiratory centre. Arch. Int. Pharmacodyn. Ther. 129:443–448; 1960.

Yamamura, Y. N-hexane polyneuropathy. Folia Psychiatr. Neurol. Jpn. 23: 45–48; 1969.

# 33

# Metals and Neurological Disease

ANTHONY J. WINDEBANK

The metals discussed in this section are not known to have biological functions. They are all toxic to some extent; nervous system toxicity is often prominent. The type of toxicity depends on the type and the chemical state of the metal. Route of ingestion or absorption also may be important in determining toxicity. All of the toxic effects of metals are reversible to some extent, and therefore it is important to determine whether a specific neurological manifestation can be linked to a metal exposure or an elevated body fluid level of a particular metal. The ubiquitous "urine heavy metal screen" obtained for every patient with peripheral neuropathy must detect hundreds of false-positive results for every true metal-induced neuropathy. Detailed reviews of the diagnostic strategies for metal toxin–induced neurological disease are available elsewhere (Windebank et al. 1984; Windebank 1987). For this review, it is assumed that a well-established diagnosis of metal-induced neurological disease has been made.

## Arsenic

Acute arsenic poisoning is almost always due to ingestion of inorganic arsenic salts. Many cases involve intentional poisoning. After a single significant dose of arsenic, the patient usually develops nausea, vomiting, and diarrhea within hours. This may proceed rapidly to death due to circulatory collapse. If the dose is not lethal, the gastrointestinal symptoms may subside within a few days. Massive but not fatal poisoning may result in a transient generalized encephalopathy with somnolence, stupor, or delirium. This delirious state may be accompanied by paranoid ideation (Danan et al. 1984; Windebank et al. 1984). These central effects clear rapidly if repeated exposure does not occur.

Skin changes, including palmar erythema and scaling, appear within days of exposure and often accompany the onset of peripheral nerve symptoms. The appearance of neuropathic symptoms may be delayed for several weeks after a single acute exposure (Le Quesne and McLeod 1977). The neuropathy may progress for days to weeks and then stabilize. It is characterized by distal to proximal progression of pain, sensory loss, and weakness that begins in the lower limbs and spreads to the upper limbs. Maximum deficit is usually established after 6 weeks.

Because of the temporal profile, an initial clinical diagnosis of acute inflammatory demyelinating polyradiculoneuropathy (Guillain-Barre syndrome) is often entertained. Arsenic neuropathy is distinguished by the distal to proximal progression and the skin and nail changes. The diagnosis should be further suspected if the cerebrospinal fluid (CSF) protein level is close to normal (<100 mg/dl) and electrophysiological changes suggest an axonal neuropathy.

The diagnosis is established by observation of elevated arsenic excretion in the urine. Blood arsenic levels increase acutely but decrease rapidly, with a half-life of 6 hours. Urine levels may be extremely high (>10,000 µg/24 hr) for the first few days after ingestion and fall to normal within several weeks (half-time for excretion is 6 to 8 days). If the patient is seen weeks after the putative exposure, then estimation of hair or nail arsenic content is useful. This estimation is particularly useful in the patient with a borderline elevation of urine arsenic levels (25 to 200 µg/24 hr). Such levels may be induced by ingestion of seafood during or immediately before urine collection. The arsenic from seafood is pentavalent, relatively nontoxic, and not deposited in the keratin of hair and nails. Reliable analytical methods are now available to distinguish between organic, nontoxic urinary arsenic (from seafood), and toxic inorganic forms of the metal.

If arsenic poisoning is diagnosed within a few days of exposure, treatment with chelating agents, such as British antilewisite (BAL) or ethylenediametetraacetic acid (EDTA), may be considered. However, if the acute systemic illness has resolved and the neuropathy is not progressing, there is probably no advantage in attempting to increase the excretion rate.

The prognosis for recovery of the neuropathy depends on the severity of nerve damage. Electrophysiological and biopsy studies confirm that the major pathological process in nerve is axonal degeneration (Dyck et al. 1968; Le Quesne and McLeod 1977). The process of recovery occurs over months to years. Maximal recovery may not be achieved for 3 to 4 years, and in severe cases, is incomplete.

## Lead

There are three main types of lead-induced neurological disease: (1) lead encephalopathy in infants due to ingestion of inorganic lead compounds; (2) lead encephalopathy in adults due to ingestion of organic lead compounds; and (3) lead neuropathy due to ingestion of inorganic lead compounds.

### Lead Encephalopathy in Infants

Encephalopathy occurs in infants who are becoming mobile and is almost invariably associated with pica. Lead is ingested from paint flakes and dust in older houses. For unknown reasons, the encephalopathy usually presents during the early summer months. Prodromal symptoms include gastrointestinal upset and headache, followed rapidly by behavioral alterations, lethargy, confusion, and coma. Physical signs during the acute illness include confusion, ataxia, and convulsions with increased intracranial pressure. The individual rate of progression through the symptoms appears to depend on the quantity of lead ingested. The mortality for children who developed frank encephalopathy with raised intracranial pressure has been high (10% to 50%) (Sachs et al. 1970). It is probable that with modern intensive care techniques and intracranial pressure monitoring, the mortality rate is significantly lower; however, there are no recent studies to confirm this.

Acute treatment involves systemic circulatory support and aggressive management of raised intracranial pressure. It is advantageous to promote lead excretion. In children with encephalopathy, BAL should be given intramuscularly (75 mg/m$^2$ every 4 hours) for 4 to 5 days, accompanied by intravenous EDTA (1500 mg/m$^2$/d) for the same period (Piomelli et al. 1984). Convulsions should be treated with phenobarbital. Many children with lead poisoning are anemic and iron deficient. This enhances the absorption of lead and should be investigated and treated appropriately. Subclinical renal impairment usually recovers without long-term sequelae.

Recovery from the acute illness is good, but 20% of children who survive may have a chronic seizure disorder or impairment of intellectual function. Long-term follow-up is extremely important to identify and manage these potential deficits. It is also important to monitor blood lead levels longitudinally. The lead exposure is environmental and tends to be more prevalent in children with fewer socioeconomic advantages. These children are at risk for significant re-exposure.

### Lead Encephalopathy in Adults

Inorganic lead salts in old paint and in environmental dust from lead-supplemented gasoline do not produce encephalopathy in adults; ionic lead does not readily cross the blood-brain barrier.

Organic lead compounds, such as tetraethyl lead, rapidly enter the brain after ingestion and produce a severe encephalopathy that has many features resembling the childhood disease. It is managed in the same way. Most cases are due to intentional ingestion, and if large quantities are absorbed, the prognosis is poor.

## Lead Neuropathy

Classic lead neuropathy due to chronic exposure to inorganic salts of lead is extremely rare. This clinical entity was common when silver was mined without protective industrial hygiene. Lead compounds were commonly found with silver deposits. The reduced use of lead in paints and plumbing materials has also contributed to the disappearance of this type of neuropathy. Occasionally, cases are seen, and the criteria for diagnosis have been described in detail elsewhere (Windebank et al. 1984).

The neuropathy is unusual because the upper limbs are affected first with prominent asymmetrical weakness of the wrist and finger extensor muscles. Peroneal weakness may be the first sign in children who develop lead neuropathy (Seto and Freeman 1964; Sachs et al. 1970). Identification and removal of the source of exposure are the most important aspects of treatment. Improvement of the neuropathy is the rule, but it may not be complete in severe cases.

## Thallium

Thallium was used therapeutically as a depilatory in the treatment of ringworm in children. Munch (1934) pointed out that the incidence of neurological side effects was extremely high. These salts are no longer used therapeutically, but they are still available in pest control products. As with arsenic, most cases of thallium intoxication are due to poisoning or intentional self-administration. The clinical effects of thallium administration are similar to those of arsenic poisoning. Severe systemic illness occurs within hours of ingestion. This may involve vomiting, diarrhea, renal impairment, circulatory collapse, and abnormalities of liver function. If the patient survives this acute illness, neuropathic symptoms begin distally after several days and spread proximally over days to weeks. The most distinct feature of thallium poisoning is hair loss, which begins 2 to 3 weeks after ingestion. This hair loss occurs over the whole body.

The best treatment of thallitoxicosis is unclear. The acute systemic illness often overshadows the neurological manifestations. Thallium appears to be less toxic than arsenic to sensory neurons in vitro (Windebank 1986). This may explain why death from systemic collapse occurs rather than survival with peripheral neuropathy (Cavanagh et al. 1974; Davis et al. 1981). Use of chelating agents has not been helpful. There is some evidence that $Tl^+$ interferes with $K^+$ metabolism, and some authors have suggested the use of intravenous potassium to accelerate thallium excretion. There is no good evidence that this helps, and it may be impractical or dangerous with renal failure. A more rational and safer therapy involves oral or nasogastric administration of potassium ferric ferrocyanide II (Prussian blue). This compound is not absorbed by the gut, but the $K^+$ is replaced by $Tl^+$, which is strongly bound and thus unabsorbable. This prevents further absorption of thallium and may lead to increased excretion through the gastrointestinal tract.

Very few cases of thallium poisoning are recognized before death, and it is probable that cases are not diagnosed even at autopsy (Cavanagh et al. 1974). If the patient survives the acute systemic illness and neurological signs develop, these may not be reversible. There is autopsy evidence that thallium produces both peripheral and central (posterior column) degeneration in humans (Cavanagh et al. 1974). This central injury is unlikely to recover.

## Gold

Gold salts are used in the treatment of rheumatoid arthritis. Evidence from animal (Katrak et al. 1980) and human studies (Meyer et al. 1978; Katrak et al. 1980) shows that these salts may produce a distal symmetrical neuropathy. It may be difficult to distinguish from neuropathy caused by the underlying rheumatoid disease. The neuropathy may be accompanied by electrophysiological evidence of myokymia. Observation of this phenomenon is distinctive for gold intoxication. If the diagnostic question cannot be resolved, then the therapy should be discontinued. Gold-induced neuropathy appears to be readily reversible.

## Mercury

The type of clinical disorder produced by mercury intoxication depends on the molecular form of the element. Chronic exposure to very low doses of short-chain alkyl mercury compounds (ethyl mercury and methyl mercury) results in prominent irreversible central nervous system damage. This includes constriction of visual fields, ataxia, dysarthria, decreased hearing, tremor, and mental impairment. Several major outbreaks of organic mercury poisoning have occurred as a result of eating grain treated with mercury-containing fungicides. A major epidemic was recognized when inorganic mercury salts in industrial effluent were discarded in Minamata Bay, Japan. These compounds were metabolized to organic mercurials by marine micro-organisms, and entered the food chain, resulting in hundreds of deaths and thousands of cases of severe permanent neurological disability (Kurland et al. 1960).

Elemental mercury exposure usually occurs through inhalation of mercury vapor. Metallic mercury is quite volatile at room temperature. In an enclosed space, exposed liquid mercury will produce toxic levels of vapor in the air. Chronic exposure may produce depression or mood changes, tremor, and occasionally a progressive motor neuropathy (Swaiman and Flagler 1971; Windebank 1987). All of these manifestations are reversible if the source of exposure is eliminated.

## Other Metals

Aluminum in the water supply has been implicated as a toxin in some individuals on chronic hemodialysis. These patients present with a rapidly progressive encephalopathy. Early signs include episodes of speech arrest, myoclonus, dysarthria, and ataxia. Once the role of aluminum is recognized, reduction in body aluminum load results in some improvement in the symptoms of "dialysis dementia." The incidence of this disorder has decreased since dialysis units started to monitor aluminum levels. Occasionally, patients with relatively normal aluminum balance present with the same clinical picture. Thus, other metabolic derangements can produce the same disorder.

Bismuth has been reported to produce an encephalopathy. Bismuth salts have been used for years in the treatment of diarrhea. They were most popular in France and Australia, and the most extensive series of case reports (Burns et al. 1974; Buge and Rancurel 1975; Supino-Viterbo et al. 1977) come from these countries. Patients were given insoluble bismuth salts (such as bismuth subgallate) by mouth but would develop high blood bismuth levels. There were various reasons suggested for the solubilization of the salts in the gastrointestinal tract. The encephalopathy presented with myoclonic jerks, dysarthria, and ataxia. It had many features in common with aluminum encephalopathy. Most patients appeared to recover when the bismuth was excreted. In an experimental study, Basinger and colleagues (Basinger et al. 1983) demonstrated that D-penicillamine is the chelating agent that most rapidly promotes bismuth excretion.

Cadmium produces hemorrhagic lesions in the brain and spinal ganglia of experimental animals. It is not known to produce any nervous system disease in humans. Itai-itai is a disease produced by chronic cadmium poisoning. It involves severe bone pain that may produce gait disorders not due to neurological involvement (Tischner 1980).

Manganese toxicity occurs almost exclusively in people who work in manganese mining, ore extraction, or smelting. There have been a number of detailed reviews concerning the metabolism and clinical manifestations produced by exposure to the dust of this metal (Mena 1979; Piscator 1979). The major features are pulmonary irritation, behavioral changes, mood changes, and an extrapyramidal syndrome. The latter is characterized by loss of postural reflexes, rigidity, masked facies, dysarthria, tremor, and occasionally dystonic posturing. The early manifestations may be reversed by removing the patient from the exposure. Once the extrapyramidal syndrome is established, it usually is not reversible. It is responsive to treatment with levodopa (Mena 1979).

Tin is not toxic in metallic or inorganic forms. Organic tin compounds, however, produce central and peripheral nervous system disorders in humans and experimental animals. The most usual toxic forms are the short-chain alkyl derivatives (e.g., dimethyl and trimethyl tin and tetraethyl tin). These compounds have widespread industrial use in plastic manufacturing and as catalysts. In animals, organotin compounds produce central nervous system demyelination in low doses and peripheral nervous system demyelination in high doses (Blaker et al. 1981). A large epidemic of organotin poisoning occurred in France in 1953. Approximately 210 people took a tin-containing remedy (probably triethyl tin) for treatment of skin infections (Alajouanine et al. 1958). One hundred people died, and autopsy demonstrated widespread intramyelinic edema (Cossa and Radermecker 1958; Foncin and Gruner 1979). Trimethyl tin intoxication (Besser et al. 1987) appears to cause neuronal damage in the central nervous system, producing a limbic-cerebellar syndrome.

Severe intoxication produces death. Patients with significant neurological deficit from trimethyl or triethyl tin do not recover, while those with only mild behavioral changes improve to normal. Besser and colleagues (Besser et al. 1987) treated three of their six patients with plasma exchange, but it was not clear if this altered the course of the disease.

**Acknowledgment.** The expert secretarial assistance of Ms. Linda A. Goldbeck is most gratefully acknowledged.

# References

Alajouanine, T.; Dérobert, L.; Thiéffry, S. Étude clinique d'ensemble de 120 cas d'intoxication par les sels organiques d'étain. Rev. Neurol. (Paris) 98: 85–96; 1958.

Basinger, M. A.; Jones, M. M.; McCroskey, S. A. Antidotes for acute bismuth intoxication. J. Toxicol. Clin. Toxicol. 20:159–165; 1983.

Besser, R.; Krämer, G.; Thümler, R.; Bohl, J.; Gutmann, L.; Hopf, H. C. Acute trimethyltin limbic-cerebellar syndrome. Neurology 37:945–950; 1987.

Blaker, W. D.; Krigman, M. R.; Thomas, D. J.; Mushak, P.; Morell, P. Effect of triethyl tin on myelination in the developing rat. J. Neurochem. 36: 44–52; 1981.

Buge, A.; Rancurel, G. Les encéphalopathies aigues myocloniques par les sels oraux de bismuth. Rev. Med. (Paris) 24:1668–1674; 1975.

Burns, R.; Thomas, D. W.; Barron, V. J. Reversible encephalopathy possibly associated with bismuth subgallate ingestion. Br. Med. J. 1:220–223; 1974.

Cavanagh, J. B.; Fuller, N. H.; Johnson, H. R. M.; Rudge, P. The effects of thallium salts, with particular reference to the nervous system changes. A report of three cases. Q. J. Med. 43:293–319; 1974.

Cossa, P.; Radermecker, J. Encéphalopathies toxiques au Stalinon (aspects anatomo-cliniques et électro-encéphalographiques). Rev. Neurol. (Paris) 98: 97–108; 1958.

Danan, M.; Dally, S.; Conso, F. Arsenic-induced encephalopathy. Neurology 34: 1524; 1984.

Davis, L. E.; Standefer, J. C.; Kornfeld, M.; Abercrombie, D. M.; Butler, C. Acute thallium poisoning: toxicological and morphological studies of the nervous system. Ann. Neurol. 10:38–44; 1981.

Dyck, P. J.; Gutrecht, J. A.; Bastron, J. A.; Karnes, W. E.; Dale, A. J. D. Histologic and teased-fiber measurements of sural nerve in disorders of lower motor and primary sensory neurons. Mayo Clin. Proc. 43:81–123; 1968.

Foncin, J. F.; Gruner, J. E. Tin neurotoxicity. In: Vinken, P. J.; Bruyn, G. W., eds. Handbook of clinical neurology. Vol. 36. New York: Elsevier North-Holland; 1979: p. 279–290.

Katrak, S. M.; Pollock, M.; O'Brien, C. P.; Nukada, H.; Allpress, S.; Calder, C.; Palmer, D. G.; Grennan, D. M.; McCormack, P. L.; Laurent, M. R. Clinical and morphological features of gold neuropathy. Brain 103: 671–693; 1980.

Kurland, L. T.; Faro, S. N.; Siedler, H. Minamata disease. The outbreak of a neurologic disorder in Minamata, Japan, and its relationship to the ingestion of seafood contaminated by mercuric compounds. World Neurol. 1:370–391; 1960.

Le Quesne, P. M.; McLeod, J. G. Peripheral neuropathy following a single exposure to arsenic. Clincal course in four patients with electrophysiological and histological studies. J. Neurol. Sci. 32:437–451; 1977.

Mena, I. Manganese poisoning. In: Vinken, P. J.; Bruyn, G. W., eds. Handbook of clinical neurology. Vol. 36. New York: Elsevier North-Holland. 1979: p. 217–237.

Meyer, M.; Haecki, M.; Ziegler, W.; Forster, W.; Schiller, H. H. Autonomic dysfunction and myokymia in gold neuropathy. In: Canal, N.; Pozza, G., eds. Peripheral neuropathies. Amsterdam: Elsevier/North-Holland Biomedical Press; 1978: p. 475–480.

Munch, J. C. Human thallotoxicosis. JAMA 102:1929–1934; 1934.

Piomelli, S.; Rosen, J. F.; Chisolm, J. J., Jr.; Graef, J. W. Management of childhood lead poisoning. J. Pediatr. 105:523–532; 1984.

Piscator, M. Manganese. In: Friberg, L.; Nordberg, G. F.; Vouk, V. B., eds. Handbook on the toxicology of metals. New York: Elsevier/North-Holland Biomedical Press; 1979: p. 485–501.

Sachs, H. K.; Blanksma, L. A.; Murray, E. F.; O'Connell, M. J. Ambulatory treatment of lead poisoning: report of 1,155 cases. Pediatrics 46:389–396; 1970.

Seto, D. S. Y.; Freeman, J. M. Lead neuropathy in childhood. Am. J. Dis. Child. 107:337–342; 1964.

Supino-Viterbo, V.; Sicard, C.; Risvegliato, M.; Rancurel, G.; Buge, A. Toxic encephalopathy due to ingestion of bismuth salts: clinical and EEG studies of 45 patients. J. Neurol. Neurosurg. Psychiatry 40: 748–752; 1977.

Swaiman, K. F.; Flagler, D. G. Penicillamine therapy of the Guillain-Barré syndrome caused by mercury poisoning. Neurology 21:456–457; 1971.

Tischner, K. Cadmium. In: Spencer, P. S.; Schaumburg, H. H., eds. Experimental and clinical neurotoxicology. Baltimore: Williams & Wilkins; 1980: p. 348–355.

Windebank, A. J. Specific inhibition of myelination by lead *in vitro;* comparison with arsenic, thallium, and mercury. Exp. Neurol. 94:203–212; 1986.

Windebank, A. J. Peripheral neuropathy due to chemical and industrial exposure. In: Matthews, W. B.,

ed. Handbook of clinical neurology: Neuropathies. Amsterdam: Elsevier Science Publishers; 1987: p. 263–292.

Windebank, A. J.; McCall, J. T.; Dyck, P. J. Metal neuropathy. In: Dyck, P. J.; Thomas, P. K.; Lambert, E. H.; Bunge, R., eds. Peripheral neuropathy. Philadelphia: W. B. Saunders Co.; 1984: p. 2133–2161.

# 34

# Neurological Effects of Chronic Alcoholism

ELLIOTT L. MANCALL

The abuse of alcohol, particularly ethyl (grain) alcohol, leads directly or indirectly to a remarkable range of neurological disorders with widely varying severities and outlooks (Adams and Victor 1989; Charness et al. 1989; Victor and Adams 1953). Many of these disorders unfortunately are treatable to only a limited extent. Although rarely fatal, they are responsible for substantial morbidity and at times permanent physical or mental incapacity.

Disorders of the central (CNS) and peripheral (PNS) nervous systems and of muscle as observed in the chronic alcoholic may be divided into those due to the direct toxic effect of ethyl alcohol, those reflecting withdrawal from alcohol, the "abstinence syndromes," and those due to concomitant and usually protracted nutritional depletion. Manifestations of the direct toxicity of alcohol may appear in occasional or accustomed drinkers if a sufficient amount of alcohol has been consumed. On the other hand, abstinence syndromes tend to appear particularly in the periodic (binge or spree) drinker, while nutritional disorders are most prominent in the steady and chronic drinker. These distinctions are useful clinically, despite their somewhat artificial character, and they are used in this chapter.

Many other neurological disorders that are not classifiable in this way occur with special frequency in an alcoholic population. Among these are the effects of craniocerebral trauma, most importantly subdural hematoma, and the many complications of liver failure, including inter alia, hepatic encephalopathy, and myelopathy; these are covered elsewhere in this book. The fetal alcohol syndrome represents a special case of direct ethanol toxicity and will be reviewed in that category. Only disorders complicating the preferential use of ethyl alcohol are considered. The consequences of ingestion of other alcohols, by accident or design, are beyond the scope of this presentation. The management of alcoholism, in a generic sense, is far removed from the parameters of this discussion. The interested reader is referred to other reviews, such as that by Peachey and Annis (1984), for a contemporary critique of the issues involved.

## Toxic Effects of Ethyl Alcohol

### Inebriation

The clinical manifestation of acute alcoholic intoxication or inebriation requires little elaboration. Alterations of mood, judgment, and alertness; blurring of vision; vertigo; nystagmus; dysarthria; incoordination of the limbs; and truncal ataxia are among the more common expressions of acute intoxication. Factors influencing the onset and severity of this syndrome include not only the amount of alcohol consumed, but also the rate of consumption, the degree of habituation or tolerance, the concomitant use of other drugs and food, genetic predisposition, and psychological attitude and expectations at the time of drinking. The extent of habituation, defining the difference between the occasional and the accustomed drinker, is of particular importance but is poorly understood. Modifications in transport of alcohol across the intestinal mucosa, induction of hepatic enzyme systems, changes in neurotransmitter and receptor site interrelationships, and morphological alterations of the neuronal lipoprotein membrane complex with resultant modifications in ion flux are among the many mechanisms that have been implicated as responses to acute or chronic ingestion of alcohol. However, the precise pathophysiological mechanism(s) basic to the development of tolerance remains unclear.

Several specific issues require particular attention concerning the inebriated person. Most important is the development of stupor and coma. Miles (1922) has pointed out that in the unaccustomed drinker, stupor appears at a blood-alcohol level of 300 mg/dl, deep coma supervenes at a level of 400 mg/dl, and death from respiratory depression occurs when the level approaches 500 mg/dl. The accustomed drinker may tolerate these high levels more effectively. In any case, the development of coma demands urgent therapeutic intervention (Mancall and Silver 1986). Hemodialysis may be life-saving. The use of the opiate antagonist naloxone has been reported to reverse coma in such patients (Lyon and Antony 1982; Mackenzie 1979); unfortunately, this is not universal, and in some studies the use of naloxone has failed to reverse the signs of intoxication (Lancet editorial 1983). Gastric lavage may be helpful in acute cases. Nonspecific stimulants, such as caffeine, are of dubious benefit. Hypertonic glucose, always administered with thiamine to preclude the development of Wernicke's encephalopathy, may be beneficial but only in the few cases in which hypoglycemia is documented.

The "alcoholic blackout" occasionally is encountered following acute ingestion of alcohol. This may be defined as a self-limited and brief period of failure of short-term memory recording,

similar clinically to transient global amnesia. The explanation for this defect is not clear. Such episodes, which often are recurrent, generally are evidence of a serious state of alcohol abuse. They require no specific therapy.

Although alcohol ordinarily is considered a sedative or depressing drug, its ingestion, even in small amounts, is sometimes followed by the development of a paradoxical state of excitement with aggressive and often violent behavior, referred to as pathological intoxication. The cause of this idiosyncratic response to ethanol is not known. There is no specific therapy, but a quiet environment and, when needed, restraints and parenteral haloperidol have a place in management. The period of agitation tends to be brief, usually ending within a few hours after a period of deep sleep. Suicide attempts are not infrequent and the patient must be monitored with this in mind.

## Myopathy

Acute alcoholic myopathy (rhabdomyolysis) most frequently appears shortly after a period of unusually excessive drinking. Although total agreement is lacking (Laureno 1979), it is widely held (Rubin 1979; Urbano-Marquez et al. 1989, 1995; Fernandez-Sola et al., 1994) that this acute disorder reflects the direct toxicity of alcohol on skeletal and cardiac muscle. The syndrome is characterized clinically by muscle weakness and pain, involving particularly the proximal muscles of the limbs, symmetrically or asymmetrically, and generally associated with severe muscle tenderness and sometimes myoedema. Myoglobinuria and elevated serum creatine kinase levels typically are encountered. Muscle biopsy demonstrates severe necrosis of muscle fibers, involving particularly type 1 fibers, with subsequent active muscle regeneration. There is no specific therapy. The disorder ordinarily is self-limited if the patient remains abstinent. Unfortunately, return of muscle function is not always complete, especially in people with very severe and widespread muscle destruction. Variable degrees of weakness and atrophy may persist indefinitely.

A more chronic form of myopathic disorder also is encountered in the alcoholic (Mancall and McEntee 1966), again involving primarily the proximal musculature but associated with less dramatic necrotic changes within muscle, a predominant type 2 fiber atrophy, absence of myoglobinuria, and only a modest rise in serum creatine kinase levels. It is uncertain whether this more indolent myopathy also reflects the direct toxicity of ethanol or, alternatively, chronic malnutrition. In this more chronic form, continued abstinence and improved nutrition ordinarily lead to restoration of function. The importance of an associated neuropathy in the pathogenesis of the acute and chronic forms of myopathy should not be underestimated.

## Fetal Alcohol Syndrome

The offspring of alcoholic women are known to exhibit a constellation of neurological abnormalities, including growth and intellectual retardation, hyperactivity, microcephaly, craniofacial anomalies, cleft palate, dislocations of the hip and a variety of other arthropathies, and many other congenital anomalies affecting the skin, heart, and urogenital system. Although the precise pathogenetic mechanisms underlying fetal alcohol syndrome (FAS) remain incompletely established, it appears to be a dose-dependent phenomenon, reflecting the quantity of alcohol consumed during pregnancy by the mother. It occurs in more than one-third of the offspring of serious alcoholics; the children of women who drink less may evidence portions of this syndrome, called fetal alcohol effects. The possible etiological significance of maternal undernutrition, smoking, and concomitant drug usage remains to be clarified, but it is likely that they play a less important role than that of ethanol itself (Charness et al. 1989).

The 10-year follow-up study by Streissguth and coworkers (1985) indicates that growth deficiency persists in FAS despite some catch-up phenomena, although the typically emaciated appearance of the younger child may disappear by adolescence. Some modifications of the craniofacial anomalies have been observed, and cardiac defects, such as atrial or ventricular septal defects and patent ductus arteriosus, assume less significance or resolve spontaneously. Osseous or dental anomalies may worsen and require surgical intervention. Defective cognitive development and attention defects remain serious problems, often attended by major social and emotional dislocations. The degree of intellectual impairment in any child appears to correlate with the severity of the

malformations and the degree of growth retardation; the best ultimate predictive factor appears to be the severity of the maternal alcoholism.

## Effects of Withdrawal

Following withdrawal, whether relative or complete, a sequence of neurological disorders appears, beginning with tremulousness and hallucinations, proceeding to seizures, and in approximately 15% of cases, to overt delirium tremens (Victor and Adams 1953). The first of these appears relatively early after reduction or elimination of ethanol, whereas delirium tends to develop later in withdrawal. Although common in combination, each of these disorders may be encountered independently; because the therapeutic and prognostic implications of each disorder vary, it is appropriate to treat them separately.

The use of psychoactive substances has been widely advocated in the management of alcohol withdrawal in general (Holloway et al. 1984; Mancall and Silver 1986) and is said to have a significant impact on outcome. Benzodiazepines, particularly chlordiazepoxide (Librium), are widely used and are claimed to effect prognosis significantly by reducing the morbidity and perhaps the mortality associated with these disorders. Unfortunately, chlordiazepoxide has a relatively long half-life (approximately 10 hours), and its metabolites, which have variable half-lives, are biologically active and are characterized by unpredictable but slow elimination; hepatic disease prolongs elimination even further. The resulting potential for benzodiazepine toxicity is significant. Oxazepam (Serax) has a shorter half-life and does not have active metabolites; therefore, it is often preferred in these circumstances. Unfortunately, the majority of benzodiazepines are available only for oral or intravenous use. Neither of these routes is ideal in an agitated negative patient in withdrawal. Because lorazepam (Ativan) is suitable for intramuscular administration, it has been particularly favored by some investigators (Rosenbloom 1986).

Other drugs advocated for use in withdrawal include diazepam (Valium), chlorpromazine (Thorazine), meprobamate, and paraldehyde. Because phenothiazines such as chlorpromazine alter seizure thresholds, they must be used with great caution. The prominence of adrenergic signs in withdrawal, reportedly related to elevated spinal fluid and cerebral levels of norepinephrine (Hawley et al. 1981), has prompted the use of propranolol (Inderal) as well.

## Alcoholic Tremulousness

Developing as soon as 6 to 8 hours after withdrawal, alcoholic tremulousness is the earliest and most benign of the abstinence syndromes. The patient exhibits prominent postural tremors of the limbs, with concomitant tremors of the face, tongue, and head. Autonomic manifestations, such as tachycardia and facial flushing, occur along with insomnia, excitement, anorexia, retching, and heightened sensitivity to external stimuli. This disorder requires no specific therapy, but its appearance should alert the observer to the potential for more serious abstinence syndromes. If the patient remains abstinent, the somatic tremors subside without incident within several days, as do the epiphenomena of tachycardia, flushing, and agitation. Many patients experience a curious inner tremor persisting for weeks; an excessive startle response also may linger.

It remains unclear whether this acute but transient movement disorder bears any relationship to the chronic postural tremor exhibited by some alcoholics or to essential tremor (Neiman et al. 1990).

## Alcoholic Hallucinosis

Within 12 to 18 hours of withdrawal, as many as 25% of patients exhibit vivid visual, auditory, or mixed hallucinations. Hallucinations are vivid and real to the patient, who often responds in an appropriate manner to these sensory experiences. They usually subside uneventfully without therapy within several days if the patient remains abstinent. In a small proportion of cases, however, the patient lapses into a stage of chronic auditory hallucinosis and may ultimately exhibit features of chronic paranoid schizophrenia. Whether this state of chronic hallucinosis is an independent process or represents a pre-existing but previously inapparent psychosis that has been unmasked by alcohol withdrawal remains unclear.

## Withdrawal Seizures

In 12% of hospitalized alcoholics (Victor and Adams 1953), generalized tonic-clonic seizures appear within 18 to 36 hours of withdrawal. Also known as alcoholic epilepsy or rum fits, these tend to occur in isolation or in a brief flurry of several seizures. Status epilepticus may occur but is very uncommon. When focal features are observed, either clinically or electroencephalographically, the possibility of other causes of late-onset seizures must be considered. The risk of developing such seizures apparently increases with repetitive bouts of detoxification (Lechtenberg and Worner 1990). Seizures also may develop during a period of active drinking, and it has been proposed that the relationship of seizures to alcohol use is dose-dependent. It has been suggested that seizures in these circumstances are due to the direct toxicity of alcohol rather than to withdrawal (Ng et al. 1988; Simon 1988); there is little general support for this theory.

The biological mechanism(s) underlying the appearance of withdrawal seizures remains unclear. There is clearly heightened epileptogenic potential during the critical period of withdrawal, as documented, for example, by unusual sensitivity to metrazol and to photic driving. Hypomagnesemia and respiratory alkalosis developing early in withdrawal and, at least in the latter instance, reflecting rebound hyperactivity of the respiratory centers of the brain stem have been implicated. Increased concentration of the excitatory neurotransmitter glutamate, increased number of postsynaptic glutamate-receptor binding sites, depressed inhibitory neurotransmitter γ-aminobutyric acid (GABA), and altered G proteins and calcium channels also have been proposed to have significant pathogenetic roles (Simon 1988).

Seizures occurring during abstinence are self-limited and generally require no specific therapeutic intervention. If status epilepticus develops, appropriate emergency management is warranted. The routine, chronic use of anticonvulsants to prevent withdrawal seizures in alcoholic patients is unnecessary because these occur only during periods of withdrawal. They commonly follow a period of binge drinking, during which time the patient is not likely to be therapeutically compliant; they are not likely to occur at other times. The use of benzodiazepines during withdrawal has been considered beneficial in reducing the frequency of seizures. The administration of an intravenous loading dose of phenytoin, followed by regular oral dosages of this agent through withdrawal, also has been advocated.

## Delirium Tremens

This syndrome of disordered sensory perceptions, hallucinations, agitation, confusion, insomnia, fever, and autonomic over-activity occurs in 5% to 15% of patients in withdrawal. It generally appears later than the other abstinence syndromes, with a peak at 72 hours after withdrawal. Its onset may be heralded by tremors, hallucinations, and seizures. Delirium tends to begin abruptly and is relatively short-lived; it ends suddenly and in less than 72 hours in more than 80% of the cases (Victor and Adams 1953).

A significant mortality rate is associated with delirium tremens, ranging up to 15% in most reported series. No single cause of death can be identified; intercurrent infections; electrolyte and other metabolic abnormalities; renal, adrenal, or hepatic failure; trauma; and acute peripheral vascular collapse have been implicated in small numbers of cases. Along with appropriate supportive management, early and vigorous use of benzodiazepines substantially reduces the morbidity and the mortality associated with this disease.

## Nutritional Disorders

In an alcoholic who drinks steadily for months or years, malnutrition becomes a major clinical threat. In the urban United States, nutritional disorders of the nervous system in adults appear most commonly in the nutritionally depleted alcoholic population. The alcoholic uses the "empty" calories of the ethanol to displace required nutrients from the diet. Although an adequate dietary history is difficult to obtain in the best circumstances and laboratory documentation of such a deficiency even more difficult, one can infer the presence of undernutrition by observing weight loss with atrophy of muscle and subcutaneous tissue, glossitis, cheilosis, angular stomatitis, and nonspecific laboratory abnormalities, such as hypochromic anemia and hypoproteinemia. However, such evidence is indirect at best, and firm documentation, especially of a specific vitamin insufficiency, is extremely problematic. Many patients manage remarkably well for extended periods of time despite a meager diet; they may develop neurological symptoms only when burdened with a superimposed metabolic demand, a sequence of events most convincingly documented in the case of Wernicke's encephalopathy.

Among these diseases, several (polyneuropathy, Wernicke-Korsakoff syndrome, amblyopia, pellagra) are of undoubted nutritional origin, with the specific deficiency reasonably well defined. The essential dietary ingredient lacking is a member of the B-vitamin group. Two others (cerebellar degeneration and Marchiafava-Bignami disease) are clearly due to undernutrition, but the nutritional lack has not been established. The role of malnutrition in the pathogenesis of central pontine myelinolysis remains a matter of dispute.

## Nutritional Polyneuropathy

Commonly referred to as alcoholic neuropathy or neuritic beriberi, nutritional polyneuropathy is the most common nutritional disorder encountered in the alcoholic population. In the series of Victor and Adams (1953), 70% of their patients were found to have features of peripheral neuropathy, although many were asymptomatic. Some investigators (Behse and Buchthal 1977) have stressed the importance of alcohol per se in pathogenesis, with or without attendant malnutrition, but there is little doubt about the fundamental importance of malnutrition in this regard. The use of the term neuritic beriberi connotes a pure thiamine deficiency, but such specificity may not be warranted in these circumstances.

Weakness, numbness, paresthesiae, and pain are the most common complaints in symptomatic individuals. The onset is insidious, and the evolution is subacute. The lower extremities invariably are involved initially; the upper extremities are involved as the disease progresses. Variable motor, sensory, and reflex changes are found on examination, generally in a distal and symmetrical distribution. In milder cases, sensory changes predominate; however, as the disease becomes more severe, motor alterations appear with progressive weakness and atrophy (Hawley et al. 1982). Cranial nerve palsies may appear and autonomic changes are frequent. Chronic skin ulcers and Charcot-like arthropathies develop, and signs of other nutritional diseases of the nervous system are common. Pain, painful paresthesiae, and dysesthesiae are among the most disabling components of the illness.

Abstinence, improved nutrition, and the supplemental use of parenteral vitamins, particularly thiamine, are fundamental to the therapy of this disorders. Analgesics may be required to control pain. Carbamazepine or amytriptyline often are of major assistance, and local application of capsaieim (Zostrix) may be helpful. Sympathetic blocks sometimes are required in very severe burning. The judicious use of physiatric techniques is an essential therapeutic ingredient.

Despite adequate therapy, recovery from nutritional polyneuropathy is slow and incomplete; however, some patients experience complete recovery with abstinence, even without vitamin supplementation (Hillborn and Wennberg 1984). Many patients note at least some improvement in sensory complaints relatively soon; at least mild degrees of sensory loss and loss of the tendon reflexes may persist indefinitely (Hawley et al. 1982). In more severely involved patients, recovery is much slower and often unsatisfactory, with significant and sometimes incapacitating sensory and motor residuals observed for months or years.

## Wernicke-Korsakoff Syndrome

Commonly considered two different disorders, Wernicke's encephalopathy and Korsakoff's psychosis in fact represent the acute and chronic phases of a single illness due to thiamine deficiency (Victor et al. 1989). The assumption that there is a definite link between the two disorders is based on the observations that the typical psychological changes of Korsakoff's psychosis may be present from the onset of Wernicke's disease or may emerge during treatment; that residual features of a prior bout of Wernicke's encephalopathy often are noted on careful examination of patients with Korsakoff's psychosis; and that the distribution of the pathological changes in the two conditions is identical, the differences noted being explicable on the basis of differences in chronology.

Wernicke's encephalopathy presents in an acute or subacute manner. Characteristic clinical features include the following: An abnormal mental status, variable in expression, occurs. In some patients, apathy, listlessness, a short attention span, and confusion appear; an hallucinatory—confusional state occurs in others; and in others, a serious memory disorder exists. Ophthalmoplegia, especially bilateral sixth nerve palsies, develop. Virtually any combination of altered ocular movements, including gaze palsies, may be encountered. Nystagmus generally is present in horizontal and vertical planes. Finally, ataxia of the trunk and gait occurs, but with little affection of the limbs. Auto-

nomic changes may appear, and although beriberi heart disease is unusual in these patients, acute peripheral vascular collapse may account for sudden death. In the series of patients with Wernicke's encephalopathy by Adams and Victor (1953), a mortality of 17% was observed, generally attributable to sepsis or hepatic failure.

The lesions of Wernicke's encephalopathy follow a regular and stereotypical pattern; particularly affected are the brain stem, cerebellum, and hypothalamus. The lesions, characteristically comprising subtotal tissue necrosis without inflammatory response, are typically found symmetrically disposed in the mammillary bodies, beneath the walls of the third ventricle, in the medial dorsal nucleus of the thalamus, in the periaqueductal gray matter of the mesencephalon, beneath the floor of the fourth ventricle in the pons and medulla, and in the superior vermis of the cerebellum. In terms of clinicopathological correlation, it is logical to consider the lesions in the periaqueductal gray matter and pontine tegmentum responsible for the ophthalmoplegias, affection of the vestibular complex for nystagmus, changes in the vermis for ataxia, and the lesions in the mammillary bodies and thalamus for the alterations in mentation.

Following the parenteral administration of thiamine, the ophthalmoplegias improve within a few hours, and complete resolution occurs in less than 1 week in most patients (Victor et al. 1989). In a smaller number of patients, particularly those exhibiting gaze palsies, 4 weeks of therapy may be required for full recovery. More time is required for resolution of ataxia and nystagmus. Vertical nystagmus disappears in most patients within 4 weeks; horizontal nystagmus, however, remains as a permanent sequela of the disease in more than half of the patients. Truncal and gait ataxia similarly improve with continued treatment with thiamine. Only 38% recover completely, even with 2 months or more of therapy; incomplete recovery is observed in 37% and no improvement in ataxia in fully 27% of the cases. It is thus clear that even prompt institution of parenteral therapy with thiamine does not necessarily result in complete recovery, particularly concerning nystagmus and ataxia.

The alterations in the mental status of Wernicke's encephalopathy respond unpredictably to thiamine. Patients who are simply confused appear to recover completely within several weeks. However, as the sensorium clears, many of these patients exhibit the amnestic dementia that is present in some from the onset and that is the typical and fundamental change of Korsakoff's psychosis.

Korsakoff's psychosis generally is characterized as an amnestic dementia with a severe disorder of memory comprising anterograde and retrograde amnesia. Cognitive functions are relatively better preserved but often are impaired to some extent. Alterations in behavioral patterns also are typical; apathy is the most prominent change. Neurological examination often demonstrates residuals of a previous perhaps unsuspected bout of Wernicke's encephalopathy, particularly horizontal nystagmus and gait ataxia.

The distribution of the pathological changes in Korsakoff's psychosis is identical to that encountered in Wernicke's encephalopathy. As noted, the lesions in the mammillary bodies and perhaps especially the thalamus appear most consistently related to the memory disorder.

In 186 patients who survived an acute bout of Wernicke's encephalopathy studied by Victor and colleagues (1989), 84% exhibited features of Korsakoff's psychosis. In 104 of these patients who were assessed for recovery of mental function for 2 months or more, four groups of roughly equal size could be discerned: 26% demonstrated no recovery; 28%, slight; 25%, significant; and only 21%, complete recovery from the amnestic state. Some patients required continued treatment for many months before gradual, and at times remarkably complete, recovery ensues. McEntee and associates (1980, 1984) have observed that the adrenergic agonist clonidine improves memory performance in Korsakoff's psychosis, and they speculate that damage to adrenergic neural systems in paraventricular brain stem and hypothalamic structures is fundamental to the memory deficit in this disorder.

Apart from the well-defined amnestic syndrome of Korsakoff, a number of chronic alcoholics exhibit a more global dementia, generally referred to as alcoholic dementia. This may represent the clinical expression of the cerebral convolutional atrophy observed pathologically in alcoholics, an atrophic process that appears at least partially reversible with abstinence as determined by magnetic resonance imaging (MRI) and computed tomography (CT) studies (Schroth et al. 1988). It may, however, reflect neurological disorders ranging from pellagra to subdural hematoma to multi-infarct dementia to Alzheimer's disease. Lishman's contention (1981, 1986) that alcoholic dementia is a neglected and perhaps subclinical form of Wernicke's encephalopathy has few adherents. Victor (1991) have recently reviewed the entire question of alcoholic dementia, stressing the primary of the Wernicks-Korsakoft syndrome in his own experience. Of some pertinence in this regard in the recent review of Harper (1998) of alcohol-specific brain damage.

## Nutritional Amblyopia

Also referred to as nutritional retrobulbar neuritis or tobacco–alcohol amblyopia, nutritional amblyopia is well established as a result of deficiency of one or several B vitamins, perhaps particularly thiamine, riboflavin, or cobalamine (Victor et al. 1960). This is an acutely or subacutely evolving disorder characterized by progressive and bilateral impairment of visual acuity and of color vision. Examination confirms bilateral impairment of visual acuity and of color vision, always with symmetrical central, cecocentral, or paracentral scotomata. In the early stages of the disease, the fundi appear normal, although optic atrophy may develop later. Pathologically one observes a symmetrical degeneration of the visual conducting system in the optic nerves, chiasm, and tracts, with involvement primarily of the papillomacular fiber bundles. It is clearly distinct from the retinal degeneration of methyl alcohol intoxication.

Treatment with B vitamins, when introduced promptly, results in complete return of visual acuity and fields. If the disease is not recognized and treatment is delayed, permanent blindness and optic atrophy result. At times, irreversible visual loss develops with remarkable speed.

## Pellagra

Pellagra is due to a deficiency of nicotinic acid or its immediate precursor, tryptophan. The fully developed syndrome of diarrhea, dermatitis, and dementia as recognized in the early part of the century is uncommonly encountered today, particularly in the West. The alcoholic population represents the most consistent reservoir of this disorder (Serdaru et at. 1988). Neurological alterations include irritability, confusion, insomnia, dementia, and amnesia. Extrapyramidal or cerebellar signs occur, and occasionally the optic nerves are affected. A polyneuropathy is common, and features of a myelopathy may appear. Widespread chromolytic changes may be found pathologically throughout the neuraxis, most prominently in the Betz cells of the motor cortex, and symmetrical degenerative changes may be found in the posterior and lateral columns of the spinal cord. Treatment with niacin often is unsatisfactory, and it has been suggested (Victor and Adams 1956) that pyridoxine deficiency and possibly deficiencies of other B vitamins may play a significant pathogenetic role.

Nicotinic acid deficiency encephalopathy is a term applied to a poorly understood syndrome involving elderly patients and characterized by confusion, stupor, and rigidity. Infantile reflexes, such as forced grasping and sucking, also are common. The disorder responds promptly to the administration of nicotinic acid. Neglected in medical writings for many years, it has recently resurfaced (Lishman, 1981) as another, generally overlooked, form of abnormal mentation in alcoholics.

## Cortical Cerebellar Degeneration

"Alcoholic" cerebellar degeneration is a frequent complication of chronic alcoholism (Victor et al. 1959) and represents the most common of the acquired cerebellar degenerations of adulthood. It develops after long-standing drinking and undernutrition. Ordinarily, patients present with ataxia of the trunk and the gait and incoordination of the lower extremities as demonstrated, for example, with the heel–knee–shin test. The symptoms are insidious in onset and slowly progressive; evolution of the disease often takes weeks to months.

On examination, patients demonstrate a serious ataxia of the trunk and of gait and incoordination of the legs. The upper extremities are spared, and little if any dysarthria or other "cerebellar signs" are seen. The pattern of clinical abnormalities remains remarkably fixed in extent, without regard to duration of the illness.

Just as the clinical symptoms and signs of alcoholic cerebellar degeneration are restricted in distribution, the pathological changes also are anatomically restricted in most cases. Alterations predominate in the superior vermis and the anterior and superior portions of the cerebellar hemispheres; occasionally, changes are found elsewhere in the cerebellar cortex, and secondary changes may be observed in the vicinity of the deep cerebellar nuclei and in the olivary complex of the medulla. All neurocellular elements of the cerebellar cortex may be involved, but Purkinje cells appear particularly vulnerable. Pathological features of other nutritional diseases, especially Wernicke's encephalopathy, may be encountered.

This form of cortical cerebellar degeneration is of nutritional origin. Its appearance has been well documented with serious nutritional depletion without the use of alcohol (Mancall and McEntee 1966). The coexistence of pathological features of Wernicke's encephalopathy in many cases and the prominence of cerebellar ataxia in otherwise uncomplicated instances of Wernicke's encephalopathy suggest that the two diseases are intimately linked. It is possible that thiamine deficiency is the basis for both disorders (Adams and Victor 1989).

Abstinence, improved nutrition, and supplemental vitamins contribute to modest improvement in the cerebellar deficit in these patients; usually an extended period of time is required, and such improvement possibly reflects improvement in other disorders that may contribute to ataxia, such as polyneuropathy. Unfortunately, such improvement is extremely limited, and all patients are left with significant cerebellar ataxia indefinitely.

## Marchiafava-Bignami Disease

This rare disorder, once thought to be a pathological curiosity, is increasingly identified using CT and MRI (Kawamura et al. 1985). Originally, it was thought to occur in middle-aged or elderly Italian men who were addicted to drinking crude red wine; with time, it has become abundantly clear that the most important pathogenetic factor is severe and chronic undernutrition (Koeppen and Barron 1978). The specific dietary lack has not been identified.

Unlike other nutritional disorders of the nervous system, the features of Marchiafava-Bignami disease are not stereotypical. The clinical sympatomatology includes dementia, psychosis, asphasia, seizures, tremor, paralysis, hypertonia, and coma. The course of the disease often is phasic. Some patients have exhibited complete remissions, but overall, the disease is progressive, usually leading to death in less than 2 years. Pathological changes comprise symmetrical degeneration of myelin with relative preservation of axons in the corpus callosum and other commissural bundles. The cerebral white matter may be involved, and similar lesions are found in the middle cerebral peduncles, the optic chiasm, and the posterior columns of the spinal cord.

No specific treatment is available for this disease, which appears to lead to death in all recognized cases, with rare exceptions (Leventhal et al. 1965).

## Central Pontine Myelinolysis

Central pontine myelinolysis (CPM) (Adams et al. 1959) is a dramatic disease characterized clinically by the rapid development of a flaccid quadriplegia with bulbar palsy, with preserved consciousness and sensation. Movements of the eyelids and globes are intact in most instances. Nystagmus has been noted. If the patient survives for more than several days, spasticity and hyper-reflexia may ensue. It is likely that mentation is intact, although difficulties in communication make cognitive function extremely difficult to assess. Neuroradiological and pathological studies have documented the existence of asymptomatic cases; the size of the pontine lesion is apparently the principal determinant of symptomatic expression.

The classic pathological change is symmetrical demyelination in the basis pontis, beginning in the midline and spreading symmetrically to either side. Axons traversing the lesion are relatively well preserved, as are the intrinsic nerve cells of the basis pontis. Extrapontine lesions have been described in areas as diverse as the subcortical white matter, basal ganglia and thalamus, cerebellar white matter, and spinal cord; the term *extrapontine myelinolysis* is sometimes applied to these cases.

Although originally considered a reflection of undernutrition in chronic and debilitated alcoholics in whom the disease was first described, it is clear that neither alcohol per se nor malnutrition play an exclusive or even essential role in pathogenesis. In many cases of CPM, significant hyponatremia is documented, and in many instances, the disease appears de novo following rapid correction of such hyponatremia (Ayus et al. 1985; Laureno and Karp 1988; Norenberg et al. 1982; Sterns et al. 1986; Tomlinson et al. 1976). It has been suggested (Ayus et al. 1987) that an increase in serum sodium to normal or hypernatremic levels in the first 48 hours and a change in the serum sodium concentration of more than 25 ml/L in the first 48 hours are important precipitating characteristics. Rapid correction of severe vasopressin-induced hyponatremia in experimental animals has been followed by the development of similar lesions (Laureno 1983). However, the majority of patients with CPM are seriously ill and often are extremely debilitated and undernourished before they develop neurological disease. Some have undergone significant hypoxic episodes; therefore, it is possible that, although not universally applicable, such might represent ancillary factors in pathogenesis. The suggestion that the demyelination reflects an osmotic shift rather than the serum sodium level per se recently has been supported by the observation by McKee and associates (1988) of serum hyperosmolality in all patients who developed CPM in association with severe burns. Attention has recently been drawn to the development of CPM following the use of cyclosporine with live transplantation (Freyer et al. 1996).

The prognosis for survival in patients with CPM who become symptomatic is extremely poor. In asymptomatic cases, the disease does not recognizably contribute to morbidity or mortality.

## References

Adams, R. D.; Victor, M.; Mancall E. L. Central pontine myelinolysis. A hitherto undescribed disease occurring in alcoholic and malnourished patients. Arch. Neurol. 81:154; 1959.

Adams, R. D.; Victor, M. Principles of neurology. 4th ed. New York: McGraw-Hill; 1989.

Ayus, J. C.; Krothapalli, R. K.; Arieff, A. I. Changing concepts in treatment of severe symptomatic hyponatremia. Am. J. Med. 78:897–902; 1985.

Ayus, J. D.; Krothapalli, R. K.; Arieff, A. I. Treatment of symptomatic hyponatremia and its relations to brain damage. N. Engl. J. Med. 317:1190–1195; 1987.

Behse, F.; Buchthal, F. Alcoholic neuropathy: clinical, electrophysiological, and biopsy findings. Ann. Neurol. 2:95; 1977.

Charness, M. E.; Simon, R. P.; Greenberg, D. A. Ethanol and the nervous system. N. Engl. J. Med. 321:442; 1989.

Fernández-Solá, J.; Estruch, R.; Grau, J. P.; et al. The relation of alcoholic myopathy to cardiomyopathy. Ann. Intern. Med. 120:529; 1994.

Fryer, J.P.; Fortier, M.V.; Metrakos, P.; et al. Central pontine myelinosis and cyclosporine neurotoxicity following liver transplantation. Transplantation 61: 658; 1996.

Harper, C. The neuropathology of alcohol-specific brain damage, or does alcohol damage the brain? I. Neuropathol. Exp. Neurol. 57:101; 1998.

Hawley, R. J.; Kurtzke, J. F.; Armbrustmacher; Saini, N.; Manz, H. The course of alcoholic–nutritional peripheral neuropathy. Acta Neurol. Scand. 66:582; 1982.

Hawley, R. J.; Major, L. F.; Schulman, E. A.; Lake, R. CSF levels of norepinephrine during alcohol withdrawal. Arch. Neurol. 38:289; 1981.

Hillbom, M.; Wennberg, A. Prognosis of alcoholic peripheral neuropathy. J. Neurol. Neurosurg. Psychiatry 47:699; 1984.

Holloway, H. C.; Hales, R. E.; Watanabe, H. K. Recognition and treatment of acute alcohol withdrawal syndromes. Psychiatr. Clin. North Am. 7:729; 1984.

Kawamura, M.; Shiota, J.; Yagishita, T.; Hirayama, K. Marchiafava-Bignami disease: computed tomographic scan and magnetic resonance imaging. Ann. Neurol. 18:103; 1985.

Koeppen, A. H.; Barron, K. D. Marchiafava-Bignami disease. Neurology 28:290; 1978.

Lancet editorial. Naloxone for ethanol intoxication. Lancet 2:145; 1983.

Laureno, R. Letter to the editor. N. Engl. J. Med. 22:1239; 1979.

Laureno, R. Central pontine myelinolysis following rapid correction of hyponatremia. Ann. Neurol. 13:232–242; 1983.

Laureno, R.; Karp, B. I. Pontine and extrapontine myelinolysis following rapid correction of hyponatremia. Lancet 1:1439; 1988.

Lechtenberg, R.; Worner, T. M. Seizure risk with recurrent alcohol detoxification. Arch. Neurol. 47:535; 1990.

Leventhal, C. M.; Baringer, J. R.; Arnason, B. G. A case of Marchiafava-Bignami disease with clinical recovery. Trans. Am. Neurol. Assoc. 90:87; 1965.

Lishman, W. A. Cerebral disorder in alcoholism: syndromes of impairment. Brain 104:1; 1981.

Lishman, W. A. Alcoholic dementia: a hypothesis. Lancet 1:1184; 1986.

Lyon, L. J.; Antony, J. Reversal of alcoholic coma by naloxone. Ann. Intern. Med 96:464; 1982.

Mackenzie, A. I. Naloxone in alcoholic intoxication. Lancet 1:733; 1979.

Mancall, E. L.; McEntee, W. J. Alterations of the cerebellar cortex in nutritional encephalopathy. Neurology 15:303; 1966.

Mancall, E. L.; McEntee, W. J.; Hirschhorn, A. M.; Gonyea, E. F. Proximal muscular weakness and atrophy in the chronic alcoholic. Neurology 16:301; 1966.

Mancall, E. L.; Silver, P. Alcohol intoxication and withdrawal. In: Johnson, R., ed. Current therapy in neurological disease. Philadelphia: B. C. Decker; 1986.

McEntee, W. J., Mair, R. G. Memory enhancement in Korsakoff's psychosis by clonidine. Ann. Neurol. 7:466; 1980.

McEntee, W. J.; Mair, R. G.; Langlais, P. J. Neurochemical patterns in Korsakoff's psychosis: implications for other cognitive disorders. Neurology 34:648; 1984.

McKee, A. C.; Winkelman, M. D.; Banker, B. Q. Central pontine myelinolysis in severely burned patients: Relationship to serum hyperosmolality. Neurology 38:1211–1217; 1988.

Miles, W. R. The comparative concentrations of alcohol in human blood and urine at intervals after ingestion. J. Pharmacol. Exp. Ther. 20:265; 1922.

Neiman, J.; Lang, A. E.; Fornazzari, L.; Carlen, P. L. Movement disorders in alcoholism: a review. Neurology 40:741; 1990.

Ng, S. K. C.; Hauser, W. A.; Brust, J. C. M.; Susser, M. Alcohol consumption and withdrawal in new-onset seizures. N. Engl. J. Med. 319:666; 1988.

Norenberg, M. D.; Leslie, K. O.; Robertson, A. S. Association between rise in serum sodium and central pontine myelinolysis. Ann. Neurol. 11:128–135; 1982.

Peachey, J. E.; Annis, H. Pharmacologic treatment of chronic alcoholism. Psychiatr. Clin. North Am. 7:745; 1984.

Rosenbloom, A. J. Optimizing drug treatment of alcohol withdrawal. Am. J. Med. 81:901; 1986.

Rubin, E. Alcoholic myopathy in heart and skeletal muscle. N. Engl. J. Med. 301:28; 1979.

Schroth, G.; Naegele, T.; Klose, U.; Mann, K.; Petersen, D. Reversible brain shrinkage in abstinent alcoholics, measured by MRI. Neuroradiology 30:385; 1988.

Serdaru, M.; Hausser-Hauw, C.; Laplane, D.; Buge, A.; Castaigne, P.; Goulon, M.; Lhermitte, F.; Hauw, J. J. The clinical spectrum of alcoholic pellagra encephalopathy. A retrospective analysis of 22 cases studied pathologically. Brain 111:829–842; 1988.

Simon, R. P. Alcohol and seizures. N. Engl. J. Med. 319:715; 1988.

Sterns, R. H.; Riggs, J. E.; Schochet, S. S. Osmotic demyelination syndrome following correction of hyponatremia. N. Engl. J. Med. 314:1535–1542; 1986.

Streissguth, A. P.; Clarren, S. K.; Jones, K. Natural history of the fetal alcohol syndrome: a 10 year follow-up of eleven patients. Lancet 2:85; 1985.

Tomlinson, B. E.; Pierides, A. M.; Bradley, W. G. Central pontine myelinolysis: two cases with associated electrolyte disturbance. Q. J. Med. 45:373; 1976.

Urbano-Marquez, A.; Estruch, R.; Navarro-Lopez, F.; Grau, J. M.; Mont, L.; Rubin, E. The effects of alcoholism on skeletal and cardiac muscle. N. Engl. J. Med. 320:409; 1989.

Urbano-Márquez, A.; Estruch, R.; Fernández-Solá, J.; et al. The greater risk of alcoholic cardiomyopathy and myopathy in women compared with men. JAMA 274:149; 1995.

Victor, M. Alcoholic dementia. Can. J. Neurol. Sci. 21:88; 1994.

Victor, M.; Adams, R. The effect of alcohol on the nervous system. Proc. Assoc. Res. Nerv. Ment. Dis. 32:526; 1953.

Victor, M.; Adams, R. D. Neuropathology of experimental vitamin B-6 deficiency in monkeys. Am. J. Clin. Nutr. 4:346; 1956.

Victor, M.; Adams, R. D.; Collins, G. H. The Wernicke-Korsakoff syndrome and related neurologic disorders due to alcoholism and malnutrition. Philadelphia: F. A. Davis; 1989.

Victor, M.; Adams, R. D.; Mancall, E. L. A restricted form of cerebellar degeneration occurring in alcoholic patients. Arch. Neurol. 1:579–688; 1959.

Victor, M.; Mancall, E. L.; Dreyfuss, D. M. Deficiency amblyopia in the alcoholic patient: a clinicopathological study. Arch. Ophthalmol. 64:1; 1960.

PART XI

# BEHAVIORAL, DEGENERATIVE, AND PAROXYSMAL DISORDERS

# 35

# Dementia and Alzheimer's Disease

MARIO F. MENDEZ AND JEFFREY L. CUMMINGS

Dementia produces cognitive and behavioral deterioration and grave disability, usually in later life. Dementia is an acquired impairment in at least two cognitive domains: memory plus language, visuospatial skills, or executive abilities (American Psychiatric Association 1994; Cummings and Benson 1992). The diagnosis is supported by cognitive impairments that are present for 6 months or more and that are severe enough to interfere with social activities, work, and activities of daily living. This disorder constitutes an immense burden not only to patients, but also to caregivers, the health care system, and society at large. Patients with dementia account for a disproportionate use of heath care resources, hospital inpatient days, and nursing home admissions. In the United States, dementia may cost over $100 billion per year, about 10% of all health care expenditures, and the average cost to families in 1990 was $18,000 per year (National Institutes on Aging 1992). With the increasing age of the population, dementia will affect greater numbers of people, and the burden of this disorder will continue to rise (Brookmeyer et al. 1998). The assessment of prognosis in dementia has important implications.

Dementia is a syndrome with many potential causes. A range of clinical and neuropathological studies indicate that Alzheimer's disease (AD) accounts for 45% to 75% of dementia patients, with most reports averaging approximately 56% to 66% (Clarfield 1988; Cummings and Benson 1992; Henderson 1990; Mendez et al. 1991). In a summary of nine clinical studies, AD was responsible for 66% of the total cases of dementia (Katzman and Rowe 1992), and a recent neuropathological series reported 62.5% AD among autopsied dementia patients (Hogan et al. 1994). In addition to the dementia syndrome, the clinical diagnosis of probable AD is based on a progressive course and the exclusion of other dementing illnesses (McKhann et al. 1984) (see Table 35-1). The definitive diagnosis of AD requires demonstration of neurofibrillary tangles and more neuritic plaques, particularly in the cerebral cortex, than expected for the patient's age (Khachaturian 1985; Mirra et al. 1991). Using clinical criteria for AD, neuropathological examination confirmed the clinical diagnosis of possible or probable AD in 90 of the first 100 patients who came to autopsy at the Johns Hopkins Alzheimer's Disease Research Center (Rasmusson et al. 1996).

Patients with dementia require a complete evaluation for the many potential causes of this disorder (see Table 35-2). Vascular dementia (VaD) is second only to AD as a basis for dementia in

**Table 35-1.** Diagnosis of Dementia and Alzheimer's Disease DSM-IV (1994) Criteria for Dementia

A. The development of multiple cognitive deficits manifested by both:
   1. Memory impairment (amnesia)
   2. One or more of the following:
      a. aphasia
      b. apraxia
      c. agnosia
      d. disturbed executive functioning
B. Cognitive deficits cause significant impairment in social or occupation functioning and represent a significant decline from a previous level of functioning.
C. The course is characterized by gradual onset and continuing cognitive decline.

NINCDS-ADRDA Criteria:  Clinically Probable Alzheimer's disease
   1. Dementia established by clinical examination (mental status testing) and documented by mental status scales (confirmed by neuropsychological testing).
   2. Deficits in two or more cognitive domains such as memory, attention, language, personality, visuospatial functions, and executive functions.
   3. Progressive deterioration in cognitive domains.
   4. No delirium (i.e., cognitive deterioration occurs in the presence of a clear sensorium).
   5. Age of onset between 40 and 90 years of age, most over 65 years of age.
   6. Negative evaluation for other causes (i.e., absence of systemic of other illnesses that affect the brain and that can produce dementia).

most Western countries, where it makes up 10% to 20% of dementias (Cummings and Benson 1992; Desmond 1996; Roman et al. 1993). In some countries, VaD may be more common than AD (Desmond 1996; Shen et al. 1994; Skoog et al. 1993). The ratio of AD to VaD in prior surveys is significantly less than 1.0 among some Asian populations (Desmond 1996) however, in more recent surveys, AD remains more common than VaD in China and Japan (Chui et al. 1998; Yamada et al. 1999). Dementia presenting with movement disturbances, especially a gait disorder, suggests dementia with Lewy bodies (DLB), Parkinson's disease, Huntington's disease, progressive supranuclear palsy, normal pressure hydrocephalus, or other basal ganglia diseases (Hughes et al. 1993; McKeith et al. 1992; Mega et al. 1996). Although the epidemiology is still undefined, DLB may surpass VaD as the second most common dementia, accounting for many patients currently diagnosed as AD (Drach et al. 1997; Mega et al. 1996). Frontotemporal dementia, or Pick's complex may account for another 10% of patients presenting with dementia, particularly if the age of onset is before age 65 (The Lund and Manchester Groups 1994). Another 5% or more of patients presenting with dementia have toxic-metabolic disorders including alcoholism and drug toxicity, metabolic changes, hepatic disease, hyponatremia, calcium disorders, vitamin $B_{12}$ deficiency, thyroid disease, and hypoglycemia. Finally, there are a range of miscellaneous dementias from infections, tumors, epilepsy, demyelination, trauma, inherited adult-onset biochemical disorders, late schizophrenia, and depressive "pseudodementia." Because dementia and AD, the most common cause of dementia, are often discussed synonymously in the literature, this chapter will focus on the prognostic aspects of de-

**Table 35-2.** Differential Diagnosis of Dementia

Alzheimer's disease
Vascular dementia and mixed Alzheimer's-vascular
Frontotemporal degenerations
Neurodegenerative movement disorders: DLBD, Parkinson's disease, Huntington's disease, and others
Normal pressure hydrocephalus
Toxic-metabolic disorders
   Anoxia and hypoglycemia
   Liver: Hepatic failure and hepatocerebral degeneration
   Kidney: Renal failure and dialysis dementia
   Vitamin deficiencies: $B_{12}$, thiamine, folate, niacin
   Endocrinopathies: thyroid, parathyroid, adrenal, pituitary
   Drugs: alcohol, cocaine, other recreational drugs, medications
   Toxins: heavy metals, organophosphates, other industrial
Infectious: AIDS, Creutzfeldt-Jakob disease, syphilis, Lyme disease, chronic meningitis
Psychiatric disease especially depression
Miscellaneous:
   Multiple sclerosis and other demyelinating diseases
   Post-traumatic and dementia pugilistica
   Inherited adult-onset biochemical disorders (e.g., metachromatic leukodystrophy, Kuf's)
   Neoplastic: gliomatosis cerebri, angioendotheliosis
   Epilepsy-related

DLBD, dementia with Lewy bodies; AIDS, acquired immune deficiency syndrome.

mentia in general, and AD in particular. The prognoses of other dementias depends, in large part, on the underlying causative disorders.

## Epidemiology

Dementia is an increasing problem in the elderly population. Worldwide, at least 7% (4% to 12%) of persons over the age of 65, and nearly half of those over the age of 85, have some form of dementing illness (Breteler et al. 1992; Evans et al. 1990; Henderson 1990; Katzman and Rowe 1992). The prevalence of dementia among the elderly is closer to 8% to 10% in developed countries where people live longer. In the Canadian Study of Health and Aging (CSHA) of over 10,000 people, the prevalence of dementia and AD were 8.0% and 5.1%, respectively, for those aged 65 and older (CSHA 1994). A recent meta-analysis of 18 studies by the U.S. General Accounting Office (GAO) found a prevalence rate for AD among Americans 65 years of age or older of 5.7% to 6.3% accounting for 1.9 to 2.1 million people (GAO Report 1998). The prevalence for moderate to severe AD was 3.3% to 4.1% accounting for 1.1 to 1.4 million older Americans likely to need active assistance with personal care (Table 35-2). With the greater longevity of the U.S. population, the numbers of people with AD may reach 3 million in the year 2015 (Table 35-3). This includes about 2 million likely to need active assistance with personal care (GAO Report 1998). In the United States, the diagnosis of AD on death certificates ranked 13th as a cause of death in 1996 (21,166 deaths), for a crude death rate of 8.0 and

an age-adjusted death rate of 2.7 (Monthly Vital Statistics Report 1997). Although death certificates greatly underestimate the number of deaths from AD (Lanska 1998), a recent re-evaluation suggests that AD is tied with cerebrovascular disease as the third leading cause of death in the United States (Ewbank 1999).

The incidence and prevalence rates for both dementia and AD rise sharply with (Table 35-3). Multiple studies show a doubling of both incidence and prevalence rates approximately every 5 years after age 60 to 65 (Bachman et al. 1993; Drachman 1994; GAO Report 1998; Jorm et al. 1987; 1991; Paykel et al. 1994). The annual incidence for dementia ranges from 0.7% to 0.9% for ages 65 to 69 to 8.5% to 11.8% for ages 85 to 89 (Bachman et al. 1993; Morgan et al. 1993; Paykel et al. 1994). The prevalence of dementia ranges from 1% to 2.5% for ages 65 to 74 to 26% to 47% for those 85 and older (CSHA 1994; Evans 1990). Some investigators found that incidence and prevalence rates for dementia and AD level off or decline beyond age 90 or 100 (Hagnell et al. 1981; Lautenschlager et al. 1996). Most studies, however, report that rates continue to rise in the oldest patients (Aronson et al. 1991; Fichter et al. 1996; Seshadri et al. 1997). In the CSHA, dementia rates rose to 58% in those 95 years and older (Ebly et al. 1994), and the recent GAO meta-analysis showed continued increases in AD for the very old (Table 35-4). Taken together, these reports suggest that the incidence of new cases of AD, in particular, continues to rise throughout late life but at a slower rate in the very old (Drachman 1994; GAO Report 1998).

**Table 35-3.** GAO Estimates of AD For Americans 65 Years of Age or Older in 1995

| Age | Any AD | | Moderate or severe AD | |
|---|---|---|---|---|
| | Number | Percent | Number | Percent |
| 65–69 | 104,785 | 1.1 | 61,815 | 0.6 |
| 70–74 | 194,716 | 2.2 | 111,111 | 1.3 |
| 75–79 | 304,399 | 4.6 | 169,549 | 2.5 |
| 80–84 | 411,363 | 9.2 | 227,757 | 5.1 |
| 85–89 | 412,764 | 17.8 | 232,726 | 10.0 |
| 90–94 | 312,509 | 31.5 | 185,516 | 18.7 |
| 95+ | 166,287 | 52.5 | 110,595 | 34.9 |
| Total | 1,906,822 | 5.7 | 1,099,069 | 3.3 |

Source: Our integration of prevalence rates from 18 studies in the literature and the U.S. Bureau of the Census population estimates in *Statistical Abstract of the United States:* 1996 (Washington, DC; 1996).

**Table 35-4.** GAO Projected Estimates for AD For Americans 65 Years or Age or Older, 1995–2015

|  | Any AD | | Moderate or severe AD | |
| --- | --- | --- | --- | --- |
| Year | Number | % Change* | Number | % Change[a] |
| 1995 | 1,906,822 | † | 1,099,069 | † |
| 2000 | 2,141,772 | +12 | 1,233,932 | +12 |
| 2005 | 2,370,615 | +24 | 1,365,085 | +24 |
| 2010 | 2,605,231 | +37 | 1,500,727 | +37 |
| 2015 | 2,872,420 | +51 | 1,656,046 | +51 |

* All percentage changes are relative to the baseline number for 1995.

† Zero by definition.

Source: The figures for 1995 are estimates based on the integration of the literature (taken from Table 35-1). The figures for the other years are projections based on the estimates and the Bureau of the Census middle series of population projections (P-25, No. 1130).

Despite the exponential increase in dementia associated with advancing age, the majority of persons are never affected with this disorder (Fig. 35-1). Since this is a disease primarily of the elderly, people who would otherwise develop AD often die of other, unrelated causes before developing dementia. Based on a longitudinal study of 2611 cognitively intact subjects, Seshadri et al. (1997) estimated the remaining lifetime risks of developing dementia from all causes and from AD. In a 65-year-old man, the remaining lifetime risk of developing a dementia was 11%, and the remaining lifetime risk of AD was 6%. Corresponding risks for a 65-year-old woman were 19% and 12%, respectively. In developed countries, the dementia-free life expectancy for men is about 14 years at age 65 and 11 years at age 70, and for women it is 17.7 years at age 65 and 14 years at age 70 (Liang et al. 1996; Perenboom et al. 1996; Ritchie et al. 1994; Sauvaget et al. 1997). These figures indicate that at least 80% of life expectancy at ages 65 or 70 are "dementia free." The percentage of life expectancy without dementia is lower for women, because of their higher total life expectancy (Sauvaget et al. 1997).

Dementia is more common among women. AD affects women at least twice as often as men (Bachman et al. 1992; Fratiglioni et al. 1997; Gao

**Figure 35-1.** Estimated percentage of total dementia patients among survivors 55 years and older. The ordinate represents percentage of those living at age 55. The abscissa represents advancing age. The total area includes survivors and is based on U.S. Census figures. The black area is the percentage of those with dementia and is based on the incidence and prevalence studies discussed in the text.

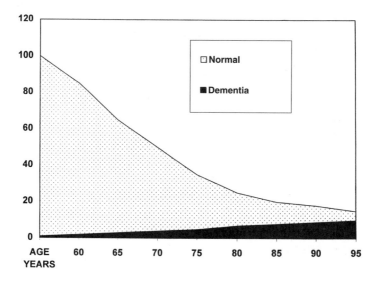

et al. 1998; Slaby and Erle 1993). The lifetime risk of AD for women at age 55 is more that twice that for men (Ott et al. 1998). This finding is partially attributable to greater longevity among women as compared to men (Jorm 1991). Greater longevity is not the complete explanation because AD is more prevalent among women at every age (GAO Report 1998). Another contributing factor is the shorter duration of AD among men as compared to women (Heyman et al. 1996). Even when this is accounted for, however, AD remains about 1.7 times as common among women as men. Additional gender differences could be accounted for by poorer education, late-life estrogen deprivation, or selective environmental exposures in women (Katzman et al. 1994).

Ethnic differences in dementia are less clear. In one autopsy series, de la Monte et al. (1989) reported a relative frequency of AD that was 2.6 times higher among whites than among blacks ($p < .001$). In contrast, other investigators report higher rates for AD among blacks than among whites (Heyman et al. 1991; Schoenberg 1985). Part of this discrepancy may be due to environmental or geographical factors. For example, some studies report relatively little AD among Africans, particularly when compared to African-Americans (Hendrie et al. 1995; Ogunniyi et al. 1992), and White et al. (1996) found that Japanese men in Hawaii were more susceptible to the development of AD than those in Japan. One study even suggests that Cherokee Indian ancestry affords some protection from AD (Rosenberg et al. 1996). Finally, surveys from different countries and ethnic groups report similar proportions of dementia patients with AD, VaD, and other dementias (Chui et al. 1998; Fillenbaum et al. 1998: Yamada et al. 1999).

The epidemiology of other dementias is not as defined as that for AD. These studies have problems related to diagnostic criteria, clinical assessments, and the availability of patients (Roman et al. 1993). The prevalence of VaD, the second most common dementia, increases linearly with age and varies greatly from country to country, ranging from 1.2% to 4.2% of people over 65 years old (Hebert and Brayne 1995). The annual incidence of VaD is about 6 to 12 cases per 1000 persons over 70 years of age and varies with the presence of cardiovascular risk factors such as hypertension (Hebert and Brayne 1995; Skoog et al. 1993). The incidence and prevalence of other dementias varies greatly depending on their underlying etiologies.

## Risk Factors

According to the threshold hypothesis of dementia, AD is an inevitable consequence of aging (Roth 1986; Roses 1995). Following the trend illustrated in Figure 35-1, everyone may develop dementia if they live to about 120 years of age. AD is a genetic disease whose individual expression is influenced by other risk factors. This means that, in addition to etiological risk factors such as family history and apolipoprotein E (APOE) genotype, there are "clinical expression" risk factors that facilitate the earlier emergence of dementia. Clinical expression factors such as history of head trauma, low educational and occupational level, and small head size reflect the underlying endowment of neurons or neural reserve (Mortimer 1988, 1992). For example, among nursing home residents who met neuropathological criteria for AD at autopsy, those who did not manifest dementia during life had higher brain weights and greater numbers of neurons in the cerebral cortex (Katzman et al. 1988). Additional proposed risk factors for which there is less supporting evidence include exposure to aluminum and other substances, maternal age at birth, a family history of Down, syndrome, depression, and thyroid disease (Table 35-5).

Other than advancing age, definite etiological risk factors for AD are family history and genetic inheritance. Among twins with at least one af-

**Table 35-5.** Risk Factors for Alzheimer's Disease

Definite risk factors
   Advanced age
   Family history of dementia in first-degree relatives
   Down's syndrome
   Presenilin mutations and the abnormal amyloid precursor protein gene
   Apolipoprotein E ε4 allele
   Head traumas, particularly in the preceding 10 years
   Low educational attainment
   Low lifelong occupational attainment
   Small head size and brain volume
Putative risk factors, not established
   Inverse association with smoking
   Alcohol or other drug abuse
   Metals such as aluminum, zinc, mercury
   Industrial solvents and pesticides
   Electromagnetic fields
   Advanced maternal age
   Maternal inheritance
   Family history of Down's syndrome
   Infectious processes
   Cerebrovascular disease
   Cardiovascular disease
   Thyroid disease

fected member, 59% to 67% of monozygotes and 22% to 40% of dizygotes were concordant for AD (Gatz et al. 1997; Nee and Lippa 1999). The risk for AD is about four times greater than that for the general population when there is an affected family member (Amaducci 1992; Breitner 1991; Graves et al. 1990; Mayeux et al. 1991; Mendez et al. 1992). In their reanalysis of 11 case-control studies, Van Duijn et al. (1991) reported an age-adjusted pooled odds ratio of 3.5 if there was a first-degree relative with dementia. The risk of AD increases with the number of affected first-degree relatives (Graves et al. 1990). The risk is similar whether siblings or parents are affected with AD (Breitner et al. 1988), but it is higher if the mother has dementia, as compared with the father (Edland et al. 1996). In other studies, of first-degree relatives of AD index cases, the lifetime risk of AD reached 39% by age 96 years (Lautenschlager et al. 1996), and the cumulative incidence of dementia ranged from 36% to 49% after age 85 years (Breitner et al. 1988; Payami et al. 1994).

About 5% of AD cases are familial and directly caused by abnormal genes on chromosomes 21, 14, or 1. Most patients with Down's syndrome develop clinical AD and the characteristic neuropathology of AD by age 40, suggesting a causative

factor on chromosome 21 (Van Duijn et al. 1994; Wisniewski et al. 1985). Indeed, AD may result from mutations of the amyloid precursor protein gene on chromosome 21 (St. George-Hyslop et al. 1987). These patients, however, belong to only about 20 known families). The majority of patients with familial AD have a defect on chromosome 14 (Kennedy et al. 1995). This "presenilin 1" mutation on chromosome 14 accounts for 50% to 70% of familial AD (100 families), and the "presenilin 2" mutation on chromosome 1 accounts for another 5% to 10% (the Volga German kindred) (Levy-Lahad et al. 1995). These presenilins produce an autosomal dominant dementia with incomplete penetrance and an early age of onset.

The remaining 95% of AD patients have a late-onset, sporadic disorder that is unrelated to presenilins but is affected by APOE genotype. APOE is a plasma protein that binds to plaques and neurofibrillary tangles (Saunders et al. 1993). Patients who are homozygous for the APOE (ε4 allele, coded on chromosome 19, are at greater risk for the expression of AD before death (Fig. 35-2). Conversely, the APOE (ε2 or ε3 genotype may delay the development of AD (Heyman et al. 1996; Royston et al. 1994). In the Framingham Study, 55% of the APOE ε4/ε4 homozygotes

**Figure 35-2.** Probability of disease for persons at high risk for Alzheimer's disease given the indicated apolipoprotein genotypes. (From Breitner 1997.)

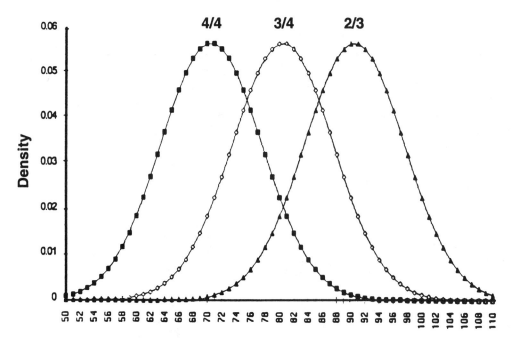

developed AD by age 80, whereas 27% of APOE ε3/ε4 heterozygotes and 9% of those without an ε4 allele developed AD by age 85 years (Myers et al. 1996). In comparison with persons without an ε4 allele, the risk ratio for AD was 3.7 (95% confidence interval [CI], 1.9 1 7.5) for APOE ε3/ε4 heterozygotes and 30.1 (95% CI, 10.7 to 84.4) for APOE ε4 homozygotes. Since the allele frequency of ε4 is about 15% in most populations (Davignon et al. 1988), only 2% of such populations are homozygous for this allele, and another 25% are heterozygous (Breitner 1997). Genetic testing for APOE and the other chromosomal abnormalities are currently available and can increase the clinical diagnostic accuracy of AD to 95% or more (Roses and Saunders 1997). Nevertheless, the APOE genotype is only a susceptibility gene for AD and not a determinative gene. Nearly 40% of AD patients with a confirmed diagnosis do not have the ε4 form of the APOE gene.

Substantial evidence implicates head trauma, either a single episode with loss of consciousness or repeated subconcussive injuries, as risk factors for dementia and AD (Amaducci et al. 1986; Heyman et al. 1984; Mortimer et al. 1985, 1991; O'Meara et al. 1997). The evidence that head injury is a risk factor is suggested from boxers who develop dementia pugilistica associated with neurofibrillary tangles in the brain (Mendez 1995). Moreover, the neuropathology of AD, including β-amyloid and neurofibrillary tangles, accumulates rapidly following severe head injuries (Roberts et al. 1991, 1994). The EURODEM collaborative reanalysis of seven case-control studies found an odds ratio of 1.82 (95% CI, 1.3 to 2.7) for head injury (Mortimer et al. 1991). When the odds ratio was limited to head traumas that occurred 10 years or less prior to the onset of dementia, the odds ratio jumped to as much as 10.0 (95% CI, 1.0 to 96.8) (Van Duijn et al. 1992). Despite these studies, controversy remains over the risk from head injury because of possible effects of recall bias or over-reporting by affected persons (Kokmen et al. 1996a; Launer et al. 1999 Mendez et al. 1992). Interestingly, the added risk of head injury may be limited to a specific subpopulation. Severe head injury accompanied by loss of consciousness may promote the onset of AD only in those carrying APOE ε4 alleles (Mayeux et al. 1995), and it may reduce the time to onset of AD among those at risk (Nemetz et al. 1999).

Lack of education and low occupational attainment are additional risk factors for both AD and other dementias. Stern et al. (1994) reported a relative risk of dementia of 2.0 in subjects with low education, 2.3 in those with low lifetime occupational attainment, and 2.9 in those with both. An uneducated individual older than 75 has about twice the risk for dementia as one who has completed at least the eighth grade (Stern et al. 1994). Studies from different countries have confirmed the independent risk for AD of both very low education and occupation with low cognitive demands (Aquero-Torres et al. 1998; Dartigues et al. 1992; Fratiglioni et al. 1991; Katzman 1993; Obadia et al. 1997; Rocca et al. 1990). Early education or lifelong intellectual activity may reflect a greater neuronal reserve that delays the clinical onset of dementia (Amaducci et al. 1992; De Ronchi et al. 1998). Snowden et al. (1996) investigated early intellectual function in 93 Catholic nuns. Low idea density, and, to a lesser extent, low grammatical complexity in autobiographies written in their early twenties were associated with low cognitive test scores at ages 75 to 95. Among the 14 who died, the neuropathology of AD was present in all of those with low idea density in early life and in none of those with high idea density. In addition, patients with a large neuronal reserve may require a large pathophysiological effect of AD in order to manifest clinical dementia. In AD, higher premorbid intellectual ability, greater years of education, and occupations with higher interpersonal skills are inversely correlated with cerebral metabolism in cortical association regions (Alexander et al. 1997; Stern et al. 1995).

The size of the head may reflect neuronal reserve. Persons born with larger head and therefore larger brains indexed by head size may have a greater neuronal buffer against pathological processes that cause dementia. Small increases in brain volume can translate into millions of excess neurons. Graves et al. (1994) examined this hypothesis among Japanese-Americans and found smaller head circumference significantly predicted cognitive impairment on the Cognitive Abilities Screening Instrument. Schofield et al. (1995) found that among 28 women with AD, those who began with larger brains on (CT) tomography exhibited dementia onset significantly later in life (10 years) than those with smaller brains. They reported an odds ratio for AD of 0.8 (95% CI, 0.7 to 0.9) for head circumference (Schofield et al. 1997). By measuring total intracranial volume with magnetic resonance imaging (MRI), Mori et al. (1997) further examined premorbid brain volume as a determinant of cognitive reserve in 60 patients with AD. The intelligence scores of these AD patients correlated positively with their premorbid brain volume and negatively with the magnitude of brain atrophy.

Many studies have evaluated environmental exposures but have not established any of them as promoting dementia or AD (Whalley et al. 1995). Investigators have proposed an inverse association between risk of AD and smoking (Van Duijn et al. 1994). Smoking could provide protection against early-onset AD in those with an APOE ε4 allele and a positive family history of dementia (Hillier and Salib 1997; Van Duijn et al. 1995). Others have not found that exposure to moderate levels of cigarette smoking decreased the risk for AD (Forster et al. 1995; Launer et al. 1999; Wong et al. 1999). Although alcohol and other drugs can destroy brain cells, it has not been consistently implicated as a risk factor for AD and moderate wine intake may even confer some protection (Fratiglioni et al. 1993; Mendez et al. 1992; Orogozo et al. 1997). Metals such as aluminum, zinc, and mercury have long been suspected of causing dementia. Although high concentrations of aluminum have been reported in neurofibrillary tangles (Perl and Brody 1980), no constant relationship exists between AD and aluminum-containing medications, antacids, antiperspirants, brewed tea, drinking water, or other sources (Amaducci et al. 1986; Graves et al. 1990; Ross 1994). Zinc may be involved in the formation of amyloid plaques; however, autopsy studies report low levels of zinc in the brain tissue of individuals with AD (Cuajungco and Lees 1997). Similarly, mercury deposits do not clearly result in neuronal degeneration. The establishment of a relation between occupational solvent exposure and AD still needs to be defined (Kukull et al. 1995). Breitner et al. (1995a) in four pairs of AD twins found that probands that had occupational histories of sewing, metal milling, welding, or sheetmetal working, whereas their siblings did not. Finally, workers who are exposed to intense and frequent levels of electromagnetic fields (EMF) in the workplace such as seamstresses, dressmakers, and tailors may be at greater risk for dementia. Sobel and colleagues (1996) reported an odds ratio of AD among workers with likely EMF exposure of 3.93 (95% CI, 1.5 to 10.6).

Many other proposed risk factors remain unconfirmed. Because of the relationship between AD and Down's syndrome, studies have investigated but not established a role for advanced maternal age in AD (Graves et al. 1990; Rocca et al. 1991). The EURODEM group found that family history of Down's syndrome had an odds ratio for AD of 2.7 (95% CI, 1.2 to 5.7) (Van Duijn et al. 1991). Schupf et al. (1994) found that only mothers who gave birth before age 35 to a child with Down's syndrome were at risk for AD, suggesting a predisposition to chromosome 21 nondisjunction. In some studies, late-life clinical depression predicts the development of dementia (Alexopoulos et al. 1993; Buntinx et al. 1996; Jorm et al. 1991; Kokmen et al. 1991, 1996a). The presence of acute-phase proteins and activated microglial cells around neuritic plaques suggests an infectious process in AD (Aisen and Davis 1994); however, the transmission of AD from human brain tissue to experimental animals has been unsuccessful. Cerebrovascular and cardiovascular changes, atherosclerosis, or high serum cholesterol levels could be risk factors for AD, particularly in the presence of an APOE ε4 allele (Aronson et al. 1990; Hoffman et al. 1997; Lopez et al. 1992; Notkola et al. 1998; Ott et al. 1997). Finally, diabetes mellitus may contribute to its occurrence but not thyroid disease (Heyman et al. 1984; Kokmen et al. 1996a; Leibson et al. 1997).

After AD, we know most about risk factors for VaD. First of all, strokes themselves are risk factors for dementia. The incidence of dementia was 8.4 per 100 person-years in a stroke group compared to 1.3 per 100 person-years in a control group (Tatemichi et al. 1994b). The odds ratio of dementia associated with stroke was 5.5 (95% CI, 2.5 to 11.1) after adjusting for demographic factors. A second stroke, along with advanced age and male sex, were significant independent predictors of dementia (Kokmen et al. 1996b; Tatemichi et al. 1994a). In the CSHA, the risk of VaD was associated with history of arterial hypertension (odds ratio, 2.08; 95% CI, 1.29 to 3.35) (Lindsay et al. 1997). Hypertensive lacunar strokes may be particular risk factor for VaD (Loeb 1995). Other significantly elevated odds ratios occurred for less than 6 years education (4.0), history of alcohol abuse (2.5), and history of a heart condition (1.7) (Lindsay et al. 1997). Similar to AD, APOE ε4 status predisposes to dementia after stroke (Tatemichi et al. 1994b). The relationship between vascular lesions and dementia includes the strategic location of the lesion such as the thalamus and the extent of cerebral atrophy and ventricular enlargement. Nevertheless, cognitive impairments correlates better with the extent of cerebral ischemia rather than with the amount of infarcted brain tissue (Meyer et al. 1994). Moreover, individuals who do not meet pathological criteria for either AD or VaD may present with intellectual impairments as a result of combined AD and vascular lesions.

## Natural History

AD is a chronic disease with a long preclinical course. Estimates of the mean survival for AD vary because of difficulty in accurately dating the onset of dementia. The mean survival after symptom onset for AD of 10.3 years may range from 2 to more than 20 years (Mann et al. 1992; Sulkava et al. 1992; Walsh et al. 1990). Barclay et al. (1985) found that the 50% survival rates from onset of the symptoms were 8.1 years for AD, 6.7 years for the VaD, and 6.2 years for mixed AD and VaD. Other studies report that dementia and AD shortens the projected lifespan by about 4.5 years (Bowen et al. 1996; Jorm et al. 1987; Kokmen et al. 1996a; Mann et al. 1992). Molsa et al. (1995) reported a 14-year survival rate for AD that was 2.4% versus an expected rate of 16.6%. Moreover, men with AD have a somewhat shorter survival time than women by about 1.5 years (Heyman et al. 1997; Moritz et al. 1997). The shortened survival of AD patients results from complications that occur in terminal stages when patients are bedbound, such as progressive debilitation, malnutrition, dehydration, pneumonia, and other infections. More effective treatments for these complications may increase the lifespan for dementia patients in the future (Rossler et al. 1995).

AD patients manifest great variability in clinical features and rate of progression. The typical patient with AD progresses through three general clinical stages (Cummings and Benson 1992). The first symptom of AD is usually an inability to incorporate new knowledge despite continued ability to retain old, established memories. A second early cognitive impairment is an inability to retrieve words. This word-finding difficulty may be so profound that speech is empty and devoid of meaningful words. Visuospatial impairment is a third early manifestation often evident as an inability to orient themselves in their surrounds or to make drawings and copy figures. In the middle stage, more prominent amnesia, aphasia, and apraxia replace early memory and word-finding difficulties. The aphasia is often a transcortical sensory type with comprehension difficulty and empty speech but with relatively preserved repetition. AD patients develop delusions, agitation, depression, and other behavioral symptoms. Throughout the first two stages, activities of daily living are progressively impaired such as driving, buying groceries, preparing meals, doing laundry, and basic functions such as walking safely and maintaining personal hygiene. In the last stage, patients are "globally" demented, motorically impaired, incontinent, and susceptible to the intercurrent illnesses that bring death.

AD does not progress linearly (Fig. 35-3). Patients in the early stages often show relatively slow cognitive deterioration. More advanced cognitive deficits are associated with a faster rate of decline. Brooks et al. (1993) have proposed an inverse "S" shaped model of decline. This "trilinear" model includes three stages beginning with an initial period of stability or plateau, most of which occurs prior to detection of clinical decline. The middle stage is characterized by a period of sharp decline. In the final stage, commonly used cognitive tests reach a floor and the patient appears relatively stable once again. Likewise, the rate of change on scales and measures in AD varies with the severity of cognitive impairment (Becker et al. 1988; Drachman et al. 1990; Morris et al. 1993). For example, the Mini-Mental State Examination (MMSE) changes 1 to 2 points per year in the first few years and 4 to 5 points per year in moderate to severe stages (Folstein et al. 1975).

Clinicians and others monitor the course of AD and other dementias with global or functional scales, mental status scales, and formal neuropsychological tests. Different aspects of AD may not progress at the same rate on these scales, and cognitive scales may not accurately reflect functional abilities. In addition, some scales emphasize some cognitive abilities over others (e.g., the MMSE is

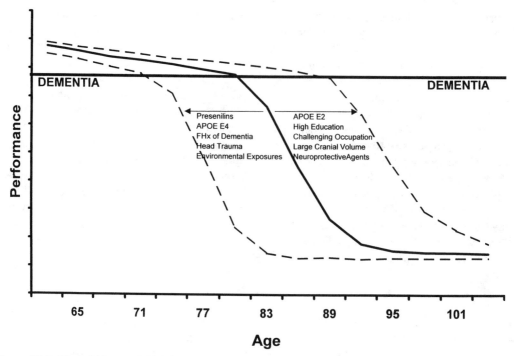

**Figure 35-3.** Natural history of Alzheimer's disease as affected by age and various risk factors. The ordinate represents cognitive and functional performance, and the top horizontal line is the threshold for dementia. The abscissa represents advancing age.

highly dependent on language (Obadia et al. 1997). Nevertheless, these scales can be useful in monitoring decline in dementia patients over time. Two widely used global scales are the Clinical Dementia Rating Scale (CDR) and the Global Deterioration Scale (GDS) (Berg et al. 1988; Reisberg et al. 1982). Following a cohort of 43 initially mild AD patients (CDR 1) for 90 months, more than 67% progressed to CDR 3 (severe) by 50 months, and more that 80% progressed to CDR 3 by 66 months (Berg et al. 1988). On the CDR, transitions between levels occur every 1 to 2 years. The GDS has up to 16 stages for characterizing progression in dementia (Reisberg et al. 1982). Commonly used mental status scales include the MMSE, the Mattis Dementia Rating Scale (DRS), and the Blessed Information-Memory-Concentration (IMC) Test (Blessed et al. 1968; Folstein et al. 1975; Mattis 1976). On average there is a yearly deterioration of 3 points (1.28 to 4.2) on the MMSE (Aquero-Torres et al. 1998; Becker et al. 1988; Boller et al. 1991; Forette et al. 1989; Katzman et al. 1988; Ortof and Crystal 1989; Salmon et al. 1990; Teri et al. 1990; Thal et al. 1988), 12 points on the DRS (Mann et al. 1992; Salmon et al. 1990), and 4

(3.2 to 4.5) points on the IMC (Salmon et al. 1990; Ortof and Crystal 1989). Salmon et al. (1990) compared these three scales in 55 community-dwelling patients with AD over 2 years. Patients had an annual rate of change of 2.8 on the MMSE, 11.38 on the DRS, and 3.24 on the IMC. On all of these scales, the standard deviations were large, and the annual rates of change in the first year were poorly correlated with the next year's rate of decline. Moreover, the rates of change determinations are less reliable when the observation is 1 year or less (Morris et al. 1993).

The natural history of other dementing illnesses varies greatly with etiology. Dementia can be subacute with death within 5 months, as in Creutzfeldt-Jakob disease, or run a course of decades, as may occur in AD. The two main cortical dementias are AD and the frontotemporal dementias such as Pick's disease. These two dementia groups differ in their cognitive and behavioral symptoms but have similar disease duration. Neocortical Lewy bodies associated with cognitive impairment, early parkinsonism, fluctuating mental status, and visual hallucinations characterize DLB. VaD patients have shorter life expectancies than both

AD patients and nondemented stroke patients (Desmond 1996; Molsa et al. 1995; Tatemichi et al. 1994b). The mean duration of VaD is around 5 years (Hebert and Brayne 1995). In one study, the 14-year survival rate for VaD it was 1.7% versus an expected 13.3% (Molsa et al. 1995). In another study, the mortality rate was 19.8 deaths per 100 person-years with VaD compared with 6.9 deaths per 100 person-years in stroke patients without dementia (Tatemichi et al. 1994b).

## Prognostic Factors

Clinicians can use some of the factors outlined here to make prognostic judgments on individual patients (Table 35-6). As expected, survival is closely related to dementia severity (Bowen et al. 1996; Walsh et al. 1990). Greater debility and functional incapacity are associated with increased mortality (Bowen et al. 1996). In addition, older patients, especially those 70 or older, are significantly more likely to die during follow-up (Becker et al. 1994; Bowen et al. 1996; Brodaty et al. 1997; Koopmans et al. 1994; Heyman et al. 1997; Reisberg et al. 1996). Male gender is also a greater risk for shorter duration to death in most but not all studies (Becker et al. 1994; Bracco et al. 1994; Bowen et al. 1996; Drachman et al. 1990; Galasko et al. 1994; Heyman et al. 1997; Jagger et al. 1995; Katzman et al. 1988; Koopmans et al. 1994; Reisberg et al. 1996).

**Table 35-6.** Prognostic Factors For Survival In Dementia and Alzheimer's Disease

Definite negative prognostic factors
   Increased dementia severity and duration
   Advanced age
   Male gender
   Comorbidity such as strokes or cardiac disease
   Alcohol or drug abuse
   Weight loss
   Increased caregiver psychological burden
   Early onset of aphasia
   Extrapyramidal signs
   Primitive reflexes
   Aggression and agitation
   Wandering and falling
   Sleep disturbances
   Sensory impairments
   Nonspecific changes on electroencephalography
   Periventricular white matter densities
   Pronounced metabolic decreases in cortex
Putative negative prognostic factors
   Late age of onset
   Low level of education
   Predominantly "posterior" cognitive deficits

In an analysis of survival time following institutionalization, men with AD survived a median of 2.1 years, compared with 4.5 years for women with AD (Heyman et al. 1997). Although earlier studies found that presenile onset was associated with a more rapid progression and shorter survival (Heyman et al. 1987; Seltzer and Sherwin 1983), most recent investigations found age of onset of symptoms had no effect on the rate of cognitive change or life expectancy in AD (Barclay et al. 1985; Bracco et al. 1994; Berg et al. 1988; Bracco et al. 1994; Drachman et al. 1990; Katzman et al. 1988; Knopman et al. 1988; Ortof and Crystal 1989; Salmon et al. 1990; Thal et al. 1988). Conversely, a later age of onset may shorten the duration of illness and is associated with more impaired functional capacity (Bayles 1991; Becker et al. 1988; Burns et al. 1991; Frisoni et al. 1995; Galasko et al. 1994; Katzman et al. 1988; Jacobs et al. 1994; Mann et al. 1992; Nyth et al. 1991; Ortof and Crystal 1989; Selnes et al. 1988; Thal et al. 1988). Ethnic background, APOE genotype, and marital status do not appear to affect survival (Corder et al. 1995), but the effect of level of education is less clear (Berg et al. 1988; Drachman et al. 1994; Katzman et al. 1993). Among 4051 elderly aged 65 to 84 years, the relative risk of death decreased in AD patients as level of education increased (0.86; 95% CI, 0.63 to 1.19) (Geerlings et al. 1997); however, others found an increased risk of death among 448 AD patients with high educational and occupational attainment (Stern et al. 1995). Some authors reported a worse prognosis associated with familial AD (Burns et al. 1991; Heston et al. 1987), but others did not find any differences from familial aggregation (Bracco et al. 1994). An increased risk of death in AD occurs with comorbidity such as heart failure, a history of heavy alcohol use, excessive weight loss, and institutionalization (Jagger et al. 1995; van Dijk et al. 1996; Wang et al. 1997). Finally, caregiver psychological morbidity may be associated with shorter survival of demented patients (Brodaty et al. 1993).

Specific clinical factors may be helpful prognostic features (Table 35-6). The early onset of aphasia predicts a rapid deterioration (Bracco et al. 1994; Faber-Langendoen et al. 1988; Goldblum et al. 1994). Severe language disability predicts death independent of dementia severity and age at onset (Bracco et al. 1994). Some studies have identified other cognitive disturbances, such as visuospatial impairments and motor apraxia, as indicating a worse prognosis (Berg et al. 1985; Burns et al. 1991; Kaszniak et al. 1978; Mortimer et al. 1992), and AD patients with a predominantly posterior pattern of cognitive impairment may have a slower deterioration than those with additional frontal lobe defects (Mann et al. 1992; Merello et al. 1994; Nyth et al. 1991). Others have not found that cognitive deficits or patterns other than aphasia predict survival (Becker et al. 1994). AD patients often develop extrapyramidal signs (EPS) such as rigidity and bradykinesia, usually at an advanced stage of dementia (Choi et al. 1994; Mayeux et al. 1985). Patients who develop EPS earlier in their course have a faster rate of cognitive and functional decline and a worse prognosis independent of dementia severity (Choi et al. 1994, 1985; Mayeux et al. 1985; Mortimer et al. 1992; Snowdon et al. 1996; Stern et al. 1994, 1997). The additional finding of primitive reflexes adds to risk of death in AD (Molsa et al. 1995). Psychiatric symptoms may be associated with a faster decline in dementia (Choi et al. 1985, 1994; Forstl et al. 1993; Mayeux et al. 1985; Mortimer et al. 1992; Stern et al. 1994, 1997).

Aggressiveness, agitation, wandering, falling, sleep disturbances, and sensory impairments predict a faster decline and an increased likelihood of death (Bowen et al. 1996; Mortimer et al. 1992; Walsh et al. 1990), but several studies in AD have failed to find that psychosis or depression accelerate the disease (Huff et al. 1987; Lopez et al. 1990; Reisberg et al. 1986). On electroencephalograms (EEG), nonspecific abnormalities may be a predictor of mortality (Kaszniak et al. 1978). Similarly, periventricular white matter hypodensity on CT are potentially significant predictors of mortality (Lopez et al. 1992; Marder et al. 1995). On functional neuroimaging, metabolic reductions in the temporal, temporoparietal, or frontal regions may correlate with cognitive decline in AD (Merello et al. 1994; Smith et al. 1992; Wolfe et al. 1995).

A specific prognostic issue in dementia is the need for institutional placement (Table 35-7). In AD, nursing home placement often occurs about 7 years into the course, and about 20%–25% of dementia years are spent in nursing homes (Heyman et al. 1997; Katzman and Rowe 1992). Among initially mild AD patients, 50% were institutionalized by 40 months and 80% by 60

months regardless of age of onset (Berg et al. 1988; Drachman et al. 1990; Katzman et al. 1988; Knopman et al. 1988; Salmon et al. 1990). Increased duration of illness, dementia severity, inability to walk, presence of EPS, and psychotic and other behavioral symptoms were factors that led to earlier institutionalization (Brandt et al. 1993; Lopez et al. 1997a, 1997b). Urinary or fecal incontinence, inability to speak coherently, and loss of skills needed for bathing and grooming were additional major determinants of institutionalization (Hutton et al. 1985). Behavioral disturbances, particularly aggression, agitation, irritability, wandering, or nocturnal behavioral problems cause great distress to caregivers and other concerned individuals, and are the most frequent reason for the acute hospitalization or institutionalization of dementia patients (Cummings and Benson 1992; Wimo et al. 1995). The presence of delusions, in particular, is a significant predictor of nursing home admission regardless of dementia severity (Magni et al. 1996). Prognostic factors to institutionalization also include the extent of social support systems. Compared to unmarried patients, those that are married are less likely to be institutionalized or may have a delay in nursing home admission by about 1 year (Hogan et al. 1994). The training and counseling of caregivers further delay nursing home admission and reduce mortality (Brodaty et al. 1997; Mittleman et al. 1996). The caregivers' physical health and ability to cope ultimately contribute to the decision to place the patient in a nursing home.

**Table 35-7.** Prognostic Factors for Institutionalization in Dementia and Alzheimer's disease

Negative Prognostic Factors
  Increased dementia severity and duration
  Inability to walk
  Extrapyramidal signs
  Psychotic symptoms, especially delusions
  Urinary and fecal incontinence
  Inability to speak coherently
  Loss of activities of daily living, especially bathing and grooming
  Aggression, agitation, and irritability
  Wandering
  Nocturnal behavioral disturbance
  Poor social support systems
  Unmarried status (particularly among men)
  Caregiver: poor health and stress
Positive Prognostic Factors
  Caregiver training and counseling
  Participation in drug trials

The prognostic factors for other dementias are less clear. Effects of aphasia and depression worsen prognosis for VaD, and increased age at presentation is associated with shorter survival in early-onset VaD (Thomas et al. 1997). Similar to AD, survival rates for VaD are less for men than for women (Thomas et al. 1997). Psychotic symptoms are associated with more severe cognitive and functional impairment in VaD (Gur et al. 1994; Lopez et al. 1997a). An abnormal EEG performed close to the first ischemic stroke may be an indicator of subsequent cognitive decline, probably because it indicates cortical involvement by the stroke or an underlying indolent cerebral degeneration (Gur et al. 1994). Silent strokes may not augur the development of VaD (Bornstein et al 1996), but VaD increases the risk of subsequent strokes and their coincident morbidity (Moroney et al. 1997).

## Prevention and Management

Interventions that delay the onset or progression of AD can have a major impact on the prevalence of this disorder (Brookmeyer et al. 1998). The prevention of head injuries and toxic exposures may also delay the onset of dementia. Although not established, current information suggests that those who continue to exercise their minds may be more likely to live longer without developing dementia. Once dementia occurs, patients benefit from a graded amount of cognitive stimulation. Maintaining a familiar, constant, and accepting environment at home can decrease agitation and other behavioral symptoms and potentially prolong the functional state of the patient. Attention should be given to other functional issues, such as safety in the home, unnecessary changes in routine, and regulation of day-night cycles. Behavioral and drug therapies are minimally effective in treating the cognitive manifestations of dementia, but the neuropsychiatric complications often respond to the judicious use of psychoactive medications. These drugs can maintain patients at home and out of the nursing home for a longer period of time. Participation in clinical drug trials can also decrease the risk of nursing home admission possibly because of the increased attention paid to patients and caregivers (Albert et al. 1997).

The clinician must consider psychosocial issues such as "care of the caregiver," education and counseling of family members, support groups, day programs and respite care, competency and conservatorship assessments, financial planning, issues of institutionalization, and others. The programs sponsored by the Alzheimer's Association are particularly valuable in providing education, referrals to community resources, and support for caregivers. When patients cannot safely be left alone in their homes, caregivers or guardians must evaluate the patients for transfer to more supervised environments or nursing homes. Once institutionalized, the patients should participate in programs that promote a reasonable amount of stimulation while maintaining their routine. Staff should help patients maintain their mobility, weight, and as much self-sufficiency as possible (Wang et al. 1997). dementia special care units may facilitate the attainment of these goals (Volicer et al. 1994).

Recent advances in understanding the clinical profile and neurobiological features of AD have led to antiacetylcholinesterase therapy and other experimental methods of treating this disorder. Early intervention with these agents may retard the expression of the disease. To date, donepezil (Aricept) and tacrine (Cognex) have been approved specifically for the treatment of dementia. Both drugs have resulted in modest improvement or a decreased rate of decline in about one-third of mild to moderate AD patients (Knapp et al. 1994; Rogers and Friedhoff 1996). This may equate to a decrease in progression of the dementia by about 6 months to 1 year. In one study, APOE genotype affected the degree of responsiveness to these drugs; 83% of ε2/ε3 AD patients improved after tacrine treatment, whereas 60% of ε4 AD patients did not (Poirier et al. 1993). The effects of hydergine are unclear, but a meta-analysis suggests that high-dose hydergine at 6 mg or more per day can result in modest symptomatic improvement (Schneider and Olin 1994).

Investigators are testing several strategies that may affect survival and prognosis in dementia and AD. Vitamin E at doses of 1000 to 2000 IU may delay the onset of AD, possibly through antioxidant effects (Aisen and Davis 1997). One study found that vitamin E and selegiline, a selective MAO-B inhibitor, were equally effective in slowing the progression of AD, but combined therapy did not confer an additional advantage (Sano et al. 1997). Other research indicates that nonsteroidal anti-inflammatory drugs (NSAIDs) can prevent or delay the onset of AD (Breitner et al. 1995b; Rogers et al. 1993). In a study of 50 sets of elderly twin pairs that included at least one with AD, the unaffected or late-affected member was four times more likely to have used glucocorticoids or NSAIDs with an average delay of 5 years and a decrease in lifetime incidence of AD by more than one-third (Breitner et al. 1994). Estrogen use in postmenopausal women may also delay the onset and decrease the risk of AD (Kawas et al 1997; Tang et al. 1996). Paginini-Hill and Henderson (1994) found that the risk of AD was significantly less common among estrogen users (15%) as compared to nonusers (30%). Recently, investigators have evaluated the efficacy of ginkgo biloba special extract EGb 761 in a 52-week trial of outpatients with mild to moderate AD or VaD (Le Bars et al. 1997). They concluded that this extract could stabilize or improve cognitive performance and social functioning for 6–12 months. Drug therapy for AD is an extremely active area of research, and many other medications that can affect the prognosis of AD may be available in the near future (Davis et al. 1993; Schneider and Tariot 1994).

**Acknowledgments** This work was supported by on NIA Alzheimer's Disease Center grant (AG10123), Alzheimer's Disease Research Center of California, and the Sidell-Kagan Foundation.

# References

Aguero-Torres, H.; Fratiglioni, L.; Guo, Z.; Viitanen, M.; Winblad, B. Prognostic factors in very old demented adults: a seven-year follow-up from a population-based survey in Stockholm. J. Am. Geriatr. Soc. 46:444–452; 1998.

Aisen, P. S.; Davis, K. L. Inflammatory mechanisms in Alzheimer's disease: implications for therapy. Am. J. Psychiatry 151:1105–1113; 1994.

Albert, S. M.; Sano, M.; Marder, K.; Jacobs, D. M.; Brandt, J.; et al. Participation in clinical trials and long-term outcomes in Alzheimer's disease. Neurology 49:38–43; 1997.

Alexander, G. E.; Furey, M. L.; Grady, C. L.; Pietrini, P.; Brady, D. R; et al. Association of premorbid intellectual function with cerebral metabolism in Alzheimer's disease: implications for the cognitive reserve hypothesis. Am. J. Psychiatry 154:165–172; 1997.

Alexopoulos, G. S.; Meyers, B. S.; Young, R. C.; Mattis, S.; Kakuma, T. The course of geriatric depression with "reversible dementia": a controlled study. Am. J. Psychiatry 150:1693–1699; 1993.

Amaducci L. Italian longitudinal study on ageing: incidence study of dementia. Neuroepidemiology 11 (suppl. 1):19–22; 1992.

Amaducci, L. A.; Fratiglioni, L.; Rocca, W. A.; Fieschi, C.; Livrea, P.; et al. Risk factors for clinically diagnosed Alzheimer's disease: a case-control study of an Italian population. Neurology 36:922–931; 1986.

American Psychiatric Association. Diagnostic and statistical manual of mental disorders. 4th ed. Washington, DC: American Psychiatric Association; 1994.

Aronson, M. K.; Ooi, W. L.; Geva, D. L.; Masur, D.; Blau, A.; Frishman, W. Dementia. Age-dependent incidence, prevalence, and mortality in the old old. Arch. Interna Med. 11:989–992; 1991.

Aronson, M. K.; Ooi, W. L.; Morgenstern, H.; Hafner, A.; Masur, D.; et al. Women, myocardial infarction, and dementia in the very old. Neurology 40:1102–1106; 1990.

Bachman, D. L.; Wolf, P. A.; Linn, R. T.; Knoefel, J. E.; Cobb, J. L.; et al. Incidence of dementia and probable Alzheimer's disease in a general population: the Framingham Study. Neurology 43:515–519; 1993.

Barclay, L. L.; Zemcov, A.; Blass, J. P.; Sansone, J. Survival in Alzheimer's disease and vascular dementias. Neurology 35:834–840; 1985.

Bayles, K. A. Age at onset of Alzheimer's disease. Relation to language dysfunction. Arch. Neurol 48:155–159; 1991.

Becker, J. T.; Boller, F.; Lopez, O. L.; Saxton, J.; McGonigle, K. L. The natural history of Alzheimer's disease. Description of study cohort and accuracy of diagnosis. Arch. Neurol. 51:585–594; 1994.

Becker, J. T.; Huff, F. J.; Nebes, R. D.; Holland, A.; Boller, F. Neuropsychological function in Alzheimer's disease. Pattern of impairment and rates of progression. Arch. Neurol. 45:263–268; 1988.

Berg, L.; Danzinger, W. L.; Storandt, M.; Coben, L. A.; Gado, M.; et al. Predictive features in mild senile dementia of the Alzheimer type. Neurology 34:563–569; 1985.

Berg, L.; Miller, J. P.; Storandt, M.; Duchek, J.; Morris, J. C.; et al. Mild senile dementia of the Alzheimer type, 11: longitudinal assessment. Ann. Neurol. 23:477–484; 1988.

Blessed, G.; Tomlinson, B. E.; Roth, M. The association between quantitative measures of dementia and of senile changes in the cerebral grey matter of elderly subjects. Br. J. Psychiatry 114:797–811; 1968.

Boller, F.; Becker, J. T.; Holland, A. L.; Forbes, M. M.; Hood, P. C.; McGonigle-Gibson, K. L. Predictors of decline in Alzheimer's disease. Cortex 27:9–17; 1991.

Bornstein, N. M.; Gur, A. Y.; Treves, T. A.; Reider-Groswasser, I.; Aronovich, B. D.; et al. Do silent brain infarctions predict the development of dementia after first ischemic stroke? Stroke 27:904–905; 1996.

Bowen, J. D.; Malter, A. D.; Sheppard, L.; Kukull, W. A.; McCormick, W. C.; et al. Predictors of mortality in patients diagnosed with probable Alzheimer's disease. Neurology 47:433–439; 1996.

Bracco, L.; Gallato, R.; Grigoletto, F.; Lippi, A.; Lepore, V.; et al. Factors affecting course and survival in Alzheimer's disease. A 9-year longitudinal study. Arch. Neurol. 51:1213–1219; 1994.

Brandt, J.; Welsh, K. A.; Breitner, J. C.; Folstein, M. F.; Helms, M.; Christian, J. C. Hereditary influences on cognitive functioning in older men. A study of 4000 twin pairs. Arch. Neurol. 50:599–603; 1993.

Breitner, J. C. S. Onset of Alzheimer's disease. Influence of genes and environmental factors, including anti-inflammatory drugs. In: progress in Alzheimer's disease and similar conditions. Washington, DC: American Psychiatric Press; 1997: p. 189–198.

Breitner, J. C. S. New epidemiologic strategies in Alzheimer's disease may provide clues to prevention and cause. Neurobiol. Aging 15(suppl.):S175–S177; 1994.

Breitner, J. C. S. Clinical genetics and genetic conseling in Alzheimer's disease. Ann. Intern. Med. 115:601–606; 1991.

Breitner, J. C. S.; Gau, B. A.; Welsh, K. A.; Plassman, B. L.; McDonald, W. M.; et al. Inverse association of anti-inflammatory treatments and Alzheimer's disease: initial results of a co-twin control study. Neurology 44:227–232; 1994.

Breitner, J. C.; Silverman, J. M.; Mohs, R. C.; Davis, K. L. Familial aggregation in Alzheimer's disease: comparison of risk among relatives of early-and late-onset cases, and among male and female relatives in successive generations. Neurology 38:207–212; 1988.

Breitner, J. C. S.; Welsh, K. A.; Gau, B. A.; McDonald, W. M.; Steffens, D. C.; et al. Alzheimer's disease in the NAS-NRC registry of aging twin veterans, III: detection of cases, longitudinal results, and twin concordance. Arch. Neurol. 52:763–771; 1995a.

Breitner, J. C. S.; Welsh, K. A.; Helms, M. J.; Gaskell, D. C.; Gau, B. A.; et al. Delayed onset of Alzheimer's disease with non-steroidal anti-inflammatory and histamine H2 blocking drugs. Neurobiol. Aging 16:523–530; 1995b.

Breteler, M. M.; Claus, J. J.; van Duijn, C. M.; Launer, L. J.; Hofman, A. Epidemiology of Alzheimer's disease. Epidemiol. Rev. 14:59–82; 1992.

Brodaty, H.; Gresham, M.; Luscombe, G. The Prince Henry Hospital dementia caregivers' training programme. Int. J. Geriatr. Psychiatry 12:183–192; 1997.

Brodaty, H.; McGilchrist, C.; Harris, L.; Peters, K. E. Time until institutionalization and death in patients with dementia. Role of caregiver training and risk factors. Arch. Neurol. 50:643–650; 1993.

Brookmeyer, R.; Gray, S.; Kawas, C. Projections of Alzheimer's disease in the United States and the public health impact of delaying disease onset. Am. J. Public Health 88:1337–1342; 1998.

Brooks, J. O.; Kraemer, H. C.; Tanke, E. D.; Yesavage, J. A.. The methodology of studying decline in Alzheimer's disease. J. Am. Geriatr. Soc. 41:623–628; 1993.

Buntinx, F.; Kester, A.; Bergers, J.; Knottnerus, J. A. Is depression in elderly people followed by dementia? A retrospective cohort study based in general practice. Age Ageing 25:231–233; 1996.

Burns, A.; Jacoby, R.; Levy, R. Progression of cognitive impairment in Alzheimer's disease. J. Am. Geriatr. Soc. 39:39–45; 1991.

Canadian Study of Health and Aging Working Group. Canadian Study of Health and Aging: study methods and prevalence of dementia. Can. Med. Assoc. J. 150:899–912; 1994.

Choi, H. C.; Lyness, S. A.; Sobel, E.; Schneider, L. S. Extrapyramidal signs and psychiatric symptoms predict faster cognitive decline in Alzheimer's disease. Arch. Neurol. 51:676–681; 1994.

Choi, H. C.; Teng, E. L.; Henderson, V. W.; Moy, A. C. Clinical subtypes of dementia of Alzheimer's type. Neurology 35:1544–1550; 1985.

Chiu, H. F.; Lam, L. C.; Chi, I.; Leung, T.; Li, S. W.; et al. Prevalence of dementia in Chinese elderly in Hong Kong. Neurology 50:1002–1009; 1998.

Clarfield, A. M. The reversible dementias: do they reverse? Ann. Intern. Med. 109:476–486; 1988.

Corder, E. H.; Saunders, A. M.; Strittmatter, W. J.; Schmechel, D. E.; Gaskell, P.C., Jr.; et al. Apolipoprotein E, survival in Aizheimer's disease patients, and the competing risks of death and Alzheimer's disease. Neurology 45:1323–1328; 1995.

Cuajungco, M. P.; Lees, G. J. Zinc and Alzheimer's disease: is there a direct link? Brain Res. 23:219–2236; 1997.

Cummings, J. L.; Benson, D. F. Dementia: a clinical approach. 2nd ed. Boston: Butterworths; 1992.

Dartigues, J. F.; Gagnon, M.; Mazaux, J. M.; Barberger-Gateau, P.; Commenges, D.; et al. Occupation during life and memory performance in non-demented French elderly community residents. Neurology 42:1697–1701; 1992.

Davignon, J.; Gregg, R. E.; Sing, C. F. Apolipoprotein E polymorphism and atherosclerosis. Arteriosclerosis 8:1–21; 1988.

Davis, R. E.; Emmerling, M. R.; Jaen, J. C.; Moos, W. H.; Spiegel, K. Therapeutic intervention in dementia. Crit. Rev. Neurobiol. 7:41–83; 1993.

de la Monte, S. M.; Hutchins, G. M.; Moore, G. W. Racial differences in the etiology of dementia and frequency of Alzheimer lesions in the brain. J. Nat. Med. Assoc. 81:644–652; 1989.

De Ronchi, D.; Fratiglioni, L.; Rucci, P.; Paternico, A.; Graziani, S.; Dalmonte, E. The effect of education on dementia occurrence in an Italian population with middle to high socioeconomic status. Neurology 50:1231–1238; 1998.

Desmond, D. W. Vascular dementia: a construct in evolution. Cerebrovasc. Brain Met. Rev. 8:296–325; 1996.

Drach, L. M.; Steinmetz, H. E.; Wach, S.; Bohl, J. High proportion of dementia with Lewy bodies in the postmortems of a mental hospital in Germany. Int. J. Geriatr. Psychiatry 12:301–306; 1997.

Drachman, D. A. If we live long enough, will we all be demented? Neurology 44: 1563–1565; 1994.

Drachman, D. A.; O'Donnell, B. F.; Lew, R. A.; Swearer, J. M. The prognosis in Alzheimer's disease. Arch. Neurol. 47:851–856; 1990.

Ebly, E. M.; Parhad, I. M.; Hogan, D. B.; Fung, T. S. Prevalence and types of dementia in the very old: results from the Canadian Study of Health and Aging. Neurology 44:1593–1600; 1994.

Edland, S. D.; Silverman, J. M.; Peskind, E. R.; Tsuang, D.; Wijsman, E.; Morris, J. C. Increased risk of dementia in mothers of Alzheimer's disease cases: evidence for maternal inheritance. Neurology 47: 254–256; 1996.

Evans, D. Estimated prevalence of Alzheimer's disease in the United States. Milbank Q. 68:267–289; 1990.

Ewbank, D. C. Deaths attributable to Alzheimer's disease in the United States. Am. J. Public Health 89:90–92; 1999.

Faber-Langendoen, K.; Morris, J. C.; Knesevich, J. W.; LaBarge, E.; Miller, J. P.; Berg, L. Aphasia in senile dementia of the Alzheimer type. Ann. Neurol. 23:365–70; 1988.

Fichter, M. M.; Schroppel, H.; Meller, I. Incidence of dementia in a Munich community sample of the oldest old. Eur. Arch. Psychiatry Clin. Neurosci. 246: 320–328; 1996.

Fillenbaum, G. G.; Heyman, A.; Huber, M. S.; Woodbury, M. A.; Leiss, J.; et al. The prevalence and 3-year incidence of dementia in older black and white community residents. J. Clin. Epidemiol. 51: 587–595; 1998.

Folstein, M.; Folstein, S.; McHugh, P. R. Minimental state: a practical method for grading the cognitive state of patients for the clinician. J. Psychiatr. Res. 12:189–198; 1975.

Forette, F.; Henry, J. F.; Orgogozo, I. M.; Dartigues, J. F.; Pere, J. J.; et al. Reliability of clinical criteria for the diagnosis of dementia. A longitudinal multicenter study. Arch. Neurol. 46:646–648; 1989.

Forster, D. P.; Newens, A. J.; Kay, D. W.; Edwardson, J. A. Risk factors in clinically diagnosed presenile dementia of the Alzheimer type: a case-control study in northern England. J. Epidiol. Community Health 49:253–258; 1995.

Forstl, H.; Besthorn, C.; Geiger-Kabisch, C.; Sattel, H.; Schreiter-Gasser, U. Psychotic features and the course of Alzheimer's disease: relationship to cognitive, electroencephalographic and computerized tomography findings. Acta Psychiatr. Scand. 87: 395–399; 1993.

Fratiglioni, L.; Ahlbom, A.; Viitanen, M.; Winblad, B. Risk factors for late-onset Alzheimer's disease: a population-based, case-control study. Ann. Neurol. 33:258–266; 1993.

Fratiglioni, L.; Grut, M.; Forsell, Y.; Viitanen, M.; Grafstrom, M.; et al. Prevalence of Alzheimer's disease and other dementias in an elderly urban population: relationship with age, sex, and education. Neurology 41:1886–1892; 1991.

Fratiglioni, L.; Viitanen, M.; von Strauss, E.; Tontodonati, V.; Herlitz, A.; Winblad, B. Very old women at highest risk of dementia and Alzheimer's disease: incidence data from the Kungsholmen Project, Stockholm. Neurology 48:132–138; 1997.

Frisoni, G. B.; Govoni, S.; Geroldi, C.; Blanchetti, A.; Calabressi, L.; et al. Gene dose of the E4 allele of apolipoprotein E and disease progression in sporadic late-onset Alzheimer's disease. Ann. Neurol. 37: 596–604; 1995.

Galasko, D.; Hansen, L. A.; Katzman, R.; Wiederholt, W.; Masliah, E.; et al. Clinical-neuropathological correlations in Alzheimer's disease and related dementias. Arch. Neurol. 51:898–895; 1994.

Gao, S.; Hendrie, H. C.; Hall, K. S.; Hui, S. The relationships between age, sex, and the incidence of dementia and Alzheimer disease: a meta-analysis. Arch. Gen. Psychiatry 55:809–815; 1998.

Gatz, M.; Pedersen, N. L.; Berg, S.; Johansson, B.; Johansson, K.; et al. Heritability for Alzheimer's disease: the study of dementia in Swedish twins. J. Gerontol 52:M117–M125; 1997.

Geerlings, M. I.; Deeg, D. J.; Schmand, B.; Lindeboom, J.; Jonker, C. Increased risk of mortality in Alzheimer's disease patients with higher education? A replication study. Neurology 49:798–802; 1997.

General Accounting Office Report. Health, Education, and Human Services Division, Alzheimer's Disease Prevalence. January 28, 1998.

Goldblum, M.-C.; Tzortzis, C.; Michot, J.-L.; Panisset, M.; Boller, F. Language impairment and rate of cognitive decline in Alzheimer's disease. Dementia 5:334–338; 1994.

Graves, A. B.; Larson, E. B.; White, L. R.; Teng, E. L.; Homma, A. Opportunities and challenges in international collaborative epidemiologic research of dementia and its subtypes: studies between Japan and the U.S. Int. Psychogeriatr. 6:209–223; 1994.

Graves, A. B.; White, E.; Koepsell, T. D.; Reifler, B. V.; van Pella, G.; et al. A case-control study of Alzheimer's disease. Ann. Neurol. 28:2766–2774; 1990.

Gur, A. Y.; Neufeld, M. Y.; Treves, T. A.; Aronovich, B. D.; Bornstein, N. M.; Korczyn, A. D. EEG as predictor of dementia following first ischemic stroke. Acta Neurol. Scand. 90:263–265; 1994.

Hagnell, O.; Lanke, J.; Rorsman, B.; Ojesjo, L. Does the incidence of age associated psychosis decrease? A prospective, longitudinal study of a complete population investigated during the 25-year period 1947–1972: the Lundby study. Neuropsychobiology 7: 201–211; 1981.

Hebert, R.; Brayne, C. Epidemiology of vascular dementia. Neuroepidemiology 14:240–257; 1995.

Henderson, A. S. Epidemiology of dementing disorders. In: Wurtman, R. J.; Browdon, J. H.; Corkin, S.; et al., eds. Alzheimer's disease. New York: Raven Press; p. 15–25. 1990.

Hendrie, H. C.; Hall, K. S.; Hui, S.; Unvrezagt, F. W.; Yu, C. E.; et al. Apoliprotein E genotypes and a community study of elderly African Americans. Ann. Neurol. 37:118–120; 1995.

Heston, L. L.; White, J. A.; Mastri, A. R. Pick's disease. Clinical genetics and natural history. Arch. Gen. Psychiatry 44:409–411; 1987.

Heyman, A.; Fillenbaum, G.; Prosnitz, B.; Raiford, K.; Burchett, B.; Clark, C. Estimated prevalence of dementia among elderly black and white community residents. Arch. Neurol. 48:594–598; 1991.

Heyman, A.; Peterson, B.; Fillenbaum, G.; Pieper, C. The consortium to establish a registry for Alzheimer's disease (CERAD). Part XIV: demographic and clinical predictors of survival in patients with Alzheimer's disease. Neurology 46:656–660; 1996.

Heyman, A.; Peterson, B.; Fillenbaum, G.; Pieper, C. Predictors of time to institutionalization of patients with Alzheimer's disease: the CERAD experience, part XVII. Neurology 48:1304–1309; 1997.

Heyman, A.; Wilkinson, V. T. E.; Hurwitz, B. J.; Helms, M. J.; Haynes, C. J.; et al. Early-onset Alzheimer's disease: clinical predictors of institutionalization and death. Neurology 37:980–984; 1987.

Heyman, A.; Wilkinson, W. E.; Stafford, J. A.; Helms, M. J.; Sigmon, A. H.; Weinberg, T. Alzheimer's disease: a study of epidemiological aspects. Ann. Neurol. 15:335–341; 1984.

Hillier, V.; Salib, E. A case-control study of smoking and Alzheimer's disease. Int. J. Geriatr. Psychiatry 12:295–300; 1997.

Hofman, A.; Ott, A.; Breteler, M. M.; Bots, M. L.; Slooter, A. J.; et al. Atherosclerosis, apolipoprotein E, and prevalence of dementia and Alzheimer's disease in the Rotterdam Study. Lancet 349:151–154; 1997.

Hogan, D. B.; Thierer, D. E.; Ebly, E. M.; Parhad, I. M. Progression and outcome of patients in a Canadian dementia clinic. Can. J. Neurol. Sci. 21:331–338; 1994.

Huff, F. J.; Growdon, J. H.; Corkin, S.; Rosen, T. J. Age at onset and rate of progression of Alzheimer's disease. J. Am. Geriatr. Soc. 35:27–30; 1987.

Hughes, A. J.; Daniel, S. E.; Blankson, S.; Lees, A. J. A clinicopathologic study of 100 cases of Parkinson's disease. Arch. Neurol. 50:140–148; 1993.

Hutton, J. T.; Dippel, R. L.; Loewenson, R. B.; Mortimer, J. A.; Christians, B. L. Predictors of nursing home placement of patients with Alzheimer's disease. Tex. Med. 81:40–43; 1985.

Jacobs, D.; Sano, M.; Marder, K.; Bell, K.; Bylsma, F.; et al. Age at onset of Alzheimer's disease: relation to pattern of cognitive dysfunction and rate of cognitive decline. Neurology 44:1215–1220; 1994.

Jagger, C.; Clarke, M.; Stone, A. Predictors of survival with Alzheimer's disease: a community-based study. Psychol. Med. 25:171–177; 1995.

Jorm, A. F. Cross-national comparisons of the occurrence of Alzheimer's and vascular dementias. Eur. Arch. Psychiatry Clin. Neurosci. 240:218–222; 1991.

Jorm, A. F.; Korten, A. E.; Henderson, A. S. The prevalence of dementia: a quantitative integration of the literature. Acta Psychiatr. Scand. 76:465–479; 1987.

Kaszniak, A. W.; Fox, J.; Gandell, D. L.; Garron, D. C.; Huckman, M. J.; Ramsey, R. G.; et al. Predictors of mortality in presenile and senile dementia. Ann. Neurol. 3:246–252; 1978.

Katzman, R. Education and the prevalence of dementia and Alzheimer's disease. Neurology 43:13–20; 1993.

Katzman, R.; Brown, T.; Thal, L. J.; Fuld, P. A.; Aronson, M.; et al. Comparison of rate of annual change of mental status score in four independent studies of patients with Alzheimer's disease. Ann. Neurol. 24:384–389; 1988.

Katzman, R.; Hill, L. R.; Yu, E. S.; Wang, Z. Y.; Booth, A.; et al. The malignancy of dementia. Predictors of mortality in clinically diagnosed dementia in a population survey of Shanghai, China. Arch. Neurol. 51:1220–1225; 1994.

Katzman, R.; Rowe, J. W. Principles of geriatric neurology. Philadelphia: F. A. Davis; 1992.

Kawas, C.; Resnick, S.; Morrison, A.; Brookmeyer, R.; Corrada, M.; et al. A prospective study of estrogen replacement therapy and the risk of developing Alzheimer's disease: the Baltimore Longitudinal Study of Aging. Neurology 48:1517–1521; 1997.

Kennedy, A. M.; Newman, S. K.; Frackowiak, R. S. J.; Cunningham, V. J.; Roques, P.; et al. Chromosome 14 linked familial Alzheimer's disease. Brain 118: 185–205; 1995.

Khachaturian, Z. S. Diagnosis of Alzheimer's disease. Arch. Neurol. 42:1097–1105; 1985.

Knapp, M. J.; Knopman, D. S.; Solomon, P. R.; Pendlebury, W. W.; Davis, C. J.; Gracons, S. I. A 30-week randomized controlled trial of high-dose tacrine in patients with Alzheimer's disease. JAMA 271:985; 1994.

Knopman, D. S.; Kitto, J.; Deinard, S.; Heiring, J. Longitudinal study of death and institutionalization in patients with primary degenerative dementia. J. Am. Geriatr. Soc. 36:108–112; 1988.

Kokmen, E.; Beard, C. M.; Chandra, V.; Offord, K. P.; Schoenberg, B. S.; Ballard, D. J. Clinical risk factors for Alzheimer's disease: a population-based case-control study. Neurology 41:1393–1397; 1991.

Kokmen, E.; Beard, C. M.; O'Brien, P. C.; Kurland, L. T. Epidemiology of dementia in Rochester, Minnesota. Mayo Clin. Proc. 71:275–282; 1996a.

Kokmen, E.; Whisnant, J. P.; O'Fallon, W. M.; Chu, C. P.; Beard, C. M. Dementia after ischemic stroke: a population-based study in Rochester, Minnesota (1960–1984). Neurology 46:154–159; 1996b.

Koopmans, R. T.; Ekkerink, J. L.; van den Hoogen, H. J.; van Weel, C. [Mortality in patients with dementia following admission to a nursing home; a 10-year analysis]. Ned. Tijdschr. Geneeskd. 138: 1169–1174; 1994.

Kukull, W. A.; Larson, E. B.; Bowen, J. D.; McCormick, W. C.; Teri, L.; et al. Solvent exposure as a risk factor for Alzheimer's disease: a case-control study. Am. J. Epidemiol. 141:1059–1079; 1995.

Lanska, D. J. Dementia mortality in the United States. Results of the 1986 National Mortality Followback Survey. Neurology 50:362–367; 1998.

Launer, L. J.; Andersen, K.; Dewey, M. E.; Letenneur, L.; Ott, A.; et al. Rates and risk factors for dementia and Alzheimer's disease: results from EURODEM pooled analyses. EURODEM Incidence Research Group and Work Groups. European Studies of Dementia. Neurology 52:78–84; 1999.

Lautenschlager, N. T.; Cupples, L. A.; Rao, V. S.; Auerbach, S. A.; Becker, R.; et al. Risk of dementia among relatives of Alzheimer's disease patients in the MIRAGE study: what is in store for the oldest old? Neurology 46:641–650; 1996.

Le Bars, P. L.; Katz, M. M.; Berman, N.; Itil, T. M.; Freedman, A. M.; Schatzberg, A. F. A placebo-controlled, double-blind, randomized trial of an extract of Ginkgo biloba for dementia. North American EGb Study Group. JAMA 278: 1327–1332; 1997.

Leibson, C. L.; Rocca, W. A.; Hanson, V. A.; Cha, R.; Kokmen, E.; et al. Risk of dementia among persons with diabetes mellitus: a population-based cohort study. Am. J. Epidemiol. 145:301–308; 1997.

Levy-Lahad, E.; Wijsman, E. M.; Nemens, E.; Anderson, L.; Goddard, K. A. B.; et al. A familial Alzheimer's disease locus on chromosome 1. Science 269: 970–973; 1995.

Liang, J.; Borawski-Clark, E.; Liu, X.; Sugisawa, H. Transitions in cognitive status among the aged in Japan. Soc. Sci. Med. 43:325–337; 1996.

Lindsay, J.; Hebert, R.; Rockwood, K. The Canadian Study of Health and Aging: risk factors for vascular dementia. Stroke 28:526–530; 1997.

Loeb, C. Dementia due to lacunar infarctions: a misnomer or a clinical entity? Eur. Neurol. 35:187–192; 1995.

Lopez, O. L.; Becker, J. T.; Rezek, D.; Weiss, J.; Boller, F.; et al. Neuropsychological correlates of cerebral white-matter radiolucencies in probable Alzheimer's disease. Arch. Neurol. 49:828–834; 1992.

Lopez, O. L.; Boller, F.; Becker, I. T.; Miller, M.; Reynolds, C. F. Alzheimer's disease and depression. Am. J. Psychiatry 147:855–860; 1990.

Lopez, O. L.; Brenner, R. P.; Becker, J. T.; Ulrich, R. F.; Boller, F.; DeKosky, S.T. EEG spectral abnormalities and psychosis as predictors of cognitive and functional decline in probable Alzheimer's disease. Neurology 48:1521–1525; 1997a.

Lopez, O. L.; Wisnieski, S. R.; Becker, J. T.; Boller, F.; DeKosky, S. T. Extrapyramidal signs in patients with probable Alzheimer disease. Arch. Neurol. 54:969–975; 1997b.

Magni, E.; Binetti, G.; Bianchetti, A.; Trabucchi, M. Risk of mortality and institutionalization in demented patients with delusions. J. Geriatr. Psychiatry Neurol. 9:123–126; 1996.

Mann, U. M.; Mohr, E.; Gearing, M.; Chase, T. N. Heterogeneity in Alzheimer's disease: progression rate segregated by distinct neuropsychological and cerebral metabolic profiles. J. Neurol. Neurosurg. Psychiatry 55:956–959; 1992.

Marder, K.; Richards, M.; Bello, J.; Bell, K.; Sano, M.; et al. Clinical correlates of Alzheimer's disease with and without silent radiographic abnormalities. Arch. Neurol. 52:146–151; 1995.

Mattis, S. Mental Staus examination for organic mental syndrome in the elderly patient. In: Bellak, L.; Karasu, T.B., eds. Geriatric psychiatry. New York: Grune & Stratton; 1976: p. 77–121.

Mayeux, R.; Ottman, R.; Maestre, G.; Ngai, C.; Tang, M. X.; et al. Synergistic effects of traumatic head injury and apolipoprotein-epsilon 4 in patients with Alzheimer's disease. Neurology 45:555–557; 1995.

Mayeux, R.; Sano, M.; Chen, J.; Tatemichi, T.; Stern, Y. Risk of dementia in first degree relatives of patients with Alzheimer's disease and related disorders. Arch. Neurol. 48:269–273; 1991.

Mayeux, R.; Stern, Y.; Spanton, S. Heterogeneity in dementia of the Alzheimer type: evidence of subgroup. Neurology 35:453–461; 1985.

McKeith, I. G.; Perry, R. H.; Fairbairn, A. F.; Jabeen, S.; Perry, E. K. Operational criteria for senile dementia of Lewy body type (SDLT). Psychol. Med. 22:911–922; 1992.

McKhann, G.; Drachman, D.; Folstein, M.; Katzman, R.; Price, D.; Stadlan, E. M. Clinical diagnosis of Alzheimer's disease: report of the NINCDS-ADRDA work group under the auspices of Department of Health and Human Services Task Force on Alzheimer's disease. Neurology 34:939–944; 1984.

Mega, M. S.; Masterman, D. L.; Benson, D. F.; Vinters, H. V.; Tomiyasu, U.; et al. Dementia with Lewy bodies: reliability and validity of clinical and pathologic criteria. Neurology 47:1403–1409; 1996.

Mendez, M. F. The neurobehavioral aspects of boxing. Int. J. Psychiatry Med. 25:243–256; 1995.

Mendez, M. F.; Mastri, A. R.; Sung, J. H.; Zander, B. A.; Frey, W. H., II. Neuropathologically confirmed Alzheimer's disease: clinical diagnoses in 394 cases. J. Geriatr. Psychiatry Neurol. 4:26–29; 1991.

Mendez, M. F.; Underwood, K. L.; Mastri, A. R.; Zander, B. A.; Frey, W. H., II. Risk factors in Alzheimer's disease: a clinicopathological study. Neurology 42:770–775; 1992.

Merello, M.; Sabe, L.; Teson, A.; Migliorelli, R.; Petracchi, M.; et al. Extrapyramidalism in Alzheimer's disease: prevalence, psychiatric and neuropsychologicat correlates. J. Neurol. Neurosurg. Psychiatry 57:1503–1509; 1994.

Meyer, J. S.; Obara, K.; Takashima, S.; Muramatsu, K.; Mortel, K. F. Problems encountered with longitudinal neurological, psychometric and cerebral CT imaging among stroke data bank patients with dementia. Neuroepidemiology 13:340–344; 1994.

Mirra, S. S.; Heyman, A.; McKeel, D.; Sumi, S. M.; Crain, B. J.; et al. The Consortium to Establish a Registry for Alzheimer's disease (CERAD). Part II. Standardization of the neuropathological assessment of Alzheimer's disease. Neurology 41:479–486; 1991.

Mittelman, M. S.; Ferris, S. H.; Shulman, E.; Steinberg, G.; Levin, B. A family intervention to delay nursing home placement of patients with Alzheimer disease. A randomized controlled trial. JAMA 276: 1725–1731; 1996.

Molsa, P. K.; Marttila, R. J.; Rinne, U. K. Long-term survival and predictors of mortality in Alzheimer's disease and multi-infarct dementia. Acta Neurol. Scand. 91:159–164; 1995.

Monthly Vital Statistics Report, Vol. 46, No. 1, suppl. 2. Hyattsville, MD: Natonal Center for Health Statistics; 1997: p. 1–6.

Morgan, K.; Lilley, J. M.; Arie, T.; Byrne, E. J.; Jones, R.; Waite, J. Incidence of dementia in a representative British sample. Br. J. Psychiatry 163:467–470; 1993.

Mori, E.; Hirono, N.; Yamashita, H.; Imamura, T.; Yoshitaka, I.; et al. Premorbid brain size as a determinant of reserve capacity against intellectual decline in Alzheimer's disease. Am. J. Psychiatry 154:18–24; 1997.

Moritz, D. J.; Fox, P. J.; Luscombe, F. A.; Kraemer, H. C. Neurological and psychiatric predictors of mortality in patients with Alzheimer disease in California. Arch. Neurol. 54:878–885; 1997.

Moroney, J. T.; Bagiella, E.; Tatemichi, T. K.; Paik, M. C.; Stern, Y.; Desmond, D. W. Dementia after stroke increases the risk of long-term stroke recurrence. Neurology 48:1317–1325; 1997.

Morris, J. C.; Edland, S.; Clark, C.; Galasko, D.; Koss, E.; et al. The consortium to establish a registry for Alzheimer's disease (CERAD). Part IV. Rates of cognitive change in the longitudinal assessment of probable Alzheimer's disease. Neurology 43:2457–2465; 1993.

Mortimer, J. A.; Ebbit, B.; Jun, S-P.; Finch, M. Predictors of cognitive and functional progression in patients with probable Alzheimer's disease. Neurology 42:1689–1696; 1992.

Mortimer, J. A.; French, L. R.; Hutton, J. T.; Schuman, L. M. Head injury as a risk factor for Alzheimer's disease. Neurology 35:264–267; 1985.

Mortimer, J. A.; van Duijn, C. M.; Chandra, V.; Fratiglioni, L.; Graves, A. B.; et al. Head trauma as a risk factor for Alzheimer's disease: a collaborative re-analysis of case-control studies. EURODEM Risk Factors Research Group. Int. J. Epidemiol. 20(suppl. 2):S28–S35; 1991.

Myers, R. H.; Schaefer, E. J.; Wilson, P. W.; D'Agostino, R.; Ordovas, J.M.; et al. Apolipoprotein E epsilon4 association with dementia in a population-based study: the Framingham Study. Neurology 46:673–677; 1996.

National Institutes on Aging. Discoveries in health of aging Americans: progress report on Alzheimer's disease. U.S. Department of Health and Human Services. Washington DC: National Institutes of Health; 1992.

Nee, L. E.; Lippa, C. F. Alzheimer's disease in 22 twin pairs—13-year follow-up: hormonal, infectious and traumatic factors. Dement. Geriatr. Cogn. Disord. 10:148–151; 1999.

Nemetz, P. N.; Leibson, C.; Naessens, J. M.; Beard, M.; Kokmen, E.; et al. Traumatic brain injury and time to onset of Alzheimer's disease: a population-based study. Am. J. Epidemiol. 149:32–40; 1999.

Notkola, I. L.; Sulkava, R.; Pekkanen, J.; Erkinjuntti, T.; Ehnholm, C.; et al. Serum total cholesterol, apolipoprotein E epsilon 4 allele, and Alzheimer's disease. Neuroepidemiology 17:14–20; 1998.

Nyth, A. L.; Gottfries, C. G.; Brane, G.; Wallin, A. Heterogeneity of the course of Alzheimer's disease: a differentiation of subgroups. Dementia 2:18–24; 1991.

Obadia, Y.; Rotily, M.; Degrand-Guillaud, A.; Guelain, J.; Ceccaldi, M.; et al. The PREMAP Study: prevalence and risk factors of dementia and clinically diagnosed Alzheimer's disease in Provence, France. Prevalence of Alzeimer's Disease in Provence. Eur. J. Epidemiol. 13:247–253; 1997.

Ogunniyi, A. O.; Osuntokun, B. O.; Lekwauwa, U. B.; Falope, Z. F. Rarity of dementia (by DSM-III-R) in an urban community in Nigeria. East Afr. Med. J. 69:64–68; 1992.

O'Meara, E. S.; Kukull, W. A.; Sheppard, L.; Bowen, J. D.; McCormick, W. C.; et al. Head injury and risk of Alzheimer's disease by apolipoprotein in E genotype. Am. J. Epidemiol. 146:373–384; 1997.

Orgogozo, J. M.; Dartigues, J. F.; Lafont, S.; Letenneur, L.; Commenges, D.; et al. Wine consumption and dementia in the elderly: a prospective community study in the Bordeaux area. Rev. Neurol. 153:185–192; 1997.

Ortof, E.; Crystal, H. A. Rate of progression of Alzheimer's disease. J. Am. Geriatr. Soc. 37:511–514; 1989.

Ott, A.; Breteler, M. M.; de Bruyne, M. C.; van Harskamp, F.; Grobbee, D. E.; Hofman, A. Atrial fibrillation and dementia in a population-based study. The Rotterdam Study. Stroke 28:316–321; 1997.

Ott, A.; Breteler, M. M.; van Harskamp, F.; Stijnen. T.; Hofman, A. Incidence and risk of dementia. The Rotterdam Study. Am. J. Epidemiol. 147:574–580; 1988.

Pagnini-Hill, A.; Henderson, V. Estrogen deficiency and risk of Alzheimer's disease in women. Am. J. Epidemiol. 140:256–261; 1994.

Payami, H.; Montee, K.; Kaye, J. Evidence for familial factors that protect against dementia and outweigh the effect of increasing age. Am. J. Hum. Genet. 54:650–657; 1994.

Paykel, E. S.; Brayne, C.; Huppert, F. A.; Gill, C.; Barkley, C.; et al. Incidence of dementia in a population older than 75 years in the United Kingdom. Arch. Gen. Psychiatry 51:325–332; 1994.

Perenboom, R. J.; Boshuizen, H. C.; Breteler, M. M.; Ott, A.; Van de Water, H. P. Dementia-free life expectancy (DemFLE) in The Netherlands. Soc. Sci. Med. 43:1703–1707; 1996.

Perl, D. P.; Brody, A. R. Alzheimer's disease: X-ray spectrometric evidence of aluminum accumulation in neurofibrillary tangle-bearing neurons. Science 208:297–299; 1980.

Poirier, J.; Davignon, J.; Bouthillier, D.; Bertrand, P.; Gauthier, S. Apolipoprotein E polymorphism and Alzheimer's disease. Lancet 342:697–699; 1993.

Rasmusson, D. X.; Brandt, J.; Steele, C.; Hedreen, J. C.; Troncoso, J. C.; Folstein, M. F. Accuracy of clinical diagnosis of Alzheimer disease and clinical features of patients with non-Alzheimer disease neuropathology. Alzheimer Dis. Assoc. Disord. 10:180–188; 1996.

Reisberg, B.; Borenstein, J.; Franssen, E.; Shulman, E.; Steinberg, G.; Ferris, S. H. Remediable behavioral symptomatology in Alzheimer's disease. Hosp. Community Psychiatry 37:1199–201; 1986.

Reisberg, B.; Ferris, S. H.; de Leon, M. J.; Crook, T. The Global Deterioration Scale for assessment of primary degenerative dementia. Am. J. Psychiatry 139:1136–1139; 1982.

Reisberg, B.; Ferris, S. H.; Franssen, E. H.; Shulman, E.; Monteiro, I.; et al. Mortality and temporal course of probable Alzheimer's disease: a 5-year prospective study. Int. Psychogeriatr. 8:291–311; 1996.

Ritchie, K.; Mathers, C.; Jorm, A. Dementia-free life expectancy in Australia. Aus. J. Public Health 18: 149–152; 1994.

Roberts, G. W.; Gentleman, S. M.; Lynch, A.; Graham, D. I. beta A4 amyloid protein deposition in brain after head trauma. Lancet 338:1422–1423; 1991.

Roberts, G. W.; Gentleman, S. M.; Lynch, A.; Murray, L.; Landon, M.; Graham, D.I. β-Amyloid protein deposition in the brain after severe head injury: implications for the pathogenesis of Alzheimer's disease. J. Neurol. Neurosurg. Psychiatry 57:419–425; 1994.

Rocca, W. A.; Bonaiuto, S.; Lippi, A.; Luciani, P.; Turtu, F.; et al. Prevalence of clinically diagnosed Alzheimer's disease and other dementing disorders: a door-to-door survey in Appignano, Macerata Province, Italy. Neurology 40:626–631; 1990.

Rocca, W. A.; van Duijn, C. M.; Clayton, D.; Chandra, V.; Fratiglioni, L.; et al. Maternal age and Alzheimer's disease: a collaborative re-analysis of case-control studies. EURODEM Risk Factors Research Group. Int. J. Epidemiol. 20(suppl. 2):S21–S27; 1991.

Rogers, J.; Kirby, L. C.; Hempelman, S. R.; Berry, D. L.; McGeer, P. L.; et al. Clinical trial of indomethacin in Alzheimer's disease. Neurology 43:1609–1611; 1993.

Rogers, S. L.; Friedhoff, L. T. The efficacy and safety of donepezil in patients with Alzheimer's disease: results of a U.S. multicentre, randomized, double-blind, placebo-controlled trial. The Donepezil Study Group. Dementia 7:293–303; 1996.

Roman, B. C.; Tatemichi, T. K.; Erkinjuntti, T.; Cummings, J. L.; Madeu, J. C.; et al. Vascular dementia: diagnostic criteria for research studies (report of the NINCDS-AIREN International Work Group). Neurology 43:250–260; 1993.

Rosenberg, R. N.; Richter, R. W.; Risser, R. C.; Taubman, K.; Prado-Farmer, I.; et al. Genetic factors for the development of Alzheimer disease in the Cherokee Indian. Arch. Neurol. 53: 997–1000; 1996.

Roses, A. D. Apolipoprotein E genotyping in the differential diagnosis, not prediction, of Alzheimer's disease. Ann. Neurol. 38:6–14; 1995.

Roses, A. D.; Saunders, A. M. Apolipoprotein E genotyping as a diagnostic adjunct for Alzheimer's disease. Int. Psychogeriatr. 9(suppl. 1):277–288; 1997.

Ross, M. Many questions but no clear answers on link between aluminum, Alzheimer's disease. Can. Med. Assoc. J. 159:68–69; 1994.

Rossler, W.; Hewer, W.; Fatkenheuer, B.; Loffler, W. Excess mortality among elderly psychiatric in-patients with organic mental disorder. Br. J. Psychiatry 167: 527–532; 1995.

Royston, M. C.; Mann, D.; Pickering-Brown, S.; Owen, F.; Perry, R.; et al. Apolipoprotein E epsilon 2 allele promotes longevity and protects patients with Down's syndrome from dementia. Neuroreport 5:2583–2585; 1994.

Roth, M. The association of clinical and neurological findings and its bearing on the classification and aetiology of Alzheimer's disease. Br. Med. Bull. 42: 42–50; 1986.

Salmon, D. P.; Thai, L. J.; Butters, N.; Heindel, W. C. Longitudinal evaluation of dementia of the Alzheimer type; a comparison of 3 standardized mental status examinations. Neurology 40: 1225–1230; 1990.

Sano, M.; Ernesto, C.; Thomas, R. G.; Klauber, M. R.; Schafer, K.; et al. A controlled trial of selegiline, alpha-tocopherol, or both as treatment for Alzheimer's disease. N. Engl. J. Med. 336:1216–1222; 1997.

Saunders, A. M.; Strittmatter, W. J.; Schmechel, D.; George-Hyslop, D. H.; Pericak-Vance, M. A.; et al. Association of apolipoprotein E allele e4 with late-onset familial and sporadic Alzheimer's disease. Neurology 43:1467–1472; 1993.

Sauvaget, C.; Tsuji, I.; Minami, Y.; Fukao, A.; Hisamichi, S.; et al. Dementia-free life expectancy among elderly Japanese. Gerontology 43:168–175; 1997.

Schneider, L. S.; Olin, J. T. Overview of clinical trials of hydergine in dementia. Arch. Neurol. 51:787–798; 1994.

Schneider, L. S.; Tariot, P. N. Emerging drugs of Alzheimer's disease. Med. Clin. North Am. 78:911–932; 1994.

Schoenberg, B. S.; Anderson, D. W.; Haerer, A. F. Severe dementia. Prevalence and clinical features in a biracial US population. Arch. Neurol. 42:740–743; 1985.

Schofield, P. W.; Logroscino, G.; Andrews, H. F.; Albert, S.; Stern, Y. An association between head circumference and Alzheimer's disease in a population-based study of aging and dementia. Neurology 49:30–37; 1997.

Schofield, P. W.; Mosesson, R. E.; Stern, Y.; Mayeux, R. The age at onset of Alzheimer's disease and an intracranial area measurement. Arch. Neurol. 52: 95–98; 1995.

Schupf, N.; Kapell, D.; Lee, J. H.; Ottman, R.; Mayeux, R.; et al. Increased risk of Alzheimer's disease in mothers of adults with Down's syndrome. Lancet 344:353–356, 1994.

Selnes, O. A.; Carson, K.; Rovner, B.; Gordon, B. Language dysfunction in early- and late-onset possible Alzheimer's disease. Neurology 38:1053–1056; 1988.

Seltzer, B.; Sherwin, I. A comparison of clinical features in early- and late-onset primary degenerative dementia: one entity or two? Arch. Neurol. 40:143–146; 1983.

Seshadri, S.; Wolf, P. A.; Beiser, A.; Au, R.; McNulty, K.; et al. Lifetime risk of dementia and Alzheimer's disease. The impact of mortality on risk estimates in the Framingham Study. Neurology 49:1498–1504; 1997.

Shen, Y. C.; Li, G.; Li, Y. T.; Chen, C. H.; Li, S. R.; et al. Epidemiology of age-related dementia in China. Chin. Med. J. 107:60–64; 1994.

Skoog, I.; Nilsson, L.; Palmertz, B.; Andreasson, L. A.; Svanborg, A. A population-based study of dementia in 85-year-olds. N. Eng. J. Med. 328:153–158; 1993.

Slaby, A. E.; Erle, S. R: Dementia and delirium. In: Stoudemire, A. ed. Psychiatric care of the medical patient. New York: Oxford University Press p. 415–455; 1993.

Smith, G. S.; de Leon, M. J.; George, A. E.; Kluger, A.; Voltow, N. D.; et al. Topography of cross-sectional and longitudinal glucose metabolic deficits in Alzheimer's disease: pathophysiologic implications. Arch. Neurol. 49:1142–1150; 1992.

Snowdon, D. A.; Kemper, S. J.; Mortimer, J. A.; Greiner, L. H.; Wekstein, D. R.; Markesbery, W. R. Linguistic ability in early life and cognitive function and Alzheimer's disease in late life. JAMA 275: 528–532; 1996.

Sobel, E.; Dunn, M.; Davanipour, Z.; Qian, Z.; Chui, H. C. Elevated risk of Alzheimer's disease among workers with likely electromagnetic field exposure. Neurology 47:1477–1481; 1996.

St. George-Hyslop, P. H.; Tanzi, R. E.; Polinsky, R. J.; Haines, J. L.; Nee, L.; et al. The genetic defect causing familial Alzheimer's disease maps on chromosome 21. Science 235:885–890; 1987.

Stern, Y.; Albert, M.; Brandt, J.; Jacobs, D. M.; Tang, M. X.; et al. Utility of extrapyramidal signs and psychosis as predictors of cognitive and functional decline, nursing home admission, and death in Alzheimer's disease: prospective analyses from the Predictors Study. Neurology 44:2300–2307; 1994.

Stern, Y.; Tang, M. X.; Albert, M. S.; Brandt, J.; Jacobs, D. M.; et al. Predicting time to nursing home care and death in individuals with Alzheimer disease. JAMA 227:806–812; 1997.

Stern, Y.; Tang, M. X.; Denaro, J.; Mayeux, R. Increased risk of mortality in Alzheimer's disease patients with more advanced educational and occupational attainment. Ann. Neurol. 37:590–595; 1995.

Sulkava, R.; Vaden, J.; Erkiniuntti, T. Survival in Alzheimer's disease (AD) and multi-infarct dementia (MID) in the 1980's. Neurology 42(suppl. 3): 143; 1992.

Tang, M. X.; Jacobs, D.; Stern, Y.; Marder, K.; Schofield, P.; et al. Effect of oestrogen during menopause on risk and age at onset of Alzheimer's disease. Lancet 348:429–432; 1996.

Tatemichi, T. K.; Paik, M.; Bagiella, E.; Desmond, D. W.; Pirro, M.; Hanzawa, L. K. Dementia after stroke is a predictor of long-term survival. Stroke 25:1915–1919; 1994a.

Tatemichi, T. K.; Paik, M.; Bagiella, E.; Desmond, D. W.; Stern, Y.; et al. Risk of dementia after stroke in a hospitalized cohort: results of a longitudinal study. Neurology 44:1885–1891; 1994b.

Teri, L.; Hughes, J. P.; Larson, E. B. Cognitive deterioration in Alzheimer's disease: behavioral and health factors. J. Gerontol. 45:58–63; 1990.

Thal, L. J.; Grundman, K.; Klauber, M. R. Dementia: characteristics of a referral population and factors associated with progression. Neurology 38:1083–1090; 1988.

The Lund and Manchester Groups. Clinical and neuropathological criteria for frontotemporal dementia. J. Neurol. Neurosurg. Psychiatry 57:416–418; 1994.

Thomas, B. M.; McGonigal, G.; McQuade, C. A.; Starr, J. M.; Whalley, L. J. Survival in early onset dementia: effects of urbanization and socio-economic deprivation. Neuroepidemiology 16:134–140; 1997.

Van Dijk, P. T.; Dippel, D. W.; Van Der Meulen, J. H.; Habbema, J. D. Comorbidity and its effect on mortality in nursing home patients with dementia. J. Nerv. Ment. Dis. 184:180–187; 1996.

Van Duijn, C. M.; Clayton, D.; Chandra, V.; Fratiglioni, L.; Graves, A. B.; et al. Familial aggregation of Alzheimer's disease and related disorders: a collaborative re-analysis of case-control studies. EURODEM Risk Factors Research Group. Int. J. Epidemiol. 20 (suppl. 2):S13–S20; 1991.

Van Duijn, C. M.; Clayton, D. G.; Chandra, V.; Fratiglioni, L.; Graves, A. B.; et al. Interaction between genetic and environmental risk factors for Alzheimer's disease: a reanalysis of case-control studies. EURODEM Risk Factors Research Group. Genet. Epidemiol. 11:539–551; 1994.

Van Duijn, C. M.; Havekes, L. M.; van Broeckhoven, C.; de Knijff, P.; Hofman, A. Apolipoprotein E genotype and association between smoking and early onset Alzheimer's disease. BMJ 310:627–631; 1995.

van Duijn, C. M.; de Knijff, P.; Wehnert, A.; de Voecht, J.; Bronzova, J. B.; et al. The apolipoprotein E ε2 allele is associated with an increased risk of early-onset Alzheimer's disease and a reduced survival. Ann. Neurol. 37:605–610; 1995.

van Duijn, C. M.; Tanja, T. A.; Haaxma, R.; Schulte, W.; Saan, R. J.; et al. Head trauma and the risk of Alzheimer's disease. Am. J. Epidemiol. 135:775–782; 1992.

Volicer, L.; Collard, A.; Hurley, A.; Bishop, C.; Kern, D.; Karon, S. Impact of special care unit for patients with advanced Alzheimer's disease on patients' discomfort and costs. J. Am. Geriatr. Soc. 42:597–603; 1994.

Walsh, J. S.; Welch, H. G.; Larson, E. B. Survival of patients with Alzheimer-type dementia. Ann. Intern. Med. 113:429–434; 1990.

Wang, H. X.; Fratiglioni, L.; Frisoni, G. B.; Viitanen, M.; Winblad, B. Smoking and the occurrence of Alzheimer's disease: cross-sectional and longitudinal data in a population-based study. Am. J. Epidemiol. 149:640–644; 1999.

Wang, S. Y.; Fukagawa, N.; Hossain, M.; Ooi, W. L. Longitudinal weight changes, length of survival, and energy requirements of long-term care residents with dementia. J. Am. Geriatr. Soc. 45:1189–1195; 1997.

Whalley, L. J.; Thomas, B. M.; Starr, J. M. Epidemiology of presenile Alzheimer's disease in Scotland (1974–88) II. Exposures to possible risk factors. Br. J. Psychiatry 167:732–738; 1995.

White, L.; Petrovich, H.; Ross, W. G.; Masaki, K. H.; Abbott, R. D.; et al. Prevalence of dementia in older

Japanese-American men in Hawaii. The Honolulu-Asia Aging Study. JAMA 276:955–960; 1996.

Wimo, A.; Asplund, K.; Mattsson, B.; Adolfsson, R.; Lundgren, K. Patients with dementia in group living: experiences 4 years after admission. Int. Psychogeriatr. 7:123–127; 1995.

Wisniewski, K. E.; Dalton, A. J.; McLachlan, C.; Wen, G. Y.; Wisniewski, H. M. Alzheimer's disease in Down's syndrome: clinicopathologic studies. Neurology 35: 957–961; 1985.

Wolfe, N.; Reed, B. R.; Eberling, J. L.; Jagust, W. J. Temporal lobe perfusion on single photon emission computed tomography predicts the rate of cognitive decline in Alzheimer's disease. Arch. Neurol. 52: 257–262; 1995.

Yamada, M.; Sasaki, H.; Mimori, Y.; Kasagi, F.; Sudoh, S.; et al. Prevalence and risks of dementia in the Japanese population: RERF's adult health study Hiroshima subjects. Radiation Effects Research Foundation. J. Am. Geriatr. Soc. 47:189–195; 1999.

# 36

# Movement Disorders

ALIREZA MINAGAR, LISA M. SHULMAN, AND WILLIAM J. WEINER

This chapter addresses the issue of prognosis in six common movement disorders. These disorders include Parkinson's disease, the most common of the neurodegenerative disorders; progressive supranuclear palsy, one of the more common atypical parkinsonian syndromes; Huntington's disease, a dominantly inherited neurodegenerative disorder with cognitive, psychiatric, and motor problems; dystonia, both generalized and focal; Tourette's syndrome, a common neurobehavioral disorder with a wide range of clinical manifestations; and tardive dyskinesia, an iatrogenic disorder caused by the administration of drugs that block dopamine receptors within the brain.

## Parkinson's Disease

James Parkinson originally described the disease that bears his name in his famous essay on the shaking palsy (Parkinson 1817). The salient clinical features of Parkinson's disease (PD) include the following: rigidity, resting tremor, bradykinesia, flexed posture, freezing phenomenon, and loss of postural reflexes.

Signs that help to distinguish idiopathic Parkinson's disease (IPD) from other parkinsonian syndromes include prominent rest tremor, significant response to levodopa, initial asymmetry of parkinsonian signs, and little or no imbalance in the first months and years of the disease. IPD accounts for 80% of all cases of parkinsonism, is of unknown etiology, and affects 1% of the population older than 60. IPD is a major cause of disability among the elderly, with peak age at onset in the sixth decade (Rajput et al. 1984). IPD is the most common movement disorder in the elderly.

## Clinical Manifestations

Of the six major clinical features of IPD, tremor is the presenting symptom in 70% of patients. Resting tremor is of insidious onset, usually begins unilaterally, and as the disease progresses becomes bilateral. Resting tremor is often accompanied by a kinetic postural tremor in the same limb. Other prominent motor signs are cogwheel rigidity and bradykinesia. Loss of postural reflexes usually appears late and is an important reason for falls in this group of patients (Jankovic and Calne 1987).

Another feature of IPD is a severe gait disorder often associated with falling. This is the most disabling and the least treatable aspect of IPD. Multiple elements including rigidity, akinesia, loss of postural reflexes, and disturbances of postural adjustment lead to postural instability in these patients. The gait abnormality usually begins with decreased arm swing and gradually evolves into short, unsteady shuffling steps. Gait initiation and turning movements become more difficult and falls become progressively frequent, which may lead to multiple fractures and other injuries.

One of the most poorly understood components of IPD is "freezing," which is an abrupt interruption in the flow of ongoing motor activity. It most often affects the gait.

Neurobehavioral abnormalities also occur in patients with PD. Depression is common and does not seem to be related to severity of disease. Dementia may occur in 25% to 30% of patients with long-standing disease. Drug-induced hallucinations occur frequently. Sensory complaints, akathisia, and restless legs syndrome can also occur. Autonomic disturbances including orthostatic hypotension, thermal dysregulation, constipation, and bladder and sexual dysfunction are frequently observed in patients with IPD (Martignoni et al. 1986; Mathers et al. 1989). Other nonmotor disturbances associated with IPD include seborrhea, fatigue, and weight loss.

Patients with IPD have facial akinesia resulting in expressionless, masked faces that leads to further hindrance of social interaction. Speech becomes hyphophonic, dysarthric, monotonous, and muffled. Drooling with excessive saliva is frequent in advanced disease.

## Etiology and Pathology

The cause of PD is unknown. Attention is focused on hereditary factors including mitochondrial genetic defects, the α-synuclein gene, and environmental toxins that could selectively injure substantia nigra cells.

Pathologically selective and severe loss of melanin-containing neurons in the ventrolateral tier of the zona compacta of the substantia nigra is characteristic of Parkinson's disease. Symmetrical bilateral lesions are more frequent than unilateral involvement. Gliosis of moderate degree, neuronal loss in locus ceruleus and dorsal vagal nucleus with variable involvement of the nucleus basalis of Mynert are also present. Lewy bodies are concentric hyaline intracytoplasmic inclusions seen in many monoaminergic and other subcortical nuclei, the spinal cord, sympathetic ganglia, and occasionally the cerebral cortex in Parkinson's disease. Lewy bodies can be observed as an incidental finding in almost 10% of aged individuals with no known neurological disorders in life.

## Treatment

Treatment of IPD is symptomatic and an individualized process. Despite our expanded knowledge of various aspects of the disease, there is still no medical or surgical treatment that can abort the progressive course of the illness. The main goal of treatment is to keep the patient functioning independently as long as possible. The most important medication that has altered the prognosis for IPD is levodopa. Levodopa markedly improves rigidity, tremor, and bradykinesia.

Direct-acting dopamine receptor agonists that stimulate striatal $D_2$-receptors and bypass degenerating nigral cells have been used in combination with levodopa or as monotherapy. The older ergot-derived agonists bromocriptine and pergolide have proven efficacy in treating the motor symptoms of PD. The newer nonergot dopamine receptor agonists pramipexole and ropinirole have efficacy in both early and advanced PD. Dopaminergic receptor agonists have also played an important part in keeping patients functional and therefore improving prognosis.

## Prognosis

The initial symptoms of unilateral resting tremor and mild bradykinesia are rarely disabling. It is important for the patient and family to understand that there will be a slow evolution of disability. There is no set rate of progression and there is tremendous individual variation. Issues of prognosis are very important to patients, and a discussion of prognosis in PD needs to focus on questions of both morbidity and mortality.

Issues of prognosis in PD relate to progression of the motor symptomatology, treatment-related problems, and effect on life span. The very gradual onset of the motor symptoms was described by James Parkinson in 1817 when he wrote: "so slight and nearly imperceptible are the first inroads of this malady, and so extremely slow is its progress, that it rarely happens, that the patient can form any recollection of the precise period of its commencement." The mean age of onset is within the sixth decade and the most common age of onset is approximately 60. Fully 20% of patients have onset before the age of 50 (Gowers 1893; Wilson 1940; Dimsdale 1946; Hoehn and Yarh 1967). The most common initial symptom is tremor, which occurs in about 70% of patients (Gowers 1893).

The natural history and progression of PD in the pre-levodopa era was divided into five stages by Hoehn and Yahn (1967). Stage I is unilateral disease, and the median duration for this stage is 3 years. Stage I symptomatology may be so mild that the disorder is not recognized by the patient or physician until it becomes bilateral or stage II. Gowers (1893) stated that the contralateral side most frequently is effected 6 months to 4 years after onset of symptoms. These patients may have bilateral tremor, bilateral rigidity and bradykinesia, facial masking, hypophonia, dysarthria, decreased arm swing, shortened stride length, and easy fatigability. Hoehn and Yahn (1967) reported that the median duration of stage II was 6 years.

Stage III PD is marked by the appearance of postural impairment. Patients may note unsteadiness, loss of balance, near falling, and actual falling. Freezing and festination may be present. Parkinson noted that festination did not appear for 10 to 12 years. The median duration of stage III is 7 years with very wide variation. Stage IV PD is defined as fully advanced, and disability in the performance of the activities of daily living are present. Surprisingly, at this stage of the illness tremor may become less severe (Gowers 1893). The median duration of stage IV is 9 years. Stage V PD is defined as severe disability with confinement to wheelchair or bed unless actively aided. The duration of this stage is dependent on the level of nursing care. Hoehn and Yahn (1967) reported that stage V median duration was 14 years with a very wide individual variation.

Many authors have commented on the rate of progression. Schwab (1960) noted that for most patients the progression from onset to fully advanced disease takes "one to several" decades. Merritt (1959) commented that it might take 10 to 15 years before a patient was disabled from a useful occupation. Prior to the levodopa era 28% of patients with disease duration up to 5 years were disabled (stage IV or V) or dead; 61% with disease duration 5 to 10 years and 83% of those with disease duration of 10 to 15 years were disabled or dead (Hoehn and Yarh 1967). Levodopa has not changed the basic rate of disease progression but it has remarkably altered the evolution to disability. Levodopa has reduced the disabled or dead percentages for each measured duration of illness two- to threefold. Hoehn (Hoehn 1983, 1985) reported that only 9% of patients in the first

5 years of illness were disabled or dead and that 22% and 51% of levodopa-treated patients with disease duration of 5 to 10 years and over 10 years were disabled or dead.

Complications of dopaminergic therapy including motor fluctuations, dyskinesias, and psychiatric dysfunction (hallucinations, delusions, psychosis) all affect prognosis in terms of quality of life and disability. Although most PD patients experience motor fluctuations and dyskinesias at some time in the course of treatment, these usually do not occur until after 2 to 3 years or longer of treatment (Nutt 1990; Marconi et al. 1994; Fahn 1974; Marsden et al. 1982; Nutt et al. 1984). Psychiatric disturbances also tend to be a late complication of therapy.

In an attempt to analyze whether or not subgroups of IPD exist in which the prognosis may be better or worse, a series of investigations involving the 800-patient cohort of the DATATOP study was conducted (Jankovic et al. 1990). Young-onset patients (<40) were compared to older onset (>70) patients with similar degree of disability at study entry. The younger patients had a longer duration of symptoms at study entry, suggesting a slower rate of progression in young-onset disease. Tremor-predominant disease was compared to postural instability and gait difficulty disease (PIGD), and tremor-predominant disease was more benign. Overall, it has been proposed that young onset with tremor-predominant disease has a better prognosis than late-onset bradykinetic PIGD forms of the disease. Others have argued that the division of PD into tremor-predominant and PIGD varients is arbitrary and that diagnostic error is introduced into such a division. In particular, patients with the PIGD form of IPD may in fact not have PD at autopsy but other forms of parkinsonism (Friedman 1998).

The effect of IPD on mortality has been discussed frequently. The indefinite time of onset, the variable rate of progression, and the uncertainty of the diagnosis have led some to speculate that the duration of disease from onset to death is much longer than usually stated (Hoehn 1990). Prior to the levodopa era the average length of life after disease onset was about 10 years (Hoehn and Yarh 1967; Brain 1955). Before levodopa, less than 25% of patients were over 75 at death, but since levodopa 60% of patients are over 75 at death. In addition, the average age of death increased by 6 years, from 67 to 73 (Hoehn 1985). Prior to levodopa the mortality from PD was three times that for the age-adjusted general population. More recent studies show mortality rates quite similar to age-adjusted comparison groups (Joseph et al. 1978; Rajput et al. 1984; Sweet and McDowell 1975; Cederbaum and McDowell 1986). Patients do not usually die of PD but of related problems such as aspiration pneumonia, urinary tract infection, decubitus ulcers, or complications of accidents and surgery.

## Progressive Supranuclear Palsy

Progressive supranuclear palsy (PSP) is often misdiagnosed as Parkinson's disease at the onset of the illness. Litvan et al. (1997) recently performed a logistic regression and classification and regression tree analysis on the clinical features that best distinguish PSP form other related disorders. The early presence of unstable gait, absence of tremor-dominant disease, and absence of a response to levodopa differentiated PSP from PD. The mean age of onset of PSP is 63 ±2 years; the mean interval from onset of symptoms to PSP diagnosis ranges from 3.6 to 3.9 years, and the mean survival from onset of symptoms to death is 5 to 6 years. The risk of developing PSP before age 50 is quite low. The risk increases with age and there is a slight male predominance (Bower et al. 1997).

### Clinical Manifestations

This late-onset neurodegenerative disease is identified by supranuclear gaze palsy, dysarthria, extensor rigidity of the neck and trunk, and dementia (Richardson et al. 1963; Steele et al. 1963; Maher and Lees 1986). Gait disorder and unsteadiness are among the first manifestations of the disease. In fact, in a large analysis of what differentiates PSP patients from related disorders it was determined that supranuclear vertical gaze palsy, moderate or severe postural instability, and falls within the first year of symptom onset correctly identified 90% of patients with PSP (Litvan et al. 1997). Early-on patients develop a low-volume dysarthria and clinical examination reveals an akinetic rigid syndrome. In PSP, in contrast to IPD, the patients do not often have tremor and have an extension posture of the head instead of increased flexion. Pseudobulbar palsy may develop during the course of the disease and a se-

vere speech disorder may ultimately result in anarthria. PSP patients frequently suffer from dysphagia, which may cause difficulties ranging from mild discomfort to malnutrition and aspiration pneumonia. Dysphagia may coexist with dysarthria in the same patient.

Dystonia is a manifestation of PSP, and limb dystonia in particular is common among these patients. In patients with dystonia in the context of PSP, dopaminergic agents should be cautiously reduced or discontinued to rule out the possibility of treatment-induced symptoms (Barclay and Lang 1997).

Almost 50% of these patients develop neurobehavioral disorders early in the course of their illness. These include apathy, depression, emotional incontinence, and slowness of intellectual processes with forgetfulness. Patients affected with PSP have difficulty with tests sensitive to frontal lobe performance and may manifest some frontal lobe features such as motor perseveration and forced grasping.

Supranuclear gaze palsy is a prominent feature of PSP. Voluntary saccades are slow and hypometric, and this primarily affects downgaze before upgaze. The supranuclear gaze palsy can be overcome by passive head movements activating the oculocephalic reflex (doll's head maneuver). Apraxia of opening and eyelid closure, blepharospasm, and decreased blink frequency are commonly seen in these patients.

Imaging studies including computed tomography (CT) scanning and magnetic resonance imaging (MRI) reveal nonspecific abnormalities such as mild to moderate cerebral atrophy, and in some patients mild enlargement of the lateral ventricles. Position emission tomography (PET) scanning reveals cortical and subcortical hypermetabolism, prominently involving the frontal cortex. Decreased levels of $N$-acetyl-aspartate in the lentiform nucleus has been demonstrated by proton MR spectroscopy (Federico et al. 1997).

### Treatment

There is no effective medical treatment for PSP. Levodopa and dopamine agonists may provide some relief in early stages. However, long-lasting motor improvement is unlikely. Other agents such as tricyclic antidepressants, methysergide, selective serotonin reuptake inhibitors (SSRIs), idoxazone, and cholinomimetic agents have been unsuccessful. A recent open-label trial of pramipexole (Weiner et al. 1998), a new dopamine receptor agonist, did not demonstrate any motor improvement in patients with PSP. Another agent, aniracetam, which is a cerebral metabolic activator that improves synaptic transmission with an acetylcholine-like effect, has not been shown to have long-lasting effects (Nagasaka et al. 1997).

## Prognosis

PSP is a progressive unrelenting illness with a very grave prognosis. Median survival time from onset of symptoms to death is approximately 5.3 to 5.9 years (Bower et al. 1997; Litvan et al. 1996). Golbe et al. (1988) reported a median survival of 9.7 years.

Variations in survival time are thought to be related to methodology involving case ascertainment. Early onset of gait disturbance, falling, and supranuclear gaze palsy are the hallmarks of PSP. The median interval from symptom onset to required gait assistance is 3.1 years. Significant dysarthria, dysphagia, and visual symptoms are present 3 1/2 to 4 years after onset of symptoms (Golbe et al. 1988). The presence of early dysphagia predicts a shorter patient survival (Litvan et al. 1996). The most frequent cause of death for these patients is pneumonia, which is probably secondary to silent aspiration. It has also been noted that patients with the most complaints related to swallowing also have the greatest cognitive impairment, perhaps overall reflecting a more malignant disease process (Litvan et al. 1997). Specific swallowing studies in PSP patients reveal that the most common abnormalities include delayed initiation of the swallowing reflex, impaired tongue motility, and pooling of secretions and food in the valleculae. It has been proposed that PSP survival time may be increased by speech pathology evaluation and concerted effort in dietary management (straws, thickening of foods) and postural modification while eating (e.g., chin tuck and head tilt).

## Huntington's Disease

Huntington's disease (HD) is an autosomal dominant progressive neurodegenerative disorder that is clinically characterized by abnormal movements, behavioral disturbances, intellectual decline, and functional deterioration (Weiner and Lang 1989).

The clinical syndrome was first described by George Huntington in 1872 under the title of "hereditary chorea" (Huntington 1872). At the beginning of the 20th century degeneration of the striatum was identified as the neuropathological marker of HD (Anton 1896; Lanois and Paviot 1897; Alzheimer 1911). The polymorphic DNA marker linked to HD was identified in 1983 (Gusella et al. 1983), and recently the mutation was characterized as an excessive number of trinucleotide CAG repeats that code for a polyglutamine [huntingtin] on chromosome 4 (Huntington's Disease Collaborating Research Group 1993). Although it is unclear what the exact upper limit of normal number of CAG repeats is, those individuals with more than 38 CAG repeats in the HD gene develop the clinical illness (Duayo et al. 1993). Patients with juvenile onset HD have increased CAG repeats. Patients who inherit their abnormal gene from their father are more likely to have early-onset disease.

### Clinical Manifestations

#### Onset of the Disease

The initial clinical manifestations and the patient's age at onset vary widely. In the majority of cases the clinical symptoms appear around age 39, but there are reported cases of symptomatic disease as early as 2 years and as late as 80 years old. The discovery of the HD gene has expanded our understanding of the wide range of phenotypic expression of the disease. The major motor manifestation of HD is chorea. Chorea derives from the Greek verb *choros* meaning "to dance." Chorea is characterized by excessive spontaneous movements that are irregularly timed, nonrepetitive, randomly distributed, and abrupt in character and that flow from one body part to another. Proximal, distal, and axial muscles are all involved. In HD, chorea is usually not disabling. Some patients with relatively severe chorea are still able to ambulate, function, and care for themselves, but in certain cases severe, uncontrollable chorea interferes with the patient's daily life (Meyers et al. 1998). Behavioral and cognitive changes are far more disabling in most patients.

As HD progresses, chorea may be replaced by dystonia and parkinsonian features such as rigidity, postural instability, and bradykinesia (Penny et al. 1990; Kremer et al. 1992; Tian et al. 1991).

Sustained dystonia, chorea, rigidity, and a chore-atic gait disorder contribute to balance problems associated with HD (Tian et al. 1991). Dysarthria and dysphagia are common in the midstages of the disease and lead to inability to communicate and swallow. Deep tendon reflexes are hyperactive. Juvenile onset cases are frequently more rapidly progressive than the older onset cases (Myers et al. 1991).

In advanced stages of HD, akinesia and rigidity may dominate the clinical picture without any chorea. Clonus and extensor plantar responses may appear.

### Psychiatric Disorders and Cognitive Decline

Psychiatric disorders are common in patients with HD. These include psychosis with visual or auditory hallucinations (approximate prevalence of 10%), mania, delusional thought disorder, apathy, obsessive behavior, and depression (Folstein 1989). Cognitive abnormalities of HD are among the earliest indicators of functional decline and can be as disabling as the motor disorders (White et al. 1992). The rate of cognitive decline varies among different individuals (MacMillan et al. 1993; Britton et al. 1995). Language function and insight may remain preserved, even in advanced stages of the disease (Kremer et al. 1992; Caine et al. 1978).

The dementia of HD is classified as subcortical and characterized by bradyphrenia and attentional and sequencing impairments without the presence of apraxia, agnosia, or aphasia (Shoulson and Fahn 1979). In terms of memory function, registration and immediate memory recall are relatively intact, while retrieval of recent and remote memories is impaired (Kennedy and Kennedy 1992, Aminoff et al. 1975, Caine et al. 1977).

### Pathology

The neurodegenerative process of HD characteristically involves the caudate nucleus, putamen and, to a lesser degree, nucleus acccumbens, globus pallidus, and substantia nigra pars reticulata (Brandt 1985). The brain weight is reduced and cortical and caudate atrophy is apparent. Microscopic examination of the striatum reveals marked loss of spiny projection neurons with preservation of the aspiny interneurons and large aspiny acetylcholinesterase-positive neurons (Von Sattel et al. 1985). These spiny neurons contain enkephaline, substance P, γ-aminobutysis acid (GABA), and dynorphin. Additional biochemical analysis of HD brains reveals reduced GABA neurons and intact somatostatin-neuropeptide γ-containing neurons (Kowall et al. 1987). MR spectroscopy demonstrates increased brain lactate in patients with HD (Beal et al. 1993).

### Epidemiology

The prevalence of HD is 5 to 10 per 100,000 in the United States. Two to four times as many individuals have inherited the mutation and are currently asymptomatic.

### Diagnosis

HD is diagnosed based on the clinical manifestations of the illness and a positive family history. MRI/CT scan of the brain may reveal prominent atrophy of the caudate nucleus that is often more obvious in patients with symptomatic disease. Neuropsychological evaluations can assess the severity of cognitive decline. Confirmation of the diagnosis can be accomplished with genetic analysis. DNA diagnostic testing for HD should be performed at special centers that provide genetic counseling services.

### Prognosis

Huntington's disease is a relentless, progressive, neurodegenerative disease that leads to death secondary to medical complications of the disabled individual. Death is most often caused by aspiration pneumonia and injury secondary to falling. The average life span is 15 to 20 years from onset to death. Early-onset cases have a more malignant course. Additional factors affecting prognosis include CAG repeat length and its relationship to age of onset. In normal alleles the range of CAG repeats may be up to 31. 31 to 38 represents an indeterminate number. HD alleles demonstrate repeat lengths greater than 38. There may be variation between laboratories as to what is considered normal CAG repeat length. There is a strong negative correlation between the number of CAG repeats and age of onset; higher repeat lengths are associated with younger onset age. However, most of this correlation is accounted for by individuals with CAG repeats over 60 and juvenile onset HD. Repeat length accounts for only 50% of variance of onset age and this points to the possible role of other factors such as environmental triggers and modifying genes that affect age of onset. Most HD alleles manifest meiotic instability that is more common in paternal transmission. The tendency for greater gene expansion of the CAG repeat in sperm rather than egg explains why juvenile cases of HD tend to be inherited paternally.

Genetic testing has led to the identification of a group of individuals who are gene positive but are currently asymptomatic. Neuropsychiatric evaluation of HD gene carriers has shown subtle subclinical cognitive and motor changes such as slower saccadic velocity and visual reaction time. This may reflect alterations of basal ganglia function before the appearance of clinical symptoms (Foroud et al. 1995). Imaging techniques have also been used to evaluate whether or not there exists anatomical or functional correlates of disease in presymptomatic gene carriers. Asymptomatic carriers may have reduced basal ganglia volume and in some cases abnormal glucose metabolism on PET studies. MR spectroscopy revealed increased cortical lactate levels in symptomatic patients, and this methodology is now being used to study asymptomatic gene carriers (Jenkins et al. 1993). Once the disease is clinically established, no specific laboratory test can predict prognosis. Extensive study of these individuals is now in progress with the intention of identifying parameters of disease progression that could be followed in clinical trials to prevent or delay disease progression.

A very useful tool to evaluate disease progression in established patients is known as the total functional capacity (TFC) score. This scale, designed by Shoulson and Fahn (1979), has been validated and is useful in clinical trials. Worldwide, there is a consistent 0.5 to 1.0 unit decrease per year in this 13-point scale in longitudinally followed populations.

## Treatment

Treatment is individualized and symptomatic. Depression is treated with antidepressants. Tegretol or valproic acid may improve manic disorder. Delusions and agitated behavior are often responsive to neuroleptics, which also decrease chorea. Dopaminergic drugs are occasionally used to improve the rigid forms of the disease, but this can worsen chorea. It is often not necessary to treat chorea unless it interferes with the patient's activities of daily living. Treatment with neuro-

leptics often worsens cognitive function and motor function.

Nutrition is an important aspect of management, since these patients may have increased caloric requirements. Dysphagia and aspiration pneumonia are of great concern in these patients and prevention should be addressed. Management of HD requires the involvement of physical, occupational, and speech therapy as well as social services (Shoulson and Fahn 1979; Ranen et al. 1993).

## Dystonia

Dystonia is a syndrome of sustained motor contractions frequently causing twisting and repetitive movements or abnormal postures. Dystonia can be classified by age of onset, anatomical distribution, and etiology. Dystonia is not common and there is some uncertainty regarding the incidence of both generalized torsion dystonia and focal dystonia. Prognosis for idiopathic (primary) dystonia both generalized and focal will be discussed. Dystonia that is secondary to other illnesses, sometimes called symptomatic dystonias (e.g., Wilson's disease), or with known etiologies (e.g., secondary to neuroleptic administration) will not be discussed. Useful clinical clues that a dystonia may be symptomatic include a history of severe head trauma, perinatal injury, encephalitis, or neuroleptic exposure and the finding of additional neurological abnormalities such as spasticity, Babinski's sign, or dementia. The early onset of speech dysfunction, hemidystonia, or abnormal imaging studies are also important to the recognition that the dystonia may be symptomatic.

Primary (idiopathic) dystonia can be either familial or sporadic. Primary dystonia is characterized by dystonia being the only neurological finding and by a normal laboratory evaluation. Idiopathic torsion dystonia (ITD), formerly known as dystonia musculorium deformans, is an autosomal dominant disorder that is characterized by reduced penetrance (approximately 30% to 40%). The abnormal gene is located on chromosome 9q34.1 and is referred to as the *DYT1* gene (Ozelius et al. 1992). This is the most common familial dystonia. There are also multiple other family groupings of dystonia that are not characterized by the *DYT1* gene and which have been identified and named including *DYT6* and *DYT7*. No doubt as additional families are identified, additional genetic abnormalities resulting in dystonia will be identified (Bentivoglio et al. 1997; Bressman et al. 1994a, 1994b; Ahmad et al. 1993).

Since the basic neuropharmacology underlying dystonia is not known (Hornykiewicz et al. 1988; Jankovic et al. 1987), the pharmacological treatment of generalized and focal dystonia is a matter of trial and error. The most successful drug treatment reported is the use of high-dose anticholinergics for generalized dystonia (Fahn 1983). Additional trials of dopaminergic, antidopaminergic, cholinergic, serotoninergic, antiserotoninergic, various anticonvulsants, benzodiazepines, and multiple other compounds have not led to a generally successful treatment. These same agents have been tried in the focal dystonias with the same results. The introduction of botulinum toxin to treat focal dystonia and some isolated aspects of generalized dystonia has been a revolution in therapy. In most patients the use of botulinum toxin (Jancovic and Brin 1991; Brin 1991) has been far more successful in treating the movement disorder than has pharmacological therapy. In very selected patients, surgical treatment of dystonia may be indicated if they have failed all other medial treatment.

### Classification and Prognosis

Prognosis in primary dystonia is very closely linked to the classification by age of onset of the symptoms and by the anatomical distribution of the abnormality. Age of onset of symptoms is the most important factor regarding prognosis (Marsden et al. 1976; Fahn 1986; Greene et al. 1995). Dystonia beginning in childhood usually starts with action dystonia in one leg. The most common age of onset in the young is between 6 and 12 years (Zeman and Dyken 1968; Herz 1944; Marsden et al. 1974). The child usually demonstrates a bizarre twisted foot (usually plantar flexed and inverted) while walking (i.e., toe walking) but not at rest or during other activities, such as walking backward or running. The prognosis for future progression to generalized dystonia is associated with two major factors: onset in childhood and onset in the legs. Marsden and Harrison (Marsden et al. 1974) found that 79% of all patients with dystonia beginning before age 11 eventually developed generalized involvement. They also found that 14 of their 15 patients whose illness began with involvement of a leg (all under 19 years at onset) progressed to develop generalized dystonia over the following 5 to 10 years. Children with onset in arm, trunk, or neck also may progress to generalized involvement; however, the illness tends to remain segmental in a larger proportion of these individuals than in those with onset in the legs. Dystonia beginning in the neck may have the greatest likelihood of remaining focal even in the young. These findings have been confirmed by Greene et al. (1995), who also demonstrated that onset of dystonia in the lower extremities is the second most important predictive factor of generalization. Dystonia is considered to be generalized in distribution when a combination of a leg involvement plus involvement of any other body part develops.

The maximum disability in more typical patients with ITD usually occurs in the first 5 to 10 years, with the disease often remaining static or improving thereafter. Usually, dystonia does not result in death, and even severe involvement can be compatible with a normal life span (Zenan and Dyken 1968; Marsden et al. 1974). On the other hand, involvement in the legs (therefore, much more often in children) and trunk frequently results in a chairbound existence. One-half of Marsden and Harrison's (Marsden et al. 1974) childhood onset patients eventually reached this state. Arm involvement may impair self-care. Dystonia of bulbar musculature may make speech unintelligible, and impair chewing, swallowing, or breathing. Blepharospasm may render a patient functionally blind, despite normal visual acuity. Rarely, the abnormal movements and prolonged dystonic spasms may be so severe as to cause muscle injury leading to myoglobinuria and even renal failure.

Dystonia that begins in adult life is almost always focal in onset and tends to remain quite localized as to affected body part. Adult-onset focal dystonia is far more common than generalized dystonia. Adult-onset focal dystonia can occur as blepharospasm, oromandibular dystonia, blepharospasm in combination with oromandibular dystonia, spasmodic dysphonia, torticollis, or involvement of an isolated foot and leg or arm. The most common of these focal dystonias is torticollis and the least common is isolated foot involvement. Although there are a few rare families where focal dystonia has a genetic basis, most focal dystonia is sporadic (Leube et al. 1996).

The focal dystonias are not life threatening but can result in significant disability. Symptom intensity may vary and physicians cannot rely solely on office examination to determine the degree of disability.

The most important consequence of blepharospasm is its effects on vision. Despite normal visual acuity, blepharospasm may render a patient functionally blind. Even those without persistent or constant blepharospasm may be so frightened of developing the symptom (which is often aggravated by sunlight) while outside, especially while crossing the road, that they remain indoors, becoming social recluses. Other complications include secondary blepharitis, excessive tearing as well as brow ptosis, dermatochalasis, levator aponeurosis, and lateral canthal tendon defects (Gillum and Anderson 1981).

Although some patients reach maximum disability in a few weeks, the course of cranial dystonia is usually one of progression over the first 1 to 4 years. Symptoms often stabilize after this; however, some may continue to worsen and progress or spread to other areas several years after the onset of symptoms. Others may demonstrate spontaneous improvement in symptoms; however, complete remissions rarely, if ever, occur in isolated adult-onset focal cranial dystonia. Patients with disabling pharyngeal dystonia, which prevents swallowing or causes recurrent aspirations, occasionally benefit from cricopharyngeal myotomy.

The course of spasmodic torticollis is usually a progressive increase in symptoms over the first 5 years. After 5 years, torticollis is usually static for the next 5 years and after that might improve slightly. Many studies indicate that approximately 14% of patients will obtain a complete remission of their symptoms and some cite figures as high as 26% (Herz and Glaser 1949; Tibbets 1971; Matthews et al. 1978; Meares 1971; Friedman and Fahn 1986). Partial or incomplete remissions may occur. These remissions are much more common in those with onset of the disease before age 40 and almost always occur within the first 4 to 5 years of the illness. Unfortunately, the vast majority of remissions are temporary. However, the duration of these is quite variable, lasting only days to weeks in some and between 20

and 40 years in others. Occasionally, patients give a history of a brief period of torticollis seemingly precipitated by emotional upset or some other trauma earlier in life, which remits after a short time but returns permanently without precipitation many years later. Individual patients may have several episodes of remission and recurrence over many years.

Torticollis may remain mild and only minimally disabling for many years. However, most patients are disabled to some extent and 10% or more are unable to continue working (Matthews et al. 1978). Although there is no good evidence for a psychiatric etiology, despite many studies suggesting the contrary, many patients demonstrate some degree of emotional disturbance. Reactive depression is extremely common, and it has been noted that fastidious individuals accommodate spasmodic torticollis very poorly (Duanne 1979). Fear of ridicule and reluctance to leave the home are present in many patients (Matthews et al. 1978).

Jahanshahi (1991) studied the disability, psychosocial aspects, and functioning of patients with cervical dystonia. One hundred patients were evaluated and 22% were labeled as permanently disabled and could not be employed. These patients had disabilities secondary to the presence of a chronic disease rather than any specific psychological disorder. The main factors in this group of patients that contributed to their disability were pain, head position, and decreased head mobility. Depression was present in one-fourth of these patients. Following treatment with botulinum toxin and improvement of cervical dystonia the patients' psychological profiles improved. This suggests that suppression of head movement and associated pain may improve disability and depression.

In summary, young onset with symptoms in the legs is a very good indication that generalized dystonia may follow. Symptom onset in adolescence, involving the neck or limb, carries a slightly better prognosis. In adult patients, with initiation of focal dystonia in neck, eyes, face, or limbs, the prognosis is better and, despite the possible spread of dystonia to other parts of body, the likelihood of developing generalized dystonia is small. During the first 5 years after onset the symptoms may fluctuate. During the first few years of focal dystonia, patients may experience transient remissions.

## Tourette's Syndrome

Gilles de la Tourette's syndrome (TS), described more than 100 years ago, is a relatively common neurobehavioral disorder, with a spectrum of neurological, behavioral, and cognitive features. Current diagnostic criteria for TS include the presence of tics, the presence of one or more vocal tics, age of onset before 21 years, and duration of symptoms for more than 1 year (Kurlan 1995). TS is commonly associated with a variety of behavioral problems including obsessive compulsive behavior and attention deficit hyperactivity disorder (ADHD) (Kurlan 1989, 1988).

### Clinical Manifestations

Tics are brief, recurrent, nonrhythmic, stereotyped movements (motor tics) or sounds that are not always present. Tics occur on a background of normal motor activity. Tics can be classified as either simple or complex. Simple motor tics are abrupt, short, sudden movements such as a head jerk, eye blink, or shoulder shrug. Complex motor tics are more coordinated and complicated and may appear to be purposeful. Touching, jumping, skipping, and teeth gnashing are examples of complex motor tics. Motor tics usually occur repetitively in the same part of body, and multiple body parts can be involved. Over the course of time individual tics wax and wane and move from one body part to another.

Simple vocal tics consist of a variety of inarticulate noises and sounds such as grunting, throat clearing, shrieking, and coughing. Complex vocal tics have linguistic meaning. Examples include coprolalia, unintelligible words, stammering, and echolalia. The wide spectrum of tic manifestations may be misinterpreted as psychological illness.

Patients frequently feel an irresistible urge to release the tic; the urge may be momentarily suppressed and controlled, but at the expense of a build-up of tension that can be relieved only by the performance of multiple tics.

### Pathogenesis

Heredity has become the focus of attention as the etiology of TS. TS and related tic disorders seem to be very importantly influenced by genetic factors. An autosomal dominant pattern with variable expression and gender-specific penetrance seem likely (Pauls and Leckman 1986). No specific gene has yet been identified.

No specific consistent anatomical abnormalities have been identified in TS brains. Although the exact neurochemical disturbances have not been identified, there is pervasive evidence that TS involves brain dopaminergic systems. This evidence includes amelioration of tics by dopamine receptor antagonists, exacerbation of tics by dopaminergic enhancers (amphetamine, methylphenidate, pemoline), and the induction of tics by chronic dopamine receptor blockade (tardive tics). There have also been reports of alterations in the dopamine metabolite homovanillic acid in the cerebrospinal fluid (CSF) of TS patients, increased density of presynaptic dopamine nerve terminals, and alterations in B-CIT single photon emission computed tomography (SPECT) results in the basal ganglia of TS patients (Singer et al. 1982, 1990; Malison et al. 1995). New directions in exploring the neurochemistry of TS include alterations in the opioid system and secondary messengers (Haber et al. 1986; Kurlan et al. 1991).

### Treatment

Treatment of TS must be individualized because of the wide range of neurological and behavioral manifestations of this syndrome. The symptoms that are most disabling should be addressed. Tics, obsessive compulsive behavior, and ADHD all have potentially different pharmacological treatment. Tics may be treated with neuroleptics (e.g., pimozide, haloperidol, risperidol), the dopamine-depleting agent tetrabenazine, clonidine, or clonazepam. Obsessive compulsive disorder is responsive to the serotonin reuptake inhibitors including fluoxetine and clomipramine, and attention deficit hyperactivity disorder may be responsive to clonidine, tricyclic antidepressants, and stimulants such as methylphenidate (Ritalin). Pharmacological agents should be started in low dose and advanced slowly to achieve therapeutic results at the lowest dosage possible. After achieving satisfactory results with a particular drug, therapy should be interrupted in 5 to 7 months to determine if drug therapy for that particular symptom is still warranted. Patients with mild TS or nondisabling symptoms may require no therapy. Psychotherapy and behavioral modification may be effective in treatment of certain selected patients with TS; this may provide further emotional support for patients and their families.

## Prognosis

The natural history of TS and particularly its prognosis remains somewhat unclear. After the initial appearance of motor tics, additional tics usually appear within several weeks to months. Early in TS there may be periods of complete remission. There is no definite time period between onset of tics and progression. Vocal tics tend to be seen after the onset of motor tics. There is extreme variability in individual patients in terms of degree and intensity of symptoms. Patients may suddenly develop "new" tics after months of stable symptoms. New tics may develop in the context of emotional stress, but patients also report going through severe emotional stress with no change or improvement in symptoms.

Although there is no clinical or laboratory evidence that can accurately establish the prognosis for an individual, there is a clinical view that TS tends to become milder with age. It is well recognized that Tourette's symptoms are often the most severe or difficult to cope with during adolescence (Brunn 1988). Tic severity in childhood has been thought to be a predictor of adult TS severity; however, Goetz et al. (1992) have recently argued that functioning during adolescence is a more important factor in predicting adult prognosis.

Erenberg et al. (1987), on the basis of a questionnaire study of 58 patients between the ages of 15 and 25, reported that 73% of the patients reported tics to be improved or virtually gone by late adolescence or early adult life. Leckman et al. (1998) also reported that a majority of TS patients displayed a consistent time course of tic severity with increasing severity for 4 to 6 years following onset of tics and then a steady decline in severity so much so that by age 18 half the patients were virtually tic free. Lucas (1970) and Nee et al. (1982) also reported gradual improvement in symptom severity with increasing age. Asam (1979) in a study of 29 patients, Singer (1985) in a review of 120 patients, Shapiro (1985) in a presentation of 650 patients, and Brunn (1988) in a study of 350 patients all report some improvement in TS as patients reach maturity and that a significant number of patients continue to improve throughout their lives. Also, many adult TS patients require less or no treatment as they grow older. Brunn suggests that one-third of patients will remit completely during late adolescence or early adulthood, another one-third will show a remarkable improvement in the severity of tics over time, and the last one-third will remain symptomatic during early adulthood and middle age (Brunn and Budman 1993).

There is even less prognostic information regarding the neurobehavioral aspects of TS to permit identification of those patients who may experience improvement of neurobehavioral symptoms. In patients with obsessive compulsive disorder, 25% will resolve, 50% will improve, and 25% will remain unaltered or even worsen over time. Regarding ADHD disorder unaccompanied by tics, almost 30% to 50% of affected children may have remaining symptoms and be diagnosed with adult residual attention deficit hyperactivity disorder (Manuzza et al. 1993).

There is no information on whether any of the drugs used to treat TS alter the natural history of the disorder. Chronic administration of neuroleptics to suppress tics may result in tardive dyskinesia, but the actual effect on long-term outcome in TS is not known. Stimulants such as methylphenidate, dextroamphetamine, and pemoline used for the management of ADHD may precipitate TS or exacerbate tics. The effect of stimulants on the long-term prognosis of TS is unknown, but there does not seem to be any evidence that stimulant use worsens the prognosis.

TS patients also need strong social and educational support, which may have a strong impact on their academic, behavioral, and psychosocial status. The early identification of learning disabilities, appropriate counseling, and understanding and parenting of children with TS can improve their educational and psychosocial outcome.

TS is not fatal or life shortening. The development of adult-onset severe behavioral problems or psychosis is quite rare (Lees 1985). However, it should be recognized that there may be long-term personality, social, and life adjustment problems associated with TS.

## Tardive Dyskinesia

In 1957, the first description of orofacial dyskinetic movements after chlorpromazine treatment was reported in the medical literature (Schonecker 1957), and since that time tardive dyskinesia (TD) has become an increasing problem. It took many years for the medical community to accept tardive dyskinesia as a consequence of chronic neuroleptic administration. Among the difficulties in recognizing TD as a movement disorder secondary to the administration of medications that block central dopamine ($D_2$) receptors is the extemely varied length of time that a patient must be exposed to the drug (weeks to years) and the extreme variation in abnormal movements produced ranging from lingual facial buccal chewing and lip-smacking movements to choreiform hand movements and truncal dystonia. In some instances the clinical syndrome develops after decreasing the dose or discontinuation of the offending drug. In some cases the signs of TD may ameliorate following increasing the dose of the $D_2$-receptor agent.

The abnormal movements in TD most often involve the oral region, with characteristic tongue protrusion, lip smacking and puckering, grimacing, and chewing. These movements may be accompanied by chorea of the hands, arms, and toes; head nodding; and pelvic rocking movements. TD is an important and relatively frequent complication of neuroleptics. Yassa and Jeste (1997) reviewed prevalence studies of TD and reported that 24% of the neuroleptic-treated population develops this disorder. They note that prevalence rates increased from 13.5% in the 1960s to 28.6% in the 1970s, finally stabilizing at 25% in the 1980s. Other reports cite prevalence figures as high as 57% in 1984 (Kane 1984). The reason for such a wide range of prevalence rates is variation in the cohort risk factors measured such as gender, age, duration of exposure, and different diagnostic criteria. It has also been postulated that the lack of standarized rating scales for TD in the 1960s as well as considering only oral buccal movements as diagnostic contributed to the widely varying prevalence rates. In one study, 64% of patients with TD had segmental dystonia, 21% had focal dystonia (primarily of head and neck), and 14% had generalized dystonia (Burke et al. 1982).

There continues to be controversy regarding the risk factors for the development of TD. More often than not increasing age and female gender are thought to be consistent risk factors (Kane et al. 1988; Jeste and Wyatt, 1982; Johnson et al. 1982). Women show an increasing prevalence of TD with age, with the prevalence rate being considerably higher over the age of 70 than under 50. Men show an increased prevalence with age but

not nearly as striking (Yassa and Jeste 1997). Whether or not psychiatric diagnosis, particularly affective disorder, is a risk factor remains controversial. In a further follow-up of the Yale Tardive Dyskinesia Study, Glazer et al. (Douchette 1997) report findings that contradict commonly held beliefs concerning TD including no relationship between gender, type of neuroleptic, depot route of administration, or diagnosis of affective disorder. These investigators also reported that the risk of developing TD as a function of previous neuroleptic treatment is very high and that two of every three patients maintained on neuroleptics for 25 years will develop TD. In addition, they report that the risk is not linear and that the greatest risk for TD is within the first 5 years of exposure.

Other less frequent complications of chronic neuroleptic treatment consist of multifocal motor and vocal tics and tardive myoclonus. Tardive akathisia may also result from treatment with antipsychotics (Gardos et al. 1987; Weiner and Luby 1983; Burke et al. 1989). These patients feel an uncomfortable internal desire to move, usually in their legs. Movements associated with akathisia include truncal rocking, complex hand movements, hair and face rubbing, scratching, shouting, and moaning (Weiner and Luby 1983). Tardive akathisia has been reported to result in increased psychotic and violent behavior in schizophrenics (Herrara et al. 1988).

Drugs that induce TD are dopamine receptor blockers, which particularly block the $D_2$-receptor subtype in the striatum. These drugs are frequently used for their antipsychotic and antiemetic properties. They are also occasionally used for the treatment of depression and hiccups and inappropriately for insomnia and anxiety. Antipsychotics such as haloperidol, perphenazine, and chlorpromazine are examples of traditional neuroleptics that can induce TD. Metoclopramide and the calcium channel blockers (cinnarizine and flunarizine) also have the capability of blocking the dopamine receptors in the striatum and inducing TD. The atypical neuroleptics (clozaril, risperidal, olanzapine, quetiapine) are effective antipsychotic agents, and because of their unique receptor affinity profile induce far less TD. If the prevalence rate of TD with these agents continues to be so low with long-term use, these agents will become standard treatment for psychosis, and the prevalence of TD should fall markedly.

The pathophysiology of TD is unknown, but supersensitivity of postsynaptic dopamine receptors due to up-regulation induced by neuroleptic receptor blockade has been suggested. This hypothesis is supported by the similarity between TD and levodopa-induced dyskinesia in idiopathic Parkinson's disease. Increased doses of neuroleptics typically suppress TD and movements in other choreic disorders. One argument against this theory is that dopamine-depleting agents, such as reserpine, do not cause TD in animals, despite their ability to increase sensitivity of dopamine receptors (Hong et al. 1987). The role of other neurotransmitters, particularly GABA, has been investigated in the pathogenesis of TD.

## Treatment and Prognosis

The most significant steps in treatment of TD are prevention, early recognition, and discontinuation of the causative agent. Treatment is often difficult and the response to therapy is suboptimal. The most crucial step is prevention. Neuroleptics should be used for the treatment of major psychotic illnesses. Patients receiving neuroleptic treatment should be examined at frequent and regular intervals for any evidence of early stages of TD, since there is evidence that early withdrawal of the etiological drug offers the best hope of reversibility of TD. In those rare circumstances when the severity of TD justifies an increase in dose of neuroleptic, the movements may improve in 75% of the patients. This is generally believed to be a poor therapeutic choice, since it means using the etiological agent as the therapy. If the symptoms of TD persist or are disabling, or if neuroleptic withdrawal is not possible, use of other pharmacological agents may be required. Dopamine-depleting agents such as reserpine and tetrabenazine are the most efficacious, and in contrast to dopamine-receptor blocking medications, they have not been reported to cause TD (Fahn 1983). The main side effects of these medications are orthostatic hypotension, parkinsonism, and depression. Doses are introduced gradually over weeks to months to help decrease these side effects.

GABA is thought to exert an inhibitory influence on nigrostriatal dopaminergic activity (Penny and Young 1983). Thus, a number of medications with GABA-enhancing activity such as sodium valproate (Fisk and York 1987), baclofen (Stewart et al 1982), clonazepam, alperazolam, and diazepam (Bobruff et al. 1981) have been tried with minimal efficacy. Electroconvulsive therapy has also been used to treat TD (Gosek and Weller 1988; Chacko et al. 1983).

Tardive dyskinesia occurs after exposure to neuroleptic medications. The resultant abnormal movements may at times be very disabling and even life threatening. The prevalence of TD is believed to increase with advanced age, female gender, and with an increasing cumulative lifetime dose of neuroleptic. Some of these risk factors remain controversial.

Prevention and early recognition of TD is crucial to prevent irreversibility of the movements (Quitkin et al. 1977). Whenever possible the offending agent should be discontinued. The earlier the discontinuation of dopamine receptor blocker after the onset of dyskinesias, the more probable is remission, and the older the patient, the less likely is remission (Klawans and Tanner 1983).

## References

Ahmad, F.; Davis, M. B.; Waddy, H. M.; Oley, C. A.; Marsden, C. D.; Harding, A. E. Evidence for locus heterogeneity in autosomal dominant torsion dystonia. Genomics 1993;15:9–12

Alzheimer, A. Uber die anatomische Grundladge der Huntingtonischen Chorea und er choreatischen Bewegungen uberhaupt [abstract]. Neurol. Cbl. 30: 891–892; 1916

Aminoff, M. J.; Marshall, J.; Smith, E. M.; Wyke, M. A. Pattern of intellectual impairment in Huntington's chorea. Psychol. Med. 5:169–172; 1975.

Anton G. Uber die Beteiligung der grossen basalen Gehringanglien bei Bewegungsstorungen und insbesondere bei Chorea. Jahrbucher. Psychiat. Neurol. (Lpz.) 14:141–181; 1896.

Asam, U. Katamnestische Untersuchung von uber jugendliche Patientente-Syndroms. Acta Paedopschiatrica 45:51–63; 1979.

Barclay, C. L.; Lang, A. E. Dystonia in progressive supranuclear palsy. J. Neurol. Neurosurg. Psychiatry 62:352–356; 1997.

Beal, M. F.; Brouillet, E.; Jenkins, B. G.; Ferrante, R. J.; Kowall, N. W.; Miller, J. M.; Storey, E.; Srivastava, R.; Rosen, B.; Hyman, B. T. Neurochemical and histologic characterization of striatal excitotoxic lesions produced by the mitochondrial toxin 3-nitropropionic acid. J. Neurosci. 13:4181–4192; 1993.

Bentivoglio, A. R.; Del Grosso, N.; Albanese, A.; Casetta, E.; Tonali, M.; Frontali, M. A large family affected by idiopathic torsion dystonia with complete penetrance not linked to DYT1. J. Neurol. Neurosurg. Psychiatry 62:357–360; 1997.

Bobruff, A.; Gaedos, G.; Tarsy, D.; et al. Clonazepam and phenobarbital in tardive dyskinesia. Am. J. Psychiatry 138:189–193; 1981.

Bower, J.; Demetrius, M.; Maraganore, M.; Shannon, K.; McDonnell, M.S.; Rocca, W. Incidence of progressive supranuclear palsy and multiple system atrophy in Olmsted County, Minnesota, 1976 to 1990. Neurology 49:1284–1288; 1997.

Brain, R. Diseases of the nervous system. London, New York, and Toronto: Oxford University Press; 1955: p. 538–550.

Brandt, J. Access to knowledge in dementia of Huntington's disease. Dev. Neuropsychol. 1:335–348; 1985.

Bressman, S. B.; Heiman, G. A.; Nygraad, T. G.; Ozelius, L. J.; Hunt, A. L.; Brin, M. F.; Goedon, M. F.; Moskowitz, C. B.; deLeon, D.; Bueke, R. E.; Fahn, S.; Risch, N. J.; Breakefield, X. O.; Kramer P. I. A study of idiopathic torsion dystonia in a non-Jewish family: evidence for genetic heterogeneity. Neurology 44:283–287; 1994a.

Bressman, S. B.; Hunt, A. L.; Heiman, G.; Brin, M. F.; Burke, R. E.; deLeon, D.; Trugman, J.; Fahn, S.; Wilhelmsen, K.; Nygraad, T. G. Exclusion of the DYT1 locus in a non-Jewish family with early dystonia. Mov. Disord. 9:626–632; 1994b.

Brin, M. F. Interventional neurology: treatment of neurological conditions with local injection of botulinum toxin. Arch. Neurobiol. 54:173; 1991.

Britton, J. W.; Uitti, R. J.; Ahlskog, J. E. Hereditory late-onset chorea without dementia: genetic evidence for substantial phenotypic variation in Huntington's disease. Neurology 45:443–447; 1995.

Brunn, R. D. The natural history of Tourette's syndrome. In: Cohen D.; Brunn, R. D.; Leckman, J. Tourette's syndrome and tics disorders. New York: John Wiley & Sons; 1988: p. 22–39.

Brunn, R. D.; Budman, C. L. The natural history of Gilles de la Tourette syndrome. In: Kurlan, R., ed. Handbook of Tourette's syndrome and related tic and behavioral disorders. New York: Marcel Dekker; 1993: p. 27–42.

Burke, R. E.; Fahn, S.; Jankovic, J. Tardive dystonia: late-onset and persistent dystonia caused by antipsychotic drugs. Neurology 32:1335–1341; 1982.

Burke, R. E.; Kang, U. J.; Jankovic, J. Tardive akathesia: an analysis of clinical features and response to open therapeutic trials. Mov. Disord. 4(2):57–75; 1989.

Caine, E. D.; Ebert, M. H.; Weingartner, H. The memory disorder of Huntington's disease. Neurology 27:1087–1092; 1977.

Caine, E. D.; Hunt, R. D.; Weingartner, H.; Ebert, M. H. Huntington's dementia: clinical and neuropsychological features. Arch. Gen. Psychiatry 35: 377–384; 1978.

Cedarbaum, J. M.; McDowell, F. H. Sixteen year follow-up of 100 patients begun on levodopa in 1968: emerging problems. In: Yahr, M. D.; Bergmann, K. J., eds. Advances in neurology: Parkinson's disease. Vol. 45. New York: Raven Press; 1986: p. 469–472.

Chacko, R. C.; Root, L. ECT and tardive dyskinesia: two cases and a review. J. Clin. Psychiatry 44:254–266; 1983.

Dimsdale, H. Changes in the parkinsonian syndrome in the twentieth century. Q. J. Med. 15:155–170; 1946.

Douchette, J. The Yale Tardive Dyskinesia Study: a prospective incidence study among long term outpatients. In: Yassa, R.; Vasavan, N. P.; Nair, N. P.; Jeste, D. V., eds. Neuroleptic Induced Movement Disorders. New York: Cambridge University Press; 1997: p. 41

Duanne, D. D. Torticollis-dystonia-tics. American College of Physicians course: Neurology for the internist. Rochester, MN; 1979.

Duayo, M.; Ambrose, C.; Myers, R.; et al. Trinucleotide repeat length instability and age of onset in Huntington's diesease. Nat. Genet. 4:387–392; 1993.

Erenberg, G.; Cruse, R. P.; Rothner, D. O.; Rothner, A. D. The natural history of Tourette's syndrome: a follow-up study. Ann. Neurol. 22:383–385; 1987.

Fahn, S. On-off phenomenon with levodopa therapy in parkinsonism. Neurology 24:431–441; 1974.

Fahn, S. High dosage anticholinergic therapy in dystonia. Neurology 33:1255–1261; 1983a.

Fahn, S. Treatment of tardive dyskinesia with dopamine depleting agents. Clin. Neuropharmacol. 6: 151–158; 1983b.

Fahn, S. Generalized dystonia: concept and treatment. Clin. Neuropharmacol. 9(suppl. 2): S37–S48; 1986.

Federico, F.; Simone, I. L.; Lucivero, V.; et al. Proton magnetic resonance spectroscopy in Parkinson's disease and progressive supranuclear palsy. J. Neurol. Neurosurg. Psychiatry 62:239–242; 1997.

Fisk, G. G.; York, S. M. The effects of sodium valproate on tardive dyskinesia. Am. J. Psychiatry 150: 542–549; 1987.

Folstein, S. E. Huntington's disease: a disorder of families. Baltimore: John's Hopkins University Press; 1989.

Fouroud, T.; Siemers, E.; Kleindorfer, D.; et al. Cognitive scores in carriers of Huntington's disease compared to non carriers. Ann. Neurol. 37:675–664; 1995.

Friedman, A.; Fahn, S. Spontaneous remissions in spasmodic torticollis. Neurology 36:398–400; 1986.

Friedman, J. H. Parkinson's disease In: Gilchrist, J., ed. Prognosis in neurology. Melbourne: Butterworth-Heineîman; 1998: p. 129–130.

Gardos, G.; Cole, J. O.; Salomon, M. Clinical forms of severe tardive dyskinesia. Am. J. Psychiatry 150: 895–902; 1987.

Gillum, W. N.; Anderson, R. L. Blpharospasm surgery. An anatomical approach. Arch. Opthalmol. 99: 1056–1062; 1981.

Goetz, C. G.; Tanner, C. M.; Stebbins, G. T.; et al. Adult tics in Tourette's syndrome: description and risk factors. Neurology 42:784–788; 1992.

Golbe, L. I.; Davis, P. H.; Schoenberg, B. S.; Duvoisin, R. C. Prevalence and natural history of progressive supranuclear palsy. Neurology 38:1031–1034; 1988.

Gosek, E.; Weller, R. A. Improvement of tardive dyskinesia associated with electroconvulsive therapy. J. Nerv. Ment. Dis. 176:120–122; 1988.

Gowers, W. R. A manual of diseases of the nervous system. 2nd ed. Philadelphia: Blakison; 1893: p. 636–657.

Greene, P.; Kang, U. J.; Fahn, S. Spread of symptoms in idiopathic torsion dystonia. Mov. Disord. 10:143–152; 1995.

Gusella, J. F.; Wexler, N. S.; Coneally, P. M.; et al. A polymorphic DNA marker genetically linked to the Huntington's disease. Nature 306:234–237; 1983.

Haber, S. N.; Kowell, N. W.; Vonsattel, J. P.; et al. Gilles de la Tourette's syndrome: a postmortem neuropathological and immunohistochemical study. J. Neurol. Sci. 75:225; 1986.

Herrara, J. N.; Sramek, J. J.; Costa, J. F. High potency neuroleptics and violence in schizophrenics. J. Nerv. Ment. Dis. 176:558–561; 1988.

Herz, E. Dystonia II. Clinical classification. Arch. Neurol. Psychiatry (Chicago) 51:319–355; 1944.

Herz, E.; Glaser, G. M. Spasmodic torticollis. II: clinical evaluation. Arch. Neurol. Psychiatry (Chicago) 61:227–239;1949.

Hoehn, M. M. Parkinsonism treated with levodopa: progression and mortality. In: Birkmayer, W.; Duvoison, R. C., eds. Extrapyramidal disorders. J. Neural Transm. Suppl. 19:253–264; 1983.

Hoehn, M. M. The result of chronic levodopa therapy and its modification by bromocriptine in Parkinson's disease. Acta Neurol. Scand. 71:97–106; 1985.

Hoehn, M. Natural history of the untreated pre-levodopa disease In: Stern, G., ed. Parkinson's disease. Baltimore: Johns Hopkins; 1990: p. 307–314.

Hoehn, M. M.; Yahr, M. D. Parkinsonism: onset, progression and mortality. Neurology 17:427–442; 1967.

Hong, M.; Jenner, P.; Marsden, C. D. Comparison of the acute actions of amine-depleting drugs and dopamine receptor antagonists on dopamine function in the brain in rats. Neuropharmacology 26: 1061–1069; 1987.

Hornykiewicz, O.; Kish, S.; Becker, L. E.; et al. Biochemical evidence for brain neurotransmitter changes in idiopathic torsion dystonia (dystonia musculorum deformans). In: Fahn, S.; Marsden, C. D.; Clone, D. B., eds. Advances in neurology: dystonia 2. Vol. 50. New York: Raven Press; 1988: p. 157–165.

Huntington, G. On chorea. Med. Surg. Rep. 26:320; 1872.

Huntington's Disease Collaborative Research Group. A novel gene containing a trinucleotide repeat that is expanded and unstable on Huntington's disease chromosomes. Cell 72:971–983; 1993.

Jahanshahi, M. Psychosocial factors and depression in torticollis. J. Psychosom. Res. 35:493–507; 1991.

Jancovic, J.; Brin, M. Therapeutic uses of botulinum toxin. N. Engl. J. Med. 324:1186; 1991.

Jankovic, J.; Calne, D. B. Parkinson's disease: etiology and treatment. In: Appel, S. H., ed. Current neurology. Chicago: Year Book Medical Publishers; 1987: p. 193–234.

Jankovic, J.; McDermott, M.; Carter, J.; Gauthier, S.; Goetz, C.; Golbe, L.; Huber, S.; Koller, W.; Olanow, C.; Shoulson, I.; Stern, M.; Tanner, C.; Weiner, W.; and the Parkinson Study Group. Variable expression of Parkinson's disease. A baseline analysis of the DATATOP cohort. Neurology 40:1529–1534; 1990.

Jankovic, J.; Svendsen, C. N.; Bird, E. P. Brain neurotransmitters in dystonia. N. Engl. J. Med. 316:278–279; 1987.

Jenkins, B.; Koroshetz, W. J.; Beal, M. F.; Rosen, B. R. Evidence of impairment of energy metabolism in vivo in Huntington's disease using localized 1H NMR spectroscopy. Neurology 43:2689–2695; 1993.

Jeste, D. V.; Wyatt, R. J. Understanding and treating tardive dyskinesia. New York: Guilford Press; 1982, p.34.

Johnson, G. F. S.; Hunt, G. E.; Rey, J. M. Incidence and severity of tardive dyskinesia increase with age. Arch. Gen. Psychiatry 39:486; 1982.

Joseph, C.; Chassan, J. B.; Koch, M. L. Levodopa in Parkinson's disease: a long term appraisal of mortality. Ann. Neurol. 3:116–118; 1978.

Kane, J. M. Tardive dyskinesia. In: Jeste, D. V.; Wyatt, R. J.; eds. Neuropsychiatric movement disorders. Washington, DC: American Psychiatric Press; 1984: p. 68.

Kane, J. M.; Woerner, M.; Lieberman, J. Tardive dyskinesia: prevalence, incidence, and risk factors. J. Clin. Psychopharmacol. 8(suppl.):52; 1988.

Kennedy, J. S.; Kenny, J. T. Cognitive disorders associated with psychiatric illnesses. In: Thal, L. J.; Moos, W. J.; Gamuz, E. R., eds. Cognitive disorders. New York: Marcel Dekker; 1992: p. 138.

Klawans, H. L.; Tanner, C. M. The reversibility of permanent tardive dyskinesia. Neurology 33(suppl. 2):163; 1983.

Kowall, N. W.; Ferrante, R. J.; Martin, J. B. Patterns of cell loss in Huntington's disease. Trends Neurosci. 10:24–29; 1987.

Kremer, B.; Weber, B.; Hayden, M. R. New insights into the clinical features. Pathogenesis and molecular genetics of Huntington's disease. Brain Pathol. 2:321–335; 1992.

Kurlan, R. What is the specturm of Tourette's syndrome? Curr. Opin. Neurol. Neurosurg. 1:294; 1988.

Kurlan, R. Tourette's syndrome current concepts. Neurology 39:1625; 1989.

Kurlan, R. Treatment of tics. In: Treatment of movement disorders. Philadelphia: J. B. Lippincott; 1995: p. 365.

Kurlan, R.; Majumdar, L.; Deeley, C.; et al. A controlled trial of propoxyphene and naltrexone in Tourette's syndrome. Ann. Neurol. 30:19; 1991.

Lanois, M.; Paviot, J. Deux cas de choree hereditaire avec autopsies. Arch. Neurol. (Paris) 4:333–334; 1897.

Leckman, J. F.; Zhang, H. P.; Vitale, A.; Lahnin, F.; Lynch, K.; Bondi, C.; Kim, Y. S.; Peterson, B. S. Course of tic severity in Tourette syndrome: the first two decades. Pediatrics 102:14–19; 1998.

Lees, A. J. Tics and related disorders. New York: Churchill Livingstone; 1985.

Leube, B.; Doda, R.; Ratzlaff, T.; Kessler, K.; Benecke, R.; Auberger, G. Idiopathic torsion dystonia: assignment of a gene to chromosome 18p in a German family with adult onset, autosomal inheritance and purely focal distribution. Hum. Mol. Genet. 5:1673–1677; 1996.

Litvan, I.; Campbell, G.; Mangone, C. A.; Verny, M.; McKee, A.; Chaudhuri, K. R.; Jellinger, K.; Pearce, B.; D'Olhaberriague, L. Which clinical features differentiate progressive supranuclear palsy (Steele-Richardson-Olszweski syndrome) from related disorders? Brain 120:65–74; 1997.

Litvan, I.; Mangone, C. A.; McKee, A.; et al. Natural history of progressive supranuclear palsy (Steele-Richardson-Olszewski syndrome) and clinical predictors of survival: a clinicopathological study. J. Neurol. Neurosurg. Psychiatry 61:615–620; 1996.

Litvan, I.; Sastry, N.; Sonies, B. C. Characterizing swallowing abnormalities in progressive supranuclear palsy. Neurology 48:1654–1662; 1997.

Lucas, A. R. Gilles de la Tourette's syndrome: an overview. N. Y. State J. Med. 70:2197–2200; 1970.

MacMillan, J. C.; Morrison, P. J.; Nevin, N. C.; et al. Identification of an expanded CAG repeat in the Huntington's disease gene in a family reported to have benign hereditary chorea. J. Med. Genet. 30:1012–1013; 1993.

Maher, E. R.; Lees, A. J. The clinical features and natural history of the Steele-Richardson-Olszewski syndrome (progressive supranuclear palsy). Neurology 36:1005–1008; 1986.

Malison, R. T.; McDougal, C. J.; van Dyck, C. H.; et al. [123 I] B-IT SPECT imaging of striatal dopamine transporter binding in Tourette's syndrome. Am. J. Psychiatry 152:1359; 1995.

Manuzza, S.; Klein, R.; Bessler, A.; et al. Adult outcome of hyperactive boys: educational achievement, occupational rank and psychiatric status. Arch. Gen. Psychiatry 50:566–576; 1993.

Marconi, R.; Lefebure-Caparros, D.; Bonnet, A. M.; et al. Levodopa induced dyskinesia in Parkinson's disease: phenomenology and pathophysiology. Mov. Disord. 9:212; 1994.

Marsden, C. D.; Harrison, M. J. G.; Bundey, S. Natural history of idiopathic torsion dystonia (dystonia musculorum deformans). A review of forty-two patients. Brain 97:793–810; 1974.

Marsden, C. D.; Harrison, M. J. G.; Bundey, S. Natural history of idiopathic torsion dystonia. Adv. Neurol. 14:177–187; 1976.

Marsden, C. D.; Parkes, J. P.; Quinn, N. Fluctuations of disability in Parkinson's disease. In: Marsden, C. D.; Fahn, S., eds. Movement disorders. London: Butterworth; 1982.

Martignoni, E.; Micieli, G.; Cavallini, A.; et al. Autonomic disorders in idiopathic parkinsonism. Neurol. Transm. 22:149–161; 1986.

Mathers, S. E.; Kempster, P. A.; Law, P. J.; et al. Anal sphincter dysfunction in Parkinson's disease. Arch. Neurol. 46:1061–1064; 1989.

Matthews, W. B.; Beasley, P.; Parry-Jones, W.; et al. Spasmodic torticollis: a combined clinical study. J. Neurosurg. Psychiatry 41:485–492; 1978.

Meares, R. Natural history of spasmodic torticollis and effect of surgery. Lancet 2:149–151, 1971.

Merritt, H. H. A textbook of neurology. Philadelphia: Lea & Febiger; 1959: p. 454–462.

Myers, R. H.; Sax, D. S.; Koroshetz, W. J.; Mastromauro, C.; Cupples, L. A.; Kiely, D. K.; Pettengeill, F.; Bird, E. D. Factors associated with a slow progression in Huntington's disease. Arch. Neurol. 48:800–804; 1991.

Myers, R. H.; Vonsattel, J. P.; Stevens, T. H.; Cupples, L. A.; Richardson, E. P.; Martin, J. B.; Bird, E. B. Clinical and neuropathologic assesment of severity in Huntington's disease. Ann. Neurol. 25:252–259; 1988.

Nagasaka, T.; Togashi, S.; Amino, A.; Nitta, K.; Shindo, K.; Shiozawa, Z. Aniracetam for treatment of patients with progressive supranuclear palsy. Eur. Neurol. 37:195–198; 1997.

Nee, L. E.; Polinsky, R. J.; Ebert, M. H. Tourrete syndrome: clinical and family studies. In: Friedhoff, A. J.; Chase, T. N. Gilles de la Tourette syndrome. New York: Raven Press; 1982.

Nutt, J. C. Levodopa induced dyskinesias. Neurology 40:340–345; 1990.

Nutt, J. G.; Woodward, W. D.; Hammerstad, J. P.; et al. The "on-off" phenomenon in Parkinson's disease: relationship to L-dopa absorption and transport. N. Engl. J. Med. 310:484–488; 1984.

Ozelius, L. J.; Kramer, P. L.; de Leon, D.; Risch, N.; Bressman, S. B.; Schuback, D. E.; Brin, M. F.; Kwiatkowski, D. J.; Burke, R. E.; Gusella, J. F.; Fahn, S.; Breakfield, X. O. Strong allelic association between the torsion dystonia gene (DYT1) and loci on chromosome 9q34 in Ashkenazi Jews. Am. J. Hum. Genet. 50:619–628; 1992.

Parkinson, J. An essay on the shaking palsy. Med. Classics 1817; 10:964, 1997.

Pauls, D. L.; Leckman, J. F. The inheritance of Gilles de la Tourette's syndrome and associated behaviors: evidence for autosomal dominant transmission. N. Engl. J. Med. 315:993; 1986.

Penney, J. B.; Young, A. B.; Shoulson, I. Huntington's disease in Venezuela: 7-year-follow-up on symptomtic and asymptomatic individuals. Mov. Disord. 5:93–99; 1990.

Penny, J. B.; Jr.; Young, A. B. Speculations on the functional anatomy of basal ganglia disorders Ann. Rev. Neurosci. 6:73–94; 1983.

Quitkin, F.; Rifkin, A.; Gochfeld, L.; et al. Tardive dyskinesia: are first signs reversible? Am. J. Psychiatry 134:84–87; 1977.

Rajput, A. H.; Offord, K. P.; Beard, C. M.; et al. Epidemiology of parkinsonism: incidence, classification, and mortality. Ann. Neurol. 16:278–282; 1984.

Ranen, N. G.; Peyser, C. E.; Folstein, S. E. A physicians guide to the management of Huntington's disease. New York: Huntington's Disease Society of America; 1993.

Richardson, J. C.; Steel, J.; Olszewski, J. Supranuclear ophthalmoplegia, psuedobulbar palsy, nuchal dystonia, and dementia. Trans. Am. Neurol. Assoc. 88: 25–27; 1963.

Schonecker, M. Ein eigentumliches syndrom in oralen Bereich bei Megphen application. Nervenarzt 28: 35–36; 1957.

Schwab, R. W. Progression and prognosis in Parkinson's disease. J. Nerv. Ment. Dis. 130:556–566; 1960.

Shapiro, A. K. Presentation at First National Clinical Symposium on Tourette's syndrome. New York; 1985.

Shoulson, I.; Fahn, S. Huntington's disease: clinical care and evaluation. Neurology 29:1–3; 1979.

Singer, H. S. Natural history of Tourette syndrome. Presentation at Tourette Syndrome Association Conference, June 1985, New York City.

Singer, H. S.; Butler, I. J.; Tune, L. E.; et al. Dopaminergic dysfunction in Tourette's syndrome. Ann. Neurol. 12:361; 1982.

Singer, H. S.; Hanh, I. -H.; Krowiak, E.; et al. Tourette's syndrome: a neurochemical analysis of postmortem cortical brain tissue. Ann. Neurol. 27:443; 1990.

Singer, H. S.; Hahn, I. -H.; Moran, T. H. Abnormal dopamine uptake sites in postmortem striatum from patients with Tourette's syndrome. Ann. Neurol. 30:558; 1991.

Steele, J. C.; Richardson, J. C.; Olszewski, J. Progressive supranulclear palsy: a heterogenerous degeneration involving the brainstem, basal ganglia and cerebellum with vertical gaze and pseudobulbar palsy, nuchal dystonia and dementia. Arch. Neurol. 2:473–486; 1963.

Stewart, R. M.; Rollins, J.; Beckham, B. Baclofen in tardive dyskinesia patients maintained on neuroleptics. Clin. Neuropharmacol. 5:365–373; 1982.

Sweet, R. D.; McDowell, F. H. Five years treatment of Parkinson's disease with levodopa: therapeutic results and survival of 100 patients. Ann. Intern. Med. 83:456–463; 1975.

Tian, J. R.; Herman, S. J.; Zee, D. S.; Folstein, S. E. Postural control in Huntington's disease (HD). Acta. Otolaryngol. Suppl. (Stockh.) 481:333–336; 1991.

Tibbetts, R. W. Spasmodic torticollis. J. Psychosom. Res. 15:461–469;1971.

Von Sattel, J. P; Myers, R. H.; Stevens, T. J. Neuropathalogical classification of the Huntington's disease. J. Neuropathol. Exp. Neurol. 44:559–577; 1985.

Weiner, W. J.; Lang, A. E. Huntington's disease. In: Movement disorder: a comprehensive survey. Mt. Kisco, NY: Futura; 1989.

Weiner, W. J.; Luby, E. D. Persistent akathsia following neuroleptic withdrawal. Ann. Neurol. 13:466–467; 1983.

Weiner, W. J.; Minagar, A.; Shulman, L. M. Pramipexole in progressive supranuclear palsy (PSP). Neurology 50:A386; 1998.

White, F. R.; Vasterling, J. J.; Koroshetz, W. J.; Myers, R. Neuropsychology of Huntington's disease. In: White, R., ed. Clinical syndromes in adult neuropsychology; the practitioner's handbook. Amsterdam: Elsevier; 1992: p. 213–248.

Wilson, S. A. K. In: Bruce, A. N., ed. Neurology. Baltimore: Williams & Wilkins; 1940: p. 787–805.

Yassa, R.; Jeste, D. Gender as a factor in the development of tardive dyskinesia. In: Neuroleptic induced movement disorders. Cambridge New York: Cambridge Univeristy Press; 1997: p. 26–40.

Zeman, W.; Dyken, P. Dystonia musculorum deformans. In Vinken, P. J.; Bruyn, G. W., eds. Handbook of clinical neurology. Vol. 6. Amsterdan: North-Holland; 1968: p. 517–543.

# 37

# Behavioral and Cognitive Disorders

ANDREW KERTESZ

Prognosis of behavioral or cognitive disorders in neurology depends on their etiology and their initial severity. Considerable experience has been accumulated with various syndromes after strokes and trauma. Much of the information concerning the aphasic syndromes will be related to the natural history of recovery from stroke. Even though each etiology is going to be treated separately there is a certain degree of commonality which is related to severity, lesion size, location, and other biological factors. The biology of recovery from cerebral damage and cortical plasticity is beyond the scope of the chapter, but it has recently been extensively studied and reviewed (Merzenich et al. 1983; Stein et al. 1995).

Aphasic syndromes are common in neurology and the knowledge of their prognosis is essential for practicing neurologists, as well as researchers. In addition to the practical aspects of recovery from aphasia, the theoretical aspects are important for knowledge of the organization of language in the brain, as well as recovery mechanisms in general. Language is a uniquely human attribute that is processed mainly in the left hemisphere, although right hemisphere language capacity has been considered important for recovery. The factors of recovery from aphasia have been extensively investigated. Some of these factors are valid

for other behavioral disorders as well, and only the differences will be pointed out subsequently. The factors listed below are inter-related and at times their interaction is as important as their distinctiveness. They will be discussed in the approximate order of their importance for prognosis.

## Severity

A major prognostic factor in recovery is initial severity (Godfrey and Douglass 1959; Schuell et al. 1964; Kertesz and McCabe 1977). Even though some studies considered the most severely affected patients or global aphasics showing little gain, whether or not they were treated (Sarno et al. 1970), there are several studies that indicate that some of these patients recover surprisingly well depending on other factors such as lesion size, location, and etiology (Kertesz 1979; Kertesz et al. 1989a). Severely affected patients have a lot of room for improvement and may show a great deal of change. However, mildly affected patients often recover completely, although the amount of gain is little. This is a "ceiling effect," which confounds recovery rates and it should be considered carefully in studies of prognosis (Kertesz and McCabe 1977). Both recovery rates and outcome measures are affected by initial severity, although in a different manner in each instance.

## Etiology

Another major factor in recovery is the etiology. Post-traumatic aphasics recover much better than patients with vascular disease (Butfield and Zangwill 1946). In our own study, we demonstrated complete recovery in more than half of our post-traumatic patients (Kertesz and McCabe 1977) and the Vietnam veterans study of aphasia outcome reached similar conclusions when their aphasics were reviewed (Ludlow et al. 1986). Some of these patients from this head injury study remained nonfluent after 30 years, particularly those who had extensive cortical and subcortical lesions. Penetrating brain lesions with a large amount of brain destruction are not really comparable to most instances of closed head injury, which have good prognosis. Even global aphasia can recover to a mild, anomic state after a closed head injury (Kertesz and McCabe 1977). Persisting, severe aphasia is unusual after a closed head injury even though dysarthria can be quite incapacitating. Memory loss and nonverbal cognitive deficits are the major problems in the severely injured motor vehicle accident population (Levin et al. 1982). There are significant personality and behavior abnormalities, common in frontal trauma, and some of this disinhibited psychopathic behavior has poor prognosis. The scatter of the extent of recovery is greater in trauma than in stroke because of the combination of contusion and concussion, and the variability of penetrating head injuries, in contrast to the rather stereotypical occurrence of vascular occlusions in the same arterial territory.

Aphasia from subarachnoid hemorrhage also shows a variability in the rate of recovery that is related to whether the patient sustained hemorrhage or an infarction and to the tissue destruction. The prognosis was predictable to some extent from the initial severity of the aphasia in our study (Kertesz and McCabe 1977). Severe, persisting jargon aphasia and global aphasia can be seen following ruptured middle cerebral artery aneurysms where the cerebral spasm produced extensive lesions. If only a hematoma occurs, absorption and recovery are usually good.

The prognosis in primary progressive aphasia (PPA) is quite different from the other etiologies discussed above. This condition was recognized to be part of Pick's diease, even though the pathology often lacks typical Pick bodies (Kertesz et al. 1994). Initially, the patients have only word-finding difficulty and are often misdiagnosed as having stroke or Alzheimer's disease (AD). However, in midstages, progressive nonfluent aphasia and eventually mutism develop in 6 to 8 years. In later stages extrapyramidal disorder or motor neuron disease may supervene, and death occurs 10 to 12 years after onset. When dysphagia or motor neuron disease occurs early, the prognosis is worse and the course of the illness leading to death is more rapid (Caselli et al. 1993).

## Type of Aphasia

Aphasia type interacts with severity. However, beyond the severity factor there is a difference between various aphasia types, which reflects the fact that various language components differ in their rate of recovery. Henry Head (1926) also observed that various aphasia types recover at different rates. Subsequent investigations indicated motor aphasia or expressive aphasia to improve the most (Weisenburg and McBride 1935; Butfield and Zangwill 1946; Messerli et al. 1976; Kertesz and McCabe 1977). Although Vignolo (1964) showed expressive disorders to have poor prognosis, Basso et al. (1982) did not find a difference between fluent and nonfluent aphasic patients in their recovery. This variation in conclusion reflects problems in classification. Vignolo's (1964) study was heavily weighted towards global aphasics with poor recovery. Other studies included aphasics with milder expressive difficulty that would produce a better prognosis. When the severity is taken into consideration and aphasia types with equal severity are compared, relatively small differences are seen between fluent and nonfluent patients; this may be the reason why Basso et al. (1982) did not demonstrate much difference. However, when we looked at a large aphasic population, we found Broca's aphasics indeed recovered somewhat better than Wernicke's aphasics of equivalent severity (Kertesz 1979, 1988).

When considering recovery from various types of aphasia, the methods of classification, the methods of measurement, and the relationship to severity must be carefully considered before comparing different studies. Most clinicians will distinguish between Broca's and Wernicke's aphasics or use the expressive/receptive dichotomy, but for the purpose of prognosis global aphasics (those who have poor or nonexisting comprehension in addition to very poor output) should be distinguished from Broca's aphasics, who may be very nonfluent but can be demonstrated to have reasonable comprehension. In fact, this preservation of comprehension makes the group, which is often called Broca's aphasia or by some speech pathologists "verbal apraxia," have good overall prognosis.

Apart from the exceptional instances of recovery in global aphasia discussed below, most global patients remain severely impaired, although about half of them recover enough comprehension to be reclassified as Broca's aphasics. Broca's aphasics have an intermediate outlook that is just about evenly divided between fair and good recovery, and in these cases lesion size and location can be helpful to predict the final outcome. Residual Broca's aphasia is often classified as anomic aphasia, except for the remaining phonological errors (Crary and Kertesz 1988). Wernicke's aphasics, when they are severely affected, often retain fluent jargon for many months, and those persisting after a year usually remain the same. Some of them, however, lose the phonemic jargon and the language deficit becomes semantic jargon with verbal substitutions and eventually anomia develops. Wernicke's aphasia may also develop towards conduction aphasia showing difficulty with repetition but improved comprehension. Anomic, conduction, and transcortical aphasics have good prognosis, and 62.5% of the conduction aphasics, 50% of transcortical aphasics, and 48% of anomic patients will have full recovery by 1 year. A common end-stage of recovery is anomic aphasia with mostly word-finding difficulty in spontaneous speech as the most significant residual symptom (Kertesz 1979).

## The Rate and Stages of Recovery

Most patients show a great deal of recovery in the first 2 weeks. This first stage of recovery is related to the absorption of hemorrhage, cellular debris, and edema, to recovery from electrolyte disturbance and cellular reaction, ionic imbalance and membrane failure and possibly to the reestablishment of the circulation in the ischemic penumbra (Astrup et al. 1981). An increase in excitability was found in brain regions surrounding lesions and also in remote areas including the contralateral hemisphere. There have been several mechanisms postulated for this, such as the

general increase in catecholamines after injury or more recently the down-regulation of GABAergic inhibition (Schiene et al. 1996) and the induction of long-term potentiation, which may facilitate learning and memory processes in second stage recovery (Hagemann et al. 1998). Second stage recovery, which takes place months, even years, after injury remains a largely unexplained process. Although axonal regrowth and collateral sprouting are important mechanisms in the peripheral and in certain instances in the central nervous system, large destructive lesions in man are probably compensated by reorganization of intact structures. This second stage process shows the greatest improvement in the first 3 months after injury.

There is considerable agreement in the literature that the steepest recovery in aphasia occurs in the first 2 or 3 months (Vignolo 1964; Culton 1969; Sarno and Levita 1971; Kertesz and McCabe 1977). After 6 months a certain amount of plateauing occurs. Typical recovery curves are asymptotic and their smoothness depends on the number of examinations performed in the study. Reproducible recovery curves can be obtained by examining the patients in the acute stage and at 3 months, at 6 months, and at a 1-year follow-up.

Many studies only use outcome measures instead of recovery rates because of the difficulty in maintaining patients for a follow-up study. If there is a great deal of attrition then the recovery curve is irregular with dips at later stages. This is often related to the milder patients being discharged and the more severe patients remaining in the rehabilitation setting where they are available for assessment.

Relatively little, if any, spontaneous recovery occurs after a year (Butfield and Zangwill 1946; Vignolo 1964; Sands et al. 1969; Kertesz and McCabe 1977). There are, however, reports of improvement under therapy many years after the injury (Marks et al. 1957; Schuell et al. 1964; Smith et al. 1972; Broida 1977), although most of these are uncontrolled studies. Some aphasics continue to improve over several years, but there are also others who decline to some extent after therapy is discontinued according to the retrospective study of Hanson et al. (1989).

The authors estimated the extent of final recovery in 1 year in an aphasic population and only found 25% to have gained enough to be considered fully recovered. We took a standard deviation below the mean, the control population as the cut-off point between normals and aphasics (Kertesz 1979). A quarter of the overall aphasic population remains severely affected, another quarter shows fair, while another 25% good recovery. What constitutes complete recovery is often relative, as slightly paraphasic speech and a slight amount of word-finding difficulty may be acceptable for most individuals but not to some, especially those who have higher education and are occupationally dependent on their full language capacity.

## Language Components

Various language functions show different rates of recovery, but a great deal depends on the actual test or type of patients tested. Altogether, there is a correlation between the recovery rates of the subtests, but at times the dissociations are important. There is a general agreement that a comprehension deficit recovers the most (Lomas and Kertesz 1978; Prins et al. 1978; Vignolo 1964). The recovery of single word comprehension tends to be good even in patients with severe, initial deficits (Sarno and Levita 1981). Selnes et al. (1985) found only very extensive left hemisphere lesions had incomplete recovery of single word comprehension and damage to Wernicke's area did not preclude the return of this. In another report, Selnes et al. (1983) indicated sentence comprehension was less likely to recover when Wernicke's area was affected. It has been suggested that single word comprehension recovers even in larger lesions because this is a function the right hemisphere is capable of assuming. There is convergent evidence from split-brain patients and hemispherectomies that the right hemisphere has the capacity to comprehend nouns in the auditory and visual modality, especially when they are concrete and imageable (Zaidel 1976). Aspects of comprehension recovery were further explored by Gainotti and Monteleone (1988). They found the degree of recovery was greater in naming and in semantic-lexical comprehension than in the other comprehension tasks concerning syntax and phonology.

Naming recovers considerably, although a residual deficit of word finding and object naming appears persistent in most residual aphasia, even when comprehension and speech output has recovered (Kertesz 1979). Among recovered patients with anterior lesions, residual phonological paraphasias, and posterior lesions, semantic paraphasias remained (Knopman et al. 1984). A residual repetition deficit was shown to be related to damage to a damaged Wernicke's area. Lesions outside of that area have good prognosis (Selnes et al. 1985). Repetition recovered to a greater extent than naming in a population of stroke aphasics (Lomas and Kertesz 1978).

The evolution of error types of expressive performance was examined by Crary and Kertesz (1988). Broca's aphasics tended to produce phonological and word omission errors when they recovered. They are usually reclassified as anomic aphasia at this stage, but the type of error distinguishes them from Wernicke's aphasics who have residual semantic and omission errors.

Writing is usually more severely affected than oral speech, and recovery of writing is often less than recovery of oral language function (Kertesz 1979, 1988). Recovery from reading disorders has been studied by Newcombe et al. (1975), who tried to quantitate errors made by eight patients over time. They found asymptotic curves plateauing around 1 year. The recovery of reading was quite parallel to the recovery of aphasia and was found to be maximum in the first 3 months in our laboratory (Kertesz 1979). Recovery of calculation was quite similar to the recovery of reading in our studies. Metabolic studies of a pure alexia showed a great deal of improvement in ipsilateral visual areas 4 months stroke after a subcortical (geniculate) infarct initially producing extensive disconnection (Silver et al. 1988).

## Lesion Size

Autopsy correlations provided frequent evidence that lesion size is correlated negatively with the extent of recovery. This has been well known not only to clinicians but also to animal behaviorists, who measured lesion size and the effect of recovery or the ability of animals to relearn tasks and give rise to the well-accepted principle of "mass effect" (Lashley 1938). However, lesion size is only one of the many complex factors, therefore, it can be misleading to look at an image of a lesion and try to establish the prognosis from the size alone. Modern neuroimaging has given us an opportunity to study lesion characteristics at the time of the stroke. Outcome measures seem to relate best to lesion size (Kertesz et al. 1979; Selnes et al. 1983, Knopman et al. 1983). Some of these studies indicated the language area of about 60 cm² was a critical mass and larger lesions resulted in relatively less recovery (Knopman et al. 1983). Small lesions under 60 cm², even though they may produce a fairly typical initial deficit, will likely recover quite well. Some residual deficit, however, often remains even with small lesions.

Recovery rates also show a trend of negative correlation with lesion size, with the exception of the recovery rate for comprehension which often shows no, or if anything positive, correlation with lesion size. This can be best understood if one looks at studies of recovery from modalities and comprehension is often the most improved component of speech (Lomas and Kertesz 1978; Knopman et al. 1983). Patients with large lesions, who had originally poor comprehension (severe Broca's aphasia or global aphasia), often show greater improvement in comprehension. Patients with smaller lesions, such as anomic aphasics, already have good comprehension; therefore, there is less room for recovery (a ceiling effect). The large lesions with more recovery and the small lesions with little change give rise to a paradoxically positive correlation. This can be eliminated to some extent by covarying the recovery rates with the initial severity (Kertesz 1988).

## Lesion Location

Lesion location interacts with lesion size closely in recovery as brain structures are not equipotential to compensate for language and cognitive deficit. There are certain crucial language areas that are important for recovery, and when these are damaged little or no recovery takes place. The study of lesion location and recovery has progressed recently because in vivo imaging techniques allow us to do reasonable follow-up studies in a larger population.

Mohr et al. (1978) emphasized large lesions with posterior extension recover very little, while lesions only in Broca's area have good prognosis. Involvement of the central structures, such as the precentral and the postcentral gyri of the face, tongue, and mouth area, in addition to Broca's area contribute to the persistence of deficit (Mohr et al. 1978; Kertesz et al. 1979; Selnes et al. 1983).

Subcortical involvement, in addition to a cortical lesion, is important in the prognosis of Broca's aphasia. Subcortical structures, when involved alone, rarely cause persisting aphasia with the exception of extensive subcortical white matter lesions. Bonhoeffer (1914) postulated these white matter lesions undercut Broca's area, preventing access. Large periventricular white matter lesions with involvement of the subcallosal fasciculus were considered important factors in persisting nonfluent aphasia (Naeser et al. 1989). We also found a few entirely subcortical white matter lesions that caused persistent global aphasia (Kertesz et al. 1989a). Mostly large lesions involving a contiguous cortical and subcortical portion of the speech areas had poor prognosis, and those with sparing of the parietotemporal area will likely recover comprehension and will have functional communication, even though residual difficulties with articulation and fluency may remain.

Global aphasics who have an anterior and posterior lesion, but the central area is spared, tend to have good prognosis (Van Horn and Hawes 1982; Ferro 1983; Tranel et al. 1987). Large temporobasal lesions seem to have poor prognosis and showed less improvement during therapy and less total recovery (Goldenberg and Spatt 1994). It was postulated that such lesions may cause a disconnection between the hippocampus and perisylvian language areas and the important pathways in language learning and memory. Patients with destruction of the hippocampal formation are still able to acquire skills by procedural learning or repeated practice of a skill. Procedural learning of language skills is a component of both language therapy and spontaneous recovery due to repeated stimulation. Lesions interfering with memory structures, such as hippocampal and language cortex connections, are assumed to prevent explicit learning of linguistic knowledge and compensatory strategies and would be less likely to benefit from linguistically oriented therapy (Goldenberg and Spatt 1994).

It appears that there are four major structures contributing to the network of elaborating articulate speech, namely, Broca's area, the anterior insula, the striatum, and the inferior central cortex. If all four are involved, the prognosis is poor for recovery of fluency. Fairly large lesions but sparing any of these four often show good recovery.

The structural correlates of prognosis in Wernicke's aphasia show lesion size is important as well as location. Poor prognosis was associated with involvement of the supramarginal and the angular gyri, in addition to the postcentral gyrus and the insula (Kertesz et al. 1993). Subcortical involvement did not appear as important for the prognosis. Naeser et al. (1987) also studied Wernicke's aphasics and they found the lesion in more than half of Wernicke's cortical area had poor recovery of auditory comprehension at 1 to 2 years following stroke onset. They defined Wernicke's area as the posterior two-thirds of the superior temporal gyrus.

Cerebral blood flow (CBF) and positron emission tomography (PET) studies of cerebral metabolism have not added much practical information to predict recovery. One CBF study showed no significant change, while clinical recovery occurred in severe aphasics (Demeurisse et al. 1983). Patients who improve more show more activation in the left hemisphere. This appears to be the consequence of the size of the lesion, which correlates with the CBF changes. Another CBF study showed better than 60% hemispheric flow in patients with good recovery (Nagata et al. 1986). Functional activation and blood flow studies with PET showed both contralateral and ipsilateral increase in metabolism recovering from aphasia (Cappa et al. 1997; Heiss et al. 1993; Weiller 1995).

The variable ability to transfer language to the right hemisphere has been suggested ever since the time of Wernicke. Clinicians have thought the right hemisphere must be responsible for the recovery of very large lesions on the left side (Nielsen 1946). Left hemispherectomies and callosal sectioned patients also indicated some degree of right hemisphere language function, which may play an important role in recovery. Dichotic listening tests showed increasing left ear advantage with recovery (Johnson et al. 1977; Pettit and Noll 1979). This increasing left ear advantage was observed in a nonfluent group, whereas a paradoxical decrease was observed in the fluent group (Castro-Caldas, and Silveira Botelho 1980).

## Age

It is often believed younger patients recover better (Wepman 1951; Eisenson 1949; Vignolo 1964). This impression may be created by including post-traumatic aphasics in a population comparing patients with mean age who are much below with those of the stroke patients who are older. A more homogenous population of stroke patients fail to show a correlation with age (Sarno and Levita 1971; Culton 1971; Smith et al. 1972; Kertesz and McCabe 1977). Some elderly patients show remarkable recovery and some of the younger patients are affected most. However, if one looks at childhood aphasia, then the issue of the plasticity of a younger organism enters the determination of prognosis. The plasticity in immature animals is called the Kennard principle, based on the dramatic recovery shown in ablation studies (Kennard 1936) It is often stated, on the basis of hemispherectomies and studies of childhood aphasia (Basser 1962), that a child will recover from an aphasic deficit by substitution until they reach a critical age, which is somewhat controversial, although most people believe puberty represents an important factor (Lenneberg et al. 1967). Not only is it more difficult to learn a new language after puberty, but it appears brain plasticity also diminishes and a lesion will result in more persisting aphasia after puberty than before. Recent studies indicated some lesions produce fairly persisting aphasia in children as well (Woods and Teuber 1978; Aram et al. 1985; Woods and Carey 1979). The previously uniformly good prognosis in childhood aphasia was related to the etiology to some extent, as infectious cases and post-traumatic cases have recovered better. Children with the Keffler-Landau syndrome appear severely affected with epilepsy, and the aphasic disturbance also appears to persist. This syndrome appears to have several etiologies but mostly it is idiopathic. At times a progressive encephalitis produces progressive or persisting aphasic symptoms.

## Sex

Recent suggestions that women have more bilateral language representation (McGlone 1977) implicated the possibility women may recover from aphasia better than men. Studies looking at recovery, however, did not show any sex difference (Basso et al. 1982; Kertesz and McCabe 1977; Kertesz 1988).

## Handedness

Subirana (1969) and Gloning et al. (1969) suggested left handers recover better from aphasias than right handers. However, the data were not based on objective language examination and subsequent studies could not confirm this. Gloning et al. (1969) also suggested left handers are likely to become aphasic, regardless of which hemisphere is damaged. Our experience is the opposite; in other words, we found less left handers among our aphasics than one would expect from the general population (Kertesz 1979). In fact, if left handers had more bilateral language distribution, then one would expect less aphasia among left handers because either hemisphere could take over from the other one.

## Intelligence and Education

Premorbid intelligence and education are often considered to influence prognosis positively. However, the study of Keenan and Brassel (1974) indicated health, employment, and age had little, if any, prognostic value and Sarno et al. (1970) also demonstrated recovery was not influenced by age, education, occupational status, and preillness language proficiency. Intelligence per se is difficult to estimate premorbidly. Higher educational achievement, which may or may not be related to higher premorbid intelligence, is considered favorable for recovery by some (Wepman 1951; Smith 1971; Darley 1972).

## Nonverbal Cognition

The recovery of right hemisphere syndromes of visuospatial deficit, neglect, anosognosia, motor impersistence and prosopagnosia, was examined by Hier et al. (1983). Age and sex did not influence recovery significantly in this older stroke group. Hemorrhages and smaller lesions tended to recover faster. Sparing of the frontal lobe seemed important for the recovery of visuospatial deficit and neglect.

## Neglect

The prognosis of neglect is not as well determined as verbal deficit. Lawson (1962) described some improvement in two cases of left visuospatial neglect over periods of time up to 2 years. Gainotti (1968) reported evidence of improvement from the initial severe involvement to complete recovery by 3 years. Persisting cases of neglect have also been described (Zarit and Kahn 1974). Camp-

bell and Oxbury (1976) examined stroke patients in the acute stage, 3 to 4 weeks, and also at 6 months after stroke with tests of copying and drawing, block design, picture completion, and cube counting. Even though neglect seemed to recover by 6 months, visuospatial deficit persisted longer. We have shown the most significant recovery from visuospatial deficit occurs in the first 3 months and plateauing occurs subsequently (Kertesz 1979). Left spatial neglect contributed significantly to the prognosis of hemiplegia (Denes et al. 1982). Both hemispheres contributed to recovery in unilateral neglect on a PET study (Perani et al. 1993). Ipsilateral cortical areas were implicated in a PET activation study of recovery of patients with primarily subcortical lesions after a 2 month rehabilitation program from neglect (Pizzamiglio et al. 1998).

## Apraxia

Recovery from ideomotor apraxia was better from anterior lesions (Basso et al. 1987). Although less than a third of their patients were followed beyond 1 year, they found improvement occurred beyond 6 months. Age, sex, lesion size, and type of aphasia did not seem to be related significantly to outcome. They found posterior temporoparietal brain regions were more often involved in persistent apraxia. We documented the recovery from apraxia in 50 aphasics and found somewhat better recovery in praxis than in the language scores in global aphasics (Kertesz 1979). The initial recovery of praxis may not be as rapid as that of language in other groups, but dissociations occurs in both directions resulting in some patients with aphasia who have no apraxia and vice versa.

## Cortical Blindness and Visual Agnosia

The prognosis of cortical blindness is usually quite good and recovery in days is often the case. There is often an improvement from cortical blindness, which may or may not be associated with denial of blindness (Anton's syndrome), through visual agnosia (impairment of recognition of objects) which then further recovers towards optic aphasia and with further recovery a residual hemianopia, or hemianopia with pure alexia may be seen. A large collection of cases of cortical blindness was analyzed by Aldrich et al. (1987), who concluded prognosis in cortical blindness is poor when caused by a stroke and bioccipital abnormalities on the computed tomographs (CT) scan are also associated with poor prognosis.

## Cognitive Recovery from Head Injury, Cardiac Arrest, Encephalitis

The major cognitive loss after these etiologies tends to be in the domain of memory. In severe head injury, cognitive recovery depends on the extent of injury as determined above all by the duration of coma and the presence or absence of penetrating injury and age (Bond 1975). Injuries are regarded as severe when post-traumatic amnesia (PTA) exceeds 24 hours and very severe if PTA is longer than 1 week. Recovery of orientation coincides well with the re-establishment of continuous memory. Mandleberg and Brooks (1975) showed less initial impairment and better recovery from verbal subtests than performance on the Wechsler Adult Intelligence Scale (WAIS) in severe closed head injury in adults. Recovery of nonverbal subtests continued after about 3 years, although a plateau was often reached at 13 months. One of the most persistent communication difficulties, dysarthria, has been treated with biofeedback successfully (Murdoch 1996). The outcome and prognosis of head injuries is further detailed in a separate chapter.

Cognitive impairment occurs after cardiac arrest and open heart surgery, such as the increasingly performed coronary artery bypass in a significant portion of patients. Particularly, delayed recall and short-term memory are impaired in about two-thirds of the patients after the arrest and in one-third 6 months later. Time to postarrest awakening was the most reliable predictor of prognosis (Sauve et al. 1996).

Cognitive recovery after encephalitis is limited. Patients often remain severely incapacitated with a Korsakoff-like amnestic syndrome after herpes simplex–induced bilateral temporal lobe destructions. Even in acyclovir-treated patients dementia is seen in 12% to 25% of cases. However, many showed improvement over several years (Hokkanen and Launes 1997).

Depression is an important factor inhibiting recovery and considered a common sequel to stroke and head injury. The treatment of depression may improve prognosis in cognitive impairment related to any cause (Robinson 1997; Satz et al. 1998).

## Therapy and Prognosis

The literature on the treatment of language disorders is the oldest but probably the most extensive, although the rehabilitation of other cognitive problems, such as neglect or memory, has recently become more widely practiced. Well-controlled, scientifically sound studies are few. There are many reasons for this, most of them social. It is very difficult to obtain untreated controls in localities where such studies are feasible. Accurate measurements of cognitive deficits are difficult to standardize. Treatment patterns are influenced by third-party payment availability.

One recent, large-scale, multicenter study of speech therapy in aphasia indicated improvement in the treated group that was significantly greater than in the untreated one in a cross-over design using the same population at different stages of their recovery (Wertz et al. 1986). Another study found no effect (Lincoln et al. 1984) using randomized controls, but a mix of etiologies and low level of treatment prevented full acceptance of this study. Some studies found no difference between aphasics treated by speech pathologists or volunteers (Meikle et al. 1979; David et al. 1982; Shewan and Kertesz 1984). Retrospective studies showing the beneficial effect of therapy had significant problems in patient selection, such as including more severely affected patients in the untreated groups and failing to control for time from onset as a factor (Basso et al. 1979). Other studies using special techniques of therapy, such as melodic intonation (Sparks et al. 1974), visual communication therapy (Glass et al. 1973; Gardner et al. 1976), visual action therapy, and sign language (Helm-Estabrooks et al. 1982; Skelly et al. 1974) described only a few selected patients. Deficit-specific training material (Shewan and Kertesz 1984; Weniger et al. 1987) has been described as more efficacious than other therapy materials chosen ad hoc or with other theoretical considerations. A more recent review of various therapies was carried out by Holland et al. (1996) and Orange and Kertesz (1998).

Robey (1998) reviewed 21 studies of the efficacy of language therapy for a meta-analysis. He concluded that individuals receiving therapy in the acute stage of recovery have a larger effect than spontaneous recovery alone and that language therapy, even after the initial stage of what is considered spontaneous recovery continues to be positive on language performance. Further conclusions were that the effect size is greater when therapy starts in the acute phase, although there is some effect even in later or more chronic stage of recovery (6 to 12 months after onset). Treatment efficacy was addressed by Holland et al. (1996). A second meta-analysis of 55 studies focused on further issues such as amount of treatment, type of treatment, and recovery factors such as severity and type of aphasia (Robey 1998). None of the studies fulfilled all the desirable requirements for efficacy analysis and there was no homogenous relations among treatment duration, time of measurement, and amount of treatment. The meta-analysis suggested that more than 2 hours per week of treatment is better than less.

Therapy for phonetic disorders or apraxia of speech has been singled out as one of the most successful models of speech therapy (Rosenbek et al. 1973). Recently, the psycholinguistic approach to aphasia therapy has attempted to develop interventions on the basis of processing models (Lesser 1987). Some approaches to therapy are based on new learning of linguistic and metalinguistic knowledge and to acquisition of explicit compensatory strategies (Huber 1991). This form of therapy is likely to add basically different cognitive elements than those that might be acquired during spontaneous recovery. However, the efficacy of linguistically oriented therapy remains to be proven.

The use of microcomputers may influence the prognosis of aphasia, but so far only uncontrolled descriptions of such use have been available (Kinsey 1986; Colby et al. 1981; Dean 1987; Katz 1986, Steele et al. 1989; Aftonomos et al. 1997). The role of microcomputers is probably most efficient in the supplementary treatment of reading (Katz 1987; Steele et al. 1989). Pharmacotherapy of aphasia with bromocriptine has been attempted, but only case descriptions are available (Albert et al. 1988). Poststroke depression occurs frequently is up to 20% of patients with left frontal injury and in about 15% after right hemispheric stroke (Robinson et al. 1984). A trial of antidepressants may improve prognosis and the success of rehabilitation.

The treatment for right hemisphere deficits, such as neglect, has been described in some detail (Diller and Gordon 1981). Perceptual remediation of visual scanning, somatosensory awareness, and size estimation improved prognosis (Gordon et al.

1985). Memory rehabilitation has become a separate entity in the last decade (Wilson 1987; Sohlberg and Mateer 1989; Kime et al. 1996). Computer retraining of cognitive deficits has also been attempted (Ben-Yishay et al. 1985; Bracy 1983). Robertson (1990) found no evidence of significant changes in memory and visuospatial function from computerized training. Sturm and Wilmes (1991) found right hemisphere–damaged patients did not benefit as much from computer training because of attentional problems.

Cognitive rehabilitation has attracted a lot of attention, but its efficacy is difficult to evaluate. Initially it was designed to remediate disorders of perception, memory, and language, but a more realistic concept is any intervention that helps patients and their families to live with these deficits. War injuries spurred on rehabilitation units. The cognitive retraining approach uses stimulation, exercise programs, and programs designed to the deficit of the patient. This approach has been criticized on various grounds. Some believe that retraining deficits does not address functional problems. Focusing on a modality fails to generalize to other deficits and it lacks theoretical underpinning (Wilson 1997). However, theoretically motivated approaches also tend to focus on treating the damage component of a model-based deficit. It has been stated that cognitive neuropsychology has learned a great deal from the study of brain damaged patients, but it is not clear that brain damaged patients have benefited from cognitive neuropsychology (Baddeley 1993). Combining cognitive and behavioral approaches is considered more effective, and emphasis on the disability and the emotional integration of the patient and family is a desirable, holistic approach (Wilson 1997).

Neuropharmacological facilitation of recovery has been attempted with numerous drugs, such as psychostimulants (dexedrine and methylphenidate), antidepressants (amitriptyline and fluoxetine), levodopa and its agonists (bromocriptine), anticonvulsants (valproate and carbamazepine), nootropics, noradrenergics (clonidine), and sympathomimetics (methylphenidate), but the results are controversial (Goldstein 1998). Drugs that may work in the laboratory may not necessarily affect prognosis in humans. Symptomatic treatment of agitation, aggression, or depression is feasible to some extent, but it improves prognosis only indirectly.

# References

Albert, M. L.; Bachman, D. L.; Morgan, A.; Helm-Estabrooks, N. Pharmacotherapy for aphasia. Neurology 38:877–879; 1988.

Aldrich, M. S.; Alessi, A. G.; Beck, R. W.; Gilman, S. Cortical blindness: etiology, diagnosis, and prognosis. Ann. Neurol. 21:149–158; 1987.

Aftonomos, L. B.; Steele, R. D.; Wertz, R. T. Promoting recovery in chronic aphasia with an interactive technology. Arch. Phys. Med. Rehabil. 78:841–846; 1997.

Aram, D. M.; Ekelman, B. L.; Rose, D. F.; Whitaker, H. A. Verbal and cognitive sequelae following unilateral lesions acquired in early childhood. J. Clin. Exp. Neuropsychol. 7:55–78; 1985.

Astrup, J.; Siesjo, B. K.; Symon, L. Thresholds in cerebral ischemia—the ischemic penumbra. Stroke 12:723–725; 1981.

Baddeley, A. D. A theory of rehabilitation without a model of learning is a vehicle without an engine: a comment on Caramazza and Hillis. Neuropsychol. Rehabil. 3:235–244; 1993.

Basser, L. S. Hemiplegia of early onset and the faculty of speech, with special reference to the effects of hemispherectomy. Brain 85:427–460; 1962.

Basso, A.; Capitani, E.; Vignolo, L. A. Influence of rehabilitation on language skills in aphasic patients: a controlled study. Arch. Neurol. 36:190–196; 1979.

Basso, A.; Capitani, E.; Moraschini, S. Sex differences in recovery from aphasia. Cortex 18:469–475; 1982.

Basso, A.; Capitani, E.; Della Sala, S.; Laiacona, M.; Spinnler, H. Recovery from ideomotor apraxia—a study on acute stroke patients. Brain 110:747–760; 1981.

Ben-Yishay, Y.; Piasetsky, E. G.; Rattok, J. A systematic method for ameliorating disorders in basic attention in Neuropsychological rehabilitation. In Meier, M. J.; Diller, L.; Benton, A. L., eds. London: Churchill Livingstone; 1985.

Bond, M. R. Assessment of psychosocial outcome after severe head injury. In: Outcome of severe damage to the central nervous system. Ciba Foundation Symposium 34 (new series), Elsevier, Amsterdam; 1975.

Bonhoeffer, K. Klinischer und anatomischer Befund zur Lehre von der Apraxie und der 'motorischen Sprachbahn'. Monatsschr. Psychiatr. Neurol. 35: 113–128; 1914.

Bracy, O. L. Computer based cognitive rehabilitation. Cognit. Rehabil. 1:7; 1983.

Broida, H. Language therapy effects in long term aphasia. Arch. Phys. Med. Rehabil. 58:248–253; 1977.

Butfield, E.; Zangwill, O. L. Re-education in aphasia: a review of 70 cases. J. Neurol. Neurosurg. Psychiatry 9:75–79; 1946.

Campbell, D. C.; Oxbury, J. M. Recovery from unilateral visuo-spatial neglect. Cortex 12:303–312; 1976.

Cappa, S. F.; Perani, D.; Grassi, F.; Bressi, S.; Alberoni, M.; Franceschi, M.; Bettinardi, V.; Todde, S.; Fazio, F. A PET follow-up of recovery after stroke in acute aphasics. Brain Lang. 56:55–67; 1997.

Caselli, R. J.; Windebank, A. J.; Petersen, R. C.; Komori, T.; Parisi, J. E.; Okazaki, H.; Kokmen, E.; Iverson, R.; Dinapoli, R. P.; Graff-Radford, N. R.; Stein, S. D. Rapidly progressive aphasic dementia and motor neuron disease. Ann. Neurol. 33:200–207; 1993.

Castro-Caldas, A.; Silveira Botelho, M. Dichotic listening in the recovery of aphasia after stroke. Brain Lang. 10:145–151; 1980.

Colby, K. M.; Christinaz, D.; Parkinson, R. C.; Graham, S.; Karpf, C. A word finding computer program with a dynamic lexical-semantic memory for patients with anomia using an intelligent speech prosthesis. Brain Lang. 14:272–281; 1981.

Crary, M. A.; Kertesz, A. Evolving error profiles during aphasia syndrome remission. Aphasiology 2:67–78; 1988.

Culton, G. L. Spontaneous recovery from aphasia. J. Speech Hear. Res. 12:825–832; 1969.

Culton, G. L. Reaction to age as a factor in chronic aphasia in stroke patients. J. Speech Hear. Disord. 36:563–564; 1971.

Darley, F. L. The efficacy of language rehabilitation in aphasia. J. Speech Hear. Disord. 37:3–21; 1972.

David, R.; Enderby, P.; Bainton, D. Treatment of acquired aphasia: speech therapists and volunteers compared. J. Neurol. Neurosurg. Psychiatry 45: 957–961; 1982.

Dean, E. C. Short report. Microcomputers and aphasia. Aphasiology 1:267–270; 1987.

Demeurisse, G.; Verhas, M.; Capon, A.; Paternot, J. Lack of evolution of the cerebral blood flow during clinical recovery of stroke. Stroke 14:77–81; 1983.

Denes, G.; Semenza, C.; Stoppa, E.; Lis, AL. Unilateral spatial neglect and recovery from hemiplegia: a follow-up study. Brain 105:543–552; 1982.

Diller, L.; Gordon, W. A. Rehabilitation and clinical neuropsychology. In: Filskov, S. B.; Boll, T. J., eds. Handbook of clinical neuropsychology. Toronto: John Wiley & Sons; 1981.

Eisenson, J. Prognostic factors related to language rehabilitation in aphasic patients. J. Speech Hear. Disord. 14:262–264; 1949.

Ferro, J. Global aphasia without hemiparesis. Neurology 33:1106; 1983.

Gainotti, G. Les manifestations de negligence et d'-inattention pour l'hemispace. Cortex 4:64–91; 1968.

Gainotti, G.; Monteleone, D. Spontaneous recovery of various aspects of language comprehension and of naming in aphasia. In: Vakil, E.; Hoofien, D.; Grosswasser, Z., eds. Rehabilitation of the brain injured. London: Freund Publishing House, Ltd.; 1988.

Gardner, H.; Zurif, E. G.; Berry, T.; Baker, E. Visual communication in aphasia. Neuropsychologia 14: 275–292; 1976.

Glass, A. V.; Gazzaniga, M. S.; Premack, D. Artificial language training in global aphasia. Neuropsychologia 11:95–103; 1973.

Gloning, I.; Gloning, K.; Haub, G.; Quatember, R. Comparison of verbal behaviour in right-handed and non-right-handed patients with anatomically verified lesion to one hemisphere. Cortex 5:53–62; 1969.

Godfrey, C. M.; Douglass, E. The recovery process in aphasia. Can. Med. Assoc. J. 80:618–624; 1959.

Goldenberg, G.; Spatt, J. Influence of size and site of cerebral lesions on spontaneous recovery of aphasia and on success of language therapy. Brain Lang. 47: 684–698; 1994.

Goldstein, L. B. Potential effects of common drugs on stroke recovery. Arch. Neurol. 55:454–456; 1998.

Gordon, W. A.; Hibbard, M. R.; Egelko, S. Perceptual remediation in patients with right brain damage. Arch. Phys. Med. Rehabil. 66:353; 1985.

Hagemann, G.; Redecker, C.; Neumann-Haefelin, T.; Freund, H-J.; Witte, O. W. Increased long-term potentiation in the surround of experimentally induced focal cortical infarction. Ann. Neurol. 44:255–258; 1998.

Hanson, W. R.; Metter, E. J.; Riege, W. H. The course of chronic aphasia. Aphasiology 3:19–29; 1989.

Head, H. Aphasia and kindred disorders of speech. Cambridge: Cambridge University Press; 1926.

Heiss, W. D.; Kessler, J.; Karbe, H.; Fink, G. R.; Pawlik, G. Cerebral glucose metabolism as a predictor of recovery from aphasia in ischemic stroke. Arch. Neurol. 50:958–964; 1993.

Helm-Estabrooks, N.; Fitzpatrick, P. M.; Barresi, B. Visual action therapy for global aphasia. J. Speech Hear. Disord. 47:385–389; 1982.

Hier, D. B.; Mondlock, J.; Caplan, L. R. Recovery of behavioral abnormalities after right hemisphere stroke. Neurology 33:345–350; 1983.

Hokkanen, L.; Launes, J. Cognitive recovery instead of decline after acute encephalitis: a prospective follow up study. J. Neurol. Neurosurg. Psychiatry 63:222–227; 1997.

Holland, A. L.; Fromm, D. S.; DeRuyter, F.; Stein, M. Treatment efficacy: aphasia. J. Speech Hear. Res. 39:S27–S36; 1996.

Huber, W. Ansätze der Aphasietherapie. Neurolinguistik 5:71–92; 1991.

Johnson, J.; Sommers, R.; Weidner, W. Dichotic ear preference in aphasia. J. Speech Hear. Res. 20:116–129; 1977.

Katz, R. C. Aphasia treatment and microcomputers. San Diego: College Hill Press; 1986.

Katz, R. C. Reply: common ground. Aphasiology 1:171; 1987.

Keenan, S. S.; Brassel, E. G. A study of factors related to prognosis for individual aphasic patients. J. Speech Hear. Disord. 39: 257–269; 1974.

Kennard, M. A. Age and other factors in motor recovery from precentral lesions in monkeys. Am. J. Physiol. 115:138–140; 1936.

Kertesz, A. Aphasia and associated disorders. New York: Grune & Stratton; 1979.

Kertesz, A. What do we learn from recovery? In: Waxman, S. G. ed. Advances in neurology, 47, functional recovery in neurological disease. New York: Raven Press; 1988 p. 279–292.

Kertesz, A.; Dennis, S.; Polk, M. Recovery from severe nonfluent aphasia: the role of lesion size and location in recovery from global and Broca's aphasia (abstract). J. Clin. Exp. Neuropsychol. 11:67; 1989a.

Kertesz, A.; Harlock, W.; Coates, R. Computer tomographic localization, lesion size and prognosis in aphasia. Brain Lang. 8: 34–50; 1979.

Kertesz, A.; Hudson, L.; Mackenzie, I. R. A.; Munoz, D. G. The pathology and nosology of primary progressive aphasia. Neurology 44:2065–2072; 1994.

Kertesz, A.; McCabe, P. Recovery patterns and prognosis in aphasia. Brain 100:1–18; 1977.

Kertesz, A.; Lau, W. K.; Polk. M. The structural determinants of recovery in Wernicke's aphasia. Brain Lang. 44:153–164; 1993.

Kime, S. K.; Lamb, D. G.; Wilson, B. A. (1996). Use of a comprehensive programme of external cueing to enhance procedural memory in a patient with dense amnesia. Brain Inj. 10:17–25; 1996.

Kinsey, C. Microcomputers speech therapy for dysphasic adults. A comparison with two conventionally administered tasks. Bri. J. Disord. Communication 21:125; 1986.

Knopman, D. S.; Selnes, O. A.; Niccum, N.; Rubens, A. B. A longitudinal study of speech fluency in aphasia: CT scan correlates of recovery and persistent nonfluency. Neurology 33:1170–1178; 1983.

Knopman, D. S.; Selnes, O. A.; Niccum, N.; Rubens, A. B. Recovery of naming in aphasia: relationship to fluency, comprehension, and CT findings. Neurology 34:1461–1470; 1984.

Lawson, I. R. Visual-spatial neglect in lesions of the right cerebral hemisphere: a study in recovery. Neurology 12:23–33; 1962.

Lashley, L. S. Factors limiting recovery after central nervous lesions. J. Nerv. Ment. Dis. 88:733–755; 1938.

Lenneberg, E. Biological foundations of language. New York: John Wiley & Sons; 1967.

Lesser, R. Cognitive neuropsychological influences on aphasia therapy. Aphasiology 1:189–200; 1987.

Levin, H. S.; Benton, A. L.; Grossman, R. G. Neurobehavioral consequences of closed head injury. New York: Oxford University Press; 1982.

Lincoln, N. B.; McGuirk, E.; Mulley, G. P.; Lendrem, W.; Jones, A. C.; Mitchell, J. R. A. The effectiveness of speech therapy for aphasic stroke patients: a randomized controlled trial. Lancet i:1197–1200; 1984.

Lomas, J.; Kertesz, A. Patterns of spontaneous recovery in aphasic groups: a study of adult stroke patients. Brain Lang. 5:388–401; 1978.

Ludlow, C.; Rosenberg, J.; Fair, C.; Buck, D.; Schesselman, S.; Salazar, A. Brain lesions associated with nonfluent aphasia fifteen years following penetrating head injury. Brain 109:55–80; 1986.

Mandleberg, I. A.; Brooks, D. N. Cognitive recovery after severe head injury. 1. Serial testing on the Wechsler Adult Intelligence Scale. J. Neurol. Neurosurg. Psychiatry 38:1121; 1975.

Marks, M. M.; Taylor, M. L.; Rusk, H. A. Rehabilitation of the aphasic patient: a summary of three years' experience in a rehabilitation setting. Arch. Phys. Med. Rehabil. 38:219–226; 1957.

McGlone, J. Sex differences in the cerebral organization of verbal functions in patients with unilateral lesions. Brain 100:775–793; 1977.

Meikle, M.; Wechsler, E.; Tupper, A.; Benninson, M.; Butler, J.; Mullhall, D.; Stern, G. Comparative trial of volunteer and professional treatments of dysphasia after stroke. Bri. Med. J. 2:87–89; 1979.

Merzenich, M. M.; Kaas, J. H.; Wall, J. T.; Nelson, R. J.; Felleman, D. Topographic reorganization in somatosensory area 3b and 1 in adult monkeys following restricted deafferentiation. Neuroscience 8:33–55; 1983.

Messerli, P.; Tissot, A.; Rodriguez, J. Recovery from aphasia: some factors of prognosis. In: 4. Recovery in aphasics. Amsterdam: Swets & Zeitlinger, B.C.; 1976.

Mohr, J. P.; Pessin, M. S.; Finkelstein, S.; Funkenstein, H. H.; Duncan, G. W.; Davis, K. R. Broca aphasia: pathologic and clinical. Neurology 28: 311–324; 1978.

Murdoch, B. E. Physiological rehabilitation of disordered speech following closed head injury. In: Uzzell, B. P.; Stonnington H. H., eds. Recovery after traumatic brain injury. Mahwah, NJ. Lawrence Erlbaum Associates, Inc., 1996: p. 163–184.

Naeser, M.; Helm-Estabrooks, N.; Haas, G.; Auerbach, S.; Srinivasan, M. Relationship between lesion extent in 'Wernicke's area' on computed tomographic scan and predicting recovery of comprehension in Wernicke's aphasia. Arch. Neurol. 44:73–82; 1987.

Naeser, M.; Palumbo, C. L.; Helm-Estabrooks, N.; Stiassny-Eder, D.; Albert, M. L. Severe nonfluency in aphasia. Role of the medial subcallosal fasciculus and other white matter pathways in recovery of spontaneous speech. Brain 112:1–38; 1989.

Nagata, K.; Yunoki, K.; Kabe, S.; Suzuki, A.; Araki, G. Regional cerebral blood flow correlates of aphasia outcome in cerebral hemorrhage and cerebral infarction. Stroke 17:417–423; 1986.

Newcombe, F.; Hiorns, R. W.; Marshall, J. C.; Adams, C. B. T. Acquired dyslexia: patterns of deficit and recovery. In: Outcome of severe damage to the central nervous system. Ciba Foundation Symposium 34. Amsterdam: Elsevier/Excerpta Medica/North-Holland; 1975.

Nielsen, J. M. Agnosia, apraxia, aphasia. New York: Hoeber; 1946.

Orange, J. B.; Kertesz, A. Efficacy of language therapy for aphasia. In: Physical medicine and rehabilitation: state of the art reviews. Vol. 12. Philadelphia: Hanley and Belfus, Inc.; 1998.

Perani, D.; Vallar, G.; Paulesu, F.; Alberoni, M.; Fazio, F. Left and right hemisphere contribution to recovery from neglect after right hemisphere damage: an [18F] FDG PET study of two cases. Neuropsychologia 31:115–125; 1993.

Pettit, J.; Noll, J. Cerebral dominance in aphasia recovery. Brain Lang. 7:191–200; 1979.

Pizzamiglio, L.; Perani, D.; Cappa, S. F.; Vallar, G.; Paolucci, S.; Grassi, F.; Paulesu, E.; Fazio, F. Recovery of neglect after right hemispheric damage. H$_2$ $^{15}$O positron emission tomographic activation study. Arch. Neurol. 55:561–568; 1998.

Prins, R. S.; Snow, C. E.; Wagenaar, E. Recovery from aphasia: spontaneous speech versus language comprehension. Brain Lang. 6:192–211; 1978.

Robertson, I. H. Does computerised cognitive rehabilitation work? A review. Aphasiology 4:381–405; 1990.

Robey, R. R. A meta-analysis of clinical outcomes in the treatment of aphasia. J. Speech Lang. Hear. Res. 41:172–187; 1998.

Robinson, R. G. Neuropsychiatric consequences of stroke. Annu. Rev. Med. 48:217–229; 1997.

Robinson, R. G.; Kubos, K. L.; Starr, L. B.; Rao, K.; Price, T. R. Mood disorders in stroke patients—importance of location of lesion. Brain 104:81–93; 1984.

Rosenbek, J. C.; Lemme, M. L.; Ahern, M. B.; Harris, E. H.; Wertz, R. T. A treatment for apraxia of speech in adults. J. Speech Hear. Disord. 38:462–472; 1973.

Sands, E.; Sarno, M. T.; Shankweiler, D. Long-term assessment of language function in aphasia due to stroke. Arch. Phys. Med. Rehabil. 50:202–207; 1969.

Sarno, M. T.; Levita, E. Natural course of recovery in severe aphasia. Arch. Phys. Med. Rehabil. 52:175–179; 1971.

Sarno, M. T.; Silverman, M.; Levita, E. Psychosocial factors and recovery in geriatric patients with severe aphasia. J. Am. Geriatr. Soc. 18:405–409; 1970.

Satz, P.; Forney, D. L.; Zaucha, K.; Asarnow, R. R.; Light, R.; McCleary, C.; Levin, H.; Kelly, D.; Bergsneider, M.; Hovda, D.; Martin, N.; Namerow, N.; Becker, D. Depression, cognition, and functional correlates of recovery outcome after traumatic brain injury. Brain Inj. 12:537–553; 1998.

Sauve, M. J.; Walker, J. A.; Massa, S. M.; Winkle, R. A.; Scheinman, M. M. Patterns of cognitive recovery in sudden cardiac arrest survivors: the pilot study. Heart Lung 25:172–181; 1996.

Schiene, K.; Bruehl, C.; Zilles, K.; et al. Neuronal hyperexcitability and reduction of GABA$_A$-receptor expressoin in the surround of cerebral photothrombosis. J. Cereb. Blood Flow Metab. 16:906–914; 1996.

Schuell, A.; Jenkins, J. J.; Pabon, J. Aphasia in adults. New York: Harper & Row; 1964.

Selnes, O. A.; Knopman, D. S.; Niccum, N.; Rubens, A. B. CT scan correlates of auditory comprehension deficits in aphasia: a prospective recovery study. Ann. Neurol. 13:553–566; 1983.

Selnes, O. A.; Knopman, D. S.; Niccum, N.; and Rubens, A. B. The critical role of Wernicke's area in sentence repetition. Ann. Neurol. 17:549–557; 1985.

Shewan, C. M.; Kertesz, A. Effects of speech and language treatment on recovery from aphasia. Brain Lang. 23:272–299; 1984.

Silver, F. L.; Chawluk, J. B.; Bosley, T. M.; Rosen, M.; Dann, R.; Sergott, R. C.; Alavi, A.; Reivich, M. Resolving metabolic abnormalities in a case of pure alexia. Neurology 38:730–735; 1988.

Skelly, M.; Schinski, L.; Smith, R.; Furst, R. S. American Indian Sign (AMERIND) as a facilitator of verbalization for the oral verbal apraxia. J. Speech Hear. Disord. 39:445–456; 1974.

Smith, A. Objective indices of severity of chronic aphasia in stroke patients. J. Speech Hear. Disord. 36: 167–207; 1971.

Smith, A.; Chamoux, R.; Leri, J.; London, R.; Muraski, A. Diagnosis, intelligence and rehabilitation of chronic aphasics. University of Michigan Department of Physical Medicine and Rehabilitation, Ann Arbor; 1972.

Sohlberg, M. M.; Mateer, C. A. Introduction to cognitive rehabilitation. New York: Guildford Press; 1989.

Sparks, R.; Helm, N. A.; Albert, M. L. Aphasia rehabilitation resulting from melodic intonation therapy. Cortex 10:303–316; 1974.

Steele, R. D.; Weinrich, M.; Wertz, R. T.; Kleczewska, M. K.; Carlson, G. S. Computer-based visual communication in aphasia. Neuropsychologia 27:409–426; 1989.

Stein, D. G.; Brailowsky, S.; Will, B. Brain repair. New York: Oxford University Press; 1995.

Sturm, W.; Willmes, K. Efficacy of a reaction training on various attentional and cognitive function in stroke patients. Neuropsychol. Rehabil. 1:259–280; 1991.

Subirana, A. Handedness and cerebral dominance. In: Vinken, P. J.; Bruyn, G. W. eds. Handbook of clinical neurology. Amsterdam: North-Holland; 1969.

Tranel, D.; Biller, J.; Damasio, H.; Adams, H. P.; Cornell, S. H. Global aphasia without hemiparesis. Arch. Neurol. 44:304–308; 1987.

Van Horn, G.; Hawes, A. Global aphasia without hemiparesis: a sign of embolic encephalopathy. Neurology 32:403–406; 1982.

Vignolo, L. A. Evolution of aphasia and language rehabilitation: a retrospective exploratory study. Cortex 1:344–367; 1964.

Weiller, C.; Issensee, C.; Riintjes, M.; Huber, W.; Muller, S.; Bier, D.; Dutschka, K.; Woods, R. P.; Noth, J.; Diener, H. C. Recovery from Wernicke's aphasia: a PET study. Ann. Neurol. 37:723–732; 1995.

Weisbenburg, T.; McBride, K. E. Aphasia: a clinical and psychological study. New York: Commonwealth Fund; 1935.

Weniger, D.; Springer, L.; Poeck, K. The efficacy of deficit-specific therapy materials. Aphasiology 3: 215–222; 1987.

Wepman, J. M. Recovery from aphasia. New York: Ronald Press; 1951.

Wertz, R. T.; Weiss, D. G.; Aten, J. L.; Brookshire, R. H.; Garcia-Bunuel, L.; Holland, A. L.; Kurtzke, J. F.; LaPointe, L. L.; Milianti, F. J.; Brannegan, R.; Greenbaum, H.; Marshall, R. C.; Vogel, D.; Carter, J.; Barnes, N. S.; Goodman, R. Comparison of clinic, home, and deferred language treatment of aphasia. A Veterans Administration cooperative study. Arch. Neurol. 43:653–658; 1986.

Wilson, B. A. Rehabilitation of memory. New York: Guildford Press; 1987.

Wilson, B. A. Cognitive rehabilitation: how it is and how it might be. J. Int. Neuropsychol. Soc. 3:487–496; 1997.

Woods, B. T.; Carey, S. Language deficits after apparent clinical recovery from childhood aphasia. Ann. Neurol. 6:405–409; 1979.

Woods, B. T.; Teuber, H. L. Changing patterns of childhood aphasia. Ann. Neurol. 3:273–280; 1978.

Zaidel, E. Auditory vocabulary of the right hemisphere following brain bisection or hemidecortication. Cortex 12:187–211; 1976.

Zarit, S. H.; Kahn, R. L. Impairment and adaptation in chronic disabilities: spatial inattention. J. Nerv. Dis. 159:63; 1974.

# 38

# Epilepsy

NANCY R. FOLDVARY AND ELAINE WYLLIE

Epilepsy, from the Greek *epilepsia,* "a taking hold of or seizing," is a chronic disorder characterized by a spontaneous tendency for recurrent unprovoked seizures. Seizures are the clinical manifestation of abnormally hyperexcitable cortical neurons. Whereas all individuals with epilepsy have seizures, many more have a single seizure during their lifetime and are not considered to have epilepsy. Epilepsy affects 6 to 7 per 1000 persons in the United States; and 30 to 50 new cases per 100,000 develop annually (Annegers 1996). The risk of epilepsy increases from approximately 1% at birth through early adulthood to 3% by age 75. The etiology is not identified in two-thirds of cases.

Seizures are classified as *focal* or *generalized* based on seizure symptomatology and electrographic manifestations (Commission on Classification and Terminology of the International League Against Epilepsy 1981). *Focal seizures* are those in which the first clinical and/or electrographic manifestations indicate initial activation of a limited population of neurons in part of one cerebral hemisphere. *Generalized seizures* have clinical and/or electrographic features that indicate initial activation of neurons in both cerebral hemispheres. Focal seizures are subdivided into *simple* and *complex* based on level of consciousness. Seizures in which consciousness is preserved

are referred to as *simple partial seizures.* Those in which consciousness is impaired are classified as *complex partial seizures.*

Generalized seizure types include *tonic-clonic, tonic, clonic, myoclonic, atonic,* and *absence.*

Epileptic syndromes are disorders characterized by specific clusters of signs and symptoms that tend to behave in a similar manner in the majority of affected individuals. Most epileptic syndromes have numerous etiologies and few have been identified as specific diseases. Proposed in 1989, the current classification of the epilepsies divides epilepsies and epileptic syndromes into three categories based on clinical history, electroencephalographic (EEG) manifestations, and etiology (Commission on Classification and Terminology of the International League Against Epilepsy 1989). Localization-related epilepsies and syndromes are characterized by seizures that originate from a localized cortical region. Generalized epilepsies and epilepsy syndromes are characterized by seizures with initial activation of neurons within both cerebral hemispheres. Finally, some patients have both focal and generalized seizures and electrographic abnormalities. These cases are classified as *undetermined.*

Epilepsies and epileptic syndromes are further classified as *idiopathic, symptomatic,* or *crypto-*

*genic* based on the presumed etiology. *Idiopathic* describes syndromes that arise spontaneously without a known cause and likely have a genetic basis. Most affected individuals have normal intelligence and neurological examinations. *Symptomatic* describes epilepsies with an identified cause such as mesial temporal sclerosis, congenital malformations, central nervous system (CNS) infection, and neoplasm. *Cryptogenic* describes syndromes that are presumed to be symptomatic, but have no known etiology. Knowledge of the epilepsy or epileptic syndrome is required to predict the natural history of the disorder; institute appropriate treatment; and counsel the patient and family on the risks of recurrence, likelihood of remission, and morbidity and mortality.

## Localization-Related (Focal) Epilepsies

### Idiopathic, Age-Related

#### Benign Focal Epilepsies of Childhood

Benign focal epilepsies of childhood are idiopathic disorders characterized by focal seizures and EEG abnormalities of unknown etiology. These are age-related syndromes that have a tendency for spontaneous remission and occur in neurologically normal children. Benign childhood epilepsy with centrotemporal spikes (BCECT) is the most common, comprising 15% of seizures in patients under the age of 15 years (Loiseau 1996). Benign epilepsy of childhood with occipital paroxysms (BCEOP) and benign psychomotor epilepsy are rare in comparison.

In BCECT, simple partial seizures of the face and oropharynx and tonic-clonic seizures sometimes followed by Todd's paralysis occur predominately during sleep. As many as 20% of affected children experience a single seizure, regardless of whether or not treatment is initiated (Loiseau 1996). Nearly two-thirds have infrequent seizures. Six percent to 24% of children have more severe epilepsy (Loiseau 1996). Earlier age of onset is associated with a longer duration of active epilepsy. Status epilepticus occurs in approximately 10% of cases. Spontaneous remission by 16 to 18 years occurs in all cases, although 1% to 2% of patients experience isolated or rare tonic-clonic seizures in adulthood (Loiseu et al. 1988). Focal seizures during adulthood are exceedingly rare and semiologically dissimilar from those seen in childhood. The

risk of tonic-clonic seizures after BCECT is ten times greater than that of the general population (Loiseau 1996).

### Symptomatic

#### Temporal, Frontal, Parietal, and Occipital Lobe Epilepsies

The symptomatic focal epilepsies include epilepsies originating from the temporal, frontal, parietal, and occipital lobes. These syndromes vary considerably in age of onset, severity, natural history, and response to treatment. Temporal lobe epilepsy (TLE) is the most common focal epilepsy presenting during adolescence and adulthood. In most cases, seizures arise from the mesial temporal structures (hippocampus, amygdala, and parahippocampal gyrus). After TLE, frontal lobe epilepsy is most common. Seizures arising from the parietal and occipital lobes are relatively rare, although the true incidence is unknown, since data are derived primarily from surgical series of intractable cases. The symptomatic focal epilepsies are characterized by simple partial, complex partial, secondary generalized seizures.

Carbamazepine and phenytoin are the recommended drugs of choice for the treatment of complex partial seizures with or without secondary generalization (Mattson et al. 1985). Phenobarbital and primidone are less effective and have a higher incidence of adverse effects. Carbamazepine and valproic acid have similar efficacy against secondary generalized seizures; however, carbamazepine is more effective for complex partial seizures and better tolerated (Mattson et al. 1992). Lamotrigine may also be used as monotherapy for partial seizures in adults. The newer anticonvulsant medications, gabapentin, topiramate, and tiagabine, produce a 50% seizure reduction in 20% to 40% of patients (Mikati and Holmes 1996). Complex partial seizures tend to be more difficult to treat than secondary generalized tonic-clonic seizures. The probability of achieving complete seizure control in the first year of treatment with standard antiepileptic drug (AED) monotherapy is approximately 70% for patients with generalized tonic-clonic seizures only, versus 21% for those with complex partial seizures only, with intermediate results for patients with both seizure types (Mattson et al. 1996). Between 60% and 70% of patients with newly diagnosed complex partial seizures achieve remission, half of whom ultimately undergo AED discontinuation (Hauser 1996). The remainder continue to have seizures despite appropriate medical management. Factors that predict a favorable outcome include a family history of epilepsy, unknown etiology, and absence of abnormalities on EEG. History of febrile seizures, onset prior to 2 years of age, high seizure frequency, IQ under 90, symptomatic etiology, and status epilepticus are associated with a lower likelihood of remission. Surgical treatment should be considered in patients with medically refractory seizures. The outcome of surgical treatment depends on the extent of resection of the area of cortex generating seizures. Surgical outcome is better in temporal than extratemporal lobe epilepsy, and in the presence of lesions visible on neuroimaging studies. Reproductive endocrine dysfunction; psychiatric disturbances such as depression, personality disorders, and anxiety; and learning disabilities are common in patints with symptomatic focal epilepsy, particularly involving the temporal lobe.

## Generalized Epilepsies

### Idiopathic, Age-Related

#### Benign Neonatal Familial and Nonfamilial Convulsions

Benign idiopathic neonatal convulsions (BINNC) and benign familial neonatal convulsions (BFNNC) are rare neonatal syndromes, characterized by seizures beginning in the first week of life. Most infants are neurologically normal, and spontaneous remission usually occurs. Seizures in BINNC consist of recurrent focal or generalized clonic seizures, apneic events, or status epilepticus occurring between the fourth and sixth day of life and remitting within the first week. In BFNNC, seizures begin on the second or third day of life and tend to recur for several months. Anticonvulsant therapy has a variable effect of the duration of seizures. Both syndromes are considered benign, although follow-up beyond early childhood has not been reported. Epilepsy develops in 11% of patients with BFNNC and 0.5% of infants with BINNC (Plouin 1992). The incidence of other abnormalities is unknown, although developmental delay and minor neurological abnormalities have been described in infants with the BINNC. Psy-

chomotor development is not affected in the familial form.

### Benign Myoclonic Epilepsy of Infancy

This syndrome is characterized by myoclonic seizures in neurologically normal children in the first or second years of life. Tonic-clonic seizures may develop during adolescence. A family history of febrile seizures or epilepsy is present in one-third of cases (Dravet et al. 1992a). In most patients, seizures are readily controlled with valproic acid. If treatment is delayed, psychomotor retardation and behavioral disturbances may result.

### Absence Epilepsy

Absence epilepsy (AE) is subdivided into childhood (CAE) and juvenile (JAE) forms. Childhood absence epilepsy presents between the ages of 4 and 8 years and comprises 80% of cases. Juvenile AE typically presents around the age of 12 years. Absence seizures occur in both disorders, sometimes as frequent as hundreds of times per day. Infrequent tonic-clonic seizures occur in approximately 30% of patients with CAE. Nearly 80% of juvenile onset cases have tonic-clonic seizures. Absence status epilepticus occurs in 10% of CAE and 40% of JAE patients. Myoclonic seizures occur in 15% of patients with JAE and are typically absent in CAE. Neurological examination and intelligence are normal. A family history of epilepsy is present in approximately 30% of patients.

Ethosuximide or valproic acid controls absence seizures in 80% of cases. Since ethosuximide is not effective against tonic-clonic seizures, valproic acid is the drug of choice in patients with both seizure types. Five percent to 20% of patients are not satisfactorily controlled on monotherapy and may benefit from a combination of ethosuximide and valproic acid, benzodiazepines, lamotrigine, or acetazolamide. Absence seizures typically remit by early adulthood, but may persist in up to 6% of cases (Loiseau 1992). Tonic-clonic seizures may persist into adulthood, but are usually infrequent and readily controlled with medication. Predisposing factors for the development of tonic-clonic seizures in CAE include age of onset after 8 years, incomplete control of absence seizures, delay in initiation of treatment, and photosensitivity. Rhythmic occipital delta activity on EEG is associated with a more favorable course and lower incidence of tonic-clonic seizures. Factors predictive of lack of remission of CAE include cognitive difficulties at the time of the diagnosis, poor control of absence seizures during the first year of treatment, absence status epilepticus, tonic-clonic or myoclonic seizures during AED therapy, background abnormalities on EEG, and seizures in first-degree relatives (Wirrell et al. 1996). In a series of patients followed for two decades, 78% of those with absence seizures only were seizure free at follow-up, compared to 35% of patients with absence and tonic-clonic seizures (Bouma et al. 1996). Infrequent tonic-clonic seizures occurred in approximately 60% of adults (Bouma et al. 1996). Adverse effects of AEDs, social prejudice, and chronicity of disease are thought to produce psychomotor slowing and behavioral disturbances that lead to poor social adaptation in 30% of patients even in the absence of active epilepsy (Loiseau 1992).

### Juvenile Myoclonic Epilepsy

Juvenile myoclonic epilepsy (JME) presents with myoclonic jerks usually of the upper extremities or generalized tonic-clonic seizures in neurologically normal adolescents between the ages of 12 and 18 years. Infrequent absence seizures are observed in up to one-third of cases. Seizures occur predominately in the early morning hours shortly after awakening and are provoked by sleep deprivation, alcohol ingestion, fatigue, and menstruation. Photosensitivity is observed in 30% of patients. Juvenile myoclonic epilepsy is a genetically determined syndrome with a gene locus on chromosome 6p. Nearly 50% of JME patients have relatives with seizures and 30% have asymptomatic relatives with generalized epileptiform abnormalities on EEG.

The prognosis of JME is favorable if appropriate treatment is initiated and precipitating factors are avoided. However, over 90% of patients experience a relapse after AED withdrawal (Wolf 1992a). Consequently, long-term AED therapy is usually recommended even in patients with long seizure-free intervals. Valproic acid has traditionally been the drug of choice and is effective in 85% to 90% of patients. Lamotrigine is also effective against the seizure types in JME. Many of the metabolic disturbances produced by valproic acid, including obesity, hyperinsulinemia, lipid abnormalities, and polycystic ovarian syndrome, may be reduced by substituting lamotrigine for valproic acid (Isojärvi et al. 1998). Phenobarbital and primidone may also be effective. Ethosuximide may be used for refractory absence seizures. Uncontrolled myoclonic seizures may respond to benzodiazepines. Neurotic personality traits and immature behavior contribute to poor psychosocial outcome in some cases (Janz 1989).

### Epilepsy with Generalized Tonic-Clonic Seizures on Awakening

This syndrome affects neurologically normal individuals during the second decade of life. Tonic-clonic seizures occur predominately or exclusively shortly after awakening or in the evening during relaxation. Myoclonic and absence seizures may also be observed. Sleep deprivation, alcohol, and sudden external arousal precipitate seizures. A family history of epilepsy exceeds that of the general population, suggesting a genetic etiology. Complete seizure control is achieved in 60% to 80% of patients (Wolf 1992b). However, over 80% of patients experience a relapse following reduction or withdrawal of medication.

## Generalized Cryptogenic or Symptomatic, Age-Related

### West Syndrome

West Syndrome is an age-dependent epilepsy characterized by infantile spasms, psychomotor retardation, and hypsarrhythmia on EEG. In 85% of cases, psychomotor retardation and spasms appear in the first year of life, the majority between 3 and 7 months. Focal motor deficits, hypotonia, microcephaly, blindness, deafness, and other seizure types are observed in some cases. Hypsarrhythmia, a chaotic pattern of high-amplitude slow waves with multifocal epileptiform discharges and poor interhemispheric synchrony, is found in over two-thirds of affected infants. Tuberous sclerosis is one of the most common causes of infantile spasms, comprising nearly 25% of symptomatic cases. Congenital malformations and perinatal brain injury each account for over 30% of case in neuropathological series (Dulac et al. 1996).

Approximately 75% of patients achieve initial seizure control with corticosteroids. Intramuscular adrenocorticotropic hormone (ACTH) is most frequently used. The response rate tends to increase with duration of therapy. However, over 50% of patients relapse after steroid treatment, typically within 2 months. In nearly three-quarters of cases, spasms respond to a second course of steroids. However, life-threatening complications of steroid treatment including cardiomyopathy and infection occur in up to 8% of patients (Dulac et al. 1996). Benzodiazepines, valproic acid, pyridoxine, immunoglobulins, and lamotrigine have shown some efficacy. Vigabatrin has produced long-term, complete suppression of spasms in some patients, particularly those with tuberous sclerosis. Favorable results have been reported following lesionectomy or hemispherectomy in patients with focal abnormalities on magnetic resonance imaging (MRI) or positron emission tomography (PET).

Infantile spasms and hypsarrhythmia tend to diminish with increasing age. By 3 years of age, hysparrhythmia typically evolves to slow spike-wave complexes or multifocal spikes and sharp waves. Complete remission of spasms occurs within 2 years in 50% of patients and by 5 years of age in 72% to 99% of cases (Dulac et al. 1996). Over 50% of patients develop Lennox-Gastaut syndrome, multifocal, or secondarily generalized epilepsy or other forms of epilepsy during childhood. Seizures after West syndrome tend to be refractory to medical management. Cerebral palsy and sensory deficits, including blindness, are observed in over 50% of cases. Mental retardation is observed in 90% of cases and is severe in over 70% (Jeavons and Livet 1992). Psychiatric disturbances including hyperkinetic syndrome and autism are not uncommon. Only 5% of patients experience spontaneous remission without neurological sequelae. The condition ultimately leads to death in 5% to 20% of patients (Jeavons and Livet 1992). Aspiration pneumonia is the major cause of death. The risk of death is significantly higher in symptomatic cases. Factors predictive of an unfavorable outcome include known etiology, delay in treatment, asymmetrical spasms, neurological and developmental deficiencies preceding the onset of spasms, abnormal neuroimaging studies, and unilateral or significantly asymmetrical EEG manifestations.

### Lennox-Gastaut Syndrome

Lennox-Gastaut syndrome is characterized by multiple seizure types, slow spike-wave complexes on EEG, and diffuse cognitive dysfunction. Atypical absence, atonic, tonic, and myoclonic seizures are observed. Onset is usually in early childhood, typically between 3 and 5 years of age. Status epilepticus, consisting of repetitive tonic seizures or fluctuating mental status lasting hours to weeks, occurs in two-thirds of patients. In approximately 70% of cases, acquired or genetic etiologies, such as congenital malformations, hypoxic ischemic encephalopathy, CNS infection, or neurocutaneous disorders, are identified. A history of West syndrome is present in one-third of cases.

The prognosis for seizure control and mental development is poor. Daily seizures occur in most patients and are usually refractory to medical therapy. Benzodiazepines and valproic acid have traditionally been the most effective agents, although the former may precipitate tonic status epilepticus. Sedation should be minimized because of the tendency for seizures to increase in sleep. Lamotrigine has been shown to be effective as adjunctive therapy. Carbamazepine, vigabatrin, the ketogenic diet, and corticosteroids may also be effective. Corpus callosotomy reduces tonic and atonic seizures in some cases. Mental retardation eventually develops in 78% to 96% of patients (Farrell 1996). Severe mental retardation is more common in patients with onset before 3 years of age and in symptomatic cases. Behavioral and personality disorders are commonly observed. In over 50% of patients, the characteristic features disappear with age but other seizure types and EEG abnormalities develop (Oguni et al. 1996). Factors predictive of a poor outcome include known etiology, onset prior to 3 years of age, history of symptomatic West syndrome, refractory tonic seizures, and recurrent status epilepticus. Seizures usually persist into adulthood, and fatal injuries related to seizures occur in 5% of cases (Beaumanoir and Dravet 1992).

### Epilepsy with Myoclonic Absences

This syndrome is characterized by rhythmic, myoclonic seizures with impairment of consciousness that begin in childhood. Seizures may last as long as 1 minute and occur many times per day. Generalized tonic-clonic seizures may also be observed. Myoclonic absences may disappear, but infrequent tonic-clonic seizures persist. Nearly 50% of patients have intellectual impairment prior to seizure onset (Tassinari et al. 1992a). Of the remainder, approximately 50% develop significant mental retardation after the appearance of seizures. Valproic acid and ethosuximide in combination may be effective, but seizures prove medically refractory in 50% of cases (Tassinari et al. 1992a).

### Epilepsy with Myoclonic-Astatic Seizures

This disorder presents as sudden drop attacks, either myoclonic or atonic in nature, in young, neurologically normal children. A family history of febrile or afebrile seizures is present in over 30% of cases (Doose 1992). Other seizure types include generalized tonic-clonic seizures, myoclonic status epilepticus, and tonic seizures. Valproic acid, ethosuximide, benzodiazepines, and ACTH produce variable results. The disorder rarely resolves spontaneously and may have a benign course. Factors predictive of a poor outcome include onset of febrile or afebrile generalized tonic-clonic seizures before 1 year of age, myoclonic-astatic status epilepticus, abnormal neurological examination, high seizure frequency, absence of normal background on EEG, nocturnal tonic seizures, and tonic-clonic seizures with shifting accentuation of motor involvement (Doose 1992). Recurrent status epilepticus, particularly in young children, commonly leads to dementia and other neurological deficits including ataxia.

## Generalized Symptomatic Epilepsies of Nonspecific Etiology, Age-Related

### Early Neonatal Myoclonic Encephalopathy

This disorder affects infants with severe neurological impairment shortly after birth. Marked psychomotor retardation and bilateral pyramidal tract signs are observed. Affected infants experience erratic fragmentary myoclonus, and generalized myoclonic, tonic, and focal motor seizures. The EEG shows a suppression-burst pattern that evolves to hypsarrhythmia or multifocal spike discharges within months. Inborn errors of metabolism and congenital malformations are present in some cases. Seizures are poorly responsive to AED therapy, and 50% of patients do not survive beyond the first year of life (Aicardi 1992).

### Early Infantile Epileptic Encephalopathy

Also known as Ohtahara's syndrome, this disorder is characterized by tonic spasms beginning in the first few months of life, a suppression-burst pattern on EEG, and rapid progression from normal to severe neurological disability. Tonic-clonic and focal motor seizures eventually develop. Hypsarrhythmia, slow spike-wave complexes, or multifocal spikes are observed beyond the neonatal period. Ohtahara's syndrome represents the first in the spectrum of age-related epileptic encephalopathies, sometimes evolving into West syndrome, followed by Lennox-Gastaut syndrome. Congenital malformations are commonly found. Seizures are poorly responsive to anticonvulsant treatment, including ACTH. Only 50% of infants survive beyond the first year of life. Survivors have severe psychomotor retardation and intractable epilepsy (Ohtahara et al. 1992).

## Epilepsies and Syndromes Undetermined as to Whether they are Focal or Generalized

### Neonatal Seizures

Seizures are a common manifestation of cerebral dysfunction in the first month of life. Hypoxic ischemic encephalopathy (HIE) is the most common etiology overall, and the most common cause of seizures during the first day of life. Other causes of seizures within the first 24 hours include bacterial meningitis, sepsis, subarachnoid hemorrhage, intrauterine infection, laceration of the tentorium or falx, drugs, and pyridoxine dependency. From 24 to 72 hours of life, additional etiologies include cerebral contusion with subdural hemorrhage, drug withdrawal, congenital malformations, and metabolic disorders. Seizures that present beyond the third day of life are usually due to inborn errors of metabolism, herpes simplex infection, kernicterus, or neonatal adrenoleukodystrophy.

The etiology, neurological examination, seizure type, and findings on serial EEGs may be used to predict outcome. The severity of background abnormalities correlates with the degree of neurological impairment (Holmes and Lombroso 1993). Infants with suppressed, undifferentiated, or suppression-burst patterns have a high incidence of neurological and developmental sequelae. Infants with normal awake and sleep background rhythms tend to have normal neurological development, regardless of the presence or absence of electrographic seizures. Isolated sharp waves are commonly seen in neurologically normal neonates without seizures, and are not predictive of seizures or subsequent epilepsy. Seizures with consistent electrographic correlates, such as focal clonic seizures, tend to be observed in infants with focal structural lesions. Over 70% of infants with clonic seizures are normal at the time of hospital discharge (Mizrahi and Kellaway 1987). Seizures without consistent EEG correlation, such as tonic posturing, myoclonus, and subtle ictal behaviors, are more commonly observed in neurologically abnormal infants. These seizure types imply more diffuse cerebral dysfunction and have been associated with hypoxic-ischemic encephalopathy, cerebral dysgenesis, and inborn errors of metabolism. Over 50% of infants with seizures that lack consistent EEG correlation are abnormal at the time of discharge, and the outcome is fatal in 20% (Mizrahi and Kellaway 1987). Antiepileptic drug therapy is recommended when recurrent clinical events are accompanied by EEG seizure patterns. In the absence of CNS pathology and significant EEG abnormalities, neurologically normal infants do not require prolonged AED therapy. Neonates with abnormal neurological examinations and focal cerebral pathology, particularly cerebral dysgenesis, are at a high risk of developing epilepsy. In infants with diffuse encephalopathy, tonic posturing and subtle behaviors not accompanied by EEG changes are thought to represent brain stem release phenomena. In these cases, treatment with AEDs is not absolutely required.

Neurological sequelae, including mental retardation and cerebral palsy, are observed in one-third of infants with neonatal seizures and epilepsy develops in approximately 25% of cases (Legido et al. 1988). In infants with seizures, an Apgar score of less than 7 at 5 minutes or later is associated with a poor outcome (Legido et al. 1988). Term infants have a better outcome than premature infants. The mortality rate for neonates with seizures is 40% for term and 50% for premature infants (Scher 1996). The incidence of permanent neurological sequelae is high in cases due to perinatal asphyxia, intraventricular hemorrhage, and cerebral dysgenesis, while most transient metabolic disturbances are associated with a better outcome and a low likelihood of epilepsy.

### Progressive Myoclonic Epilepsies

The progressive myoclonic epilepsies (PMEs) represent a group of disorders of various etiologies that collectively account for 1% of all epilepsy

syndromes (Berkovic et al. 1993). The natural history varies with the specific disorder from mild neurological impairment to severe disability progressing to death in early childhood. Onset is typically during childhood or adolescence, although some of the disorders may present at any age. The PMEs are characterized by progressive myoclonus, seizures, variable degrees of cognitive impairment, and other neurological deficits. Myoclonus is commonly precipitated by action, sustained posture, or sensory stimulation, and varies from mild to debilitating depending on the specific disorder. Dementia is characteristic of many of the PMEs, but is not a universal feature. The severity of intellectual deterioration is related to the degree of cortical loss and varies between individuals affected with the same disorder. Other neurological findings include ataxia, spasticity, visual impairment, hearing loss, peripheral neuropathy, and extrapyramidal signs. Tonic-clonic seizures are the most common seizure type, although atypical absences and focal seizures are observed in some disorders.

Unverricht-Lundborg disease, or Baltic myoclonus, is the prototype of the PMEs. Tonic-clonic seizures and severe myoclonus develop in the later half of the first decade. Dementia and ataxia may develop late in the course and are generally mild. Most affected individuals survive into the sixth or seventh decade, although death within a few years of onset has been described. Myoclonic epilepsy with ragged red fibers (MERRF) is now one of the most common forms of PME. This is a mitochondrial disorder with a highly variable course. Affected individuals have severe, debilitating myoclonus, tonic-clonic seizures, and ataxia. Less common features include dementia, myopathy, neuropathy, deafness, optic atrophy, dysarthria, short stature, and axial lipomas. Other causes of PME include Lafora's disease, neuronal ceroid lipofuscinoses, and the sialidoses.

Myoclonus responds best to valproic acid and benzodiazepines, particularly clonazepam; L-tryptophan, 5-hydroxytryptophan with carbidopa, and piracetam may also be effective. Valproic acid, clonazepam, phenobarbital, and lamotrigine may be used to control seizures. Phenytoin commonly exacerbates ataxia and myoclonus in subjects with Unverricht-Lundbourg disease and should be avoided.

## Severe Myoclonic Epilepsy in Infancy

This disorder presents in the first year of life with prolonged, recurrent febrile seizures in previously neurologically normal infants. A family history of epilepsy is common. Atypical absence, myoclonic, partial, and tonic-clonic seizures and myoclonic status epilepticus may appear in early childhood. By the second year of life, infants develop psychomotor retardation often accompanied by ataxia, pyramidal signs, and myoclonus. Seizures are poorly responsive to anticonvulsant medications. In one series, the mortality rate was 16% at a mean age of follow-up of 11 years (Dravet et al. 1992b). The remainder of infants were severely disabled.

## Acquired Epileptic Aphasia

Acquired epileptic aphasia, or the Landau-Kleffner syndrome, is characterized by an auditory verbal agnosia and reduction of spontaneous speech in children younger than 6 years, after the initial acquisition of verbal language. Seizures are observed in 75% of cases. Approximately one-third of affected children experience a single seizure or episode of status epilepticus. The remainder have infrequent seizures that are nocturnal and readily controlled with AEDs. The EEG shows temporoparieto-occipital epileptiform discharges during sleep. Psychomotor disturbances or personality disorders occur in 70% of patients. Seizures and EEG abnormalities tend to remit spontaneously by 15 years of age, and speech typically recovers by adulthood. However, nearly 50% of patients experience neuropsychological or academic deficiencies due to the prolonged aphasia (Beaumanoir 1992). Onset after 6 years of age and early speech therapy are associated with a more favorable prognosis. Outcome is not affected by seizure frequency or seizure type. Administration of intravenous diazepam may produce dramatic but transient improvements in language and EEG abnormalities. The benefit of long-term anticonvulsant therapy has not been demonstrated. Early treatment with high doses of corticosteroids and multiple subpial transections have been efficacious in some cases.

## Epilepsy with Continuous Spike Waves During Slow-Wave Sleep

Also known as electrical status epilepticus during slow-wave sleep (ESES), this syndrome is characterized by spike-wave discharges occupying 85% or more of slow-wave sleep in children. Unilateral or generalized clonic, atonic, and tonic seizures, absence seizures, and absence status epilepticus begin in early childhood. Seizures occur daily in the majority of cases. Benzodiazepines, valproic acid, corticosteroids, and ethosuximide produce partial but transient improvements in the EEG. Prior to the occurrence of epilepsy with continuous spike waves during slow-wave sleep (CSWS), approximately 50% of children exhibit abnormal psychomotor development. Psychomotor retardation, reduction in language function, behavioral problems, and worsening seizures occur with the onset of CSWS. Seizures typically disappear before or with resolution of the EEG abnormality. In a minority of cases, rare tonic-clonic or absence seizures persist after the cessation of CSWS. The EEG abnormality resolves during the early part of the second decade of life and normalization of the EEG gradually occurs over a few years. However, persistent focal EEG abnormalities have been described. Neuropsychological status improves with the cessation of continuous spiking, but persistent deficits are observed in over 50% of cases (Tassinari 1992b).

## Special Situations

### The First Seizure

Approximately 6% of the population will experience an afebrile seizure at least once in their lifetime (So 1993). The decision to initiate AED therapy after a single seizure is based on the risk of recurrence versus that of treatment. Over 30% of treated patients experience adverse effects requiring medication discontinuation (Mattson et al. 1985). Recurrence rates after single unprovoked seizures range from 23% to 71% (Berg and Shinner 1991). Factors predictive of seizure recurrence include neurological abnormality on examination or neuroimaging studies, symptomatic etiology, epileptiform abnormalities on EEG, and focal seizures, particularly if followed by a Todd's paralysis (Berg et al. 1991). The risk of recurrence increases with the number of risk factors present. Treatment with AEDs reduces the risk of recurrence. In one series, the risk of recurrence after a first unprovoked tonic-clonic seizure during the next 24 months was 25% among treated subjects and approximately 50% for untreated subjects (First Seizure Trial Group 1993). However, the probability of achieving remission for 1 and 2 years was the same whether treatment was initiated after the first or second seizure (Musicco et al. 1997). Once a second seizure has occurred, the risk of a third seizure is over 90% (So 1993). After a single unprovoked seizure, the majority of recurrences take place within 6 months, and more than 80% happen within 2 years (Berg and Shinner 1991). Treatment with AEDs should be considered in patients with abnormal neurological examination or neuroimaging studies, or focal seizures. Hyponatremia, hypoglycemia, withdrawal from alcohol, barbiturates, and benzodiazepines, and medications are common causes of isolated seizures, particularly in hospitalized patients. Medications that precipitate tonic-clonic seizures include tricyclic antidepressants, antipsychotics, anticholinergics, antihistamines, methylxanthines, and some antibiotics. Treatment with anticonvulsant medication is not required in subjects with isolated seizures due to medications, alcohol and drug withdrawal, and metabolic disturbances. If the decision to treat with AEDs is made, therapy is generally continued for a period of 1 to 2 years, after which medication is gradually withdrawn if seizures have not recurred and negative predictors are absent.

### Remission and Relapse and the Effects of AED Withdrawal in Chronic Epilepsy

Approximately 70% to 80% of patients with newly diagnosed seizures achieve lasting remission (Sander 1993). The remainder continue to have seizures despite adequate treatment with AEDs. In a community-based study of patterns of seizure remission, 65% of patients entered long-term remission, 25% had chronic active epilepsy from the onset, and 12% had a remitting and relapsing course (Shorvon and Sander 1986). Most patients who enter remission do so within 2 years of initiation of treatment. With time, the chance of achieving remission decreases if seizures persist with treatment. The likelihood of remission is lower in patients with neurological deficits, focal seizures, multiple seizure types, psychiatric disturbances, high seizure frequency before treatment, and epileptiform features on EEG. Once a 2-year remission is achieved, drug withdrawal is usually considered.

Knowledge of the epilepsy syndrome is imperative in choosing the appropriate anticonvulsant drug and determining whether medication withdrawal should be considered, since the risk of relapse varies with the specific syndrome. The selection of an AED is based on its established efficacy against specific seizure types and the potential for adverse effects. The goal of treatment is to control seizures using a single agent maintained at serum concentrations that do not produce adverse effects. If seizures persist, the dosage is gradually increased until seizure control is achieved or intolerable side effects occur. A second agent is introduced only after an adequate trial of the first drug has failed. In many cases, seizures persist because an agent that is not considered first-line is chosen, or an appropriate medication is administered in inadequate doses.

The probability of relapse after AED withdrawal ranges from 11% to 41% (Sander 1993). However, patients at high risk for relapse, such as those with JME and structural brain lesions, tend to be excluded from studies evaluating medication withdrawal. In one large randomized series of patients experiencing two or more definite seizures without a progressive disease, 41% of patients who discontinued AEDs relapsed after a 2-year remission, compared to 22% of patients who continued treatment (Medical Research Council Antiepileptic Drug Withdrawal Study Group 1991). Most relapses occurred within the first year of drug withdrawal. One-third experienced a single recurrence and the remainder experienced two or more seizures during a 5-year follow-up (Chadwick et al. 1996). By 5 years after a single relapse, 90% of patients experienced another 2-year remission. Of the group having a second relapse, only 25% remained seizure free during the 5-year follow-up. Treatment with AEDs did not alter the proportion of patients seizure free 1 and 2 years after relapse. Shorter lengths of remission, history of tonic-clonic seizures, and polytherapy are associated with a higher relapse rate.

### Febrile Seizures

Febrile seizures are events associated with fever that occur in infancy or childhood usually between 3 months and 5 years of age, in the absence of intracranial infection or a defined cause. They occur in 2% to 5% of infants and children, representing the most common seizure disorder in this age group (Nelson and Ellenberg 1976). Secondary causes are more common in patients who present with a first febrile seizure before 6 months and after 5 years of age. Simple febrile seizures, which are single, generalized convulsions lasting less than 15 minutes, comprise 80% to 90% of cases. Seizures that exceed 15 minutes in duration, occur more than once in a 24-hour period, or have focal manifestations, are classified as complex febrile seizures. Approximately 30% of patients will experience a single recurrence, and of this group, half will experience multiple febrile seizures (Freeman 1980). The risk of recurrent febrile seizures is 50% in infants experiencing the first seizure before 1 year of age as compared to 20% in children over the age of 3 years (Duchowny 1996). The risk of afebrile seizures is 1.5% to 9% in infants and children with febrile seizures. Those with abnormal neurological examinations or development, family history of afebrile seizures, and complex febrile seizures are at an increased risk for developing epilepsy. The incidence of epilepsy is 11% to 18% when two or more risk factors are present versus 1% to 2% in their absence (Nelson and Ellenberg 1976: Freeman 1980). The risk of developing epilepsy is greatest in the first few years after febrile seizures. Nearly 50% of children with recurrent, prolonged, and focal febrile seizures develop epilepsy (Duchowny 1996). Infants with severe and very prolonged febrile hemiconvulsions followed by permanent hemiplegia have a high incidence of subsequent epilepsy, a condition referred to as the hemiconvulsion-hemiplegia-epilepsy syndrome. Status epilepticus constitutes approximately 8% of initial febrile seizure cases. The risk of permanent disability or death following febrile status epilepticus is low. Isolated febrile seizures do not adversely affect neuropsychological status. The risk of seizures in family members of patients with febrile seizures is two to three times that of the general population. Prophylactic anticonvulsants are usually not recommended because of the high incidence of neurobehavioral adverse effects and their failure to reduce the risk of epilepsy.

## Epilepsy During Pregnancy

Epilepsy is the most common neurological disorder encountered by obstetricians. In most women with epilepsy, seizure frequency during pregnancy parallels preconception seizure control. Breakthrough seizures are usually due to noncompliance, stress, or sleep deprivation. The incidence of status epilepticus is not increased. Obstetrical

and neonatal outcome is normal in over 90% of cases (Yerby 1991). Proper nutrition, regular prenatal care, folate supplementation, and optimal seizure control improve the chance of a favorable outcome. When possible, women should be treated with the single AED at the lowest possible dose that best controls seizures, since the incidence of fetal malformations increases with polytherapy and high serum concentrations. The risk of major and minor malformations in offspring is 6% to 8% (Delgado-Escueta and Janz 1992). No single AED is believed to be more teratogenic than the others. Major malformations, including neural tube defects, cleft lip-palate, congenital heart, and urogenital defects, have been reported in offspring of women taking phenytoin, carbamazepine, phenobarbital, valproic acid, and primidone. The incidence of neural tube defects associated with the use of carbamazepine and valproic acid is 1% and 2%, respectively. Folate deficiency is one proposed mechanism for congenital malformations and spontaneous abortions. The recommended dose of folate for pregnant women with epilepsy is 1 mg daily. Women with prior pregnancies complicated by or family history of neural tube defects should take 4 mg daily.

Most pregnant women with epilepsy have normal spontaneous vaginal deliveries. Inductions of labor, mechanical rupture of membranes, forceps-assisted deliveries, cesarean sections, toxemia, pre-eclampsia, bleeding, placental abruption, premature labor, and spontaneous abortion occur more commonly in women with epilepsy than their nonepileptic counterparts. The indications for cesarean section include repeated tonic-clonic seizures during labor that cannot be controlled and poor maternal cooperation. Two percent to 4% of women with epilepsy experience a tonic-clonic seizure during labor or the immediate postpartum period. Total and free serum AED levels should be obtained periodically throughout pregnancy to ensure adequate serum concentrations, particularly during labor and delivery. Vitamin $K_1$ should be administered to the mother during the last month of pregnancy to protect the infant from bleeding disorders due to AED exposure, which have a mortality rate of over 30% (Delgado-Esqueta and Janz 1992). At the time of birth, 1 mg of vitamin $K_1$ is administered intramuscularly to the infant. In general, breast-feeding is not contraindicated. However, sedating AEDs can produce lethargy, failure to thrive, and irritability in the newborn.

New-onset seizures may be the initial manifestation of a host of diseases that present during pregnancy. Ischemic stroke, vascular anomalies, paradoxical embolus, vasculitis, and metastatic choriocarcinoma may present at any time during pregnancy. The risk of bleeding due to arteriovenous malformations and aneurysms increases as pregnancy progresses. Eclampsia, oxytocin-induced water intoxication, toxicity of local anesthetics, amniotic fluid embolus, thrombotic thrombocytopenic purpura, cerebral venous thrombosis, pheochromocytoma, and subarachnoid hemorrhage may produce seizures in the peripartum period.

### Nonepileptic Seizures

Non-epileptic, or psychogenic, seizures are spells of altered awareness, abnormal movements, or abnormal sensations that share some features of epileptic seizures but are caused by emotional distress. They occur in individuals with conversion disorders, anxiety, panic disorder, depression, post-traumatic stress disorder, schizophrenia, and personality disorders. Over two-thirds of subjects have a history of childhood sexual or physical abuse and 10% to 60% also have epilepsy (Lesser 1996). The majority of affected patients are women. Psychotherapy and pharmacological treatment of psychiatric disease is indicated in most cases. Factors associated with better outcome include shorter duration of seizures, normal psychiatric evaluation, psychiatric intervention in appropriate cases, absence of epileptic seizures, and more independent lifestyle. With treatment, seizures remit in 40% to 60% of cases (Lesser 1996).

### Status Epilepticus

Status epilepticus (SE) is defined as continuous clinical or electrical seizure activity or repetitive seizures from which consciousness is not regained for 30 minutes or longer. An estimated 126,000 to 195,000 episodes of status epilepticus occur in the United States annually, resulting in 22,000 to 42,000 deaths (DeLorenzo et al. 1996). The incidence is higher in infants under 1 year of age and adults over the age of 60 years. In the pediatric population, systemic infection, subtherapeutic drug levels, and congenital malformations are the most common causes. Acute or subacute stroke, low anticonvulsant levels, remote CNS

insults, alcohol, and anoxia account for the majority of cases in adults. Approximately 20% of all SE cases occur in epileptic patients during medication adjustment or as a result of noncompliance. In one-third of patients, the cause for SE is undetermined.

In adults, the most common type of SE is secondary generalized convulsive SE (GCSE). The manifestations change over time such that discrete convulsions give way to increasingly subtle clinical manifestations, a condition known as subtle SE. Generalized convulsive activity produces a variety of systemic effects including hypoxia; hyperpyrexia; blood pressure instability; cerebral dysautoregulation; and metabolic derangements including respiratory and metabolic acidosis, hyperazotemia, hypokalemia, hyponatremia, and alterations in blood glucose. Rhabdomyolysis may produce myoglobinuria, acute tubular necrosis, and renal failure. Aspiration pneumonia and neurogenic pulmonary edema can occur.

Status epilepticus is a medical emergency that demands prompt diagnosis and treatment to minimize severe neurological sequelae and death. Despite improvements in medical management, the incidence of significant morbidity and mortality remains high. Status epilepticus may result in permanent neurological deficits, intellectual decline, recurrent seizures, and death. The majority of deaths are due to the underlying etiology as opposed to the status itself. Mortality rates ranging from 8% to 32% have been reported (DeLorenzo et al. 1992). Morbidity and mortality are largely dependent on the speed of intervention, age of the patient, and etiology. Subtle SE and GCSE exceeding 1 hour is associated with a higher mortality rate (34.8%) than episodes of shorter duration (3.7%) (DeLorenzo et al. 1992). The mortality rate is lower in children (3%) than adults (26%), and increases with advancing age. Infants under 1 year of age have a particularly high mortality rate (DeLorenzo et al. 1996). The outcome is favorable in SE due to pre-existing epilepsy and low anticonvulsant levels, drugs and alcohol, and when no cause is identified. The mortality rate is highest among those with acute symptomatic SE due to anoxic encephalopathy. Within 24 hours of resolution of SE, a normal EEG portends an excellent prognosis, whereas the mortality rate exceeds 50% in subjects with burst suppression, rhythmic discharges unaccompanied by clinical manifestations, and periodic lateralized epileptiform discharges (Jaitly et al. 1997). The morbidity and mortality of absence, simple partial, and complex partial SE is not entirely known. While significant neurological sequelae are less common, several cases of death and permanent cognitive or memory impairment have been reported after prolonged complex partial SE. Treatment with benzodiazepines and intravenous loading with phenytoin is effective in terminating over 90% of cases of GCSE. If seizures persist, elective intubation followed by administration of phenobarbital is generally performed. Only 6% of cases prove refractory to this approach and require pharmacological coma.

### Mortality and Sudden Death in Epilepsy

Compared to the general population, patients with epilepsy have an increased mortality rate. The overall standardized mortality ratio (SMR) in patients with definite epilepsy is 3.0 (Cockerell et al. 1997). The risk is greatest in patients with remote symptomatic seizures, severe neurological deficits, and frequent, poorly controlled seizures. The SMR is 4.3 for patients with remote symptomatic epilepsy and 1.6 for those with idiopathic epilepsy. Causes of death include accidents, particularly drowning, aspiration pneumonia, new CNS insults, status epilepticus, and suicide. Sudden death in epilepsy (SUDEP) is sudden, unexpected, and nonaccidental death (excluding status epilepticus) in patients with epilepsy in whom there is no obvious medical cause. There is often evidence of a seizure near the time of death. The incidence of SUDEP is estimated at nearly 1 per 200 per year in patients with severe epilepsy, a relative risk that is 40 times greater than that of the general population. In the epilepsy population as a whole, the incidence of SUDEP is between 1 in 500 and 1 in 1000 individuals (O'Donoghue and Sander 1997). Risk factors for SUDEP include poorly controlled seizures, generalized tonic-clonic seizures, symptomatic epilepsy, male gender, and medication noncompliance. Sudden death is more common in adolescents and young adults than in other age groups. The pathophysiology of SUDEP is unknown, although central apnea and seizure-induced cardiac arrhythmias have been suggested and pulmonary edema is a constant pathological finding.

### Epilepsy Surgery

Surgical treatment is considered when seizures prove refractory to adequate medication trials and a well-defined epileptogenic focus is identified, the resection of which is unlikely to result in significant neurological impairment. Patients with idiopathic generalized epilepsy, benign childhood epilepsy, progressive diseases, and significant medication noncompliance are not considered surgical candidates. Mental retardation, psychiatric disease, and the coexistence of epileptic and nonepileptic seizures are not absolute contraindications. Dominant hemisphere seizure origin, bilateral or multifocal epileptic discharges on EEG, and neurological deficits on examination should not preclude surgical consideration. Rarely, surgery is considered in patients with seizures arising from more than one epileptogenic focus. Surgery should be performed as early as possible, since intractable seizures portend a poor prognosis for seizure remission and psychosocial outcome. Once adequate trials of several first-line AEDs prove ineffective, the likelihood of improvement with adjunctive agents is low.

Anterior temporal lobectomy is the most common surgical procedure for the treatment of intractable epilepsy in adolescents and adults. The resection typically includes the anterior 3.0 to 3.5 cm of the inferior and middle temporal gyri, uncus, part of the amygdala, and the anterior 2.0 to 3.0 cm of the hippocampus and adjacent parahippocampal gyrus. In patients with mesial temporal sclerosis, selective amygdalohippocampectomy is an alternate surgical approach. Lesionectomy, with preservation of the mesial temporal structures, may be indicated in patients with temporal lobe lesions without evidence of mesial temporal involvement. Language mapping is required when lesions are located in or near the language cortex. A seizure-free state is achieved in 60% to 70% of patients, although auras may persist (Engel et al. 1993). Material-specific memory deficits are common after unilateral temporal lobectomy and are dependent on the functional adequacy of the resected hippocampus (Chelune 1995). The risk of significant verbal memory impairment after dominant temporal lobectomy is greatest in patients with intact memory function preoperatively and normal hippocampal tissue on pathology. Decrements in nonverbal memory after nondominant temporal lobe resection are less consistently observed and tend to be milder or clinically asymptomatic. Transient dysphasia is observed in 12% of patients after dominant temporal lobe resection (Popovic et al. 1995). A contralateral superior quadranopsia after temporal lobectomy is observed in over 50% of cases, but this is typically asymptomatic. Rare complications include hemiparesis that is usually transient, psychiatric disturbances, hematoma, meningitis, and diplopia due to third or fourth cranial neuropathy.

The procedure of choice for patients with extratemporal epilepsy is the complete resection of the lesion producing seizures and the surrounding epileptogenic cortex. This is the most common type of epilepsy surgery performed during infancy and early childhood. Subtotal removal of a structural lesion is associated with a lower likelihood of seizure remission. Patients with nonlesional extratemporal epilepsy generally require intracranial monitoring to delineate the epileptogenic zone, and cortical mapping if the proposed resection is located in or near eloquent cortex. Surgical outcome in these cases depends on the certainty with which the epileptogenic zone is defined and the completeness of the resection (Lüders and Awad 1991). Only 25% to 35% of patients with nonlesional epilepsy become seizure free and another 20% to 45% have a significant reduction in seizures (Benbadis et al. 1996). After complete resection of tumors and vascular malformations (lesionectomy), two-thirds of patients become seizure free, over 20% are significantly improved, and approximately 12% are unchanged (Engel 1993). Resections of the perirolandic region can produce motor and sensory deficits of the face and extremities. Transient or permanent aphasia is produced following resections in or near Broca's area. Supplementary sensorimotor area resection may produce transient mutism and paralysis. In these cases, cortical mapping is performed to identify eloquent areas so that deficits are minimized.

Hemispherectomy is indicated in patients with intractable partial and secondary generalized seizures in whom an entire hemisphere is considered epileptogenic, with little or no remaining functional cortex. The procedure is usually performed in patients with Rasmussen's encephalitis, Sturge-Weber syndrome, hemimegancephaly, or large hemispheric infarctions. Functional hemispherectomy is the removal of the central region and temporal lobe with complete disconnection of the remaining cortex and corpus callosum. This procedure is an alternative to total hemispherectomy and has a lower risk of complications. In patients with intact visual fields and some motor function of the contralateral limbs, homonymous hemianopsia and hemiplegia are usually produced. Hemorrhage, hydrocephalus, and infection in the immediate postoperative period occur rarely after hemispherectomy. Superficial cerebral hemosiderosis is a late, and sometimes fatal, complication of a total hemispherectomy, occurring in 15% to 30% of patients (Villemure 1996). The incidence of late hydrocephalus after total hemispherectomy is 18% (Villemure 1996). Seizures are completely abolished in nearly 80% of patients and significantly reduced in 15% (Villemure 1996). Significant improvements in psychosocial development are observed, particularly in those rendered seizure free.

Corpus callosotomy should be considered in patients with medically refractory secondary generalized tonic-clonic, tonic, and atonic seizures that lead to falls and injuries when focal cortical resection and hemispherectomy are not options. This procedure is most commonly performed in patients with multiple seizure types, such as in the Lennox-Gastaut syndrome. The goal of the procedure is to disrupt the major central pathways necessary for the propagation of generalized seizures. Complete callosal section may result in mutism, apraxia, or frontal lobe dysfunction. For this reason, the procedure is often performed in two stages beginning with sectioning of the anterior two-thirds followed by transection of the remainder of the corpus callosum, if necessary. Postoperative complications include aseptic or bacterial meningitis, hydrocephalus, superior sagittal sinus tear with bleeding, cerebral edema, and frontal lobe venous infarction. Approximately two-thirds of patients experience a significant reduction in seizures but only 11% are rendered seizure free (Wyler 1996).

## References

Aicardi, J. Early myoclonic encephalopathy. In: Roger, J.; Bureau, M.; Dravet, C.; Dreifuss, F. E.; Perret, A.; Wolf, P., eds. Epileptic syndromes in infancy, childhood, and adolescence. 2nd ed. London: John Libbey & Company Ltd.; 1992: p. 13–24.

Annegers, J. F. The epidemiology of epilepsy. In: Wyllie, E., ed. The treatment of epilepsy: principles and practice. 2nd ed. Baltimore: Williams & Wilkins; 1996; p. 165–177.

Beaumanoir, A. The Landau-Kleffner syndrome. In: Roger, J.; Bureau, M.; Dravet, C.; Dreifuss, F. E.; Perret, A.; Wolf, P., eds. Epileptic syndromes in infancy, childhood, and adolescence. 2nd ed. London: John Libbey & Company Ltd.; 1992: p. 231–243.

Beaumanoir, A.; Dravet, C. The Lennox-Gastaut syndrome. In: Roger, J.; Bureau, M.; Dravet, C.; Dreifuss, F. E.; Perret, A.; Wolf, P., eds. Epileptic syndromes in infancy, childhood, and adolescence. 2nd ed. London: John Libbey & Company Ltd.; 1992: p. 115–132.

Benbadis, S. R.; Chelune, G. J.; Stanford, L. D.; et al. Outcome and complications of epilepsy surgery. In: Wyllie, E., ed. The treatment of epilepsy: principles and practice, 2nd ed. Baltimore: Williams & Wilkins; 1996; p. 1103–1118.

Berg, A. T.; Shinnar S. The risk of seizure recurrence following a first unprovoked seizure: a quantitative review. Neurology 41:965–972; 1991.

Berkovic, S. F.; Cochius, J.; Andermann, E. Progressive myoclonus epilepsies: clinical and genetic aspects. Epilepsia 34(suppl. 3):19–30; 1993.

Bouma, P. A. D.; Westendrop, R. G. J.; van Dijk, J. G. The outcome of absence epilepsy: a meta-analysis. Neurology 47:802–808; 1996.

Chadwick, D.; Taylor, J.; Johnson, T. Outcomes after seizure recurrence in people with well-controlled epilepsy and the factors that influence it. Epilepsia 37:1043–1050; 1996.

Chelune, G. J. Hippocampal adequacy versus functional reserve: predicting memory functions following temporal lobectomy. Arch. Clin. Neuropsychol. 10:413–432; 1995.

Cockerell, O. C.; Johnson, A. L.; Sander, J. W. A. S.; et al. Prognosis of epilepsy: a review and further analysis of the first nine years of the British General Practice Study of Epilepsy, a prospective population-based study. Epilepsia 38:31–46; 1997.

Commission on Classification and Terminology of the International League Against Epilepsy. Proposal for revised clinical and electrographic classification of epileptic seizures. Epilepsia 22:489–501; 1981.

Commission on Classification and Terminology of the International League Against Epilepsy. Proposal for revised classification of epilepsies and epileptic syndromes. Epilepsia 30:389–399; 1989.

Delgado-Escueta, A. V.; Janz, D. Consensus guidelines: preconception counseling, management, and care of the pregnant woman with epilepsy. Neurology 42 (suppl. 5):149–160; 1992.

DeLorenzo, R. J.; Hauser, W. A.; Towne, A. R. A prospective, population-based epidemiologic study of status epilepticus in Richmond, Virginia. Neurology 46:1029–1035; 1996.

DeLorenzo, R. J.; Towne, A. R.; Pellock, J. M. Status epilepticus in children, adults, and the elderly. Epilepsia 33(suppl. 4):15–25; 1992.

Doose, H. Myoclonic-astatic epilepsy of early childhood. In: Roger, J.; Bureau, M.; Dravet, C.; Dreifuss, F. E.; Perret, A.; Wolf, P., eds. Epileptic syndromes in infancy, childhood, and adolescence. 2nd ed. London: John Libbey & Company Ltd.; 1992: p. 103–114.

Dravet, C.; Bureau, M.; Guerrini, R.; et al. Severe myoclonic epilepsy in infancy. In: Roger, J.; Bureau, M.; Dravet, C.; Dreifuss, F. E.; Perret, A.; Wolf, P., eds. Epileptic syndromes in infancy, childhood, and adolescence. 2nd ed. London: John Libbey & Company Ltd.; 1992b: p. 75–88.

Dravet, C; Bureau, M; Roger, J. Benign myoclonic epilepsy in infancy. In: Roger, J.; Bureau, M.; Dravet, C.; Dreifuss, F. E.; Perret, A.; Wolf, P., eds. Epileptic syndromes in infancy, childhood, and adolescence. 2nd ed. London: John Libbey & Company Ltd.; 1992a: p. 67–74.

Duchowny, M. Febrile seizures in childhood. In: Wyllie, E., ed. The treatment of epilepsy: principles and practice. 2nd ed. Baltimore: Williams & Wilkins, 1996; p. 622–628.

Dulac, O.; Plouin, P.; Schlumberger, E. Infantile spasms. In: Wyllie, E., ed. The treatment of epilepsy: principles and practice. 2nd ed. Baltimore, Williams & Wilkins, 1996: p. 540–572.

Engel, J., Jr.; Van Ness, P. C.; Rasmussen, T. B.; et al. Outcome with respect to epileptic seizures. In: Engel, J., Jr., ed. Surgical treatment of the epilepsies. 2nd ed. New York: Raven Press; 1993: p. 609–621.

Farrell, K. Symptomatic generalized epilepsy and Lennox-Gastaut syndrome. In: Wyllie, E., ed. The treatment of epilepsy: principles and practice. 2nd ed. Baltimore: Williams & Wilkins, 1996: p. 530–538.

First Seizure Trial Group. Randomized clinical trial of the efficacy of antiepileptic drugs in reducing the risk of relapse after a first unprovoked tonic-clonic seizure. Neurology 43:478–483; 1993.

Freeman, J. M. Febrile seizures: a consensus of their significance, evaluation, and treatment. Pediatrics 66:1009–1012; 1980.

Hauser, W. A.; Herdorffer, D. C. The natural history of seizures. In: Wyllie, E., ed. The treatment of epilepsy: principles and practice. 2nd ed. Baltimore: Williams & Wilkins, 1996: p. 173–178.

Holmes, G. L.; Lombroso, C. T. Prognostic value of background patterns in the neonatal EEG. J. Clin. Neurophysiol. 10:323–352; 1993.

Isojärvi, J. I.; Raättyä, J.; Myllylä, V. V.; et al. Valproate, lamotrigine, and insulin-mediated risks in women with epilepsy. Ann. Neurol. 43:446–451; 1998.

Jaitly, R.; Sgro, J. A.; Towne, A. R.; et al. Prognostic value of EEG monitoring after status epilepticus: a prospective adult study. J. Clin. Neurophysiol. 14:326–334; 1997.

Janz, D. Juvenile myoclonic epilepsy. Cleve. Clin. J. Med. 56 (suppl. 1):23–33; 1989.

Jeavons, P. M.; Livet, M. O. West syndrome: infantile spasms. In: Roger, J.; Bureau, M.; Dravet, C.; Dreifuss, F. E.; Perret, A.; Wolf, P., eds. Epileptic syndromes in infancy, childhood, and adolescence.

2nd ed. London: John Libbey & Company Ltd.; 1992: p. 53–65.

Legido, A.; Clancy, R. R.; Berman, P. H. Recent advances in the diagnosis, treatment, and prognosis of neonatal seizures. Pediatr. Neurol. 4:79–86; 1988.

Lesser, R. Psychogenic seizures. Neurology 46:1499–1507; 1996.

Loiseau, P. Childhood absence epilepsy. In: Roger, J.; Bureau, M.; Dravet, C.; Dreifuss, F. E.; Perret, A.; Wolf, P., eds. Epileptic syndromes in infancy, childhood, and adolescence. 2nd ed. London: John Libbey & Company Ltd.; 1992: p. 135–150.

Loiseau, P. Benign focal epilepsies of childhood. In: Wyllie, E., ed. The treatment of epilepsy: principles and practice. 2nd ed. Baltimore: Williams & Wilkins, 1996: p. 442–450.

Loiseau, P.; Duché, B.; Cordova, S. Prognosis of benign childhood epilepsy with centrotemporal spikes: a follow-up study of 168 patients. Epilepsia 29:229–235; 1988.

Lüders, H. O.; Awad, I. Conceptual considerations. In: epilepsy surgery. Lüders, H., ed. New York: Raven Press; 1991: p. 51–62.

Mattson, R. H.; Cramer, J. A.; Collins, J. F.; et al. Comparison of carbamazepine, phenobarbital, phenytoin, and primidone in partial and secondarily generalized tonic-clonic seizures. N. Engl. J. Med. 313:145–151; 1985.

Mattson, R. H.; Cramer, J. A.; Collins, J. F.; et al. A comparison of valproate with carbamazepine for the treatment of complex partial seizures and secondarily generalized tonic-clonic seizures in adults. N. Engl. J. Med. 327:765–771; 1992.

Mattson, R. H.; Cramer, J. A.; Collins, J. F.; et al. Prognosis for total control of complex partial and secondarily generalized tonic clonic seizures. Neurology 47:68–76; 1996.

Medical Research Council Antiepileptic Drug Withdrawal Study Group. Randomized study of antiepileptic drug withdrawal in patients in remission. Lancet 337:1175–1180; 1991.

Mikati, M.; Holmes, G. Temporal lobe epilepsy. In: Wyllie, E., ed. The treatment of epilepsy: principles and practice. 2nd edition. Baltimore, Williams & Wilkins, 1996: p. 401–414.

Mizrahi, E. M.; Kellaway, P. Characterization and classification of neonatal seizures. Neurology 37:1837–1844; 1987.

Musicco, M.; Beghi, E.; Solari, A.; et al. treatment of first tonic-clonic seizure does not improve the prognosis of epilepsy. Neurology 49:991–998; 1997.

Nelson, K. F.; Ellenberg, J. H. Predictors of epilepsy in children who have experienced febrile seizures. N. Engl. J. Med. 295: 1029–1033; 1976.

O'Donoghue, M. F.; Sander, J. W. A. S. The mortality associated with epilepsy, with particular reference to sudden unexpected death: a review. Epilepsia 38 (suppl. 11): S15–S19; 1997.

Oguni, H.; Hayashi, K.; Osawa, M. Long-term prognosis of Lennox-Gastaut syndrome. Epilepsia 37 (suppl. 3): 44–47; 1996.

Ohtahara, S.; Ohtsuka, Y.; Yamatogi, Y. In: Roger, J.; Bureau, M.; Dravet, C.; Dreifuss, F. E.; Perret, A.; Wolf, P., eds. Epileptic syndromes in infancy, childhood, and adolescence. 2nd ed. London: John Libbey & Company Ltd.; 1992: p. 25–34.

Plouin, P. Benign idiopathic neonatal convulsions. In: Roger, J.; Bureau, M.; Dravet, C.; Dreifuss, F. E.; Perret, A.; Wolf, P., eds. Epileptic syndromes in infancy, childhood, and adolescence. 2nd ed. London: John Libbey & Company Ltd.; 1992: p. 3–12.

Popovic, E. A.; Fabinyi, G. C. A.; Brazenor, G. A.; et al. Temporal lobectomy for epilepsy: complications in 200 patients. J. Clin. Neurosci. 2:238–244; 1995.

Sander, J. W. A. S. Some aspects of prognosis in the epilepsies: a review. Epilepsia 34:1007–1016; 1993.

Scher, M. S. Neonatal seizures. In: Wyllie, E., ed. The treatment of epilepsy: principles and practice. 2nd ed. Baltimore: Williams & Wilkins, 1996: p. 600–621.

Shorvon, S. D.; Sander, J. W. A. S. Temporal patterns of remission and relapse in patients with severe epilepsy. In: Schmidt, D.; Morceli, P., eds. Intractable epilepsy. New York: Raven Press; 1986: p. 13–23.

So, N. K. Recurrence, remission, and relapse of seizures. Cleve. Clin. J. Med. 60:439–444; 1993.

Tassinari, C. A.; Bureau, M.; Thomas P. Epilepsy with myoclonic absences. In: Roger, J.; Bureau, M.; Dravet, C.; Dreifuss, F. E.; Perret, A.; Wolf, P., eds. Epileptic syndromes in infancy, childhood, and adolescence. 2nd ed. London: John Libbey & Company Ltd.; 1992a: p. 151–160.

Tassinari, C. A.; Bureau, M.; Dravet, C.; et al. Epilepsy with continuous spikes and waves during sleep. In: Roger, J.; Bureau, M.; Dravet, C.; Dreifuss, F. E.; Perret, A.; Wolf, P., eds. Epileptic syndromes in infancy, childhood, and adolescence. 2nd ed. London: John Libbey & Company Ltd.; 1992b: p. 245–256.

Villemure, J. G. Hemispherectomy: techniques and complications. In: Wyllie, E., ed. The treatment of epilepsy: principles and practice. 2nd ed. Baltimore: Williams & Wilkins, 1996: p. 1081–1086.

Wirrell, E. C.; Camfield, C. S.; Camfield, P. R. Long-term prognosis of typical childhood absence epilepsy: remission or progression to juvenile myoclonic epilepsy. Neurology 47:912–918; 1996.

Wolf, P. Juvenile myoclonic epilepsy. In: Roger, J.; Bureau, M.; Dravet, C.; Dreifuss, F. E.; Perret, A.; Wolf, P., eds. Epileptic syndromes in infancy, childhood, and adolescence. 2nd ed. London: John Libbey & Company Ltd.; 1992a: p. 313–327.

Wolf, P. Epilepsy with grand mal on awakening. In: Roger, J.; Bureau, M.; Dravet, C.; Dreifuss, F. E.; Perret, A.; Wolf, P., eds. Epileptic syndromes in infancy, childhood, and adolescence. 2nd ed. London: John Libbey & Company Ltd.; 1992b: p. 329–341.

Wyler, A. R. Corpus callosotomy. In: Wyllie, E., ed. The treatment of epilepsy: principles and practice. 2nd ed. Baltimore: Williams & Wilkins, 1996: p. 1097–1102.

Yerby, M. Pregnancy and epilepsy. Epilepsia. 32 (suppl. 6):S51–S59; 1991.

# 39

## Sleep Disorders

ANTONIO CULEBRAS

Sleep is a function of the brain, and disorders of sleep are mostly disorders of brain function. Sleep and its disorders have become a clinical discipline, in part because of growing research into the sources of sleep as a function of the brain, and in part because of recent therapies that restore quality to nocturnal sleep and the ensuing daytime vigilance. Job performance, work productivity, and transportation safety depend largely on mind alertness, an attribute of consciousness subsidiary to nocturnal sleep. Sleep medicine revolves around the sleep center. In a typical laboratory the largest contingent of patients is referred for evaluation of snoring and sleep apnea (70%), while excessive somnolence represents 10%, insomnia 10%, and the rest are miscellaneous conditions where parasomnias and alleged seizure disorders predominate. Erectile impotence is only studied in specialized laboratories. Pediatric sleep medicine is a highly specialized section that can only be practiced under the leadership of a trained pediatrician. The assortment of patients is served by sleep specialists with different backgrounds. The American Sleep Disorders Association (ASDA) (renamed American Academy of Sleep Medicine, June 1999) documented in 1998 the following breakdown of primary specialization for sleep specialists: pulmonary medicine 36%, neurology 24%, psychiatry 7%, otolaryngology 8%, psychology 5%, dentistry 4%, pediatrics 3%, internal medicine 10%, and other 3%.

### Sleepiness: Causes and Consequences

Sleepiness is defined as the tendency to fall asleep. Sleepiness is the physiological consequence of sleep deprivation and the pathological manifestation of various sleep disorders. When excessive, undesirable, inappropriate, or unexplained, sleepiness often indicates a clinical disorder. The patient with sleepiness tends to be passive and compliant, unlike the patient with insomnia who is angry and vocal about the frustration with sleep. Inappropriate and excessive somnolence erodes professional achievement, reduces productivity, disturbs social liaisons, affects family life, and prevents academic advancement. Furthermore, it can lead to traffic accidents and increase the risk of work-related injuries. Inappropriate sleepiness and excessive sleep or hypersomnia should be considered manifestations of neurological dysfunction and a psychosocial handicap that can be identified and measured by polysomnography and the multiple sleep latency state (MSLT).

The clinician confronted with a patient complaining of excessive sleepiness must consider the diagnoses listed in Table 39-1 in the differential diagnosis of its causes and probably resort to polysomnography for a proper resolution of the diagnostic dilemma. Some patients suffer excessive daytime sleepiness and appear to need more sleep than the norm for reasons that are not obvious. Their hypersomnia is the result of some disorder of the central nervous system (CNS) that eludes us. These patients have primary hypersomnia that should be distinguished from other disorders also featuring hypersomnia that are clearly the consequence of a factor external to the sleep mechanisms. Narcolepsy, idiopathic hypersomnia, and the periodic hypersomnias are examples of primary conditions, whereas the sleepiness of the sleep apnea syndrome and that associated with sleep deprivation are classical examples of secondary hypersomnias.

The sleep specialist tends to see more patients with excessive daytime sleepiness than with insomnia despite the fact that the prevalence of the insomnias is higher. This trend is an indication of the patient's concern about his or her ability to function, the chronic discomfort suffered, and the perceived danger when driving. It has been estimated that excessive daytime sleepiness occurs in 2% to 10% of the population or 5 to 25 million persons in the United Sates (Lemmi 1995).

Chronic sleep deprivation as a result of insufficient nocturnal sleep may be the most common cause of subtle and even moderately excessive somnolence in the productive years of life. Sleep loss may be total, partial, or stage-specific; the immediate manifestation is sleepiness. The effect of rapid-eye-movement (REM) sleep deprivation on

**Table 39-1.** Diagnostic Symptoms Associated With Sleepiness

| | | |
|---|---|---|
| Poor sleep hygiene | ----> | Sleep deprivation |
| Very loud snoring | ----> | Sleep apnea |
| Nap dreaming | ----> | Narcolepsy |
| Cataplexy | ----> | Narcolepsy |
| Unrefreshing naps | ----> | Idiopathic hypersomnia |
| Intermittent sleepiness | ----> | Periodic hypersomnia |
| Very late hours | ----> | Phase-delayed syndrome |
| Head trauma | ----> | Post-traumatic hypersomnia |
| Neurological disorder | \| | |
| Psychiatric alteration | \|-----\ secondary | |
| Medical disorder | \|-----/ hypersomnia | |
| Pharmacological abuse | \| | |

From Culebras (1996b).

mental functions and personality characteristics is elusive. Some studies have shown enhanced drive of food and sexual appetite, increased aggression and restlessness, but no psychopathology. Animal tests have shown that REM sleep deprivation results in decreased memory retention, but human tests have been less explicit.

Selective deprivation of slow-wave sleep (SWS) causes a rebound of stage 4 on the first recovery night (Agnew et al. 1964) and, interestingly, an increase in REM sleep on the second and third night, a phenomenon that might have some parallels in clinical practice. Tests have failed to show a decrement in daytime performance following SWS deprivation.

The person deprived of total sleep develops over time a decrease in alertness and performance that is modulated by the circadian rhythm. Mood changes including irritability, fatigue, difficulty in concentration, and disorientation are commonly reported. Short-term memory alterations also appear as a result of decreased attention, concentration lapses, decreased motivation, and general difficulty to encode elements presented to memory. Early manifestations of psychopathology are more pronounced in individuals with a premorbid personality. Illusions, hallucinations, visual misperceptions and paranoid ideation are thus observed with sleep loss. Subtle neurological manifestations such as horizontal nystagmus, intermittent slurring of speech, hand tremor, increased deep tendon reflexes, and increased sensitivity to pain have been described following more than 205 hours of sleep deprivation (Kollar et al. 1968). Under such conditions the electroencephalogram (EEG) has shown unsustained alpha rhythms (Naitoh et al. 1969) and lack of facilitation of alpha activity with eye closure, along with modest increases of intermixed slowing in the theta and delta range. Microsleeps have been identified by performance errors associated with episodes of slowing of the EEG.

Partial sleep loss studies in humans suggest that the main sleep requirement can be accomplished with 4 to 5 hours of sleep every 24 hours. Further decrements of sleep accumulated over several weeks begin to erode motor and mental performance. There is a difference between the required amount of sleep, perhaps 4 to 5 hours, and the desired amount that in most individuals revolves around 8 to 9 hours per 24 hours. It has been estimated that 17 hours of sustained wakefulness decrease performance as much as a blood alcohol concentration of 0.05 per cent, or two 45-ml drinks of spirits (Dawson and Reid 1997). This concentration marks the legal limit for driving in some European countries.

A poor sleep hygiene, continued detraction of nocturnal sleep, loss of circadian rhythmicity, and lack of respect for the sleep needs eventually lead to a state of sleep debt that is manifested by chronic fatigue and sleepiness. Twenty million night-shift workers in the United States are probably sleep deprived and suffer the manifestations of chronic sleepiness. The number of people who are sleep deprived because of poor sleep hygiene is unknown. Teenagers and college students are particularly vulnerable. It has been estimated that 40% of high-school and college students are seriously sleep deprived (Carskadon and Dement 1981; Carskadon 1990).

Sleepiness may lead to transportation and industrial accidents. A study in Great Britain estimated that 27% of drivers who lost consciousness while driving and had an accident had fallen asleep and that these drivers accounted for 83% of fatalities (Parsons 1986). In New York State 25% of 1000 drivers randomly polled in 1994 admitted falling asleep while driving at some point in their lifetime (The New York State Governor's Task Force on Sleepiness/Fatigue and Driving 1994; McCartt et al. 1996). Half of the group admitted driving very often in a state of drowsiness during the previous year. Only a small percentage (4.7%) were involved in a crash, but extrapolation of the figures suggests that 2500 accidents per year in New York alone are caused by mental fatigue and drowsiness. Nationwide, the National Highway Traffic Safety Administration reported 50,000 crashes in 1992 or 1% of the total caused by drowsiness (National Highway Traffic Safety Administration General Estimates System 1992), a figure that likely falls short of reality, since drowsiness can only be determined indirectly by exclusion of other factors such as weather conditions, alcohol intoxication, medication effect, rage, and so on. Furthermore, traffic officers are not conventionally trained to identify mental fatigue as a probable cause of accident. The profile of the driver who falls asleep at the wheel, the circumstances of the accident and the factors that lead to it have been defined in various studies

(The New York State Governor's Task Force on Sleepiness/Fatigue and Driving 1994; National Highway Traffic Safety Administration General Estimates System 1992). Drivers are usually young (62% <30 years), male (77%), driving alone (66%) for over 4 hours, at night or following the night shift. Shift workers, hospital staff, and commercial drivers are at higher risk than other workers. A study in long-haul truck drivers has shown that the greatest vulnerability to sleep or sleep-like states occurs in the late night and early morning (Mitler et al. 1997).

Commercial drivers suffer fewer accidents, but when it happens the scope of the accident is of larger magnitude; 4800 fatal accidents involve trucks each year in the United States and 57% are probably caused by mental fatigue or performance failure highly suggestive of drowsiness (National Transportation Safety Board 1990). Obese long-haul truck drivers have two times more accidents per mile driven than nonobese truck drivers, a phenomenon that suggests a background factor, perhaps sleep apnea, causing excessive sleepiness in obese drivers (Stoohs et al. 1994).

Patients with sleep disorders such as sleep apnea and narcolepsy constitute a small segment of the population with a high risk of accident. In a review of 424 adults with a sleep disorder and sleep-related accidents compared with 70 adults who suffered a sleep-related accident but had no sleep disorder, Aldrich (1989) found that the hypersomnolent group had a 1.5 to 4 times greater risk of being involved in an accident. Narcoleptics had the highest incidence of accidents.

## Narcolepsy

Gélineau a French neuropsychiatrist described the condition in 1880 (Gélineau 1880a, 1880b) and called it narcolepsy, meaning in Greek "seized by somnolence." Narcolepsy is a disorder dominated by persistent, unrelenting daytime sleepiness that is alleviated transiently by short naps. Patients with narcolepsy may have other manifestations that include cataplexy or abrupt generalized muscle weakness triggered by emotions; hallucinations upon falling asleep or waking up; sleep paralysis and, ironically may present to their physician complaining of inability to maintain nocturnal sleep.

The etiology of narcolepsy remains unknown. Predisposing genetic factors are evidenced by the fact that 85% or more of all narcoleptic patients with definite cataplexy share a specific HLA allele, HLA-DQB10602, most often in combination with HLA-DR2 (human leukocyte antigen) (Mignot 1998). One percent to 2% of first-degree relatives of narcolepsy patients manifest the sleep disorder, which is 10 to 40 times higher than in the general population. Environmental factors must also be important when epidemiological studies indicate that only 25% to 31% of monozygotic twins are concordant for narcolepsy (Mignot 1998).

The family history of narcoleptics is commonly positive for excessive daytime sleepiness, but when relatives are objectively tested only 3% show polygraphic evidence of narcolepsy (Guilleminault et al. 1989). The risk of developing narcolepsy in children of one narcoleptic parent is 1%. Some patients with narcolepsy have associated diseases of an immunoallergic nature such as asthma and lupus erythematosus leading to the suspicion of an autoimmune disorder. This relationship is reinforced by the linkage that exists between narcolepsy and the antigen HLA-DR2, the strongest association between this antigen and any disorder so far discovered (Kramer et al. 1987). Some patients with narcolepsy lack either antigen, indicating that it is not necessary for expression of the disease.

With a prevalence estimated at 1 in 3000 individuals in North America, narcolepsy may be more common than multiple sclerosis. The condition remains underdiagnosed despite expanding publicity and increasing general perception of sleepiness as a clinical alteration. It takes more than three physician referrals to diagnose the condition. Most sleep laboratories record the experience of diagnosing narcolepsy in old persons who recount a history of sleepiness going back to their teenage years. Narcolepsy is more commonly diagnosed in North America, where public education in sleep disorders is more prevalent and sleep laboratory evaluations are more available. Men and women are equally affected and the age of onset occurs in the second or third decade of life. Narcolepsy may appear in prepubertal children as young as 2 years. In a recent study (Guilleminault and Pelayo 1998) prepubertal narcolepsy represented 5% of the total narcoleptic database. This group is particularly vulnerable to misdiagnoses, depression, and behavioral problems.

**Clinical Manifestations**

The sleepiness of narcolepsy is similar to the sleepiness of other disorders of sleep. The difference is that patients with narcolepsy may become dysfunctional with sleepiness and actually fall asleep more often against their desire, creating a risk of accident or contravening common rules of behavior. Falling asleep at work, while talking on the phone, or when eating at the table is unacceptable and may generate unfortunate lasting consequences. Despite persistent sleepiness, patients with narcolepsy do not exhibit excessive time asleep.

Chronic sleepiness is responsible for poor job performance, scholastic failure, family pathology, and accidents. Like other individuals with unsatisfied sleep needs, patients with narcolepsy show irritability, lack of motivation, unexplained mood changes, and general social decline. Patients with severe forms of sleepiness may continue functioning at a low level of performance in automatic behavior that underlies occurrences such as irrational notes taken by a sleepy student in class, or the unexplained packing of laundry in the dishwasher by a confused housewife. Automatic behavior is not exclusive of narcolepsy but is a common experience in untreated patients. Nocturnal insomnia is paradoxically common in patients with narcolepsy and nocturnal sleep is fragmented and unrefreshing in many, a phenomenon that undoubtedly contributes to daytime sleepiness. Patients with narcolepsy frequently complain of restlessness at night and some show early REM sleep without atonia that facilitates motor activity and acting out of dreams.

The risk of being involved in a traffic accident is high as a result of falling asleep at the wheel, an occurrence acknowledged by two-thirds of patients with narcolepsy. In a comparison of driving records performed in 1984, narcoleptics exhibited poorer outcomes than epileptics (Broughton et al. 1984). In a separate study Broughton et al. (1981) noted 37% of accidents reported by narcoleptics versus 5% by control subjects. Some legislations have regulated the conditions under which patients with narcolepsy may drive commercial and noncommercial vehicles (Pakola et al. 1995). In California a driver's license may be revoked if narcolepsy is out of control. In six states (California, Maryland, North Carolina, Oregon, Texas, and Utah) there are regulations for commercial and noncommercial drivers regarding narcolepsy. Commercial drivers with a history of narcolepsy are prohibited from operating a vehicle in Texas. Oregon has regulated that patients may not drive until the condition has been satisfactorily controlled as judged by a physician. The legislation regarding sleepiness and specifically narcolepsy is in a state of flux and concerned drivers should check with the Motor Vehicles Department.

Cataplexy is the sudden loss of muscle tone associated with weakness involving all voluntary muscles of the body except the oculomotor muscles and diaphragm. Episodes of cataplexy last a few seconds to several minutes and are not accompanied by loss of consciousness. Typically, cataplectic events are precipitated by laughter, excitement, emotion, stress, and startle. Severe events are followed by sleep and vivid dreaming. Patients may suffer as many as four or five episodes daily, or as few as one or two per month. Cataplexy is absent in *monosymptomatic narcolepsy,* although some patients may still develop cataplexy as many as 40 years after the onset of sleepiness.

Sleep paralysis is the inability to move during sleep or upon awakening lasting a few seconds to a few minutes. Patients are aware and struggle to escape the uncomfortable feeling. Sleep paralysis may be associated with hallucinations that are called hypnagogic if occurring at sleep onset and hypnopompic if at termination of sleep. Sleep paralysis may occur in the absence of narcolepsy.

Hypnagogic and hypnopompic hallucinations are classically associated with narcolepsy but are not specific for the disorder and may occur in other sleep disorders. A recent epidemiological study conducted in the United Kingdom found that 41% of the general population reported having hypnagogic hallucinations and 12% hypnopompic hallucinations at least once per year (Ohayon et al. 1996).

Failing grades, work impairment, a history of falling asleep on the job, and loss of productivity punctuate the history of psychosocial decline or arrested advancement, so common in patients with narcolepsy. Depression has a prevalence of 30% (Kales et al. 1982), perhaps as a by-product of the psychosocial impact of suffering the condition.

Patients with narcolepsy may be misdiagnosed as schizophrenics if the complaints of hallucinations are taken out of context. The psychosocial impact of narcolepsy is worse if the condition remains undiagnosed and untreated. With appropriate intervention the negative impact on students can be minimized (Douglas 1998). Socioeconomic effects at the workplace include decreased quality of work, reduced earning capacity, lack of promotion, and actual dismissal. In a study of 50 narcoleptics with sleep attacks and cataplexy (Godbout and Montplaisir 1986) 92% reported work-related problems, 80% had fallen asleep at work on several occasions according to their own testimony, while 24% quit their job and 18% said they had been fired. Marital strife has been reported in 72% of subjects with narcolepsy (Kales et al. 1982) and 20% attributed their divorce to the direct effects of the condition on family life.

*Symptomatic narcolepsy* is rare and associated with lesions of the upper brain stem and floor of the third ventricle (Aldrich and Naylor 1989). Imaging studies have shown a variety of lesions invading the diencephalon including glioma, glioblastoma, gliosis, sarcoidosis, surgical ablation of craniopharyngioma, adenoma, colloid cyst of the third ventricle, and infarct. A recent case report of arteriovenous malformation invading the third ventricle and affecting the hypothalamus described symptomatic improvement following successful treatment of the malformation (Clavelou et al. 1995). The long-term prognosis of patients with symptomatic narcolepsy is dependent on the underlying disorder. Excessive somnolence and inappropriate daytime sleep can occur in patients with multiple sclerosis (Berg and Hanley 1963). In some individuals excessive daytime sleepiness and sleep attacks occur in conjunction with cataplexy, sleep paralysis, and hypnagogic hallucinations leading to a diagnosis of narcolepsy. Midbrain plaques in the hypothalamic periventricular region are often cited as a potential cause of narcolepsy but are seldom seen in multiple sclerosis (Castaigne and Escourolle 1967).

Narcolepsy may develop following a closed head injury in previously asymptomatic patients, a condition that has been termed *secondary narcolepsy* (Lankford et al. 1994). Genetic susceptibility in some patients suggests a dormant condition brought to full clinical expression by the head trauma. However, there are patients who develop excessive daytime somnolence following head trauma who do not have narcolepsy and the specter of litigation obscures the diagnosis (Guilleminault et al. 1983).

All patients newly diagnosed with narcolepsy should undergo a full neurological examination. Brain imaging studies are indicated should focal or lateralizing signs of neurological alteration be present, or when the natural history of the disease takes an unconventional course. Polysomnography is the principal test for the evaluation and diagnosis of narcolepsy. Patients should undergo a nocturnal polygraphic evaluation followed by an MSLT. Using strict criteria, the MSLT has a sensitivity for the diagnosis of narcolepsy of 61% (Aldrich et al. 1995), and a specificity of 97% (Chervin and Aldrich 1995), being similar for narcolepsy with and without cataplexy. Patients clinically suspected of having narcolepsy who do not meet diagnostic criteria on initial polysomnography should undergo additional testing at a subsequent time.

## Treatment

Making an accurate diagnosis enables the physician to counsel the patient and relatives, while avoiding difficulty obtaining stimulant drug treatment from reluctant physicians. Occupational and career counseling should be offered to young patients so that they understand the importance of avoiding sedentary, monotonous work and jobs that involve hazard should they fall asleep.

Behavioral counseling should include a discussion on vehicle driving and sleep hygiene. Patients should understand that if adequately treated, driving is permitted, but only for short distances and limited to daytime hours. When the need arises to drive a long distance, patients are authorized to increase the administration of stimulant medication while making highway stops at 1-hour intervals to take naps if necessary. Some patients with narcolepsy have fragmented nocturnal sleep and prefer to be active at night, taking nocturnal jobs that camouflage their inadequate cycles. Fifteen- to 20-minute naps are refreshing for most narcoleptics if taken at times when the pressure to fall asleep is most intense such as midmorning, after lunch, in midafternoon, and after dinner. Napping regularly cuts down on the amount of stimulant medication required and decreases unscheduled falling asleep. If needed, naps should be prescribed

formally in a prescription form so that patients can present it to their supervisors.

In the absence of major controlled clinical therapeutic trials the treatment of narcolepsy is largely based on consensus of opinions and to a certain extent on the results of a few small studies assessing the effect of drugs on the MSLT and Maintenance of Wakefulness Test (MWT) (Mitler 1994).

In the United States excessive daytime sleepiness is most commonly treated with methylphenidate (Ritalin), dextroamphetamine (Dexedrine), pemoline (Cylert) and modafilin (Provigil). Pemoline is less effective in controlling somnolence as measured by objective MSLT and MWT assessments (Mitler 1994), but has the advantage of not being a controlled drug. It is generally prescribed for patients with mild to moderate forms of excessive sleepiness. In 65% of patients treated with pemoline alone (60 to 200 mg/d) sleepiness was markedly or moderately reduced (Honda and Hishikawa 1980).

Methylphenidate is perhaps the most commonly prescribed drug for narcolepsy in the United States. Doses higher than 65 mg/d provide more stimulant effect but may cause behavioral changes, along with irritability and insomnia that are dose dependent. Tolerance tends to develop with prolonged use of the medication; it can be delayed by starting at the lowest possible dose and escalating slowly over the ensuing months or years. Drug holidays are effective in decreasing tolerance but increase the risk of accident and constitute an annoyance to implement for most patients. According to a 1991 medication survey of the American Narcolepsy Association, 48% of patients with narcolepsy took methylphenidate, versus 28% dextroamphetamine and 17% pemoline (Fry 1998). Marked or moderate improvement in sleep tendency has been experienced by 92% of patients taking methylphenidate (Honda et al. 1979).

Other drugs used in narcolepsy are dextroamphetamine sulfate, methamphetamine, selegiline, and protryptiline also effective in cataplexy. In late 1998 modafinil was approved by the Food and Drug Administration and released for clinical use in the United States to treat somnolence in narcolepsy. The authorized dose is 200 mg taken in the morning to avoid nocturnal fragmentation of sleep.

Despite definite subjective and functional improvement, sleepiness as measured by the MWT and the Epworth Sleepiness Scale (ESS) is not completely normalized with medication in subjects with narcolepsy (Mitler and Hajdukovic 1991). It has been estimated using group means that therapeutic efficacy with amphetamine or methylphenidate reaches 80% of normal values, whereas modafinil reaches 55% and pemoline 53%.

CNS stimulants when taken in large doses may cause side effects that include insomnia, irritability, headache, and in some instances paranoid behavior with rare delusions indistinguishable from paranoid psychosis. The sympathomimetic effects of the amphetamines and derivatives include systolic and diastolic hypertension, variations in heart rate, rarely cardiac arrhythmias, mydriasis, and hyperthermia; at therapeutic doses side effects are rare (Mitler et al. 1993). Intracranial hemorrhage, brain infarction, myocardial infarction, and hypertensive crisis have been reported in drug abusers (Derlet et al. 1989).

Cataplexy is most effectively controlled with tricyclic antidepressants. Protryptiline, (5 to 15 mg in divided doses) is effective in approximately 80% of patients with cataplexy (Aldrich 1992). In Europe, clomipramine (25 to 200 mg/d) is the treatment of choice. Imipramine and fluoxetine are secondary choices. Abrupt discontinuation of anticataplectic drugs may lead to a rebound increase in cataplexy or even to continuous incapacitating cataplexy also known as *status cataplecticus.*

Nocturnal disruption of sleep is a common complaint of many narcoleptics. If the complaint is not resolved by reducing the dose of medication, clonazepam 0.5 mg may be helpful taken at bedtime. In some patients with severely disrupted nocturnal sleep, zolpidem 5–10 mg at bedtime may be tried for short periods of time in an attempt to consolidate nocturnal sleep. γ-Hydroxybutyrate appears to control nocturnal disruption of sleep better than other medications, but the effect is irregular and the substance is not available in the United States.

Some of the behavioral manifestations reported by narcoleptics may be attributed to adverse effects of the medication they take. Guilleminault et al. (1974) noted complaints of decreased libido and disturbed erection in 67% of 50 men treated with imipramine or desipramine. Patients on high doses of stimulant medication report personality

changes in as many as 48% of cases (Broughton et al. 1981).

## Idiopathic Central Nervous System Hypersomnia

This disorder is characterized by the inability to obtain sufficient sleep despite prolonged sleep episodes. Episodes of daytime sleepiness are followed by prolonged nonrestorative naps devoid of dream content. Sleepiness dominates the life of the individual and modifies the behavior. Complaints suggestive of autonomic imbalance are also common; these include nonspecific headaches, orthostatic syncope, and Raynaud's phenomenon.

The cause of the disorder is unknown and its prevalence is variable depending on the criteria used to diagnose it. Some clinicians estimate that 10% of patients referred with a complaint of sleepiness have idiopathic hypersomnia, whereas others indicate that they rarely observe the condition. Idiopathic CNS hypersomnia usually starts in adolescence or early adult life affecting equally men and women. The rate of the familial to the sporadic cases remains unknown.

The diagnosis is made with the help of polysomnography (Bové et al. 1994). Patients with idiopathic hypersomnia may develop secondary psychophysiological manifestations and depression that complicate the diagnostic definition. Post-traumatic hypersomnia may be clinically indistinguishable from idiopathic hypersomnia.

The management of idiopathic hypersomnia follows the same clinical guidelines as in narcolepsy. Counseling is desirable for this lifelong disorder that may be disabling and is poorly responsive to treatment. CNS stimulants pemoline, methylphenidate and dextroamphetamine provide relief of sleepiness, but the response is more irregular and less predictable than in narcolepsy. Complete relief of sleepiness is hardly ever achieved. Naps are not refreshing, but in their absence the patient may feel more sleepy and uncomfortable; proper rules of sleep hygiene should be followed to avoid worsening.

## Snoring and Sleep Apnea

There is a strong liaison between sleep and breathing, such that while the individual is asleep, the pneumotaxic centers of the brain stem assume total control of respiration. Were this to fail, the individual would die asphyxiated in a matter of minutes, an extraordinarily rare occurrence in the adult person. The CNS has interfaced a series of safeguard mechanisms destined to preserve vital functions among which prevails the immediate awakening should respiration be threatened. Ironically, these essential mechanisms reduce the quality of sleep in individuals predisposed to the development of sleep-related respiratory dysfunction.

## Habitual Primary Snoring

Snoring is the act of breathing during sleep with a rough hoarse noise. Habitual snoring occurs in 9% to 24% of middle-aged men and 4% to 14% of middle-aged women (Koskenvuo et al. 1985). Snoring occurs with the turbulent passage of air through a narrow oropharynx causing rough vibration of soft tissues. There is a continuum between heavy snoring and obstructive sleep apnea syndrome. The factors that force the conversion from asymptomatic snoring to sleep apnea have not been worked out, but there is strong evidence that weight gain, alcohol ingestion, drug administration, and progressive age play a significant role. Snoring of loud intensity, persistent occurrence, and irregular quality may be a marker of the sleep apnea syndrome and in consequence a manifestation of disease. As the sleep apnea syndrome worsens and episodes of obstruction become increasingly prolonged, snoring may become intermittent and more sparse.

Snoring is aggravated while sleeping supine and made worse by rhinitis, smoking, alcohol ingestion, administration of CNS depressants, and sleep deprivation. It acquires maximal intensity in stage 4 of sleep and tends to be softer during REM sleep, perhaps because the negative pressures provoked by the effort of the diaphragm are less forceful during REM stage. A similar dissociation is observed in patients with neuromuscular disorders who may have severe sleep apnea syndrome but soft snoring.

Snorers often have to endure marital friction when asked to leave the bed or when abandoned at night by a sleepless spouse. Snoring may be embarrassing particularly when it alters the sleep of other persons in the household and even of neighbors who complain of incessant noise at night.

An association between habitual snoring and hypertension was noted in epidemiological studies conducted in the Republic of San Marino (Lugaresi et al. 1980). When snoring was combined with other risk factors such as male sex, smoking, and obesity, the risk of hypertension was 4.2 times greater and for heart disease 2.0 times greater (Mondini et al. 1983). Snoring has been considered an independent risk factor for stroke and myocardial infarction, perhaps because of the profound hemodynamic alterations that appear with the increased negative intrathoracic pressures of inspiration (Palomaki et al. 1992).

The treatment of snoring should address all risk factors that intervene (obesity, smoking, alcohol ingestion, sedatives, hypnotics, hypothyroidism, acromegaly, and chronic rhinitis). For individuals who snore predominantly while sleeping on their back, a snore ball that trains individuals to sleep on their side is recommended. Oral appliances may be tried in individuals who do not respond to more conservative measures of risk factor control.

*Laser-assisted uvulopalatoplasty (LAUP)* is an office-based procedure for the treatment of habitual snoring that uses carbon dioxide laser beam to vaporize the uvula and adjacent soft-palate tissues. The Standards of Practice Committee of the ASDA has published recommendations shown in Table 39-2 (Standards of Practice Committee of the American Sleep Disorders Association 1994).

*Uvulopalatopharyngoplasty (UPPP)* for the alleviation of snoring in adult patients who have not responded to other less invasive procedures is controversial. In children with loud snoring and

**Table 39-2** Standards of Practice Recommendations for Use of Palatoplasty

---

1. LAUP is not recommended for the treatment of obstructive sleep apnea syndrome for lack of validated data.
2. Surgical candidates for LAUP as a treatment for snoring should undergo nocturnal polysomnography to detect underlying sleep-related breathing disorders.
3. Patients should be informed that the risks, benefits, and complications have not been established.
4. Patients should be informed that snoring is a marker of sleep apnea and its elimination may reduce the chances of diagnosing the disorder at a future time, unless evaluations are performed periodically.
5. The use of narcotics, alcohol, sedatives, and sleeping pills may pose a hazard to patients following the operation, that becomes more pronounced in the immediate postoperative period.

---

From Standards of Practice Committee of the American Sleep Disorders Association (1994).

tonsillar and adenoidal hypertrophy, tonsillectomy and adenoidectomy are followed by a satisfactory and lasting response. Maxillofacial reconstruction is reserved for special circumstances of retrognathia, micrognathia, and stenosis of the hypopharynx with inveterate loud snoring.

## Sleep Apnea Syndromes

Sleep apnea events, whether complete or partial, occur in virtually all men past the age of 45 years and in many women. Disease occurs whenever the frequency and depth of respiratory alterations disturbs sleep architecture, modifies oxygen saturation of circulating hemoglobin, alters cardiac function, or reduces the quality of subsequent vigilance. Some authors (Guilleminault and Partinen 1990) predicate that five or more episodes of apnea, lasting 9 seconds or more, per hour of nocturnal sleep, constitute the threshold beyond which normalcy disappears. However, most patients fail to exhibit clinical manifestations until the frequency of apnea events reaches or surpasses 30 episodes per hour of sleep.

The increasing evidence that advanced obstructive sleep apnea syndrome reduces the quality of life, increases the risk of accident, and constitutes a risk factor for the development of cardiovascular and cerebrovascular disease justifies fully the evaluation of patients suspected of harboring the disorder. Furthermore, available treatments are efficacious and their administration cannot be ignored or missed whenever the opportunity arises.

The most common alteration determining a syndrome of sleep apnea is the partial or complete obstruction of the upper respiratory airway during sleep. Most patients with sleep apnea syndrome breathe without difficulty while awake. Upon falling asleep, one or more factors converge to occlude the upper airway usually at the oropharyngeal level.

Some patients exhibit congenital stenosis of the oropharyngeal opening that diminishes the pharyngeal lumen, or retrognathia that reduces the diameter of the hypopharynx. In other instances the obstructive lesion is acquired, like tonsillar hypertrophy in children, or redundant soft palate and pharyngeal tissues in obese adults. Patients with sleep apnea have more adipose tissue adjacent to the airway than normal subjects, contributing to compression and narrowing of the upper airway (Shelton et al. 1993). Sometimes macroglossia, as observed in hypothyroidism or in acromegaly, may determine the occlusion. But even in the face of anatomical lesions or anomalies, one has to explain why the manifestations of obstruction occur exclusively at night while the individual is asleep. Failure of proper dilation of pharyngeal muscles during the inspiratory act in sleep is the final common pathway upon which converge the factors that determine obstructive sleep apnea syndrome.

### Obstructive Sleep Apnea

This is characterized by the occurrence during sleep of repetitive episodes of respiratory interruption generally associated with a decrease in oxygen saturation of the oxyhemoglobin. Motor restlessness in sleep is a hallmark of the advanced sleep apnea syndrome and patients sometimes fall out of bed, an event that is virtually unique to the condition. Bed partners usually move out of the bedroom to regain the ability to sleep, a situation that leads to family pathology. Ingestion of alcohol, central sedatives, and all hypnotics aggravate all nocturnal manifestations of the patient with sleep apnea syndrome.

In advanced forms, patients may get out of bed and walk out in a state of automatism. Some are found asleep in uncomfortable positions in areas of the house where they do not belong at night. In the morning, patients have difficulty waking up, feeling lethargic and unrefreshed. Morning headaches lasting 30 to 60 minutes are reported by some patients with severe forms of sleep apnea syndrome. Some patients complain of sore throat perhaps due to the incessant snoring, and others report dry mouth that leads to repetitive drinking of water during the night. During daytime hours patients are plagued by excessive somnolence that is hardly satisfied with naps and leads to inappropriate episodes of falling asleep particularly during monotonous sequences. As the condition advances patients relate falling asleep in situations increasingly inopportune and bizarre such as when talking to clients, on the phone, eating at the table, or more ominously while driving a car. Lethargy and sleepiness are aggravated by apathy and depression that interfere with productivity at work and with family life at home. Inability to concentrate and poor memory force patients to stop reading even newspapers and cease in their studies. Finally, an automobile accident, the loss of a job, or a determined spouse induce a reluctant patient to seek consultation.

Recent weight gain in overweight or morbidly obese patients is a common phenomenon that can be associated with a recent worsening of symptoms, perhaps the same that brought the patient to the attention of the physician. Sexual impotence along with affective depression are common findings in patients with advanced disorder.

Recent population-based studies conducted in North America indicate that the prevalence of sleep disordered breathing is 9% for women and 24% for men (Young et al. 1993). The combination of sleep-disordered breathing and daytime hypersomnia constitutes the sleep apnea syndrome that occurs in 2% of women and 4% of men (Young et al. 1993). Most patients are male (8:1) and past the age of 45 years; a familial occurrence has been noted perhaps due to the inheritance of pharyngeal structural anomalies, though most cases are sporadic. In some patients, a neuromuscular disorder is found.

Children with sleep apnea syndrome are commonly afflicted by apathy that may be mistaken with laziness. They may show difficulty with concentration and poor memory leading to poor grades in school and behavioral changes, often misdiagnosed as attention deficit disorder or minimal brain defect.

### Sleep Apnea and Cardiovascular Disease

Obstructive sleep apnea syndrome may have serious cardiovascular consequences. In patients with five episodes or more of apnea-hypopnea per hour of sleep, mean blood pressures are significantly higher both during wakefulness (>9 mm Hg systolic/5 mm Hg diastolic) and in sleep (>9/4 mm Hg) (Hla et al. 1994). Transient elevations of blood pressure lasting 3.5 seconds during the recovery phase from apnea may reach above 200 mm Hg in REM sleep. This phenomenon has been attributed to the arousal at the termination of the apnea. During the apneic episode there are high negative intrathoracic pressures, progressive desaturation of oxyhemoglobin, and even hypercapnia that contribute to elevate the blood pressure. Transcranial ultrasound techniques have revealed a decrease of blood flow velocity in the middle cerebral artery with obstructive hypopnea and apnea events attributed to the hemodynamic alteration secondary to negative intrathoracic pressure (Netzer et al. 1998). Repeated bouts of hypertension, night after night, in patients with untreated sleep apnea may eventually lead to sustained hypertension through unknown mechanisms (Millman et al. 1991). Successful treatment of obstructive sleep apnea with tracheostomy or nasal continuous positive air pressure (CPAP) results in a stepwise reduction of blood pressure levels (Guilleminault et al. 1981; Rauscher et al. 1992).

The cardiac response to prolonged apnea consists of a reduction of stroke volume, decreased heart rate, and reduced cardiac output (Garpestad et al. 1992). In patients with advanced obstructive sleep apnea, cardiac arrhythmias occur when the oxyhemoglobin saturation falls below 65%. Consequences of untreated obstructive sleep apnea are left ventricular hypertrophy, pulmonary hypertension, nocturnal myocardial ischemia, myocardial infarction, stroke, and vascular death. Increased mortality in patients with sleep apnea syndrome has been attributed to the development of hypertension (Lavie et al. 1995).

### Sleep Apnea and Stroke

Obstructive sleep apnea may be a risk factor for stroke, although definitive epidemiological evidence is still lacking. Several authors have remarked on the association but the presence of confounding factors such as obesity, hypertension, smoking, and age have complicated the analysis. In one study (Partinen and Guilleminault 1990), 198 patients with sleep apnea were divided in two groups; group A received tracheostomy and group B a recommendation to reduce weight. Seven years later two patients had suffered myocardial infarction or stroke in the group receiving a tracheostomy, whereas in the conservatively treated group 15 patients had suffered a myocardial infarction or stroke. Cardiac dysrhythmias commonly seen in patients with advanced sleep apnea (Guilleminault and Connolly 1983) may increase the risk of cardioembolic strokes.

During REM sleep cerebral blood flow normally increases, whereas REM sleep related atonia of the dilator muscles in the oropharynx result in more prolonged episodes of obstructive apnea. Morbidly obese patients with globular abdomens and patients with neuromuscular disorders have a mechanically disadvantaged diaphragm that aggravates even further the apneic phenomena. In patients whose cerebral circulation is compromised by atherosclerosis these hemodynamic changes may precipitate irreversible ischemic changes in areas of the brain with poor hemodynamic reserve, in particular borderzone regions and terminal artery territories. Neurophysiological studies of auditory event-related potentials in patients with sleep apnea syndrome before and after treatment with CPAP found no improvement in abnormal P3 wave latencies (Neau et al. 1996) suggesting a structural pathological substrate in the white matter of the hemispheres perhaps as a result of chronic hemodynamic changes and nocturnal hypoxemia.

## Sleep Apnea After Stroke

Studies of the prevalence of sleep-disordered breathing in patients with ischemic stroke (Good et al. 1996) using overnight oximetry and nocturnal polysomnography have indicated that functional outcome at 3 months, at 12 months, and at discharge as measured by the Barthel Index is worse in patients with oxygen desaturations and sleep apnea. Mortality is also increased in these patients. Such studies suggest that the prognosis for stroke recurrence and functional recovery may be negatively modified by the occurrence of sleep apnea events. Identification and elimination of sleep apnea in patients recovering from stroke may improve the functional outcome of stroke victims.

## Nonobstructive (Central) Sleep Apnea Syndrome

Central or nonobstructive sleep apnea is characterized by the cessation of respiration that may be associated with hypoxemia. In contrast with obstructive sleep apnea, there is no inspiratory effort during the respiratory pause. Patients complain of choking and gasping at night with insomnia and prolonged awakenings. During daytime hours they complain of lassitude and fatigue, and exhibit excessive somnolence.

Only 10% of patients attending sleep centers with complaints referable to sleep-disordered respiration have central sleep apnea. It is somewhat more common in men and tends to increase in prevalence as age advances. Habitual, loud snoring is not as common or manifest, but cardiac dysrhythmias are present. Patients afflicted with central sleep apnea are not obese and the physical examination fails to reveal occluding lesions in the oropharynx.

In patients with predominant or pure forms of central sleep apnea syndrome the physician should suspect a CNS or a neuromuscular disorder affecting the neural control of sleep respiration. Such is the case in patients with autonomic dysfunction as in the Shy-Drager syndrome, familial dysautonomia, and diabetes mellitus. Disorders of the brain stem of any nature can affect the automatic control of respiration in sleep as occurs in mild forms of bulbar poliomyelitis (Plum and Swanson 1958) and in the early postpolio syndrome. The bulbar centers of ventilation may be altered also by stroke (Levin and Margolis 1977), encephalitis, tumor, and cervical cordotomy. In neurological and neuromuscular disorders affecting ventilation, the sleep-related function is affected much earlier than the awake system of respiration, a phenomenon to be taken in consideration when assessing the global diagnosis.

## Upper Airway Resistance Syndrome

Patients with loud snoring and excessive daytime sleepiness may exhibit many nocturnal arousals in the polysomnogram despite minimal polygraphic evidence of obstructive sleep apnea and few, if any, oxygen desaturations. This combination of findings suggests the upper airway resistance syndrome (Guilleminault and Stoohs 1991). Patients tend to be nonobese with a triangular face, malocclusion, and retrognathia indicative of a small space behind the base of the tongue. In the polysomnogram, patients exhibit many short arousals in relation to snoring but no changes in oxygen saturation. A therapeutic trial with CPAP mask and a pressure between 4 and 8 cm $H_2O$ may have diagnostic value if the arousals disappear and the sleepiness comes under control.

## Neuromuscular Disorders

Patients with neuromuscular disorders are at high risk for the development of sleep-related respiratory disorders and respiratory failure mostly as a result of diaphragmatic weakness and failure. Chest wall weakness along with restrictive lung disease caused by chest-wall deformities and kyphoscoliosis contribute to hypoventilation both in REM and non-REM sleep. Weakness of the pharyngeal wall compounded with obesity of sedentary origin and craniofacial maldevelopment may facilitate the development of obstructive sleep apneas. The most profound alterations are observed during REM sleep. Conditions to be considered are poliomyelitis and postpolio syndrome, myasthenia gravis, myotonic dystrophy, congenital and metabolic myopathies, neuropathy, and phrenic nerve paralysis (Culebras 1996a). Patients with neuromuscular disorder developing a sleep-related respiratory alteration will present with nocturnal restlessness, frequent unexplained awakenings, and loud snoring punctuated by occasional episodes of awakening gasping for breath. Subjects report difficulty awakening in the morning and prolonged sleep inertia that interferes with morning activities. During the day these patients may present somnolence, fatigue, and inappropriate napping, that underlie failure to thrive in the very young and poor school grades or declining work performance at later ages. Some patients develop nocturnal cyanosis, severe insomnia, morning lethargy, headaches, vomiting, and leg edema that indicate the insidious but relentless occurrence of acute respiratory failure and cor pulmonale. Polysomnographic evaluation with the sleep apnea protocol followed by a multiple sleep latency test is necessary to distinguish among the different causes of sleep disturbance and to assess the severity of the disorder. Nocturnal CPAP or bilevel positive airway pressure (Bi-PAP) application corrects sleep apnea, improves hypoventilation, and assists diaphragmatic failure. BiPAP is better tolerated by patients with a neuromuscular disorder. Supplemental oxygen bled into the mask may be required in some cases.

## Cognitive Function and Sleep Apnea Syndrome

Patients with sleep apnea syndrome commonly report poor memory, confusion, and irritability along with daytime sleepiness. These cognitive changes may lead to low scholarly achievement and poor job performance that reduce the quality of life of the patient. Poor performance immediately following arousal is called sleep inertia and ranges from a few seconds to 30 minutes (Dinges 1989), being worse after awakening from stage 4 of sleep. Using the MWT, Mitler (1993) made the interesting observation that among patients with excessive somnolence, patients with sleep apnea syndrome were the most impaired on cognitive tasks. Sleep apnea syndrome is a potentially treatable factor contributing to mental decline in old age.

## Driving and Traffic Crashes in Patients With Sleep Apnea

Patients with sleep apnea syndrome represent a small segment of society but, within the group, the traffic crash rate is higher. The condition, if untreated, should be considered a risk factor for the occurrence of highway accidents. Patients with severe sleep apnea syndrome have two to three times more automobile accidents than other drivers (Strohl 1994; Findley et al. 1989). A survey of 253 patients with a driver's license referred to a sleep disorders center in California indicated that 31% of sleep apnea patients had suffered motor vehicle accidents, whereas only 15% of the non–sleep apnea group had been involved in accidents. Falling asleep at inappropriate times and driving past destination points with no recollection were considered indicators of risk of motor vehicle accidents (Wu and Yan-Go 1995). Commercial drivers suffer fewer accidents than noncommercial drivers, only 3% of the total, but their scope is of larger magnitude and some are spectacular because of the lives lost or the destruction caused (Knipling and Wierwille 1994). Obese drivers have a higher prevalence of excessive daytime sleepiness, and this ominous symptom is likely the result of sleep-disordered breathing. In a study of long-haul truck drivers, Stoohs et al. (1994) found a clear trend of a higher accident frequency in truck drivers with sleep-disordered breathing. Two states, California and Texas, have legislation with guidelines restricting the operation of vehicles by patients with sleep apnea, and one state, Maine, has proposed legislation (Pakola et al. 1995).

## Treatment of Sleep Apnea Syndromes

Obesity is a prime factor that contributes importantly to the development and progression of obstructive sleep apnea; unfortunately, it responds poorly to treatment. Patients with obstructive sleep apnea should discontinue the consumption of alcohol-containing beverages in the evening along with sedative medications. Smoking that irritates the oropharynx and contributes to reduce the oropharyngeal opening should be eliminated.

Protryptiline has a modest stimulant effect on neurogenic mechanisms that intervene in the maintenance of dilator glossopharyngeal muscle tone during sleep. This effect contributes to reduction of snoring and of sleep apnea (Brownell et al. 1982). The beneficial action of protriptyline tends to disappear gradually in 2 to 3 months, thereby serving only as an adjunct to the management of mild to moderate forms of obstructive sleep apnea that do not respond to other more efficacious forms of treatment.

In patients with nonobstructive central sleep apnea syndrome, Diamox 250 mg at bedtime may be tried. There are instances when episodes of central sleep apnea disappear with the administration of oxygen via nasal cannula (Gold et al. 1986).

Central stimulants such as mehthylphenidate, pemoline, or dextroamphetamine may be required to maintain safe levels of alertness in patients with any form of sleep apnea. Stimulants provide temporary help and should serve only as an adjunct to the main treatment.

The application of CPAP during sleep is the treatment of choice for obstructive sleep apnea syndrome. The apparatus consists of a mask adapted to the face covering the nose that delivers air at a continuous specified pressure with the objective to overcome the negative pressures created during inspiration that tend to collapse the upper airway (Abbey et al. 1989). Excessive daytime somnolence disappears or improves vastly with only one night of therapeutic intervention, but progressive improvement in alertness may be seen over the ensuing weeks (Lamphere et al. 1989). Complications, adverse reactions, and side effects are benign but annoying to patients. CPAP application should be discontinued following head trauma until there is assurance that cerebrospinal fluid (CSF) leakage is not present.

Successful elimination of apneas and hypopneas with the application of CPAP mask is sometimes associated with the emergence of periodic leg movements during non-REM sleep variably associated with arousals (Fry et al. 1989). Whether this is a de novo occurrence or the unveiling of a subclinical phenomenon is not clear. If the clinical judgment is that periodic limb movements of sleep (PLMS) affect quality of sleep, drug treatment may be warranted.

The application of CPAP to patients with sleep apnea syndrome and advanced COPD or congestive heart failure should be carefully monitored in the laboratory (Krieger et al. 1983). Increased thoracic pressure and consequent diminished venous return could compromise cardiac function and output. Extreme caution should be exercised in patients with bullous emphysema or cystic lung lesions that might be ruptured by the delivery of external air pressures. Oxygen via the mask may be required by some patients

CPAP tolerance is good or excellent in 80% of patients with moderate or advanced obstructive sleep apnea syndrome. Compliance declines in 25% to 30% of all patients treated who show an initial good response. Approximately 20% of patients drop the use of the apparatus within the first year of therapy and 30% report that applications are not taken nightly (Nino-Murcia et al. 1989). Young patients tend to contemplate with disgust the perspective of a life-long dependency on the apparatus especially if they are unattached and socially active. However, they may accept its temporary use as a compromise while they lose weight and explore other therapeutic modalities. In children with obstructive sleep apnea syndrome secondary to structural anomalies, CPAP application may be the only viable therapeutic alternative until craniofacial growth has been completed and surgical reconstruction is acceptable. In general, tolerance and compliance to CPAP increase with severity of the sleep apnea syndrome and of daytime sleepiness. Consistent use on consecutive nights is recommended and desirable, since there is suggestive evidence of continued improvement of various parameters after several weeks of optimal use of CPAP (Lamphere et al. 1989). Indeed, blood pressure measurements tend to decrease after several weeks of treatment (Mayer et al. 1991). The mask should not be used if there is a risk of vomiting leading to aspiration of gastric contents, a consideration particularly important in weakened individuals or patients with neuromuscular disorders. The apparatus should have incorporated a safety system to deliver fresh air in case of power failure.

The Bi-PAP apparatus delivers differential inspiratory positive air pressure (IPAP) and expiratory positive air pressure (EPAP). The Bi-PAP apparatus is useful in patients with restrictive neuromuscular disorders, kyphoscoliosis, or when CPAP is indicated but not tolerated. It is likewise indicated in bullous and cystic lung conditions where high pressures could traumatize the lungs. Finally, Bi-PAP is the alternative of choice when the expiratory effort against CPAP pressure causes discomfort and arousals, or prevents sleep.

Patients with nonobstructive central sleep apnea syndrome deserve a trial on CPAP and Bi-PAP. Bi-PAP is indicated in patients with central sleep apnea intolerant of CPAP and in patients exhibiting a prominent central apnea component after elimination of the obstructive portion of the apneas with CPAP. Patients with loud snoring and daytime sleepiness suspected of having the upper airway resistance syndrome (Shepard 1993) should undergo a test with CPAP with the goal to eliminate nocturnal arousals and snoring and eventually excessive sleepiness.

*Tracheostomy* was originally performed in patients with advanced obstructive sleep apnea to bypass the pharyngeal obstruction. Tracheostomy is socially unacceptable and difficult to maintain free of complications, posing a risk of chronic infection. Today, tracheostomy is rarely used, remaining as a backup intervention for severe cases with high risk of death. *Nasal reconstruction* may be required in patients with septal deviation and turbinate hypertrophy interfering with the adequate passage of air delivered by CPAP. *Tonsillectomy* is indicated in children with sleep apnea syndrome and hypertrophic tonsils. *UPPP* was originally introduced to alleviate snoring and later on the indications were extended to obstructive sleep apnea syndrome. The results obtained have been irregular, although proper selection of patients improves the outlook. Pain associated with the intervention in adults, and the risk of development of permanent deficits are serious complications. Patients who benefit most are those with obstructive sleep apneas and large tonsils, those with redundant lateral pharyngeal walls, and those with long soft palate. Some centers report that with careful selection 87% of patients experience at least a 50% reduction in respiratory events (Sher et al. 1985); others indicate that less than 50% of patients show at least a 50% reduction in the sleep apnea/hypopnea index following the intervention (Pelausa and Tarhis 1989). Complications usually relate to postoperative swelling or excessive reduction of tissue, and include nasal reflux that is transient in most patients (Powell et al. 1994), partial wound dehiscence, and rarely palatal incompetence. Failure to alleviate sleep apnea occurs in patients with multiple sites of obstruction that had remained occult prior to the operation (Nordlander 1993).

*Mandible, tongue and hyoid reconstructions are* interventions intended to improve the airflow at the base of the tongue in the hypopharynx. Patients are selected on the basis of radiographic analysis and cephalometric measurements showing stenosis of the hypopharynx. Advancement of the mandible 1 or 2 mm may be sufficient to improve airflow. Patients who benefit most from these operations are young, with moderate to severe sleep apnea syndrome and loud snoring caused by hypopharyngeal stenosis, frequently with associated craniofacial malformations, retrognathia, or malocclusions. The procedures are specialized maxillofacial interventions available only in selected centers. Complications appear to be small in number and range from surgical edema of the floor of the mouth, to mental nerve dysesthesias. Contraindications are psychiatric disorders, old age, and drug dependency.

As many as 13 *oral and dental appliances* have been introduced in clinical practice for the treatment of snoring and mild to moderate sleep apnea. The objective is to eliminate snoring and improve sleep apnea by changing the dynamics of the mandible, intraoral cavity, and upper airway sufficiently to improve the passage of air while the subject is asleep. Oral appliances have been devised to move the mandible forward, lift the soft palate, and/or move the tongue forward. Early results with SNOAR (Sleep and Nocturnal Obstructive Apnea Reductor) that advances the mandible up to 9 mm indicate a reduction in respiratory disorder index from 45.5 to 9.7 along with elimination of snoring (Viscomi et al. 1988). Snore Guard has been marketed for the treatment of snoring only. Snoring is reduced in 60% and eliminated in 40% (Schmidt-Nowara et al. 1991); compliance appears to be acceptable. The tongue retaining device may be useful in some patients with macroglossia (Cartwright and Samelson 1982). In general, oral appliances are safe and may be considered in individuals with snoring and in patients with obstructive sleep apnea syndrome of any degree of severity who refuse or do not tolerate CPAP. The ASDA recommends that patients with moderate to severe obstructive sleep apnea receive follow-up polysomnography, or another objective measure of respiration during sleep, with the appliance in place, to ensure satisfactory therapeutic benefit (Practice Parameters for the Treatment of Snoring and Obstructive

Sleep Apnea with Oral Appliances 1995). The precise indications for dental appliances have not been validated with reliable clinical studies.

## Parasomnias and Motor Disorders of Sleep

### Arousal Disorders

The arousal disorders are disturbances of the waking mechanism that result in a delay or blockage of full control of volitional motor activity. When awakened the individual appears slow, with memory impairment, poor judgment, and inappropriate behavior. Typical arousal disorders are confusional arousals, sleep terrors, and sleepwalking.

*Confusional arousals* or sleep drunkenness generally occur in the process of waking up in predisposed individuals who are deprived of sleep or whose sleep is so profound that full vigilance is not restored with sufficient rapidity. As a result, the person appears confused and sleepy in transitions to wakefulness out of deep sleep. In this state the subject can walk, climb stairs, move about, get dressed, and even drive a car. Violence and assault may take place driven by a distorted perception of reality (Bonkalo 1974), though planning and premeditation are not possible. Rarely, homicides have been committed during confusional arousals (Klawans 1991) but acts appear more irrational than malicious. Most often events are limited to simple acts like picking up a lamp instead of a ringing phone or mumbling incoherently in response to a question. Children under 5 years of age are universally prone to develop confusional arousals when awakened from deep sleep. As age advances, the frequency diminishes and in the adult years confusional arousals are limited to predisposed individuals who are severely sleep deprived. Patients with sleep apnea, narcolepsy, and idiopathic hypersomnia are especially vulnerable and may develop confusional arousals with more frequency than the rest of the population. The individual in a state of confusional arousal may become aggressive if challenged. A sleepwalking event may turn into a confusional arousal. Treatment is best achieved by avoiding a sleep debt and preventing falling into a deep, prolonged sleep. Susceptible individuals should avoid CNS depressants such as alcohol, antihistaminic preparations, hypnotics, sedatives, and tranquilizers.

*Sleep terrors* appear almost exclusively in children between the ages of 4 and 12 years. The prevalence is 3% in children, being more frequent in boys, sometimes showing a familial incidence (Kales et al. 1980). Episodes are characterized by a sudden awakening out of deep sleep, preceded by a chilling scream that interrupts abruptly the sleep of parents. Children sit up in bed crying inconsolably and agitated, with dilated pupils, rapid respirations, and a fast pulse. If forcibly awakened children act confused and incoherent, but soon fall asleep having no recollection of the event on the following morning. With the passage of time episodes tend to disappear spontaneously.

When sleep terrors appear once or more times per week management consists of eliminating precipitating factors while reducing the level of daytime stress and reassuring the parents of the benign character of the condition. In some cases, benzodiazepines that reduce the cortical arousal component may be administered at bedtime (e. g., diazepam 2 to 5 mg). Rare sleep terrors that persist into adulthood are commonly associated with psychopathology, and the response to treatment is weaker requiring the complement of psychotherapy in most instances.

*Somnambulism or sleepwalking* is common in children over 4 years of age. It is characterized by ambulation during slow wave sleep in the first third of the night. Sleepwalking occurs in 30% of children with sleep terrors; a sex predominance is not identified, but a familial incidence is commonly observed (Kales et al. 1980). Up to 15% of the general population has had at least one episode of sleepwalking in childhood. Peak prevalence occurs between 4 and 8 years, disappearing spontaneously by the age of 15 years. Past that age only 0.5% of adults retain occasional sleepwalking episodes. The risk of serious accidents like falling down the stairs or exiting through a window is high. Motor activity does not suggest planning. Precipitating factors are those that promote deep sleep including sleep deprivation, fever, excessive tiredness, hypnotics, and some neuroleptics. Psychopathology is common in the adult sleepwalker but not in the child. In the young adult the differential diagnosis should be made with episodic wandering, while in the third and fourth decades with epileptic fugues, and in the old person with REM sleep behavior disorder. In the demented old person nocturnal wandering may simulate sleepwalking.

Violence in the course of sleepwalking occupies a special category (Broughton et al. 1994). The sleepwalker has the potential to drift into a confusional arousal, a state in which violence and assault are likely. Malingering can be ruled out when the violent act appears irrational without malicious or premeditated intent and there is a past history of nocturnal events supporting an arousal disorder.

Management consists of protecting the patient from harm by closing windows and locking doors, blocking stairs, and securing balconies. Daytime stress should be reduced and relaxation techniques tried. Sleep deprivation should be avoided and a regular sleep hygiene maintained. Administration of small doses of benzodiazepines, like diazepam 2 to 10 mg at bedtime, reduces the number and intensity of episodes. Medication should be considered when the episodes are frequent and pose a risk to the patient.

### REM Sleep-Related Parasomnias

REM sleep is characterized by dream content and muscle atonia. Abnormalities of these phenomena determine most of the parasomniac experiences of REM sleep.

*Nightmares* are dream anxiety attacks that frighten patients. The element of fright is intrinsic to the nightmare and not a mere reaction to the dream experience. Memory of the event is vivid and independent of awakenings terminating the sequence. Children may suffer nightmares starting at the age of 3 years. It is probable that up to one half of the population has experienced nightmares at some point (Hartmann 1984). By age 6 years nightmares begin to subside and gradually disappear. The few adolescents and adults who continue to report nightmares are often women harboring a schizoid or borderline personality disorder with fragile emotional structure and predisposition to develop mental illness (Kales et al. 1980). Frightening and intense real-life experiences may precipitate recurrent nightmares in vulnerable adults, as in the post-traumatic stress syndrome (Lavie et al. 1979).

Treatment is not necessary unless nightmares are frequent, recurrent, and disturbing to the patient and parents or immediate relatives. Stress avoidance and discontinuation of drugs that promote nightmares should be considered along with a disciplined sleep hygiene. Psychotherapy is helpful in individuals with borderline personality disorders. Medications that suppress REM sleep also suppress nightmares. A useful regimen is the administration of protryptiline 10 mg at bedtime.

*REM sleep behavior disorder (RSBD)* is characterized by a history of bizarre motor acts during nocturnal sleep associated with polygraphic evidence of loss of muscle atonia. Clinical manifestations range from simple motor deeds to complex forms of organized activity in REM stage. Motor overactivity driven by a dream (phantasmagoria) may lead to physical injuries to the patient or spouse. The frequency of episodes ranges from one or more nightly to once per month. RSBD predominates in old persons and in males (Schenck and Mahowald 1990). In Schenck and Mahowald's series, neurological disorders were identified in 42.9% of patients neurologically examined. These authors noted the following conditions associated with RSBD: olivopontocerebellar degeneration, ischemic cerebrovascular disorder, multiple sclerosis, Parkinson's disease, Guillain-Barre syndrome, brain stem astrocytoma, narcolepsy, dementia, Shy-Drager syndrome, and alcoholism. RSBD may precede by as long as 12 years the onset of Parkinson's disease. Up to 15% of patients with Parkinson's disease report episodes of RSBD (Comella and Nardine 1997). In Schenck and Mahowald's series 42 patients were studied with magnetic resonance imaging (MRI) of the head and the incidence of abnormalities of likely clinical importance was 14.6%.

Episodes commonly result in injury to the patient or spouse. The diagnosis of RSBD in an older patient should elicit suspicion of an underlying neurological disorder, in particular cerebrovascular or degenerative in nature. An MRI of the head is recommended (Culebras and Moore 1989). RSBD could be the presenting complaint of small vessel arteriopathy involving the brain stem, Parkinson's disease, or of the Shy-Drager syndrome (Sforza et al. 1988). Patients should be followed neurologically to detect potential neurological problems. Clonazepam, 0.5 mg at bedtime, is generally sufficient to suppress episodes and the associated violent dreams.

### Restless Legs Syndrome and Periodic Movements of Sleep

Restless legs syndrome (RLS) has been a relatively well-known though poorly understood neurological condition since the early accounts by

Ekbom in 1945 (Ekbom 1945). Later reports noted a familial incidence (Godbout et al. 1987) and the association with various metabolic, neurological, and vascular disorders. In 1953 Symonds (1953) described myoclonic jerks upon falling asleep persisting through the night that he called nocturnal myoclonus. Based on polysomnographic evaluations, Lugaresi et al. (1972) established the association between RLS and nocturnal myoclonus. Subsequent studies by Coleman et al. (Coleman et al. 1980) defined in more detail nocturnal myoclonus and proposed the term *periodic movements in sleep* to separate the disturbance from true myoclonic alterations. PLMS is considered a common cause of sleep disturbance, particularly in the elderly.

Patients with RLS complain of unpleasant, crawling sensations in both legs, occasionally alternating extremities. Symptoms occur only while the patient is at rest, particularly in the evening and at night. Long periods of rest at any time during the day precipitate symptoms, and fatigue worsens the manifestations. The discomfort may continue or reappear after the patient goes to bed, provoking sleeplessness. The urge to move the limbs and pace the floor for as long as 30 minutes may, in fact, become irresistible.

Upon falling asleep 70% to 80% of patients with RLS (Montplaisir et al. 1992) develop involuntary, repetitive, periodic movements of the lower limbs (PLMS) characterized by a partial flexion at the ankle, knee, and sometimes the hip with extension of the big toe, followed by slow recovery of the extended posture. Patients are generally unaware of the disturbance that is brought to their attention by the awakened bedmate who hears the rumble under the sheets.

RLS plus PLMS disturbs sleep either by preventing its occurrence or by provoking multiple awakenings. The resultant sleep deprivation causes excessive daytime somnolence and tiredness. Depression, emotional distress, and other psychological dysfunctions often appear along with insomnia and daytime somnolence. Families with many affected members have been reported by various authors and as many as half of the cases may be of familial origin (Godbout et al. 1987).

A variety of neurological, metabolic, and vascular disorders are associated with RLS and PLMS, although the latter may occur in otherwise healthy individuals and remain asymptomatic. These include iron deficiency anemia and folate deficiency, chronic renal failure, hypothyroidism, rheumatoid arthritis, and various neurological disorders such as poliomyelitis, peripheral neuropathy in particular of diabetic origin, chronic myelopathy, and Parkinson's disease. Caffeine abuse, barbiturate withdrawal, and the intake of a variety of drugs including antidepressants, tricyclic compounds, phenothiazines, lithium, and calcium channel blockers are a risk factor for development of RLS plus PLMS. RLS is considered idiopathic when there are no other associated disorders known to cause or increase the risk of developing the alteration.

The prevalence of RLS is uncertain. Ekbom cited a prevalence of 5% (Ekbom 1945) of the general population including all ranges of symptom intensity. RLS plus PLMS occur in any age group but increase in frequency as age advances without sex preference. By age 65 years and older perhaps 30% of the population has a significant number of PLMS (Ancoli-Israel et al. 1991). Severe forms of RLS plus PLMS persist during the lifetime of the individual and progress in intensity with remissions and exacerbations without identifiable cause. If untreated, RLS plus PLMS impair the quality of life. At least in one study RLS was a significant predictor of death in elderly subjects (Pollack et al. 1990).

Therapy is indicated when the movement disorder alters the ability to initiate or maintain sleep. The treatment of RLS plus PLMS revolves around pharmacotherapy with benzodiazepines, dopaminergic drugs, and opioids, individually or in combination. A few, mostly small, controlled treatment trials have been conducted within the last 15 years (Walters et al. 1988, 1993; Brodeur et al. 1988) but much of the evidence is based on experts' opinions. Tolerance, habituation, and even addiction are risks that can be decreased by rotating medications or administering interrupted doses in mild cases. Nonetheless, most patients derive benefit and tolerate the drugs satisfactorily. A panel of international experts with a collective experience based on the treatment of 1065 patients with RLS responded to a questionnaire to determine treatment practices (Hening et al. 1995). Twelve of 19 started treatment when the patient was impaired in his sleep and daily function. As drug of choice, 11 used carbidopa/levodopa (regular or CR), five used clonazepam, one used both, and another one used clonidine.

Recent clinical studies with dopamine agonist agents have shown great efficacy in RLS and PLMS. Montplaisir et al. (1999b) showed that pramipexole reduced the PLMS index to normal values as well as the periodic leg movement index during wakefulness. Wetter et al. (1999) evaluated the efficacy of pergolide and found that when given as a low to medium bedtime dose in combination with domperidone it relieved sensorimotor symptoms and improved sleep disturbances in patients with RLS.

## Fatal Familial Insomnia

This is a rare familial disorder with relentless loss of neuroendocrine regulation and of vegetative circadian rhythms starting in middle age (Lugaresi et al. 1986). Prominent manifestations are severe progressive insomnia with frequent awakenings, autonomic disturbances, and daytime stupor alternating with wakefulness. In the terminal stages of the disease there is increasing agitation, confusion, disorientation, progressive stupor from which the patient is only transiently arousable, and coma. Death occurs 1 to 1 1/2 years after the manifestations begin. At autopsy there is severe degeneration and gliosis of the anterior and dorsomedial nuclei of the thalamus. Recent investigations indicate a prion etiology (Medori et al. 1992), akin to Creutzfeldt-Jakob disease.

Very recently Mastrianni et al. (1999) described a sporadic form of fatal insomnia with clinical features typical of fatal familial insomnia and death 16 months after the onset of symptoms. Laboratory studies revealed that the patient carried a strain of prions similar to that in fatal familial insomnia but without the PRNP gene mutation that causes it.

## Conclusions

Sleep disorders cause chronic misery and reduction of quality of life that may be reversed. Serious social decline and poor scholastic performance are commonplace for persons with intrinsic hypersomnias. Indirect morbidity and mortality are also a cause for concern in sleep pathology. Severe sleep apnea may be a risk factor for vascular disease and cognitive deficit. A large number of high-

way crashes and work-related accidents are the result of sleepiness and loss of vigilance, conditions that could probably have been improved with the help of sleep specialists. Some parasomnias provoke bizarre and violent behavior with resultant accidents. Thus, long-term health consequences, loss of work productivity, reduced income, poor health, and even risk of violent accidents and dying as a result of sleep disorders, or of poor sleep hygiene, are considerations to be entertained when making a decision to evaluate these patients vigorously, since treatment is available. The prognosis of some of the prevailing sleep disorders such as narcolepsy has improved and the natural history of conditions such as sleep apnea may have been favorably changed by the introduction of therapeutic techniques based on pathogenetic mechanisms.

The future calls for a pivotal intervention of sleep centers and specialists in the prevention of mental fatigue and sleep-related accidents; development of countermeasures where there is loss of work productivity resulting from poorly designed work shifts; as well as active participation in the correction of family pathology, scholastic decline, social disruption, and general loss of quality of life that afflicts people in a state of subvigilance and chronic somnolence. State-wide studies are uncovering the endemic somnolence that underlies automobile and commercial vehicle accidents (McCartt et al. 1996), the pervasive sleep deprivation that undermines shift workers, as well as those who work excessive number of hours, and in general individuals who do not follow a proper sleep hygiene. Advances in these fronts may go beyond the improvement of an individual prognosis for some conditions and reach the physical and mental health of vast segments of the population.

## References

Abbey, N. C.; Cooper, K. R.; Kwentus, J. A. Benefit of nasal CPAP in obstructive sleep apnea is due to positive pharyngeal pressures. Sleep 12:420–422; 1989.

Agnew, H. W.; Webb, W. B.; Williams, R. L. The effects of stage 4 sleep deprivation. Electroencephalogr. Clin. Neurophysiol. 17:68–70; 1964.

Aldrich, M. S. Automobile accidents in patients with sleep disorders. Sleep 12:487–494; 1989.

Aldrich, M. S.; Naylor, M. W. Narcolepsy associated with lesions of the diencephalon. Neurology 39:1505–1508; 1989.

Aldrich, M. Narcolepsy. Neurology 42(suppl. 6):S34–S43; 1992.

Aldrich, M. S.; Chervin, R. D.; Malow, B. A. Sensitivity of the Multiple Sleep Latency Test (MSLT) for the diagnosis of narcolepsy. Neurology 45(suppl.): A432; 1995.

Ancoli-Israel, S.; Kripke, D. F.; Klauber, M. R.; et al. Periodic limb movements in sleep in community-dwelling elderly. Sleep 14:496–500; 1991.

Berg, O.; Hanley, J. Narcolepsy in two cases of multiple sclerosis. Acta Neurol. Scand. 39:252–257; 1963.

Bonkalo, A. Impulsive acts and confusional states during incomplete arousal from sleep: criminological and forensic implications. Psychiatry Q. 48: 400–409; 1974.

Bové, A.; Culebras, A.; Moore, J. T.; Westlake, R. E. Relationship between sleep spindles and hypersomnia. Sleep 17:449–455; 1994.

Brodeur, C.; Montplaisir, J.; Godbout, R.; et al. Treatment of restless legs syndrome and periodic movements during sleep with L-DOPA: a double-blind controlled study. Neurology 38:1845–1848; 1988.

Broughton, R.; Ghanem, Q.; Hishikawa, Y.; Sugita, Y.; Nevsimalova, S.; Roth, B. Life effects of narcolepsy in 180 patients from North America, Asia and Europe compared to matched controls. Can. J. Neurol. Sci. 8:299–304; 1981.

Broughton, R.; Guberman, A.; Roberts, J. Comparison of the psychosocial effects of epilepsy and narcolepsy/cataplexy: a controlled study. Epilepsia 25:423–433; 1984.

Broughton, R.; Billings, R.; Cartwright, R.; et al. Homicidal somnambulism: a case report. Sleep 17: 253–264; 1994.

Brownell, L. G.; West, P.; Sweatman, P.; et al. Protriptyline in obstructive sleep apnea. A double blind trial. N. Engl. J. Med. 307:1037–1042; 1982.

Carskadon, M. A.; Dement, W. C. Cumulative effects of sleep restriction on daytime sleepiness. Psychophysiology 18:107–113; 1981.

Carskadon, M. A. Patterns of sleep and sleepiness in adolescents. Pediatrician 17:5–12; 1990.

Cartwright, R.; Samelson, C. The effects of a non-surgical treatment for obstructive sleep apnea—the tongue retaining device. JAMA 248:705–709; 1982.

Castaigne, P.; Escourolle, R. Etude topographique des lesions anatomiques dans les hypersomnies. Rev. Neurol. 116:547–584; 1967.

Chervin, R. D.; Aldrich, M. S. Specificity of the Multiple Sleep Latency Test (MSLT) for the diagnosis of narcolepsy. Neurology 45(suppl. 4):A432; 1995.

Clavelou, P.; Tournilhac, M.; Vidal, C.; et al. Narcolepsy associated with arteriovenous malformation in the diencephalon. Sleep 18:202–205; 1995.

Coleman, R. M.; Pollak, C. P.; Weitzman, E. D. Periodic movements in sleep (nocturnal myoclonus): relation to sleep disorders. Ann. Neurol. 8:416–421; 1980.

Comella, L. C.; Nardine, T. M. Sleep-related violence, injury and REM sleep behavior disorder in Parkinson's disease. Neurology 48:A359; 1997.

Culebras, A.; Moore, J. T. Magnetic resonance findings in REM sleep behavior disorder. Neurology 39: 1519–1523; 1989.

Culebras, A. Sleep and neuromuscular disorders. Neurolo. Clin. 14:791–805; 1996.

Culebras, A. Clinical handbook of sleep disorders. Boston: Butterworth/Heinemann; 1996b.

Dawson, D.; Reid, K. Fatigue, alcohol and performance impairment. Nature 388:235; 1997.

Derlet, R. W.; Rice, P.; Horowitz, B. Z.; Lord, R. V. Amphetamine toxicity: experience with 127 cases. J. Emerg. Med. 7:157–161; 1989.

Dinges, D. F. Napping patterns and effects in human adults. In: Dinges, D. F.; Broughton, R. J., eds. Sleep and alertness chronobiological, behavioral, and medical aspects of napping. New York: Raven Press; 1989: p. 171–204.

Douglas, N. J. The psychosocial aspects of narcolepsy. Neurology 50(suppl. 1):S27–S30; 1998

Ekbom, K. A. Restless legs: a clinical study. Acta Med. Scand. Suppl. 158:1–122; 1945.

Findley, L. J.; Fabrizio, M.; Thommi, G.; Suratt, P. M. Severity of sleep apnea and automobile crashes. N. Engl. J. Med. 320:868–869; 1989.

Fry, J. Treatment modalities for narcolepsy. Neurology 50(suppl. 1):S43–S48; 1998.

Fry, J. M.; DiPhillipo, M. A.; Pressman MR. Periodic leg movements in sleep following treatment of obstructive sleep apnea with nasal continuous positive airway pressure. Chest 96:89–91; 1989.

Garpestad, E.; Katayama, H.; Parker, J. A.; et al. Stroke volume and cardiac output decrease at termination of obstructive apneas. J. Appl. Physiol. 73(5):1743–1748; 1992.

Gélineau, J. De la narcolepsie. Gaz. Hop. (Paris) 53:626–628; 1880a.

Gélineau, J. De la narcolepsie. Gaz. Hop. (Paris) 54:635–637; 1880b.

Godbout, R.; Montplaisir, J. All-day performance variations in normal and narcoleptic subjects. Sleep 9:200–204; 1986.

Godbout, R.; Montplaisir, J.; Poirier, G. Epidemiological data in familial resless legs syndrome. Sleep Res. 16:338; 1987.

Gold, A. R.; Schwartz, A. R.; Bleecker, E. R.; Smith, P. L. The effect of chronic nocturnal oxygen administration upon sleep apnea. Am. Rev. Respir. Dis. 134:925–929; 1986.

Good, D. C.; Henkle, J. Q.; Gelber, D.; Welsh, J.; Verhuls, S. Sleep-disordered breathing and poor functional outcomes after stroke. Stroke 27:252–759; 1996.

Guilleminault, C.; Carskadon, M.; Dement, W. C. On the treatment of rapid eye movement narcolepsy. Arch. Neurol. 30:90–93; 1974.

Guilleminault, C.; Simmons, F. B.; Motta, J.; et al. Obstructive sleep apnea syndrome and tracheostomy. Long-term follow-up experience. Arch. Intern. Med. 141:985–988; 1981.

Guilleminault, C.; Faull, K. F.; Miles, L.; Van den Hoed, J. Post-traumatic excessive daytime sleepiness: a review of 20 patients. Neurology 33:1548–1549; 1983.

Guilleminault, C.; Connolly, S. J. Cardiac arrhythmia and conduction disturbances during sleep in 400 patients with sleep apnea syndrome. Am. J. Cardiol. 52:490–494; 1983.

Guilleminault, C.; Mignot, E.; Grumet, F. C. Familial patterns of narcolepsy. Lancet 2:1376–1379; 1989.

Guilleminault, C.; Partinen, M. Introduction. In: Guilleminault, C.; Partinen, M., eds Obstructive sleep apnea syndrome. New York: Raven Press; 1990.

Guilleminault, C.; Stoohs, R. Upper airway resistance syndrome. Am. Rev. Respir. Dis. 143:A589; 1991.

Guilleminault, C.; Pelayo, R. Narcolepsy in prepubertal children. Ann. Neurol. 43:135–142; 1998.

Hartmann, E. The nightmare: the psychology and biology of terrifying dreams. New York: Basic Books; 1984.

Hening, W. A.; Walters, A. S.; Chokroverty, S. Treatment of the restless legs syndrome: current practices of sleep experts. Neurology 45(suppl. 4):A285; 1995.

Hla, M. K.; Young, T. B.; Bidwell, T.; et al. Sleep apnea and hypertension. Ann. Intern. Med. 120:382–388; 1994.

Honda, Y.; Hishikawa, Y.; Takahashi, Y. Long term treatment of narcolepsy with methylphenidate (Ritalin®). Curr. Ther. Res. 25:288–298; 1979.

Honda, Y.; Hishikawa, Y. A long-term treatment of narcolepsy and excessive daytime sleepiness with pemoline (Betanamin®). Curr. Ther. Res. 27:429–441; 1980.

Kales, A.; Soldatos, C. R.; Bixler, E. O.; et al. Hereditary factors in sleep walking and night terrors. Br. J. Psychiatry 137:111–118; 1980.

Kales, A.; Soldatos, C. R.; Caldwell, A. B.; et al. Nightmares: clinical characteristics and personality patters. Am. J. Psychiatry 137:1197–1201; 1980.

Kales, A.; Soldatos, C. R.; Bixler, E. O.; et al. Narcolepsy-cataplexy. II. Psychosocial consequences and associated psychopathology. Arch. Neurol. 39:169–171; 1982.

Klawans, H. L.; ed. The Sleeping Killer. In: Trials of an expert witness. Boston: Little, Brown & Co.; 1991: p. 130–137.

Knipling, R. R.; Wierwille, W. W. Vehicle-based drowsy driver detection: current status and future prospects. Proceedings of the Fourth Annual Meeting of IVHS America. IVHS America; 1994.

Kollar, E. J.; Namerow, N.; Pasnau, R. O.; Naitoh, P. Neurological findings during prolonged sleep deprivation. Neurology 18:836–840; 1968.

Koskenvuo, M.; Kaprio, J.; Partinen, M.; et al. Snoring as a risk factor for hypertension and angina pectoris. Lancet 1:893–895; 1985.

Kramer, R. E.; Dinner, D. S.; Braun, W. E.; Zachary, A.; Teresi, G. A. HLA-DR2 and narcolepsy. Arch. Neurol. 44:853–855; 1987.

Krieger, J.; Weitzenblaum, E.; Monassier, J. P.; et al. Dangerous hypoxemia during continuous positive airway pressure treatment of obstructive sleep apnea. Lancet 2:1429–1430; 1983.

Lamphere, J.; Roehrs, T.; Wittig, R.; et al. Recovery of alertness after CPAP in apnea. Chest 96:1364–1367; 1989.

Lankford, D. A.; Wellman J. J.; Ohara, C. Post-traumatic narcolepsy in mild to moderate closed head injury. Sleep 17:S25–S28; 1994.

Lavie, P.; Hefez, A.; Halpern, G.; et al. Long-term effects of traumatic war related events on sleep. Am. J. Psychiatry 136:1175–1178; 1979.

Lavie, P.; Herer, P.; Peled, R.; Berger, J.; Yoffe, N.; Zomer, J.; et al. Mortality in sleep apnea patients: a multivariate analysis of risk factors. Sleep 18:149–157; 1995.

Lemmi, H. Excessive daytime sleepiness: is it narcolepsy? Sleep Med. Rev. 3:1–2; 1995.

Levin, B.; Margolis, G. Acute failure of autonomic respirations secondary to unilateral brainstem infarct. Ann. Neurol. 1:583–586; 1977.

Lugaresi, E.; Coccagna, G.; Montovani, M.; et al. Some periodic phenomena arising during drowsiness and sleep in man. Electroencephalogr. Clin. Neurophysiol. 32:701–705; 1972.

Lugaresi, E.; Cirignotta, F.; Coccagna, G.; et al. Some epidemiological data on snoring and cardiocirculatory disturbances. Sleep 3:221–224; 1980.

Lugaresi, E.; Medori, R.; Montagna, P.; et al. Fatal familial insomnia and dysautonomia with selective degeneration of thalamic nuclei. N. Engl. J. Med. 315:997–1003; 1986.

Mastrianni, J. A.; Nixon, R.; Layzer, R.; Telling, G. C.; Han, D.; DeArmond, S. J.; Prusiner S. B. Prion protein conformation in a patient with sporadic fatal insomnia. N. Engl. J. Med. 340:1630–1638; 1999.

Mayer, J.; Becker, H.; Brandenburg, U.; et al. Blood pressure and sleep apnea: results of long-term nasal continuous positive airway pressure therapy. Cardiology 79:84–92; 1991.

McCartt, A. T.; Ribner, S. A.; Pack, A. I.; Hammer, M. C. The scope and nature of the drowsy driving problem in New York State. Accid. Anal. Prev. 28:511–517; 1996.

Medori, R.; Tritschler, H. J.; LeBlanc, A.; et al. Fatal familial insomnia is a prion disease with a mutation at codon 178 of the prion disease. N. Engl. J. Med. 326:444–449; 1992.

Mignot, E. Genetic and familial aspects of narcolepsy. Neurology 50(suppl. 1):S16–S22; 1998.

Millman, R. P.; Redline, S.; Caelisle, C. C.; et al. Daytime hypertension in obstructive sleep apnea. Prevalence and contributing risk factor. Chest 99:861–866; 1991.

Mitler, M. M.; Hajdukovic, R. Relative efficacy of drugs for the treatment of sleepiness in narcolepsy. Sleep 14:218–220; 1991.

Mitler, M. M. Daytime sleepiness and cognitive functioning in sleep apnea. Sleep 16:S68–S70, 1993.

Mitler, M. M.; Hajdukovic, R.; Erman, M. K. Treatment of narcolepsy with methamphetamine. Sleep 16:306–317; 1993.

Mitler, M. M. Evaluation of treatment with stimulants in narcolepsy. Sleep 17:S103–S106; 1994.

Mitler, M. M.; Miller, J. C.; Lipsitz, J. J.; Walsh, J. K.; Wylie, C. D. The sleep of long-haul truck drivers. N. Engl. J. Med. 337:755–761; 1997.

Mondini, S.; Zucconi, M.; Cirignotta, F.; et al. Snoring as a risk factor for cardiac and circulatory problems: an epidemiological study. In: Guilleminault, C.; Lugaresi, E., eds. Sleep wake disorders: natural history, epidemiology and long-term evolution. New York: Raven Press; 1983: p. 99–105.

Montplaisir, J.; Lapierre, O.; Warnes, H.; et al. The treatment of the restless legs syndrome with or without periodic leg movements of sleep. Sleep 15:391–395; 1992.

Montplaisir, J.; Nicolas, A.; Denesle, R.; Gómez-Mancilla, B. Restless legs syndrome improved by pramipexole. A double-blind randomized trial. Neurology 52:938–943; 1999.

Naitoh, P.; Kales, A.; Kollar, E. J.; et al. Electro-encephalographic activity after prolonged sleep loss. Electroencephalogr. Clin. Neurophysiol. 27:2–11; 1969.

National Highway Traffic Safety Administration General Estimates System. Statistical Report for 1992.

National Transportation Safety Board: Safety study: fatigue, alcohol, other drugs, and medical factors in fatal-to-the-driver heavy truck crashes. Vols. 1 & 2. Washington, DC; NTSB/SS-90/01 & 02; 1990: p. 1–447.

Neau, J. P.; Paquereau, J. C.; Meurice, J. C.; Chavagnat, J. J.; Pinon-Vignaud, M. L.; Vandel, B.; et al. Auditory event-related potentials before and after treatment with nasal continuous positive airway pressure in sleep apnea syndrome. Eur. J. Neurol. 3:29–35; 1996.

Netzer, N.; Werner, P.; Jochums, I.; Lehmann, M.; Strohl, H. P. Blood flow of the middle cerebral artery with sleep-disordered breathing. Correlation with obstructive hypopneas. Stroke 29:87–93; 1998.

Nino-Murcia, G.; McCann, C. C.; Bliwise, D. L.; et al. Compliance and side effects in sleep apnea patients treated with continuous positive airway pressure. West. J. Med. 150:165–169; 1989.

Nordlander, B. Long-term studies addressing success of surgical treatment for sleep apnea syndrome. Sleep 16:S100–S102; 1993.

Ohayon, M.; Priest, R. G.; Caulet, M.; Guilleminault, C. Hypnagogic and hypnopompic hallucinations: pathological phenomena? Br. J. Psychiatry 169:459–467; 1996.

Pakola, S. J.; Dinges, D. F.; Pack, A. I. Driving and sleepiness. Review of regulations and guidelines for commercial and noncommercial drivers with sleep apnea and narcolepsy. Sleep 18:787–796; 1995.

Palomaki, H.; Partinen, M.; Erkinjuntti, T.; Kaste, M. Snoring, sleep apnea syndrome, and stroke. Neurology 42(suppl. 6):75–82; 1992.

Parsons, M. Fits and other causes of loss of consciousness while driving. Q. J. Med. 58:295–303; 1986.

Partinen, M., Guilleminault, C. Daytime sleepiness and vascular morbidity at seven-year follow-up in obstructive sleep apnea patients. Chest 97:27–32; 1990.

Pelausa, E. O.; Tarhis, L. M. Surgery for snoring. Laryngoscope 99:1006–1010; 1989.

Plum, F.; Swanson, A. G. Abnormalities in central regulation of respiration in acute and convalescent poliomyelitis. Arch. Neurol. Psychiatry 80:267–285; 1958.

Pollack, C. P.; Perlick, D.; Linsner, J. P.; et al. Sleep problems in the community elderly as predictors of death and nursing home placement. J. Community Health 15:123–135; 1990.

Powell, N. B.; Guilleminault, C.; Riley, R. W. Surgical therapy for obstructive sleep apnea. In: Kryger, M. H.; Roth, T.; Dement, W. C. Principles and practice of sleep medicine. 2nd ed. London: WB Saunders Co.; 1994: p. 706–721.

Practice Parameters for the Treatment of Snoring and Obstructive Sleep Apnea with Oral Appliances. An American Sleep Disorders Association Report. Sleep 18:511–513; 1995.

Rauscher, H.; Pormanek, D.; Popp, W.; et al. The effects of nasal CPAP and weight loss on daytime hypertension in obstructive sleep apnea (abstract). Am. Rev. Respir. Dis. 145:442A; 1992.

Schenck, C. H.; Mahowald, M. W. Polysomnographic, neurologic, psychiatric, and clinical outcome report on 70 consecutive cases with REM sleep behavior disorder (RBD): sustained clonazepam efficacy in 89.5% of 57 treated patients. Cleve. Clin. J. Med. 57(suppl.):9–23; 1990.

Schmidt-Nowara, W.; Meade, T.; Hays, M. Treatment of snoring and obstructive sleep apnea with a dental orthosis. Chest 99:1378–1385; 1991.

Sforza, E.; Zucconi, M.; Petronelli, R.; Lugaresi, E.; Cirignotta, F. REM sleep behavioral disorders. Eur. Neurol. 28:295–300; 1988.

Shelton, K. E.; Woodson, H.; Gay, S. B.; Suratt, P. M. Adipose tissue deposition in sleep apnea. Sleep 16: S103–S105; 1993.

Shepard, J. W. Excessive daytime sleepiness, upper airway resistance, and nocturnal arousals. Chest 104: 665–666; 1993.

Sher, A. E.; Thorpy, M. J.; Shrintzen, R. J.; et al. Predictive value of Muller maneuver in selection of patients for uvulopalatopharyngoplasty. Laryngoscope 95:1483–1487; 1985.

Standards of Practice Committee of the American Sleep Disorders Association. Practice parameters for the use of laser-assisted uvulopalatopharyngoplasty. Sleep 17:744–748; 1994.

Stoohs, R. A.; Guilleminault, C.; Itoi, A.; Dement, W. C. Traffic accidents in commercial long-haul truck drivers. The influence of sleep-disordered breathing and obesity. Sleep 17(7):619–623; 1994.

Strohl, K. P. Overview of the problem: sleepiness, its assessment and the players in the equation. In: Legal implications of sleep disorders handout. 8th Annual APSS Meeting, June 4, Boston; 1994.

Symonds, C. P. Nocturnal myoclonus. J. Neurol. Neurosurg. Psychiatry 16:166–171; 1953.

The New York State Governor's Task Force on Sleepiness/Fatigue and Driving. Albany, NY; 1994.

Viscomi, V.; Walker, J.; Farney, R.; Tooney, K. Efficacy of a dental appliance in patients with snoring and sleep apnea (abstract). Sleep Res. 17:266; 1988.

Walters, A.; Hening, W. A.; Kavey, N.; et al. A double blind randomized cross-over trial of bromocriptine and placebo in the restless legs syndrome. Ann. Neurol. 24:455–458; 1988.

Walters, A. S.; Wagner, M. L.; Hening, W. A.; et al. Successful treatment of the idiopathic restless legs syndrome in a randomized double-blind trial of oxycodonoe versus placebo. Sleep 16:327–332; 1993.

Wetter, T. C.; Stiasny, K.; Winkelmann, J.; Buhlinger, A.; Brandenburg, U.; Penzel, T.; Medori, R.; Rubin, M.; Oertel, W. H.; Trenkwalder, C. A randomized controlled study of pergolide in patients with restless legs syndrome. Neurology 52:944–950; 1999.

Wu, H.; Yan-Go, F. L. The association of sleep apnea syndrome and risk of motor vehicle accidents. Neurology 45(suppl. 4):A269; 1995.

Young, T. B.; Palta, M.; Dempsey, J.; et al. The occurrence of sleep-disordered breathing among middle-aged adults. N. Engl. J. Med. 328:1230–1235; 1993.

# CONGENITAL, GENETIC-METABOLIC, AND DISORDERS OF PREGNANCY

# 40

# Neurofibromatosis

DAVID H. GUTMANN AND VINCENT M. RICCARDI

A discussion of the prognosis of neurofibromatosis (NF) is a challenge. First, there is more than one type of neurofibromatosis, necessitating a discussion of each type as a separate entity. Second, each type of neurofibromatosis is extremely variable in its manifestations, so a discussion about prognosis concerns the individual types of manifestations and their cumulative importance. This chapter deals with two primary categories of NF: NF1 and NF2 (Riccardi 1982, 1989a; Riccardi and Eichner 1986; Huson and Hughes 1994; Gutmann and Collins 1995). For both of these categories, the prognosis for the major complications of the respective disorders will be considered separately.

## NF1

NF1 is also known as von Recklinghausen's NF (Gutmann and Collins 1995; Huson and Hughes 1994; Riccardi 1981, 1992) to reflect the original observations of Frederick von Recklinghausen, who first recognized the syndrome. NF1 is inherited as an autosomal dominant trait and affects 1 in 3000 individuals worldwide without regard for gender, race, or ethnic background. Significant advances in our understanding of the molecular genetics of NF1 have resulted from the identification of the genetic locus on the proximal long arm of chromosome 17 (Collins et al. 1989; Fountain et al. 1989; O'Connell et al. 1989) and subsequently the *NF1* gene (Cawthon et al. 1990; Viskochil et al. 1990; Wallace et al. 1990).

The defining features of NF1 include multiple café-au-lait spots, skinfold freckling, neurofibromas, and iris Lisch nodules (Lewis and Riccardi 1981). The diagnosis of NF1 is made in an individual based on established diagnostic criteria which include two or more of the following features: (1) six or more café-au-lait macules (>0.5 cm before puberty and >1.5 cm after puberty), (2) axillary or inguinal (skinfold) freckling, (3) two or more Lisch nodules (iris hamartomas), (4) two or more neurofibromas or one plexiform neurofibroma, (5) optic pathway gliomas, (6) distinctive bony lesions such as sphenoid wing dysplasia or dysplasia of the long bones, and (7) a first-degree relative with NF1 diagnosed using the above diagnostic criteria (Gutmann et al. 1997). Other features are commonly associated with NF1 but are not sufficiently specific enough to warrant inclusion as diagnostic criteria. Individuals with NF1 often manifest with macrocephaly, short stature, hyperintense $T_2$ abnormalities on brain magnetic resonance imaging (MRI), and learning disabilities.

## Overview

NF1 is potentially serious because patients with NF1 can be significantly compromised in many ways, and this compromise may be delayed for years or even decades (Reynolds and Pineda 1988). The prognosis for any individual affected with NF1 is heavily dependent on the clinical features in that individual. There is no correlation between the severity of the disorder and the type of genetic mutation, the prior clinical history of the individual, or the severity of NF1 in affected family members. The only exception to the lack of genotype-phenotype correlation in NF1 are patients with large deletions involving the entire *NF1* gene (Kayes et al. 1992). These patients present with large numbers of neurofibromas often from early childhood, mental retardation, and dysmorphic facies.

Although NF1 can have severe manifestations, many patients with NF1 lead wholesome and relatively normal lives. Moreover, the serious complications considered here are distributed over the entire NF1 population: No one patient will develop all of the complications of the disorder. The following discussion considers the anatomical and functional complications resulting from NF1 with respect to the degree of associated functional impairment. It is worth noting that the prognosis for individuals affected with NF1 is often influenced to a greater extent by other coexisting medical disorders such as spina bifida or diabetes mellitus, than by the complications of NF1 itself.

## Mild Impairment

The defining features of NF1 include café-au-lait spots, skinfold freckling, neurofibromas, and Lisch nodules. These are likely to be present in all patients with the disorder if they live long enough. However, it is rare that a patient is so free of neurofibromas as to preclude some element of moderate compromise.

Various types of headache affect many patients with NF1 and include (1) typical "tension" headaches and those associated with chronic nasal sinus congestion; (2) migraine types of headache, suggesting a vascular pathogenesis; and (3) infrequently, headaches, presenting as an initial symptom of a brain tumor, hydrocephalus. or cerebrovascular compromise (Clementi et al. 1996). It is important to obtain a detailed headache history and perform a neurological examination upon initial evaluation of any individual with NF1 and headaches. A change in the character of the headaches or the development of neurological abnormalities should warrant an aggressive evaluation for underlying intracranial pathology. The prognosis for the first two types of headaches is relatively good in that they are readily managed and are almost always associated with minimal to mild morbidity. The third type of headache, which is not always easily distinguished from the other two types, may indicate pathological processes that may significantly alter the patient's long-term prognosis. Brain MRI in these cases is very useful in excluding intracranial pathology.

## Moderate Impairment

Learning disabilities occur in at least 40% to 60% of patients with NF1 (Denckla 1987; Eliason 1986, 1988; Riccardi 1984; Riccardi and Eichner 1986; Varnhagen et al. 1988; North et al. 1994, 1995, 1997). Although the burden of this clinical problem can be relatively modest, it is the most common focus of attention in the NF clinical program and warrants aggressive intervention (Zigmond 1995). It tends to be extremely disruptive of the affected child's household and social life. The primary problems involve poor attention span, impulsivity, poor visual-motor skills, and a diminished information-processing capability. In addition, there is often generalized incoordination (Dunn and Roos 1988; Riccardi and Eichner 1986). Delayed gross motor development and infantile muscular hypotonia appear to be reasonably accurate harbingers of this type of NF1 school performance problem. IQ scores generally are within the normal range; however, the mean IQ scores of some children with NF1 are shifted to the left (Riccardi 1984). Brain MRI has demonstrated the presence of hyperintense lesions on $T_2$-weighted scans, termed unidentified bright objects (UBOs). Although the clinical significance of these lesions is not known (DiPaolo et al. 1995), several studies have demonstrated a correlation between the presence of these lesions and IQ scores (North et al. 1994; Moore et al. 1996). Further studies will be required to confirm and extend these suggestive findings.

Many types of speech impediments without any feature accounting for all patients are seen in many patients with NF1. Velopharyngeal incompetence appears to be a common problem

(Pollack and Shprintzen 1981) and involvement of the oral, oropharyngeal, or nasopharyngeal structures by the direct or indirect effects of strategically located neurofibromas frequently contribute to this problem. The speech defect often is characterized as hypernasal, breathy, and monotonous (Riccardi and Eichner 1986). Compromise of expressive and receptive prosody skills is a major element of this clinical problem. Language skills also may be affected.

Cosmetic defects of varying degrees probably develop at some time in the life of at least half of all patients with NF1. They may result from three mechanisms: (1) localized or segmental hypertrophic growth of plexiform neurofibromas, especially cranial or facial tumors and large tumors of the trunk, buttocks, or limbs (Reed et al. 1986); (2) cutaneous neurofibromas because of the large numbers or strategic (e. g., facial) location; and (3) skeletal deformities, including kyphoscoliosis, sphenoid wing dysplasia, or tibial pseudarthrosis. For many of the neurofibroma-associated distortions, surgery is one approach to treatment. However, it is generally unsatisfactory if the perceived goal is restoration of a totally normal appearance.

A heavy psychosocial burden (i.e., an excessive emotional and social discomfiture resulting from the stigmatization of a chronic and progressive disease, the dread of an unknown future, and the cosmetic and other handicaps) is present in a large proportion of patients with NF1. Teenagers and young adults are particularly likely to experience this complication of NF1, even if transiently. An excess of unmarried or childless men with moderately severe NF1 (compared to similarly affected women) probably reflects the magnitude of this aspect of the disorder (Crowe et al. 1956; Riccardi and Eichner 1986). Discussions with knowledgeable clinicians, input from social workers or family counselors, and psychotherapy can help alleviate this problem (Roback et al. 1981).

Plexiform neurofibromas in the sites previously considered and elsewhere can also be associated with much less severe outcomes (see below). With respect to the neurofibroma, the determinants of growth and size are unknown, with the exception of the potential contribution of trauma (Riccardi 1989b). Surgery for tumors in strategic locations or to reduce burdensome mass is frequently required and often more than once.

Short stature, other than that associated with chiasm optic gliomas, occurs in a significant proportion of patients with NF1 (Riccardi and Haeberlin 1989). Alone, this aspect of NF1 is not particularly serious, but when added to school performance problems, various types of disfigurement, and other clinical tribulations, short stature can be an important aspect of the overall clinical picture. On the other hand, short stature does not necessarily implicate a chiasm glioma or other neuroanatomical basis. More likely, the short stature is another manifestation of the disease.

Other skeletal abnormalities, including cranial vault defects (Mann et al. 1983), nondystrophic scoliosis, pectus excavatum, angulation deformities at the knees (genu varum, genu valgum), ankle valgus, and pes planus are relatively common in patients with NF1. Although most are relatively trivial in terms of their clinical impact, some patients may require surgical treatment or prolonged bracing.

Renovascular hypertension occurs in a significant portion of patients with NF1 (Craddock et al. 1988; Elias et al. 1985; Finley and Dabbs 1988; Lassmann 1988; Pollard et al. 1989). Although the exact frequency of this feature is not known, it is included in this section because the frequency may be higher than 5% and should be suspected in all age groups, particularly the early and middle teenage years. Pregnancy may represent another epoch of time when renovascular hypertension presents as a feature of NF1 (Edwards et al. 1983). The prognosis of renovascular hypertension may be greatly improved by timely surgical intervention (Baxi et al. 1981; Gardiner et al. 1988; Mallmann and Roth 1986).

Precocious puberty occurs in NF1 with a frequency of no more than 0.5% and its presence virtually always indicates the presence of a progressing optic chiasm glioma (Laue et al. 1985; Tertsch et al. 1979). Delay in the onset of progression of puberty is less often a complication of NF1. Aggressive management by an experienced neurooncologist and endocrinologist is often required.

Cerebrovascular disturbances as part of the clinical picture of NF1 probably occur more commonly than appreciated (DeKersaint et al. 1980). Individuals may present with fixed neurological deficits from cerebral ischemia or transient neurological impairment mimicking a complicated migraine. However, an estimate of 0.5% is probably consistent with its clinical detectability. In general, when recognized on the basis of clinical problems, the overall prognosis for the disorder is considerably worse than when no such problems are seen.

Spinal arachnoid cysts in patients with NF1 (Erkulvrawatr et al. 1979; Kaiser et al. 1986; O'Neill et al. 1983) are more likely to occur in association with the various types of scoliosis, and particularly with lordoscoliosis (Dickson 1985). Accurate frequency figures are not available. However, in a portion of patients with this feature of NF1 there may be substantial amounts of localized back pain that has no alternative explanation.

**Major Morbidity**

NF1 can cause serious long-term handicaps in many ways. Neurological compromise is the most frequent cause. Paraspinal neurofibromas, particularly in the cervical region, may result in quadriparesis or quadriplegia. At least a portion of intracranial tumors, particularly astrocytomas of the optic pathway or the posterior fossa, can lead to serious disability. Cerebrovascular disturbances leading to stroke or hydrocephalus can also cause long-term functional compromise. Peripheral neuropathies resulting from direct involvement by neurofibromas or from surgical complications are common. A variety of pain syndromes usually associated with large neurofibromas or spinal arachnoid cysts may be a source of major clinical distress. Skeletal dysplasias or hypertrophic overgrowth of congenital plexiform neurofibromas are the second most frequent cause of major disabilities. Among the skeletal dysplasias, kyphoscoliosis, sphenoid wing dysplasia, or tibial pseudarthrosis account for a significant portion of long-term physical handicaps. Congenital plexiform neurofibromas that lead to chronic disability include those involving the upper midline of the body from the retropharyngeal region to the lower reaches of the mediastinum and those involving the limb girdles or face.

Optic pathway gliomas occur in 15% of patients with NF1 with the vast majority presenting in children under the age of 6 years (Lewis et al. 1984; Listernick et al. 1989, 1997). Of those patients with optic gliomas, approximately half are symptomatic from these tumors at the time of diagnosis. The clinical problems range from unilateral visual acuity decreases (i.e., associated with a unilateral optic nerve glioma) (Coyle et al. 1988; Duffner and Cohen 1988) to total blindness, hydrocephalus, precocious puberty, and diencephalic syndrome (Adornato and Berg 1977) and other endocrine disturbances (i.e., associated with chiasmal tumors). Although some controversy remains concerning the efficacy of treatment of patients detected before irreversible damage is done (Gould et al. 1987; Hoyt and Baghdassarian 1969; Imes and Hoyt 1986; Weiss et al. 1987), an increased consensus suggests that early detection and properly timed treatment can be important in enhancing the progn osis for patients with this complication of NF1 (Chung and McCrary 1988; Easley et al. 1988; Packer et al. 1988). At present, there is an emerging role for chemotherapy, as opposed to radiation therapy, in the management of these tumors (Listernick et al. 1997). Without question, optic pathway gliomas are among the most important of the early childhood complications of NF1 (Cohen and Duffner 1983; Cohen et al. 1986). There has been some suggestion that the prognosis is better for patients with an optic glioma as part of NF1 compared to similar isolated tumors (Stern et al. 1979, 1980; Alvord and Lofton 1988; Borit and Richardson 1982).

Kyphoscoliosis affects approximately 5% of patients with NF1. In virtually all instances, the onset of the spinal distortion occurs in the first decade of life. Most often the process becomes apparent between ages 6 and 10, but occasionally an earlier onset is noted. Especially for the latter group, a localized or diffuse vertebral dysplasia is the underlying basis for the more serious types of disfigurement (Cimino et al. 1986; Yaghmai 1986). A useful clinical sign of the propensity to develop clinically important, progressive kyphoscoliosis is a distortion of the hair pattern along the midline of the back (Flannery and Howell 1987). When the kyphoscoliotic process has been detected, the prognosis can be improved greatly by prompt and aggressive treatment, primarily using spinal fusion, often with internal fixation, such as Harrington rods or similar devices (Chaglassian et al. 1976). External bracing generally only temporizes, but this might be useful as part of a strategy to allow maximum vertical growth before surgery is performed. Only sometimes are neurofibromas associated with the kyphoscoliotic process, but when they are present, the surgical approach and follow-up must take them into account.

Congenital glaucoma probably occurs in 0.5% to 1% of patients with NF1 (Bost et al. 1985; Grant and Walton 1968). All at-risk newborns must be examined with this feature of the disorder in mind. A protruding ocular globe, frank buphthalmos, or even persistent crying may be a helpful clinical sign. Loss of vision in the involved eye is likely and enucleation may be necessary.

Seizures of all types occur in approximately 5% of patients with NF1. Although most often they are readily managed with anticonvulsant medications, they are listed as "serious complications" to emphasize that for some patients, especially with a neonatal or infantile onset, seizures may be associated with a serious prognosis. Myoclonic jerks (infantile spasms with hypsarrhythmia) fall into this category (Goldberg et al. 1985; Terada et al. 1986). In addition, the later onset of seizures may indicate the development of hydrocephalus or the progression of a previously quiescent astrocytoma.

Tibial pseudarthrosis occurs in 0.5% to 1% of patients with NF1. This lesion usually is unilateral, but bilateral cases are well documented. Conservative treatment with casting and bracing may be sufficient treatment, but often surgical treatment (DeBoer et al. 1988) or amputation is required. The recent availability of the Ilizarov bone-lengthening technology (Dal Monte and Donzelli 1987; Green 1988) may significantly improve the prognosis for patients with the more serious forms of this complication of NF1. Less serious forms of this problem, involving bowing of the tibia, are associated with a much better prognosis. In addition, similar lesions can occur in many other sites, including any of the long bones and clavicles (Ali and Hooper 1982; Bayne 1985).

Sphenoid wing dysplasia occurs in approximately 2% to 3% of patients with NF1. Severity ranges from trivial findings on radiographic studies to serious problems, including facial disfigurement and pulsating enophthalmos associated with herniation of a portion of the brain into the orbit (DeVilliers 1982; Grenier et al 1984). It is important to recognize that this is a dysplastic lesion of the bone (i.e., it is not the result of a local plexiform neurofibroma, which also may be present) and that it will progressively worsen. Surgical reconstruction of the posterior orbital wall ultimately may be indicated.

Plexiform neurofibromas are congenital lesions, but their detection in infancy may require a high level of clinical suspicion (Bourgouin et al. 1988). The presence of overlying hyperpigmentation may facilitate detection, and if the hyperpigmentation reaches the midline of the body, involvement of the neuraxis should be presumed. Conservatively, 2% to 3% of patients with NF1 ultimately will have serious problems resulting from such tumors. Those involving the second and third branches of the trigeminal nerve may have particularly adverse effects in terms of cosmetic disfigurement and compromise of ocular and oral structures. Plexiform neurofibromas involving the retropharyngeal regions and upper mediastinum may seriously compromise the upper respiratory tree and deglutition, and they may be associated with kyphoscoliosis, thoracic wall tumor growth, or both. Similar tumors involving the limb girdles and proximal limbs may lead to joint destruction and limited use of the limb. These may require amputation, often in the teen or young adult years, for effective management (Match and Leffert 1987). Deeper involvement of the intrathoracic space or the retroperitoneal space must be considered for such tumors. Plexiform neurofibromas with massive overgrowth involving the distal extremities also are a significant cause of major compromise of ambulation or manual dexterity and may require disfiguring surgery or amputation.

Paraspinal neurofibromas (Burk et al. 1987; Castelein and MacEwen 1984; Levy et al. 1986; Lewis and Kingsley 1987), particularly in the cervical region, may have a grave prognosis (Adekeye et al. 1984). Massive cervical paraspinal neurofibromas are among the most common causes of serious long-term morbidity in NF1. Destruction of adjacent vertebrae (Ferner et al. 1988), centripetal growth into and around the spinal cord, and centrifugal growth with consequent compromise of nerve roots and proximal nerve trunks can lead to quadriparesis (or quadriplegia) combined with peripheral neuropathies. The course is slowly but inexorably progressive and frequently leads to premature death. Involvement of the thoracic and lumbosacral regions with neurofibromas can lead to paraparesis (or paraplegia) in a similar manner. Chronic, relatively intense pain is more likely to accompany the lumbosacral lesions than those higher up the vertebral column.

Cerebral, brain stem, and posterior fossa astrocytomas (distinct from astrocytomas of the optic pathways) are a definite part of the NF1 tumor spectrum, but the frequency is unclear (Miller 1975; Gray and Waimann 1987; Molloy et al. 1995). Moreover, the consequences of such tumors are variable. However, little is known about the natural history of these tumors. In some instances, for unknown reasons, they may become aggressive and lead to serious brain compromise and death (Hochstrasser et al. 1988; Sorensen et al. 1986). It is critically important to distinguish tumors (i.e., lesions showing a breakdown of the blood-brain barrier and a "mass effect") from the hyperintense $T_2$-weighted signal lesions commonly seen frequently on MRI scans of the brains of patients with NF1. These foci have limited and arguable prognostic significance (Bognanno et al. 1988; Brown et al. 1987; Duffner et al. 1989; Dunn and Rons 1988; DiPaolo et al. 1995). Several studies have examined the relationship between cognitive impairment and the presence of UBOs (Denckla et al. 1996; Moore et al. 1996; North et al. 1997). Further analyses will be required to determine if the presence of the lesions has clinical value in the management of individuals with NF1.

Hydrocephalus may be seen in approximately 0.5% of patients with NF1 (Riviello et al. 1988). Although occasionally hydrocephalus may be the result of a demonstrable brain tumor, usually a chiasmal glioma or Chiari malformation (Afifi et al. 1988), in many instances the exact pathogenesis is unclear. In some cases, there is stenosis of the aqueduct of Sylvius. Prompt recognition and treatment can minimize the potential for a seriously worsened prognosis.

## Fatal Complications of NF1

Individuals with NF1 can die of complications directly related to their disease. Most commonly, these are the result of metastatic disease or local effects of a benign tumor. For the most part, the tumors seen in individuals with NF1 are benign tumors. However, less commonly, malignancies can arise in NF1 (Hope and Mulvihill 1981; Matsui et al. 1993). These include astrocytomas, pheochromocytomas, rhabdomyosarcomas, juvenile myeloid leukemias and malignant peripheral nerve sheath tumors (MPNSTs). Astrocytomas can lead to death by local invasion of normal brain tissue and result in prolonged seizures or serious neurological deficits. Pheochromocytomas and rhabdomyosarcomas are treatable tumors but have significant associated mortality. In contrast, MPNSTs and leukemias can be rapidly fatal. Lastly, pronounced kyphoscoliosis or local invasion by a benign plexiform neurofibroma may have fatal consequences.

MPNSTs occur in approximately 6% of patients with NF1 (Riccardi and Eichner 1986), although some authors portray the risk as higher or lower. Typically, MPNSTs do not occur until the end of the first decade or thereafter, and tend to cluster in the second, third, and fourth decades (D'Agostino et al. 1963a, 1963b). The most consistent clinical indicator of an MPNST is pain. Therefore, the development of pain in a preexisting plexiform neurofibroma must be considered to indicate an MPNST until proven otherwise. Additional clinical indicators are the sudden appearance of a new mass, the rapid growth of a previously quiescent neurofibroma, or the unexplained development of a focal neurological deficit. The prognosis for patients with NF1 and an MPNST is bleak unless amputation can completely remove the tumor from the patient's body. In general, local surgery, irradiation, and chemotherapy only temporize at best (Bolton et al. 1989; Goldman et al. 1977). MPNSTs represent one of the most important causes of untimely death among young patients with NF1. Moreover, in individuals with NF1, MPNSTs behave more aggressively than MPNSTs seen in the general population and represent highly metastatic malignancies.

The frequency of pheochromocytomas is generally overestimated among patients with NF1 (Healy and Mekalatos 1958; Nakamura et al. 1986). The actual frequency is approximately 0.5% to 1%. Nonetheless, pheochromocytomas are critically important because unappreciated tumors can lead to an untimely and probably unnecessary death, sometimes in association with otherwise minor or trivial surgery (Riccardi and Eichner 1986). Routine screening of patients with NF1 using measurements of catecholamines in 24-hour urine specimens has not been helpful (Riccardi and Eichner 1986). However, the slightest clinical suspicion of a pheochromocytoma (e.g., excessive sweating, palpitations, episodic headaches) should lead to a prompt and vigorous effort to discount or confirm the presence of this tumor.

## NF2

NF2, previously known as bilateral acoustic/vestibular NF or central NF, is different from NF1. Its clinical burden is determined by central nervous system (CNS) tumors (schwannomas and meningiomas) and by paraspinal neurofibromas (Martuza and Eldridge 1988; Mulvihill et al. 1990). NF2 is inherited as an autosomal dominant trait. Genetically, NF2 is localized to a different chromosome than NF1. The *NF2* gene located on the long arm of chromosome 22 (Rouleau et al. 1987, 1993; Seizinger et al. 1986; Trofatter et al. 1993; Wertelecki et al. 1988) was identified by positional cloning. Despite occasional confusion, the diagnosis of NF1 and NF2 can be readily made based on established diagnostic criteria (Gutmann et al. 1997).

The original National Institutes of Health (NIH) Consensus Development Conference diagnostic criteria for NF2 included (1) bilateral eighth-nerve masses visualized by MRI or (2) a first-degree relative with NF2 and either unilateral eight nerve masses or any two of the following: neurofibroma, meningioma, glioma, schwannoma, or juvenile posterior subcapsular lenticular opacity (Mulvihill et al. 1992). Recently, new criteria have been suggested (Gutmann et al. 1997). Individuals with definite (confirmed) NF2 have bilateral vestibular schwannomas or a first-degree relative with NF2 plus (1) a unilateral vestibular schwannoma presenting before age 30 or (2) any two of the following including meningioma, glioma, schwannoma, juvenile posterior subcapsular lenticular opacities/juvenile cortical cataract. Individuals with presumptive (probable) NF2 require further evaluation and are classified as those with (1) a unilateral vestibular schwannoma presenting before age 30 plus at least one of the following including meningioma, glioma, schwannoma, juvenile posterior subcapsular lenticular opacities/juvenile cortical cataract or (2) multiple meningiomas (1 or more) plus a unilateral vestibular schwannoma or one of the following including glioma, schwannoma, juvenile posterior subcapsular lenticular opacities/juvenile cortical cataract.

The prognosis of patients with NF2 also is different from that of NF1 (Fickel 1989; Martuza and Eldridge 1988; Huson and Hughes 1994) but, as with NF1, the clinical course is variable and dictated by tumor burden, surgical management, and associated complications. There are individuals with NF2 who escape the serious effects of the CNS tumors or the paraspinal neurofibromas and generally have a milder course and a good prognosis (Parry et al. 1996; Ruttledge et al. 1996). In contrast, other patients with NF2 who become symptomatic from these tumors at an early age are likely to be seriously compromised and have a relatively poor prognosis. These individuals tend to present with tumors earlier in life and manifest greater numbers of tumors and a more fulminant clinical course. The majority of patients with NF2 have few or no problems during the first decade of life. However, by the end of the third decade, one or more tumors manifest. Typically, the age of onset of clinical symptoms is between 18 and 22 years. Posterior subcapsular cataracts may be detected with increasing frequency as the patient ages (Kaiser-Kupfer et al. 1989; Pearson-Webb et al. 1986). Some of these cataracts may result in visual compromise (Ragge et al. 1995). Although patients with NF2 have few café-au-lait spots or cutaneous neurofibromas, cutaneous schwannomas are not uncommonly detected on routine skin examination.

Deafness can present acutely but most commonly occurs insidiously with a lag in hearing deficits between the two ears. There are patients in whom a fluctuating course with episodes of sudden hearing loss is followed by complete or partial recovery. In addition, facial weakness, visual abnormalities, and painful peripheral neuropathies may occur as a result of tumor growth. Unlike NF1, the average age of death in individuals with NF2 is 36 years, with a 15-year mean survival from diagnosis.

Schwannomas involve the CNS of patients with NF2 in three ways. First, the hallmark lesion is the vestibular schwannoma, more commonly known as an acoustic neuroma. In NF2, vestibular schwannomas virtually always are bilateral but not necessarily simultaneous in terms of presentation or as causes of clinical problems (Curati et al. 1986a, 1986b; House et al. 1986; Martuza and Ojemann 1982; Mazzoni 1987; Stack et al. 1988). Most often, progressive growth leads to compression of the auditory or vestibular portion of the eighth cranial nerve, resulting in varying degrees of deafness or balance problems. In addition, surgical manipulation completes or adds to the deafness and frequently results in an ipsilateral facial palsy. Second, schwannomas also may develop on the fifth cranial nerve in 25% of individuals (McCormack et al. 1988). Third, schwannomas may develop within the substance of the spinal cord and on dorsal nerve roots, leading to focal spinal cord deficits. Upwards of 80% of NF2 patients will harbor these spinal schwannomas.

Meningiomas may develop virtually anywhere within the cranial vault or along the length of the spinal cord. They are detected in half of the individuals affected with NF2. Occasionally, these tumors may masquerade as optic pathway gliomas and affect vision. Careful radiographic evaluation usually distinguishes optic pathway gliomas from meningiomas. Frequently, more than one meningioma complicates the clinical picture for a patient with NF2. These tumors may be among the most troublesome for patients with NF2. While astrocytomas of the optic pathway are virtually unheard of in NF2, spinal astrocytomas are a hallmark of NF2.

Ependymomas represent a distinctive lesion seen in NF2. They may occur within the cranial vault or within the spinal cord and may result in serious compromise and death. Paraspinal neurofibromas and schwannomas are often an unappreciated feature of NF2 (Levy et al. 1986). Nonetheless, they are a major aspect of this disorder and may lead to serious motor and sensory deficits, and at times, they may be associated with local kyphoscoliosis. For these reasons, baseline spinal MRI scans are often recommended in the initial evaluation of an individual at risk for NF2 (Gutmann et al. 1997).

## Treatment Strategies

Surgery is the mainstay of treatment for NF1 and NF2. Decreasing each tumor's bulk and the effects of its impingement on local structures are the primary goals of surgery (Briggs et al. 1994; Kelly et al. 1988; Nadol et al. 1992; Ojemann 1993; Pickard and Rose 1988; Slattery et al. 1998). This approach may have dramatic results in the short term, but the long-term results are less than satisfactory. Laser technology for surgical approaches (Katalinic 1987; Roenigk and Ratz 1987) probably offers no unique advantages. Recently, stereotactic radiosurgery (gamma knife) has emerged as a possible alternative to conventional surgery in selected patients with vestibular schwannomas (Linskey et al. 1992).

The medical treatment of other benign tumors, such as optic gliomas (Packer et al. 1988; 1992) or acoustic neuromas and other schwannomas, is now emerging as an alternative to radiation therapy (Jahrsdoerfer and Benjamin 1988). Given the fact that most children with NF1 and optic pathway gliomas are under the age of 6 years, radiation therapy is often associated with neurocognitive sequelae, hypothalamic dysfunction, and the development of cerebral vascular abnormalities ("moya-moya" syndrome) (Kestle et al. 1993). Similarly, the medical treatment of malignant tumors (primarily MPNSTs) that complicate NF1 and NF2 is less than satisfactory (Goldman et al. 1977). As mentioned above, the most satisfactory results obtained with MPNSTs is seen in individuals with MPNSTs localized to an extremity treated with radical excision or amputation and without evidence of metastasis.

Remediation to overcome some of the physical and social handicaps of NF may be especially useful. Programs to assist in school performance, prostheses and hearing aids (including brain stem implants), and communication devices (computers) may be especially useful (Brody 1989). NF2 patients with hearing difficulties should be referred to an audiologist for training in optimizing hearing and speech, including lip-reading, sign language, and hearing aids. Counseling should also be provided to individuals with NF2, especially with regard to balance problems to avoid drowning or near-drowning caused by underwater disorientation.

Dialogue for treatment includes genetic counseling. Each person with NF1 or NF2 is told of the 50% risk for transmitting the mutant gene to each offspring and that prenatal diagnosis may be available for selected patients with NF1 (i.e., those with multiple generations affected) (Crandall et al. 1988; Hofman et al. 1992). Educational counseling clarifying the various types of NF-related problems that may arise is especially important (Powell 1988a, 1988b). Support groups, such as those provided in the context of the National Neurofibromatosis Foundation, regional NF chapters; Neurofibromatosis Inc., and the Acoustic Neuroma Association may be especially helpful to patients and families dealing with the tribulations and trials of NF. Social counseling may be of particular benefit as may psychotherapy (Messner et al. 1985; Messner and Smith 1986). Enhancing self-esteem and sense of control may be specific goals in this regard.

## Molecular Testing

NF1 and NF2 remain largely clinical diagnoses (Gutmann et al. 1997). Individuals with NF1 desiring prenatal testing can be provided with molecular testing in the setting of genetic counseling. For families with two or more affected individuals, linkage analysis can be performed. Other testing modalities, such as the protein truncation assay, are unproven as stand-alone tests. The greatest limitation to molecular testing for NF1 is the inability to predict severity in at-risk individuals. This inability to predict clinical severity significantly limits the usefulness of present molecular prenatal diagnostic testing for NF1.

Molecular testing for individuals at risk for NF2 also involves linkage analysis using flanking polymorphic markers in families with two or more affected individuals. Standard mutation detection is time-consuming and expensive, but may one day provide predictive information. Preliminary genotype-phenotype correlations have been established for NF2. Individuals with severe clinical disease tend to harbor mutations or deletions that disrupt the *NF2* gene (Parry et al. 1996; Ruttledge et al. 1996). Unfortunately, exceptions to these genotype-phenotype correlations have been reported (Scoles et al. 1996). With future refinements in genetic testing, molecular analysis of at-risk individuals with NF2 may become an adjunct to the clinical evaluation.

## References

Adekeye, E. O; Abiose, A.; Ord, R. A. Neurofibromatosis of the head and neck: clinical presentation and treatment. J. Maxillofac. Surg. 12:78–85; 1984.

Adornato, B.; Berg, B. Diencephalic syndrome and von Recklinghausen's disease. Ann. Neurol. 2:159–160; 1977.

Afifi, A. K.; Dolan, K. D.; Van Gilder, J. C.; Fincham, R. W. Ventriculomegaly in neurofibromatosis I: association with Chiari-I malformation. Neurofibromatosis 1:229–305; 1988.

Ali, M. S.; Hooper, G. Congenital pseudarthrosis of the ulna due to neurofibromatosis. J. Bone Joint Surg. 64:600–602; 1982.

Alvord, E. C., Jr.; Lofton, S. Gliomas of the optic nerve or chiasm: outcome by patient's age, tumor site and treatment. J. Neurosurg. 68:85–98; 1988.

Baxi, R.; Epstein, H. Y.; Abitbol, C. Percutaneous transluminal renal artery angioplasty in hypertension associated with neurofibromatosis. Radiology 139:583–584; 1981.

Bayne, L. G. Congenital pseudarthrosis of the forearm. Hand Clin. 1:457–465; 1985.

Bognanno, J. R.; Edwards, M. K.; Lee, T. A.; Dunn, P. W.; Roos, K. L.; Klatte, E. C. Cranial MR imaging in neurofibromatosis. AJR 151:381–388; 1988.

Bolton, J. S.; Vauthey, J. N.; Farr, G. H. Jr.; Sauter, E. I.; Bowen, J. C., III; Kline, D. G. Is limb-sparing surgery applicable to neurogenic sarcomas of the extremities? Arch. Surg. 124:118–121; 1989.

Borit, A.; Richardson, E. P., Jr. The biological and clinical behavior of pilocytic astrocytomas of the optic pathways. Brain 105:161–187; 1982.

Bost, M.; Mouillon, M.; Romanet, J. P.; Deiber, M.; Navoni, F. Congenital glaucoma and von Recklinghausen's disease. Pediatric 40:207–212; 1985.

Bourgouin, P. M.; Shepard, J. A. O.; Moore, E. H.; McCloud, T. C. Plexiform neurofibromatosis of the mediastinum: CT appearance. Am. J. Roentgenol. Radial. Ther. Nucl. Med. 151:461–463; 1988.

Briggs, R. J. S.; Brackmann, D. E.; Baser, M. E.; Hitselberger, W. E. Comprehensive management of bilateral acoustic neuromas. Arch. Otolaryngol. Head Neck Surg. 120:1307–1314; 1994.

Brody, H. The great equalizer: PCs empower the disabled. P. C. Computing 2(7):82–93; 1989.

Brown, E. W.; Riccardi, V. M.; Mawad, M.; Handel, S.; Goldman, A.; Bryan, R. N. Magnetic resonance imaging of optic pathways in patients with neurofibromatosis. AJNR Am. J. Neuroradiol. 8:1031–1036; 1987.

Burk, D. L., Jr.; Brunberg, J. A.; Kanal, E.; Latchaw, R. E. Spinal and paraspinal neurofibromatosis: surface coil MR imaging at 1.5T. Radiology 162:797–801; 1987.

Castelein, R. M.; MacEwen G. D. A dumbbell (hourglass) neurofibroma of the spine in a patient with von Recklinghausen's disease. A case report with twelve year follow up. Arch. Orthop. Trauma Surg. 102:216–220; 1984.

Cawthon, R. M.; Weiss, M.; Xu, G.; Viskochil, D.; Culver, M.; Stevens, J.; Robertson, M.; Dunn, D.; Gesteland, R.; O'Connell, P.; White, R. A major segment of the neurofibromatosis type 1 gene: cDNA sequence, genomic structure, and point mutations. Cell 62: 193–201; 1990.

Chaglassian, J. H.; Riseborough, E. J.; Hall, J. E. Neurofibromatous scoliosis: natural history and results of treatment in thirty-seven cases. J. Bone Joint Surg. 58A:695–702; 1976.

Chung, S. M.; McCrary, J. A., III. Management of pregeniculate anterior visual pathway gliomas. Neurofibromatosis 1:240–247; 1988.

Cimino, P. M.; Roberts, J. M.; King, A. G.; Burke, S. W.; Larocca, S. H. Dystrophic scoliosis and neurofibromatosis. Is myelogram indicated? Orthop. Trans. 10:580; 1986.

Clementi, M.; Battistella, P. A.; Rizzi, L.; Boni, S.; Tenconi, R.; Headache in patients with neurofibromatosis type 1. Headache 36:10–13; 1996.

Cohen, M. E.; Duffner, P. K. Visual-evoked responses in children with optic gliomas, with and without neurofibromatosis. Child's Brain 10:99–111; 1983.

Cohen, M. E.; Duffner, P. K.; Kuhn, J. P.; Seidel, F. G. Neuroimaging in neurofibromatosis. Ann. Neurol. 20:444; 1986.

Collins, F. S.; Ponder, B. A. J.; Seizinger, B. R.; Epstein, C. J. The von Recklinghausen neurofibromatosis region on chromosome 17— Genetic and physical maps come into focus. Am. J. Hum. Genet. 44:1–5; 1989.

Coyle, J. T.; Seiff, S. R.; Hoyt, W. F. Orbital optic glioma in neurofibromatosis. Arch. Ophthalmol. 106:718–723; 1988.

Craddock, G. R., Jr.; Challo, V. R.; Dean, R. W. Neurofibromatosis and renal artery stenosis: a case of familial incidence. J. Vasc. Surg. 8:489–494; 1988.

Crandall, K. A.; Edwards, J. G.; Riccardi, V. M. Attitudes of individuals affected with neurofibromatosis toward prenatal diagnosis. Am. J. Hum. Genet. 43: A165; 1988.

Crowe, F. W.; Schull, W. J.; Neel, J. V. A clinical, pathological, and genetic study of multiple neurofibromatosis. Springfield, IL: Charles C. Thomas; 1956.

Curati, W. L.; Graif, M.; Kingsley, D. P. E.; King, T.; Scholtz, C. L.; Steiner, R. E. MRI in acoustic neuroma: a review of 35 patients. Neuroradiology 28: 208–214; l986a.

Curati, W. L.; Graif, M.; Kingsley, D. P. E.; Niendorf, H. P.; Young, I. R. Acoustic neuromas: Gd-DTPA enhancement in MR imaging. Radiology 158:447–451; 1986b.

D'Agostino, A. N.; Soule, E. H.; Miller, R. H. Primary malignant neoplasms of nerves (malignant neurilemmomas) in patients with manifestations of multiple neurofibromatosis (von Recklinghausen's disease). Cancer 16:1003–1014; 1963a.

D'Agostino, A. N.; Soule, E. H.; Miller, R. H. Sarcomas of peripheral somatic tissue associated with multiple neurofibromatosis (von Recklinghausen's disease). Cancer 16:1015–1027; 1963b.

Dal Monte, A.; Donzelli, O. Tibial lengthening according to Ilizarov in congenital hypoplasia of the leg. J. Pediatr. Orthop. 7:135–138; 1987.

DeBoer, H. H.; Verbout, A. J.; Nielsen, H. K.; van der Eijken, J. W. Free vascularized fibular graft for tibial pseudarthrosis in neurofibromatosis. Acta Orthop. Scand. 59:425–429; 1988.

DeKersaint Gilly, A.; Zenthe, L.; Dabouis, G.; Mussini, J. M.; Lajat, Y.; Robert, R.; Picard, L. Abnormalities of the intracerebral vasculature in a case of neurofibromatosis. J. Neuroradiol. 7:193–198; 1980.

Denckla, M. B. Cognitive impairments in neurofibromatosis. Dysmorphol. Clin. Genet. 1:49–57; 1987.

Denckla, M. B.; Hofman, K.; Mazzocco, M. M. M.; Melhem, E.; Reiss, A. L.; Bryan, E. N.; Harris, E. L.; Lee, J.; Cox, C. S.; Schuerholz, L. J. Relationship between T2-weighted hyperintensities (unidentified bright objects) and lower IQs in children with neurofibromatosis-1. Am. J. Med. Genet. 67:98–102; 1996.

De Villiers, J. C. Neurofibromatous orbitocranial dysplasia in childhood. S. Afr. J. Surg. 20:137–144; 1982.

Dickson, R. A. Thoracic lordoscoliosis in neurofibromatosis: Treatment by a Harrington rod with sublaminar wiring. Report of two cases. J. Bone Joint Surg. 67:822–823; 1985.

DiPaolo, D. P.; Zimmerman, R. A.; Rorke, L. B.; Zackai, E. H.; Bilaniuk, L. T.; Yachnis, A. T. Neurofibromatosis type 1: pathological substrate of high signal intensity foci in the brain. Radiology 195:721–724; 1995.

Duffner, P. K.; Cohen, M. E. Isolated optic nerve gliomas in children with and without neurofibromatosis. Neurofibromatosis 1:201–211; 1988.

Duffner, P. K.; Cohen, M. E.; Seidel, F. G.; Shucard, D. W. The significance of MRI abnormalities in children with neurofibromatosis. Neurology 39:373–378; 1989.

Dunn, D. W.; Roos, K. L. RI evaluation of learning disability and incoordination in neurofibromatosis. Neurofibromatosis 2:1–5, 1988.

Easley, J. D.; Scharf, L.; Chou, J. L.; Riccardi, V. M. Controversy in the management of optic pathway gliomas. 29 patients treated at the Baylor College of Medicine from 1967 through 1987. Neurofibromatosis 1:248–251; 1988.

Edwards, J. N.; Fooks, M.; Davey, D. A. Neurofibromatosis and severe hypertension in pregnancy. Br. J. Obstet. Gynecol. 90:528–531; 1983.

Elias, D. L.; Ricketts, R. R.; Smith, R. B. Renovascular hypertension complicating neurofibromatosis. Am. J. Surg. 51:97–106; 1985.

Eliason, M. J. Neurofibromatosis: implications for learning and behavior. J. Dev. Behav. Pediatr. 7: 175–179; 1986.

Eliason, M. J. Neuropsychological patterns: neurofibromatosis compared to developmental learning disorders. Neurofibromatosis 1:17–25; 1988.

Erkulvrawatr, S.; Gammal, T. E.; Hawkins, J.; Green, J. B.; Srinivasan, G. Intrathoracic meningoceles and neurofibromatosis. Arch. Neurol. 36:557–559; 1979.

Ferner, R. E.; Honovar, M.; Gullan, R. W. A spinal neurofibroma presenting as atlanto-axial subluxation in von Recklinghausen neurofibromatosis (NF-1). Neurofibromatosis 2:43–46; 1988.

Fickel, G. Acoustic Neuroma Association annual meeting report: NF-2 update. Neurofibromatosis 2:57–66; 1989.

Finley, J. L.; Dabbs, D. J. Renal vascular smooth muscle proliferation in neurofibromatosis. Hum. Pathol. 19:107–110; 1988.

Flannery, D. B.; Howell, C. G. Confirmation of the Riccardi sign. Proc. Greenwood Genet. Ctr. 6:161; 1987.

Fountain, J. W.; Wallace, M. R.; Bruce, M. A.; Seizinger, B. R.; Menon, A. G.; Gusella, J. F.; Michels, V. V.; Schmidt, M. A.; Dewald, G. W.; Collins, F. S. Physical mapping of a translocation breakpoint in neurofibromatosis. Science 244:1085–1087; 1989.

Gardiner, G. A., Jr.; Freedman, A. M.; Shlansky-Goldberg, R. Percutaneous luminal angioplasty: delayed response in neurofibromatosis. Radiology 169:79–80; 1988.

Goldberg, A.; Kohelet, D.; Mundel, G. Congenital neurofibromatosis presenting as neonatal cerebral damage with hypsarrhythmia. Harefuah 108:332–333; 1985.

Goldman, R. L.; Jones, S. L.; Heusinkveld, R. S. Combination chemotherapy of metastatic malignant schwannoma with vincristine, adriamycin, cyclophosphamide, and imidazole carboxamide. Cancer 39:1955–1958; 1977.

Gould, R. J.; Hilal, S. K.; Chutorian, A. M. Efficacy of radiotherapy in optic gliomas. Pediatr. Neurol. 3:29–32; 1987.

Grant, W. M.; Walton, D. S. Distinctive gonioscopic findings in glaucoma due to neurofibromatosis. Arch. Ophthalmol. 79:127–134; 1967.

Gray, J.; Swaimann, K. F. Brain tumors in children with neurofibromatosis: computed tomography and magnetic resonance imaging. Pediatr. Neurol. 3: 335–341; 1987.

Green, S. A. Ilizarov external fixation. Technical and anatomic considerations. Bull. Hosp. Jt. Dis. Orthop. Inst. 28:28–35; 1988.

Grenier, N.; Guibert Tranier, F.; Nicholau, A.; Caille, J. M. Contribution of computerized tomography to the study of spheno-orbital dysplasia in neurofibromatosis. J. Neuroradiol. 11:201–211; 1984.

Gutmann, D. H.; Collins, F. S.; von Recklinghausen neurofibromatosis. In: Scriver, C.; Beaudet, A.; Sly, W.; Valle, D. The metabolic and molecular bases of inherited disease. 7th ed. New York: McGraw Hills; 1995: p. 667–696.

Gutmann, D. H.; Aylsworth, A.; Carey, J. C.; Korf, B.; Marks, J.; Pyeritz, R. E.; Rubinstein, A.; Viskochil, D. The diagnostic evaluation and multidisciplinary management of neurofibromatosis 1 and neurofibromatosis 2. JAMA 278:51–57; 1997.

Healy, F. H., Jr.; Mekalatos, C. J. Pheochromocytoma and neurofibromatosis. N. Engl. J. Med. 258:540–546; 1958.

Hochstrasser, H.; Boltshauser, E.; Valavanis, A. Brain tumors in children with neurofibromatosis. Neurofibromatosis 1:233–239; 1988.

Hofman, K. J.; Boehm, C. D.; Familial neurofibromatosis type 1: clinical experience with DNA testing. J. Pediatr. 120:394–398; 1992.

Hope, D. G.; Mulvihill, J. J. Malignancy in neurofibromatosis. Adv. Neurol. 29:33–55; 1981.

House, J. W.; Waluch, V.; Jackler, R. K. Magnetic resonance imaging in acoustic neuroma diagnosis. Ann. Otol. Rhinol. Laryngol. 95:16–20; 1986.

Hoyt, W. F.; Baghdassarian, S. A. Optic glioma of childhood: natural history and rationale for conservative management. Br. J. Ophthalmol. 53:793–798; 1969.

Huson, S. M.; Hughes, R. A. C. The neurofibromatoses: a pathogenetic and clinical overview. Cambridge: Chapman and Hall; 1994.

Imes, R. K.; Hoyt, W. F. Childhood chiasmal gliomas: update on the fate of patients in the 1969 San Francisco Study. Br. J. Ophthalmol. 70:179–182; 1986.

Jahrsdoerfer, R. A.; Benjamin, R. S. Chemotherapy of bilateral acoustic neuromas. Otolaryngol. Head Neck Surg. 98:273–282; 1988.

Kaiser, M. C.; De Slegte, R. G.; Crezee, F. C.; Valk, J. Anterior cervical meningoceles in neurofibromatosis. Am. J. Neuro. Radiol. 7:1105–1110; 1986.

Kaiser-Kupfer, M. I.; Freidlin, V.; Datiles, M. B.; Edwards, P. A.; Sherman, J. L.; Parry, D.; McCain, L. M.; Eldridge, R. The association of posterior capsular lens opacity with bilateral acoustic neuromas in patients with neurofibromatosis type 2. Arch. Ophthalmol. 107:541–544; 1989.

Katalinic, D. Therapy of neurofibromatosis with the argon laser. Lasers Surg. Med. 7:128–135; 1987.

Kayes, L. M.; Riccardi, V. M.; Burke, W.; Bennett, R. L.; Stephens, K. Large de novo DNA deletion in a patient with sporadic neurofibromatosis, mental retardation and dysmorphism. J. Med. Genet. 29:686; 1992.

Kelly, D. L., Jr.: Britton, B. H.: Branch, C. L., Jr. Cooperative neuro-otologic management of acoustic neuromas and other cerebellopontine angle tumors. South. Med. J. 81:557–561; 1988.

Kestle, J. R. W.; Hoffman, H. J.; Mock, A. R. Moyamoya phenomenon after radiation for optic glioma. J. Neurosurg. 79:32–35; 1993.

Lassmann, G. Vascular dysplasia of arteries in neurocristopathies: a lesson for neurofibromatosis. Neurofibromatosis 1:281–293;1988.

Laue, L.; Comite, F.; Hench, K.; Loriaux, D. L.; Cutler, G. B., Jr.; Pescovitz, 0. H. Precocious puberty associated with neurofibromatosis and optic gliomas. Treatment with luteinizing hormone releasing hormone analogue. Am. J. Dis. Child. 139:1097–1100, 1985.

Levy, W. J.; Latchaw, J.; Hahn, J. F.; Sawhny, B.; Bay, J.; Dohn, D. F. Spinal neurofibromas: a report of 66 cases and a comparison with meningiomas. Neurosurgery 18:331–334;1986.

Lewis, R. A.; Riccardi, V. M. Von Reck-linghausen neurofibromatosis: prevalence of iris hamartomata. Ophthalmology 88:348–354;1981.

Lewis, R. A.; Riccardi, V. M.; Gerson, L. P.; Whitford, R.; Axelson, K. A. Von Recklinghausen neurofibromatosis: II. Incidence of optic nerve gliomata. Ophthalmology 91:929–935;1984.

Lewis, T. T.; Kingsley, D. P. Magnetic resonance imaging of multiple spinal neurofibromata—neurofibromatosis. Neuroradiology 29:562–564;1987.

Linskey, M.; Lunsford, D.; Flickinger, J. Tumor control after stereotactic radiosurgery in the treatment of patients with bilateral acoustic tumors. Neurosurgery 31:829–838;1992.

Listernick, R.; Louis, D. N.; Packer, P. J.; Gutmann, D. H. Optic pathway gliomas in children with neurofibromatosis 1: consensus statement from the NF1 optic pathway glioma task force. Ann. Neurol. 41: 143–149;1997.

Listernick, R.; Charrow, J.; Greenwald, M. J.; Esterly, N. B. Optic glioma in children with neurofibromatosis type I. J. Pediatr. 114:788–792; 1989.

Mallmann, R.; Roth, F. J. Treatment of neurofibromatosis associated renal artery stenosis with hypertension by percutaneous transluminal angioplasty. Clin. Exp. Theory Pract. 8:893–899; 1986.

Mann, H.; Kozic, Z.; Medinilla, 0. R. Computed tomography of lambdoid calvarial defect in neurofibromatosis. Neuroradiology 25:175–176; 1983.

Martuza, R. L.; Eldridge, R. Neurofibromatosis 2 (bilateral acoustic neurofibromatosis), N. Engl. J. Med. 318:684–688; 1988.

Martuza, R. L.; Ojemann, R. G. Bilateral acoustic neuromas: clinical aspects, pathogenesis, and treatment. Neurosurgery 10:1–12; 1982.

Match, R. M.; Leffert, R. D. Massive neurofibromatosis of the upper extremity with paralysis. J. Hand Surg. [Am] 12:718–722; 1987.

Matsui, I.; Tanimura, M.; Kobayashi, N.; Sawada, T.; Nagahara, N.; Akatsuka, J.-I. Neurofibromatosis type 1 and cancer. Cancer 72:746–754; 1993.

Mazzoni, A. Pitfalls in the diagnosis of acoustic neuroma. The ABR-CT protocol. Adv. Otorhinolaryngol. 37:91–92; 1987.

McCormick, P. C.; Bello, J. A.; Post, K. D. Trigeminal schwannoma. Surgical series of 14 cases with review of the literature. J. Neurosurg. 69:850–860; 1988.

Messner, R. L.; Messner, M. R.; Lewis, S. J. Neurofibromatosis; a familial and family disorder. J. Neurosurg. Nurs. 17:221–229; 1985.

Messner, R. L.; Smith, M. N. Neurofibromatosis; relinquishing the masks; a quest for quality of life. J. Adv. Nurs. 11:459–464;1986.

Meyer, G. W.; Griffiths, W. J.; Welsh, J.; Cohen, L.; Johnson, L.; Weaver, M. J. Hepatobiliary involvement in von Recklinghausen's disease. Ann. Intern. Med. 97:722–723; 1982.

Miller, N. R.; Optic nerve glioma and cerebellar astrocytoma in a patient with von Recklinghausen's neurofibromatosis. Am. J. Ophthalmol. 79:582–588; 1975.

Molloy, P. T.; Bilaniuk, L. T.; Vaughan, S. N.; Needle, M. N.; Liu, G. T.; Zackai, E. H.; Phillips, P. C. Brainstem gliomas in patients with neurofibromatosis type 1: a distinct clinical entity. Neurology 45:1897–1902; 1995.

Moore, B. D.; Slopis, J. M.; Schomer, D.; Jackson, E. F.; Levy, B. M. Neuropsychological significance of areas of high signal intensity on brain MRIs of children with neurofibromatosis. Neurology 46:1660–1668; 1996.

Mulvihill, J. J.; Parry, D. M.; Sherman, J. L.; Pikus, A.; Kaiser-Kupfer, M. I.; Eldridge, R. Neurofibromatosis 1 (Recklinghausen disease) and neurofibromatosis 2 (bilateral acoustic neurofibromatosis): an update. Ann. Intern. Med. 113:39–52; 1990.

Nadol, J.; Chiong, C.; Ojemann, R. Preservation of hearing and facial nerve function in resection of acoustic neuroma. Laryngoscope 102:1153–1158; 1992.

Nakamura, H.; Koga, M.; Sato, B.; Noma, K.; Morimoto, Y.; Kishimoto, S. Von Recklinghausen's disease with pheochromocytoma and nonmedullary thyroid cancer. Ann. Intern. Med. 105:796–797; 1986.

North, K.; Joy, P.; Yuille, D.; Cocks, N.; Mobbs, E.; Hutchins, P.; McHugh, K.; de Silva, M. Specific learning disability in children with neurofibromatosis type 1: significance of MRI abnormalities. Neurology 44:878–883; 1994.

North, K.; Joy, P.; Yuille, D.; Cocks, N.; Hutchins, P. Cognitive function and academic performance in children with neurofibromatosis type 1. Dev. Med. Child Neurol. 37:427–436; 1995.

North, K. K.; Riccardi, V.; Samango-Sprouse, C.; Ferner, R.; Moore, B.; Legius, E.; Ratner, N.; Denckla, M. B. Cognitive function and academic performance in neurofibromatosis 1: consensus statement from the NF1 Cognitive Disorders Task Force. Neurology 48:1121–1127; 1997.

O'Connell, P.; Leach, R.; Cawthon, R. M.; Culver, M.; Stevens, J.; Viskochil, D.; Fournier, R. E. K.; Rich, D. C.; Ledbetter, D. H.; White, R. two NP-I translocations map within a 600-kilobase segment of 17q11.2. Science 244:1087–1088; 1989.

Ojemann, R. G. Management of acoustic neuromas (vestibular schwannomas). Clin. Neurosurg. 40:489–535; 1993.

O'Neill, P.; Whatmore, W. J.; Booth, A. E. Spinal meningoceles in association with neurofibromatosis. Neurosurgery 13:82–84;1983.

Packer, R. J.; Bilaniuk, L. T.; Cohen, B. H.; Braffman, B. H.; Obringer, A. C.; Zimmerman, R. A.; Siegel, K. R.; Sutton, L. N.; Savino, P. J.; Zackai, E. H.; Meadows, A. T. Intracranial visual pathway gliomas in children with neurofibromatosis. Neurofibromatosis 1:212–222; 1988.

Packer, R. J.; Lange, B.; Ater, J. Carboplatinum and vincristine for progressive low grade gliomas of childhood. J. Clin. Oncol. 11:850–857; 1992.

Packer, R. J.; Sutton, L. N.; Bilaniuk, L. T.; Radcliffe, J.; Rosenstock, J. G.; Siegel, K. R.; Bunin, G. R.; Savino, P. J.; Bruce, D. A.; Schut, L. Treatment of chiasmatic/hypothalamic gliomas of childhood with chemotherapy: an update. Ann. Neurol. 23:79–85; 1988.

Parry, D. M.; MacCollin, M. M.; Kaiser-Kupfer, M. I.; Pulaski, K.; Nicholson, H. S.; Bolesta, M.; Eldridge, R.; Gusella, J. F. Germ-line mutations in the neurofibromatosis 2 gene: correlations with disease severity and retinal abnormalities. Am. J. Hum. Genet. 59:529–539; 1996.

Pearson-Webb, M. A.; Kaiser-Kupfer, M. I.; Eldridge, R. Eye findings in bilateral acoustic (central) neurofibromatosis: association with presenile lens opacities and cataracts, but absence of Lisch nodules. N. Engl. J. Med. 315:1553–1554; 1986.

Pickard, L. R.; Rose, J. E. Avoidable complications of resection of major nerve trunk neurofibromas and schwannomas. Neurofibromatosis 1:43–49; 1988.

Pollack, M. A.; Shprintzen, R. J. Velopharyngeal insufficiency in neurofibromatosis. Int. J. Pediatr. Otorhinolaryngol. 3:257–262; 1981.

Pollard, S. G.; Hornick, P.; Macfarlane, R.; Caine, R. Renovascular hypertension in neurofibromatosis. Postgrad. Med. J. 65:31–33; 1989.

Powell, P. P. An overview of childhood von Reckling-hausen neurofibromatosis for parents. Neurofibro-matosis 1:50–53; 1988a.

Powell, P. P. Schematic representation of von Reck-linghausen neurofibromatosis (NF-1): an aid for patient and family education. Neurofibromatosis 1: 164–165; 1988b.

Ragge, N.K.; Baser, M.E.; Klein, J.; Nechiporuk, A.; Sainz, J.; Pulst, S.-M.; Riccardi, V. M. Ocular ab-normalities in neurofibromatosis 2. Am. J. Ophthal-mol. 120:634–641; 1995.

Reed, D.; Robertson, W. D.; Rootman, J.; Douglas, G. Plexiform neurofibromatosis of the orbit: CT evalu-ation. AJNR Am. J. Neurol 7:259–263; 1986.

Reynolds, R. L.; Pineda, C. A. Neurofibromatosis: review and report. J. Am. Dent. Ass. 117:735–737; 1988.

Riccardi, V. M. Von Recklinghausen neurofibromato-sis. N. Engl. J. Med. 305:1617–1627; 1981.

Riccardi, V. M. Neurofibromatosis: clinical hetero-geneity. Curr. Probl. Cancer 7(2):1–34; 1982.

Riccardi, V. M. Neurofibromatosis as a model for in-vestigating hereditary vs. environmental factors in learning disabilities. The developing brain and its disorders. Tokyo: University of Tokyo Press; 1984.

Riccardi, V. M. Neurofibromatosis: a spectrum of dis-orders. In: Wetterberg, L., ed. Genetics of neuropsy-chiatric disease, London; MacMillan Press; 1989a; p.235–248.

Riccardi, V. M. Trauma and wound-healing in the patho-genesis of birth defects. Proc. Greenwood Genet. Ctr. 8:152–153; 1989b.

Riccardi, V. M.; Eichner, J. E. Neurofibromatosis: phenotype, natural history, and pathogenesis. Balti-more: Johns Hopkins University Press; 1986.

Riccardi, V. M.; Haeberlin, V. Disjoining of height and head circumference in patients with NF-1; implica-tions for CNS pathogenesis. Am. J. Hum. (Genet. 44: A60; 1989.

Riccardi, V. M. Neurofibromatosis: phenotype; natural history and pathogenesis. 2nd ed. Baltimore: Johns Hopkins University Press; 1992.

Riviello, J. J.; Marks, H. G.; Lee, M. S.; Mandell, G. A. Aqueductal stenosis in neurofibromatosis: a report of two cases. Neurofibromatosis 1:312–317, 1988.

Roback, H. B.; Kirshner, H.; Roback, E. Physical self-concept changes in a mildly facially disfigured neurofibromatosis patient following communication skill training. Int. J. Psychiatr. Med. 11:137–143; 1981.

Roenigk, R. K.; Ratz, J. L. Carbon dioxide laser treat-ment of cutaneous neurofibromas J. Dermatol. Surg. Oncol. 13:187–190; 1987.

Rouleau, G. A.; Merel, P.; Lutchman, M.; Sanson, M.; Zucman, J.; Marineau, C.; Hoang-Xuan, K.; Dem-czuk, M.; Desmaze, C.; Plougastel, B.; Pulst, S. M.; Lenoir, G.; Bijisma, E.; Fashold, R.; Dumanski, J.; de Jong, P.; Parry, D.; Eldrige, R.; Aurias, A.; Delattre, O.; Thomas, G. Alteration in a new gene encoding a putative membrane-organizing protein causes neuro-fibromatosis type 2. Nature 363:515–521; 1993.

Rouleau, G. A.; Wertelecki, W.; Haines, J. L.; Hobbs, W. J.; Trofatter, J. A.; Seizinger, B. R.; Martuza, R. L.; Superneau, D. W.; Conneally, P. M.; Gusella, J. F. Genetic linkage of bilateral acoustic neurofi-bromatosis to a DNA marker on chromosome 22. Nature 329:246–248; 1987.

Ruttledge, M. H.; Andermann, A. A.; Phelan, C. M.; Claudio, J. O.; Han, F.-Y.; Chretien, N.; Rangarat-nam, S.; MacCollin, M.; Short, P.; Parry, D.; Michels, V.; Riccardi, V. M.; Weksberg, R.; Kita-mura, K.; Bradburn, J. M.; Hall, B. D.; Propping, P.; Rouleau, G. A. Type of mutation in the neurofibro-matosis type 2 gene (NF2) frequently determines severity of disease. Am. J. Hum. Genet. 59:331–342; 1996.

Scoles, D. R.; Baser, M. E.; Pulst, S.-M. A missense mutation in the neurofibromatosis 2 gene occurs in patients with mild and severe phenotypes. Neuro-logy 47:544–546; 1996.

Seizinger, B. R.; Martuza, R. L.; Gusella, J. F. Loss of genes on chromosome 22 in tumorigenesis of human acoustic neuroma. Nature 322:644–647; 1986.

Slattery, W. H.; Brackmann, D. E.; Hitselberger, W. Hearing preservation in neurofibromatosis type 2. Am. J. Otol. 19:638–643; 1998.

Sorensen, S. A.; Mulvihill, J. J.; Nielsen, A. Nation-wide follow-up of Recklinghausen neurofibromato-sis: survival and malignant neoplasms. N. Engl. J. Med. 314:1010–1015; 1986.

Stack, J. P.; Ramsden, R. T.; Antoun, N. M.; Lyle, R. H.; Isherwood, I; Jenkins, J. P. Magnetic reso-nance imaging of acoustic neuromas: The role of gadolinium-DTPA, Br. J. Radiol. 61:800–805; 1988.

Stern, J. D.; DiGiacinto, G. V.; Housepian, E. M. Neuro-fibromatosis and optic glioma: clinical and morpho-logical correlations. Neurosurgery 4:524–528; 1979.

Stern, J.; Jakobiec, F. A.; Housepian, E. M. The archi-tecture of optic nerve gliomas with and without neuro-fibromatosis. Arch. Ophthalmol. 98:505–511; 1980.

Terada, H.; Mimaki, T.; Takiyama, N.; Tagawa, T.; Tanaka, J.; Itoh, N.; Yabuuchi, H. A case of infantile spasms with multiple neurofibromatosis. Brain Dev. 8:145–147; 1986.

Tertsch, D.; Schon, R.; Ulrich, F. E.; Alexander, H.; Herter, U. Pubertas precox in neurofibromatosis of the optic chiasma. Acta. Neurochir. 28:413–415; 1979.

Trofatter, J. A.; MacCollin, M. M.; Rutter, J. L.; Mur-rell, J. R.; Duyao, M. P.; Parry, D. M.; Eldridge, R.; Klay, N.; Menon, A. G.; Pulaski, K.; Haase, V. H.; Ambrose, C. M.; Munroe, D.; Bove, C.; Haines, J. L.; Martuza, R. L.; MacDonald, M. E.; Seizinger, B. R.; Short, M. P.; Buckler, A. J.; Gusella, J. F. A novel moesin-, ezrin-, radixin-like gene is a candi-date for the neurofibromatosis 2 tumor suppressor. Cell 72:1–20; 1993.

Varnhagen, C. K.; Lewin, S.; Das, J. P.; Bowen, P.; Ma, K.; Klimek, M. Neurofibromatosis and psycho-logical processes. Dev. Behav. Pediatr. 9:257–265; 1988.

Viskochil, D.; Buchberg, A. M.; Xu, G; Cawthom, R. M.; Stevens, J.; Wolff, R. K.; Culver, M.; Carey, J. C.; Copeland, N. G.; Jenkins, N. A.; White, R.; O'Connell, P. Deletions and a translocation interrupt a cloned gene at the neurofibromatosis type 1 locus. Cell 62:187–192; 1990.

Wallace, M. R.; Marchuk, D. A.; Andersen, L. B.; Letcher, R.; Odeh, H. M.; Saulino, A. M.; Fountain, J. W.; Brereton, A.; Nicholson, J.; Mitchell, A. L.; Brownstein, B. H.; Collins, F. S. Type 1 neurofibromatosis gene: identification of a large transcript disrupted in three NF1 patients. Science 249:181–186; 1990.

Weiss, L.; Sagerman, R. H.; King, G. A.; Chung, C. T.; Dubowy, R. L. Controversy in the management of optic nerve glioma. Cancer 59:1000–1004; 1987.

Wertelecki, W.; Rouleau, G. A.; Superneau, D. W.; Forehand, L. W.; Williams, J. P.; Haines, J. L.; Gusella, J. F. Neurofibromatosis 2: Clinical and DNA linkage studies of a large kindred. N. Engl. J. Med. 319:278–283; 1988.

Yaghmai, I. Spine changes in neurofibromatosis. Radiographics 6:261–285; 1986.

Zigmond, N. Models for the delivery of special education services to students with learning disabilities in public school. J. Child. Neurol. 10:886–892; 1995.

# 41

# Progressive Genetic-Metabolic Diseases

ISABELLE RAPIN

Many neurologists view genetic-metabolic and degenerative diseases of the brain, most of which will ultimately have a fatal outcome, as a most discouraging part of their field. The number of different diseases and variants of diseases is daunting. The number of those whose molecular biology and clinical pathology are understood is exploding. Although bold new technologies are opening the door to potentially effective treatments and to prevention, incompletely understood and untreatable diseases far outnumber the others. Also, the lag between full elucidation of the biology of a disease and the devising of a specific therapy is frustratingly long. Yet the momentum of accelerating understanding has removed much of the pall on this chapter of neurology.

This chapter cannot attempt to deal with all of these diseases, many of which are diseases of infants and young children well covered in recent textbooks of neurology and child neurology, for example, *Merritt's Textbook of Neurology, 10th edition* (Rowland 1999); Swaiman and Ashwal's *Pediatric Neurology* (1999); *Menkes' Textbook of Child Neurology, 5th edition* (1995); as well as Lyon, Adams, and Kolodny's (1996) *Neurology of Hereditary Metabolic Diseases of Children, 2nd edition* and Baraitser's (1997) *Genetics of Neurological Disorders, 3rd edition*. Better still,

readers are referred to McKusick's (1999) *Online Mendelian Inheritance in Man (OMIM)* for up-to-date and continuously updated computerized information on the molecular biology of genetic diseases, including brief clinical sketches and pertinent literature references. Consult the *Metabolic and Molecular Bases of Inherited Disease, 7th edition* (Scriver et al. 1995) for detailed biochemical and molecular information.

The tables in this chapter consist of lists of diseases, their prognoses, and some available treatments, with no attempt to cover either their clinical or their biochemical basis, nor to be exhaustive. Information about treatment and prognosis provided here should be viewed with caution: what is believed to be true today is likely to require modification tomorrow.

The chapter focuses on diseases whose biological basis is at least partially understood and for which a specific and variably effective treatment has been tried. It also mentions some symptomatic and palliative treatments that affect prognosis and longevity in many diseases because patients can now be maintained almost indefinitely in a vegetative state. Like the new treatments based on progress in molecular approaches, these palliative treatments raise thorny ethical questions about the appropriateness of therapeutic interventions.

## New Advances in Genetics and Molecular Biology

Spectacular advances in genetics and molecular biology have both complicated and clarified the nosology of mendelian genetic diseases and have profound implications for the development of novel therapies. Multiple allelic point mutations of any particular disease-causing gene is the rule, not the exception, with variable consequences for the synthesis, molecular configuration, stability, and enzymatic activity of the protein it encodes. Compound heterozygotes for two allelic recessive mutations or for a point mutation and a deletion are frequent. To complicate matters, insertions, inversions, deletions, and other rearrangements may affect parts of chromosomes rather than single genes. In addition to mutations that inactivate a particular enzyme directly, enzymes may be inactivated indirectly by mutations in genes for interacting proteins that act as transporters, activators, and protectors (e.g., Ito et al. 1993; Gieselmann et al. 1994; Burkhardt et al. 1997; Bargal and Bach 1997). The end result is increased phenotypic variation, which may be extreme for some diseases, ranging from death in infancy to lack of symptoms into adulthood or even, in some cases, old age.

In addition to single base substitutions, amplification of trinucleotides that may be repeated a few dozen to several thousand times are now known to be the cause of many neurological conditions ranging from the spinocerebellar degenerations to Huntington's disease, fragile X syndrome, and others. Another new concept in mendelian genetics is genetic imprinting, where the paternal or maternal origin of both copies of a chromosome, gene, or group of genes determines two distinct phenotypes, for example, Prader-Willi and Angelman syndromes. Paternal uniparental disomy has been reported in neonatal methylmalonic acidemia with diabetes mellitus (Abramowitz et al. 1994). Finally, the now classic concept of mitochondrial DNA inheritance has altered our concept of genetic-metabolic diseases profoundly and explains its strictly maternal inheritance affecting both sexes. Heteroplasmy (i.e., the variable number of mitochondria with defective DNA in various tissues) accounts for phenotypic variability and explains the threshold effect and a galtonian distribution of phenotypes rather than the familiar mendelian patterns of inheritance.

## Factors that Influence Prognosis

The pace of the illness and the extent of disease in the nervous system, together with the severity of its systemic manifestations, are major factors influencing prognosis. In general, diseases in which lack of enzymatic activity is complete or near complete have the most severe phenotype. Their victims may be symptomatic at birth or in infancy and reduced to a vegetative state the earliest. Because it is now possible to maintain many patients in a vegetative state for a decade or more with the use of antibiotics to treat infections and the insertion of feeding gastrostomies with fundal plication to ensure adequate nutrition, the endpoint of disease is probably best thought of in terms of reaching a vegetative state rather than death.

It is relatively easy to prognosticate in the case of a second affected child in a family because, with exceptions—in particular some dominant and mitochondrially inherited diseases, or cases where one of the affected siblings has inherited two distinct but interacting mutations—recessive disease in sibs is likely to run a fairly predictable course. But because genetic heterogeneity is so prevalent, one must exercise the utmost caution in providing prognostic information when the proband does not present with the most classical clinical picture. Heterogeneity highlights the critical importance of obtaining fibroblasts or immortalized white cells from patients for later study, and of securing autopsies in undiagnosed patients, as modern pathology often provides the key to the discovery and unraveling of new heretofore unsuspected diseases.

## Symptomatic and Palliative Treatments

### Health Maintenance

Adequate nutrition and general care determine the longevity of many seriously handicapped persons. Some of them cannot be maintained at home and are cared for in a variety of institutional settings. The quality of care in these facilities has clearly improved as a result of earlier, widely publicized scandals in institutions for the severely handicapped. Many fewer patients develop decubitus ulcers, they receive more habilitative services, and their hygiene and nutrition are superior to what they typically were in the past (Rubin and Crocker 1989). The continued strong trend toward deinstitutionalization has continued in an attempt to reduce costs, and as a result of greater recognition of the rights of the handicapped for an optimal quality of life. Even severely affected persons, especially while they are children, are now maintained at home, often with the help of visiting nurses and the provision of needed appliances and services. Many of the patients are bused to day programs in the community where attempts are made to occupy them meaningfully, teach them self-help skills, and provide them with recreation and socialization, and their caretakers with relief. The nutrition of home-based patients tends to be better than that of the institutionalized, not only because devoted family members spend adequate time feeding them, but because feeding by gastrostomy has become more acceptable. Provision of physiotherapy to minimize joint contractures and recognition of the importance of weight bearing, even strapped to a board, have reduced spontaneous fractures, a significant hazard for immobilized patients. Frequent turning to prevent decubiti, avoidance of bowel impaction, and keeping the child out of bed and within the family circle enhances quality of life. Regular health maintenance visits to a physician willing to care for the handicapped is another measure that has had favorable effects on longevity. Whether longevity is a blessing for patients who have reached a vegetative state and for their families is debatable and needs to be discussed openly when offering therapeutic options.

## Treatment of Intercurrent Illnesses

Most patients with genetic-metabolic diseases of the brain do not die of the disease but of an intercurrent illness. This used to be pneumonia, urosepsis, or some other unrecognized infectious illness. Availability and liberal prescription of broad-spectrum antibiotics for nonspecific febrile episodes has minimized infectious causes of death. Nonetheless, aspiration remains a significant and often lethal hazard.

## Treatment of Seizures

Many diseases, especially those affecting the gray matter and certain subcortical nuclei, carry a substantial risk of seizures and myoclonus. Vigorous treatment of these seizures with appropriate drugs, monitoring of anticonvulsant blood levels, and avoidance of oversedation and of therapy with multiple drugs have substantially altered prognosis, although death during unobserved seizures remains fairly common.

## Treatment of Hydrocephalus

Some diseases, in particular Hurler's disease (mucopolysaccharidosis [MPS] type I), some of the other MPS, Alexander's disease, and a few others cause true hydrocephalus—as opposed to hydrocephalus ex vacuo, either by obstructing the aqueduct or by involvement of the leptomeninges. Shunting improves the quality of these children's lives by increasing alertness, and by regaining, or avoiding the loss of some motor and cognitive skills compromised by hydrocephalus. Bone marrow grafting may prevent the development of hydrocephalus in some diseases.

## Treatment of Spasticity and Musculoskeletal Deformities

Many of the diffuse genetic metabolic diseases of the brain cause increasingly severe spasticity with immobility and joint contractures. Drugs such as baclofen and diazepam have a modestly beneficial effect on spasticity, more so than dantrolene, which tends to increase weakness. Botulinum toxin injections and chronic intraspinal delivery of baclofen with a refillable pump may be viable alternatives, especially for children who are alert and in whom spasticity presents a major problem (Armstrong et al. 1997, Zelnik et al. 1997). Selective dorsal rhizotomy is most often offered to children with spastic cerebral palsy, but it may have a place in progressive diseases with a long life expectancy (Chicoine et al. 1997). Physiotherapy to avoid joint contractures and even the surgical release of contractures to improve mobility or facilitate perineal care, and scoliosis surgery to minimize lung compression may be justified in patients with a slowly progressive disease. Awareness and, in some cases, surgical correction of potentially lethal skeletal complications such as atlanto-occipital instability and pending cord compression may greatly affect prognosis in some of the MPS. Treatment of dystonia and other movement disorders may be urgently needed but frustratingly difficult.

## Treatment of Pain

Most of the metabolic diseases of the nervous system do not produce pain unless there is severe dystonia or spasticity or a small fiber neuropathy, a fact that should be pointed out to patients' families. The lancinating pain of the neuropathy of Fabry's disease may respond to phenytoin, carbamazepine, gabapentin, or tricyclic antidepressants. Some severely spastic vegetative patients who lie in opisthotonos may be fretful because of the pain of muscle spasms and seem to gain some relief from muscle relaxants and other treatments for spasticity.

## Treatment of Psychic Pain

Families of progressively neurologically impaired persons of all ages, and the non demented affected older children and adults themselves, experience great anguish and are often chronically depressed. It is critical to provide them with emotional support, including psychiatric counseling and antidepressants when indicated. Families may desperately need the help of home attendants or practical nurses. Families require the free time provided by temporary respite facilities. As parents age, full-time placement in a long term care facility or nursing home may be inevitable, although those for children are almost nonexistent. Introducing families with similar problems to one another and to support groups is often very helpful. One must also remember to help families cope with the financial demands of the illness.

Enlisting the family in a partnership to investigate an illness for which there is currently no treatment by admitting our ignorance and bringing them up to date with new scientific developments often does a great deal to alleviate their pain and frustration. Parent groups such as those of patients with leukodystrophies, Jewish diseases, MPS, Rett's syndrome, and many others have not only raised monies for research but have disseminated information about "their" rare disease, for example by developing a home page on the Internet. Several parent groups organize yearly meetings with scientists and other parents. They thus become extremely knowledgeable about new scientific developments and often enter into active partnership with investigators. They insist that the physicians who care for their children be aware of every new potential therapy. They have facilitated research by getting family members to agree to biopsies and blood tests, and by helping recruit new patients into patient registries and clinical trials. Parents are often the most militant proponents of experimen-

tal treatments such as bone marrow transplantation or dietary trials, and of postmortem examination so as to provide tissue for research. They understand that careful clinical and pathological description is the stepping stone to the advances in genetics, molecular biology, and biochemistry required to develop specific and innovative treatments.

## Specific Treatments

### Dietary Manipulation

There are a few diseases where avoidance of a nutrient that cannot be metabolized—if possible together with its increased excretion, provision of pharmacological doses of a cofactor such as a vitamin to accelerate or bypass a metabolic block, or a combination of these approaches—has totally altered prognosis (Table 41-1). In the most successful cases (e.g., restriction of phenylalanine in phenylketonuria [PKU], of chlorophyl-containing foods rich in phytanic acid in Refsum's disease, and of dietary copper coupled with copper chelation in Wilson's disease), treatment is so successful as to prevent the appearance of the disease altogether, provided a diagnosis is made before irreversible damage has taken place (Anonymous 1994; Claridge et al. 1992; Scheinberg and Sternlieb 1984). The administration of chenodeoxycholic acid in cerebrotendinous xanthomatosis lowers cholestanol and is associated with significant regression of clinical signs (Berginer et al. 1984; van Heijst et al. 1998). Unfortunately, avoidance of long-chain fatty acids and administration of erucic acid improves the fatty acid profile of the blood in adrenoleukodystrophy and some of the other peroxisomal disorders, with only marginal clinical benefit. Widespread neonatal testing for treatable disorders of amino acid metabolism, galactosemia, biotinidase deficiency, and congenital hypothyroidism has dramatically decreased some of these causes of severe neurological morbidity. Intrauterine treatment of prenatally diagnosed diseases may become a reality (Evans et al. 1993, 1997). Physician education has heightened awareness of acute lethal disorders causing hyperammonemia, hypoglycemia, and organic acidemia in neonates. Prognosis has improved substantially for some of the urea cycle defects with the combination of a low-protein diet and the prescription of metabolites that promote the excretion of nitro-

**Table 41-1.** Dietary Treatments

| Disease | Treatment | Efficacy |
|---|---|---|
| Aminoacidurias, organic acidurias | Restrict unmetabolized amino acids + provide missing metabolites + provide vitamin cofactors | Satisfactory in PKU, fair to satisfactory in MSUD and other branched chain aminoacidurias, poor to fair in organic acidurias |
| Urea cycle defects | Low protein diet + sodium benzoate and phenylacetate/butyrate | Poor to fair |
| Galactosemia | Galactose restriction | Satisfactory |
| Glycogenosis type I | Continuous feeding of cornstarch | Fair to satisfactory |
| Fatty acid β-oxidation deficiencies | Avoid fasting | Fair to satisfactory |
| Mitochondrial disorders of carbohydrate metabolism | Cofactors of mitochondrial metabolism | Poor to fair |
| Abetalipoproteinemia | Tocopherol, other lipid-soluble vitamins | Satisfactory |
| Cerebrotendinous xanthomatosis | Chenodeoxycholic acid | Fair to satisfactory |
| Sjögren-Larsson syndrome | Low-fat diet + medium chain triglycerides | ? |
| Adrenoleukodystrophy | Erucic acid + restrict very long chain fatty acids | Ineffective |
| Refsum's disease | Phytanic acid restriction | Fairly satisfactory, does not improve the retinopathy and deafness |
| Carbohydrate-deficient glycoprotein syndrome | Mannose (+ low glucose?) | Questionable |
| Juvenile neuronal ceroid lipofuscinosis | Polyunsaturated fatty acids | ? |
| Wilson's disease | Low copper diet, copper chelation | Satisfactory |

geneous waste via an alternate pathway to the urea cycle (Batshaw 1984; Maestri et al. 1996). Prenatal treatment, by providing large doses of cobalamin to mothers known to carry a fetus with vitamin $B_{12}$-responsive methylmalonic aciduria (Zass et al. 1995; Evans et al. 1997) and placing women with PKU on a phenylalanine-free diet before conception or in very early pregnancy can prevent the birth of a retarded child (Anonymous 1994).

## Enzyme Replacement Therapy

This approach depends on the delivery of sufficient amounts of a missing enzyme to the affected tissue. It has become standard treatment for systemic (type I) Gaucher's disease, where a recombinant DNA-modified form of glucocerebrosidase has replaced the placentally derived form of the enzyme, and has reduced organomegaly and bony involvement dramatically (Morales 1996). Genetic engineering techniques such as this have brightened the prospect for synthesis of some enzymes in therapeutically realistic amounts for other diseases. Problems such as rapid turnover, the development of antibodies to the enzyme, and the need for specific markers to target the enzyme

to particular tissues have not yet been fully satisfactorily addressed. Enzyme replacement therapy for diseases of the nervous system is complicated by the existence of the blood-brain and blood-nerve barriers. Experimental attempts to overcome this problem have included infusion of hyperosmolar agents to open the barrier temporarily, the encasement of quanta of the enzyme in lipid-soluble coats (liposomes), and infusion of enzyme directly into the cerebrospinal fluid (CSF) using an indwelling catheter with a subcutaneous refillable reservoir. These promising techniques have yet to achieve significant clinical application.

## Transplantation

Another approach to enzyme replacement is the engrafting of enzyme-producing tissue from an HLA-matched donor. This procedure, which carries a mortality of 10% if an HLA-identical sibling is available, and 20% to 25% if less than fully matched tissue is used (Hoogerbrugge et al. 1995), also has significant later morbidity because of the requirement for long-term immunosuppression. Promising ways to avoid immunological intolerance are the grafting of fetal tissue (Scaggiante et al.

1987) or pluripotent hematopoietic stem cells from cord blood (Krivit et al. 1998), and autologous transplantation of the patient's own cells genetically engineered ex vivo. Intrauterine cell grafting into the peritoneal cavity is also being investigated.

Liver transplantation has been life-saving in a few patients with Wilson's disease presenting with fulminant liver failure. Such patients are among the best candidates for transplantation, since they often have not yet developed central nervous system (CNS) damage and since there is an effective treatment for Wilson's disease. They require continuation of a copper-restricted diet and use of copper-chelating agents, which means that liver grafting represents organ replacement and not enzyme replacement in this disease (Rakela et al. 1986). In Fabry's disease renal failure is alleviated, although the new kidney does not always provide adequate enzyme replacement and eventually may become diseased as well. However, this approach has prolonged survival with improved quality of life in some patients (Friedlaender et al. 1987, Van Loo et al. 1996).

Bone marrow transplantation is an attractive option for systemically symptomatic diseases, especially if autologous transplantation of hematopoietic cells transfected ex vivo is achieved, thus avoiding the need for immunosuppression (Kaye 1995). Bone marrow grafting alleviates some symptoms due to storage in cerebral perivascular spaces and the leptomeninges, for example, hydrocephalus in Hurler's disease (e. g., Whitley et al. 1993; Belani et al. 1993). In order to affect storage in neurons, enzyme producing cells—which appear to be microglia derived from marrow macrophages—must penetrate the parenchyma, which is protected by the blood-brain barrier (Krivit et al. 1995b). Transplantation of enzymatically competent bone marrow (Walkley et al. 1994) and neural progenitor cells (Snyder and Wolfe. 1996) has successfully prevented the development of neurological symptoms in immature animal models. In humans, transplantation is unlikely to prove effective in conditions like infantile Tay-Sachs disease where neuronal storage is already substantial at 20 weeks gestation and for which meaningful prognostic improvement would require prenatal enzyme replacement or engraftment (Zlokovic and Apuzzo 1997).

Worldwide, bone marrow transplantation has been performed with variable success in probably over 1000 patients affected by a variety of genetic-metabolic diseases of the brain (Krivit et al. 1995a), yet its long-term effects require further evaluation. It seems to be most effective for presymptomatically detected diseases or for those that have not yet produced severe cognitive impairment in which it may stabilize or slow deterioration and reverse troublesome somatic signs (Kaye 1995). Because transplantation is extremely expensive and technically demanding, because the identification of a suitable and willing donor is so difficult and the results may be disappointing, transplantation is unlikely to become a widely viable option unless very significant further technical progress is achieved. Before recommending grafting for a metabolic disease, it is necessary to weigh its high financial cost, the child's burden of suffering, and the limited efficacy of current transplants for mitigating CNS disease in the face of the still "sobering morbidity and mortality rates" of allogenic transplantation (Clark 1990; Rappeport and Ginns 1984).

Transplantation has been publicized widely and, unfortunately, this has raised great hope in parents of severely affected patients. Transplantation may be justified on a research basis in more advanced cases of a lethal disease, provided the family (and patient if capable of it) gives informed consent and fully understands the potential burden of caring for a severely handicapped individual much longer than would have been the case if the child had been left untreated. So far transplantation in children with the severe early variants of storage diseases such as infantile Gaucher's, Niemann-Pick, Krabbe's, and I-cell diseases, and late infantile metachromatic leukodystrophy have been discouraging. Table 41-2 summarizes currently available information on some of the diseases for which transplantation has been tried and the results achieved thus far.

## The Lysosomal Storage Diseases

Lysosomes are cellular organelles with an acid pH in which catabolism of many cellular constituents takes place. Absence or inactivity of lysosomal enzymes results in the storage within lysosomes of undegradable products of metabolism. This storage may result in swelling and distortion of the geometry and function of cells or even in cell death. In some cases, for example, infantile Gaucher's disease and Krabbe's disease, there is also an accumulation of toxic metabolites

**Table 41-2.** Transplantation Results*

| Disease | Type of Transplantation | Results |
|---|---|---|
| Krabbe's, metachromatic leukodystrophy | Bone marrow, stem cells | Somewhat effective if offered early or in presymptomatic children |
| Fabry's | Kidney | Successful in some but not all cases |
| Niemann-Pick type A | Liver | Ineffective |
| Niemann-Pick type C/D | Bone marrow | Decreased visceral storage |
| Swedish neuronopathic Gaucher | Bone marrow | Decreased visceral storage, no effect on CNS? |
| Hurler's | Bone marrow | Visceral and joint improvement, CNS stabilized |
| Hunter's, Sanfilippo's | Bone marrow | Questionable to unsatisfactory |
| Morquio's, Maroteaux-Lamy | Bone marrow | Some visceral and joint improvement |
| Adrenoleukodystrophy | Bone marrow, stem cells | Effective in preclinical cases? stabilizes early cases |
| Wilsons's disease with acute hepatic failure | Liver | Successful but requirement for copper restriction and chelation persists |

* Bone marrow transplantation is currently being tried in other diseases, but evaluation of results is not yet possible, nor are results of more advanced transplantation strategies such as transplantation of stem or genetically engineered cells available.

generated in an alternate degradative pathway (Suzuki 1998). Although truly effective treatment for the neurological manifestations of these diseases has not yet been achieved, enzymatic and, for most, molecular diagnosis, carrier detection, and prenatal diagnosis are available. Genetic screening in a high-risk population like Ashkenazi Jews for Tay-Sachs disease has greatly decreased the number of affected infants and is available for many diseases to prevent the birth of a second affected child. Although each of the diseases may

be rare, in the aggregate they are much more frequent than appreciated before molecular biology made it possible to detect atypical variants *in vivo*.

One of the prototypical groups of these disorders, the glycogen storage diseases, is not discussed here because they are covered in the chapter on muscle diseases.

### The Sphingolipidoses

Table 41-3 belies the complexity of these disorders. For example, there are at least three enzy-

**Table 41-3.** Sphingolipidoses

| Disease | Variants* | Prognosis |
|---|---|---|
| GM$_2$ gangliosidosis | Infantile (Tay-Sachs disease) | Death in the preschool years |
| | Juvenile | Death in adolescence |
| | Adolescent and adult | Survival for variable number of years |
| | Chronic | Survival for decades |
| GM$_1$ gangliosidosis | Infantile | Death in late infancy |
| | Childhood | Death in adolescence |
| | Adult | Variable |
| | Dystonic | Survival into young adulthood |
| Fabry's disease | | Death in adulthood |
| Niemann-Pick disease | Group A (infantile) | Death in the preschool years |
| | Group C/D (heterogeneous) | Varies from death in adolescence to prolonged survival |
| Gaucher's disease | Infantile (type II) | Death in infancy |
| | Juvenile neuronopathic (type III) | Death in childhood or adolescence |
| Farber's disease | Infantile | Death in late infancy or early childhood |
| Krabbe's disease | Infantile | Death in infancy or early childhood |
| | Later onset forms | Death after several years |
| | Adult | Chronic paraparesis |
| Metachromatic leukodystropy | Late infantile | Death in school years |
| | Juvenile | Death in adolescence |
| | Adult | Death after protracted course |
| | Multiple sulfatase deficiency | Death in early childhood |

* A number of variants are due to the deficiency of prosaposin or saposin (spingolipid activator proteins) deficiencies.

matic variants of $GM_2$ gangliosidosis: classic infantile Tay-Sachs disease in Ashkenazi and French Canadian infants (lack of hexosaminidase A [hex-A] because of the lack of the hexosaminidase $\alpha$ chain coded on chromosome 15); Sandhoff disease (lack of hex-A and -B because of lack of the hexosaminidase $\beta$ chain coded on chromosome 5), and the AB variant in which hexosaminidase is present but there is deficiency of a saposin (sphingolipid activator protein) coded on chromosome 5. Furthermore, multiple allelic mutations affecting the hex-A gene means that there are many more genetic than enzymatic variants. The statement that early clinical disease heralds a shorter and more severe course, while generally true, suffers many exceptions. For example, three Ashkenazi siblings, compound heterozygotes for hex-A deficiency, became ataxic in the preschool years, yet two of the three lived into their forties (Rapin et al. 1976). They had normal or near normal intelligence but had severe signs of corticospinal, basal ganglia, cerebellar, sensory, autonomic, and motor neuron involvement, without seizures or retinal involvement. There are even a few asymptomatic (presymptomatic?) adult carriers of hexosaminidase deficiency.

Prognosis is particularly difficult in adult variants of the sphingolipidoses, as our knowledge rests mostly of single case reports of patients with unusual phenotypes who were carriers of rare mutations. Not all the sphingolipidoses produce an early dementing illness. There are variants of the gangliosidoses with the phenotype of motor neuron disease or cerebellar degeneration (Federico et al. 1991; Johnson 1993), others with dystonia (Goldman et al. 1981). Adult metachromatic leukodystrophy (MLD) masquerades as schizophrenia (Baumann et al. 1991) and adult-onset Krabbe's disease as spastic paraplegia (Satoh et al. 1997). Niemann-Pick disease type A, due to one of several dozen mutations of the acid sphingomyelinase gene, presents in infancy with severe hepatosplenomegaly, neurological impairment, and death in early childhood, whereas Niemann-Pick disease type C/D, which is due to an error in intracellular trafficking of exogenous cholesterol, has a much more indolent course, with little or no organomegaly, although there is bone marrow storage in "sea-blue" histiocytes. Down-gaze ophthalmoplegia, ataxia, dystonia, and mild to moderate mental retardation dominate the clinical picture in type C/D in which survival into adulthood is the rule (Schiffman 1996). Type C/D may also present in adults as a psychosis (Turpin et al. 1991) and there may be neurofibrillary tangles identical to those in Alzheimer's disease (Love et al. 1995). In short, extreme phenotypic heterogeneity and absence in some variants of visceral storage highlights the need to consider unsuspected metabolic disorders in patients with even very slow unexplained neurological or psychiatric regression and dictates caution in offering prognostic information.

Whereas enzyme replacement is now the accepted and efficacious treatment for non-neuronopathic Gaucher's disease (type I), it is ineffective, even when it is injected directly into the CSF, in other sphingolipidoses. Renal grafting in Fabry's disease has improved renal function in some but not all cases (Clement et al. 1982; Van Loo et al. 1996). Bone marrow transplantation has had mixed results. It reduces splenomegaly and may slow or even prevent further cognitive deterioration in children with Swedish type III neuronopathic Gaucher's disease (Svennerholm et al. 1991; Tsai et al. 1992). In symptomatic infantile Krabbe's and late infantile MLD it may slow deterioration and improve the neuropathy (Krivit et al. 1995a); although this is encouraging, more prolonged survival of a vegetative child is of questionable benefit to the child and family. Bone marrow transplantation in a presymptomatic infant with Krabbe's disease has markedly slowed symptoms of the disease, and successful hematopoietic stem-cell or compatible marrow engraftment reversed or stabilized children with later onset disease (Krivit et al. 1998).

## The Mucopolysaccharidoses

The mucopolysaccharidoses (Table 41-4) are due to lack of cleavage in lysosomes of sulfated sugars from acid mucopolysaccharides (glycosaminoglycans). Their enzymatic deficiencies and molecular biology are well understood. Patients excrete a variety of MPS degradation products in their urine, which is helpful for diagnostic screening. As a group, they are characterized by dwarfing and prominent storage in connective tissue, skeleton, and viscera, including, in some variants, the cornea, middle ear, and leptomeninges. There is massive hepatosplenomegaly in Hurler's disease, while visceral involvement is less striking in

**Table 41-4.** Mucopolysaccharidoses

| Type | Chromosome | Eponym | Age of Onset | Prognosis |
|---|---|---|---|---|
| I-H | 4p16.3 | Hurler's | Infancy | Death in first decade |
| I-H/S | " | Hurler/Scheie | Childhood | Survival to adulthood |
| I-S | " | Sheie's | Adolescence/adulthood | Survival for decades |
| II-A | Xq28 | Severe Hunter | Early childhood | Death in adolescence |
| II-B | " | Mild Hunter's | Preschool | Survival to adulthood |
| III-A to D | * | Sanfilippo's | Childhood | Death in teens or early adulthood |
| IV-A | 16q24.3 | Morquio's | Early childhood | Survival to teens or adulthood |
| IV-B | 3p21-23 | Morquio's | Early childhood | Survival to teens or adulthood |
| VI-A | 5q11-q13 | Maroteaux-Lamy | Early childhood | Death in teens or early adulthood |
| VI-B & C | " | Maroteaux-Lamy | Later childhood | Survival for decades |
| VII | 7q21.11 | Sly's | Early childhood | Survival to adulthood |

\* Sanfilippo A: 17q25.3; B: 17q21; C: 14; D: 12q14

other variants. Compression of the spinal cord characterizes Maroteaux-Lamy disease and entrapment of peripheral nerves because of storage in ligaments is dramatic in many variants. Accumulation of ganglioside in neurons contributes to the dementia of Hurler's and Sanfilippo's diseases. The cause of death is often heart failure, especially in Hurler's disease. It may be respiratory failure due in part to thickening of the walls of the airway in Hunter's disease. Sudden death due to compression of the cervical cord by an unstable odontoid peg occurs in Morquio's disease and may take place during anesthesia in any of the MPS unless special precautions are taken (Belani et al. 1993).

The drastic differences in phenotype and prognosis resulting from allelic mutations responsible for the severe Hurler's and much milder Scheie's diseases illustrates different consequences for the enzymatic activity of one product protein, L-iduronidase. In dramatic contrast, a single clinical subtype, San filippo's disease, can arise from any one of four enzymatically and genetically distinct deficits responsible for the accumulation of one substrate, heparan sulfate.

Aggressive treatment of symptoms such as hydrocephalus, nerve entrapments, and spinal problems, together with the wearing of hearing aids enhances the quality of life of patients with MPS and should be provided. The largest experience with bone marrow transplantation is in Hurler's disease (e.g., Vellodi et al. 1997), where it improves systemic storage in the viscera, meninges, bones, joints, and heart valves. Whether it decreases neuronal storage of ganglioside is less clear. Thus far engraftment has had modest effects

at best on the signs of central nervous system compromise, especially in Sanfilippo's disease, where dementia is more severe than peripheral storage.

## The Mucolipidoses

This group of lysosomal diseases is characterized by storage of glycoproteins in various tissues, excretion of oligosaccharides in the urine and, as is the case in the MPS, glycolipid accumulation in neurons (Table 41-5). Once again there is considerable genetic and phenotypic heterogeneity, some disorders arising from a variety of mutations in hydrolases, others from mutations in other proteins that affect the activity or transport of these hydrolases into lysosomes. In addition to central nervous system damage, several induce a neuropathy and deafness.

The geographic distribution of the mucolipidoses (ML) is uneven, with the very slowly progressive aspartylglucosaminuria a relatively common cause of mental deficiency in Finland (Arvio 1993a, 1993b), whereas Italians are prone to carry the genes for fucosidosis and the cherry-red spot myoclonus variant of sialidosis (Tiberio et al. 1995). This latter very chronic disorder, which is due mutations in the sialidase gene (Pzhehetsky et al. 1997), is compatible with survival into middle age without dementia but with a devastating and virtually untreatable myoclonus. A second subtype, galactosialidosis, lacks activity of both sialidase and β-galactosidase; it is due to any one of several mutations in cathepsin A, a serine protease that protects both these enzymes from degradation (Okamura-Oho et al. 1994; Bonten et al. 1996). What determines its very variable phenotype is the residual amount of enzyme activity in

**Table 41-5.** Mucolipidoses

| Type | Chromosome | Variants | Age of Onset | Prognosis |
|---|---|---|---|---|
| Sialidosis | 6p21.3 | Infantile | Birth | Death in early infancy |
| | 6p21.3 | Cherry-red spot myoclonus | School-age | Survival to adulthood |
| Galactosialidosis (mostly Japanese) | 20q13.1 | Early infantile | Birth | Death in late infancy |
| | | Late infantile | Toddler | Survival to adulthood |
| | | Childhood (mucolipidosis I) (several types) | Infancy/ childhood | Death in childhood/ adolescence |
| Mucolipidosis II | 4q21-23 | I-cell | Birth | Death in infancy or early childhood |
| Mucolipidosis III | ? (several) | Pseudopoly-dystrophy | Early childhood | Survival to adulthood |
| Mucolipidosis IV | ? | — | Infancy | Survival to adulthood |
| Fucosidosis | lp34 | Severe | Infancy | Death in childhood |
| | | Mild | Childhood | Survival to early adulthood |
| α-Mannosidosis | 19cen.q12 | Several clinical types | Early childhood | Variable, death in childhood to survival to adulthood |
| β-Mannosidosis | 4q22-25 | Several clinical types | Childhood | Survival to adulthood |
| Aspartylgluco-saminuria | 4q32-33 | Early childhood | Childhood | Survival to adulthood |
| Carbohydrate-deficient glycoprotein | Several | Several clinical types | Early childhood | Variable, survival to adulthood in some individuals |

each of the two deficient enzymes, depending on the particular mutation of the cathepsin A gene (Kleijer et al. 1996). This variant is reported mostly from Japan, with phenotypes ranging from hydrops fetalis with kidney involvement, to nephrosialidosis associated with bony changes and a cherry red spot with death in childhood, to late infantile variants (mucolipidosis I), which may be associated with a neuropathy and death in childhood or adolescence, or a very chronic course with survival into adulthood with crippling, mental retardation, deafness, coarse features, and organomegaly. This latter variant shares with Fabry's, disease and some subtypes of fucosidosis and neuroaxonal dystrophy inguinal angiokeratomatosis of the skin.

ML II and ML III were confused at first with the MPS which they resemble by their clinical features and by the presence of inclusions in fibroblasts, but they differ by the lack of MPS in the urine. Both diseases are due to deficiency of enzymes that attach the phosphomannosyl residues required by a number of cytosolic hydrolases to enter lysosomes. The result is high levels of these hydrolases in the blood with correspondingly deficient intracellular levels. Prognosis is dismal in ML II, but is more variable in ML III.

ML IV (Folkerth et al. 1995) is a disease of Ashkenazi Jews in which clouding of the cornea presents early but, for unclear reasons, fluctuates in intensity and responds somewhat to the frequent instillation of artificial tears. There is severe mental and motor deficiency, with pigmentary degeneration of the retina and hearing loss, but no clinical storage in the viscera or skeleton. It has a very protracted course and is probably often missed because it is mistaken for undifferentiated mental deficiency. It has recently been shown to be due to defective endocytosis and excessive transport into lysosomes of glycolipids and phospholipids for degradation (Bargal and Bach 1997; Chen et al. 1998).

The carbohydrate-deficient glycoprotein diseases are a group of autosomal recessive multisystem disorders in which there is inadequate cellular transport because of inadequate incorporation of mannose into glycoproteins or lipid-linked oligosaccharides (Dupre et al. 1999; Antoun et al. 1999; Young and Driscoll 1999). The clinical manifestations are more severe in younger children, in whom it may be lethal, than in adolescents. The disorder may present as hydrops fetalis, congenital nephrotic syndrome, cardiomyopathy, or a coagulopathy with stroke-like episodes. Children are mentally retarded, may have a characteristic facies with almond-shaped eyes, strabismus, cataracts, inverted nipples, fat pads above the buttocks, dysostosis multiplex, and brachydactyly. They are retarded, often epileptic, and ataxic with ponto-cerebellar atrophy on MRI. Results of short-term treatment with dietary mannose were unsuccessful despite correction of the defect in vitro (Kjaergaard et al. 1998; Korner et al 1998).

There is no specific treatment for any of these diseases. Again, bone marrow transplantation has been tried but in too few patients to enable appraisal of its efficacy. Prenatal diagnosis and carrier detection are possible.

## The Neuronal Ceroid Lipofuscinoses

Table 41-6 summarizes the clinically and genetically defined variants of Batten's disease or neuronal ceroid lipofuscinoses (CLN), almost all of which are recessive. Only 80% fall into the classical infantile (CLN1), late infantile (CLN2), juvenile (CLN3), and adult variants (CLN4) (Nardocci, et al., 1995; Mole 1999). Molecular genetics are required to sort out the 20% atypical cases which overlap the classical variants (Wisniewski et al. 1997, 1998; Lauronen et al. 1999). CLN2 and CLN3 are cerebromacular degenerations that are by far the most prevalent subtypes in the United States and Europe, whereas the CLN1 and CLN5 variants are particularly frequent in Finland. Great progress has been made in the past decade toward clarifying the molecular basis of the ceroid lipofuscinoses. Deficiency of palmitoyl-protein thioesterase characterizes the classic devastating infantile CLN1 variant which is most prevalent in Finland but also some allelic variants in preschool and older children with a more protracted course.

Storage in these variants, as well as in the non-allelic CLN5 late infantile variant, consists of granular osmiophilic deposits made up of polyunsaturated fatty acids and activator proteins (saposins) A and D (Vesa et al. 1995; Tyynela et al., 1995). The fluorescent storage material is made up of subcellular organelle membranes, which are curvilinear in CLN2, have a fingerprint pattern in CLN3, and are of both types in CLN6 (Sharp et al. 1997; Sleat et al. 1997; Savukoski et al. 1998; Kremmidiotis et al. 1999; Rawlings and Barrett 1999). Variation in types of mutations and sizes of deletions provide a partial explanation for the clinical and ultrastructural variability in CLN3 (Munroe et al. 1997). Prenatal molecular diagnosis is now possible in all defined subtypes, but all too often a family is complete before the oldest affected sib, especially with one of the juvenile variants, becomes overtly symptomatic, resulting in many multiplex families.

The ceroid lipofuscinoses are characterized ultrastructurally by membrane-bound fluorescent lipoprotein inclusions in neurons and many peripheral tissues, including skin where they are diagnostically helpful. Although there is some structural overlap among variants, the lysosomal inclusions are granular in NCL1 and some atypical variants where they may be associated with extraneuronal pigment deposition (Goebel et al. 1995). Inclusions are curvilinear in NCL2, have a fingerprint pattern in NCL3, and are mixed in atypical and some adult variants.

Prominent macular degeneration is regularly the presenting sign of NCL3, in which signs of dementia, motor deficit, and seizures may not appear for 4 to 6 years after loss of central vision. Patients with NCL3 may remain ambulatory and able to attend school until their late teens, although perhaps a quarter of them die in their teens after a more

**Table 41-6.** Ceroid—lipofuscinoses*

| Variants | Chromosome | Age of Onset | Prognosis for Survival | Severity of Illness |
|---|---|---|---|---|
| CLN 1 **Infantile** (Finnish) | 1p32 | Infancy | Death in first decade | Devastated in late infancy |
| CLN 2 **Late infantile** | 11p15.5 | Preschool | Death in first decade | Devastated in 2–3 years |
| vCLN 1 Variant late infantile | 1p32 | Preschool | Death in first decade/teens | Devastated in a few years |
| vCLN 5 Variant late infantile (Finnish) | 13q21 | Preschool | Death in first decade | Devastated in a few years |
| vCLN 6 Variant late infantile | 11q21-23 | Preschool | Death in first decade | Devastated in a few years |
| CLN 3 **Juvenile** | 16p12.1 | Early school-age | Death in teens or twenties | Devastated in late teens |
| vCLN 1 Variant Juvenile | 1p32 | School-age | Death in teens/adulthood | Later visual loss than CLN3 |
| CLN 4 **Adult** | ? | Adulthood | Death within a decade | Severe, not blind |
| Other atypical variants | — | — | — | — |

*The classically described variants are indicated in bold.

rapidly dementing course with prominent seizures. Blindness also characterizes the NCL1 and NCL2 variants, which are usually fatal before the end of the first decade, whereas macular degeneration is usually not a feature of some of the atypical childhood cases and of adult cases which, rarely, are dominantly inherited. NCL2 presents with disabling myoclonus with drop seizures and a subacute dementia. NCL1 produces such rapid and severe neuronal devastation as to render the cortex virtually aneuronal and the electroencephalogram (EEG) flat by 3 to 4 years.

There is no effective treatment beyond attempting to control seizures and providing children with the juvenile variant with an education suitable for the blind. Results of bone marrow transplantation and the administration of polyunsaturated fatty acids are too preliminary to judge their effectiveness (Bennett et al. 1994). Clonazepam and valproate are the drugs of choice in the late infantile variant. Phenytoin should be avoided as long as possible in NCL3, as it seems to worsen ataxia.

## Other Disorders of Lipid Metabolism

This is a heterogeneous group of disorders a few of which are now treatable (Table 41-7), notably some disorders of fatty acid oxidation discussed later. Wolman's disease is a lysosomal storage disease of early infancy due to acid lipase deficiency. It is characterized by massive storage of cholesteryl esters in the liver. Death occurs before 1 year of age (Wolman 1995). Administration of the cholesteryl-lowering agent lovastatin and an attempt at liver transplantation failed to alter the prognosis. Tangier's disease, like Wolman's and Niemann-Pick disease type C, is characterized by deposition of cholesterol in the tissues, in this case because of hypercatabolism of high-density lipoproteins (Remaley et al. 1997). It produces enlarged orange tonsils in adolescence, early cardiovascular disease with low levels of high-density lipoproteins in blood, and a neuropathy that generally does not become symptomatic until adulthood.

Early treatment with large doses of vitamin E prevents or reverses most of the neurological symptoms of abetalipoproteinemia with acanthocytosis (Bassen-Kornzweig [B-K] disease) if started early. B-K is characterized by ataxia, a neuropathy, retinal degeneration, and cognitive deficits that appear in adolescence and progress gradually over a decade or so if untreated. It is due to the deficiency of protein disulfide-isomerase (Ricci et al. 1995) resulting in inability of the gut

**Table 41-7.** Other Disorders of Lipid Metabolism

| Disease | Age of Onset | Prognosis for Survival (Untreated) | Disability (Untreated) | Treatment | Effectiveness* |
|---------|--------------|-----------------------------------|------------------------|-----------|----------------|
| Wolman's disease | Early infancy | Death before 1 year | Devastating | — | — |
| Tangier's disease | Teens, adulthood | Survival for decades, early atherosclerosis | Mild to moderate | — | — |
| Abetalipoproteinemia | Early childhood | Survival to adulthood | Mild to moderate | Vitamin E | Satisfactory |
| Pelizaeus-Merzbacher | Infancy | Survival to teens or young adulthood | Moderate to severe | — | — |
| Familial spastic paraplegia | Childhood to adulthood | Long-term survival | Moderate to severe | — | |
| Sjögren-Larsson | Early childhood | Survival to adulthood | Severe | Low fat, MCT oil | Fair |
| Marinesco-Sjögren | Infancy | Death in childhood (?) | Severe | — | — |
| Cerebrotendinous xanthomatosis | Teens, adulthood | Survival for decades | Moderate to severe | Chenodeoxycholic acid | Fair to satisfactory |
| Orthochromatic leukodystrophy | Childhood | Death within a decade | Severe | — | — |

* Depends on severity at inception of treatment.

to secrete apolipoprotein B. The consequence is early-onset chronic diarrhea and malabsorption of fat-soluble vitamins (Du et al. 1996). B-K is related to the chorea-acanthocytosis syndrome and other disorders resulting in vitamin E deficiency and impaired resistance to oxidative stress (Rubio et al., 1997; Copp et al. 1999).

Pelizaeus-Merzbacher (P-M) disease, an X-linked trait, presents with striking nystagmus in infancy and a "tigroid" orthochromatic leukodystrophy with long tract and cerebellar signs and moderate mental deficiency (Seitelberger 1995). Its course is a very slowly progressive but eventually results in severe spastic ataxia. Most patients survive to young adulthood. The disease is due to any one of many mutations of the gene for proteolipid protein, which is a major component of myelin that is also deficient in one of two forms of X-linked recessive familial spastic paraplegia (Kobayashi et al. 1996; Hodes et al. 1999). The other X-linked recessive form of familial spastic paraplegia, which involves the gene for the neural cell adhesion molecule L1, is allelic with X-linked hydrocephalus. There are also at least one autosomal recessive and several genetically distinct autosomal dominant forms of spastic paraplegia, most of which start in adults and are slowly progressive (Bruyn et al. 1997).

Sjögren-Larsson syndrome, which is most prevalent in northern Sweden, presents with spastic quadriplegia precluding ambulation, mental deficiency, retinopathy, and ichthyosis. It was recently found to be due to the deficiency of fatty aldehyde dehydrogenase (De Laurenzi et al. 1996; van Domburg et al. 1999). It is said to improve with dietary restriction of fat and supplementation with medium chain triglycerides.

Marinesco-Sjögren syndrome is a rare and as yet untreatable chronic disease of early childhood producing ataxia, mental deficiency, cataracts, muscular weakness with characteristic rimmed vacuoles in muscle fibers, and pituitary insufficiency responsible for growth failure and hypogonadism (Suzuki et al. 1997). Its chemical pathology is not understood.

Cerebrotendinous xanthomatosis, a cholestanol lipidosis, shares some symptoms with Marinesco-Sjögren syndrome except that it does not become symptomatic until the teens at the earliest, and often not until middle age. It is often mistaken for multiple sclerosis or some other ataxic syndrome

with mild dementia (Berginer 1984). The giveaway is thickening of the Achilles tendon, other tendinous xanthomas, and cataracts, often with a history of chronic diarrhea. Untreated, most patients die of myocardial infarction or bulbar palsy in middle life, following decades of a slowly progressive deterioration affecting peripheral nerves, the spinal cord, and the brain. Treatment with chenodeoxycholic acid improves all the manifestations of the disease substantially, provided it is started before they become severe (Soffer et al. 1995).

Orthochromatic leukodystrophy encompasses a heterogeneous group of diseases whose molecular basis is not yet understood and which may be inherited as autosomal recessive or dominant traits (Knopman et al. 1996; Constantinidis and Wisniewski 1991). A number of cases, which overlap with adult ceroid lipofuscinosis, are associated with pigmented autofluorescent inclusions in macrophages and oligodendroglia, which may explain the myelin destruction visible on magnetic resonance imaging (MRI). Most cases present in adulthood with a progressive dementia with spasticity, ataxia, and extrapyramidal signs. The course varies from a few years to several decades and there is no known treatment.

## The Peroxisomal Diseases

Peroxisomes are subcellular organelles that contain a variety of cytosolic and membrane-bound enzymes, in particular very long chain fatty acid (VLCFA) acyl-CoA $\beta$-oxidases whose end products are $H_2O_2$, which is toxic and is broken down by catalase, and medium chain fatty acids that are transported to mitochondria for further $\beta$ oxidation. Peroxisomes are also involved in the synthesis of plasmalogens and metabolism of bile acids, oxalate, and other substrates. Peroxisomal diseases are divided into three groups (Table 41-8) (Moser 1996). The first encompasses a single enzyme deficiency with normal appearing peroxisomes, of which adrenoleukodystrophy is the main example. The second group, epitomized by Zellweger's disease, encompasses disorders of peroxisomal biogenesis associated with multiple enzyme deficiencies in neonates or infants who have dysmorphic features and severe multiorgan involvement. In rhizomelic chondrodysplasia punctata, a third variant, peroxisomes are normal appearing but lack multiple enzymes. It is a some-

**Table 41-8.** Peroxisomal Diseases

| Diseases | Age of Onset | Prognosis for Survival | Disability |
|---|---|---|---|
| Diseases with single peroxisomal enzyme deficiencies | | | |
| Adrenoleukodystrophy | Childhood (ALD) | Death in teens | Severe |
| | Adulthood (AMN) | Prolonged, variable in AMN | Moderate to severe |
| | Adult carrier females | Good | None to moderate |
| Pseudo-Zellweger's + several others | Birth | Death in infancy to childhood | Total or severe |
| Refsum's | Adolescence | Survival to adulthood | Moderate to severe (untreated) |
| Diseases of peroxisomal biogenesis with multiple enzyme deficiencies | | | |
| Zellweger's | Birth | Death in early infancy | Total |
| Neonatal ADL | Birth | Death in infancy or preschool | Severe |
| Infantile Refsum's | Birth | Survival into childhood | Severe |
| Pipecolatacidemia | Infancy | Death in infancy or preschool | Severe |
| Disease with normal peroxisomal morphology but multiple enzyme deficiencies | | | |
| Rhizomelic chondro-dysplasia punctata | Infancy | Survival into childhood | Severe |

ALD, adrenoleukodystrophy; AMN, adrenomyeloneuropathy.

what less severe disease of early childhood characterized by dysmorphic features, short limbs, cataracts, and mental deficiency. Clinical diagnosis in the infantile disorders is complicated by the fact that there are several severe diseases with single enzyme defects whose phenotypes are reminiscent of Zellweger's disease, a disorder in which the organelle fails to form (Goldfisher et al. 1973), and other less severe disorders of peroxisomal biogenesis in which peroxisomes are small and reduced in number. Assay of VLCFA in plasma is the most effective test to screen for peroxisomal disorders (Moser et al. 1999).

The most common peroxisomal disease is juvenile X-linked adrenoleukodystrophy (ALD), which is due to the deficiency of acyl-CoA synthetase, an ATP transsporter. It is characterized by the accumulation of $C_{26}$ and longer fatty acids that can be seen ultrastructurally as flat leaflets in the adrenal gland, testis, Schwann cells, and oligodendroglia. The classic neurological picture is one of dementia starting insidiously before age 10 years in a boy who will subsequently develop cortical blindness and deafness, long tract signs, and in some cases seizures (Moser 1997). The computed tomography (CT) and MRI scans show large areas of demyelination that spread from the occipital region forward, less often from the frontal region backwards. Virtually all these boys die within a decade or less of the diagnosis, often after several years in a vegetative state. Carrier testing and prenatal diagnosis are available (Boehm et al. 1999).

Some affected male members in families of children with classic ALD do not become symptomatic until adulthood, when they present with signs of a chronic myelopathy and neuropathy (adrenomyeloneuropathy). Occasional individuals remain asymptomatic or develop only adrenal insufficiency. Reasons for this extremely variable prognosis are baffling, as family members, who presumably carry the same mutation, may run the gamut of courses, suggesting the possibility of an as yet undefined gene interaction. Obligate carrier females often develop a mild to moderate spastic paraparesis in middle life and, rarely, a progressive dementia.

As a result of research by the father of a boy with the disease, an experimental dietary treatment has undergone clinical trial (Moser and Borel 1995). The diet involves avoiding foods containing long-chain fatty acids and administering glycerol trioleate and $C_{22}$ oils (erucic acid). It decreases blood levels of VLCFA dramatically but its efficacy, even in presymptomatic boys, has been disappointing. Other treatments under investigation are the administration of immunoglobulin G (Cappa et al. 1994), interferon-$\beta$ (Korenke et al. 1997), thalidomide (which affects tumor necrosis factor), and other immunomodulators (Pahan et al. 1998). These attempts at immunomodulation are based on the observation that once demyelination starts, it often spreads subacutely and that there is an inflammatory reaction at its margins. Double-blind studies are in progress, but preliminary results are not very encouraging. At least several dozen boys have undergone bone marrow transplantation, in some combined with the erucic acid diet. Although transplantation does not arrest the disease and should not be offered in advanced cases, it may slow progression if performed early, and the hope is that it may prevent the disease in presymptomatic boys (Krivit et al. 1995a).

Refsum's disease, which is autosomal recessive, is due to the lack of phytanoyl-CoA hydroxidase, which breaks down phytanic acid, mainly in mitochondria. The phenotype varies depending on the particular mutation and on how much phytanic acid, which comes from chlorophyll, the diet contains. It usually becomes symptomatic in adolescence with pigmentary degeneration of the retina and hearing loss associated with a slowly progressive ataxic polyneuritic gait. The neurological, but not the retinal or cochlear, deficits are largely reversible over a period of months of a phytanic acid–restricted diet, which is preventive if administered early enough. Intermittent plasmapheresis can be used to hasten recovery and allows patients a respite from their monotonous diet (Dickson et al. 1989).

Zellweger's disease or the cerebrohepatorenal syndrome is the prototypical and most severe of the infantile disorders of peroxisomal biogenesis. These are characterized by various combinations of the accumulation of $>C_{24}$ VLCFA, phytanic acid, and pipecolic acid, abnormalities of plasmalogen synthesis, and elevated bile acid intermediates. A characteristic of many of these disorders, which are autosomal recessive and genetically heterogeneous, is that they are recognizable clinically because they are associated with a variety of developmental somatic and brain anomalies. The infants with Zellweger's disease are severely hypotonic, have a characteristic facies, and visceromegaly with multiorgan dysfunction. In the brain there are disorders of neuronal migration, some detectable with MRI, which no doubt account in part for the severe cognitive deficits, seizures, and neurological findings to which altered fatty acid composition and impaired mitochondrial function also contribute (Kamei et al. 1993). The biochemical pathogenesis of the constellation of anomalies of the kidneys, liver, heart, muscles, bones, eyes, ears, and brain that characterize the infantile peroxisomal disorders is not fully understood. The clinical and biochemical phenotypes of the other infantile peroxisomal disorders overlap with Zellweger's syndrome (Poggi-Travert et al. 1995). Thus far, no treatment has helped infants with Zellweger's disease who die in infancy.

Results of bone marrow transplantation and the administration of certain medium chain polyunsaturated fatty acids to some of the children with the less severe phenotypes are awaited.

## The Mitochondrial Cytopathies

These disorders are not discussed here because they are covered in the chapter on neuromuscular diseases, even though many present with signs of a progressive encephalopathy due to disorders of energy metabolism or fatty acid β-oxidation. As is well known, many are mendelian and due to nuclear DNA mutations, whereas those due to mitochondrial DNA mutations are maternally inherited. Their clinical manifestations and course are extraordinarily varied (De Vivo 1993, Shanske and DiMauro 1997). More of them may become specifically treatable as their biochemical pathophysiology is better understood.

## Aminoacidurias, Hyperammonemias, and Organic Acidurias

The most effective dietary therapies have been devised for some of these disorders of early life although, as is shown in Tables 41-1, 41-9, and 41-10, much remains to be done. Nyhan and Sakati's (1987) book remains a classic and useful reference on the aminoacidurias and organic acidurias and their management. The key to avoiding death or severe damage to the brain in these rare disorders is a high index of suspicion in sick neonates and prompt referral to centers with extensive experience in their acute and long-term management. Such centers have the resources to study patients at the metabolic and molecular level. This is essential because there are multiple variants of the classic disorders whose prognosis and treatment may differ substantially. These centers can also provide prenatal diagnosis for the many disorders for which it is available. It is again generally the case that the severity of the phenotype depends on the amount of residual enzyme activity which, in turn, is determined by the particular allelic mutation/deletion.

Except for Lesch-Nyhan disease, Lowe's disease, and ornithine transcarbamylase (OTC) deficiency, which are X-linked recessive, all these disorders are inherited as autosomal recessive traits and therefore appear sporadic until an affected sib

**Table 41-9.** Some Disorders of Amino Acid and Urea Metabolism

| Disease | Age at Onset | Prognosis for Survival (Untreated) | Disability (Untreated) | Treatment (Key Elements) | Effectiveness of Treatment |
|---|---|---|---|---|---|
| Phenylketonuria (PKU) | Birth | Good | Severe, some milder variants | Phenylalanine restriction | Satisfactory |
| PKU with tetrahydro-biopterin deficiency (several variants) | Variable | Good | Variable, some severe | Phenylalanine restriction, tetrahydrobiopterin, $B_{12}$ IM, levodopa, etc. | Depends on variant |
| Maple syrup urine (MSUD) | Birth | Death in infancy | Very severe | Branched chain amino acid restriction, thiamine | Reasonably good |
| MSUD variants | Variable | Variable | Mild to severe | Branched chain amino acid restriction, thiamine | Satisfactory |
| Homocystinuria | Infancy | Fair | Severe | Methionine restriction, cysteine, folate, $B_{12}$ IM | Poor to fair |
| Homocystinuria $B_6$ responsive | Infancy | Good | Variable | Methionine restriction, $B_6$, folic acid, betaine | Fair to good |
| Homocystinuria with methylmalonic aciduria | Infancy / Childhood | Poor to fair / Fair to good | Severe / Severe | $B_{12}$, betaine, carnitine | Poor to fair / Fair to good |
| Lowe's syndrome | Birth | Survive to teens or adulthood | Severe | Vitamin D, alkali | Poor, except for renal function |
| Hartnup's disease | Childhood | Good | Moderate, intermittent | Niacin | Good |
| Urea cycle | Birth | Poor | Severe to very severe | Low-protein diet, sodium benzoate, phenyl acetate/butyrate | Fair |
| OTC* carrier females | Early childhood | Fair to good | Mild to moderate | Ditto | Good |

*OTC: ornithine transcarbamylase deficiency.

| Disease | Age at onset | Prognosis for survival (untreated) | Disability (untreated) | Treatment | Effectiveness of treatment |
|---|---|---|---|---|---|
| Propionic aciduria type I (ketotic hyperglycinemia) | Neonate | Death in infancy | Severe (most variants) | Branched chain amino acid restriction | Poor to satisfactory |
| Type II—late onset | Childhood | Guarded | Severe—intermittent or progressive | | |
| Methylmalonic aciduria B₁₂ responsive | Neonate | Generally poor | Severe | Branched chain amino acid restriction, B₁₂ IM | Fair to satisfactory |
| Methylmalonic aciduria B₁₂ unresponsive | Neonate | Death: infancy/early childhood | Severe | Tube feeding low-protein branched chain amino acid restriction, carnitine, metronidazole | Fair |
| | Infancy/toddler | Death in childhood | | | |
| Isovaleric aciduria | Neonate | Death in childhood | Severe | Leucine restriction; L-glycine administration | Poor to fair |
| Glutaric aciduria type I | Infancy | Death in childhood | Severe | Lysine and tryptophan restriction, riboflavin, carnitine | Poor to fair |
| Fatty acid acyl CoA deficiency (long, medium, and short chain) | Infancy to childhood | Variable, including death | Variable—precipitated by fasting or other metabolic stress | Avoid fasting, high-dose biotin, carnitine | Good |
| Multicarboxylase deficiency | Neonate | Death in infancy | Severe | Biotin | Fair to good |
| Biotinidase deficiency | Infancy to childhood | Infancy or childhood, intermittent | Variable | Biotin | Good |
| Pyridoxine dependency | Infancy | Variable, including death | Variable | Lifelong pyridoxine | Good |
| Lactic acidosis (mitochondrial defects) | Neonate to childhood | Death in neonate or infant | Generally severe—variably progressive or intermittent thereafter | Carnitine, thiamine, biotin, coenzyme Q, lipoic acid (depends on variant) | Questionable |
| Lesch-Nyhan disease | Infancy | Death in teens or adulthood | Severe | None specific; allopurinal, colchicine for gout; carbidopa, tetrabenazine, risperidone for the movement disorder and self-injury | Poor |
| Nonketotic hyperglycinemia | Neonate | Death in infancy or early childhood | Severe | Sodium benzoate, dextromethorphan, ketamine | Poor |
| Canavan's disease | Infancy | Death in childhood or teens | Severe | — | — |
| Alexander's disease | Infancy | Severe | Death in childhood | — | — |
| | Childhood or teens | Severe | Death in teens or early adulthood | | |

is born. The most severe neonatal diseases, such as the urea cycle defects, maple syrup urine disease (MSUD), and some of the organic acidurias and acute mitochondrial encephalopathies (De Vivo 1993) present with progressive lethargy, vomiting, and often seizures, going on to brain swelling, coma, and death. Affected infants are usually normal at birth and become symptomatic soon after feeding has been started. In critically ill neonates, it may not be enough to stop feedings and empirically administer glucose with carnitine and pharmacological doses of vitamins that act as coenzymes (e.g., thiamine, riboflavine, pyridoxine, cobalamine, and biotin) it may be necessary to perform an emergency exchange transfusion or hemodialysis while awaiting the results of analyses of blood gases, serum glucose, lactate, and ammonia, and gas liquid chromatography/mass spectrometry of the blood, urine, or CSF to guide further management. Long-term results in the most severe neonatal encephalopathies are often unsatisfactory, with survival of a child with a profoundly damaged brain. Again, early diagnosis requires a high degree of suspicion in a lethargic or comatose infant with or without seizures for a disorder other than neonatal asphyxia.

In the case of PKU and MSUD, preventive treatment consists of a synthetic diet deficient in phenylalanine in the case of PKU and of branched amino acids on the case of MSUD. How long to continue the diet is controversial. For classical PKU due to phenylalanine hydroxylase (PAH) deficiency, which presents somewhat later and less acutely than the acute neonatal encephalopathies, the original recommendation was to continue the diet up to age 4 years when major tracts are myelinated, as myelin bears the brunt of the disorder. However, a report indicates that 32 of 34 asymptomatic adequately treated children and young adults had persistent white matter changes on MRI, the severity of which was correlated with their level of hyperphenylalaninemia. Therefore, hyperphenylalaninemia may not be completely innocuous, even at that age (Thompson 1993). Several reports indicate that there may be modest declines in IQ and academic achievement and the emergence of some behavior problems after the diet is discontinued (e.g., Koch 1997). In a national collaborative study of 125 10-year-old children with PKU, there was a significant relationship between blood phenylalanine levels between ages 3 1/2 and 10 years and cognitive outcome variables, suggesting that the diet be continued until 10 years (Michals et al. 1988). A comprehensive discussion of treatment issues can be found in supplement 407 of *Acta Paediatrica* (Anonymous 1994). There are more than 100 alleles of the PAH gene, and the severity of the phenotype and amount of PAH residual activity varies (Trefz et al. 1993). Non-PKU-hyperphenylalaninemia does not require treatment (Weglage et al. 1996). In contrast, there are at least four different mutations responsible for atypical PKU associated with tetrahydrobiopterin deficiency whose clinical phenotype varies in severity. These disorders affect catecholamine metabolism, and may require replacement therapy with $B_{12}$, 5-hydroxytryptophan or Levodopa because of the block in catecholamine metabolism, in addition to phenylalanine restriction (Goldstein et al. 1995, Blau et al. 1996).

Women homozygous for PKU need to go back on a phenylalanine-restricted diet prior to conception in order to avoid bearing retarded children because dietary restriction started in the first or second trimester of pregnancy is not as effective in preventing mother's hyperphenylalaninemia from damaging the fetus' brain (Cipcic-Schmidt et al. 1996, Hanley et al. 1996). Intrauterine treatment of the fetus is also indicated in biotin-responsive multiple carboxylase deficiency and $B_{12}$-responsive methylmalonic aciduria (Zass et al. 1995; Evans et al. 1997).

Avoidance of profound mental deficiency and achievement of normal or near normal intelligence by dietary means in promptly diagnosed PKU has led to mandatory neonatal screening programs for this and other treatable metabolic disorders such as MSUD, galactosemia, biotinidase deficiency, and hypothyroidism. Dietary restriction may have to be continued indefinitely in the severe form of MSUD (Korein et al. 1994). Critically ill neonates with MSUD may benefit from prompt dialysis, hemofiltration, or other measures (Jouvet et al. 1997; Nyhan WL et al. 1998; Yoshimo et al. 1999). Patients with some milder forms of MSUD may not need continuous treatment but, like those with severe variants, are at risk for an acute encephalopathy at the time of intercurrent febrile illnesses.

Homocystinuria affects $B_{12}$ metabolism and produces megaloblastic anemia, ectopic lenses, and affects all caliber blood vessels with resulting strokes and, in over half of the children, mental deficiency. A low methionine cysteine-supplemented diet with administration of pyridoxine and intramuscular $B_{12}$ is modestly effective (Wilcken and Wilcken 1997). Combined homocystinuria and methylmalonic aciduria presents in early infancy and has a variable prognosis depending on the particular mutation, ranging from death in infancy to survival with mental deficiency and a movement disorder, despite treatment with $B_{12}$, carnitine, and betaine (Rosenblatt et al. 1997).

Vigorous treatment of the renal defect in Lowe's syndrome with alkali and of its rickets with vitamin D enables many boys to survive to adult life. This treatment does not prevent the mental deficiency or the cataracts, which are present at birth but may be ameliorated with the compulsive instillation of ascorbic acid eye drops (Hayasaka et al. 1997). Hartnup's disease presents with intermittent ataxia and a facial rash, and responds to the administration of niacin.

There are numerous other rare disorders of amino acid metabolism, many of them associated with mental deficiency (Kaye and Hyland 1998). Screening for these rare disorders is now possible with high-performance automated methodologies and is indicated in children with unexplained neurological deficits and inadequate cognitive development, especially if they present with associated physical abnormalities as some may be treatable. These medical oddities have helped elucidate many metabolic pathways and in a few cases to devise a therapy. Molecular methods that regularly demonstrate multiple mutations of any given gene help explain some of the bewildering variability of phenotypes.

Outcome in the neonatal disorders of the urea cycle is variable, with significant mortality and mental deficiency. The most common is OTC deficiency which is X-linked. Some success has been achieved in the emergency treatment of hyperammonemic coma, followed by protein restriction and the chronic administration of sodium benzoate, phenylbutyrate, citrulline or arginine, and biotin to activate an alternate pathway for the excretion of waste products of nitrogen metabolism (Batshaw 1984). Successfully treated children remain at high risk for developing hyperammonemic coma and dying during the course of intercurrent infections. Acute dialysis and liver transplantation have been offered to a few infants with OTC deficiency with some success if performed before mental retardation has developed (Busuttil et al. 1998). Carrier

females of OTC who present with migraine headaches, ill-defined episodes of lethargy, or frank hyperammonemic coma, also require treatment (Batshaw et al. 1980; Maestri et al. 1996) or even liver transportation (Kasahara et al. 1998). Hyperammonemia is not specific to the disorders of the urea cycle but also occurs in transient hyperammonemia of the newborn, which requires treatment but has a good prognosis, and in many acute mitochondrial disorders and organic acidemias.

The most prevalent of the organic acidemias listed in Table 41-10 result from inadequate β-oxidation of fatty acids in mitochondria. Many present in early infancy with a hyperammonemic/hypoketotic/hypoglycemic encephalopathy with dicarboxylic aciduria and carnitine deficiency. They require the emergency treatments already discussed. Some are precipitated by fasting or other physical stress and may be intermittently symptomatic (De Vivo 1993). Some have become treatable, but outcome depends on the level of enzymatic activity and, consequently, age at presentation. Even in adequately treated surviving infants, outcome is often unsatisfactory because of a variety of motor signs, seizures, and mental deficiency, and recurrent acute encephalopathic episodes (e.g., van der Meer et al. 1994). New disorders and variants are regularly being described (Ozand et al. 1994). Specific and prompt biochemical diagnosis is essential to rational management. There are some clinical clues to diagnosis. For example, lucency of the basal ganglia on MRI strongly suggests a mitochondrial disease, methylmalonic, combined methylmalonic/homocystinuric, or propionic acidemia; megalencephaly points to glutaric aciduria, Alexander's or Canavan's disease, a rash to a disorder of biotin metabolism, and hair abnormality to Menkes' disease, homocystinuria, or biotin deficiency.

Lesch-Nyhan disease, a disorder of purine metabolism, can arise as a result of many different mutations inactivating hypoxanthine guanine phosphoribosyltransferase (Nyhan 1997). Once again, the amount of residual enzyme activity determines the severity of the phenotype and its prognosis. Prognosis in the classic infantile variant is poor, with all affected boys manifesting a movement disorder in infancy that precludes ambulation, the majority having significant mental deficiency, and all mutilating themselves, often to a grotesque degree (Nyhan and Sakati 1987). Treatment with allopurinol may postpone death from uricemic nephropathy and gouty arthropathy is alleviated with colchicine, but these treatments do not affect the basic defect and its neurological consequences. Carbidopa and tetrabenazine seem to provide a modest amelioration of the movement disorder (Jankovic et al. 1988) and risperidone may have a role in treating both self-injury and the abnormal movements. There are variants of the disease with hyperuricemia and deafness without the movement disorder or self-mutilation; they are due to other purine enzyme deficiencies.

There is no effective specific treatment yet for invariably fatal disorders such as nonketotic hyperglycinemia and spongy degeneration of the brain (Canavan's disease) (Traeger and Rapin 1998). Survival in a vegetative or near vegetative state may extend to the second decade, notably in Canavan's disease. A trial of intraventricular administration of genetically engineered cells to children with Canavan's disease is reportedly ineffective. In nonketotic hyperglycinemia, sodium benzoate lowers glycine levels in the blood and CSF and may provide some control for the intractable seizures and myoclonus, but it does not seem to influence the children's profound mental deficiency (Wolff et al. 1986). More recently, the $N$-methyl-D-aspartete (NMDA) antagonist dextromethorphan and ketamine have been tried, with limited success (Kure et al. 1997; Hamosh et al. 1998).

Prognosis is variable in Alexander's disease, a clinically and genetically heterogeneous white matter disease of unknown cause for which there is no treatment. It may present subacutely in infancy, as a more chronic illness lasting some 5 years in preschool children, whereas it may last a decade or more in adolescents or adults in whom bulbar signs may predominate (Reichard et al. 1996). The diagnosis can be suspected in young children on the basis of megalencephaly and characteristic lucency of the white matter with periventricular and periaqueductal hyperintensity on MRI, but there is currently no specific test short of demonstrating eosinophilic Rosenthal inclusions in fibrous astrocytes.

## Other Disorders

Table 41-11 lists some miscellaneous diseases whose genetic/biochemical basis is well understood in some but not others, with an increasing number becoming diagnosable in utero and treatable. With the exception of copper malabsorption syndrome (Menkes' disease), which is X-linked, and acute intermittent prophyria, which is dominant, they are inherited as autosomal recessive traits.

Prognosis in Wilson's disease, which is due to copper storage, has been revolutionized by the introduction of a low-copper diet and administration of copper chelating agents. Treated early, before the occurrence of irreversible cavitation of the basal ganglia or death from fulminant hepatic failure, Wilson's disease is compatible with indefinite survival, regression of many or all neurological and psychiatric signs, and even with successful pregnancy (Scheinberg and Sternlieb 1984; Shilsky 1996). Liver transplantation has been occasionally used successfully in children with acute hepatic failure unresponsive to more conservative treatments. The disease is due to lack of a copper-transporting ATPase critical for copper excretion by the liver, whereas the analogous but distinct enzymatic defect in Menkes' disease precludes copper absorption from the gut and results in a copper deficiency disease.

Menkes' or kinky hair disease is at the other therapeutic extreme because, despite a recent report of provention of some of its consequences with parenteral copper histidine replacement, prognosis remains poor (Kaler et al. 1996; Christodoulou et al. 1998). The infants are symptomatic from birth and die in infancy or in a vegetative state in the preschool years (Tumer and Horn 1997). There are multiple mutations affecting enzyme activity, including two that result in a less severe phenotype (Proud et al. 1996). Prenatal diagnosis is available.

Acute intermittent porphyria, which rarely becomes symptomatic before puberty, is more common in women than men. It is due to porphobilinogen deaminase deficiency. Attacks are invariably associated with increased porphobilinogen in the urine which turns brown on standing. Its manifestations vary a great deal and may include acute autonomic crises with abdominal pain, constipation and vomiting, hypertension, tachycardia, inappropriate antidiuretic hormone secretion, and fever, seizures, psychosis, and in some cases an acute or subacute neuropathy that can resemble Guillain-Barré syndrome (Tefferi et al. 1994). Attacks that last a number of days

**Table 41-11.** Other Disorders

| Disease | Age of Onset | Prognosis for Survival | Disability (Untreated) | Specific Treatment | Effectiveness of Treatment |
|---|---|---|---|---|---|
| Wilson's | Childhood to early adulthood | Variable | Severe | Low-copper diet + chelation | Satisfactory |
| Menkes' (copper malabsorption) | Early infancy | Death in infancy or early childhood | Devastated | Copper + histidine | Poor; fair if early in mild variant |
| Acute intermittent porphyria | Adolescence | Generally good | Intermittently severe | Avoid precipitants; IV heme, gabapentin, cimetidine | Satisfactory |
| Lafora's | Mid-childhood | Death within a decade | Severe | — | — |
| Baltic myoclonus | Mid-childhood | Survival to adulthood | Moderate to severe | Antioxidants, L-cysteine | ? |
| Neuroaxonal dystrophy | Infancy | Death in childhood | Severe | — | — |
| Hallervorden-Spatz | Childhood or later | Most survive to adulthood | Severe | — | — |
| Ataxia-telangiectasia | Early childhood | Survival to teens, adulthood | Moderate to severe | IgA, prophylactic antibiotics | Fair |
| Cockayne's syndrome | Infancy | Death in childhood or teens | Severe | — | — |
| Xeroderma pigmentosum | Infancy | Most survive to adulthood | Severe | Sun screens | Fair |
| Familial dysautonomia | Infancy | Survival to early adulthood, some early deaths | Moderate to severe | Bethanechol, midodrine | Fair |

may be precipitated by barbiturates or alcohol, menstruation, intercurrent illnesses, starvation, and dehydration. A new treatment of severe attacks with intravenous infusion of heme together with parenteral nutrition with carbohydrates has improved their prognosis (Kaupipinen 1998; Grandchamp 1998). Because gabapentin is not metabolized in the liver, it can be used safely as an anticonvulsant (Zandra et al. 1998). Cimetidine may be useful both to treat acute attacks and for prophylaxis (Rogers 1997). Prognosis is favorable if the acute attack is diagnosed correctly and treated appropriately, and long-term prognosis is good if precipitants are avoided. The major risk is missing the diagnosis and using drugs that will worsen the crisis, with occasionally fatal results. Many patients have had to endure multiple hospital admissions for unneeded abdominal surgery or psychiatric symptoms before the correct diagnosis is made. There may be a significant long-term risk for hepatocarcinoma, at least in northern Sweden (Andersson et al. 1996). Variegate porphyria has cutaneous manifestations as well as similar, but usually less severe, neurological symptoms. Hereditary coproporphyria may present as a psychosis in adolescence. Both have increased porphyrins in the stool as well as the urine.

Of the two forms of familial myoclonus, Lafora's disease is the more severe, resulting in death in 6 to 10 years, whereas so-called Baltic/ Mediterranean myoclonus or Unverricht-Lundborg disease is compatible with survival into adulthood. Unverricht-Lundborg disease is due to mutations in the cystatin-B gene and treatment with antioxidants and N-acetylcysteine may be beneficial (Hurd et al. 1996) and Lafora's disease is due to mutations in the protein tyrosine phosphatase gene (Serratosa et al. 1999). No curative treatment is available for either disease and the myoclonus does not necessarily respond to klonopin or valproate. Dementia is more severe and occurs earlier in Lafora's disease, in which there are widespread polyglucosan inclusions in neurons, and also in sweat glands, which is helpful for diagnosis.

Progress is being made in sorting out the group of diseases characterized by spheroids in axon terminals which contain collections of mitochondria and other bodies (Halliday 1995). In infantile and late infantile neuroaxonal dystrophy (NAD), spheroids are found in the peripheral as well as ubiquitously in the central nervous system (Itoh et al. 1993). In Hallervorden-Spatz disease (HSD), spheroids predominate in the basal ganglia where there is extensive iron storage giving them an orange color at autopsy and a distinctive "tiger-eye" appearance on MRI. The infantile and late infantile variants present with spasticity, ataxia, dystonia, optic atrophy, and in some cases acanthocytosis and pigmentary degeneration of the retina. HSD has a similar phenotype with a slower, more protracted course (Taylor et al. 1996b). A recently identified new variant of NAD that may present in infancy or adults is characterized by angiokeratoma of the skin (Wang et al. 1994). It is characterized by α-$N$-acetylgalactosaminidase deficiency (α-NAGA) and glycopeptiduria, which suggests its classification with the mucolipidoses. No treatment is known for any of these diseases. Children with early NAD succumb in a vegetative state during the school years, while those with HSD, who may not become symptomatic until their teens, may survive for a decade or more and may not be severely demented despite their devastating motor deficits.

Ataxia telangiectasia presents in the preschool years with an unsteady gait and may be falsely labeled "ataxic cerebral palsy" (Boder 1985). Neurological deterioration is slowly progressive and is compatible with survival into young adulthood provided immunological incompetence does not result in respiratory failure following severe sinopulmonary infection or in the occurrence of a lymphoma or other malignancy. Infusion of fresh frozen plasma to raise the level of IgA may be beneficial in the 90% of immunologically incompetent patients but has no effect on the neurological symptoms. These patients often have multiple endocrine deficiencies, including diabetes mellitus, and are exquisitely sensitive to radiation and to radiomimetic drugs, which precludes effective therapy of the malignancies that kill 20% of them, often in their teens (Taylor et al. 1996a). Blacks are three times as likely as whites to die of a malignancy. Variability in the manifestations of the disease is accounted in part by genetic heterogeneity (Gilad et al. 1998), with some patients surviving into their fifties with only moderate neurological handicap. Heterozygote carriers are at substantially increased risk of harboring a malignancy, especially breast cancer.

Cockayne's syndrome is an untreatable severe disease producing extreme dwarfing with profound microcephaly, mental deficiency, ataxia, spasticity, neuropathy, deafness, and retinopathy, but a surprisingly pleasant personality and ability to speak despite a brain that may weigh only 600 to 900 g (Nance and Berry 1992). Death tends to occur in the second decade, although occasional patients survive to the end of the third. Genetic heterogeneity is marked, with seven complementation groups described so far. A very severe form of Cockayne's disease is associated with xeroderma pigmentosum and results in early death (Moriwaki et al. 1996). Like ataxia telangiectasia, Cockayne's syndrome and xeroderma pigmentosum are associated with defects in DNA repair. Xeroderma pigmentosum, a genetically heterogeneous dermatological condition characterized by extreme sensitivity to ultraviolet light resulting in multiple carcinomas and melanomas of the skin, is associated in 18% of cases with ataxia, neuropathy, mental deficiency, hearing loss, and endocrine abnormalities (Kraemer et al. 1987). Probability of survival in xeroderma pigmentosum is 90% at age 13 years, 80% at age 28 years, 70% at age 40 years, with death occurring on average 30 years earlier than in the general population. Cancer is responsible for a third of the deaths.

Prognosis in familial dysautonomia, a recessive disease of Ashkenazi Jews, has been greatly improved by vigorous treatment of the malignant hyperthermia and gastrointestinal and hypertensive crises that threatened survival, even of infants. Among 227 patients described by Axelrod and Abularrage (1982), a third were 20 years or older. Long-term survival into the late thirties and early forties and even pregnancy are being achieved in optimally managed patients in whom dysautonomic crises are treated vigorously with chlorpromazine, bethanechol, and diazepam. Troublesome postural hypotension and heart rhythm abnormalities respond to midodrine (Axelrod et al. 1995) and severe problems with swallowing, gastric immobility, and reflux may require fundal plication and gastrostomy in some children (Szold et al. 1996). While survivors may be normally intelligent, they tend to be somewhat less so than their sibs and to have difficult personalities.

## References

Abramowicz, M. J.; Andrien, M.; Dupont, E.; et al. Isodisomy of chromosome 6 in a newborn with methylmalonic acidemia and agenesis of pancreatic beta cells causing diabetes mellitus. J. Clin. Invest. 94:418–421; 1994.

Al-Essa, M.; Bakheet, S.; Patay, Z.; et al. [18]Fluoro 2-deoxyglucose ([18]FDG) PET scan of the brain in propionic acidemia: clinical and MRI correlations. Brain Dev. 21:312–317; 1999.

Andersson, C.; Bjersing, L.; Lithner, F. The epidemiology of hepatocellular carcinoma in patients with acute intermittent porphyria. J. Intern. Med. 240:195–201; 1996.

Anonymous. Phenylketonuria—past, present, future. Acta Paediatr. Suppl. 407:1–129; 1994.

Antoun, H.; Villeneuve, N.; Gelot, A.; et al. Cerebellar atrophy: an important feature of carbohydrate deficient glycoprotein syndrome type I. Pediatr. Radiol. 29:194–198; 1999.

Armstrong, R. W.; Steinbok, P.; Cochrane, D. D. Intrathecally administered baclofen for treatment of children with spasticity of cerebral origin. J. Neurosurg. 87:409–414; 1997.

Arvio, M. Follow-up in patients with aspartylglucosaminuria. Part I. The course of intellectual functions. Acta Paediatr. 82:468–471; 1993a.

Arvio, M. Follow-up in patients with aspartylglucosaminuria. Part II. Adaptive skills. Acta Paediatr. 82:590–594; 1993b.

Axelrod, F. B.; Abularrage, J. J. Familial dysautonomia: a prospective study of survival. J. Pediatr. 101:234–236; 1982.

Axelrod, F. B.; Krey, L.; Glickstein, J. S.; et al. Preliminary observations on the use of midodrine in treating orthostatic hypotension in familial dysautonomia. J. Autonom. Nerv. Syst. 55:29–35; 1995.

Bargal, R.; Bach, G. Mucolipidosis IV: abnormal transport of lipids to lysosomes. J. Inherit. Metab. Dis. 20:625–632; 1997.

Baraitser, M. genetics of neurological disorders 3rd ed. Oxford: Oxford University Press; 1997.

Batshaw, M. L. Hyperammonemia. Curr. Probl. Pediatr. 14 (11):1–69; 1984.

Batshaw, M. L.; Roan, Y.; Jung, A. L.; et al. Cerebral dysfunction in asymptomatic carriers of ornithine transcarbamylase deficiency. N. Engl. J. Med. 302:482–485; 1980.

Baumann, M.; Masson, M.; Carreau, V.; et al. Adult forms of metachromatic leukodystrophy: clinical and biochemical approach. Dev. Neurosci. 13:211–215; 1991.

Belani, K. G.; Krivit, W.; Carpenter, B. L.; et al. Children with mucopolysaccharidosis: perioperative care, morbidity, mortality, and new findings. J. Pediatr. Surg. 28:403–408; 1993.

Bennett, M. J.; Gayton, A. R.; Rittey, C. D.; et al. Juvenile ceroid-lipofuscinosis: developmental progress after supplementation with polyunsaturated fatty acids. Dev. Med. Child Neurol. 36:630–638; 1994.

Berginer, V. M.; Salen, G.; Shefer, S. Long-term treatment of cerebrotendinous xanthomatosis with chenodeoxycholic acid. N. Engl. J. Med. 311:1649–1652; 1984.

Blau, N.; Thony, B.; Spada, M.; et al. Tetrahydrobiopterin and inherited hyperphenylalaninemias. Turk. J. Pediatr. 38:19–35; 1996.

Boder, E. Ataxia-telangiectasia: an overview. In: Gatti, R. A.; Swift, M. eds. Ataxia-telangiectasia: genetics, neuropathology, and immunology of a degenerative disease of childhood. New York: Alan R. Liss; 1985: p. 1–63.

Boehm, C. D.; Cutting, G. R.; Lachtermacher, M. B.; et al. Accurate DNA-based diagnostic and carrier testing for X-linked adrenoleukodystrophy. Mol. Gen. Metab. 66:128–136; 1999.

Bonten, E.; van der Speol, A.; Fornerod, M.; et al. Characterization of human lysosomal neuraminidase defines the molecular basis of the metabolic storage disorder sialidosis. Genes Dev. 10:3156–3169; 1996.

Bruyn, R. P.; van Veen, M. M.; Kremer, H.; et al. Familial spastic paraplegia: evidence for a fourth locus. Clin. Neurol. Neurosurg. 99:87–90; 1997.

Busuttil, A. A.; Goss, J. A.; Seu, P.; et al. The role of orthotopic liver transplantation in the treatment of ornithine transcarbamylase deficiency. Liver Transplant. Surg. 4:350–354; 1998.

Burkhardt, J. K.; Huttler, S.; Klein, A.; et al. Accumulation of sphingolipids in SAP-precursor (prosaposin)-deficient fibroblasts occurs in intralysosomal membrane structures and can be completely reversed by treatment with human SAP-precursor. Eur. J. Cell Biol. 73:10–18; 1997.

Cappa, M.; Bertini, E.; del Balzo, P.; et al. High dose of immunoglobulin IV treatment in adrenoleukodystrophy. J. Neurol. Neurosurg. Psychiatry 57 (suppl.): 69–70; 1994.

Chen, C. S.; Bach, G.; Pagano, R. E. Abnormal transport alont the lysosomal pathway in mucolipidosis, type IV disease. Proc. Nat. Acad. Sci. USA 95:6373–6378; 1998.

Chicoine, M. R.; Park, T. S.; Kaufman, B. A. Selective dorsal rhizotomy and rates of orthopedic surgery in children with spastic cerebral palsy. J. Neurosurg. 86:34–39; 1997.

Christodoulou, J.; Danks, D. M.; Sarkar, B.; et al. Early treatment of Menkes disease with parental copper-histidine: long-term follow-up of four treated patients. Am. J. Med. Genet. 76:154–164; 1998.

Cipcic-Schmidt, S.; Trefz, F. K.; Funders, B.; et al. German maternal phenylketonuria study. Eur. J. Pediatr. 155(suppl. 1):S173–S176; 1996.

Claridge, K. G.; Gibberd, T. B.; Sidey, M. C. Refsum disease: the presentation and ophthalmic aspects of Refsum disease in a series of 23 patients. Eye 6:371–375; 1992.

Clark, J. G. The challenge of bone marrow transplantation. Mayo Clin. Proc. 65:111–114; 1990.

Clement, M.; McGonigle, R. J. S.; Monkhouse, P. M.; et al. Renal transplantation in Anderson-Fabry disease. J. R. Soc. Med. 75:557–560; 1982.

Constantinidis, J.; Wisniewski, T. M. The dominant form of the pigmentary orthochromatic leukodystrophy. Acta Neuropathol. 82:483–487; 1991.

Copp, R. O.; Wisniewski, T.; Hebtati, F.; et al. Localization of alpha-tocopherol transfer protein in the brains of patients with ataxia with vitamin E deficiency and other oxidative stress related neurodegenerative disorders. Brain Res. 822:80–87; 1999.

De Laurenzi, V.; Rogers, G. R.; Hanrock, D. J.; et al. Sjögren-Larsson syndrome is caused by mutations in the fatty aldehyde dehydrogenase gene. Nat. Genet. 12:52–57; 1996.

De Vivo, D. C. The expanding clinical spectrum of mitochondrial diseases. Brain Dev. 15:1–22; 1993.

Dickson, N.; Mortimer, J. G.; Faed, J. M.; et al. A child with Refsum disease: successful treatment with diet and plasma exchange. Dev. Med. Child Neurol. 31:92–97; 1989.

Du, E. Z.; Wang, S. L.; Kayden, H. J. Translocation of apolipoprotein B across the endoplasmic reticulum is blocked in abetalipoproteinemia. J. Lipid Res. 37:1309–1315; 1996.

Dupré, T.; Ogier-Denis, E.; Moore, S. E.; et al. Alteration of mannose transport in fibroblasts from type I carbohydrate deficient glycoprotein patients. Biochim. Biophys. Acta 1453:169–177; 1999.

Evans, M. I.; Duquette, D. A.; Rinaldo, P.; et al. Modulation of B12 dosage and response in fetal treatment of methylmalonic aciduria (MMA): titration of treatment dose to serum and urine MMA. Fetal Diagn. Ther. 12:21–23; 1997.

Evans, M. I.; Pryde, P. G.; Reichler, A.; et al. Fetal drug therapy. West. J. Med. 159:325–332; 1993.

Federico, A.; Palmeri, S.; Malandrini, A.; et al. The clinical aspects of adult hexosaminidase deficiencies. Dev. Neurosci. 13:280–287; 1991.

Folkerth, R. D.; Alroy, J.; Lomakina, I; et al. Mucolipidosis IV: morphology and histochemistry of an autopsy case. J. Neuropathol. Exp. Neurol. 54:154–164; 1995.

Friedlaender, M. M.; Kopolovic, J.; Rubinger, D.; et al. Renal biopsy in Fabry's disease. Clin. Nephrol. 27:206–211; 1987.

Gieselmann, V.; Zlotogora, I. I.; Harris, A.; et al. Molecular genetics of metachromatic leukodystrophy. Hum. Mutat. 4:233–242; 1994.

Gilad, S.; Chessa, L.; Khosravi, R.; et al. Genotype-phenotype relationships in ataxia-telangiectasia and variants. Am. J. Hum. Genet. 62:551–561; 1998.

Goebel, H. H.; Gullotta, F.; Bajanowski, T.; et al. Pigment variant of neuronal ceroid-lipofuscinosis. Am. J. Med. Genet. 57:155–159; 1995.

Goldfisher, S. L.; Moore, C. L.; Johnson, A. B.; et al. Peroxisomal and mitochondrial defects in the cerebro-hepato-renal syndrome. Science 182:62–64; 1973.

Goldman, J. E.; Katz, D.; Rapin, I.; et al. Chronic $GM_1$-gangliosidosis presenting as dystonia. I. Clinical and pathological features. Ann. Neurol. 9:465–475; 1981.

Goldstein, D. S.; Hahn, S. H.; Holmes, C.; et al. Monoaminergic effects of folinic acid, L-DOPA, and 5-hydroxytryptophan in dihydropteridine reductase deficiency. J. Neurochem. 64:2810–2813; 1995.

Grandchamp, B. Acute intermittent porphyria. Semin. Liver Dis. 18:17–24; 1998.

Halliday, W. The nosology of Hallervorden-Spatz disease. J. Neurol. Sci. 134(suppl.):84–91; 1995.

Hamosh, A.; Maher, J. F.; Bellus, G. A.; et al. Long-term use of high-dose benzoate and dextromethorphan for the treatment of nonketotic hyperglycinemia. J. Pediatr. 132:709–713; 1998.

Hanley, W. B.; Koch, R.; Levy, H. L.; et al. The North American Phenylketonuria Collaborative Study, developmental assessment of the offspring: preliminary report. Eur. J. Pediatr. 155(suppl. 1):S169–S172; 1996.

Hayasaka, S.; Yamada, T.; Nitta, K.; et al. Ascorbic acid and amino acid values in aqueous humor of a patient with Lowe's syndrome. Graefe's Arch. Clin. Exp. Ophthalmol. 235:217–221; 1997.

Hodes, M. E.; Zimmerman, A. W.; Aydanian, A.; et al. Different mutations in the same codon of the proteolipid protein gene, PLP, may help in correlating genotype with phenotype in Pelizaeus-Merzbacher disease/X-linked spastic paraplegia. Am. J. Med. Genet. 82:132–139; 1999.

Hoogerbrugge, P. M.; Brouwer, O. F.; Bordigoni, P.; et al. Allogenic bone marrow transplantation for lysosomal storage diseases. The European Group for Bone Marrow Transplantation. Lancet 345:1382–1383; 1995.

Hurd, R. W.; Wilder, B. J.; Helverston, W. R. Treatment of four siblings with progressive myoclonus epilepsy of the Unverricht-Lundborg type with N-acetylcysteine. Neurology 47:1264–1268; 1996.

Ito, K.; Takahashi, N.; Takahashi, A.; et al. Structural study of the oligosaccharide moieties of sphingolipid activator proteins, saposin A, C and D obtained from the spleen of a Gaucher patient. Eur. J. Biochem. 215:171–179; 1993.

Itoh, K.; Negishi, H.; Obayashi, C.; et al. Infantile neuroaxonal dystrophy—immunohistochemical and ultrastructural studies on the central and peripheral nervous systems in infantile neuroaxonal dystrophy. Kobe J. Med. Sci. 39:133–146; 1993.

Jankovic, J.; Caskey, T. C.; Stout, J. T.; et al. Lesch-Nyhan syndrome: a study of motor behavior and cerebrospinal fluid neurotransmitters. Ann. Neurol. 23:466–469; 1988.

Johnson, W. G. Motor neuron diseases resulting from hexosaminidase deficiency. Semin. Neurol. 13:369–374; 1993.

Jouvet, P.; Poggi, F.; Rabier, D.; et al. Continuous venovenous haemofiltration in the acute phase of neonatal maple syrup urine disease. J. Inherit. Metab. Dis. 20:463–472; 1997.

Kaler, S. G.; Das, S.; Levinson, B.; et al. Successful early copper therapy in Menkes disease associated with a mutant trancript containing a small in-frame deletion. Biochem. Mol. Med. 57:37–46; 1996.

Kamei, A.; Houdou, S.; Takashima, S.; et al. Peroxisomal disorders in children: immunohistochemistry and neuropathology. J. Pediatr. 122:573–579; 1993.

Kasahara, M.; Kiuchi, T.; Uryuhara, K.; et al. Treatment of ornithine transcarbamylase (OTC) deficiency in girls by auxilliary liver transplantation: conceptual changes in a living-donor program. J. Pediatr. Surg. 33:1753–1756; 1998.

Kauppinen, R. Management of acute porphyria. Photoderm. Photoimmunol. Photomed. 14:48–51; 1998.

Kaye, E. M. Therapeutic approaches to lysosomal storage diseases. Curr. Opin. Pediatr. 7:650–654; 1995.

Kaye, E. M.; Hyland, K. Amino acids and the brain; too much, too little, or just inappropriate use of a good thing? Neurology 51:668–670; 1998.

Kjaergaard, S.; Kristiansson, B.; Stibler, H.; et al. Failure of mannose therapy of patients with carbohydrate-deficient glycoprotein syndrome type IA. Acta Paediatr. 87: 884–888; 1998.

Kleijer, W. J.; Geilen, G. C.; Janse, H. C.; et al. Cathepsin A deficiency in galactosialidosis: studies of patients and carriers in 16 families. Pediatr. Res. 39:1067–1071; 1996.

Knopman, D.; Sung, J. H.; Davis, D. Progressive familial leukodystrophy of late onset. Neurology 46:429–434; 1996.

Kobayashi, H.; Garcia, C. A.; Alfonso, G.; et al. Molecular genetics of familial spastic paraplegia: a multitude of responsible genes. J. Neurol. Sci. 137:131–138; 1996.

Koch, R.; Fishler, K.; Azen, C.; et al. The relationship of genotype to phenotype in phenylalanine hydroxylase deficiency. Biochem. Mol. Med. 60:92–101; 1997.

Korein, J.; Sansaricq, C.; Kalmijn, M.; et al. Maple syrup urine disease: clinical, EEG, and plasma amino acid correlations with a theoretical mechanism of acute neurotoxicity. Int. J. Neurosci. 79:21–45; 1994.

Korenke, G. C.; Christen, H. J.; Kruse, B.; et al. Progression of X-linked adrenoleukodystrophy under interferon-beta therapy. J. Inherit. Metab. Dis. 20:59–66; 1997.

Korner, C.; Lehle, L.; von Figura, K. Carbohydrate-deficient glycoprotein syndrome type I: correction of the glycosylation defect by deprivation of glucose or supplementation with mannose. Glycoconj J. 15: 499–505; 1998.

Kraemer, K. H.; Lee, M. M.; and Scotto, J. Xeroderma pigmentosum: cutaneous, ocular, and neurologic abnormalities in 830 published cases. Arch. Dermatol. 123:241–250; 1987.

Kremmidiotis, G.; Lesink, I. L.; Bilton, R. L.; et al. The Batten disease gene product (CLN3p) is a Golgi integral membrane protein. Hum. Mol. Genet. 8:523–531; 1999.

Krivit, W.; Lockman, L. A.; Watkins, P. A.; et al. The future for treatment by bone marrow transplantation for adrenoleukodystrophy, metachromatic leukodystrophy, globoid cell leukodystrophy and Hurler syndrome. J. Inherit. Metab. Dis. 18:398–412; 1995a.

Krivit, W.; Sung, J. H.; Shapiro, E. G.; et al. Microglia: the effector cell for reconstitution of the central nervous system following bone marrow transplantation for lysosomal and peroxisomal storage diseases. Cell Transplant. 4:385–392; 1995b.

Krivit, W.; Shapiro, E. G.; Peters, C.; et al. Hematopoietic stem-cell transplantation in globoid-cell leukodystrophy. N. Engl. J. Med. 338:1119–1126; 1998.

Kure, S.; Tada, K.; Narisawa, K. Nonketotic hyperglycinemia: biochemical, molecular, and neurological aspects. Jpn. J. Hum. Genet. 42:13–22; 1997.

Lauronen, L.; Munroe, P. B.; Jarvels, I.; et al. Delayed classic and protracted phenotypes of compound heterozygous juvenile neuronal ceroid lipofuscinosis. Neurology 52:360–365; 1999.

Love, S.; Bridges, L. R.; Case, C. P. Neurofibrillary tangles in Niemann-Pick disease type C. Brain 118:119–129; 1995.

Lyon, G.; Adams, R. D.; Kolodny, E. H. Neurology of hereditary metabolic diseases of children 2nd ed. New York: McGraw-Hill; 1996.

Lauronen, L.; Munroe, P. B.; Jarvels, I.; et al. Delayed classic and protracted phenotypes of compound heterozygous juvenile neuronal ceroid lipofuscinosis. Neurology 52:360–365; 1999.

Maestri, N. E.; Brusilow, S. W.; Clissold, D. B.; et al. Long-term treatment of girls with ornithine transcarbamylase deficiency. N. Engl. J. Med. 335:855–859; 1996.

McKusick, W. A. On-line mendelian inheritance in man, OMIM (TM). Baltimore: Johns Hopkins University and Bethesda, MD, National Center for Biotechnology Information, National Library of Medicine. Web URL: http://www3.ncbi.nlm.nih.gov; 1999.

Menkes, J. H. Textbook of child neurology 5th ed. Baltimore: Williams & Wilkins; 1995.

Michals, K.; Azen, C.; Acosta, P.; et al. Blood phenylalanine levels and intelligence of 10-year-old children with PKU in the National Collaborative Study. J. Am. Diet. Assoc. 88:1226–1229; 1988.

Mole, S. Neuronal ceroid lipofuscinoses (Gene table). Eur. J. Paediatr, Neurol. 3:43–44; 1999.

Morales, L. E. Gaucher's disease: a review. Ann. Pharmacother. 30:381–388; 1996.

Moriwaki, S.; Stefanini, M.; Lehmann, A. R.; et al. DNA repair and ultraviolet mutagenesis in cells from a new patient with xeroderma pigmentosum group G and Cockayne syndrome resemble xeroderma pigmentosum cells. J. Invest. Dermatol. 107:647–653; 1996.

Moser A. B.; Kreiter, N.; Bezman, L.; et al. Plasma very long chain fatty acids in 3,000 peroxisome disease patients and 29,000 controls. Ann. Neurol. 45:100–110; 1999.

Moser, H. W. Peroxisomal disorders. Semin. Pediatr. Neurol. 3:298–304; 1996.

Moser, H. W. Adrenoleukodystrophy: phenotype, genetics, pathogenesis and therapy. Brain 120:1485–1508; 1997.

Moser, H. W.; Borel, J. Dietary management of X-linked adrenoleukodystrophy. Annu. Rev. Nut. 15:379–397; 1995.

Munroe, P. B.; Mitchison, H. M.; O'Rawe, A. M.; et al. Spectrum of mutations in the Batten disease gene, CLN3. Am. J. Med. Genet. 61:310–316; 1997.

Nance, M. A.; Berry, S. A. Cockayne syndrome: review of 140 cases. Am. J. Med. Genet. 42:68–84; 1992.

Nardocci, N.; Verga, M. L.; Binelli, S.; et al. Neuronal ceroid-lipofuscinosis; a clinical and morphological study of 19 patients. Am. J. Med. Genet. 57:137–141; 1995.

Nyhan, W. L. The recognition of Lesch-Nyhan syndrome as an inborn error of purine metabolism. J. Inherit. Metab. Dis. 20:171–178; 1997.

Nyhan, W. L.; Rice-Kelts, M.; Barshop, B. A. Treatment of acute crisis in maple syrup urine disease. Arch. Pediat. Adolesc. Med. 152:593–598; 1998.

Nyhan, W. L.; Sakati, N. O. Diagnostic recognition of genetic disease. Philadelphia; Lea & Febiger; 1987.

Okamura-Oho, Y.; Zhang, S.; Callahan, J. W. The biochemistry and clinical features of galactosialidosis. Biochim. Biophys. Acta 1225:244–254; 1994.

Ozand, P. T.; Fukuyama, Y.; Brismar, J.; et al., eds. Organic acidemias. Brain Dev. 16(Suppl.):1–144; 1994.

Pahan, K; Kha, M.; Singh I. Therapy for X-adrenoleukodystrophy; normalization of very long chain fatty acids and inhibition of induction of cytokines by cAMP J. Lipid Res. 39:109–1100; 1998.

Poggi-Travert, F.; Fournier, B.; Poll-The, B. T.; et al. Clinical approach to inherited peroxisomal disorders. J. Inherit. Metab. Disord. 18(Suppl. 1):1–18; 1995.

Proud, V. K.; Mussell, H. G.; Kaler, S. G.; et al. Distinctive Menkes disease variant with occipital horns: delineation of natural history and clinical phenotype. Am. J. Med. Genet. 65:44–51; 1996.

Pshehetsky, A. V. Richard, C.; Michaud, L.; et al. Cloning, expression and chromosomal mapping of human lysosomal sialidase and characterization of mutations in sialidosis. Nat. Genet. 15:316–320; 1997.

Rakela, J.; Kurtz, S. B.; McCarthy, J. T.; et al. Fulminant Wilson's disease treated with post dilution hemofiltration and orthotopic liver transplantation. Gastroenterology 90:2004–2007; 1986.

Rapin, I.; Suzuki, K.; Suzuki, K.; et al. Adult (chronic) GM$_2$ gangliosidosis. atypical spinocerebellar degeneration in a Jewish sibship. Arch. Neurol. 33:120–130; 1976.

Rappeport, J. M.; Ginns, E. I. Bone-marrow transplantation in severe Gaucher's disease. N. Engl. J. Med. 311:84–88; 1984.

Rawling, N. D.; Barrett, A. J. Tripeptidyl-peptidase is apparently the CNL2 protein absent in classical late-infantile neuronal ceroid lipofuscinosis. Biochim. Biophys, Acta 1429:496–500; 1999.

Reichard, E. A.; Ball, W. S., Jr.; Bove, K. E. Alexander disease: a case report and review of the literature. Pediatr. Pathol. Lab. Med. 16:327–343; 1996.

Remaley, A. T.; Schumacher, U. K.; Stonik, J. A.; et al. Decreased reverse cholesterol transport in Tangier disease fibroblasts. Acceptor specificity and effect of brefeldin on lipid efflux. Arterioscler. Thromb. Vas. Biol. 17:1813–1821; 1997.

Ricci, B.; Sharp, D.; O'Rourke, E.; et al. A 30-amino acid truncation of the microsomal triglyceride transfer protein subunit disrupts its interaction with protein disulfide-isomerase and causes abetalipoproteinemia. J. Biol. Chem. 270:14281–14285; 1995.

Rogers, P. D. Cimetidine in the treatment of acute intermittent porphyria. Ann. Pharmacother. 31:365–367; 1997.

Rosenblatt, D. S.; Aspler, A. L.; Shevell, M. I.; et al. Clinical heterogeneity and prognosis in combined methylmalonic aciduria and homocystinuria (cblC). J. Inherit. Metab. Dis. 20:528–538; 1997.

Rowland, L. P.; ed. Merritt's textbook of neurology. 9th ed. Baltimore: Williams & Wilkins; 1995.

Rubin, I. L.; Crocker, A. C. Developmental disabilities: delivery of medical care for children and adults. Philadelphia: Lea & Febiger; 1989.

Rubio, J. P.; Danek, A.; Stone, C.; et al. Chorea-acanthocytosis: genetic linkage to chromosome 9q21. Am. J. Hum. Genet. 61:899–908; 1997.

Satoh, J.-I.; Tokumoto, H.; Kurohara, K.; et al. Adult-onset Krabbe disease with homozygous T1854C mutation in the galactocerebrosidase gene: unusual findings of corticospinal tract demyelination. Neurology 49:1392–1399; 1997.

Savukoski, M.; Klochars, T.; Homberg, V.; et al. CLN5, a novel gene encoding a putative transmembrane protein mutated in Finnish variant late infantile neuronal ceroid lipofuscinosis. Nat. Genet. 19:286–288; 1998.

Scaggiante, B.; Pineschi, A.; Bembi, B.; et al. Successful therapy of Niemann-Pick disease by implantation of human amniotic membrane. Transplantation 44:59–61; 1987.

Scheinberg, I. H.; Sternlieb, I. Wilson's disease. Philadelphia: W. B. Saunders Co.; 1984.

Schiffman, R. Niemann-Pick disease type C: from bench to bedside. JAMA 276:561–564; 1996.

Schilsky, M. L. Wilson disease: genetic basis for copper toxicity and natural history. Semin. Liver Dis. 16:1683–1695; 1996.

Scriver, C. R.; Beaudet, A. L.; Sly, W. S.; Valle, D.; eds. The metabolic and molecular bases of inherited disease. 7th ed. New York: McGraw-Hill; 1995.

Seitelberger, F. Recent history of Pelizaeus-Merzbacher disease. Brain Pathol. 5:267–273; 1995.

Serratosa, J. M.; Gomez-Garre, P.; Gallardo, M. E.; et al. A novel protein phosphatase gene is mutated in progressive myoclonus epilepsy of the Lafora type (EPM2). Hum. Mol. Genet. 8:345–352; 1999.

Shanske, S.; DiMauro, S. Diagnosis of the mitochondrial encephalomyopathies. Curr. Opin. Rheumatol. 9:496–503; 1997.

Sharp, J. D.; Wheeler, R. B.; Lake, B. D.; et al. Loci for classical and a variant late infantile neuronal ceroid lipofuscinosis map to chromosomes 11p15 and 15q21–23. Hum. Mol. Genet. 6:591–595; 1997.

Sleat, D. D.; Donnelly, R. J.; Lackland, H.; et al. Association of mutations in a lysosomal protein with classical late-infantile neuronal ceroid lipofuscinosis. Science 277:1802–1805; 1997.

Snyder, E. Y.; Wolfe, J. H. Central nervous system cell transplantation: a novel therapy for storage diseases? Curr. Opin. Neurol. 9:126–136; 1996.

Soffer, D.; Benharroch, D.; Berginer, V. The neuropathology of cerebrotendinous xanthomatosis revisited: a case report and review of the literature. Acta Neuropathol. 90:213–220; 1995.

Suzuki, K. Twenty five years of the "psychosine hypothesis": a personal perspective of its history and present status. Neurochem. Res. 23:251–259; 1998.

Suzuki, Y.; Murakami, N.; Goto., Y.; et al. Apoptotic nuclear degeneration in Marinesco-Sjögren syndrome. Acta Neuropathol. 94:410–415; 1997.

Svennerholm, L.; Erikson, A.; Groth, C.; et al. Norbottnian type Gaucher disease—clinical, biochemical, and marrow transplantation. Dev. Neurosci. 13:345–351; 1991.

Swaiman, K. F.; Ashwal, S., eds. Pediatric Neurology: principles and practice. St Louis: Mosby; 1999 (in press).

Szold, A.; Udassin, R.; Maayan, C.; et al. Laparoscopic-modified Nissen fundoplication in children with dysautonomia. J. Pediatr. Surg. 31:1560–1562; 1996.

Taylor, A. M.; Metcalfe, J. A.; Thick, J.; et al. Leukemia and lymphoma in ataxia telangiectasia. Blood 87:423–438; 1996a.

Taylor, T. D.; Litt, M.; Kramer, P.; et al. Homozygosity mapping of Hallervorden-Spatz syndrome to chromosome 20p12.3–p13. Genet. 14:479–481; 1996b.

Tefferi, A.; Colgan, J. P.; Solberg, L. A., Jr. Acute intermittent porphyrias: diagnosis and management. Mayo Clin. Proc. 69:991–995; 1994.

Thompson, A. J.; Tillotson, S.; Smith, I.; et al. Brain 116:811–821; 1993.

Tiberio, G.; Filocamo, M.; Gatti, R.; et al. Mutations in fucosidosis gene: a review. Acta Genet. Med. Gemellol. 44:223–232; 1995.

Traeger, E. C.; Rapin, I. The clinical course of Canavan disease. Pediatr. Neurol. 18:207–212; 1998.

Trefz, F. K.; Burgard, P.; Konig, T.; et al. Genotype-phenotype correlations in phenylketonuria. Clin. Chim. Acta 217:15–21; 1993.

Tsai, P.; Lipton, J.; Sahev, I.; et al. Allogenic bone marrow transplantation in severe Gaucher disease. Pediatr. Res. 31:503–507; 1992.

Tumer, Z.; Horn, N. Menkes disease: recent advances and new aspects. J. Med. Genet. 34:265–274; 1997.

Turpin, J. C.; Masson, M.; Baumann, N. Clinical aspects of Niemann-Pick type C disease in the adult. Dev. Neurosci. 13:304–306; 1991.

Tyynela, J.; Baumann, M.; Henseler, M.; et al. Spingolipid activator proteins (SAPs) are stored together with glycosphingolipids in the infantile neuronal ceroid-lipofuscinosis (INCL). Am. J. Med. Genet. 57:294–297; 1995.

van der Meer, S. B.; Poggi, F.; Spada, M.; et al. Clinical outcome of long-term management of patients with vitamin B12-unresponsive methylmalonic acidemia. J. Pediatr. 125:903–908; 1994.

van Domburg, P. H.; Willemsen, M. A.; Rotteveel, J. J.; et al. Sjögren-Larsson syndrome: clinical and MRI/MRS findings in FALDH-deficient patients. Neurology 52:1345–1352; 1999.

van Heijst, A. F.; Verrips, A.; Wevers, R. A.; et al. Treatment and follow-up of children with cerebrotendinous xanthomatosis. Eur. J. Pediatr. 157:313–316; 1998.

van Loo, A.; Vanholder, R; Madsen, K.; et al. Novel frameshift mutation in a heterozygous woman with Fabry disease and end-stage renal failure. Am. J. Nephrol. 16:352–357; 1996.

Vellodi, A.; Young, E. P.; Cooper, A.; et al. Bone marrow transplantation for mucopolysaccharidosis type I: experience of two British centres. Arch. Dis. Child. 76:92–99; 1997.

Vesa, J.; Hellsten, E.; Verkruyse, L. A.; et al. Mutations in the palmitoyl protein thioesterase gene causing infantile neuronal ceroid lipofuscinosis. Nature 376:584–587; 1995.

Walkley, S. U.; Thrall, M. A.; Dobrenis, K. Bone marrow transplantation corrects the enzyme defect in neurons of the central nervous system in a lysosomal storage disease. Proc. Natl. Acad. Sci. USA 91:2970–2974; 1994.

Wang, A. M.; Kanzaki, T.; Desnick, R. J. The molecular lesion in the alpha-N-acetylgalactosaminidase gene that causes angiokeratoma corporis diffusum with glycopeptiduria. J. Clin. Invest. 94:839–845; 1994.

Weglage, J.; Ullrich, K.; Pietsch, M.; et al. Untreated non-phenylketonuric-hyperphenylalaninemia: intellectual and neurological outcome. Eur. J. Pediatr. 155(suppl. 1):S26–S28; 1996.

Whitley, C. B.; Belani, K. G.; Chanag, P. N. Long-term outcome of Hurler syndrome following bone marrow transplantation. Am. J. Med. Genet. 46:209–218; 1993.

Wilcken, D. E.; Wilcken, B. The natural history of vascular disease in homocystinuria and the effects of treatment. J. Inherit. Metab. Dis. 20:295–300; 1997.

Wisniewski, K. E.; Connell, F.; Kaczmarski, W.; et al. Palmitoyl-protein thioesterase deficiency in a novel granular variant of LINCL. Pediatr. Neurol. 18:119–123; 1998.

Wisniewski, K. E.; Zhong, N.; Kida, E.; et al. Atypical late infantile and juvenile forms of neuronal ceroid lipofuscinosis and their diagnostic difficulties. Folia Neuropathol. 35:73–79; 1997.

Wolff, J. A.; Kulovich, S.; Yu, A. L.; et al. The effectiveness of benzoate in the management of seizures in nonketotic hyperglycinemia. Am. J. Dis. Child. 140:596–602; 1986.

Wolman, M. Wolman disease and its treatment. Clin. Pediatr. 34:207–212; 1995.

Yoshino, M.; Aoki, K.; Akeda, H.; et al. Management of acute metabolic decompensation in maple syrup urine disease: a multi-center study. Pediatr. Int. 41:132–137; 1999.

Young, G.; Driscoll, M. C. Coagulation abnormalities in the carbohydrate-deficient glycoprotein syndrome: case report and review of the literature. Am. J. Hemat. 60:66–69; 1999.

Zadra, M.; Grandi, R.; Erli, L. C.; et al. Treatment of seizures in acute intermittent porphyria; safety and efficacy of gabapentin. Seizure 7:415–416; 1998.

Zass, R.; Leupold, D.; Fernandez, M. A.; et al. Evaluation of prenatal treatment in newborns with cobalamin-responsive methylmelanic acidaemia. J. Inherit. Metab. Dis. 18:100–101; 1995.

Zelnik, N.; Giladi, I.; Keren, G.; et al. The role of botulinum toxin in the treatment of lower limb spasticity in children with cerebral palsy. Isr. J. Med. Sci. 33:129–133; 1997.

Zlokovic, B. V.; Apuzzo, M. L. Cellular and molecular neurosurgery: pathways from concept to reality—part I: target disorders and concept approaches to gene therapy of the central nervous system. Neurosurgery 40:803–804; 1997.

# 42

# Inherited Ataxias

S. H. SUBRAMONY

The inherited ataxias comprise a group of diverse disorders that result from a variety of gene mutations inherited in a number of different fashions; however, they share a number of clinical features, the most prominent of which is progressive imbalance related to abnormalities in the cerebellum and its afferent and efferent connections. In addition to the ataxia, the phenotype of these disorders includes a variety of other abnormalities in varying combinations. Until molecular genetic studies disclosed the enormous genetic heterogeneity of these disorders, it was not even clear whether these disorders represented single genetic entities or many. Thus, earlier studies in these disorders deal with clinically and genetically heterogeneous disorders grouped together often as single entities, and there is not much information on the natural history and prognosis of well-defined entities. This is being rapidly corrected as patient groups with well-defined gene mutations are being studied in a longitudinal fashion and the course of illness defined. In spite of being related to diverse gene mutations, the diseases do share many clinical features and overall their natural history is similar.

The difficulty with recognizing the different genotypes based on phenotype alone is related not only to the phenotypic overlap among different genetic entities but also to the variable pheno-type related to the same gene mutation. This variability in clinical features related to the same gene mutation is also reflected in considerable variability in the natural history and prognosis of the disorder in different patients with the same gene mutation. Molecular genetics has greatly increased our understanding of this variability; most of the progressive inherited ataxias are the result of unstable trinucleotide expansions and the variability of clinical features as well as natural history appears to be related to a significant degree to the instability of the gene mutation involved. This chapter will summarize the natural history and overall prognosis of the various inherited ataxias. It should be pointed out that in many families with inherited ataxias, the gene mutations are as yet unknown and the natural history and prognosis of these disorders remain to be defined.

## Autosomal Recessive Ataxias

The autosomal recessive (AR) ataxias result from the inheritance of two copies of the mutated gene, one from each of the parents who themselves are carriers and have no phenotypic abnormalities. The most common AR ataxias are Friedreich's ataxia (FA) and ataxia telangiectasia (AT).

## Friedreich's Ataxia

Friedreich's ataxia is an autosomal recessive disease related to the unstable expansion of an intronic GAA repeat in the gene X25 on chromosome 9 (Campuzano et al. 1996). The expansion involves both copies of the gene in a homozygous fashion, though the size of the expansion is often different in the two alleles. Classically, the disorder was characterized as having an age of onset below 25 (Harding 1981a). The typical disease presents with increasing ataxia, dysarthria, and loss of deep tendon reflexes. In addition, systemic features occur in a variable number of affected persons and include cardiomyopathy usually of the hypertrophic type, diabetes, and skeletal deformities including scoliosis and pes cavus. Direct mutation analyses of large series of patients have revealed a much broader range for age of onset and an even more variable course of the disease than was previously realized.

The age of onset of molecularly defined FA varies from 2 to 51 years. An age of onset over 21 is seen in close to 20% of the patients (Filla et al. 1996; Durr et al. 1996a; Montermini et al. 1997, Geschwind et al. 1997; Lamont et al. 1997; Monros et al. 1997). Even within the same family the age of onset can vary by a mean of 4.7 years (Mueller-Felber et al. 1993). Overall, the disease tends to progress gradually; the rate of progression can also vary enormously. In general, earlier age of onset is associated with more rapid progression (Filla et al. 1990). This has been more quantitatively examined by Klockgether et al. (1998), who found that each year that the onset of disease was postponed decreased the risk of losing ambulation in a significant manner (Klockgether et al. 1998). In the series of Mueller-Felber et al. (1993), the mean variability in duration of the disease at loss of ambulation within families was 8 years, with a range of 0 to 17 years. Much of the data on the natural history of this illness come from earlier clinical series and deal with more classical cases, which perhaps account for about 80% of the molecularly defined cases. In the series of Harding (1981a), the patients became chairbound from 3 to 44 years after onset; the mean age at loss of ambulation was 25 ± 16 years. The mean duration of disease at this time was 15.5 years. In a series of 80 patients reported by Filla et al. (1990), the mean age at loss of ambulation was 26.7 ± 7.8 years and

the mean duration of disease at loss of ambulation was 13.8 years. In the same series, significant enough clinical deficits to create some dependency and inability to work occurred at a mean age of 20.8 years (range, 14 to 30 years).

The age at death in an early autopsy series (Hewer 1968) was from 5 to 71 years with a mean of 37 years, not very different from the clinical series of Harding (1981a); 56% of the deaths were related to cardiac failure and the others were due to a variety of reasons including pneumonia and diabetes.

The major factor that affects the variable phenotypic features and the prognosis appears to be the unstable nature of the GAA expansion. This may be related to the fact that repeat expansion of variable sizes may allow a variable amount of frataxin to be produced. The age of onset is inversely correlated with the number of GAA repeats; the correlation is better with the size of the smaller allele (Filla et al. 1996, Monros et al. 1997; Durr et al. 1996a) as well as the mean of the two alleles (Lamont et al. 1997). In the study by Filla et al. (1996) about 50% of the variability in age of onset could be related to the size of the smaller allele; thus the mean size of the smaller allele in patients with age of onset below 10 was 856; in patients with age of onset between 11 and 20 the mean repeat size was 755 and in those with age of onset above 20, it was 462. In the study of Monros et al. (1997), the mean repeat size of the smaller allele in patients with late-onset disease was 351 as opposed to 700 for patients with classical disease. Thus, the majority of patients with late onset (i.e., onset after 20 years) have repeat size smaller than 500 and those with the typical childhood onset have larger repeats. Nevertheless, the significant scatter in age of onset for a given repeat size makes it hazardous to predict the age of onset from the repeat size alone in a given patient. There is also a correlation between the repeat size and disease progression as measured by time to loss of ambulation (Filla et al. 1996; Montermini et al. 1997). The repeat size also influences other phenotypic features that can affect the prognosis. In particular, the presence of cardiomyopathy may be correlated with larger repeat sizes. In the study of Durr et al. (1996a), only 44% of the patients with fewer than 520 repeats had a cardiomyopathy; 83% of patients with repeats larger than 780 had cardiomyopathy. Similar correlations were reported by Filla et al. (1996) and Monros et al. (1997) as well. In fact, in a recent echocardiographic study, left ventricular wall thickness was related to the repeat size (Isnard et al. 1997). Filla et al. (1996) also noted that repeat sizes were larger in patients with diabetes, a finding not corroborated by Durr et al. (1996a). In the latter study, scoliosis and pes cavus were related to larger repeat sizes. Progressive scoliosis that can adversely affect prognosis tends to occur in children with age of onset earlier than 12. Genetic factors other than the repeat size alone may have some role to play in the prognosis. The Acadian patients with FA tend to have a slower course and a lower incidence of cardiomyopathy, despite having repeat sizes similar to those in classical FA (Montermini et al. 1992). The Acadian patients from both Louisiana and Canada share an extended haplotype surrounding the FA gene, suggesting that this population has a "founder effect" (Richter et al. 1996); nevertheless, other polymorphic variations in the FA gene itself could not account for the milder disease in the Acadians (Montermini et al. 1997).

In terms of management, patients with FA need to be monitored for those features that adversely affect prognosis. Neurological deficits that adversely affect prognosis include the overall impairment in mobility, the severity of bulbar deficits, alterations in cough mechanisms, and abnormalities of sphincter control. Many features such as dysphagia as well as problems like visual loss and hearing loss appear to be related to the duration of the disease rather than the repeat size (Durr et al. 1996a). There should be a periodic search for systemic problems that can result in morbidity and mortality, such as skeletal deformity, cardiomyopathy, and diabetes. Many nonambulatory patients with cardiac problems may not develop the classic symptoms of cardiac failure and may need periodic laboratory assessment of cardiac function.

Given the genetic nature of the disease, management may also involve genetic counseling, including possible carrier detection in relatives. It is reasonable to have a geneticist or genetic counselor involved in such procedures.

## Ataxia Telangiectasia

This disorder tends to begin earlier than FA with ataxia and truncal instability around the age of 12 to 14 months. During the first decade there is progressive ataxia associated with other neurological features such as choreoathetosis, hypotonia, bradykinesia, and a prominent abnormality of saccadic eye movements (Swift et al. 1993). Typical oculocutaneous telangiectasia develop between 3 and 6 years. Many of these children are susceptible to malignancies especially of the lymphoreticular type and also may have an associated immune deficiency.

The natural history of AT is again one of progression and no therapy directed at the basic abnormality is as yet available. Prognosis is related to both the neurological disability as well as the systemic abnormalities. Most of the patients lose ambulation by 10 or 11 years (Boder 1985). Patients tend to lose their reflexes and develop some muscle wasting and weakness by the second to third decade. The major cause of death is sinopulmonary infections, accounting for about 50% of the cases; in about 25%, death is related to complications of malignancy and in the rest there is a combination of the two (Boder 1985). The pulmonary infections are related to both the neurological disability and the immune deficiency. With better treatments available for infections, malignancies, and immune deficiencies, death often does not occur till the fourth and fifth decades of life.

Overall, the degree of phenotypic variability in AT is less than that observed in FA. This may be related to the fact that the disease is related to a number of different point mutations that affect a large gene, labeled ATM on chromosome 11 (Savitsky et al. 1995). Even though the mutations involved in each family may be different, nearly all of them inactivate the protein. Some variant types of AT have been described, that include a later age of onset, a longer disease course, reduced radiosensitivity, or the lack of sensitivity to infections (Gilad et al. 1998; Stankovic et al. 1998). In such patients, the mutations present may allow the synthesis of some amount of protein unlike the typical null mutations found in typical AT patients (Gilad et al. 1998).

The management of these patients again involves close monitoring for those features that can lead to increased morbidity and mortality and speedy management of these features. Thus, periodic assessments for malignancies and immune function may be needed. Appropriate rehabilitation measures directed at the neurological disability also may be helpful. It should be pointed out that these patients are very radiosensitive and treatment of malignancies should not involve radiation.

Genetic counseling in AT has features similar to those in FA, though mutation detection is more difficult. There is some evidence that heterozygous carriers of the AT gene may have an increased susceptibility to cancer (Swift et al. 1987).

## Other Autosomal Recessive Ataxias

Harding (1981b) coined the term *early-onset cerebellar ataxia with retained tendon reflexes* for a group of patients with onset and manifestations of ataxia similar to that of FA but with the difference that the tendon reflexes were retained (Harding 1981b). Many of these patients are now known to have the FA mutation and are grouped together as Friedreich's ataxia with retained reflexes (FARR). The other patients with this syndrome that do not have the FA mutation are likely to be genetically heterogeneous. Overall they tend to have slower progression, with loss of ambulation about 21 to 33 years after onset. In a recent series of 30 patients with this syndrome no effect of age of onset was seen in the progression rate contrary to the findings in FA (Klockgether et al. 1998).

## Autosomal Dominant Ataxias

These disorders result from mutations in just one of the two copies of the gene involved, and the family tree shows affected individuals in each generation. Molecular genetic studies have significantly improved our understanding of this group of disorders within the past decade. These diseases are characterized by both phenotypic heterogeneity within a given genotype and by genotypic heterogeneity with a given phenotype. As such, the genotypic recognition of these disorders is dependent on mutation analysis because clinical recognition of the underlying genotype can be very inaccurate. Both the clinical overlap among the different disorders and the varied manifestations of specific disorders can be to a large extent explained by the finding that all the mutations so far described for progressive dominant ataxias have been unstable CAG expansions. These disorders share many clinical features including several that may have prognostic significance; therefore, assessment of prognosis involves the evaluation of several features that can be dealt with as a whole for the dominant ataxias. First of all, unlike in the common recessive ataxias, none of the dominant ataxias have any major systemic features that may have any bearing on prognosis. Thus, prognosis is solely determined by the progression of neurological deficits as well as the type

of neurological abnormalities that occur in a given patient. Earlier onset of disease is associated with more rapid progression (Currier et al. 1982). Other clinical features that may result in poorer prognosis include prominent bulbar dysfunction, dysphagia, tongue atrophy, and poor cough mechanism. There is certainly some involvement of the lower motor neuron in these disorders with possible affliction of the respiratory muscles. The occurrence of significant bladder dyscontrol may also have an adverse effect on prognosis. Nutritional problems often occur in the advanced stage of the illness because of dysphagia; but in addition, in many of these disorders there may be weight loss unexplained by dysphagia alone. Thus, in any given patient, the degree of bulbar, respiratory, bladder, and nutritional involvement may all have a bearing on the future prognosis.

In addition, both the specific gene mutation involved as well as the severity of the mutation clearly affect the prognosis. In the following sections the available data on the prognosis of the specific disorders are briefly discussed. It should be remembered that from 30% to 40% of the dominant ataxias have not yet been characterized at a genetic level.

### Spinocerebellar Ataxia1

This dominant ataxia is related to an unstable expansion of a CAG repeat sequence within the ataxin 1 gene on chromosome 6 (Orr et al. 1993). The disease typically begins in the third and fourth decades, though both childhood onset and old age onset are known. The disease is characterized by progressive ataxia associated in its early stages with upper motor neuron signs and dysarthria. Progressive disease causes loss of ambulation, further abnormalities of eye movements, and bulbar function and death.

The natural history of spinocerebellar ataxia (SCA 1) is one of gradual progression. The duration of illness from onset to death has been reported in a limited number of patients and shows a wide range from 5 to 38 years (Nino et al. 1980; Zoghbi et al. 1988; Sasaki et al. 1996; Schut 1950). Age at death has also been variable from 12 to 72 years (Nino et al. 1980; Zoghbi et al. 1988; Matilla et al. 1993; Goldfarb et al. 1989). Death usually results from pulmonary problems related to bulbar and respiratory muscle involvement often complicated by nutritional problems.

The clinical signs of the disease evolve in a predictable fashion. Saccadic eye movements become slower and gaze palsies may develop. As the ataxia becomes more severe, a peripheral polyneuropathy develops associated with sensory loss and ankle areflexia. Increasing bulbar problems are characterized by severe dysarthria, dysphagia, and poor cough mechanisms. Some dystonia tends to occur in the late stages. Disease progression may be somewhat faster in SCA 1 than in SCA 2 and SCA 3, but this is not significant (Klockgether et al. 1998). This study did find that earlier age of onset was significantly associated with earlier age at chairbound status and death.

The variable number of repeats in the mutated allele accounts for some of the variability in clinical features, and this has a bearing on prognosis. Normal alleles have 6 to 40 CAG repeats; disease causing alleles have 39 to 82 repeats. Abnormal alleles can be distinguished from normal alleles with the same number of repeats by the presence of CAT interruptions within the CAG repeat sequence in the latter (Chung et al. 1993). Age of onset is inversely correlated with the number of repeats in the abnormal allele (Orr et al. 1993; Ranum et al. 1994a; Jodice et al. 1994; Duborg et al. 1995; Giunti et al. 1994). Some variability between different families in age of onset cannot be entirely attributable to the number of repeats alone (Ranum et al. 1994a). A correlation between disease progression rate and the number of repeats has been noted by some but not others (Jodice et al. 1994; Klockgether et al. 1998). There is also a correlation between larger repeat size and shorter duration of disease before death (Jodice et al. 1994; Ranum et al. 1994a). However, these correlations tend to be weaker than correlations with age of onset. Thus, genetic factors other than the CAG repeat size or environmental factors may have a role to play in disease progression. Goldfarb et al. (1996) examined the relation between the repeat size and a number of phenotypic features in a large cohort of patients from Siberia and found that the severity of cerebellar ataxia was primarily correlated with the duration of the disease; however, certain other features such as dysphagia, tongue atrophy, and skeletal muscle atrophy were related to the presence of larger repeats. Patients with over 52 repeats were significantly disabled by 5 years into the illness in this study. A correlation between tongue atrophy and CAG repeat size was

also noted by Sasaki et al. (1996). In the series of Goldfarb et al. (1996), two homozygous persons had a disease onset and severity no different from what would have been predicted by the larger allele alone. Goldfarb et al. (1996) also have suggested that the disease may have a lower penetrance in females.

## Spinocerebellar Ataxia 2

SCA 2 is a dominant ataxia that was originally described from the eastern provinces of Cuba and subsequently shown to be linked to markers on chromosome 12 (Orozco et al. 1990). The mutation involves an unstable CAG expansion in the ataxin 2 gene. The clinical picture of SCA 2 is very similar to that of SCA 1; however, the occurrence of very slow eye movements in the early stages of the disease as well as the loss of deep tendon reflexes may be clues to SCA 2.

Overall, the natural history and progression rate of SCA 2 are similar to those of SCA 1 and SCA 3 (Klockgether et al. 1998). Klockgether et al. (1998) also found that females with the disease had a significantly higher risk for entering advanced stages of the disease. The duration of illness from onset to death has varied from 7 to 32 years among the limited number of patients that have been published (Orozco et al. 1989; Belal et al. 1994). Age at death varied from 20 to 82 years. These figures reflect the great variability in the age of onset as well as progression rate that seems to be intrinsic features of the CAG expansion disorders in general. Though earlier age at onset may be associated with more rapid progression of disease, Klockgether et al. (1998) did not find this in a series of 56 SCA 2 patients that were retrospectively analyzed.

The unstable CAG expansion in the ataxin 2 gene accounts for some of the variability noted. Normal alleles carry 14 to 31 repeats, though, the majority have 22 repeats (Pulst et al. 1996; Imbert et al. 1996, Sanpei et al. 1996; Cancel et al. 1997). The expanded alleles have 36 to 59 repeats and there is a strong negative correlation between the number of repeats and the age of onset. This relation is particularly steep between 36 and 45 repeats; as an example, in the series of Imbert et al. (1996), four patients with 37 repeats had age of onset of 45 to 60. Three patients with 46 to 50 repeats had ages of onset between 13 and 18 years. Once again, though, one cannot accurately predict the age of onset from a given repeat size. Cancel et al. (1997) estimated that for every increase in repeat size, the age of onset diminished by 3.24 years. Many clinical signs that adversely affect prognosis, such as dysphagia and extrapyramidal deficits, were primarily related to duration of disease (Cancel et al. 1997). However, in this series, CAG repeat size was related to the presence of dystonia, myokymia, and myoclonus. Occasionally, asymptomatic, but at-risk persons have had 34 or 35 repeats and the significance of these numbers need to be determined yet (Schols et al. 1997; Cancel et al. 1997).

## Spinocerebellar Ataxia 3 (Machado-Joseph disease; SCA 3/MJD)

This disorder was originally described among the Portuguese Azorean emigrants to the United States and was characterized by remarkable variability in the clinical picture between different families as well as within families (Nakano et al. 1972, Rosenberg et al. 1976; Coutinho and Andrade 1978). In 1994, the causative mutation for MJD was shown to be an unstable CAG expansion within the MJD1 gene on chromosome 14 in Japanese patients (Kawaguchi et al. 1994). The same mutation was quickly confirmed not only among the Azorean patients (Silveira et al. 1996) but also in many other families worldwide who were often not clinically diagnosed as having MJD (Matilla et al. 1995; Ranum et al. 1995; Sasaki et al. 1995; Durr et al. 1996b; Takiyama et al. 1995; Cancel et al. 1995; Schols et al. 1996). Many of these families lacked the typical phenotypic variability seen among the Portuguese families and were diagnosed as having SCA 3. Thus, SCA 3 and MJD result from the same mutation.

The age of onset is variable, ranging from childhood to 70 years (Sequeiros and Coutinho 1993). The mean age of onset in many series is in the mid to upper thirties (Sequeiros and Coutinho 1993; Watanabe et al. 1996; Durr et al. 1996b; Cancel et al. 1995). The clinical picture is similar to that in SCA 1 and SCA 2; initial findings include a combination of ataxia and upper motor neuron signs. Patients become increasingly disabled by ataxia and often develop a variety of oculomotor disturbances including nystagmus, slow saccades, and gaze palsies. Increasing dysphagia, peripheral amyotrophy, and areflexia develop later. This clinical picture has been labeled as the type II phenotype and is the most common. Some patients with younger age of onset initially have a syndrome

that comprises spasticity and rigidity as well as bradykinesia (type I phenotype). Others with later adult onset have a combination of ataxia and muscle wasting and areflexia (type III phenotype). The mean age of onset among Portuguese patients with type I disease was 24.7 years; with type II, it was 40.3 and with type III, 47.1 years (Sequeiros and Coutinho 1993). The disease is one of relentless progression, but the age of onset may not influence progression rate (Klockgether et al. 1998). Klockgether et al. (1998) noted that female sex was associated with faster progression rate.

Among 36 patients who died of the disease, the mean duration from onset to death was 15.6 years (Sequeiros and Coutinho 1993), with a range of 7 to 29 years. The median survival in the series of Sudarsky et al. (1992) was 20 years.

As with other SCAs, a major factor in the variability in the clinical picture and course of this disease is the polymorphic nature of the repeat expansion. The normal number of CAG repeats in the MJD1 gene varies from 12 to 43 (Matilla et al. 1995; Ranum et al. 1995; Sasaki et al. 1995; Matsumura et al. 1996; Takiyama et al. 1995.) The abnormal range is 65 to 86 (Ranum et al. 1995; Matilla et al. 1995; Silveira et al. 1996; Schols et al. 1996, Zhou et al. 1997). There is a significant inverse correlation between age of onset and the number of repeats in the mutated allele. The number of CAG repeats also correlates with faster progression rate (Klockgether et al. 1998). Patients with 73 or fewer repeats have the type III phenotype (Schols et al. 1996; Matsumura et al. 1996). Type I phenotype often is associated with larger repeat sizes; 58% to 70% of the variability in age of onset can be ascribed to the repeat size.

The unstable CAG expansion often expands on intergenerational transmission, which accounts for some of the anticipation observed between generations. The mean anticipation has been around 12 years and is often greater with paternal than maternal inheritance (Takiyama et al. 1995).

## Spinocerebellar Ataxia 6

SCA 6 results from a relatively small CAG expansion in the gene encoding the $\alpha$-subunit of the calcium channel protein (CACNL1A4) and was described by Zuchenko et al. in 1997. It differs from SCA 1, 2 and 3 and from SCA 7 in many respects. The clinical picture is predominantly cerebellar with only mild involvement if any of the upper motor neuron pathways, peripheral nerves, and the bulbar muscles. The disease is much milder in its course.

The age of onset is usually later than in the other SCAs. Though the range is wide from the mid twenties to early seventies, the mean age of onset is in the fifties (Riess et al. 1997; Ikeuchi et al. 1997). The progression rate appears slower and compatible with a normal life span in many. In one of the families described, three persons died of the disease 16 to 33 years after onset (Subramony et al. 1996). The mean age of death in the patients described by Gomez et al. (1997) was 80 years (62 to 94 years). The mean time to need a walker was 15 to 17 years, and six patients were still walking 15 to 30 years after onset.

The normal number of CAG repeats in this gene is from 4 to 18 (Zuchenko et al. 1997; Matsuyama et al. 1997; Ikeuchi et al. 1997; Schols et al 1997, Gomez et al. 1997). The expanded range in affected persons is 21 to 28. Overall, there is a negative correlation between the age of onset and the number of repeats (Riess et al. 1997; Matsuyama et al. 1997; Ikeuchi et al. 1997). In the series of Riess et al. (1997), patients with 26 to 28 repeats had age of onset between 30 and 40. With 22 and 23 repeats, the age of onset was always over 50. Though there is a scatter in the age of onset in many families with the appearance of genetic anticipation, this cannot be accounted for by any instability of the expanded repeat because the repeat size tends to be the same in all affected persons within a family (Gomez et al. 1997; Schols et al. 1998). The effects of a homozygous expansion has been debatable but probably results in an earlier age of onset (Matsuyama et al. 1997; Ikeuchi et al. 1997).

## Spinocerebellar Ataxia 7

This dominant ataxia is associated with progressive visual failure related to a maculopathy. Perhaps this disorder has the greatest phenotypic variability among the dominant ataxias. The age of onset appears to be bimodal with both adult- and childhood-onset cases occurring in the same family (Jampel et al. 1961; Foster et al. 1962; Colan et al. 1981; Enevoldson et al. 1994). The disorder can present with either ataxia or visual loss; in some both are evident at presentation. In some, visual problems can be subtle and can be detected only with color vision tests or electroretinograms (To et al. 1993). Childhood disease, which may occur before the affected parent becomes sympto-

matic, is characterized by ataxia, visual loss, upper motor neuron signs, intention tremor, seizures, myoclonus, and dementia. Adult onset disease is characterized by ataxia, variable visual loss, brisk reflexes and spasticity, and very slow saccades. Recently, the SCA 7 mutation has been shown to be a very unstable CAG expansion in the ataxin 7 gene on chromosome 3. (David et al. 1997; Johansson et al. 1998; Del-Favero et al. 1998).

The natural history of the disease is one of progression. The progression is rapid in childhood cases, with death often occurring before the age of 5 (De Jong and Hoppenreijs 1991). Adult-onset cases have lengthier courses ranging from 5 to 41 years. There is a strong negative correlation between the length of the expanded CAG repeat and age of onset. The normal number of repeats at this locus has varied from 4 to 18. The expanded range is from 38 to 130 repeats. The disorder also shows remarkable anticipation, which may be related to the instability of the mutation. Early-onset cases usually have a paternal origin (Enevoldson et al. 1994).

## Other dominant ataxias

Spinocerebellar ataxias 4 and 5 have had their chromosomal loci identified, but the mutations themselves are not known (Flanigan et al. 1996; Ranum et al. 1994b). SCA 4 is characterized by progressive ataxia and a prominent polyneuropathy with associated proprioceptive defects. SCA 5 has almost a pure cerebellar presentation. Both may be more benign than SCA 1, 2, 3, or 7, but large numbers of families have not been identified and analyzed.

More recently two additional dominant genotypes have been identified (Koob et al. 1999; Matsuura et al. 1999; Zu et al. 1999). SCA-8 (Koob et al. 1999) has a mean age of onset around 39, causes a progressive ataxia with dysarthria and nystagmus, and has a slow progression rate. It appears to be related to an expansion of an untranslated CTG repeat located on chromosome 13q21. SCA-10 (Matsuura et al. 1999; Zu et al. 1999) is characterized by progressive ataxia associated with seizures. Linkage studies localize this to chromosome 22q13.

## Genetic Counseling in Dominant Ataxias

Each offspring of an affected person has a 50% risk of acquiring the mutated gene. Because of the adult onset of many of these diseases, many persons at risk may seek predictive testing before making decisions regarding marriage, reproduction, or career. Such predictive testing carries many of the ethical issues raised in the case of Huntington's disease (Hersch et al. 1994) and is best done in the setting of a formal predictive testing protocol. Such protocols involve a team effort among neurologists, psychiatrists or psychologists, geneticists, and genetic counselors. Of course, such testing is possible only if the causative mutation in the family has already been identified. These issues point to an important aspect of genetic diseases in general: such diseases carry an enormous significance for the family as a whole and the clinician needs to be aware of this.

## References

Belal, S.; Cancel, G.; Stevanin, G.; et al. Clinical and genetic analysis of a Tunisian family with autosomal dominant cerebellar ataxia type 1 linked to the SCA 2 locus. Neurology 44:1423–1426; 1994.

Boder, E. Ataxia telangiectasia: an overview. In: Gatti, R. A.; Swift, M. S., eds. Ataxia telangiectasia. Genetics, neuropathology and immunology of a degenerative disease of childhood. Kroc Foundation Series 19:1–63; 1985.

Campuzano, V.; Montermini, L.; Molto, M. D.; et al. Friedreich's ataxia: autosomal recessive disease caused by an intronic GAA triplet repeat expansion. Science 271:1423–1427; 1996.

Cancel, G.; Abbas, N.; Stevanin, G.; Durr, A.; Chneiweiss, H.; Duyckaerts, C.; Penet, C.; Cann, H. M.; Agid, Y.; Brice, A. Marked phenotypic heterogeneity associated with expansion of a CAG repeat sequence at the spinocerebellar ataxia 3/Machado-Joseph disease locus. Am. J. Hum. Genet. 57:809–816; 1995

Cancel, G., Durr, A.; Didierjean, O.; Imbert, G.; Burk, K.; et al. Molecular and clinical correlations in spinocerebellar ataxia 2: a study of 32 families. Hum. Mol. Genet. 6(5):709–715; 1997.

Chung, M-y; Ranum, L. P. W.; Divuc, L.; et al. Analysis of the CAG repeat expansion in spinocerebellar ataxia type 1: evidence for a possible mechanism predisposing to instability. Nat. Genet. 5:254–258; 1993.

Colan, R. V.; Snead, O. C.; Ceballos, R. Olivopontocerebellar atrophy in children: a report of seven cases in two families. Ann. Neurol. 10:355–363; 1981.

Coutinho, P.; Andrade, C. Autosomal dominant system degeneration in Portuguese families of the Azores Islands. Neurology 28:703–709; 1978.

Currier, R. D.; Jackson, J. F.; Meydrech, E. F. Progression rate and age at onset are related in autosomal dominant neurologic diseases. Neurology 32:907–909; 1982.

David, G.; Abbas, N.; Stevanin, G.; Durr, A.; Yvert, G.; et al. Cloning of the SCA 7 gene reveals a highly unstable CAG repeat expansion. Nat. Genet. 17: 65–70; 1997.

Del-Favero, J.; Krols, L.; Michalik, A.; Theuns, J.; Lofgren, A.; et al. Molecular genetic analysis of autosomal dominant cerebellar ataxia with retinal degeneration (ADCA type II) caused by CAG triplet repeat expansion. Hum. Mol. Genet. 7(2):177–186; 1998.

De Jong, P. T. V. M.; Hoppenreijs, V. P. T. Olivopontocerebellar atrophy and retinal degeneration. In: de Jong, J. M. B. V., ed. Handbook of clinical neurology. Vol. 16(60): Hereditary neuropathies and spinocerebellar atrophies. Amsterdam: Elsevier Science Publishers; 1991: p. 505–509.

Duborg, O.; Durr, A.; Cancel, G.; Stevanin, G.; Chneiweiss, H.; Agid, Y.; Brice, A. Analysis of the SCA-1 CAG repeat in a large number of families with dominant ataxia: clinical and molecular correlations. Ann. Neurol. 37:176–180; 1995.

Durr, A.; Cossee, M.; Agid, Y.; Campuzano, V., Mignard, C.; et al. Clinical and genetic abnormalities in patients with Friedreich's ataxia. N. Engl. J. Med. 335:1169–1175; 1996a.

Durr, A.; Stevanin, G.; Cancel, G.; Duyckaerts, C.; Abbas, N.; et al. Spinocerebellar ataxia 3 and Machado-Joseph disease: clinical, molecular and neuropathological features. Ann. Neurol. 39:490–499; 1996b.

Enevoldson, T. P.; Sanders, M. D.; Harding, A. E. Autosomal dominant cerebellar ataxia with pigmentary macular dystrophy. A clinical and genetic study of eight families. Brain 117:445–460; 1994.

Filla, A.; De Michele, G.; Caruso, G.; et al. Genetic data and natural history of Friedreich's disease: a study of 80 Italian patients. J. Neurol. 237:345–351; 1990.

Filla, A.; De Michele, G.; Cavalcanti, F.; et al. The relationship between tricnucleotide (GAA) repeat length and clinical features in Friedreich's ataxia. Am. J. Hum. Genet. 59:554–560; 1996.

Flanigan, K.; Gardner, K.; Alderson, K.; Galster, B.; et al. Autosomal dominant spinocerebellar ataxia with sensory axonal neuropathy (SCA 4): clinical description and genetic localization to chromosome 16q22.1. Am. J. Hum. Genet. 59:392–399; 1996.

Foster, J. B.; Ingram, T. T. S. Familial cerebro-macular degeneration and ataxia. J. Neurol. Neurosurg. Psychiatry 25:63–68; 1962.

Geschwind, D. H.; Perlman, S.; Grody, W. W., Telatar, M.; Montermini, L.; et al. Friedreich's ataxia GAA repeat expansion in patients with recessive or sporadic ataxia. Neurology 49:1004–1009; 1997.

Gilad, S.; Chessa, L.; Khosravi, R.; Russell, P.; Galanty, Y.; et al. Genotype-phenotype relationships in ataxia-telangiectasia and variants. Am. J. Hum. Genet. 62:551–561; 1998.

Giunti, P.; Sweeney, M. G.; Spadaro, M.; Jodice, C.; Novelletto, A.; et al. The trinucleotide repeat expansion on chromosome 6p (SCA 1) in autosomal dominant cerebellar ataxia. Brain 117:645–649; 1994.

Goldfarb, L. G.; Chumakov, M. P.; Petrov, P. A.; Fedorova, N. I.; Gajdusek, D. C. Olivopontocerebellar atrophy in a large Iakut kinship in eastern Siberia. Neurology 39:1527–1530; 1989.

Goldfarb, L. G.; Vasconcelos, O.; Platonov, F. A.; Lunkes, A.; Kipnis, V.; et al. Unstable triplet repeat and phenotypic variability of spinocerebellar ataxia type 1. Ann. Neurol. 39:500–506; 1996.

Gomez, C. M.; Thompson, R. M.; Gammack, J. T.; Perlman, S. L.; Dobyns, W. B.; et al. Spinocerebellar ataxia type 6: gaze-evoked and vertical nystagmus, Purkinje cell degeneration, and variable age of onset. Ann. Neurol. 42: 933–950; 1997.

Harding, A. Friedreich's ataxia: a clinical and genetic study of 90 families with an analysis of early diagnostic criteria and intrafamilial clustering of clinical features. Brain 104:589–620; 1981a.

Harding, A. E. Early onset cerebellar ataxia with retained tendon reflexes: a clinical and genetic study of a disorder distinct from Friedreich's ataxia. J Neurol. Neurosurg. Psychiatry 44:502–508; 1981b.

Hersch, S.; Jones, R.; Koroshetz, W.; Quaid, K. The neurogenetic genie: testing for Huntington's disease mutation. Neurology 44:1369–1373; 1994.

Hewer, R. L. Study of fatal cases of Friedreich's ataxia. Br. Med. J. 3:649–652; 1968.

Ikeuchi, T.; Takano, H.; Koide, R.; Horikawa, Y.; Honma, Y,; et al. Spinocerebellar ataxia type 6: CAG repeat expansion in $a_{1A}$ voltage-dependent calcium channel gene and clinical variations in Japanese population. Ann. Neurol. 42:879–884; 1997.

Imbert, G.; Saudou, F.; Yvert, G.; Devys, D.; et al. Cloning of the gene for spinocerebellar ataxia 2 reveals a locus with high sensitivity to expanded CAG/glutamine repeats. Nat. Genet. 14:285–291; 1996.

Isnard, R.; Kalotka, H.; Durr, A.; Cossee, M.; Schmitt, M.; et al. Correlation between left ventricular hypertrophy and GAA trinucleotide repeat length in Friedreich's ataxia. Circulation 95(9):2247–2249; 1997.

Jampel, R. S.; Okazaki, H.; Bernstein, H. Ophthalmoplegia and retinal degeneration associated with spinocerebellar ataxia. Arch. Ophthalmol. 66:247–259; 1961.

Jodice, C.; Malaspina, P.; Perischettie, F.; Novelletto, A.; Spadaro, M.; et al. Effect of trinucleotide on repeat length and parental sex on phenotypic variation in spinocerebellar ataxia I. Am. J. Hum. Genet. 54:959–965; 1994.

Johansson, J.; Forsgren, L.; Sandgren, O.; Brice, A.; Holmgren, G.; Holmberg, M. Expanded CAG repeats in Swedish spinocerebellar ataxia type 7 (SCA 7) patients: effect of CAG repeat length on the clinical manifestation. Hum. Mol. Genet. 7(2):171–176; 1998.

Kawaguchi, Y.; Okamoto, T.; Taniwaki, M.; Aizawa, M.; Inoue, M.; et al. CAG expansion in a novel gene for Machado-Joseph disease at chromosome 14q32.1. Nat. Genet. 8: 221–228; 1994.

Klockgether, T.; Ludtke, R.; Kramer, M., Abele, K.,; Burk, L.; et al. The natural history of degenerative ataxia: a retrospective study in 466 patients. Brain 121:589–600; 1998.

Koob, M. D.; Moseley, M. L.; Schut, L. I., Benzow, K. A.; Bird I. D.; Day, J. V.; Ranum, L. P. An un-translated CTG expansion causes a novel form of spinocerebellar ataxia (SCA8). Nat. Genet 21: 379–384; 1999.

Lamont, P. J.; Davis, M. B.; Wood, N. W. Identification and sizing of the GAA trinucleotide repeat expansion of Friedreich's ataxia in 56 patients. Clinical and genetic correlates. Brain 120:673–680; 1997.

Matilla, T.; Volpini, V.; Genis, D.; Rosell, J.; Corral, J.; et al. Presymptomatic analysis of spinocerebellar ataxia type 1 (SCA 1) via the expansion of the SCA 1 CAG repeat in a large pedigree displaying anticipation and parental male bias. Hum. Mol. Genet. 2(12):2123–2128; 1993.

Matilla, T.; McCall, A.; Subramony, S. H.; et al. Molecular clinical correlations in spinocerebellar atxia type 3 and Machado-Joseph disease. Ann. Neurol. 38:68–72; 1995.

Matsumura, R.; Takayanagi, T.; Fujimoto, Y.; Murata, K.; Mano, Y.; Horikawa, H.; Chuma, T. The relationship between trinucleotide repeat length and phenotypic variation in Machado-Joseph disease. J. Neurol. Sci. 139:52–57; 1996.

Matsuura, T.; Achari, M; Khajavi, M.; Bachinski, L. L.; Zoghbi, H. Y.; Ashizawa, T. Mapping of the gene for a novel spinocerebellar ataxia with pure cerebellar signs and epilepsy. Ann. Neurol. 45(3):407–411; 1999.

Matsuyama, Z.; Kawakami, H.; Maruyama, H.; Izumi, Y.; Komure, O.; et al. Molecular features of the CAG repeats of spinocerebellar ataxia 6 (SCA 6). Hum. Mol. Genet. 6(8):1283–1287; 1997.

Monros, E.; Molto, M. D.; Martinez, F.; Canizares, J.; Blanca, J.; et al. Phenotype correlation and intergenerational dynamics of the Friedreich ataxia GAA trinucleotide repeat. Am. J. Hum. Genet. 61:101–110; 1997.

Montermini, L.; Richter, A.; Morgan, K.; Justice, C. M.; Julien, D.; et al. Phenotypic variability in Friedreich ataxia: role of the associated CAA triplet repeat expansion. Ann. Neurol. 41:675–682; 1997.

Mueller-Felber, W.; Rossmanith, T.; Spes, C.; et al. The clinical spectrum of Friedreich's ataxia in German families showing linkage to FRDA locus on chromosome 9. Clin. Invest. 71:109–114; 1993.

Nakano, K. K.; Dawson, D. M.; Spence, A. Machado disease: a hereditary ataxia in Portuguese emigrants to Massachusetts. Neurology 22:49–55; 1972.

Nino, H. E.; Noreen, H. J.; Dubey, D. P.; Resch, J. A.; Namboodiri, K.; et al. A family with hereditary ataxia: HLA typing. Neurology 30:12–20; 1980.

Orozco, G.; Astride, R.; Perry, T.; Arena, J.; et al. Dominantly inherited olivopontocerebellar atrophy from eastern Cuba. Clinical, neuropathological and biochemical findings. J. Neurol. Sci. 93:37–50; 1989.

Orozco, G.; Nodarse, A.; Cordoves, R. C.; et al. Autosomal dominant cerebellar ataxia: clinical analysis of 263 patients from a homogeneous population in Holguin, Cuba. Neurology 40:1369–1375; 1990.

Orr, H.; Chung, M-y; Banfi, S.; et al. Expansion of an unstable trinucleotide (CAG) repeat in spinocerebellar ataxia type I. Nat. Genet. 4:221–226; 1993.

Pulst, S. M.; Nechiporuk, A.; Nechiporuk, T.; Gispert, S.; et al. Moderate expansion of a normally biallelic trinucleotide repeat in spinocerebellar ataxia type 2. Nat. Genet. 14:269–276; 1996.

Ranum, L. P. W.; Chung, M-y: Banfi, S.; et al. Molecular and clinical correlations in spinocerebellar ataxia type I (SCAA-1): evidence for familial effects on age of onset. Am. J. Hum. Genet. 55:244–252; 1994a.

Ranum, L. P. W.; Schut, L. J.; Lundgren, J. K.; et al. Spinocerebellar ataxia type V in a family descended from the grandparents of President Lincoln maps to chromosome 11. Nat. Genet. 8:280–284; 1994b.

Ranum, L. P. W.; Lundgren, J. K.; Schut, L. J.; et al. Spinocerebellar ataxia type 1 and Machado-Joseph disease: incidence of CAG expansions among adult-onset ataxia patients from 311 families with dominant, recessive or sporadic ataxia. Am. J. Hum. Genet. 57:603–608; 1995.

Richter, A.; Poirier, J.; Mercier, J.; Julien, D.; Morgan, K.; et al. Friedreich ataxia in Acadian families from eastern Canada: clinical diversity with conserved haplotypes. Am. J. Med. Genet. 64:594–601; 1996.

Riess, O.; Schols, L.; Bottger, H.; Nolte, D.; Vieira-Saecker, A. M. M.; et al. SCA 6 is caused by moderate CAG expansion in the $a_{1A}$-voltage-dependent calcium channel gene. Hum. Mol. Genet. 6(8):1289–1293; 1997.

Rosenberg, R. N.; Nyhan, W. L.; Bay, C.; Shore, P. Autosomal dominant striatonigral degeneration. Neurology 26:703–714; 1976.

Sanpei, K.; Takano, H.; Igarashi, S.; Sato, T.; et al. Identification of the spinocerebellar ataxia type 2 gene using a direct identification of repeat expansion and cloning technique, DIRECT. Nat. Genet. 14:277–284; 1996.

Sasaki, H.; Wakisaka, A.; Fukazawa, T.; Iwabuchi, K.; Hamada, T.; et al. CAG repeat expansion of Machado-Joseph disease in the Japanese: analysis of the repeat instability for parental transmission, and correlation with disease phenotype. J. Neurol. Sci. 133:128–133; 1995.

Sasaki, H.; Fukazawa, T.; Yanagihara, T.; Hamada, T.; Shima, K.; et al. Clinical features and natural history of spinocerebellar ataxia type 1. Acta Neurol. Scand. 93: 64–71; 1996.

Savitsky, K.; et al. A single ataxia telangiectasia gene with a gene product similar to PI-3 kinase. Science 268:1749–1753; 1995.

Schols, L.; Amoiridis, G.; Epplen, J. T.; et al. Relations between genotype and phenotype in German patients with Machado-Joseph disease mutation. J. Neurol. Neurosurg. Psychiatry 61:466–470; 1996.

Schols, L.; Gispert, S.; Vorgerd, M.; Vieira-Saecker, A. M. M.; Blanke, P.; et al. Spinocerebellar ataxia type 2. Arch. Neurol. 54:1073–1080; 1997.

Schols, L.; Kruger, R.; Amoiridis, G.; Przuntek, H.; Epplen, J. T.; Riess, O. Spinocerebellar ataxia type 6: genotype and phenotype in German kindreds. J. Neurol. Neurosurg. Psychiatry 64:67–73; 1998.

Schut, J. W. Hereditary ataxia: clinical study through six generations. Arch. Neurol. Psychiatry 63:535–568; 1950.

Sequeiros, J.; Coutinho, P. Epidemiology and clinical aspects of Machado-Joseph disease: In: Harding, A. E.;

Duefel, T., eds. Advances in neurology. Vol. 61. New York: Raven Press, 1993: p. 139–153.

Silveira, I.; Lopes-Cendes, I.; Kish, S.; et al. Frequency of spinocerebellar ataxia type 1, dentatorubrual-pallidoluysian atrophy and Machado-Joseph disease mutations in a large group of spinocerebellar ataxia patients.. Neurology 46:214–218; 1996.

Stankovic, T.; Kidd, A. M. J.; Sutcliffe, A.; McGuire, G. M.; Robinson, P.; et al. ATM mutations and phenotypes in ataxia-telangiectasia families in the British Isles: expression of mutant ATM and the risk of leukemia, lymphoma, and breast cancer. Am. J. Hum. Genet. 62:334–345; 1998.

Subramony, S. H.; Fratkin, J. D.; Manyam, B. V.; Currier, R. D. Dominantly inherited cerebello-olivary atrophy is not due to a mutation at the spinocerebellar ataxia-1, Machado-Joseph disease, or dentatorubro-pallidoluysain atrophy locus. Mov. Disord. 11(2): 174–180; 1996.

Sudarsky, L.; Corwin, L.; Dawson, D. M. Machado-Joseph disease in New England: clinical description and distinction from the olivopontocerebellar atrophies. Mov. Disord. 7(3):204–208; 1992.

Swift, M.; Reitnauer, P. J.; Morrell, D.; Chase, C. L. Breast and other cancers in families with ataxia-telangiectasia. N. Engl. J. Med. 316:1289–1294; 1987.

Swift, M. S.; Heim, R. A.; Lench N. J. Genetic aspects of ataxia telangiectasia. Adv. Neurol. 61:115–126; 1993.

Takiyama, Y.; Igarashi, S.; Rogaeva, E. A.; Endo, K.; Rogaev, E. I.; et al. Evidence for intergenerational instability in the CAG repeat in the MJD1 gene and for conserved haplotypes at flanking markers amongst Japanese and Caucasian subjects with Machado-Joseph disease. Hum. Mol. Genet. 4(7): 1137–1146; 1995.

To, K. W.; Adamian, M.; Jakobiec, F. A.; Berson, E. L. Olivopontocerebellar atrophy with retinal degeneration. Ophthalmology 100(1):15–23; 1993.

Watanabe, M.; Abe, K.; Aoki, M.; Kameya T.; Kaneko, J.; et al. Analysis of CAG trinucleotide expansion associated with Machado-Joseph disease. J. Neurol. Sci. 136:101–107; 1996.

Zhou, X. Y.; Takiyama, Y.; Igarashi, S.; Li, Y. F.; Zhou, B. Y.; et al. Machado-Joseph disease in four Chinese pedigrees: molecular analysis of 15 patients including two juvenile cases and clinical correlations. Neurology 48: 482–485; 1997.

Zhuchenko, O.; Bailey, J.; Bonnen, P.; Ashizawa, T.; et al. Autosomal dominant cerebellar ataxia (SCA 6) associated with small polyglutamine expansions in the $a_{1A}$-voltage-dependent calcium channel. Nature Genetics 15:62–68, 1997.

Zoghbi, H. Y.; Pollack, M. S.; Lyons, L. A.; Ferrell, R. E.; Daiger, S. P.; Beaudet, A. L. Spinocerebellar ataxia: variable age of onset and linkage to human leukocyte antigen in a large kindred. Ann. Neurol. 23:58–584; 1988.

Zu, L.; Figueroa, K.P.; Grewal, R.; Pulst, S.M. Mapping of a new autosomal dominant spinocerebellar ataxia to chromosome 22. Am. J. Hum. Genet. 64: 594–599;1999.

# 43

# Pregnancy

BARNEY J. STERN, JANE L. GILMORE, PAGE B. PENNELL,
AND JACQUELINE WASHINGTON

Physicians caring for the pregnant woman need to consider the effects of pregnancy on a particular disease, the effects of a disease on pregnancy, and the effects of any interventions on the fetus or neonate. There are many changes in maternal physiology during pregnancy and the postpartum period that require changes in the way many situations are approached as compared to the nonpregnant state. Finally, since pregnancy is often a fairly predictable event, measures can be taken prospectively to address medical concerns.

## Epilepsy

Pregnancy for women with epilepsy (WWE) has not always been acceptable. As recently as 1986 state laws have allowed for the prevention of persons with epilepsy from reproducing and even marrying. Today, WWE are still often discouraged from childbearing or they are given erroneous information. A national survey of neurologists and obstetricians found that many of the respondents did not know the accurate risk of birth defects (Krauss et al. 1996). Approximately 1 million women of childbearing age in the United States have epilepsy and give birth to some 20,000 babies each year (Devinsky and Yerby 1994). Current information indicates that

over 90% of the pregnancies in WWE occur without complications. Because there are potential increased complications to both the mother and the fetus during pregnancy, however, careful planning and management of any pregnancy in a woman with epilepsy is essential.

## Effects of Pregnancy on Epilepsy

The effect of pregnancy on seizure frequency is variable and unpredictable between patients. Seventeen percent to 20% will have an increase in seizures, 4% to 25% a decrease, and 60% to 83% no significant change in seizure frequency (Cantrell et al. 1997; Gjerde et al. 1988; Otani 1985; Svigos 1984; Tanganelli and Regesta 1992). Unfortunately, which route an individual's course will take is impossible to know and cannot be predicted based on factors such as age, ethnic origin, number of pregnancies, seizure type(s), antiepileptic drugs (AEDs), and seizure frequency during a previous pregnancy (Cantrell et al. 1997; Devinsky and Yerby 1994).

Pregnancy is associated with several physiological and psychological changes that can alter seizure frequency, including changes in sex hormone concentrations, changes in metabolism, sleep deprivation, and new stresses. Plasma levels of estrogen and progesterone increase gradually throughout pregnancy and peak during the last trimester. It may be that during pregnancy, women who have a relatively greater increase in estrogen than progesterone are more likely to have a worsening of their seizures, while those with a higher progesterone to estrogen ratio have improvement in their seizures (Backstrom 1976; Ramsay 1987). No studies have adequately addressed this question. Also, plasma chorionic gonadotropin levels rise during the first trimester before falling again, and animal studies suggest that this may contribute to increases in seizures during the first trimester (Loiseau et al. 1974). Metabolic changes include increased weight, fluid and sodium retention, compensated respiratory alkalosis, and hypomagnesemia. There has been no convincing evidence linking these factors to seizure control, however (Devinsky and Yerby 1994).

In studies analyzing the WWE who experience an increase in seizures during pregnancy, sleep deprivation or noncompliance played a clear role in 40% to 90% of the women (Otani 1985; Schmidt et al. 1983). Noncompliance with medications is common during pregnancy and is in large part due to the strong message that any drugs during pregnancy are harmful to the fetus. Teratogenic effects of AEDs are well described, but risks to the fetus are often exaggerated or misrepresented. Proper education about the risks of AEDs versus the risks of seizures can be very helpful in assuring compliance during pregnancy.

Levels of AEDs need to be monitored closely throughout pregnancy and the postpartum period. Plasma AED concentrations decrease during pregnancy despite steady or increasing doses (Table 43-1) (Yerby et al. 1992). A similar effect has been reported in a case study of lamotrigine (LTG); the dose/plasma concentration ratio was 5.8 times higher at delivery than the ratio at

**Table 43-1.** Proportionate Decline (%) in Levels of AEDs During the Full Pregnancy and During the Trimester With the Greatest Decline

| AED | Overall (Total/Free) | Trimester (Total/Free) |
|---|---|---|
| CBZ | 42 / 28% | 3rd: 52 / 83% |
| PHT | 56 / 31% | 1st: 66 / 102% |
| PB | 55 / 50% | 1st: 80 / 98% |
| VPA | 39 / +25% | Consistent throughout |

Adapted from Yerby et al. (1992).

CBZ, carbamazepine; PHT, phenytoin; PB, phenobarbital; VPA, valproic acid.

5 months postpartum (Tomson et al. 1997). The total AED levels generally decline more than the free levels (Yerby et al. 1992). Several factors contribute to the decline in AED levels during pregnancy (Yerby and Devinsky 1994). Impaired absorption is one cause, though relatively uncommon. The volume of distribution increases throughout pregnancy, but this would not account for the relatively lesser reduction in free levels compared to total levels. The most important contributing mechanisms are thought to be decreased albumin concentration, reduced plasma protein binding, and increased drug clearance. The decline in albumin concentration and plasma protein binding creates an increased percentage of unbound AED, which in turn provides an increased proportion of the drug available for metabolic degradation. Additionally, the increased sex steroid hormone levels may cause an induction of the hepatic microsomal enzymes and contribute to the increased clearance of AEDs.

The optimal approach to monitoring AED levels during pregnancy is one that measures free levels of the AED on a monthly basis (Report of the Quality Standards Subcommittee of the American Academy of Neurology [AAN] 1998). Although the ratio of free to bound drug increases during pregnancy, the amount of free AED still declines for all major AEDs except valproate (Yerby et al. 1992). The changes in total and free AEDs during pregnancy can vary widely and are not predictable for the individual based on reported group changes or total levels only.

## Effects of Epilepsy on Pregnancy

Women with epilepsy do have a slightly increased risk of certain obstetrical complications. There is an approximate twofold increased risk of vaginal bleeding, anemia, hyperemesis gravidarum, abruptio placentae, eclampsia, and premature labor (Yerby 1992). Weak uterine contractions have been described in women taking AEDs, which may account for the twofold increased use of interventions during labor and delivery including induction, mechanical rupture of membranes, forceps or vacuum assistance, and cesarean sections (Yerby et al. 1985).

Fetal death (fetal loss at >20 weeks gestational age) is another increased risk for pregnancies of WWE. Reported stillbirth rates vary between 1.3% and 14.0% for WWE compared to rates of

1.2% to 7.8% for women without epilepsy (Yerby and Collins 1997). Perinatal death rates appear to be also slightly increased for WWE (1.3% to 7.8%) compared to controls (1.0% to 3.9%). In contrast, spontaneous abortions (<20 weeks gestational age) do not appear to occur more frequently in WWE (Yerby and Collins 1997).

### Effects of Epilepsy and AEDs on the Fetus

Infants of epileptic mothers (IEMs) are at an increased risk for minor anomalies, major congenital malformations, developmental disability, microcephaly, and intrauterine growth retardation (Lindhout and Omtzigt 1992, 1994; Yerby 1994; Yerby and Devinsky 1994). These features in various combinations have often been referred to as the "fetal anticonvulsant syndrome." Minor anomalies are defined as structural deviations from the norm that do not constitute a threat to health and occur in less than 4% of the population. Minor anomalies are reported in 6% to 20% of infants of epileptic mothers. Major malformations are defined as an abnormality of an essential anatomical structure present at birth that interferes significantly with function and/or requires major intervention. Major malformations affect 4% to 6% of IEMs, compared to 2% of the general population.

Some component of the "fetal anticonvulsant syndrome" may be due to traits carried by mothers with epilepsy, but there is also a definite contribution from AEDs. The syndrome has been described for phenobarbital (PB), phenytoin (PHT), carbamazepine (CBZ), and valproic acid (VPA). Consensus guidelines from a workshop and symposium in 1990 concluded that, based on the available data, each of these four AEDs carried a similar teratogenic risk (Delgado-Escueta and Janz 1992). Trimethadione (Triodione) is considered contraindicated during pregnancy due to a high prevalence of severe birth defects (Delgado-Escueta and Janz 1992). The AAN practice parameter summary statement in 1998 recommended that "the AED most appropriate for seizure type and the drug producing optimal control with least side effects remains the AED of choice for WWE" (Report of the Quality Standards Subcommittee of the American Academy of Neurology [AAN] 1998). As of yet, there is no convincing evidence for teratogenicity for gabapentin (GBP), tiagabine (TGB), or vigabatrin (VGB), but experience with

these agents during pregnancy has been exceptionally limited. Information from the lamotrigine pregnancy registry (Glaxo-Wellcome 1997) indicates that congenital defects have occurred at similar frequencies to older AEDs (approximately 5% of live births) in the 81 prospectively collected cases thus far. Additional retrospective cases indicate that some of the cases with major malformations did involve women on LTG monotherapy (Glaxo-Wellcome 1997). Rodent studies have shown limb agenesis with TPM, but this is a common finding with other carbonic anhydrase inhibitors without apparent similar effects in humans. (Topiramate prescribing information package 1996). It is clear that the risk increases with the number of AEDs that the fetus is exposed to during pregnancy, especially during the first trimester. Previous studies have reported major malformations in 25% of IEMs using four or more AEDs (Lindhout and Omtzigt 1992).

Children of WWE, including those born to mothers on no AEDs, tend to have slightly more minor anomalies than controls or children of men with epilepsy (Lindhout et al. 1992). The minor anomalies may be outgrown in the first several years of life. They include distal digital and nail hypoplasia and the craniofacial anomalies, including ocular hypertelorism, broad nasal bridge, short upturned nose, altered lips, epicanthal folds, abnormal ears, and low hairline (Lindhout and Omtzigt 1992, 1994; Yerby 1994; Yerby and Devinsky 1994).

Major congenital malformations (Table 43-2) associated with AEDs include congenital heart disease, cleft lip/palate, neural tube defects, and urogenital defects (Lindhout et al. 1992; Lindhout and Omtzigt 1992, 1994; Yerby 1994; Yerby and Devinsky 1994). Urogenital defects

**Table 43-2.** Major Malformations in IEMs Compared to the General Population

| | General Population | IEMs |
|---|---|---|
| Congenital heart | 0.5% | 1.5–2% |
| Cleft lip/palate | 0.15% | 1.4% |
| Neural tube defect | 0.1% | 1–2% (VPA) |
| | | 0.5–1% (CBZ) |
| Urogenital defects | | 1.7% |

IEMs, infants of epileptic mothers; VPA, valproic acid; CBZ, carbamazepine.

occur in 1.7% of IEMs and commonly involve glandular hypospadias (Lindhout et al. 1992). The congenital heart defects include atrial septal defect, ventricular septal defect, tetralogy of Fallot, coarctation of the aorta, patent ductus arteriosus, and pulmonary stenosis. The neural tube defects usually consist of spina bifida and not anencephaly, but tend to be severe open defects frequently complicated by hydrocephaly and other midline defects (Lindhout et al. 1992). CBZ and VPA are associated with neural tube defects at a rate of 10 and 20 times the general population, respectively. A recent paper pooling data from five prospective studies suggested that the absolute risk of IEMs treated with VPA monotherapy may be as high as 3.8%, and that offspring of WWE receiving more than 1000 mg/d of VPA were at particularly increased risk (Samren et al. 1997). PB monotherapy also showed a trend for increased risk of major malformations with increasing dose, but the differences were not significant.

Results of studies investigating psychomotor retardation in IEMs have been as varied as the protocols employed, but the majority of studies report a two- to sevenfold increased risk of mental deficiency, affecting 1.2% to 6.2% of IEMs (Ganstrom and Gaily 1992). Verbal scores on neuropsychometric measures may be selectively more involved (Yerby and Collins 1997). An association has been found between cognitive impairment in IEMs and in utero AED exposure, seizures, a high number of minor anomalies, major malformations, decreased maternal education, impaired maternal-child relations, and maternal partial seizure disorder (Meador 1996).

Microcephaly has also been associated with all AEDs (Yerby and Collins 1997). Low birth weight (<2500 g) and prematurity have been reported in IEMs at rates of 7% to 10% and 4% to 11%, respectively (Yerby and Collins 1997).

Teratogenicity by AEDs is thought to be mediated by several mechanisms, including folate deficiency, AED free radical intermediates, and oxidative metabolites. Antifolate effects are well established for PHT, PB, and primidone, while VPA and CBZ have also been implicated (Dansky et al. 1992). GBP does not have any obvious antifolate properties. Low serum and red blood cell folate levels are associated with an increased incidence of spontaneous abortions and malfor-

mations in animal and human epilepsy studies (Dansky et al. 1992). Folate supplementation provides a 72% protective effect for offspring of high-risk nonepileptic women (MRC Vitamin Study Research Group 1991) and reduces the incidence of other major malformations (except cleft lip and palate). The maximal benefit of folate is achieved, however, only with folate supplementation beginning prior to and continuing after conception. The gestational age at which many of the major malformations develop is prior to diagnosis of pregnancy (Table 43-3). The optimal folate dosage has not been established for WWE, and recommendations vary between 0.4 and 5 mg/d.

Prenatal screening can detect major malformations. High-resolution ultrasound and maternal serum α-fetoprotein can detect greater than 94% of neural tube defects (Delgado-Escueta and Janz 1992), as well as oral clefts, limb defects, and heart anomalies (Yerby 1994). Amniocentesis with measurements of α-fetoprotein and acetylcholinesterase may be required, especially if an ultrasound and serum α-fetoprotein measurements are not conclusive.

For those women with epilepsy who have seizures during pregnancy, the risk of seizures to the fetus is important. Maternal seizures of all types in the first trimester have been associated with a higher malformation rate of 12.3% compared to a malformation rate of 4% for IEMs not exposed to seizures during the first trimester (Lindhout et al. 1992). With regard to type of epilepsy, no significant differences in malformation rates were observed between offspring of women with different epilepsy syndrome classifications (Lindhout et al. 1992; Samren et al. 1997).

Trauma secondary to seizures can result in ruptured fetal membranes, which increases the risk of infection, premature labor, and even fetal death

**Table 43-3.** Relative Timing and Developmental Pathology of Certain Malformations

| Tissues | Malformations | Time after LMP |
|---------|---------------|----------------|
| CNS | Meningomyelocele | 28 days |
| Heart | Ventricular septal defect | 6 weeks |
| Face | Cleft lip | 36 days |
| | Cleft maxillary palate | 10 weeks |

Adapted from Delgado-Escueta and Janz (1992).

LMP, first day of last menstrual period; CNS, central nervous system.

(Yerby and Devinsky 1994). If membranes rupture before 24 weeks' gestation, pulmonary hypoplasia and orthopedic deformities can occur. Abruptio placentae occurs after 1% to 5% of minor and 20% to 50% of major blunt injuries of all causes (Pearlman et al. 1990).

Generalized tonic-clonic seizures (GTCSs) can cause maternal and fetal hypoxia and acidosis. After a single GTCS, miscarriages and stillbirths have been reported. Status epilepticus is an uncommon complication of pregnancy, but when it does occur it carries a high maternal and fetal mortality rate. One series of 29 cases reported nine maternal deaths and 14 infant deaths (Teramo and Hiilesmaa 1982). A single brief tonic-clonic seizure has been shown to cause depression of fetal heart rate for more than 20 minutes (Teramo et al. 1979), and longer or repetitive tonic-clonic seizures are incrementally more hazardous to the fetus as well as the mother.

The risk of epilepsy in children of WWE is higher (relative risk, 3.2) compared to controls. Children of fathers with epilepsy do not demonstrate this same degree of increased risk. This may be related to the finding that the occurrence of maternal seizures during pregnancy, but not AED use, confers an increased risk of seizures in the offspring (relative risk, 2.4) (Ottman et al. 1988).

A hemorrhagic disorder can occur during the neonatal period due to deficiency of vitamin K–dependent clotting factors. It has been reported with CBZ, PHT, PB, ethosuximide (ESX), primidone (PRM), diazepam, mephobarbital, and amobarbital (Nelson and Ellenberg 1982; Yerby and Collins 1997). Infant mortality from this bleeding disorders is greater than 30% and is usually due to bleeding in the abdominal and pleural cavities leading to shock. The mechanism is unknown. These effects can be overcome by large concentrations of vitamin K. Prophylactic treatment consists of vitamin $K_1$ administered orally as 20 mg to the mother during the last month of pregnancy and 1 mg administered intramuscularly or intravenously to the newborn at birth (Krumholz 1992).

## Summary of Management of Epilepsy and Pregnancy

WWE considering pregnancy should be on supplemental folate and, if possible, AED monotherapy utilizing the medication that is the best choice for their seizure type and epilepsy syndrome (Report of the Quality Standards Subcommittee of the American Academy of Neurology [AAN] 1998). However, if a woman has a family history of neural tube defects, then VPA and CBZ should be avoided. The lowest effective plasma level for seizure control should be used. The risk of teratogenicity may increase with higher doses of all AEDs, as has been shown for VPA and spina bifida (Omtzigt et al. 1992). If large daily doses are needed, then frequent smaller doses may be helpful to avoid high peak levels. Seizure control remains an important goal during pregnancy in WWE.

## Eclampsia

The constellation of hypertension and proteinuria or edema associated with pregnancy characterizes pre-eclampsia (Kaplan and Repke 1994). If convulsions develop without another apparent cause, eclampsia is said to occur. Other neurological manifestations of eclampsia include cortical visual loss, ischemic and hemorrhagic infarction, and coma. The posterior leukoencephalopathy syndrome, characterized by headache, emesis, confusion, convulsions, and visual abnormalites, is associated with eclampsia (Donnan 1996; Hinchey et al. 1996).

Pre-eclampsia is a systemic disease, characterized by hypoperfusion, hypercoagulability, and dysfunctional vascular endothelium (Roberts 1997). Physiological changes associated with pre-eclampsia are apparent weeks prior to clinical presentation. Although the precise cause of pre-eclampsia is unknown, there is a heritable component.

The neurological sequelae of eclampsia may follow a pathophysiological process similar to that of hypertensive encephalopathy, with failure of cerebral autoregulation (Donaldson 1994; Kaplan and Repke 1994). Diffusion-weighted magnetic resonance imaging (MRI) has demonstrated vasogenic edema in an eclamptic patient, consistent with the hypertensive encephalopathy hypothesis (Schaefer et al. 1997). Brain computed tomography (CT) reveals foci of reversible white matter hypodensities and MRI demonstrates areas of reversible increased $T_2$-weighted signal in eclampsia (Digre et al. 1993). Digre et al. (1993) further characterize severe pre-eclamptic MRI findings as being limited to deep cerebral white matter changes and eclamptic MRI changes as also involving cortical/subcortical foci or cortical edema or hemorrhage. Using transcranial Doppler, eclamptic patients have higher mean flow velocities and lower average pulsatility indexes compared to normotensive pregnant women, whereas pre-eclamptic women had lower pulsatility indexes but similar mean flow velocities when compared to normotensive women (Qureshi et al. 1996). Magnetic resonance angiography may demonstrate reversible vasospasm during eclampsia (Kanayama et al. 1993), as can conventional angiography. The electroencephalogram (EEG) often shows background slowing during eclampsia, at times accompanied by spikes and sharp waves (Thomas et al. 1995). These changes typically resolve over time, especially the background slowing.

Sibai et al. examined the outcome of 254 eclamptic pregnancies (Sibai et al. 1992). Only one patient died acutely of eclampsia. None of his surviving patients had neurological deficits or seizures after 2 to 13 years of follow-up. All 14 pre-eclamptic or eclamptic women with cortical blindness reported by Cunningham et al. had resolution of their deficit after 4 hours to 8 days (Cunningham et al. 1995).

Lucas et al. randomized hypertensive women in labor to either magnesium sulfate or phenytoin therapy (Lucas et al. 1995). None of the 1049 women given magnesium sulfate had a seizure as compared to 10 of the 1089 women treated with phenytoin ($p = .004$). This study demonstrated the efficacy of magnesium sulfate treatment for the prevention of eclampsia. Magnesium sulfate therapy for hypertensive women in labor may prevent one eclamptic maternal death for every 5000 women treated (Saunders and Hammersley 1995). The Eclampsia Trial Collaborative Group (1995) found that fewer eclamptic women treated with magnesium sulfate compared to diazepam had recurrent seizures (13.2% vs. 27.9%; a 52% risk reduction) as well as when magnesium sulfate was compared to phenytoin (5.7% vs. 17.1%; a 67% risk reduction).

## Stroke

Although results vary by locale, time of study, and methodology, data from the urban/suburban United States mid-Atlantic region suggest an attributable risk of 8.1 per 100,000 pregnancies for ischemic stroke or intracerebral hemorrhage during pregnancy or within 6 weeks after delivery (Kittner et al. 1996). The relative risk of ischemic infarction is 0.7 during pregnancy and 8.7 for the 6 weeks after delivery. The relative risk of intracerebral hemorrhage is 2.5 during pregnancy and 28.3 for the 6 weeks after delivery. Lanska et al., using data from the National Hospital Discharge Survey, defined a risk for venous thrombosis of 8.9 to 11.4 per 100,000 deliveries (Lanska and Kryscio 1997, 1998).

Pregnancy-associated ischemic stroke can be caused by any of the many etiologies of stroke in the young (Stern and Wityk 1996). There are, however, several conditions unique to pregnancy that can lead to stroke. These include peripartum cardiomyopathy, peripartum vasculopathy, and "idiopathic" ischemic events attributed to the hypercoagulable state of pregnancy. In one series, only 24% of women with ischemic infarction and 14% with intracerebral hemorrhage had eclampsia (Kittner et al. 1996). Predisposing risk factors for stroke are frequently absent, and for the vast majority of women in Kittner's study "there is little to suggest that medical intervention could have prevented these strokes." A similar conclusion was reached by Witlin et al. (1997). Presumably, women with known stroke risk factors were managed in such a way as to decrease stroke risk. Although there is no consensus as to optimal use of antiplatelet or anticoagulant therapy during pregnancy, these medications can be used successfully to diminish ischemic stroke risk (Gilmore et al. 1998).

One group of disorders deserves special mention. Various vasculopathies, including vasospasm and vasculitis, can have similar angiographic appearances. Presumptive vasospasm has been documented in association with eclampsia (Trommer et al. 1988; Will et al. 1987). Postpartum hypertension, not associated with eclampsia, can also cause angiographic vasospasm (Garner et al. 1990; Geraghty et al. 1991). At times, the distinction between postpartum eclampsia and isolated hypertension can be difficult (Raps et al. 1993). A possibly hormonally mediated intimal hyperplasia may cause segmental arterial narrowing (Brick 1988). The feature common to all of these patient reports is the reversible nature of the angiographic finding. Hypertension, associated with or independent of eclampsia, may be a precipitant in many of the patients. These patients may fall within the rubric of "benign angiopathy of the central nervous system (CNS)" as defined by Calabrese et al., and should be distinguished from a primary, progressive angiitis of the CNS (Calabrese et al. 1992). Importantly, the "vasospasm" in these patients is reversible, and patients seem to stabilize with blood pressure control and perhaps a short course of calcium channel antagonists and steroids.

There is little information on stroke outcome within the context of pregnancy and the puerperium. Since the prognosis of a patient with stroke is dependent on the etiology of the event, it would be optimal to have data on the functional outcome and risk of recurrence relative to the many causes of pregnancy-associated stroke. Unfortunately, for the most part, this information is not readily available (Grosset et al. 1995).

Lanska et al., using National Hospital Discharge Survey data, reported that the in-hospital case fatality rates were 0% for intracranial venous thrombosis and 2.2% for peripartum stroke (Lanska and Kryscio 1997, 1998). On the other hand, seven of 24 women (29.2%) in the Witlin et al. study of all stroke types died; all of these individuals had a hemorrhagic event or hypertensive encephalopathy. Ten of the surviving 17 women had "residual neurologic deficits" (Witlin et al. 1997). Data from the first National Health and Nutrition Examination Survey Epidemiology Follow-up Study suggested that women with six or more pregnancies had a subsequent adjusted relative risk for stroke of 1.3, with an ischemic stroke relative risk of 1.3 (Qureshi et al. 1997).

There is no convincing evidence that the functional outcome of a pregnancy-associated stroke is any different from that of a stroke not associated with pregnancy. A critical, often asked question, concerns the risk of ischemic stroke recurrence during a subsequent pregnancy. Natural history data are sparse and probably dependent on the etiopathogenesis of the index event. Some representative outcomes of ischemic stroke in young patients are a mortality rate of less than 10% and stroke recurrence rates of less than 2% annually (Hindfelt and Nilsson 1992; Kappelle

et al. 1994). Presumably, therapeutic interventions can modify these risks, though there is no consensus as to optimal management to prevent recurrent stroke (Gilmore et al. 1998).

Horton et al. reviewed the Massachusetts General Hospital experience regarding hemorrhage from an untreated arteriovenous malformation (AVM) in a cohort of women referred for proton beam therapy (Horton et al. 1990). The risk of first hemorrhage during pregnancy in this select group of patients was 3.5% and did not differ from the risk in nonpregnant women. In an oft-quoted article, Robinson et al. observed in their referral population that if a woman with an AVM becomes pregnant, the "likelihood" of subarachnoid hemorrhage is 87% (Robinson et al. 1974). However Horton et al. interpret the Robinson et al. data as indicating "that when an AVM becomes clinically evident in association with pregnancy, a hemorrhage will be the first manifestation in 87% of cases"; their data suggest that for a similar 61% of their patients, hemorrhage was the initial manifestation of an AVM during pregnancy (Horton et al. 1990). Forster et al. evaluated a group of women referred for AVM radiosurgery with a gamma knife (Forster et al. 1993). During "pregnancy years" the rate of hemorrhage was 9.3% compared to a rate of 4.5% when not pregnant. The likelihood of bleeding was greatest in the second trimester, and no woman bled during labor, delivery, or the puerperium. Dias and Sekhar could not define a significant reduction in maternal or fetal mortality with surgical treatment of an AVM; maternal mortality was 23% to 32% and fetal mortality was 0% to 23% (Dias and Sekhar 1990). Long-term mortality from an AVM is estimated to be approximately 20% (Barrow and Reisner 1993), thus implying that pregnancy-associated AVM hemorrhage carries a substantive short-term maternal risk. Pregnancy may be associated with an increased likelihood of growth or bleeding from a cavernous angioma (Pozzati et al. 1996).

Aneurysmal rupture tends to occur during the second or third trimesters, as well as postpartum, with a mortality rate of 35% (Dias 1994). Dias states that the risk of recurrent hemorrhage from an untreated aneurysm is 33% to 50%; the mortality rate then rises to 50% to 68%. In 1990, Dias and Sekhar reported that maternal mortality with surgical aneurysmal treatment during pregnancy was 11%, compared with a rate of 63% in the nonsurgically treated group (Dias and Sekhar 1990). Furthermore, fetal mortality decreased from 27% to 5% with aneurysm surgery, though with adjustment for maternal clinical grade statistical significance was not achieved.

It is difficult to extrapolate the relatively high maternal morbidity and mortality rates quoted in the literature (Dias 1994) to what might be more timely values given current neurointensive care support, interventional neuroradiological procedures, and surgical techniques. Stereotactic radiosurgery would not be expected to be a viable treatment option for intrapartum AVM treatment, since there is a substantial time lag before the AVM is obliterated. There seems to be a general consensus that "decisions about whether and when to operate on an aneurysm or AVM should be the same as for the non-gravid patient; that is, the decision should be based on neurosurgical rather than obstetric considerations" (Dias 1994). Furthermore, "cesarean delivery should be reserved for obstetric indications" (Dias 1994), though some authors advocate cesarean delivery for an AVM (Sharma et al. 1995; Uchide et al. 1992).

## Multiple Sclerosis

Studies of the overall influence of pregnancy on patients with multiple sclerosis (MS) have had some conflicting results. The preponderance of the evidence supports the idea that there is no overall change in the relapse rate during the period of pregnancy and the first 6 months postpartum. However, there is a relative decreased risk of an exacerbation during pregnancy while the risk is increased postpartum (Abramsky 1994; Cook et al. 1994; Sadovnick et al. 1994; Worthington et al. 1994). Long-term disability also does not seem to be altered by pregnancy (Runmarker and Anderson 1995; Stenager et al. 1994; Verdru et al. 1994).

MS has not been shown to have significant adverse effects on fertility, pregnancy, labor, or delivery. Women who are taking disease-modifying drugs at the time of conception, such as the interferons or glatiramer acetate, should be advised to discontinue them, as spontaneous abortions have been reported during treatment. No systematic assessment of the impact of these therapies on pregnancy has been done (Gilmore et al.

1998). Other, less frequently used agents, such as cyclophosphamide and methotrexate, have been associated with an increase in congenital malformations, prematurity, and low birth weight (Weinreb 1994). Symptomatic therapies used need to be assessed for their potential for toxicity. The risk of urinary tract infections may increase due to the pressure of the gravid uterus on what may already be a dysfunctional bladder (Cook et al. 1994; Weinreb 1994). Women who have received corticosteroids to treat a relapse in the later months of pregnancy may require stress doses of hydrocortisone to prevent adrenal insufficiency. Methods of delivery and anesthesia are based on obstetrical grounds (Gilmore et al. 1998).

## Headache

Primary headache disorders, such as migraine and tension-type, may occur for the first time during pregnancy, or pre-existing headaches may improve, worsen, or remain unchanged. Maggioni et al. surveyed 430 women 3 days after delivery about headaches before and during pregnancy. Using IHS criteria, 126 (29.3%) had primary headaches, 81 of whom had migraine without aura, 12 migraine with aura, and 33 tension-type headache. In all groups, approximately 80% showed a complete remission or greater than 50% decline in the attack frequency during pregnancy. The improvement was more evident after the first trimester. Only one primary headache disorder developed during pregnancy in this series. Multiparous women maintained this pattern of improvement in subsequent pregnancies in half of the cases, while the other half had a worsening in parallel with successive pregnancies. These primary headaches were not found to be associated with greater pregnancy or delivery risks, nor infant mortality (Maggioni et al. 1997).

Pharmacological therapy for headaches during pregnancy must be done judiciously. Many medications are potentially hazardous to the fetus, such as sumatriptan, nonsteroidal anti-inflammatory agents, and ergot alkaloids. Prophylaxis is considered when attacks are frequent, prolonged, unresponsive to symptomatic therapy, and may result in dehydration and fetal distress. Prophylactic drug use may have adverse effects on the developing fetus and requires a full discussion of the risks and benefits (Gilmore et al. 1998).

Primary headaches must be distinguished from secondary headaches, such as those caused by infection, vascular disease, or neoplasm. Pituitary tumors, choriocarcinoma, eclampsia, stroke, venous thrombosis, and subarachnoid hemorrhage may present with headache, and may occur more commonly with pregnancy than at other times (Silberstein 1997). The choice of diagnostic studies should be primarily based on the likelihood serious secondary causes exist, and what tests are most likely to be definitive. MRI is preferable to CT due to lack of radiation; however, MRI would be inappropriate to evaluate a suspected acute subarachnoid hemorrhage. Radiological testing with exposure to ionizing radiation should not be excluded solely because of pregnancy. Therapy for secondary headaches is directed to the underlying cause (Gilmore et al. 1998).

## Tumors

Pregnancy is not associated with an increased incidence of primary brain tumors (Simon 1988). Additionally, the relative frequency of the different types of primary brain tumors is not changed: gliomas predominate followed by meningiomas and acoustic neuromas (Weinreb 1994).

The progression of gliomas and acoustic neuromas is probably not altered by pregnancy. Meningiomas and pituitary adenomas tend to enlarge, particularly during the latter months of pregnancy, and then improve again postpartum (Weinreb 1994). This may be due to increases in cell size or vascularity. Meningiomas have both estrogen and progesterone receptors, with the latter predominating. Although meningiomas tend to increase during the latter months of pregnancy when progesterone levels are the highest, neither estrogen nor progesterone agonists or antagonists have been effective in altering meningioma cell growth in vitro (Yahr et al. 1991). A definitive relationship between progesterone and any of the brain tumors is yet to be established (Roelvink et al. 1987; Simon 1988). The physiological effects of the normal increase in extracellular and intracellular fluid compartments may be just as likely to contribute to the appearance of symptoms from intracranial and intraspinal tumors during pregnancy (Yahr et al. 1991).

During pregnancy, the risk of clinically significant pituitary microadenoma enlargement is only 1.6% to 5.5%, but the risk for macroadenoma enlargement is much higher at 15.5% to 35.7% (Molitch 1985). The risk is reduced if the woman is treated with irradiation or surgery prior to pregnancy. If the woman with symptomatic worsening is 34 weeks or greater IUP, then labor may be induced, as these tumors often shrink rapidly after delivery (Weinreb 1994). Often, prolactinomas are treated with bromocriptine. Its safety on the fetus is not established, but preliminary studies have not demonstrated an increase in spontaneous abortions or congenital malformations (Hammond et al. 1983; Robinson and Nelson 1983). However, when the pregnancy is planned, it is suggested that the drug be discontinued prior to conception if possible.

Choriocarcinomas are of trophoblastic origin and are highly invasive. They often present with irregular vaginal bleeding or uterine enlargement following a molar pregnancy or an abortion. Choriocarcinomas can even occasionally occur during or following normal pregnancies (Weinreb 1994). Cerebral metastases have been reported to occur in 3% to 28% of patients (Weed and Hunter 1991). The cerebral metastasis can present as a solitary mass lesion or as a cerebrovascular event (ischemic infarction, intraparenchymal hemorrhage, or subdural hematoma) due to the propensity of the trophoblastic tissue to infiltrate and proliferate within vascular spaces. Choriocarcinoma metastases can also present neurologically as local invasion of the lumbosacral plexus or the vertebral bodies with cauda equina or extradural cord compression (Weinreb 1994).

## Neuromuscular Disorders

Neuromuscular disorders during pregnancy may be classified according to peripheral nervous system anatomy and the time of occurrence during pregnancy. Peripheral neuropathies that may present during the antenatal period include carpal tunnel syndrome, meralgia paresthetica, iliohypogastric neuropathy, Bell's palsy, and Guillain-Barre syndrome. Peripheral neuropathies at the puerperium include postpartum foot drop, and femoral, obturator, and pudendal neuropathies. Myasthenia gravis poses special considerations during the antenatal, puerperal, and postpartum periods. Polymyositis also calls for special considerations during pregnancy but occurs rarely. Low back pain is a common accompaniment of pregnancy due to various neuromuscular and musculoskeletal causes.

## Peripheral Nerve Disorders During the Antenatal Period

### Carpal Tunnel Syndrome

The incidence of carpal tunnel syndrome is increased during pregnancy. Carpal tunnel syndrome occurs in 2% to 25% of pregnant women (Ekman-Orderberg et al. 1987; Gould and Wissinger 1978; McLennan et al. 1987; Stahl et al. 1996). The syndrome occurs most frequently during the third trimester of pregnancy (Stahl et al. 1996). Clinical features that increase the risk of carpal tunnel syndrome during pregnancy include older age, excessive weight gain, edema, toxemia of pregnancy, and a history of carpal tunnel syndrome in previous pregnancies. Clinical symptoms of numbness, tingling, and pain at night frequently affect both upper extremities and are exacerbated by use of the hands. Physical examination may reveal the presence of Tinel's or Phalen's sign. Objective sensory loss and weakness are rare.

The recommended approach to therapy is conservative because symptoms usually resolve spontaneously following delivery. Wrist splints worn at night are effective and may result in improvement of symptoms as early as 1 week after splinting (Courts 1995). Symptoms usually resolve completely and at times dramatically soon after delivery. Complete relief of symptoms was reported in 95% of patients in one series by the second postpartum week (Ekman-Orderberg et al. 1987). The benign course of disease in the majority of patients dictates the need for conservative management.

### Meralgia Paresthetica

Compression of the lateral femoral cutaneous nerve at the inguinal ligament may lead to the symptom complex of meralgia paresthetica. Risk factors for the development of the syndrome include obesity with a protuberant abdomen and diabetes. The symptoms of pain, tingling, and numbness of the lateral anterior thigh usually occur after the 30th week of gestation. Symptoms may be bilateral in many cases (Donaldson 1992). Pain and numbness typically resolve within 3 months of delivery (Massey 1988). Conservative management is recommended. Local injection of anesthetic at the site of nerve entrapment may aid diagnosis and

usually provides symptomatic relief. Tricyclic antidepressant therapy may be useful in the treatment of residual postpartum symptoms.

### Iliohypogastric Neuropathy

Entrapment of the iliohypogastric nerve occurs during pregnancy due to rapid expansion of the growing uterus (Racz and Hagstrom 1992). During pregnancy the uterus stretches the abdominal wall, placing tension on the iliohypogastric nerve as it exits the internal oblique, external oblique, and transverse abdominus muscles. The syndrome of severe, persistent pain of the lower abdominal quadrant, flank, or inguinal region is frequently associated with hyperpathia in the same region. The diagnosis can be confirmed by iliohypogastric nerve block. Injection of bupivocaine at the site of entrapment results in complete pain relief within minutes (Carter and Racz 1994).

### Bell's Palsy

Idiopathic facial neuropathy or Bell's palsy occurs with an increased frequency during pregnancy that is three times that of nongravid women of childbearing age (Hilsinger et al. 1975). During the third trimester of pregnancy the incidence rises to ten times that of nongravid women of childbearing age. Prognosis for recovery is excellent, with complete recovery without treatment in 75% of patients. Improvement is expected in the majority of patients in 2 to 4 weeks. Treatment with high-dose prednisone may accelerate recovery and reduce the incidence of aberrant regeneration (Wolf et al. 1978). Herpes simplex virus type 1 is the probable etiological agent for "idiopathic" facial paralysis (Murakami et al. 1996). Antiviral agents such as ganciclovir and acyclovir have been used to treat Bell's palsy but are designated class C for use during pregnancy. The potential for teratogenicity should be weighed against the potential benefit when these agents are considered.

### Landry-Guillain-Barré Syndrome

Landry-Guillain-Barré syndrome or acute immune-mediated inflammatory demyelinating polyradiculoneuropathy may occur during pregnancy. The incidence of disease during pregnancy of 0.7 to 1.9 per 100,000 is comparable to the general population (Clifton 1992). Guillain-Barré syndrome during pregnancy poses significant risks to mother and fetus but is similar to the general population with regard to course, therapy, and prognosis.

Supportive care and careful monitoring of the patient's respiratory, cardiovascular, and hemodynamic status are the mainstays of management. Plasmapheresis and intravenous immunoglobulin (IVIG) therapy are both effective in gravid and nongravid patients. Experience with plasmapheresis has been shown to be associated with a low complication risk (Clifton 1992). Experience with use of IVIG in pregnancy is less well documented.

There is no significant adverse effect of Guillain-Barré syndrome on pregnancy, and pregnancy has no significant effect on the course of illness. Spontaneous delivery without prolonged labor is expected in the majority of patients. Assistance during the second stage of labor may be necessary if abdominal muscles are weak.

## Peripheral Nerve Disorders at the Puerperium

### Postpartum Foot Drop

Postpartum foot drop is the most common peripheral neuropathy that occurs at the puerperium. Foot drop is most commonly due to compression of the lumbosacral trunk by the fetal brow as it passes the brim of the pelvis (Massey 1988). Postpartum foot drop has rarely been associated with distal peroneal neuropathy after prolonged squatting during natural childbirth (Reif 1988) and positioning of the knees in hyperflexion during delivery (Colachis et al. 1994).

### Femoral Neuropathy

Femoral neuropathy occurs during the puerperium as a result of compression of the intrapelvic portion of the nerve by the fetal head. This neuropathy may occur following vaginal or cesarean delivery (Montag and Mead 1981). The neuropathy is not common during pregnancy. Risk factors for development include primiparity, prolonged labor, and cephalopelvic disproportion.

### Obturator Neuropathy

Postpartum neuropathy due to compression of the obturator nerve has been rarely reported (Linder et al. 1997). The syndrome consists of hypoesthesia of the medial thigh and weakness of thigh adductors. Obturator neuropathy may be associated with postpartum femoral neuropathy.

### Pudendal Neuropathy

Traumatic vaginal delivery may result in local damage to the pudendal nerves. Pudendal nerve damage may result in urinary and fecal incontinence. Patients with vaginal delivery of a large fetus and those with a long second stage of labor were shown to have electrophysiological abnormalities in pudendal nerve function following delivery (Sulton et al. 1994).

### Prognosis of Puerperal Nerve Injury

In general, prognosis for return of function is determined by the degree of axonal involvement. Those nerves that are readily available to neurophysiological techniques should be studied 2 to 3 weeks following the injury to determine the degree of axonal involvement. Recovery is expected in neuropractic injuries 6 to 8 weeks following injury.

## Neuromuscular Disorders that Occur During the Antenatal, Puerperal, and Postpartum Periods

### Myasthenia Gravis

Myasthenia gravis is a relatively uncommon disorder that occurs most frequently in women of childbearing age and elderly males. Myasthenia gravis during pregnancy poses unique maternal and fetal therapeutic considerations. Symptoms from myasthenia gravis may worsen, improve, or remain unchanged during pregnancy. Plauche reported rates of 41% relapse, 28.6% remission and 29.8% postpartum exacerbation in a series of 322 pregnancies in 225 myasthenic mothers. The same report documented 4% maternal mortality and perinatal mortality of 68 in 1000 (Plauche 1991).

Treatment of myasthenia gravis during pregnancy may be symptomatic or corrective. Corrective therapy includes immunosuppression and immunomodulation. Corticosteroids are the agents of choice for immunosuppression during pregnancy. Care must be taken in the institution of corticosteroid therapy in myasthenia gravis to prevent acute exacerbation of symptoms. Plasmapheresis and intravenous immunoglobulin therapy are treatment options for severe exacerbation when an immediate response is required. Plasmapheresis has been used effectively in pregnancy and is not associated with an increased rate of complication (Watson et al. 1990). There is less experience in the use of intravenous immunoglobulin during pregnancy. Prior early thymectomy has been associated with less frequent worsening of symptoms during pregnancy (Eden and Gall 1990).

Special consideration at the time of delivery is necessary. The intrapartum period will increase fatigue in the mother and may precipitate crises. The second stage of labor may be aided by the intravenous administration of neostigmine. Cesarean section may be indicated in some patients. Narcotic and sedative medications may be used with careful and continuous assessment. The use of magnesium sulfate for the prevention of seizures during preeclampsia and the treatment of seizures during eclampsia in myasthenic patients is contraindicated. Magnesium interferes with neuromuscular transmission and thus results in a worsening of weakness (Duff 1979). Seizures associated with eclampsia should be treated with more traditional anticonvulsants with close patient observation for complications of depressed mental status.

## Effect of Maternal Myasthenia Gravis on the Infant

Effects of maternal myasthenia gravis on progeny may be permanent or transient in nature. Permanent effects result from inadequate fetal movement as a result of weakness. Congenital arthrogryposis has been reported in progeny of symptomatic and asymptomatic myasthenic mothers (Duff 1979). Antenatal myasthenia gravis can also manifest as polyhydramnios, due to inadequate swallowing and pulmonary hypoplasia (Verspyck et al. 1993).

Neonatal myasthenia is a transient effect of maternal myasthenia gravis. Neonatal myasthenia gravis occurs in 10% to 21% of infants of myasthenic mothers. The symptoms of sucking, swallowing, and respiratory difficulties are the most common. Generalized weakness, feeble cry, and floppiness are additional symptoms. Affected infants demonstrate evidence of these symptoms within the first 3 days of life. Diagnosis is confirmed by administration of edrophonium. Neonatal myasthenia gravis resolves spontaneously in the majority of patients, but may persist for weeks. Eighty percent of affected patients require supportive management and anticholinesterase agents prior to feeding (Papazian 1992).

## Polymyositis

Polymyositis/dermatomyositis during pregnancy is a rare occurrence because the onset of disease

is typically after the traditional childbearing period. Prognosis is different in patients with pre-existing disease and those with disease presentation during pregnancy. Those with pre-existing controlled disease rarely have exacerbations, but deterioration does occur during the third trimester of pregnancy. Initial presentation during pregnancy is associated with active disease throughout gestation (Rosenzweig et al. 1989). Symptoms tend to improve during the postpartum period in both groups. Reported complications during pregnancy include abruptio placentae, uterine atony, preterm labor, intrauterine growth retardation, and spontaneous abortion. The effects of the disease on the fetus are significant, with fetal death having been reported in 21% to 50% of cases (Gutierrez et al. 1984).

Corticosteroid therapy may be necessary to manage exacerbations. The use of antimetabolites during pregnancy is relatively contraindicated because use has been frequently associated with fetal malformation and spontaneous abortion.

## Low Back Pain

Back pain is common during pregnancy, with an incidence of 49% to 67% (Alexander and McCormick 1993; Orvieto et al. 1994; Rungee 1993). The pain may be severe in nature and frequently occurs later in the day or at nighttime (Hainline 1994). Common etiologies include sacroiliac joint dysfunction, muscle strain, muscle spasm, and lumbar disc disease. The incidence of lumbar disc disease during pregnancy is not known. Risk factors for development of back pain during pregnancy include increased age and parity. Diagnostic imaging is indicated when back pain is associated with acute paralysis or bowel and/or bowel dysfunction. Conservative management of low back pain during pregnancy should be guided by the clinical knowledge of the specific etiology.

## References

Abramsky, O. Pregnancy and multiple sclerosis. Ann. Neurol. 36 (suppl.):S38–S41; 1994.

Alexander, J.; McCormick, P. Pregnancy and discogenic disease of the spine. Neurosurg. Clin. North Am. 153–159; 1993.

Backstrom, T. Epileptic seizures in women related to plasma estrogen and progesterone during the menstrual cycle. Acta Neurol. Scand. 54:321–347; 1976.

# 726 CONGENITAL, GENETIC-METABOLIC, AND DISORDERS OF PREGNANCY

Barrow, D.; Reisner, A. Natural history of intracranial aneurysms and vascular malformations. Clin. Neurosurg. 40:3–39; 1993.

Brick, J. Vanishing cerebrovascular disease of pregnancy. Neurology 38:804–806; 1988.

Calabrese, L.; Furlan, A.; Gragg, L.; Ropos, T. Primary angiitis of the central nervous system: diagnostic criteria and clinical approach. Cleve. Clin. J. Med. 59:293–306; 1992.

Cantrell, D.; Riela, S.; Ramus, R.; Riela, A. Epilepsy and pregnancy: a study of seizure frequency and patient demographics. Epilepsia 38(suppl. 8):231; 1997.

Carter, B.; Racz, G. Iliohypogastric nerve entrapment in pregnancy: diagnosis and treatment. Anesth. Analg. 79:1193–1194; 1994.

Clifton, E. Guillain-Barre syndrome, pregnancy, and plasmapheresis. J. Am. Osteopath. Assoc. 92:1279–1282; 1992.

Colachis, S.; Pease, W.; Johnson, E. A preventable cause of foot drop during childbirth. Am. J. Obstet. Gynecol. 171:270–272; 1994.

Cook, S.; Troiano, R.; Bansil, S. Multiple sclerosis and pregnancy. In: Devinsky, O.; Feldmann, E.; Hainline, B., eds. Neurological complications of pregnancy. New York: Raven Press; 1994: p. 83–94.

Courts, R. Splinting for symptoms of carpal tunnel syndrome during pregnancy. J. Hand Ther. 8:31–34; 1995.

Cunningham, F.; Fernandez, C.; Hernandez, C. Blindness associated with preeclampsia and eclampsia. Am. J. Obstet. Gynecol. 172:1291–1298; 1995.

Dansky, L.; Rosenblatt, D.; Andermann, E. Mechanisms of teratogenesis: folic acid and antiepileptic therapy. Neurology 42 (suppl. 5):32–42; 1992.

Delgado-Escueta, A.; Janz, D. Consensus guidelines: preconception counseling, management, and care of the pregnant woman with epilepsy. Neurology 42(suppl. 5):149–160; 1992.

Devinsky, O.; Yerby, M. Women with epilepsy. Neurol. Clin. 12:479–495; 1994.

Dias, M. Neurovascular emergencies in pregnancy. Clin. Obstet. Gynecol. 37:337–354; 1994.

Dias, M.; Sekhar, L. Intracranial hemorrhage from aneurysms and arteriovenous malformations during pregnancy and the puerperium. Neurosurgery 27:855–865; 1990.

Digre, K.; Varner, M.; Osborn, A.; Crawford, S. Cranial magnetic resonance imaging in severe preeclampsia vs eclampsia. Arch. Neurol. 50:399–406; 1993.

Donaldson, J. Pregnancy. In: Evans, R.; Baskin, D.; Yatsu, F., eds. Prognosis of neurological disorders. New York: Oxford University Press; 1992: p. 673–679.

Donaldson, J. Eclampsia. In: Devinsky, O.; Feldmann, E.; Hainline, B., eds. Neurological complications of pregnancy. New York: Raven Press: 1994: p. 25–33.

Donnan, G. Posterior leucoencephalopathy syndrome. Lancet 347:988; 1996.

Duff, G. Preeclampsia and the patient with myasthenia gravis. Obstet. Gynecol. 54:355–358; 1979.

Eden, R.; Gall, S. Myasthenia gravis and pregnancy: a reappraisal of thymectomy. Obstet. Gynecol. 62:328; 1990.

Ekman-Orderberg, G.; Slageback, S.; Ordeberg, G. Carpal tunnel syndrome in pregnancy: a prospective study. Acta Obstet. Gynecol. Scand. 66:233–235; 1987.

Forster, D.; Kunkler, I.; Hartland, P. Risk of cerebral bleeding from arteriovenous malformations in pregnancy: the Sheffield experience. Stereotact. Funct. Neurosurg. 61 (Suppl. 1):20–22; 1993.

Ganstrom, M.; Gaily, E. Psychomotor development in children of mothers with epilepsy. Neurology 42(suppl. 5):144–148; 1992.

Garner, B.; Burns, P.; Bunning, R.; Laureno, R. Acute blood pressure elevation can mimic arteriographic appearance of cerebral vasculitis (a postpartum case with relative hypertension). J. Rheumatol. 17:93–97; 1990.

Geraghty, J.; Hoch, D.; Robert, M.; Vinters, H. Fatal puerperal cerebral vasospasm and stroke in a young woman. Neurology 41:1145–1147; 1991.

Gilmore, J.; Pennell, P.; Stern, B. Medication use during pregnancy for neurologic conditions. Neurol. Clin. North Am. 16:189–206; 1998.

Gjerde, I.; Strandjord, R.; Ulstein, M. The course of epilepsy during pregnancy: a study of 78 cases. Acta Neurol. Scand. 78:198–205; 1988.

Glaxo-Wellcome. International lamotrigine pregnancy registry, interim report. 1997.

Gould, J.; Wissinger, H. Carpal tunnel syndrome in pregnancy. South. Med. J. 71:144–145; 1978.

Grosset, D.; Ebrahim, S.; Bone, I.; Warlow, C. Stroke in pregnancy and the puerperium: what magnitude of risk? J. Neurol. Neurosurg. Psychiatry 58:129–131; 1995.

Gutierrez, G.; Dagnino, R.; Mintz, G. Polymyositis/dermatomyositis and pregnancy. Arthritis Rheum. 27:291–294; 1984.

Hainline, B. Low-back pain in pregnancy. In: Devinski, O.; Feldmann, E.; Hainline, B., eds. Neurological complications of pregnancy. New York: Raven Press; 1994: p. 65–76.

Hammond, C.; Haney, A.; Land, M.; vanderMerwe, J.; Ory, S.; Wiebe, R. The outcome of pregnancy in patients with treated and untreated prolactin-secreting pituitary tumors. Am. J. Obstet. Gynecol. 147(2):148–157; 1983.

Hilsinger, R.; Adour, K.; Doty, H. Idiopathic facial paralysis, pregnancy, and the menstrual cycle. Ann. Otol. 84:433–442; 1975.

Hinchey, J.; Chaves, C.; Appignani, B.; Breen, J.; Pao, L.; Wang, A.; Pessin, M.; Lamy, C.; Mas, J.-L.; Caplan, L. A reversible posterior leukoencephalopathy syndrome. N. Engl. J. Med. 334:494–500; 1996.

Hindfelt, B.; Nilsson, O. Long-term prognosis of ischemic stroke in young adults. Acta Neurol. Scand. 86:440–445; 1992.

Horton, J.; Chambers, W.; Lyons, S.; Adams, R.; Kjellberg, R. Pregnancy and the risk of hemorrhage from cerebral arteriovenous malformations. Neurosurgery 27:867–872; 1990.

Kanayama, N.; Nakajima, A.; Maehara, K.; Halim, A.; Kajiwara, Y.; Isoda, H.; Masui, T.; Terao, T. Magnetic resonance imaging angiography in a case of eclampsia. Gynecol. Obstet. Invest. 36:56–58; 1993.

Kaplan, P.; Repke, J. Eclampsia. Neurol. Clin. 12:565–582; 1994.

Kappelle, L.; Adams, H.; Heffner, M.; Torner, J.; Gomez, F.; Biller, J. Prognosis of young adults with ischemic stroke: a long-term follow-up study assessing recurrent vascular events and functional outcome in the Iowa Registry of Stroke in Young Adults. Stroke 25:1360–1365; 1994.

Kittner, S.; Stern, B.; Feeser, B. Pregnancy and the risk of stroke. N. Engl. J. Med. 335:768; 1996.

Krauss, G.; Brandt, J.; Campbell, M.; Plate, C.; Summerfield, M. Antiepileptic medication and oral contraceptive interactions: A national survey of neurologists and obstetricians. Neurology 46:1534–1539; 1996.

Krumholz, A. Epilepsy in pregnancy. In: Goldstein, P.; Stern, B., eds. Neurological disorders of pregnancy. Mount Kisco, NY: Futura Publishing Co.; 1992: p. 25–50.

Lanska, D.; Kryscio, R. Peripartum stroke and intracranial venous thrombosis in the National Hospital Discharge Survey. Obstet. Gynecol. 89:413–418; 1997.

Lanska, D.; Kryscio, R. Stroke and intracranial venous thrombosis during pregnancy and puerperium. Neurology 51:1622–1628;1998.

Linder, A.; Shulte-Mattler, W.; Zierz, S. Post partum obturator neuropathy: case report and review of nerve compression syndromes during pregnancy and delivery. Zentralbl. Gynakol. 119:93–99; 1997.

Lindhout, D.; Meinardi, H.; Meijer, J.; Nau, H. Antiepileptic drugs and teratogenesis in two consecutive cohorts: changes in prescription policy paralleled by changes in pattern of malformations. Neurology 42:94–110; 1992.

Lindhout, D.; Omtzigt, J. Pregnancy and the risk of teratogenicity. Epilepsia 33:S41–S48; 1992.

Lindhout, D.; Omtzigt, J. Teratogenic effects of antiepileptic drugs: implications for the management of epilepsy in women of childbearing age. Epilepsia 35:S19–S28; 1994.

Lindhout, D.; Omtzigt, J.; Cornel, M. Spectrum of neural-tube defects in 34 infants perinatally exposed to antiepileptic drugs. Neurology 42 (suppl. 5):111–118; 1992.

Loiseau, P.; Legroux, M.; Henry, P. Epilepsies et grossesses. Bordeaux Med. 7:1157–1164; 1974.

Lucas, M.; Leveno, K.; Cunningham, F. A comparison of magnesium sulfate with phenytoin for the prevention of eclampsia. N. Engl. J. Med. 333:201–205; 1995.

Maggioni, F.; Alessi, C.; Maggino, T.; Zanchin, G. Headache during pregnancy. Cephalalgia 7:765–769; 1997.

Massey, E. Mononeuropathies in pregnancy. Semin. Neurol. 8:193–196; 1988.

McLennan, H.; Oats, J.; Walstab, J. Survey of hand symptoms in pregnancy. Med. J. Aust. 147:542–544; 1987.

Meador, K. Cognitive effects of epilepsy and of antiepileptic medications. In: Wyllie, E., ed. The treatment of epilepsy: principles and practice. Baltimore: Williams & Wilkins: 1996: p. 1121–1130.

Molitch, M. Pregnancy and the hyperprolactinemic woman. N. Engl. J. Med. 312:1364–1370; 1985.

Montag, T.; Mead, P. Postpartum femoral neuropathy. J. Reprod. Med. 26:563–566; 1981.

MRC Vitamin Study Research Group. Prevention of neural-tube defects: results of the Medical Research Council Vitamin Study. Lancet 338:131–137; 1991.

Murakami, S.; Mizobuchi, M.; Nakashiro, Y.; Doi, T.; Hato, N.; Ynagihara, N. Bell palsy and herpes simplex virus: identification of viral DNA in endoneurial fluid and muscle. Ann. Intern. Med. 125:698–699; 1996.

Nelson, K.; Ellenberg, J. Maternal seizure disorder, outcome of pregnancy, and neurologic abnormalities in the children. Neurology 32:1247–1254; 1982.

Omtzigt, J.; Los, F.; Grobbee, D.; Pijpers, L.; Jahoda, M.; Brandenburg, H.; Stewart, P.; Gaillard, H.; Sachs, E.; Wladimiroff, J. The risk of spina bifida aperta after first-trimester exposure to valproate in a prenatal cohort. Neurology 42 (suppl. 5):119–125; 1992.

Orvieto, R.; Achiron, A.; Zion, B.; Gerlernter, I.; Achiron, R. Low back pain of pregnancy. Acta Obstet. Gynecol. Scand. 723:209–214; 1994.

Otani, K. Risk factors for the increased seizure frequency during pregnancy and the puerperium. Folia Psychiatr. Neurol. Jpn. 39:33–42; 1985.

Ottman, R.; Annegers, J.; Hauser, W.; Kurland, L. Higher risk of seizures in offspring of mothers than fathers with epilepsy. Am. J. Hum. Genet. 43:357–364; 1988.

Papazian, O. Transient neonatal myasthenia gravis. J. Child Neurol. 7:135–141; 1992.

Pearlman, M.; Tintinalli, J.; Lorenz, R. Blunt trauma during pregnancy. N. Engl. J. Med. 323:1609–1613; 1990.

Plauche, W. Myasthenia gravis in mothers and their newborns. Clin. Obstet. Gynecol. 34:82; 1991.

Pozzati, E.; Acciarri, N.; Tognetti, F.; Marliani, F.; Giangaspero, F. Growth, subsequent bleeding, and de novo appearance of cerbral cavernous angiomas. Neurosurgery 38:662–670; 1996.

Qureshi, A.; Frankel, M.; Ottenlips, J.; Stern, B. Cerebral hemodynamics in preeclampsia and eclampsia. Arch. Neurol. 53:1226–1231; 1996.

Qureshi, A.; Giles, W.; Croft, J.; Stern, B. Number of pregnancies and risk for stroke and stroke subtypes. Arch. Neurol. 54:203–206; 1997.

Racz, G.; Hagstrom, D. Iliohypogastric and ilioinguinal nerve entrapment: diagnosis and treatment. Pain Digest 2:43–48; 1992.

Ramsay, R. Effect of hormones on seizure activity during pregnancy. J. Clin. Neurophysiol. 4:23–25; 1987.

Raps, E.; Galetta, S.; Broderick, M.; Atlas, S. Delayed peripartum vasculopathy: cerebral eclampsia revisited. Ann. Neurol. 33:222–225; 1993.

Reif, M. Bilateral common peroneal nerve palsy secondary to prolonged squatting in natural childbirth. Birth 15:100–102; 1988.

Report of the Quality Standards Subcommittee of the American Academy of Neurology. Practice parameter: management issues for women with epilepsy (summary statement). Report of the Quality Standards Subcommittee of the American Academy of Neurology (AAN). Neurology 51:944–948; 1998.

Roberts, J. Prevention or early treatment of preeclampsia. N. Engl. J. Med. 337:124–125; 1997.

Robinson, A.; Nelson, P. Prolactinomas in women: current therapies. Ann. Intern. Med. 99:115–118; 1983.

Robinson, J.; Hall, C.; Sedzimir, C. Arteriovenous malformations, aneurysms, and pregnancy. J. Neurosurg. 41:63–70; 1974.

Roelvink, N.; Kamphorst, W.; vanAlphen, H.; Rao, B. Pregnancy-related primary brain and spinal tumors. Arch. Neurol. 44:209–215; 1987.

Rosenzweig, B.; Rotmensch, S.; Binnette, S.; Phillippe, M. Primary idiopathic polymyositis and dermatomyositis complicating pregnancy: diagnosis and management. Obstet. Gynecol. Surv. 44:162–170; 1989.

Rungee, M. Low back pain during pregnancy. Orthopedics 16:1339–1344; 1993.

Runmarker, B.; Anderson, O. Pregnancy is associated with a lower risk of onset and a better prognosis in multiple sclerosis. Brain 118 (1). 253–261; 1995.

Sadovnick, A.; Eisen, K.; Hashimoto, S. Pregnancy and multiple sclerosis: a prospective study. Arch. Neurol. 51:1120–1124; 1994.

Samren, E.; vanDuijn, C.; Koch, S.; Hiilesmaa, V.; Klepa, H.; Bardy, A.; Mannagetta, G.; Deichl, A.; Gaily, E.; Granstrom, M.; Meinardi, H.; Grobbee, D.; Hofman, A.; Janz, D.; Lindhout, D. Maternal use of antiepileptic drugs and the risk of major congenital malformations: a joint European prospective study of human teratogenesis associated with maternal epilepsy. Epilepsia 38(9):981–990; 1997.

Saunders, N.; Hammersley, B. Magnesium for eclampsia. Lancet 34:788–789; 1995.

Schaefer, P.; Buonanno, F.; Gonzalez, R.; Schwamm, L. Diffusion-weighted imaging discriminates between cytotoxic and vasogenic edema in a patient with eclampsia. Stroke 28:1082–1085; 1997.

Schmidt, D.; Canger, R.; Avanzini, G.; Battino, D.; Cusi, C.; Beck-Mannagetta, G.; Koch, S.; Rating, D.; Janz, D. Change of seizure frequency in pregnant epileptic women. J. Neurol. Neurosurg. Psychiatry 46(8):751–755; 1983.

Sharma, S.; Herrera, E.; Sidawi, J.; Leveno, K. The pregnant patient with an intracranial arteriovenous malformation: cesarean or vaginal delivery using regional or general anesthesia? Reg. Anesth. 20: 455–458; 1995.

Sibai, B.; Sarinoglu, C.; Mercer, B. Eclampsia: VII. Pregnancy outcome after eclampsia and long-term prognosis. Am. J. Obstet. Gynecol. 166:1757–1763; 1992.

Silberstein, S. Migraine and pregnancy. Neurol. Clin. 15:209–230; 1997.

Simon, R. Brain tumors in pregnancy. Semin. Neurol. 8:214–221; 1988.

Stahl, S.; Blumenfeld, Z.; Yarnitsky, D. Carpal tunnel syndrome in pregnancy: indications for early surgery. J. Neurol. Sci. 136:182–184; 1996.

Stenager, E.; Stenager, E.; Jensen, K. Effect of pregnancy on the prognosis for multiple sclerosis: a 5-year follow-up investigation. Acta Neurol. Scand. 9:305–308; 1994.

Stern, B.; Wityk, R. Stroke in the young. In: Gilman, S.; Goldstein, G.; Waxman, S., eds. Neurobase, CD-ROM. LaJolla, CA: Arbor Publishing Corp.; 1996.

Sulton, A.; Kamm, M.; Hudson, C. Pudendal nerve damage during labor: prospective study before and after childbirth. Br. J. Obstet. Gynaecol. 101:22–28; 1994.

Svigos, J. Epilepsy and pregnancy. Aust. N. Z. J. Obstet. Gynaecol. 24:182–185; 1984.

Tanganelli, P.; Regesta, G. Epilepsy, pregnancy and major birth anomalies: an Italian prospective, controlled study. Neurology 42 (suppl. 5):89–93; 1992.

Teramo, K.; Hiilesmaa, V. Pregnancy and fetal complications in epileptic pregnancies: review of the literature. In: Janz, D.; Bossi, L.; Dam, M., ed. Epilepsy, pregnancy and the child. New York: Raven Press; 1982: p. 53–59.

Teramo, K.; Hiilesmaa, V.; Bardy, A.; Saarikoski, S. Fetal heart rate during a maternal grand mal epileptic seizure. J. Perinat. Med. 7(1):3–6; 1979.

Thomas, S.; Somanathan, N.; Radhakumari, R. Interictal EEG changes in eclampsia. Electroencephalogr. Clin. Neurophysiol. 94:271–275; 1995.

The Eclampsia Trial Collaborative Group Which anticonvulsant for women with eclampsia? Evidence from the Collaborative Eclampsia Trial. Lancet 345:1455–1463: 1995.

Tomson, T.; Ohman, I.; Vitols, S. Lamotrigine in pregnancy and lactation: a case report. Epilepsia 48:1039–1041; 1997.

Topframate prescribing information package insert. McNeil Pharmaceutical, Ortho Pharmaceutical Corporation 1996.

Trommer, B.; Homer, D.; Mikhael, M. Cerebral vasospasm and eclampsia. Stroke 19:326–329; 1988.

Uchide, K.; Terada, S.; Akasofu, K.; Higashi, S. Cerebral arteriovenous malformations in a pregnancy with twins: case report. Neurosurgery 31:780–782; 1992.

Verdru, P.; Theys, P.; D'Hooghe, M.; Carton, H. Pregnancy and multiple sclerosis: the influence on long-term disability. Clin. Neurol. Neurosurg. 96:38–41; 1994.

Verspyck, E.; Maldebrot, L.; Dommergues, M.; Huon, C.; Woimant, F.; Baumann, C.; Vernet-DerGarabedian, B. Myasthenia gravis with polyhydramnios in the fetus of an asymptomatic mother. Prenat. Diagn. 13:539–542; 1993.

Watson, W.; Katz, V.; Bowes, W. Plasmapheresis during pregnancy. Obstet. Gynecol. 76:451–457; 1990.

Weed, J.; Hunter, V. Diagnosis and management of brain metastasis from gestational trophoblastic disease. Oncology 5:48–49; 1991.

Weinreb, H. Demyelinating and neoplastic diseases in pregnancy. Neurol. Clin. 12:509–526; 1994.

Will, A.; Lewis, K.; Hinshaw, D.; Jordan, K.; Cousins, L.; Hasso, A.; Thompson, J. Cerebral vasoconstriction in toxemia. Neurology 37:1555–1557; 1987.

Witlin, A.; Friedman, S.; Egerman, R.; Frangieh, A.; Sibai, B. Cerebrovascular disorders complicating pregnancy—beyond eclampsia. Am. J. Obstet. Gynecol. 176:1139–1148; 1997.

Wolf, S.; Wagner, J.; Davidson, S.; Forsythe, A. Treatment of Bell's palsy with prednisone: a prospective, randomized study. Neurology 28:158–161; 1978.

Worthington, J.; Jones, R.; Crawford, M. Pregnancy and multiple sclerosis: a 3-year prospective study. J. Neurol. 241:228–233; 1994.

Yahr, M.; Ellis, S.; Gudesblatt, M.; Cohen, J. Neurological complications of pregnancy. In: Cherry, S.; Merkatz, I., eds. Complications of pregnancy: medical surgical, gynecologic, psychosocial, and perinatal. Baltimore: Williams & Wilkins; 1991: p. 1008–1022.

Yerby, M. Risks of pregnancy in women with epilepsy. Epilepsia 33:S23–S27; 1992.

Yerby, M. Pregnancy, teratogenesis and epilepsy. Neurol. Clin. 12:749–771; 1994.

Yerby, M.; Collins, S. Teratogenicity of antiepileptic drugs. In: Engel, J.; Pedley, T., ed. Epilepsy, a comprehensive textbook. Philadelphia: Lippincott-Raven Publishers; 1997: p. 1195–1203.

Yerby, M.; Devinsky, O. Epilepsy and pregnancy. In: Devinsky, O.; Feldmann, E.; Hainline, B., eds. Neurological complications of pregnancy. New York: Raven Press; 1994: p. 45–64.

Yerby, M.; Friel, P.; McCormick, K. Antiepileptic drug disposition during pregnancy. Neurology 42 (suppl. 5): 12–16; 1992.

Yerby, M.; Koepsell, T.; Daling, J. Pregnancy complications and outcomes in a cohort of women with epilepsy. Epilepsia 26:631–635; 1985.

Zahn C. Neurologic care of pregnant women with epilepsy. Epilepsia 39(suppl. 8):S26–S31; 1998.

# Index